SURGICAL PATHOLOGY

Surgical pathology

Lauren V. Ackerman, M.D.

*Professor Emeritus of Surgical Pathology and Pathology,
Washington University School of Medicine, St. Louis, Mo.;
Professor of Pathology, State University of New York at Stony Brook,
Stony Brook, Long Island, N. Y.;
Consultant to the Armed Forces Institute of Pathology*

Juan Rosai, M.D.

*Associate Professor of Pathology, Washington University School
of Medicine, St. Louis, Mo.; Associate Surgical Pathologist,
Barnes and Affiliated Hospitals, St. Louis, Mo.*

With 1329 figures

FIFTH EDITION

THE C. V. MOSBY COMPANY

St. Louis   1974

FIFTH EDITION

Copyright © 1974 by The C. V. Mosby Company

All rights reserved. No part of this book may be reproduced in any manner without written permission of the publisher.

Previous editions copyrighted 1953, 1959, 1964, 1968

Printed in the United States of America

Distributed in Great Britain by Henry Kimpton, London

Library of Congress Cataloging in Publication Data

Ackerman, Lauren Vedder, 1905-
   Surgical pathology.

    1. Pathology, Surgical. I. Rosai, Juan, 1940-
joint author. II. Title. [DNLM: 1. Pathology,
Surgical. WO142 A182s 1974]
RD57.A2 1974   617′.07   73-12725
ISBN 0-8016-0044-8

CB/CB/B 9 8 7 6 5 4 3 2

To the men and women who have worked with me in Surgical
Pathology over the past twenty-five years

Harlan, Walter, Malcolm, Ron D., Dick K., Sid S., Ruy, John
K., and Fred K.; Barbara, Elsbeth, Emily, Geraldine, Hemprova,
Margaret, and Nadya; all the Williams (B., B., C., H., H., M.,
S., S., T., and W.), the Roberts (A., F., O., and S.), the
Thomases (H., T., T., and V.), the Johns (E., K., M., S.,
and T.), the Guses (A., D., R., and R.); Eli, Dave E.,
Dave S., Jules, Gene, Dick P., Dick R., Sid A., Dieter,
Rene, Juan, Carlos R., Carlos P.-M., Humberto,
Jesus, Jacques, Ferrucio, Bo, Yvon, Fumikazi,
Luis, Prometeo, Manuel, Victor, Hector,
Francisco, Pradit, J. D., Jason, Vernon,
Dan, James, Joel, Colin, Chick,
Larry, Rex, Quinton, Ron A.,
Dale, Mike, Harrison, Mor-
ton, Max, Oscar, Henry,
Charles, Steve, Leon-
ard, Lawrence S.,
and Boris   —L.V.A.

And with both of us over the past five years

Cassim, Paul, Julio, Richard, Gerald, Philip,
Landy, Jerry, Hertzel, Kun, William,
Bradley, Louis, David, Bruce,
Kavous, Fred, Clinton, Enrique,
Sam, Neil, John, José,
Scott, Steve, Hatton,
Jung, and
Raul   —L.V.A. and J.R.

Preface
TO FIFTH EDITION

Surgical pathology has now been in print since 1953, when the first edition was published. With the passage of time and particularly with the advent of this edition, it seemed to me that another younger and fresh viewpoint was needed to give the book a new spark and spirit. Fortunately, my choice for co-author, Dr. Juan Rosai, was not only willing to undertake this responsibility but was also enthusiastic and offered constructive criticism in every aspect of this revision. He saw many areas that needed change which I could no longer visualize. Large sections of this book have been completely rewritten by him. With the next edition, he will assume the major responsibility.

Portions of the manuscript have been reviewed by our colleagues who are more expert than we in certain areas—Dr. John Kissane in renal pathology, Dr. Joseph Grisham in liver pathology, and Dr. Richard M. Torack and Dr. William Schlaepfer in neuropathology. Dr. Walter C. Bauer and Dr. Malcolm H. McGavran (now Professor of Pathology at the Pennsylvania State University School of Medicine in Hershey) have continued to take the responsibility for the chapter on ultrastructure and surgical pathology, and Dr. McGavran has again assumed the responsibility for the sections on dermatoses and tumors in the chapter on the skin. Dr. Rosai has entirely rewritten the section on tumors in the chapter on the central nervous sys-tem. Dr. Morton E. Smith has taken over the complete responsibility for the chapter on the eyes and ocular adnexa. We are indebted to Dr. Harvey R. Butcher, Jr., Dr. Frederick T. Kraus, Mrs. Eleanor V. Paul, Dr. David E. Smith, and Dr. Lorenz E. Zimmerman for their previous contributions.

Exfoliative cytology has become an extremely important area of knowledge to the pathologist. Dr. Michael Kyriakos, who is in charge of this discipline in our Department, has written short sections on this subject where applicable.

We have continued to use examples of how electron microscopy has been helpful to us in making diagnoses. Other techniques, such as immunofluorescence and histochemistry, also are mentioned when considered particularly relevant.

As with the text, the references have undergone thorough revision. Those no longer pertinent have been deleted and hundreds of new ones added. Further, approximately 300 new figures, some additions and some substitutions, have been included in this edition.

It is to be hoped that this book, under the new joint authorship, will continue to be useful in the constantly expanding field of surgical pathology.

Lauren V. Ackerman
St. Louis, Mo.
APRIL, 1973

vii

Preface
TO FIRST EDITION

This book can be only an introduction to the vast field of surgical pathology: the pathology of the living. It does not pretend to replace in any way the textbooks of general pathology, its purpose being merely to supplement them, assuming that the reader has a background in or access to those texts. The contents are not as complete as they might be because emphasis has been placed on the common rather than the rare lesions and are, to a great extent, based on the author's personal experiences.

This book has been written for the medical student as well as for those physicians who are daily intimately concerned with surgical pathology. This must of necessity include not only the surgeon and the pathologist, but also those physicians in other fields who are affected by its decisions, such as the radiologist and the internist. Gross pathology has been stressed throughout with an attempt to correlate the gross findings with the clinical observations. The many illustrations have been selected as typical of the various surgical conditions, although in a few instances the author has been unable to resist showing some of the more interesting rare lesions he has encountered. Concluding each chapter there is a bibliography listing those references which are not only relatively recent and readily available, but also those which will lead the reader to a more detailed knowledge of the subject.

Dr. Zola K. Cooper, Assistant Professor of Pathology and Surgical Pathology, has written one of the sections on Skin, and Dr. David E. Smith, Assistant Professor of Pathology and Surgical Pathology, has written the chapter on Central Nervous System. Both of these members of the Department are particularly well qualified for their respective roles because of their background and present responsibilities in these fields. Their efforts on my behalf are most gratefully acknowledged.

Many members of the Surgical Staff at Barnes Hospital have given much help both knowingly and unwittingly. I am particularly grateful to Dr. Charles L. Eckert, Associate Professor of Surgery, for letting me bother him rather constantly with my questions and for giving freely of his experience. Dr. Richard Johnson, who succeeded me as Pathologist at the Ellis Fischel State Cancer Hospital, agreeably made available all the material there, and Dr. Franz Leidler, Pathologist at the Veterans Hospital, has been most cooperative.

Thanks must be given to Dr. H. R. McCarroll, Assistant Professor of Orthopedics, for constructively criticizing the chapter on Bone and Joint, and to Dr. C. A. Waldron for helping me with the chapters related to the Oral Cavity. Among other faculty friends and colleagues who were especially helpful, I would like to mention Dr. Carl E. Lischer, Dr. Eugene M. Bricker, Dr. Heinz Haffner, Dr. Thomas H. Burford, Dr. Carl A. Moyer, Dr. Evarts A. Graham, Dr. Robert Elman, Dr. Edward H. Reinhard, Dr. J. Albert Key, Dr. Glover H. Copher, Dr. Margaret G. Smith, and Dr. Robert A. Moore.

Mr. Cramer K. Lewis, of our Department of Illustration, has been very patient with my demands, and his efforts and skill have been invaluable. Miss Marion Murphy, in charge of our Medical Library, and her associates gave untiringly of their time.

Because of recent advances in anesthesia, antibiotics, and pre- and postoperative care, modern surgery permits the radical excision of portions or all of various organs. There is a need today for contemplative surgeons, men with a rich background in the fundamental sciences, whether chemistry, physiology, or pathology. The modern surgeon should not ask himself, "Can I get away with this operation?" but rather, "What does the future hold for this patient?" It is hoped that this book may contribute in some small fashion toward the acquisition of this attitude.

Lauren V. Ackerman
St. Louis, Mo.

Contents

SURGICAL PATHOLOGY

1 Introduction

Surgical pathology and surgical pathologist

The department of pathology in large medical centers should have a division of surgical pathology closely affiliated with the department of surgery. In the past, the diagnosis of tissue removed from a living patient often was delegated to a resident, and reports emanating from the department of pathology not only were delayed but also often indicated only whether the tissue was benign or malignant. These circumstances sometimes forced clinicians to direct some branch of surgical pathology. Under these conditions, the clinician's diagnoses and recommendations were better than those of the experienced, uninterested pathologist. Although it is mandatory for the clinician to have some knowledge of surgical pathology, it is difficult, if not impossible, to be both a competent clinician and a skillful pathologist. Nor is it rational for the surgical pathologist to believe himself capable of doing radical mastectomies as a sideline. There are exceptional persons who are not trained pathologists but who have made fundamental contributions to pathology in their respective fields of interest. However, the most profitable arrangement is to have an experienced pathologist with a clinical background working with clinicians interested in pathology.

Surgical pathology implies surgery, but actually the surgical pathologist is closely affiliated with all branches of medicine. A peripheral lymph node may show unexpected malignant lymphoma and resolve a difficult diagnosis for the internist. An aspiration biopsy of the liver may clarify a diagnostic problem for the pediatrician. Close cooperation with the department of radiology is essential.

The surgical pathologist has the unique opportunity of bridging the gap between the beginning of disease and its end stages, and he should take advantage of this circumstance. He can do this only after a solid foundation of study at the autopsy table, where the ravages of cancer, tuberculosis, ulcerative colitis, and other diseases are all too clear. With this background, he can then correlate the initial stages of disease seen in specimens from living patients in the surgical pathology laboratory. With this objective in mind, the student may make many fundamental contributions to knowledge. With the integration of clinical findings, pathologic anatomy is still a living science. Only by understanding the pathology of disease as a whole can the pathologic process affecting a given organ be understood. This is the main reason a clinician cannot hope to deal adequately with some small branch of surgical pathology. Disease does not cooperate by remaining neatly confined to an anatomic system.

The surgical pathologist not only must know his own field thoroughly, but he also must have a rich background in clinical medicine. He must be in a position to advise the clinicians about the biopsy or the

1

excised material he receives. It is not sufficient for him to be able to say whether a lesion is benign or malignant. He must be able to tell the surgeon the extent of the disease, the adequacy of the excision, and other pertinent information. He can do this only if the clinician supplies him with all clinical and laboratory data. There are still pathologists who pride themselves on being able to render an opinion and make recommendations for treatment without clinical information. The pathologist makes enough errors without trying to be dramatic.

By the very nature of the material submitted to him, the surgical pathologist makes mistakes. He sees the earliest subtle and sometimes bewildering changes in Hodgkin's disease. He may very well not recognize that the minimal granulomatous response in a lymph node is really a peripheral manifestation of histoplasmosis. The surgical pathologist must continue to haunt the postmortem table, for there his diagnoses are confirmed or his errors are made painfully clear. The necessity of follow-up on the patient in whom the diagnosis is not certain is mandatory. Time is often a better diagnostician.

The surgeon we choose to operate has not only technical dexterity (a fairly common commodity) but also, more important, good *judgment* and a personal concern for his patient's welfare. The surgeon with a prepared mind and a clear concept of the pathology of disease invariably is the one with good judgment. Without this background of knowledge, he will not recognize specific pathologic alterations at operation nor will he have a clear concept of the limitations of his knowledge, and therefore he will not know when to call the pathologist to help him. Without this basic knowledge, he may improve his technical ability but never his judgment. You might say that with time his ignorance is refined rather than his knowledge broadened.

Although the study of radiology deals with shadows and the study of pathology with substance, the correlation of those shadows with the gross substance strengthens the diagnostic skill of the radiologist, explains errors in radiologic interpretation, and instills humility rather than dogmatism. The radiotherapist, too, can learn much from the study of surgical pathology, particularly the effects of irradiation on normal tissue and radiosensitive neoplasms. Furthermore, explanations for the success or failure of irradiation therapy may become apparent by the study of surgical specimens.

Biopsy

The interpretation of a biopsy is one of the most important duties of the surgical pathologist. Certain generalizations must be mentioned even though they are obvious.

Material obtained by cautery is usually unsatisfactory for biopsy because the cautery chars and distorts the tissue and prevents clear staining. If the tumor shows a central ulceration, removal of a small biopsy from the center may show only necrosis and inflammation. The biopsy should be taken with a cold knife from the margin of the ulcer and should include both normal and ulcerated tissue. In a mass of lymph nodes, a deep-seated node may be of diagnostic value whereas a superficial node is not. We have seen bone biopsies taken near the lesion but not through it. *The pathologist cannot make a diagnosis of a disease from material that is not representative.* The surgeon should be equipped with the proper instruments to obtain the best possible biopsy, whether it be from the esophagus, the bronchus, the nasopharynx, the endometrium, or even the stomach.

The size of the biopsy may range from the smallest wisp of tissue to a large excision. It is imperative that the small biopsies be quickly placed in good fixative. Although 10% formalin is not the best, it is the one most commonly used. For some types of tissue or techniques, special fixatives may be needed. Testicular biopsies are best preserved in Bouin's fixative. Zenker's or Helly's fixatives are preferable for tissues of endocrine glands such as pituitary and Langerhans' islets. If examination by electron microscopy is contemplated, small fragments of tissue should be placed in 3% buffered glutaraldehyde immediately after excision. Freezing of fresh specimens is important if a biochemical study is contemplated, especially in cases of secretory endocrine neoplasms. An imprint taken from the cut surface of a tumor made prior to fixation can be extremely useful, especially for lesions of the hematopoietic system. It is unfortunate if tissue that has been carefully and tediously obtained by the surgeon is mishandled, allowed to dry, or poorly fixed.

Aspiration biopsy

There are two ways of handling an aspiration biopsy. The material obtained is either smeared on a slide or placed in a fixative and sectioned as a small tissue biopsy.[5] Although a diagnosis may be made on smeared material, the skill and effort entailed in making a diagnosis by smear are great. We therefore recommend placing the material in fixative and cutting it as a small biopsy because under these conditions the architecture is maintained. If the biopsy is positive, the diagnosis is assuredly accurate, and surgery can be undertaken without delay. If the diagnosis is negative or if the material is insufficient, cancer may still be present. The value of a negative biopsy depends, to a great extent, upon the skill of the person taking the biopsy.[7]

The merits and indications for incisional and aspiration biopsy for the various organs are more fully discussed in the respective chapters.

Frozen section

Frozen section technique is a procedure of great value to the surgeon.[8] The only reason for frozen section is to *make a therapeutic decision*.[1] A frozen section should be accurate, rapid, and reliable. We believe that the responsibility for frozen section diagnosis should be that of a senior pathologist and that such a person should be experienced, be conservative in attitude, and, above all, have judgment. We do not favor using the pathologist as a technician to satisfy the surgeon's intellectual curiosity or to prove that the pathologist is in the hospital. Frozen section diagnosis should not be a method used routinely in every specimen removed at the operating table but should be reserved for those in-

Table 1 Frozen section diagnosis in 2,240 consecutive cases at Barnes Hospital, St. Louis, Mo.*†

Organ	Cases	Benign lesions	Malignant lesions	False positives	False negatives	Diagnosis deferred
Breast	679	437	202	0	3 (0.5%)	6 (0.9%)
Soft tissues	298	135	163	1 (0.3%)	1 (0.3%)	7 (2.3%)
Gastrointestinal tract	251	192	59	0	3 (1.2%)	6 (2.4%)
Lymph nodes	232	108	124	0	1 (0.4%)	0
Lung	169	49	120	2 (1.2%)	0	0
Thyroid gland	112	100	12	0	0	5 (4.4%)
Central nervous system	112	18	94	1 (0.9%)	2 (1.8%)	4 (3.6%)
Bone and joints	79	42	37	0	1 (1.3%)	5 (6.3%)
Liver and gallbladder	73	29	44	0	0	1 (1.4%)
Pancreas and bile ducts	45	22	23	0	2 (4.4%)	0
Parathyroid glands	44	44	0	0	0	0
Skin	51	18	33	0	0	0
Miscellaneous	135	73	62	1 (0.7%)	0	4 (3.0%)
Total	2,240	1,267	973	5 (0.2%)	13 (0.6%)	38 (1.7%)

*Adapted from Elsner, B.: La biopsia por congelación: su valor asistencial y en la educación médica del patólogo, Prensa Med. Arg. **55:**1741-1749, 1968.

†Ear, nose, and throat and gynecologic cases excluded.

stances in which a therapy will be affected. The indications and limitations of this method of diagnosis vary from organ to organ and have been detailed in the respective chapters. Although the pathologist must be conservative, he must not be so conservative as not to make some decision. Otherwise his value to the surgeon is diminished tremendously. Inasmuch as he is using his knowledge to the limit, rare errors may be made (Table 1).

Frozen section diagnosis demands of a pathologist a well-balanced clinical background coupled with skillful interpretation and an awareness of the limitations of the method. The pathologist should enter the operating room thoroughly briefed on the clinical history of the patient and should consult with the surgeon as to the best area to biopsy. He must then have skill in selecting from the removed material the piece to be frozen and stained. Various stains can be used. The cryostat is being used increasingly because of the technical excellence of the sections obtained.

In cancer, there are only three possible diagnoses: positive for cancer, negative for cancer, or no diagnosis made. At times, more than one frozen section is required. The diagnosis is most important because upon it may rest the decision to remove a breast, to amputate a leg, to remove a lung, or to terminate an operation. It is evident that a surgeon with only a slight knowledge of pathology is not equipped to interpret a frozen section, nor are pathologists with little clinical knowledge qualified to undertake frozen section diagnosis.

Exfoliative cytology

Exfoliative cytology has become extremely popular particularly in the United States, and in many departments of pathology in which this technique is used, the diagnosis of cytologic material usually is based on the apparent presence or absence of cancer cells. The decision is, of course, of great significance. In some instances, the method has become discredited because poorly trained pathologists, gynecologists, and technicians have been handling the material and making definitive diagnoses that prove to be incorrect. The cytologist will make a certain number of false negative diagnoses depending on the source of the material, but false positive diagnoses should practically never occur, for they will in themselves invalidate the method.

In writing the cytology reports, we have made it our policy whenever possible to use the same terminology as that used for the microscopic sections instead of employing the original grading system of Papanicolaou. A cytologic diagnosis of "squamous cell carcinoma" rendered on a sputum specimen gives the surgeon a better idea about the nature of a pulmonary mass than one of "cytology Grade IV." There is a proportion of cases in which we cannot be certain whether the cells present are malignant or not. We report them as "suspicious" and ask for further material.

Under most circumstances we feel that a determined effort must be made to substantiate the diagnosis by a conventional biopsy procedure before decisive treatment is carried out. For instance, if a cytologic diagnosis of cancer is obtained from a cervical smear, irradiation or surgical treatment should not be started until a positive formal biopsy is at hand. Of course, exceptions to this rule occur. A patient may have a shadow in the right lung field and a negative bronchoscopic biopsy but the sputum shows cancer cells. We believe this finding is reliable enough to recommend thoracotomy with lobectomy or pneumonectomy without benefit of frozen section (see lung, p. 230). In this instance, the weight of a positive cytologic diagnosis is added to the clinical and radiologic evidence of carcinoma and helps make the decision to resect the lung.

Exfoliative cytology is of little value for lesions that are readily accessible to incisional biopsy, such as the skin or the oral cavity. Neither does it seem advisable to use this time-consuming method as a

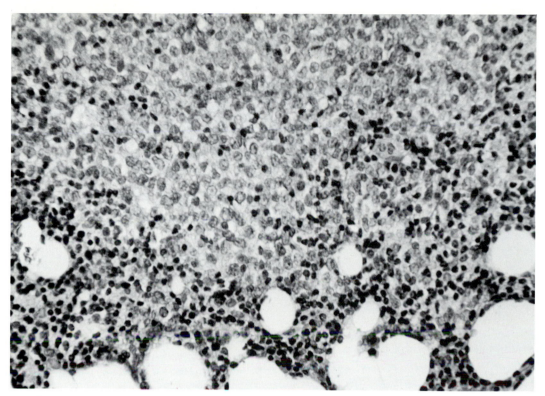

Fig. 1 Bone marrow biopsy showing infiltration by histiocytic lymphoma. Smear was non-diagnostic. (×350; WU neg. 70-5708.)

screening procedure for asymptomatic patients except under special circumstances. It is logical to screen cytologically selected groups of patients in whom the statistical chance of finding a carcinoma is high enough to warrant the time and expense. This might include patients with pernicious anemia and those over 40 years of age with achlorhydria. In the latter group, there is a heightened chance of the patient having cancer of the stomach, and gastric cytology would be of value. It has been well demonstrated now by Boyes et al.[3] that screening for cancer of the cervix is an extremely useful and practical method for finding early carcinoma of the cervix. It must be remembered, however, that only a positive result has value, and a negative finding does not necessarily indicate that cancer is not present. Special techniques are often helpful.[2] The indications and limitations of this method are discussed further in the individual chapters.

Bone marrow biopsy

Microscopic examination of tissue sections derived from bone marrow biopsy or aspirated material is a useful and often essential adjunct to the examination of marrow smears in the diagnosis of diseases involving the hemopoietic system. It aids in assessing the cellularity of the marrow provided the age of the patient and the site of biopsy are known.[9] The conditions in which tissue sections are mandatory or nearly mandatory for diagnosis include aplastic anemia, granulomatous diseases of the marrow (including sarcoidosis, miliary tuberculosis, and fungal diseases), malignant lymphoma (including Hodgkin's disease), myelofibrosis, myelophthisic anemias due to primary or metastatic malignant disease,[4] multiple myeloma, and thrombotic thrombocytopenic purpura[6] (Fig. 1). Difficulty or failure to aspirate marrow may be the result of leukemia with a "packed marrow" or of myelofibrosis. In the latter disease, silver stains will demonstrate increased reticulin formation associated with myelocytic and megakaryocytic hyperplasia.

In the past, Zenker's or Helly's fixatives have been recommended for bone marrow biopsies. We have now discarded these in favor of neutral buffered formalin, which has proved most satisfactory. The hematoxylin and eosin stain is used routinely. Perls' Prussian blue reaction is employed to assess iron stores in the marrow. These will be low or absent in iron-deficiency anemias and be increased, often markedly, in sideroachrestic anemias.

There is no doubt that the combination of bone marrow biopsy sections and aspiration smears stained with Wright's stain or May-Grünwald-Giemsa stain provides the most valuable information. A detailed review of the bone marrow findings is not warranted in a book of this type.

REFERENCES

1 Ackerman, L. V., and Ramirez, G. A.: Indications for and limitations of frozen section diagnosis; a review of 1269 consecutive frozen section diagnoses, Br. J. Surg. **46:**336-350, 1959.
2 Bernhardt, H., Gourley, R. D., Young, J. M., Shepherd, M. C., and Killian, J. J.: A modified membrane-filter technic for detection of cancer cells in body fluids, Am. J. Clin. Pathol. **36:** 462-464, 1961.
3 Boyes, D. A., Fidler, H. K., and Lock, D. R.: Significance of in situ carcinoma of the uterine cervix, Br. Med. J. **1:**203-210, 1962.
4 Contreras, E., Lawrence, D. E., and Lee, R. E.: Value of the bone marrow biopsy in the diagnosis of metastatic carcinoma, Cancer **29:** 234-239, 1972.
5 Hajdu, S. I., and Melamed, M. R.: The diagnostic value of aspiration smears, Am. J. Clin. Pathol. **59:**350-356, 1973.
6 Liao, K. T.: The superiority of histologic sections of aspirated bone marrow in malignant lymphomas, Cancer **27:**618-628, 1971.
7 Meatheringham, R. E., and Ackerman, L. V.: Aspiration biopsy of lymph nodes; critical review of results of 300 aspirations, Surg. Gynecol. Obstet. **84:**1071-1076, 1947.
8 Nakazawa, H., Rosen, P., Lane, N., and Lattes, R.: Frozen section experience in 3000 cases, Am. J. Clin. Pathol. **49:**41-51, 1968.
9 Wintrobe, M. M.: Clinical hematology, ed. 6, Philadelphia, 1967, Lea & Febiger.

2 Ultrastructure and surgical pathology*

Walter C. Bauer, M.D.
Malcolm H. McGavran, M.D.

Introduction

The study of thin sections of biologic material with the electron microscope has opened a new realm of structure. The eventual place of electron microscopy in surgical pathology, particularly its diagnostic role, is difficult to assess at present, for only tentative beginnings have been made in its application to the everyday practice of diagnostic pathology. The power of the technique is obvious. Improvements in methodology of fixation,[8] embedding,[3] and sectioning of tissues, of differential cell fractionation,[11] of negative staining,[1] and of fine structure localization of cytochemical[4, 9] and immunochemical reactions[5, 6] are bound to have their impact on the electron microscopy problems of surgical pathologists.

Electron microscopy has already made important, if only limited, contributions to diagnostic surgical pathology. Using formalin-fixed postosmicated material, it has been possible to resolve certain troublesome diagnostic problems. The differential diagnosis between melanoma and anaplastic carcinomas, atypical carcinoid tumor, and adenocarcinoma and the osseous lesions of myeloma, histiocytic lymphoma, and metastatic carcinoma has been settled by electron microscopy.[7] The presence of tonofilaments and typical desmosomes in tumor cells in a cervical lymph node established the diagnosis of metastatic poorly differentiated carcinoma rather than malignant lymphoma (Figs. 2 and 3). A clinically unrecognized nasopharyngeal primary lesion was found subsequent to the electron microscopic report. Zimmerman et al.[14] have found electron microscopy useful in the differential diagnosis of ocular lesions such as glial and retinal tumors, ciliary body tumors, and skeletal muscle neoplasms. The study of suspected melanocytic lesions can be especially rewarding. The presence of reaction product in electron micrographs of nonpigmented tumor cells subjected to controlled dopa reaction after glutaraldehyde fixation made possible the diagnosis of melanoma (Fig. 4) and illustrates the benefits of combining other

*This work was supported in part by a grant from the John A. Hartford Foundation.

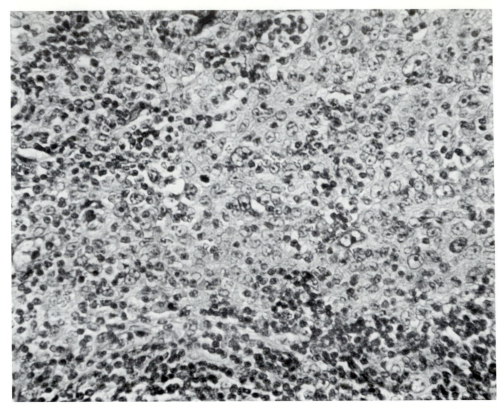

Fig. 2 Undifferentiated tumor in cervical lymph node of 12-year-old boy. Exact diagnosis was difficult. Electron microscopic examination was done on material from this node (Fig. 3). (×350; WU neg. 67-5666A.)

techniques with electron microscopy for diagnostic purposes. The study of fine structure changes in human renal disease has provided significant information relating to prognosis and treatment.[2, 12, 13] Electron microscopy is an essential part of the tissue diagnostic work-up.[10]

Special problems in electron microscopy

It should be emphasized at the onset that in terms of laboratory time required for adequate training and mastery of techniques, the maintenance of equipment, and the investigation of the problems of pathology, electron microscopy is more than a simple extension of light microscopy. Much valuable information is available in an excellent review of techniques for electron microscopy by Pease.[24]

Many of the difficult aspects of electron microscopy of tissues arise from the employment of special preparative procedures and techniques and, paradoxically, from the high resolution of the instrument. Proper fixation and embedding of the tissues are of utmost importance—the examination of beautifully cut, carefully stained, dirt-free, thin sections of badly fixed material is a disappointment of the worst possible sort. A casual attitude on the part of the pathologist toward the fixation of surgically traumatized tissue excised under conditions of severe local anoxia has disastrous results on fine structure. Careful planning and the closest cooperation of the surgeon must be obtained in order that preparative artifacts be minimized. The best results with human tissues usually are obtained when a small biopsy, taken with a sharp knife prior to ligation of blood vessels, is immediately sub-

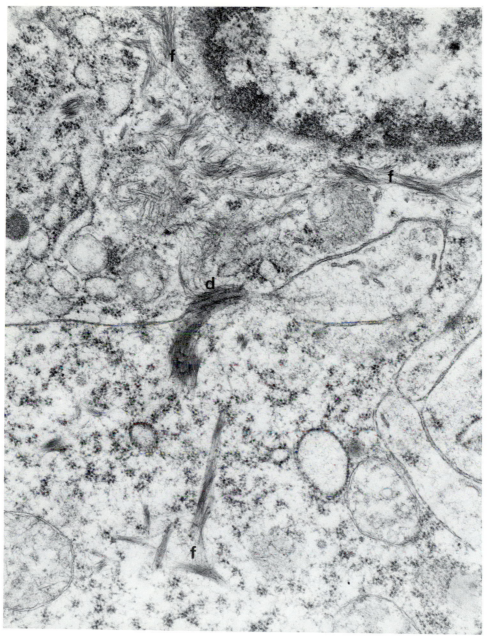

Fig. 3 Electron micrograph that resolved diagnostic difficulty of lesion shown in Fig. 2. Biopsy was variously interpreted as reticulum cell sarcoma and undifferentiated carcinoma metastatic from nasopharynx (Fig. 2). Ultrastructural features of many tonofilaments, **f,** and desmosomes, **d,** prove that lesion is poorly differentiated carcinoma. Subsequent examination and blind biopsies of nasopharynx disclosed primary lesion. (Uranyl acetate–lead citrate; ×45,000.)

divided into minute fragments and put into a suitable fixative. Special clamps for muscle biopsies[26] and special procedures for handling[25] and orienting[27] small intestinal biopsies have been devised. It may be necessary to devise other special procedures in some situations to achieve the best results.

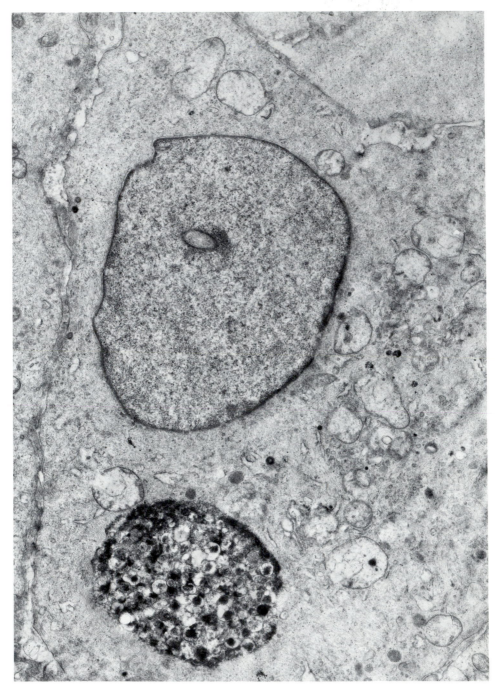

Fig. 4 Amelanotic malignant melanoma that had been fixed in glutaraldehyde, incubated with dopa, and then embedded. Black reaction product of tyrosinase activity represents melanin. It is present in individual melanosomes as well as in large aggregate of vesicles below nucleus. (Uranyl acetate–lead citrate; ×10,000; courtesy Dr. H. Rodriguez, Mexico City, Mexico.)

However, it should be emphasized also that the nature and rapidity of changes in fine structure attendant upon the removal, fixation, and embedding of tissues may not be ruinous for diagnostic purposes. It seems clear that certain cells, such as liver, maintain a remarkable stability in fine structure for time periods up to fifteen minutes at 37° C.[33-35] This provides the basis for hope that human material may be satisfactorily prepared under less stringent but carefully chosen conditions.

Of the several aldehydes explored for use as fixatives,[30] buffered glutaraldehyde gives excellent preservation of fine structure and is now widely used.[18] Postfixation in osmium tetroxide is the rule. Occasional deleterious effects of the two-step procedure of fixation with glutaraldehyde and osmium tetroxide can be minimized by combining the two reagents into one fixative.[32]

We have not found glutaraldehyde useful as a routine fixative for all tissues in the laboratory because of poor penetration, hardness of the tissue blocks, and poor staining quality with periodic acid–Schiff.[28] Fresh methanol-free formaldehyde prepared from paraformaldehyde provides tissue preservation that is not significantly different from that obtained with glutaraldehyde.[22, 24] When used as an s-collidine–buffered fixative coupled with postosmication and rapid embedment in either Epon 812 or Maraglas, specimens with reasonable preservation for both light and electron microscopy may be obtained within twenty-four hours.[21] Epon 812,[20] Araldite,[19] Maraglas,[17] and modifications of the foregoing with triallyl cyanurate[37] are widely used for embedding media because of the greatly reduced polymerization damage and improved stability of the thin sections in the electron beam.

It is possible to obtain information from thin section examination of tissues initially prepared for light microscopy in situations in which the light microscopic findings are not diagnostic yet suggest that electron microscopic study would provide clues as to the nature of the lesion. Zimmerman et al.[38] described methods for reprocessing paraffin-embedded tissues. In several instances, they were able to establish the identity of tumors with puzzling light microscopic features. As an example, a tumor of the ciliary body originally thought to have a ganglion cell component was found to be of skeletal muscle origin by virtue of finding myofilaments and glycogen particles. We have had similar experiences with amelanotic tumors thought possibly to be melanoma or undifferentiated carcinoma. The electron micrographs of reprocessed tissue showed organelles consistent with that of premelanosomes.

To those accustomed to good ultrastructure preservation, the examination of conventionally processed tissues may seem impossible. In the modern surgical pathology laboratory, every effort should be made to preserve tissues in a manner that will permit thin section examination if needed. It also should be recognized that in appropriate circumstances diagnostic clues may be obtained from the material at hand that can have great meaning and value in treatment and prognosis.

The high resolving power of the electron microscope has made possible visualization of the most minute structures and, in consequence, has also greatly restricted the area that can be examined in a reasonable length of time. Pease[24] estimated that days and even months would be required to examine what the pathologist sees in a few moments on a single slide. The benefits, then, of a closer look are often offset by sampling problems, particularly in the study of sequential changes in nonhomogeneous tissues and organs.

In all instances, careful light and electron microscopic correlation is invaluable. To provide a reassuringly familiar light microscopic image for orientation, $\frac{1}{2}\mu$ thick sections of osmium-fixed, plastic-embedded material may be stained with hematoxylin-eosin, toluidine blue, or PAS.[15, 23, 36]

Alternatively, similar "thick" sections may be examined in the phase microscope (Figs. 5 and 536). Such images are

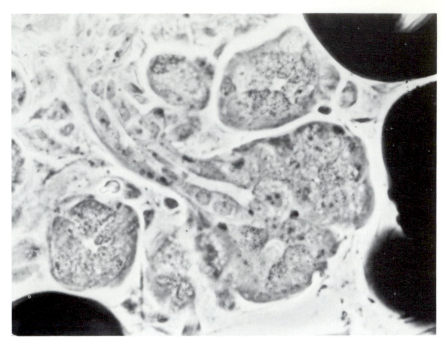

Fig. 5 Phase contrast micrograph of osmium-fixed, Epon-embedded human salivary gland tissue showing terminal duct and acini of secretory cells. Both topography of tissue and cytology of cells are easily appreciated. Peripheral black masses are fat cells. Thin sections for electron microscopy may be cut from such specific areas by careful trimming of block face. (×500.)

equally pleasing and suitable for orientation and possess additional advantages such as the following:

1 May be examined immediately without further staining

2 Provide an image with black and white contrasts similar to those seen in the electron microscope

3 Possess sufficient resolution at highest magnifications to make some judgments as to the preservation of fine structure, thus permitting more efficient use of the electron miscroscope

With either method, appropriate areas of the tissue may be selected for thin sections by careful trimming of the face of

Fig. 6 Plasma cell from normal human bone marrow showing cytoplasm rich in ergastoplasm, **e,** with stacks of ribosome-studded membranes oriented concentrically around nucleus, **N.** Homogeneously distributed, moderately electron-dense material can be seen in ergastroplasmic sacs. Many unattached ribosomes (RNP particles), **r,** can be seen between ergastoplasm and in other areas of cytoplasm. Large Golgi zone with several Golgi structures, **gi,** is present adjacent to nucleus. These are typically composed of stacks of agranular sacs sometimes seen in cup-shaped profiles and associated with many vesicles. Material of varying electron density fills these vesicles. Several mitochondria, **m,** with spaced transverse cristae can be seen in lower portion. Few very dense intramitochondrial granules dot each mitochondrion. Nucleus is delimited by definite double membrane, outer one often studded with ribonucleoprotein particles. Several nuclear "pores" are indicated (arrows). Chromatin material of nucleus can be seen as fine clumps on inhomogeneously distributed material that is focally concentrated at nuclear margins. Nucleolus, **nu,** occupies more central position. Dense continuous membrane (plasmalemma), **pm,** sharply delimits cytoplasmic boundaries, and narrow gap separates cell from neighboring cells. (Uranyl acetate—lead citrate; ×24,800; courtesy Dr. G. D. Sorensen, Hanover, N. H.)

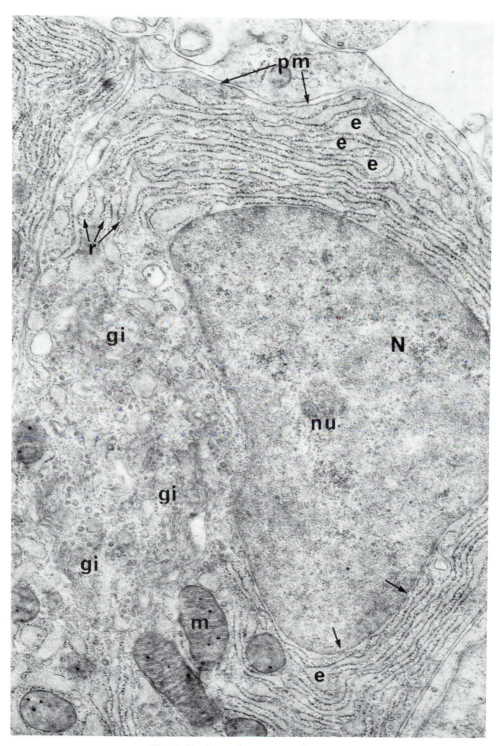

Fig. 6 For legend, see opposite page.

the block. With appropriate techniques, it is even possible to obtain electron micrographs of the same cells selected for study by light microscopy.[29, 31] A rapid method for preparing isolated cells for ultrastructural study was described by Collan and Sainio.[16]

Cell membrane and its specializations

The cytoplasm is limited by an uninterrupted membrane approximately 75Å in width (Fig. 6). High resolution electron microscopy has shown that the membrane may be resolved into 25Å dense lines separated by a 25Å space.[44] Such a structure has been termed a "unit" membrane and is believed to be the basic structure for all membranes. The relationship of the plasmalemma to other cytoplasmic membranous components is still unclear for most cells, but direct connections between the sarcolemma of striated muscle and the intermediate component of the sarcoplasmic triad system have been shown.[43, 47] Such connections play an important role in the passage of the excitation wave initiating contraction into the interior of the muscle cell.

Seen near the plasmalemma of mesenchymal derivatives and in the endothelium of capillaries are numerous thin-walled round or oval vesicles (400Å to 800Å) that tend to line up along the cell membrane (Fig. 7). A constricted or flasklike opening may be seen in the cell membrane leading into the interior of the vesicle. These pinocytotic vesicles arise by invagination of the cell membrane, thereby enclosing a small amount of the extracellular environment. Thus pinocytosis is regarded as an important cellular mechanism for the imbibition of fluid, particulate matter,[40] and proteins[45] from the extracellular space.

Many small villous projections (microvilli) of the cell membrane are found on the luminal surfaces of epithelial cells (Fig. 8). Especially well-developed microvilli comprise the brush borders of cells such as those lining the intestinal tract and the tubular cells of the kidney. Electron microscopic abnormalities, consisting of deformed, stunted, and sparse microvilli, are seen in small intestinal biopsies from patients suffering from primary malabsorption syndromes (Fig. 9). Similar findings also have been found in patients with primary small intestinal malignancies.[46] Although normal morphologic microvillus structure returns following successful dietary therapy, the role of microvilli in alimentary absorption is not yet known.

Another specialization of the cell membrane occurs at the base of tubular cells of the kidney and consists of deep invaginations of the basilar plasma membrane. At points of contact between neighboring cells, the invaginations of one cell interdigitate closely with evaginations of another. The invaginated basilar plasma membranes create a potential extracellular space bounded by the basement membrane below. This potential space is capable of enlarging to a considerable degree under experimental conditions, producing polyuria.[41] Folded basilar membranes and interdigitated processes similar to those of the kidney tubule are found in the duct cells of the salivary gland (Fig. 10), in the secretory cells of eccrine sweat glands, and in the salt gland cells of the albatross —all involved in water transport.

The plasma membranes of neighboring cells are not in direct contiguity but rather are separated by a space of 100Å to 300Å. Specialized zones of attachment known as desmosomes are often present (Figs. 19 and 20). In the epidermis, where desmosomes are numerous, localized thickenings of the opposing plasma membranes occur, and into these thickenings tonofilaments insert. Three electron opaque lines, the central one more prominent, are visualized between the thickened plasma membranes.[42] What lies between these densities and what the forces of adhesion or attraction are is unknown. About the necks of epithelial cells lining the intestine and glands elsewhere, attachments called terminal bars are seen (Fig. 8). These are larger than des-

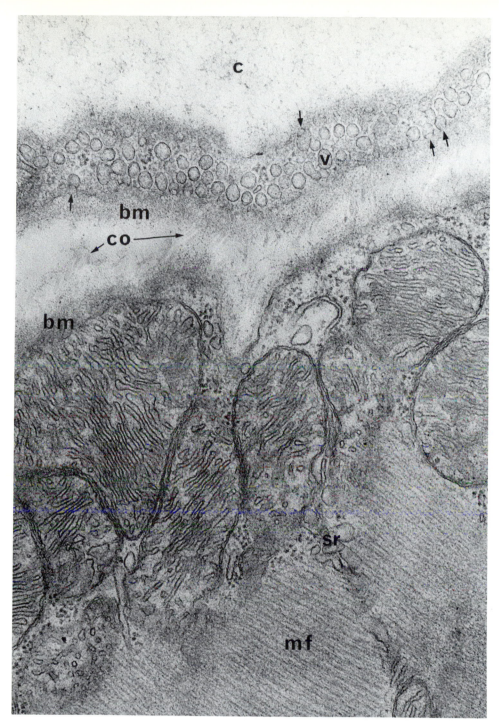

Fig. 7 Surface of striated muscle cell and nearby capillary with lumen labeled **c.** Layer of basement membrane, **bm,** is closely applied to external surfaces of both muscle and endothelial cell. Few collagen fibers, **co,** are embedded in this basement membrane material. Attenuated endothelial cytoplasm is crowded with thin-walled vesicles, **v.** Such vesicles are thought to arise by pinocytosis and to play role in transport across endothelium. In this somewhat tangential section, flasklike opening of several of these pinocytotic vesicles can be seen (arrows). Myofilaments, **mf,** as well as profiles of sarcoplasmic reticulum, **sr,** can be seen in lower portion. Fine structure of numerous mitochondria in this area can easily be seen. (Uranyl acetate–lead citrate; ×64,000.)

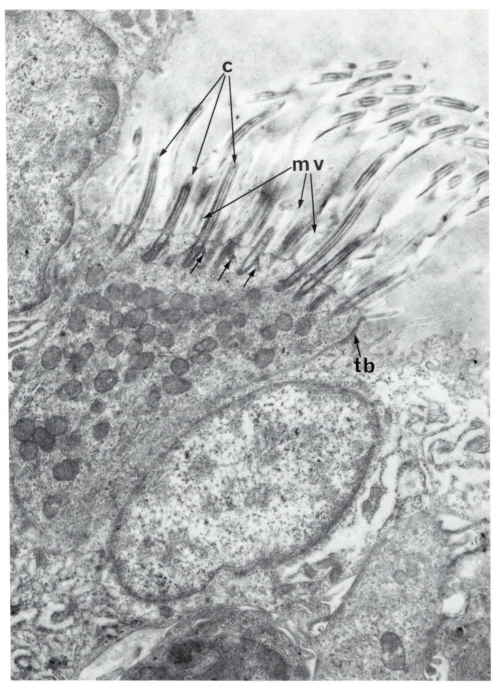

Fig. 8 Numerous cilia, **c,** arising from apex of thyroid epithelial cell, as well as microvilli, **mv,** can be seen. Longitudinal fine filaments can be seen in free portion of cilia. These filaments undergo fusion and further differentiation at cell surface, where they then pass into apical cytoplasm to form base of cilium. Lateral projections in this region are termed rootlets (arrows). Terminal bar, **tb,** can be seen at apical border of two adjoining cells. (Uranyl acetate–lead citrate; ×15,000; courtesy Dr. T. Murad, Atlanta, Ga.)

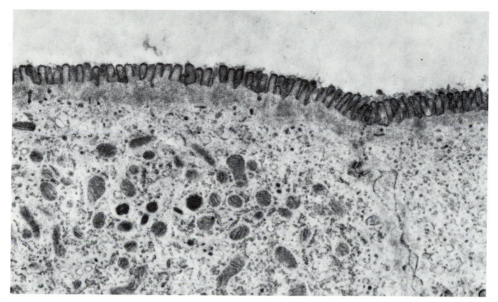

Fig. 9 Severely atrophic microvilli on cells from apical portion of flattened jejunal villus. Patient had celiac sprue that responded to gluten-free diet. (Uranyl acetate–lead citrate; ×9,000.)

mosomes but have a similar ultrastructure. Epidermoid carcinoma cells are found to have fewer desmosomes when compared with the number usually found in the spiny layer of the skin.[39]

Cytoplasmic organelles

Before describing the organelles, it should be kept in mind that a wide variety of substances are present in the cytoplasm, not all of which are limited by electron-opaque membranes. Use of the negative staining procedure devised by Horne[59] shows that the spaces between the membranes can be filled with phosphotungstic acid, an electron-opaque material, and what appeared as dense lines in osmium-fixed tissues appears as lucid lines. The use of other preparatory techniques such as freeze drying and the making of replicas shows comparable structures.

Ribosomes and endoplasmic reticulum

The basophilia of the cytoplasm is due to the presence of ribosomes (Figs. 6 and 11). These are minute (150Å to 300Å) round particles composed of ribonucleo-

protein. They may occur free as single particles or aggregated as polyribosomes or be attached in orderly arrays to the major membranous component of the cytoplasm, the endoplasmic reticulum. Two forms of endoplasmic reticulum are found. One is a rough-surfaced endoplasmic reticulum, ergastoplasm, in which ribosomes are attached to the outer surface of flattened membranous sacs or cisternae. These sacs are about 50 mμ in width and several microns in length (Fig. 11). In the acinar cells of the pancreas, about 50% of the total ribonucleic acid content of the cells is accounted for by the ergastoplasm. Isolated ergastoplasm is able to incorporate labeled amino acid into protein.[65] Separation of the ribosomes from the membranous component has shown that virtually all of the ribonucleic acid content and the ability to incorporate labeled amino acids into proteins are associated with the particulate fraction, whereas most of the protein nitrogen, phospholipid content, and glucose-6-phosphatase activity resides with the membrane fraction.[71]

Labeled amino acids incorporated into

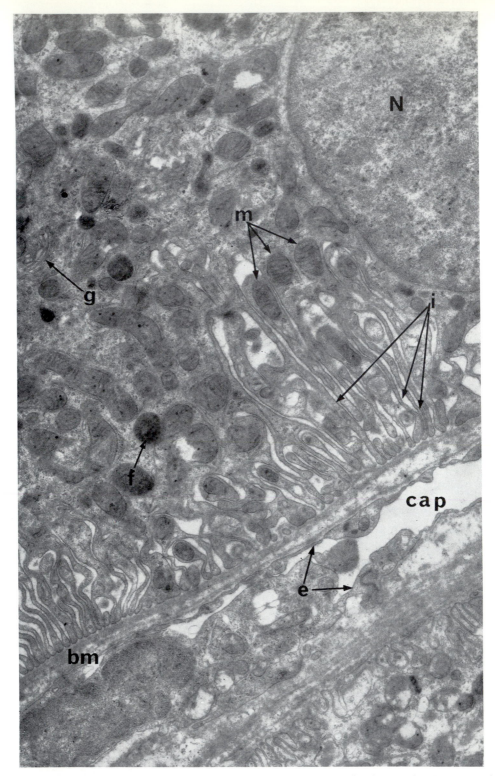

Fig. 10 Basilar portion of cell lining intercalated duct in parotid salivary gland. Repeated infoldings, **i,** of basilar plasma membrane and imbrications of these processes with those of adjacent cells are specialization of cell membrane that occurs at sites of active fluid transport (e.g., renal tubular epithelium). Proximity of capillary, **cap,** attenuation of its endothelial lining, **e,** and basement membrane, **bm,** are shown. Other cytoplasmic organelles are present and may be identified as follows: mitochondria, **m,** within batonets of cytoplasm; fat globules, **f;** Golgi apparatus, **g;** and nucleus, **N.** (Uranyl acetate–lead citrate; ×18,000.)

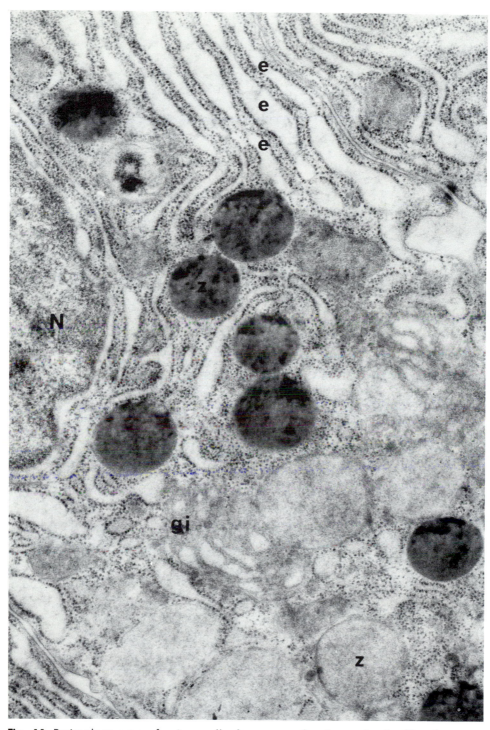

Fig. 11 Perinuclear area of acinar cell of pancreas showing variously dilated ergasto-plasm, **e,** with their ribosome-studded membranous sacs in more or less parallel array. Golgi zone, **gi,** composed of agranular membranous sacs and vesicles, can be seen in vicinity of nucleus, **N,** and associated with zymogen granules, **z,** in various stages of formation. (Uranyl acetate–lead citrate; ×31,700; courtesy Dr. B. L. Munger, Hershey, Pa.)

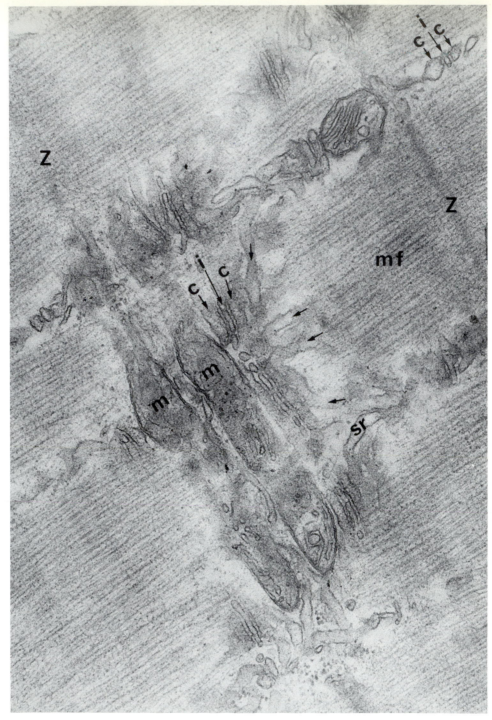

Fig. 12 Highly complex differentiation of endoplasmic reticulum found in striated muscle. **Z** line of myofibril can be seen in upper right with myofilaments, **mf.** As plane of section passes out of myofibril at about middle of sarcomere, longitudinal elements of sarcoplasmic reticulum, **sr,** are encountered (arrows). These converge to join transverse sarcoplasmic cisterna, **c,** first element of "triad." "Intermediate" component, **i,** of triad can be seen next as row of elongated vesicles. Last element of triad can then be seen as cisterna, **c,** similar to first. Portions of "triad" structures are visible in other areas and can be seen in cross section in upper right corner. Precise positioning of "triad" structure on either side of two mitochondria, **m,** straddling **Z** line level (upper left) can be seen. (Uranyl acetate–lead citrate; ×64,500.)

zymogen granules of the pancreas are found first associated with the ribosomes, then in the membranous sacs of the ergastoplasm, and later in the Golgi vesicles. Present concepts hold that protein synthesis occurs within the ergastoplasm, followed by transport of protein moieties to the Golgi apparatus, where they are packaged for storage or secretion.

The other form of endoplasmic reticulum is the agranular or smooth-surfaced type that is found in the cytoplasm of virtually all animal and plant cells. It forms tubules, vesicles, and anastomosing flattened sacs. Transitions between smooth-surfaced and rough-surfaced reticulum, as well as continuity between the agranular form of reticulum and the outer membrane of the nuclear envelope, are found. A remarkable specialization of smooth-surfaced endoplasmic reticulum occurs in striated muscle. Some of the details of this sarcotubular system may be seen in Fig. 12. Some cells associated with steroid hormone metabolism have large numbers of endoplasmic tubules or vesicles in areas of their cytoplasm.

Glycogen

Glycogen from human tissues is a spheroidal particle measuring 180Å to 300Å in diameter, with subunit filaments measuring 30Å. In this form, it is found as a component of the cytoplasm and, less commonly, the nucleus of many different cells. In the liver cell, an aggregated or "rosette" form occurs in proximity to the smooth endoplasmic reticulum and its associated glucose-6-phosphatase activity.[68] This spatial arrangement of substrate and membrane with enzyme activity suggests a mechanism in morphologic terms of glucose release from the liver.[50]

Both aggregated and nonaggregated forms are heavily stained with lead hydroxide. Glycogen rosettes from diseased liver stain unpredictably with uranyl acetate and phosphotungstic acid, resulting in difficulty in distinguishing glycogen from polyribosomes and viral particles.[50]

Mitochondria

Mitochondria are cylindrical rods large enough to be visible with the light microscope in appropriately stained preparations and with the phase microscope in 0.5μ to 1μ thick sections of osmium-fixed, plastic-embedded tissues. Their ultrastructure is characteristic. They are bounded by a double membrane. Infoldings of the inner membrane form an array of shelves (cristae) traversing the core of the mitochondrion[64] (Fig. 7). High resolution studies of negatively stained mitochondria have shown regular arrays of spherical particles (80Å in diameter) attached to the inner mitochondrial membrane by slender stalks (50Å long).[56, 72] This inner membrane subunit is a specific structural component of the mitochondrion and may be important in the oxidative phosphorylative function of this organelle.[67] Autoradiographs of animal and plant tissues treated with tritiated thymidine show localization of the label over both nucleus and mitochondria.[73, 74] Mitochondria from chick embryos show internal fibers in the matrix with the morphologic and cytohistochemical characteristics of DNA. Such studies indicate that structural and biochemical components of DNA reside within mitochondria.[62]

Variations in the numbers and size of mitochondria are found in neoplastic and embryonic cells. Abnormalities in mitochondrial size and cristae have been shown in hepatic mitochondria of rats made thyrotoxic[57] or riboflavin deficient.[61] The abnormal numbers of mitochondria found in oxyphilic cells (oncocytes) of the thyroid and Warthin's tumor (Figs. 13 and 532) are unexplained. In the oncocytoma illustrated in Fig. 13, the stacking of the cristae is reminiscent of grana in chloroplasts. The intramitochondrial aggregates of glycogen are perhaps evidence of metabolic aberrations.

Golgi apparatus

The Golgi apparatus is often located near the nucleus and in secretory cells is supra-

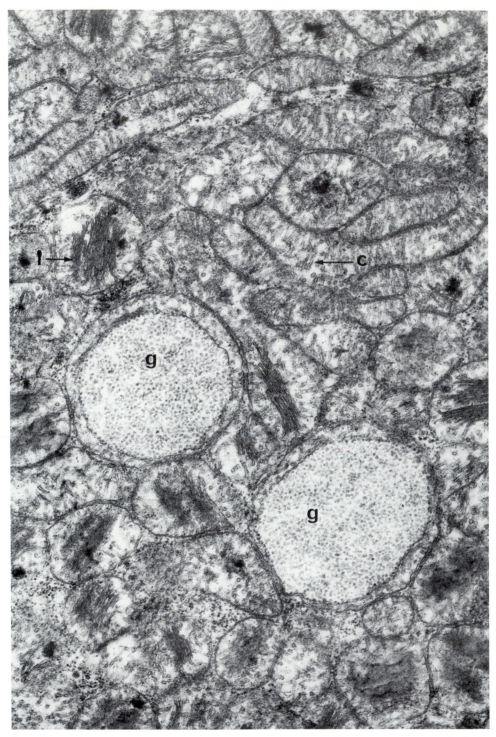

Fig. 13 Portion of oncocyte from oncocytoma of submandibular salivary gland. Entire cytoplasm is filled with mitochondria. Mitochondrial cristae, **c,** are prominently displayed and form stacked lamellae, **l,** in some areas. Two aggregates of glycogen, **g,** are present apparently within mitochondria. (Uranyl acetate–lead citrate; ×25,000.)

nuclear. It is composed of stacks of flattened agranular cisternae associated with round or oval vesicles. In certain planes of section, the lamellar cisternae are cup shaped (Fig. 6). This organelle is quite conspicuous in secretory cells or cells active in the synthesis of protein for use outside the cell.

The formative stages of zymogen granules of the acinar cell of the pancreas (Fig. 11), of the secretory granules of the pituitary and parathyroid glands, and of alpha and beta islet cells are seen in association with the Golgi vesicles.[66] For these reasons, this region of the cell is thought to be a processing or packaging area for products synthesized by the cell ultimately destined for use outside the cell. Thus the prominent Golgi apparatus of the liver cell and plasma cell is related to the production of plasma proteins. Cells with synthetic mechanisms devoted primarily to producing proteins with intracellular functions (i.e., striated and smooth muscle and epidermis) possess compact and rather inconspicuous Golgi bodies.

Filaments

Areas of cytoplasm containing dispersed or partially oriented fine filaments (80Å) may be found in many diverse cells such as astrocytes, myoepithelial cells, smooth muscle cells, beta cells of pancreatic islets, axons, hepatic cells, myxoma cells, epidermal and endothelial cells, and many tumor cells. The chemical composition and function of these filaments are as yet unknown, and it is not certain that they are the same in all the cells mentioned. However, in the cells of the epidermis, in which bundles of filaments (tonofilaments) are found coursing through the cytoplasm and attached to desmosomes (Fig. 20), they are considered precursors of keratin. In the process of keratinization, the cytoplasm becomes progressively filled with tonofilaments.[51] When keratinization is complete, only tightly packed tonofilaments, a few ribosomal particles, and occasional nuclear fragments may be found.[70]

In striated muscle, a striking orientation and disposition of filaments occur[60] (Figs. 12 and 14). Each myofibril is made up of two types of filaments arranged in a precise periodic manner along the longitudinal axis. The I (isotropic) band of classical light microscopy is comprised of longitudinally oriented parallel arrays of "thin" filaments (50Å to 60Å) that are attached to a centrally positioned, very dense Z line. The A (anisotropic) band is made up of similarly disposed "thick" filaments (100Å), each possessing a thickened region in the middle of the length of the filament that is responsible for the M line. The thick and thin filaments interdigitate along a portion of their length in the manner of a close-packed hexagonal array in which each thick filament is surrounded by six equidistant "thin" filaments. Muscle contraction, in Huxley and Hanson's view,[60] results from the "sliding" of thin filaments past "thick" filaments until interdigitation along the full length of the filaments is obtained at maximal shortening. In this process, the I band disappears and reappears when relaxation occurs, and the thick and thin filaments partially slide apart. Differential extraction procedures[60] have provided evidence that the thin filaments consist of the protein actin and that the thick filaments consist of myosin.

Filaments of the "thin" variety are present in smooth muscle cells but do not exhibit the orderly orientation, distribution, or banding observed in skeletal muscle.[69] Hanson and Lowry[58] showed that actin filaments have been identified in all types of muscle examined thus far.

Lysosomes

A particulate fraction of liver homogenate (lysosomes) has been found to contain high levels of acid phosphatase and other hydrolytic enzymes.[52] Single membrane-limited structures containing membrane fragments, rounded or irregular densities, granular materials, and altered or distorted pieces of other cytoplasmic organelles contain acid phosphatase as dem-

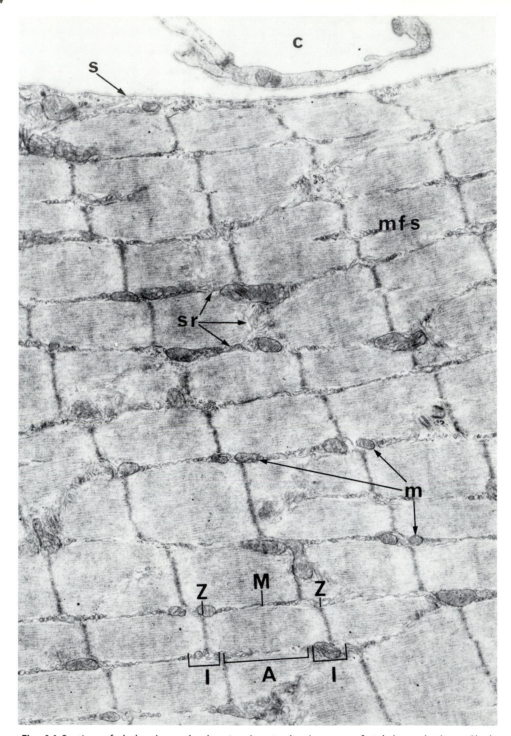

Fig. 14 Section of skeletal muscle showing longitudinal arrays of tightly packed myofibrils, **mfs,** separated one from another by sheath of tubules (**Sr,** sarcoplasmic reticulum). Within myofibrils can be seen myofilaments oriented longitudinally and characteristically cross-banded into **A** and **I** bands. Dense **Z** line is situated in center of **I** band, and **M** line can be seen in middle of **A** band. Interfibrillar mitochondria, **m,** occupy positions on either side of **Z** lines. Sarcolemma, **s,** can be seen at top with small capillary, **c,** nearby. (Uranyl acetate–lead citrate; ×16,600.)

onstrated by ultrastructural histochemical methods.[54, 63] Such structures, variously termed cytosomes and cytosegresomes ("autophagic vacuoles"), are involved in the storage, degradation, and intracellular digestion of different endogenous and exogenous materials.[52] Although the mechanisms by which cytosomes and cytosegresomes are formed and by which they acquire enzymatic activity are complex and not fully understood,[53, 63] it appears that inherent cellular defects in their function are found in human disease, such as glycogen storage disease, type II,[49] and metachromatic leukodystrophy.[48] Microbodies containing enzymes of the peroxisome complex and lacking acid phosphatase are not considered part of the lysosomal system.

Other cytoplasmic organelles

Lipids are seen as membrane-limited spheres of homogenous material of varying electron opacity. Due to the difference in density of the lipid and the cytoplasm, they are often cut unevenly. A variety of other bodies, such as microbodies, multivesicular bodies, myelin figures, and siderosomes, occur in the cytoplasm.

Cilia have a characteristic ultrastructure across a wide range of genera and species.[55] They are formed of nine peripheral and two central filaments. The intracytoplasmic extension or rootlet has, within limits, structural similarities to the centriole. On occasion, cilia have been found in seemingly unlikely sites such as the adenohypophysis and the pancreas.

Nucleus

The nucleus is surrounded by a double membrane that is interrupted at intervals by discontinuities termed nuclear pores.[77] Several pores may be seen in the electron micrographs of the normal and neoplastic plasma cell (Figs. 6 and 15). The fine structure of chromatin material is disappointing in osmium-fixed material and is usually observed as variously sized aggregates of dark particles. Cells in the process of division are occasionally encountered with clumps of chromatin material distributed in broad bands reminiscent of the chromosomal strands of light microscopy. Thin "spindle" fibers also may be seen. The double limiting nuclear membrane disappears in the early stages of nuclear division and re-forms again in the later stages. Such a stage is depicted in the electron micrograph of a dividing cell from a human malignant lymphoma (Fig. 16).

The nucleolus is seen as a spongelike meshwork composed principally of zones of closely packed fibrils, 50Å in width and of variable length, contiguous with poorly defined regions of aggregated dense granules (100Å to 150Å)[75] (Figs. 6 and 20). Dispersion and disassociation of nucleolar components are noted under experimental conditions affecting the synthesis of ribosomal precursors or messenger ribonucleic acid.[76] The nucleoli of tumor cells often are very large and give the impression of being formed from tangled threads or skeins of material (Figs. 15 and 535).

Formed extracellular elements

The intercellular ground substance that bathes the cells and formed elements of connective tissue is a structureless electron lucid matrix. The precursors of collagen are formed in fibrocytes, are secreted, and assume the structure of collagen in the extracellular space. Native collagen seen in longitudinal sections has a characteristic banding at intervals of 640Å to 700Å (Fig. 17). In cross section, fine microfibrils are seen interspersed between the larger collagen bundles. Another form of collagen occurs with banding at 1,200Å to 2,800Å.[78] It is called fibrous or long-spacing collagen. Bone is formed by the deposition of crystals of apatite on osteoid, which is collagen. This deposition occurs first at the banding of the collagen. Reticulum is minute collagen fibers. Its argyrophilia is unexplained.

Elastic tissue, in contrast to collagen, is a relatively lucid and structureless mate-

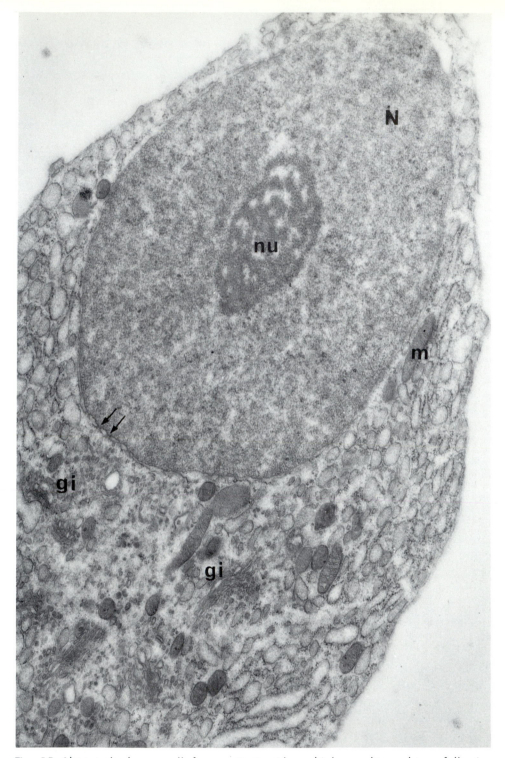

Fig. 15 Abnormal plasma cell from patient with multiple myeloma shows following changes. Large central nucleolus, **nu,** can be seen in nucleus, **N.** Cytoplasm is largely filled with vesiclular profiles of endoplasmic reticulum that are sparsely studded with ribosomes. Golgi apparatuses, **gi,** are compact and somewhat small. Mitochondria, **m,** are also diminished in size. Nuclear "pores" are indicated by arrows. (Uranyl acetate–lead citrate; ×28,000; courtesty Dr. G. D. Sorenson, Hanover, N. H.)

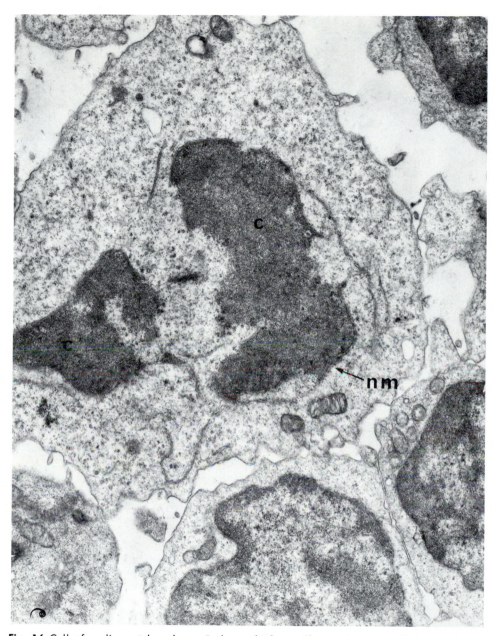

Fig. 16 Cell of malignant lymphoma in late telophase. Chromatin, **c,** is still dispersed, and nuclear membrane, **nm,** is incomplete. Few mitochondria and membranous profiles can be seen in cytoplasm among numerous ribosomes. (Uranyl acetate–lead citrate; ×14,000.)

rial in epoxy resin-embedded specimens. Fine microfibrils, thought by some to be collagenous, are found within and about the elastic fibers.

Basement membranes (Figs. 535 and 635) are a structural enigma. They are formed by a variety of cells (epithelial, mesothelial, and endothelial) and appear to function both as footholds and as filters. Histochemically, they are PAS positive and contain large amounts of mucopolysaccharide. Although structural differentiation in basement membrane material is not seen by electron microscopy, there may be func-

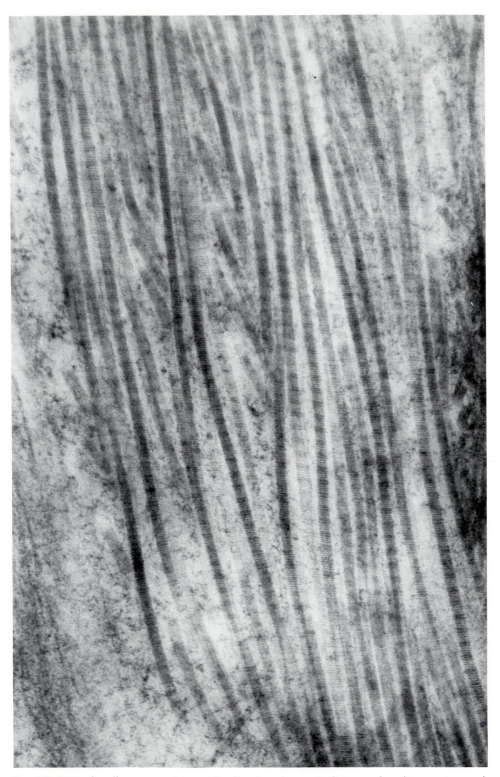

Fig. 17 Dermal collagen cut longitudinally. Regular periodicity or banding at intervals of 640Å units can be readily seen. (Uranyl acetate–lead citrate; ×69,000.)

tional differentiation. A high level of cholinesterase activity can be demonstrated in basement membrane material in the region of the neuromuscular junction.[79]

Neoplastic cells

Many studies have been made in an attempt to discover some difference between normal and neoplastic cells. The findings were reviewed by Mercer[87] and Oberling and Bernhard,[88] and the consensus fails to demonstrate specific structural features in cancer cells that are not also present in normal cells.

Thus far, the main differences described have been of numbers and configuration of cellular structures, all of which are found in the normal parent cell. In keeping with light microscopic observations, the nuclei are large and pleomorphic, with deep invaginations of the nuclear membrane. Where the light microscope shows regular round nuclei, such as those seen in malignant lymphoma and seminoma, the electron microscopic picture is the same (Fig. 7). The nuclei of some tumors, particularly lymphomas, show the presence of remarkable outpouchings or "blebs." Such undulations of the nucleus are not usually seen in normal cells and imply an unusual nuclear characteristic. The nucleoli are frequently found enlarged, with the dense nucleolar material arranged in a skeinlike pattern[80] (Figs. 15 and 535). In many cancer cells, the organization of cytoplasmic organelles is much less complex than in the cells of origin. In very anaplastic cells, the intracytoplasmic membranous components consist of little more than a few scattered segments of endoplasmic reticulum, inconspicuous Golgi bodies, and few small mitochondria. Unattached ribosomes make up the bulk of the formed elements in the scanty cytoplasm. The "sameness" in fine structural appearance of many malignant cells has led to the impression that these cells resemble each other more than do their fully differentiated parent cells.[80]

Exceptions have been noted, however,

particularly in brain tumors and endocrine tumors (Fig. 311). Oligodendrogliomas may have increased numbers of mitochondria, often greatly enlarged.[85] Eosinophilic adenomas of the pituitary gland, pheochromocytomas, and carcinoid tumors have many secretory granules in their cytoplasm. Specific secretory granules have been demonstrated in functioning beta, alpha, and D cell tumors of the pancreas.[82, 83, 86]

The centriole pair of normal cells possess a constant orthogonal spatial relationship one to another. Furthermore, centrioles of adjacent groups of cells display a symmetrical spatial periodicity pattern along a given axis. Cancer cells show evidence of intracellular disorder in the spindle mechanism that manifests itself in a random orientation of one centriole to another. There is some evidence that the intercellular centriolar periodicity pattern is maintained.[89, 90]

An observation of possible significance has been the absence or attenuation of the basement membrane in invasive squamous cancer of the cervix[84] and oral cavity[81] as contrasted with the intact basement membrane of most specimens of carcinoma in situ.

The fine structural appearance of embryonic cells has invited a comparison with neoplastic cells.[88] Scanty endoplasmic reticulum, scattered ribosomes, compact Golgi bodies, and small mitochondria are often noted in the early stages of differentiating cells (Fig. 18). Large bizarre nucleoli also may be seen. In the opinion of Bernhard,[80] the similarities that exist between embryonic and neoplastic cells are only superficial—cancer cells are somehow a caricature of the embryonic cell.

Viruses and tumors

The possibility that viruses are among the causes of neoplasia has attracted attention for many years. Long before the appearance of the electron microscope, which now makes viruses visible, the induction and transmission of certain tumors by viruses in animals were established

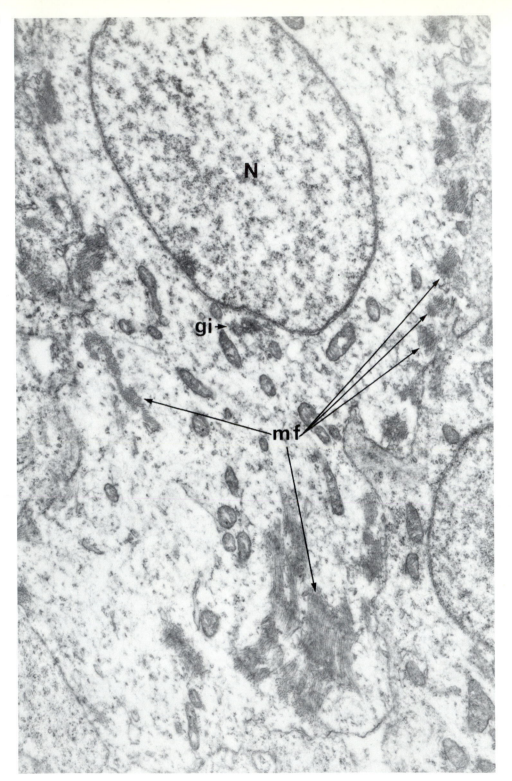

Fig. 18 Small bundles of myofilaments, **mf,** can be seen in periphery of cytoplasm in chick myoblast. Z band formation is suggested in lower portion of figure. Note small numbers of ribosomes and endoplasmic reticulum. Ergastoplasm is absent. Inconspicuous compact Golgi apparatus, **gi,** can be seen adjacent to nucleus, **N.** Many widely scattered fine filaments can be seen in cytoplasm. (Uranyl acetate–lead citrate; ×18,300.)

(e.g., the Shope papilloma and the Rous sarcoma). A host of transmissible tumors of animals are now known.[104] Ultrastructural studies of neoplasms induced by viruses are appearing in increasing numbers. The emphasis has been on the leukemias and mammary carcinoma of mice,[96, 100] the chicken leukosis complex,[98] the Rous sarcoma,[99] the Shope papilloma,[95] and the variety of tumors induced in several species by the polyoma virus.[94]

Of human tumors, only warts, molluscum contagiosum, and squamous papillomas of the larynx are known to be due to viruses. Sporadic reports have appeared of the finding of viruslike particles in electron micrographs of isolated cases of multiple myeloma,[103] leukemia,[93, 101] breast cancer,[97] and gastric carcinoma.[102] The identification of morphologically characteristic virus in tumor cells does not, however, prove their etiologic relationships. The problem is further complicated in that similar nucleolar changes have been found in certain virus-infected cells and Hodgkin's disease,[92] as well as in lead poisoning.[91] Even in the virus-induced neoplasms of animals, the mechanisms by which the viruses cause neoplasia are not elucidated by the electron microscope. Certainly, detailed surveys of a greater variety of human neoplasms are warranted. However, the absence of artificial models and experimental hosts for some of the known and probably for the unknown oncongenic viruses and the possibility of latent infection present great problems in the attempt to study viral oncogenesis.

REFERENCES

Introduction

1 Horne, R. W., and Whittaker, V. P.: The use of the negative staining method for the electron microscopic study of subcellular particles from animal cells, Z. Zellforsch. **58**:1-16, 1962.

2 Kimmelstiel, P., Kim, O. J., and Beres, J.: Studies on renal biopsy specimens with the aid of the electron microscope. I. Glomeruli in diabetes, Am. J. Clin. Pathol. **38**:270-279, 1962.

3 Luft, J. H.: Improvements in epoxy resin embedding methods, J. Biophys. Biochem. Cytol. **9**:409-414, 1961.

4 Maul, G. G., and Romsdahl, M. M.: Ultrastructural comparison of two human malignant melanoma cell lines, Cancer Res. **30**:2782-2790, 1970.

5 Metzger, J. F., and Smith, C. W.: The application of immune electron microscopy to the demonstration of antigenic sites in biologic systems, Lab. Invest. **11**:902-911, 1962.

6 Nakane, P. K., and Pierce, G. B.: Enzyme-labelled antibodies for light and electron microscopic localization of tissue antigens, J. Cell Biol. **33**:307-318, 1967.

7 Rosai, J., and Rodriguez, H. A.: Application of electron microscopy to the differential diagnosis of tumors, Am. J. Clin. Pathol. **50**:555-562, 1968.

8 Sabatini, D. D., Bensch, K., and Barrnett, R. J.: Cytochemistry and electron microscopy; the preservation of cellular ultrastructure and enzymatic activity by aldehyde fixation, J. Cell Biol. **17**:19-58, 1963.

9 Scarpelli, D. G., and Kanczak, N. M.: Ultrastructural cytochemistry: principles, limitations and applications, Int. Rev. Exp. Pathol. **4**:55-126, 1965.

10 Seymour, A. E., Spargo, B. G., and Penksa, R.: Contributions of renal biopsy studies to the understanding of disease, Am. J. Pathol. **65**:550-588, 1971.

11 Siekevitz, P.: The cytological basis of protein synthesis in the cytochemistry of enzymes and antigens, Exp. Cell. Res. (suppl. 7), pp. 90-110, 1959.

12 Steiner, J. W., Slater, R. J., and Movat, H. Z.: Studies on lipoid nephrosis in children and adolescents. I. The fine structural changes in "pure" nephrosis, Lab. Invest. **10**:763-786, 1961.

13 Trump, B. F., and Benditt, E. P.: Electron microscopy studies of human renal disease; observations of normal visceral glomerular epithelium and its modification in disease, Lab. Invest. **11**:753-781, 1962.

14 Zimmerman, L. E., Font, R. L., and T'so, M. O. M.: Application of electron microscopy to histopathologic diagnosis, Trans. Am. Acad. Ophthalmol. Otolaryngol. **76**:101-107, 1972.

Special problems in electron microscopy

15 Chang, S. C.: Hematoxylin-eosin staining of plastic-embedded tissue sections, Arch. Pathol. **93**:344-351, 1972.

16 Collan, Y., and Sainio, P.: Rapid standardized method for preparing isolated cells for ultrastructural study, Acta Cytol. **14**:603-606, 1970.

17 Erlandson, R. A.: A new Maraglas D.E.R. 732 embedment for electron microscopy, J. Cell Biol. **22**:704-708, 1964.

18 Fahimi, H. D.: Perfusion and immersion fixation of rat liver with glutaraldehyde, Lab. Invest. **16**:736-750, 1967.

19 Glauert, A. M., and Glauert, R. H.: Araldite as an embedding medium for electron microscopy, J. Biophys. Biochem. Cytol. **4**:191-194, 1958.

20 Luft, J. H.: Improvements in epoxy resin embedding methods, J. Biophys. Biochem. Cytol. **9**:409-414, 1961.

21 Lynn, J. A., Marlin, J. H., and Race, G. J.: Recent improvements of histologic techniques for the combined light and electron microscopic examination of surgical specimens, Am. J. Clin. Pathol. **45**:704-713, 1966.

22 Maunsbach, A. B.: The influence of different fixatives and fixation methods on the ultrastructure of rat kidney proximal tubule cells. I. Comparison of different perfusion fixation methods and of glutaraldehyde, formaldehyde and osmium tetroxide fixatives, J. Ultrastruct. Res. **15**:242-282, 1966.

23 Munger, B. L.: Staining methods applicable to sections of osmium-fixed tissue for light microscopy, J. Biophys. Biochem. Cytol. **11**:502-506, 1962.

24 Pease, D. C.: Histological techniques for electron microscopy, ed. 2, New York, 1964, Academic Press, Inc.

25 Pittman, F. E., and Pittman, J. C.: Electron microscopy of intestinal mucosa; some notes on techniques, Arch. Pathol. **81**:398-401, 1966.

26 Price, H. M., Howes, E. L., Sheldon, D. B., Hutson, O. D., Fitzgerald, R. T., Blumberg, J. M., and Pearson, C. M.: An improved biopsy technique for light and electron microscopic studies of human skeletal muscle, Lab. Invest. **14**:194-199, 1965.

27 Rangan, S. R.: A method of orientation of biological specimens for electron microscopy, J. Roy. Micr. Soc. **79**:377-378, 1961.

28 Rosai, J., and Rodriguez, H. A.: Application of electron microscopy to the differential diagnosis of tumors, Am. J. Clin. Pathol. **50**:555-562, 1968.

29 Rossi, G. L., Luginbühl, H., and Probst, D.: A method for ultrastructural study of lesions found in conventional histological sections, Virchows Arch. [Pathol. Anat.] **350**:216-224, 1970.

30 Sabatini, D. D., Bensch, K., and Barnett, R. J.: Cytochemistry and electron microscopy; the preservation of cellular ultrastructure and enzymatic activity by aldehyde fixation, J. Cell Biol. **17**:19-58, 1963.

31 Sparvoli, E., Gay, E., and Kaufmann, B. P.: Open-face, epoxy embedding of single cells for ultra-thin sections, Stain Technol. **40**:83-88, 1965.

32 Trump, B. F., and Bulger, R. E.: New ultrastructural characteristics of cells fixed in a glutaraldehyde–osmium tetroxide mixture, Lab. Invest. **15**:368-379, 1966.

33 Trump, B. F., Goldblatt, P. J., and Stowell, R. E.: An electron microscopic study of early cytoplasmic alterations in hepatic parenchymal cells of mouse liver during necrosis in vitro (autolysis), Lab. Invest. **11**:986-1015, 1962.

34 Trump, B. F., Goldblatt, P. J., and Stowell, R. E.: Studies on necrosis of mouse liver in vitro; ultrastructural alterations in the mitochondria of hepatic parenchymal cells, Lab. Invest. **14**: 343-371, 1965.

35 Trump, B. F., Goldblatt, P. J., and Stowell, R. E.: Studies of necrosis in vitro of mouse hepatic parenchymal cells; ultrastructural alterations in endoplasmic reticulum, Golgi apparatus, plasma membranes and lipid droplets, Lab. Invest. **14**:2000-2028, 1965.

36 Trump, B. F., Smuckler, E. A., and Benditt, E. P.: A method for staining epoxy sections for light microscopy, J. Ultrastruct. Res. **5**: 343-348, 1961.

37 Winborn, W. B.: Dow epoxy resin with triallyl cyanurate, and similarly modified Araldite and Maraglas mixtures, as embedding media for electron microscopy, Stain Technol. **40**: 227-231, 1965.

38 Zimmerman, L. E., Font, R. L., and T'so, M. O. M.: Application of electron microscopy to histopathologic diagnosis, Trans. Am. Acad. Ophthalmol. Otolaryngol. **76**:101-107, 1972.

Cell membrane and its specializations

39 Abercrombie, M., and Ambrose, J. J.: The surface properties of cancer cells: a review, Cancer Res. **22**:525-548, 1962.

40 Farquhar, M. G., and Palade, G. E.: Incorporation of electron-opaque tracers by cells of the renal glomerulus. In Fifth International Congress for Electron Microscopy, vol. 2, LL-3 (Breese, S. S., Jr., editor), New York, 1962, Academic Press, Inc.

41 Latta, H., Sergio, A. B., Knigge, K. M., and Madden, S. C.: Extracellular compartments in renal tubules associated with polyuria from glucose imbibition, Lab. Invest. **11**:569-579, 1962.

42 Odland, G. R.: The fine structure of the interrelationship of cells in the human epidermis, J. Biophys. Biochem. Cytol. **4**:423-433, 1958.

43 Reger, J. F.: The fine structure of triads from swimmerette muscle of A. salinus. In Fifth International Congress for Electron Micros-

copy, vol. 2, TT-4 (Breese, S. S., Jr., editor), New York, 1962, Academic Press, Inc.

44 Robertson, J. D.: The ultrastructure of cell membranes and their derivatives, Biochem. Soc. Symp. **16**:3, 1959.

45 Roth, T. F., and Porter, K. R.: Specialized sites on the cell surface for protein uptake. In Fifth International Congress for Electron Microscopy, vol. 2, LL-4 (Breese, S. S., Jr., editor), New York, 1962, Academic Press, Inc.

46 Shearman, D. J., Girdwood, R. H., Williams, A. W., and Delamore, I. W.: A study with the electron microscope of the jejunal epithelium in primary disease, Gut **3**:16-25, 1962.

47 Smith, D. S.: The sarcoplasmic reticulum of insect muscles. In Fifth International Congress for Electron Microscopy, vol. 2, TT-3 (Breese, S. S., Jr., editor), New York, 1962, Academic Press, Inc.

Cytoplasmic organelles

48 Austin, J., McAfee, D., Armstrong, D., O'Rourke, M., Shearer, L., and Bachhawat, B.: Abnormal sulphatase activities in two human diseases (metachromatic leucodystrophy and gargoylism), Biochem. J. **93**:15C-17C, 1964.

49 Bauduin, P., Hers, H. G., and Loeb, H.: An electron microscopic and biochemical study of type II glycogenosis, Lab. Invest. **13**:1139-1152, 1964.

50 Biava, C.: Identification and structural forms of human particulate glycogen, Lab. Invest. **12**:1179-1197, 1963.

51 Brody, I.: The ultrastructure of the tonofibrils in the keratinization process of normal human epidermis, J. Ultrastruct. Res. **4**:264-297, 1960.

52 de Duve, C.: Functions of lysosomes, Ann. Rev. Physiol. **28**:435-492, 1966.

53 Ericsson, J. L., and Glinsmann, W. H.: Observations on the subcellar organization of hepatic parenchymal cells. I. Golgi apparatus, cytosomes, and cytosegresomes in normal cells, Lab. Invest. **15**:750-761, 1966.

54 Ericsson, J. L., and Trump, B. F.: Electron microscopic studies of the epithelium of the proximal tubule of the rat. I. The intracellular localization of acid phosphatase, Lab. Invest. **13**:1427-1456, 1964.

55 Fawcett, D.: Cilia and flagella. In Brachet, I., and Mirsky, A. E., editors: The cell, vol. 2, New York, 1961, Academic Press, Inc., p. 217.

56 Fernández-Morán, H.: Cell membrane ultrastructure, Circulation **26**:1039-1065, 1962.

57 Greenwalt, J. W., Foster, G. V., and Lehninger, A. L.: The observation of unusual membranous structures associated with liver mitochondria in thyrotoxic rats. In Fifth International Congress for Electron Microscopy, 00-5 (Breese, S. S., Jr., editor), New York, 1962, Academic Press, Inc.

58 Hanson, J., and Lowry, J.: Actin in contractile systems. In Fifth International Congress for Electron Microscopy, vol. 2, 0-9 (Breese, S. S., Jr., editor), New York, 1962, Academic Press, Inc.

59 Horne, R. W.: The examination of small particles. In Kay, D., editor: Techniques for electron microscopy, Springfield, Ill., 1961, Charles C Thomas, Publisher, pp. 150-165.

60 Huxley, H. E., and Hanson, J.: The molecular basis of contraction in cross-striated muscle, In Bourne, G. H., editor: Structure and function of muscle, vol. 1, New York, 1960, Academic Press, Inc., pp. 183-227.

61 Luse, S. A., Burch, H. B., and Hunter, F. E., Jr.: Ultrastructural and enzymatic changes in the liver of the riboflavin deficient rat. In Fifth International Congress for Electron Microscopy, VV-5 (Breese, S. S., Jr., editor), New York, 1962, Academic Press, Inc.

62 Nass, M. M. K., and Nass, S.: Intramitochondrial fibers with DNA characteristics, J. Cell Biol. **19**:593-611, 1963.

63 Novikoff, A. B., and Essner, E.: Cytolysosomes and mitochondrial degeneration, J. Cell Biol. **15**:140-146, 1962.

64 Palade, G. E.: Electron microscopy of mitochondria and other cytoplasmic structures. In Gaebler, O. H., editor: Enzymes: units of biologic structure and function, New York, 1956, Academic Press, Inc., p. 185.

65 Palade, G. E., and Siekevitz, P.: Pancreatic microsomes: an integrated morphological and biochemical study, J. Biophys. Biochem. Cytol. **2**:671-690, 1956.

66 Palay, S. L.: The cytology of secretion. In Palay, S. L., editor: Frontiers in cytology, New Haven, 1958, Yale University Press, pp. 305-342.

67 Parsons, D. F.: Recent advances correlating structure and function in mitochondria, Int. Rev. Exp. Pathol. **4**:1-54, 1965.

68 Revel, J. P., Napolitano, L., and Fawcett, D. W.: Identification of glycogen in electron micrographs of thin tissue sections, J. Biophys. Biochem. Cytol. **8**:575-589, 1960.

69 Rhodin, J. A. G.: Fine structures of vascular walls in mammals with special reference to smooth muscle component, Physiol. Rev. **42** (suppl. 5):48-81, 1962.

70 Roth, S. I., and Helwig, E. B.: The zone of keratinization in the internal root sheath of the mouse hair. In Fifth International Congress for Electron Microscopy, vol. 2, T-3

(Breese, S. S., Jr., editor) New York, 1962, Academic Press, Inc.

71 Siekevitz, P., and Palade, G. E.: A cytochemical study on the pancreas of the guinea pig. V. In vivo incorporation of leucine-1-C^{14} into the chymotrypsinogen of various cell fractions, J. Biophys. Biochem. Cytol. **7**:619-630, 1960.

72 Stoeckenius, W.: Some observations on negatively stained mitochondria. J. Cell Biol. **17**:443-454, 1963.

73 Stone, G. E., and Miller, O. L., Jr.: A stable mitochondrial DNA in Tetrahymena pyriformis, J. Exp. Zool. **159**:33-37, 1965.

74 Swift, H., Kislev, N., and Bogorad, L.: Evidence for DNA and RNA in mitochondrion and chloroplasts, J. Cell Biol. **23**:91A, 1964.

Nucleus

75 Bruni, C., and Porter, K. R.: The fine structure of the parenchymal cell of the normal rat liver. I. General observations, Am. J. Pathol. **46**:691-755, 1965.

76 Miyai, K., and Steiner, J. W.: Fine structure of interphase liver nuclei in acute ethionine intoxication, Lab. Invest. **16**:677-692, 1967.

77 Watson, M. L.: Further observations on the nuclear envelope in the animal cell, J. Biophys. Biochem. Cytol. **6**:147-156, 1959.

Formed extra-cellular elements

78 Rohen, J. W.: Ueber das Ligamentum pectinatum der Primaten, Z. Zellforsch. Mikrosk. Anat. **58**:403-421, 1962.

79 Zacks, S. I., and Blumberg, J. M.: Observations on the fine structure and cytochemistry of mouse and human intercostal neuromuscular junctions, J. Biophys. Biochem. Cytol. **10**:517-528, 1961.

Neoplastic cells

80 Bernhard, W.: Some problems of fine structure in tumor cells. In Homburger, F., editor: Progress in experimental tumor research, vol. 3, New York, 1962, Hafner Publishing Co., Inc., pp. 1-34.

81 Frithiof, L.: Ultrastructure of the basement membrane in normal and hyperplastic human oral epithelium compared with that in pre-invasive and invasive carcinoma, Acta Pathol. Microbiol. Scand. **200**(suppl.):1-25, 1969.

82 Greider, M. H., and Elliot, D. W.: Electron microscopy of human pancreatic tumors of islet cell origin, Am. J. Pathol. **44**:663-678, 1964.

83 Lacy, P. E., and Williamson, J. R.: Electron microscopy and fluorescent antibody studies of islet cell adenomas, Anat. Rec. **136**:227-228, 1960.

84 Luibel, F. J., Sanders, E., and Ashworth, C. T.: An electron microscopic study of carcinoma-in-situ and invasive carcinoma of the cervix uteri, Cancer Res. **20**:357-361, 1960.

85 Luse, S. A.: Ultrastructural characteristics of normal and neoplastic cells. In Homburger, F., editor: Progress in experimental tumor research, vol. 2, New York, 1961, Hafner Publishing Co. Inc., pp. 1-35.

86 McGavran, M. H., Unger, R. H., Recent, L., Polk, H. C., Kilo, C., and Levin, M. E.: A glucagon-secreting-alpha cell carcinoma of the pancreas, N. Engl. J. Med. **274**:1408-1413, 1966.

87 Mercer, E. H.: The cancer cell, Br. Med. Bull. **18**:187-192, 1962.

88 Oberling, C., and Bernhard, W.: The morphology of cancer cells. In Brachet, J., and Mirsky, A. E., editors: The cell, vol. 5, New York, 1961, Academic Press, Inc., pp. 405-496.

89 Schafer, P. W.: Centrioles of a human cancer: intercellular order and intracellular disorder, Science **164**:1300-1303, 1969.

90 Schafer, P. W.: Centrioles: intercellular order in normal and malignant cells, J. Thorac. Cardiovasc. Surg. **63**:472-477, 1972.

Viruses and tumors

91 Beaver, D. L.: The ultrastructure of the kidney in lead intoxication with particular reference to intranuclear inclusions, Am. J. Pathol. **39**:195-208, 1961.

92 Bernhard, W., Febvre, H. L., and Cramer, R.: Mise en evidence en microscope electronique d'un virus dans des cellules infectés in vitro par l'agent de polyome, C. R. Acad. Sci. [D.] (Paris) **249**:483-485, 1959.

93 Dmochowski, L., Grey, C. E., Sykes, J. A., Shullenberger, C. C., and Howe, C. D.: Studies on human leukemia, Proc. Soc. Exp. Biol. Med. **101**:686-690, 1959.

94 Dourmashkin, R. R.: Electron microscopy of polyoma virus: a review. In Dalton, A. J., and Haguenau, F., editors: Tumors induced by viruses, New York, 1962, Academic Press, Inc., pp. 151-182.

95 Febvre, H.: The Shope fibroma virus of rabbits. In Dalton, A. J., and Haguenau, F., editors: Tumors induced by viruses, New York, 1962, Academic Press, Inc., pp. 79-112.

96 Gross, L.: Oncogenic viruses, New York, 1961, Pergamon Press, Inc.

97 Haguenau, F.: Le cancer mammaire de la souris et de la femme: étude comparative au microscope electronique, Pathol. Biol. (Paris) **7**:989-1015, 1959.

98 Haguenau, F., and Beard, J. W.: The avian sarcoma-leukosis complex: its biology and

ultrastructure. In Dalton, A. J., and Haguenau, F., 1962, Academic Press, Inc., pp. 1-60.

99 Hollman, K. N.: Infectious papillomatosis of
rabbits (Shope): biology and ultrastructure.
In Dalton, A. J., and Haguenau, F., editors:
Tumors induced by viruses, New York, 1962,
Academic Press, Inc., pp. 61-78.

100 Moore, D. H.: The milk agent. In Dalton, A.
J., and Haguenau, F., editors: Tumors induced by viruses, New York, 1962, Academic Press, Inc., pp. 113-150.

101 Saraiva, L. G., Bourroul, C. P., Silveira, M.,
Prospero, J. D., and Angulo, J. J.: Cytoplasmic inclusions in acute hemocytoblastic leukemia: case report, Blood 17:334-344, 1961.

102 Schipkey, F. H., Geer, J. D., Allen, B. R., and
Moore, D. H.: Observation of the fine struc-
ture of some human tumors. Fifty-eighth
Meeting of the American Association of Pa-
thologists and Bacteriologists, Chicago, 1961,
Program Abstract, p. 54.

103 Sorenson, G. D.: Electron microscopic observations of viral particles in the myeloma cells
of man, Exp. Cell. Res. 25:219-221, 1961.

104 Stewart, H. L., Snell, K. C., Dunham, L. J.,
and Schlyen, S. M.: Transplantable and transmissible tumors of animals. In Atlas of tumor
pathology, Sect. XII, Fasc. 40, Washington,
D. C., 1959, Armed Forces Institute of Pathology.

3 Skin

Dermatoses Malcolm H. McGavran, M.D.
Tumors Malcolm H. McGavran, M.D.
Nevi and malignant melanoma

Dermatoses

Malcolm H. McGavran, M.D.

Introduction to dermatopathology

The entities described in this section are a select group taken from the large number of diseases that affect the skin. They have been chosen to encompass the types of nonneoplastic material generally seen in laboratories of surgical pathology. Many of the infrequently biopsied, histologically nonspecific, and rare dermatoses are excluded. Their characteristics are described in texts devoted wholly to dermatopathology and in the dermatologic literature.[1-10]

Isolated morphologic analysis has distinct limitations. These are even more evident in the evaluation of the reactive processes associated with diseases of the skin than in certain other organs. Therefore, it is imperative that all the information (clinical history, differential diagnosis, gross and microscopic observations) be correlated and from this synthesis an opinion rendered.

Only when this is done, and it requires some mental and occasionally physical exertion, may one expect to contribute meaningfully to the care of the patient.

Biopsies, usually small, are the commonly submitted specimens. The gross changes in them are minimal and of little moment. For evaluation of the gross changes, it is far better to see the lesions on the patient, preferably with the dermatologist. In lieu of this optimal form of examination, an accurate description of the characteristics, the sites of involvement, and a clinical differential diagnosis should accompany each biopsy. All biopsies should be taken from grossly characteristic areas. It is a waste of time and money to biopsy ruptured bullae, secondarily infected or heavily scratched areas, the incipient or involuting lesion. Multiple biopsies may be advisable when the lesions present differing forms and stages. Formalin, 10% buffered, is an adequate and available fixative. Bouin's and Zenker's fixatives may be used but have no unique merits. Incisional and punch biopsies can be kept from curling during fixation by placing them on a piece of file card prior to immersion. When the specimen is 0.6 cm or less in size, and most punch biopsies are, it is best processed into paraffin in one piece. It may then be sampled at various levels in the block. This prevents loss of tissue during the facing-up of the block and allows more adequate sampling. These technical niceties prevent delays, mishaps, and some mistakes.

Skin

The integument is formed by the epidermis and dermis. Within the dermis are the adnexa: the eccrine and apocrine sweat glands, sebaceous glands, and hair follicles. The regional variations in distribution of the adnexa and the character of the epidermis should be remembered.

Epidermis

The epidermis is formed by several layers of cells that differentiate to form the outer protective layer of keratin. Alterations in the pattern and process of keratinization are often produced by disease. All of the epidermal cells are derived from the layer of basal cells. Thus the presence of mitotic figures therein, the favorite cytologic observation of neophytes, is of interest but seldom of diagnostic significance. These basal cells are set upon, interdigitate with, and are attached to a basement membrane by hemidesmosomes. The dermoepidermal junction is thrown into undulating folds of interlocking ridges of epidermis, *rete ridges*, and dermal papillae. Thus the undersurface of the epidermis seen in whole mounts presents an anastomosing and reticulate pattern of ridges and valleys.[12] The pattern and size of these ridges vary from area to area. With age, they diminish in size, and the dermoepidermal junction becomes flattened.

The basal cells have a moderately basophilic cytoplasm in which, in contrast to the other epidermal cells, melanin pigment is present. As the cells differentiate, they enter the *stratum spinosum*, lose most of the melanin pigment, and become amphophilic and then eosinophilic. This correlates with the intracytoplasmic accumulation of filaments, which are the precursors of keratin, and a diminution of ribosomes. The cells of the epidermis are attached to each other by focal specializations of their walls called desmosomes (Figs. 19 and 20). When, due to fixation and dehydration or intercellular edema, the cells are separated, these areas of attachment are seen via the light microscope as fine spiny bridges (Fig. 21). The epidermal cells are not a syncytium, and "intercellular bridges" do not exist. Destruction of these attachments causes the cells to lose their cohesiveness. This process, termed *acantholysis*, is seen in pemphigus vulgaris and in some other bullous diseases.

Above the stratum spinosum is a layer of cells containing basophilic keratohyaline granules, the *granular layer*. Immediately above the granular layer, without transition forms, the *stratum corneum* begins. It

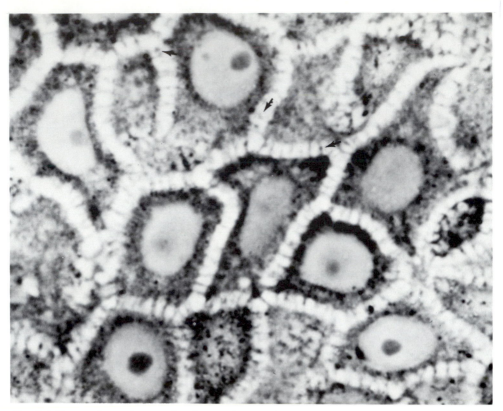

Fig. 19 Phase photomicrograph of spiny layer of slightly edematous epidermis. Nucleolar and nuclear outlines are distinct. Small black dots and rods in cytoplasm are mitochondria. Attachment plaques, desmosomes, may be seen (arrows) as increased densities on spines between cells. Compare with Fig. 20. (×2,200.)

is formed by flattened eosinophilic ghosts of cells that lack nuclei, keratohyaline granules, and other cytoplasmic organelles. Abnormal keratinization may be manifest by *hyperkeratosis,* in which the stratum corneum is thickened, usually in association with a more prominent granular layer, or by *parakeratosis,* in which the cells of the stratum corneum retain their nuclei and the granular layer is diminished or absent.

Certain descriptive terms are applied to alterations in the pattern of the epidermis. It may become *atrophic* or thinned with age or disease. It may be thickened, and as it proliferates the rete ridges extend deeper into the dermis. This is *acanthosis.* Excessive acanthosis produces a disorganized pattern at the dermoepidermal junction and is termed *pseudoepitheliomatous* *hyperplasia.* Outward overgrowth of the epidermis accompanied by elongation of the dermal papillae is *papillomatosis.* A degenerative process in which the basal cells become vacuolated, separated, and disorganized is called *liquefaction degeneration.* Various combinations of these changes are seen in the dermatoses, and this descriptive jargon allows succinct communication.

The melanocytes are specialized neuro-ectodermal derivatives that produce melanin. They are interspersed among the basal cells and are present in albinotic, vitiliginous, white, or dark skin. The amount of pigment they produce is determined by genetic, humoral, and physical factors. These cells have clear cytoplasm and fine dendritic processes, demonstrable in silver-stained sections, that extend between the

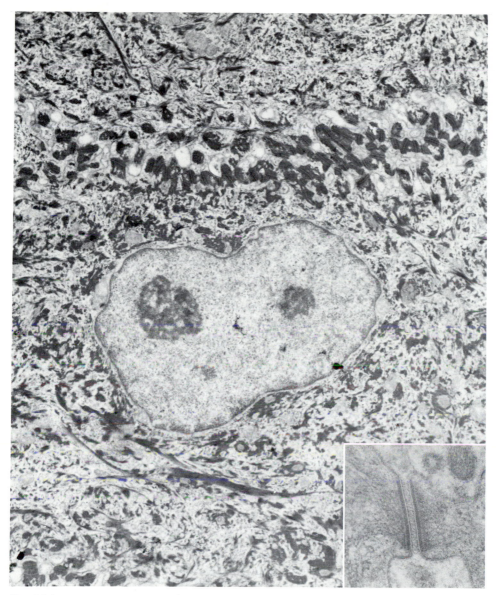

Fig. 20 Low stratum spinosum showing extensive desmosomal attachments, bundles of filaments in cytoplasm, nucleus, and two nucleoli. **Inset** shows details of desmosome. (Uranyl acetate–lead citrate; ×8,000; **inset,** ×80,000.)

epidermal cells.[11, 13] The melanocytes are dopa positive, whereas cells that contain but do not form melanin, such as basal cells and macrophages, are dopa negative. Such cells are *melanophages. Melanophores* are specialized cells, found in amphibians and reptiles, that are concerned with the humorally controlled distribution of pigment. *Melanoblasts* are the embryonic precursors of melanocytes.

Within the interphase nuclei of female cells, be they epidermal or of other epithelial origin, the sex chromatin body described by Moore and Barr[14] can be seen. This is a small, approximately 1μ, planoconvex, basophilic, Feulgen-positive mass applied to the nuclear membrane (Fig. 21). Thus genetic sex can be determined on skin biopsies.[16] For diagnostic use, however, we prefer the buccal smear, and for

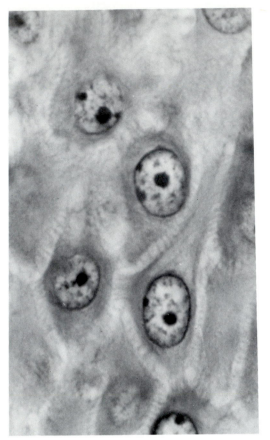

Fig. 21 Barr chromatin bodies are dark, plano-convex bodies impinging on nuclear membrane. "Intercellular bridges" are spiny lines between cells. (×1,500; WU neg. 55-6045.)

the refined chromosomal studies, leukocyte cultures are required.[15]

Dermis

The dermis supports and nourishes the epidermis and adnexa. It contains a sizable vascular plexus and network of sensory and vasomotor nerves that play significant roles in the homeostasis of the orgaism.[22] The dermis is divided into a superficial papillary layer and a deep reticular layer. Both contain interwoven bands of collagen and elastic fibers bathed in ground substance.[18] Two vascular plexuses are found, one at the junction of the dermis and subcutis and the other in the papillary layer. From the superficial vascular plexus capillary loops extend into the

dermal papillae. The details of the anatomic complexities, regional variations, and neurogenic control of the vessels of the skin may be found in the works of Horstman[19] and Winkelmann.[24]

With age, and more so in areas exposed to sunlight, the collagen and elastica undergo structural and tinctorial changes called basophilic degeneration of the collagen and senile elastosis, respectively[21, 23] (Fig. 22). These changes should not be attributed to some suspect disease and should be differentiated from pathologic connective tissue changes.

The dermis is the site of inflammatory reactions. In normal skin, a few fibrocytes, macrophages, mast cells, and lymphocytes are present. The perivascular and periadnexal spaces and the papillary layer of the dermis are the usual sites in which inflammatory cells aggregate. Certain dermatoses, such as lichen planus and chronic discoid lupus erythematosus, have distinct patterns of inflammatory reaction. Others, such as urticaria pigmentosa, have a specific cellular population. Changes in the nerves, visible in sections stained with hematoxylin-eosin, are infrequent but when present are of note (see leprosy, p. 45).

The epidermal adnexa are seldom the sites of primary changes. However, diagnostic changes do occur: heterotopias as in nevus sebaceous of Jadassohn, in which apocrine glands are found in the scalp; pigmentation of eccrine gland basement membranes in argyria and hemochromatosis; atrophy, as in scleroderma; duct obstruction with subsequent retention, as in the various forms of miliaria[20]; and deposition of aggregates of granules of mucoprotein in the eccrine gland cells in myxedematous patients.[17]

Inflammatory diseases
of known cause
Viral diseases

The histologically commonly seen viral lesions are warts. However, the vesiculobullous lesions caused by herpes simplex and herpes zoster and the varicelliform

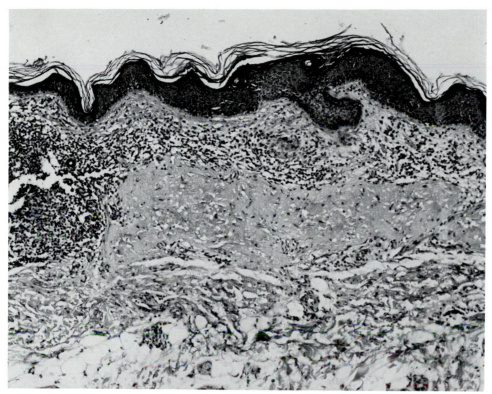

Fig. 22 Collagen is clumped and smudged and stains pale blue in this skin from face of 65-year-old woman. Mild lymphocytic infiltrate surrounds "basophilic degeneration." (×87; WU neg. 62-8937.)

eruption following vaccination of atopic individuals may occasionally be biopsied. These lesions are formed by ballooning and reticular degeneration of the epidermal cells. The fine points of differentiation are described by Ebert and Otsuka.[26] More recently, Williams et al.[33] were able to identify the viruses of *herpes, vaccinia,* and *warts* directly from vesicular fluid or tissue using the technique of negative staining and the electron microscope.

Warts

Several variants of warts occur. *Verruca vulgaris,* the common (hence vulgar) wart, usually occurs on the hands. It is an elevated, hard, rough, flesh-colored lesion. The top may be peeled off, leaving a pink granular surface. *Verruca plantaris* occurs on the sole of the foot and is covered by a callus. It is painful. *Verruca plana* is, as its name indicates, a flatter

lesion usually seen in crops or clusters on the face and hands. *Condyloma acuminatum,* "venereal wart," occurs around the anus and vulva and on the glans penis.

The histologic characteristics of these lesions are those of focal epidermal hyperplasia manifest by hyperkeratosis and parakeratosis, varying degrees of acanthosis, and papillomatosis (Fig. 23). Papillomatosis does not occur in verruca plana. Distinct vacuolization of the cells in the upper portion of the stratum spinosum is a feature in early lesions. These vacuolated cells have pyknotic nuclei and may be seen in the lower portions of the thickened stratum corneum. In condyloma acuminatum, acanthosis may be florid, and tangential cuts can show isolated nests of squamous cells surrounded by inflamed dermis. Care should be taken not to overdiagnose such lesions as squamous carcinoma.

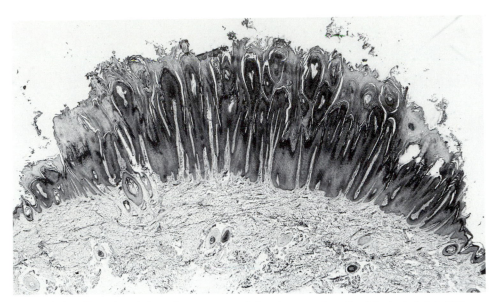

Fig. 23 Wart from hand that shows some of the changes described in text. (×14; WU neg. 62-8600.)

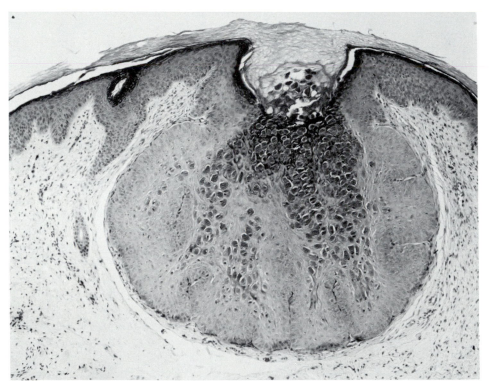

Fig. 24 Progressive differentiation of molluscum bodies can be readily seen. (×85; WU neg. 62-8601.)

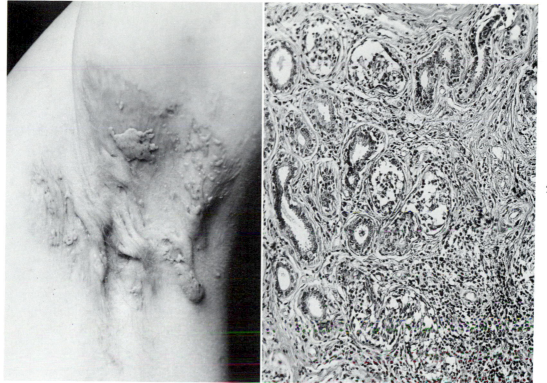

25

26

Fig. 25 Hidradenitis suppurativa of axilla showing nodules, sinuses, and scars. (WU neg. 52-4428.)

Fig. 26 Inflammatory reaction about and involving apocrine sweat glands. (WU neg. 52-4407.)

The viral etiology and transmission of warts by cell-free filtrates have been known for a long time.[32] Almeida et al.[25] have shown that the virus is formed in the nucleus and produces crystalline arrays of virus particles. The virus measures 55 mμ in diameter. These nuclear inclusions are basophilic, Feulgen positive, and DNA-ase resistant. The eosinophilic cytoplasmic masses are not viral but rather accumulations of tonofilaments. The virus of human warts is a member of the papova group.[30]

Molluscum contagiosum

Molluscum contagiosum is a skin disease characterized by small, firm, usually multiple nodules that, when fully developed, have central cores from which white keratinous material can be expressed. The microscopic picture is characteristic (Fig. 24). The dermis is indented by a sharply

delimited and lobulated mass of proliferating epidermis. As the epidermal cells differentiate within this mass, their cytoplasm gradually is filled by a faintly granular eosinophilic inclusion that displaces the nucleus and enlarges the cells.[27] These molluscum bodies are formed of viral particles that are similar in size and mode of formation to the poxviruses.[31]

Herpes zoster

A painful disease, herpes zoster is caused by the same virus that causes chickenpox (varicella). It may vary from relatively benign pruritic lesions on the trunk, usually unilateral and in the distribution of a single dermatome, to severe involvement of the first division of the trigeminal nerve with herpetic keratitis and corneal ulceration.[29] Postherpetic neuralgia is the unpleasant sequela. Patients with leukemia

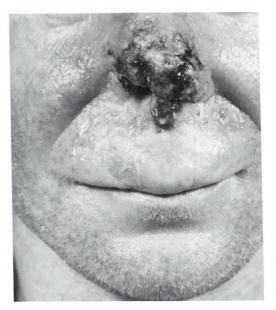

Fig. 27 Patient had lupus vulgaris for many years and eventually developed epidermoid carcinoma. (WU neg. 57-5443.)

and malignant lymphoma develop herpes zoster more frequently.[28]

Bacterial diseases
Hidradenitis suppurativa

Hidradenitis suppurativa is due to staphylococcal or streptococcal infection in and about apocrine sweat glands, usually in the axilla but occasionally involving the perineum.[35] Abscesses, sinuses, and perianal fistulas occur with subsequent scarring (Figs. 25 and 26). The process tends toward chronicity, and in refractory cases excision of the involved skin may be required.[38] Shelley and Cahn[41] suggested that the follicles into which the apocrine glands open are plugged by keratin and that infection develops following stasis. The end stages are similar to those of severe acne vulgaris and the more chronic disfiguring lesions of acne aggregata seu conglobata, in which squamous carcinoma may eventuate.[36]

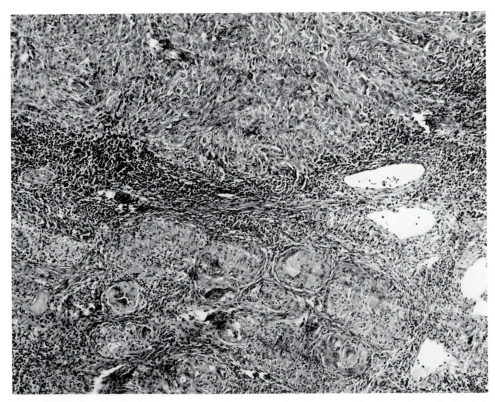

Fig. 28 Poorly differentiated epidermoid carcinoma (above) and tuberculosis (below) in biopsy taken from patient shown in Fig. 27. (×100; WU neg. 63-76.)

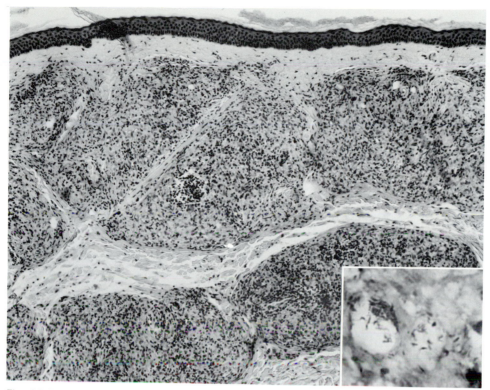

Fig. 29 Lepromatous leprosy wherein lepra cells are plentiful in dermis. **Inset** shows acid-fast bacilli in lepra cells. (×90, WU neg. 67-4411; **inset,** acid-fast stain; ×1,000; WU neg. 67-4414.)

Tuberculosis

Cutaneous tuberculosis is an uncommon disease in the United States. It has various clinical and morphologic forms depending on the mode of entry and whether it is a primary or secondary infection.[39, 40]

Lupus vulgaris is a reactivation type of tuberculosis. It generally involves the face, and the lesions are formed of red patches in which small, firm nodules reside. When pressed with a glass slide (diascopy), these nodules have a pale tan color, distastefully described as resembling apple jelly. Typically, noncaseous tubercles are found in the dermis. Acid-fast bacilli are difficult to demonstrate but may be found. Cultures are recommended. Ulceration of the skin, an uncommon feature in sarcoid and secondary bacterial infection, occurs. In longstanding cases, frank squamous carcinoma may arise in conjunction with lupus vulgaris (Figs. 27 and 28).

Leprosy

In the United States, leprosy is a rarity. However, the pathologist should consider it in his differential diagnosis of dermal granulomas[34] and histiocytic tumors.[37] In lepromatous leprosy the lepra cells, filled with acid-fast bacilli, are plentiful (Fig. 29), but in tuberculoid leprosy bacilli are all but absent. The only way to differentiate the noncaseous granulomatous reaction from sarcoidosis is to find neural involvement. Of course, the Matsuda and Kveim tests are valuable differential diagnostic adjuncts.

Fungal diseases
Tinea (dermatophytoses)

In the dermatophytoses, tinea of various sites, the fungal spores and hyphae are found in the stratum corneum and in or about hair shafts.[45] Mild epidermal changes such as focal intercellular edema and varying amounts of dermal inflammation may be seen. The fungal elements are readily seen in sections stained by the periodic acid–Schiff or Gomori's methenamine silver methods. Occasionally, atypical clinical forms of tinea are biopsied, and the fungi are readily missed if not sought. Bacterial folliculitis and perifolliculitis may be superimposed on tinea of the scalp and beard. These lesions are known as *kerion celsi* and *sycosis barbae*, respectively, and may, on occasion, be mistaken for infected tumors. Histologically, cellulitis, abscesses, pseudo-epitheliomatous hyperplasia, and a few fungi in the hair follicles and adjacent tissues are seen.

North American blastomycosis

Isolated cutaneous blastomycosis is an uncommon lesion. Usually the skin lesion is secondary to pneumonic involvement, which may be subclinical.[46] The causative

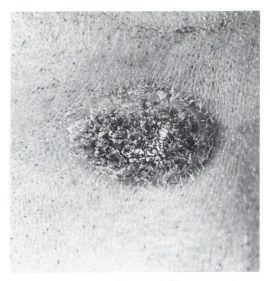

Fig. 30 Verrucous plaque of blastomycosis on neck. (WU neg. 54-6088.)

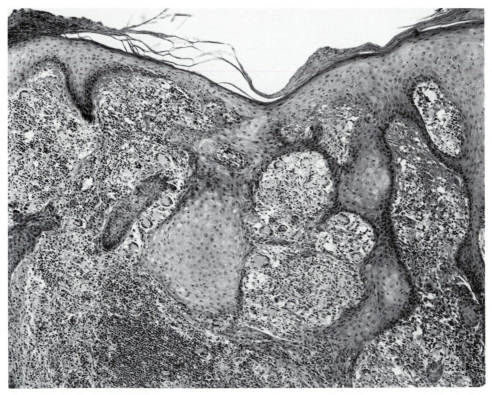

Fig. 31 Mixed granulomatous and acute inflammatory reaction of blastomycosis and pseudoepitheliomatous hyperplasia of epidermis. (×150; WU neg. 63-77.)

organism, *Blastomyces dermatitidis,* is a spherical, double-contoured $12\mu \pm 4\mu$ yeast. It reproduces by budding, and this characteristic allows its identification in sec-

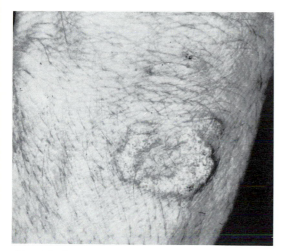

Fig. 32 Chromoblastomycosis on forearm.

tions. The skin lesions are slowly enlarging verrucous plaques in which numerous small abscesses are present (Fig. 30). Microscopically, they are characterized by marked pseudoepitheliomatous hyperplasia and a mixed granulomatous and acute polymorphonuclear infiltrate[43] (Fig. 31). The organism is generally found in giant cells. Smears and cultures are, of course, recommended diagnostic adjuncts.

Chromoblastomycosis

An indolent cutaneous disease, chromoblastomycosis is usually misdiagnosed clinically as carcinoma and excised[44, 48] (Fig. 32). Morphologically, identical fungi may be found in small subcutaneous abscesses.[47] Hematogenous dissemination occurs very rarely.[42] The spores are brown, hence their name, and the tissue reaction is similar to that seen in blastomycosis (Fig. 33). These fungi, closely related species of *Phialophora*

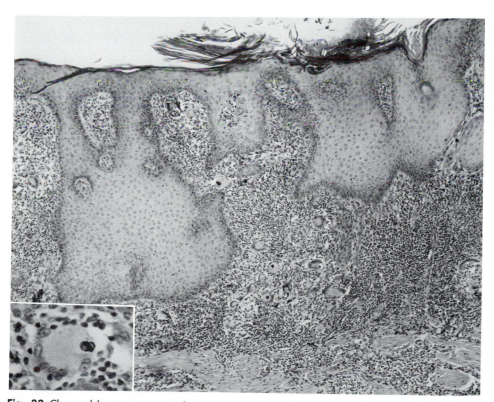

Fig. 33 Chromoblastomyces can be seen in giant cells surrounded by granulomatous reaction and acanthosis. **Inset** shows cross wall. (×85; WU neg. 62-8603; **inset,** ×340; WU neg. 62-8604.)

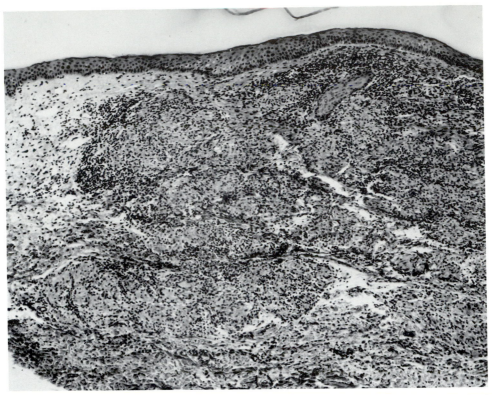

Fig. 34 Biopsy taken six weeks after injection of Kveim antigen. Noncaseating epithelioid granulomas are evident. (×85; WU neg. 62-8935.)

and *Fonsecaea* and *Cladosporium*, multiply by cross wall formation and splitting. Their color, cross walls, and lack of budding differentiate them from *Blastomyces dermatitidis.*

Miscellaneous diseases
Sarcoid

An etiologic enigma, sarcoid affects the skin as well as the lymph nodes and viscera. We have seen sarcoidlike reactions in lymph nodes draining sites of carcinomas and nonspecific inflammatory processes. Nonetheless, distinct clinical syndromes, both systemic and dermatologic, exist.[49, 52] They are presently called sarcoidosis.

The histopathologic pictures of the varying skin manifestations are similar. The dermis is infiltrated by nests and clusters of noncaseating epithelioid tubercles all but devoid of associated inflammatory cells. Langhans' giant cells are few. The often-mentioned asteroids, seen in giant cells, and the calcified Schaumann bodies are uncommon and nonspecific.

The Kveim test is often used to diagnose sarcoid. Sterilized brei of sarcoid tissue, usually spleen, is injected intradermally, and six weeks later the area is biopsied.[53] The presence of a typical sarcoidal reaction is considered a positive test (Fig. 34). Israel and Goldstein's paper[51] deals with the pitfalls and details of this test. When the antigen is potent, the test is reliable, and very few false positive results are found. However, foreign body and nonspecific inflammatory reactions do occur following injections of the Kveim antigen. Hurley and Shelley[50] reported the formation of sarcoid granulomas in five of fifty normal individuals following the inoculation of PPD. Thus the reaction must be typical and the clinical findings consistent for the diagnosis of a positive Kveim test.

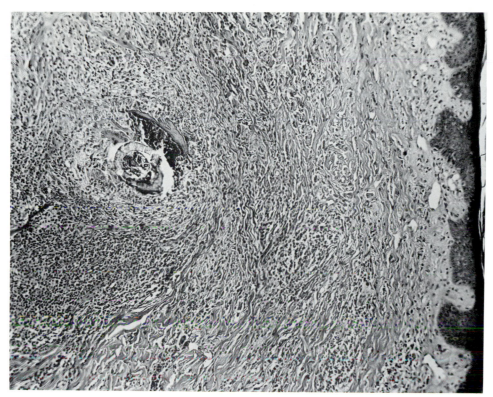

Fig. 35 Tick bite in which portion of head of tick was found surrounded by pronounced inflammatory reaction. (×100; WU neg. 52-4508.)

Foreign body reaction

Silica, talc, exogenous lipids, zirconium, and beryllium induce granulomatous reactions within the dermis.[55, 57-59] Residual particles of talc, silica, and lipids are demonstrable in tissue by routine or polariscopic microscopy. Beryllium, previously a component of the phosphorus in fluorescent lights, induces a distinct necrotizing and granulomatous reaction.[56] Shelley and Hurley[59] described the allergic origin of the zirconium deodorant granulomas. Insect bites may, on occasion, cause inflammatory and granulomatous reactions that can be mistaken for lymphomas[54] (Fig. 35).

Inflammatory diseases of unknown cause
Psoriasis

Psoriasis is one of the commoner dermatoses. Estimates of its incidence vary between 0.5% and 1.5% of the population.[61] It is a chronic, bilaterally symmetrical, non pruritic lesion formed by erythematous plaques covered by fine silvery scales. Typically, it involves the extensor surfaces such as the elbows, the knees, the back, and the scalp. Generalized lesions also occur (Fig. 36). Considerable effort has been expended in studying psoriasis from many aspects. Biochemical, histochemical, enzymatic, epidemiologic, and ultrastructural studies have failed so far to determine its cause. The morphologic characteristics are those of incomplete keratinization manifest as parakeratosis resulting from a markedly shortened turnover time.[63] Acanthosis in which there is a regular elongation of the rete ridges, seen as pegs in two dimensions, is prominent. Above the tips of the dermal papillae, the layer of epidermal cells is distinctly thinned —"suprapapillary thinning." Within the dermal papillae, the capillaries are promi-

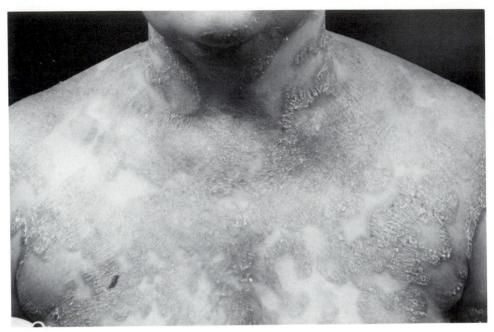

Fig. 36 Generalized psoriasis. (WU neg. 56-1398.)

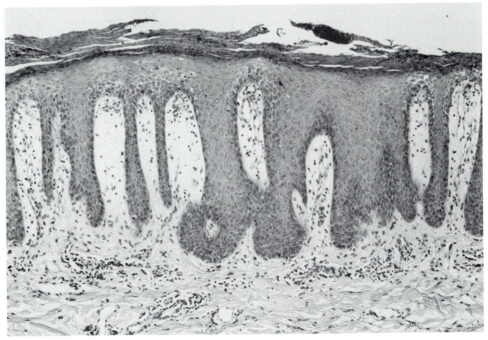

Fig. 37 Biopsy of psoriasis showing regular acanthosis, parakeratosis, Munro abscesses, and capillary dilatation. Suprapapillary edema is apparent. (×90; WU neg. 67-4142.)

nent. Transmigration of polymorphonuclear leukocytes through the reactive epidermis into the parakeratotic scale results in the formation of Munro microabscesses[62] (Fig. 37).

Typical psoriasis is seldom biopsied. The atypical cases often are and they create diagnostic difficulties. These are due to the fact that irritated epidermis, be it from lichen simplex chronicus, florid seborrheic dermatitis, or other causes, can develop comparable morphologic changes. Certain fine points of differentiation, such as the extent of suprapapillary thinning, the regularity of the acanthosis, and the lack of hyperkeratosis, may be used but are not absolute. Again, synthesis of all the information is required. The skin lesions of Reiter's syndrome are psoriasiform.[60]

Exfoliative dermatitis and erythroderma

Our experience with exfoliative dermatitis and erythroderma[65] is summarized in Table 2. It must be emphasized that the dermatopathic lymphadenitis (lipomelanotic reticulosis) associated with these skin diseases should not be confused with malignant lymphoma. It is probable that such confusion accounts for the greater incidence of lymphomas associated with erythroderma, other than chronic lymphocytic leukemia, in the literature. Usually, the histologic changes in the skin are nonspecific.[64]

Table 2 Exfoliative dermatitis and erythroderma in sixty-eight patients at Washington University School of Medicine, 1942-1958*

Cause	Patients	%
Unknown	23	34
Chronic lymphocytic leukemia†	12	18
Contact dermatitis	10	15
Drug sensitivity‡	9	13
Miscellaneous§	8	10
Psoriasis	6	9

*Tombridge, T. L.: Personal communication.

†The leukemia in many of these patients had an atypically benign course.

‡Includes four patients with sensitivity to arsenic.

§Eczematoid, seborrheic, and neurodermatitis.

Lichen planus

Lichen planus is a pruritic, violaceous, subacute to chronic, papulosquamous dermatitis. It usually involves the flexor surfaces of the arms and the legs (Fig. 38) but occurs elsewhere as well.[67] Lesions may be confined to the oral mucosa,[66] or they may precede or accompany the skin changes. Lumpkin and Helwig[68] describe isolated skin lesions. Histologically, the well-developed lesions are rather distinct (Fig. 39). The epidermis is hyperkeratotic, the granular layer is prominent, and the hyperplastic epithelium forms irregular acanthotic pegs. The papillary dermis is heavily infiltrated by lymphocytes and histiocytes that form a bandlike infiltrate which involves and destroys the dermoepidermal junction. On occasion, subepidermal cleavage occurs with the formation of bullae. The border of the inflammatory infiltrate is sharply delimited so that the reticular dermis is uninflamed. The oral lesions are readily mistaken for leukoplakia. Histologically, the absence of atypia and dyskeratotic cells in oral lichen planus assists in differentiating it from leukoplakia. *Lichen nitidus* occurs in a small percentage of patients with lichen planus and may be a variant thereof.[69]

Chondrodermatitis helicis

Chondrodermatitis helicis is characterized by tender hyperkeratotic nodules that occur preferentially on the helix and rarely on the anthelix of the ear.[70] In carefully blocked specimens, a small ulcer rimmed with hyperplastic and hyperkeratotic epidermis is found. The dermis is inflamed and contains numerous capillaries. The perichondrium of the aural cartilage may show proliferative and inflammatory changes, and on occasion the underlying cartilage is altered in appearance.[71] Excision may be necessary for cure.[72] Many of the lesions are excised as small carcinomas or actinic keratoses.

Granuloma faciale

Granuloma faciale occurs on the face of adults.[76] It is a thickened, purplish

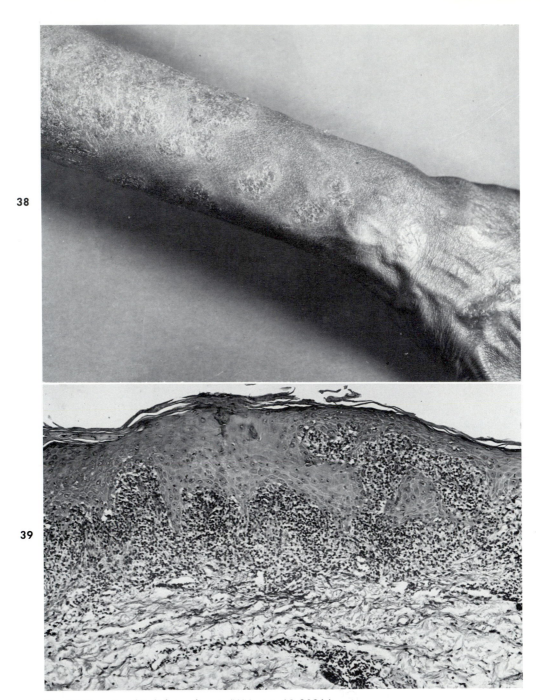

Fig. 38 Hypertrophic lichen planus. (WU neg. 60-3086.)
Fig. 39 Biopsy of lichen planus showing hyperkeratosis and infiltrate that hugs irregularly acanthotic epidermis. (×87; WU neg. 62-8938.)

patch usually clinically thought to be something other than granuloma faciale (e.g., infected nevus, tumor, sarcoid). For this reason, it is often excised or biopsied, and an acquaintance with its histologic appearance is helpful. The epidermis is unaltered, except in unusual circumstances, and is separated from the zone of dermal inflam-

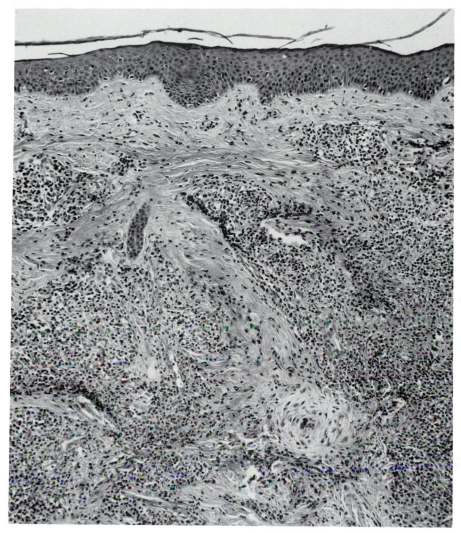

Fig. 40 Mixed infiltrate of granuloma faciale is well demarcated and separated from epidermis by narrow band of uninvolved dermis. (×85; WU neg. 62-8605.)

mation by a narrow band of uninvolved dermis (Fig. 40). The inflammatory reaction is formed by lymphocytes, histiocytes, and large numbers of eosinophilic leukocytes. The latter may be concentrated about the vessels and a mild to moderate vasculitis observed.[75] Granuloma faciale differs from the tumor stage of mycosis fungoides by the absence of the characteristic epidermal involvement, the Pautrier microabscesses, and atypical monocytes. Infected insect bites may have considerable eosinophilic infiltrate but seldom occur on the face.[73] Benign lymphocytic infiltration

of the skin lacks the variety of inflammatory cells and may, in fact, contain lymphoid follicles.[74]

Erythema nodosum

The painful, red, subcutaneous lesions that characterize erythema nodosum occur on the anterior surface of the legs. They involve within a few days or weeks, leaving slightly depressed pigmented areas. They do not ulcerate as do the lesions of erythema induratum. The pathogenesis is unknown. Studies by Vesey and Wilkinson[79] show that in a British population with

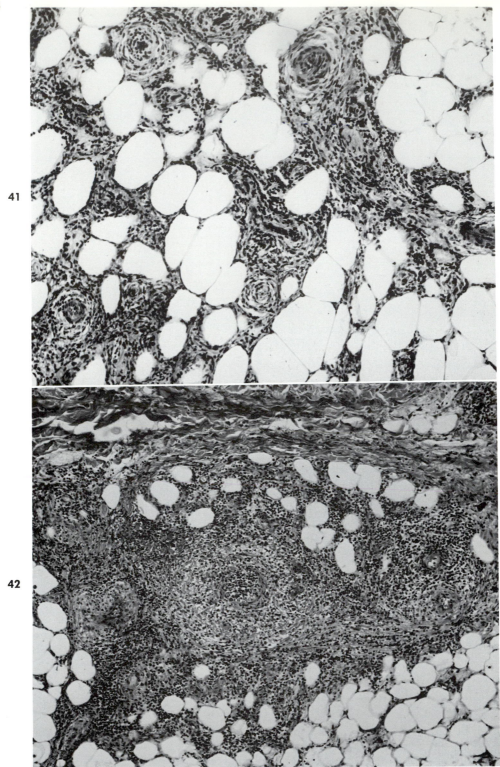

Fig. 41 Subacute inflammatory reaction almost limited to connective tissue septa in erythema nodosum. (×150; WU neg. 62-8606.)
Fig. 42 Obliterative vasculitis within subcutis from thigh of woman with nodular vasculitis. (×85; WU neg. 62-8939.)

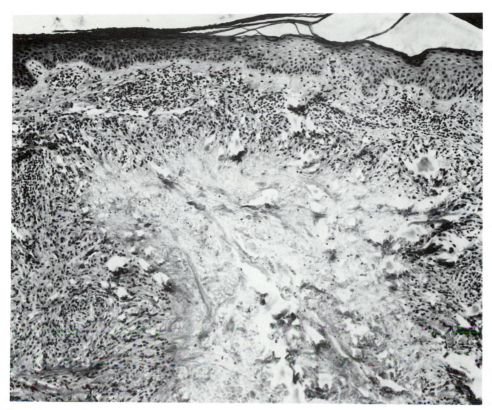

Fig. 43 Granuloma annulare showing necrotic core of collagen surrounded by zone of radially oriented epithelioid cells and lymphocytes. (×85, WU neg. 62-8607.)

erythema nodosum, 45% of the patients had antecedent streptococcal infections, 6% had tuberculosis, 36% had sarcoid, and 13% had a variety of lesions. In the endemic areas of the United States, coccidioidomycosis is a common antecedent.

Histologically, the junction of the dermis and the subcutis is inflamed. A subacute infiltrate extends along the fibrous septa between the fat and about the vessels of the dermis (Fig. 41). Fat necrosis, caseation, and tubercles are not seen. Varying degrees of vasculitis, chiefly of the veins, may be seen. Other nodular lesions of the leg that are probably results of antigen-antibody precipitates with ensuing vasculitis are nodular vasculitis[77] (Fig. 42) and subacute nodular migratory panniculitis.[78]

Granuloma annulare

Granuloma annulare occurs most frequently on the dorsum of the hands and arms as circinate or grouped clusters of pink nodules with slight central depressions. Histologically, a well-demarcated zone of necrotic collagen is found in the mid-dermis surrounded by a cuff of radially oriented fibroblasts admixed with lymphocytes and histiocytes (Fig. 43). Occasional foreign body giant cells may be found, and mucin is present in the areas of altered collagen. In some lesions, the necrotic collagen is not so distinctly demarcated. No associated symptoms or diseases are known.[84]

The subcutaneous nodules of rheumatoid arthritis and rheumatic fever are histologically similar. The details of differentiation are set forth by Wood and Beerman.[85] Isolated, large, necrobiotic nodules or giant granuloma annulare are seen chiefly on the extremities and occiput in children.[81, 82] Rubin and Lynch[83] suggest that this condition is not so uncommon as

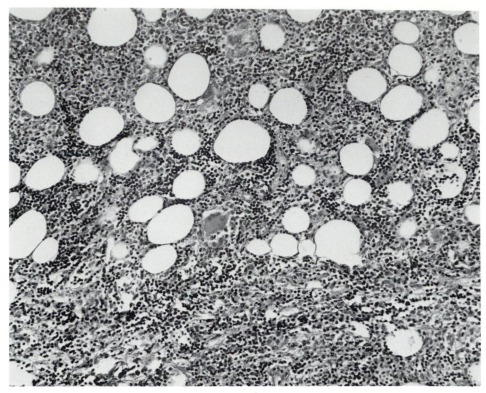

Fig. 44 Weber-Christian disease in which destruction of fat cells and inflammatory infiltrate with giant cells are apparent. (×120; WU neg. 62-8664.)

reports indicate, and in two of their five patients characteristic granuloma annulare involvement of the skin ensued. The children do not develop rheumatic or rheumatoid disease, and prolonged prophylaxis is not indicated. Occasionally, siblings may be affected.[80]

Necrobiosis lipoidica

Necrobiosis lipoidica is characterized by atrophic, yellow, depressed plaques that involve the legs most often but may occur in atypical sites and without clinical diabetes. Studies by Muller and Winkelmann,[88] Bauer and Levan,[86] and Fisher and Danowski[87] show that it is possible to distinguish, on histologic grounds, lesions in patients with and without diabetes mellitus. In the lesions associated with diabetes, the necrobiotic zones are surrounded by more prominent palisading, mucinous deposits, and capillary thickening. This differential is not absolute.

Weber-Christian disease

The changes seen in Weber-Christian disease are acute to subacute inflammation of the subcutaneous adipose tissue with necrosis of fat cells (Fig. 44) and resolution by macrophagic ingestion and subsequent fibrosis. The lesions are tender and usually accompanied by malaise and remittent fever.[89, 91] In contrast, the lipogranulomatosis subcutanea of Rothmann and Makai has no associated systemic symptoms and does not appear in crops.[90]

Urticaria pigmentosa

Although urticaria pigmentosa usually has its onset during childhood, the disease may make its first appearance in adults. The brown macules may be diffusely distributed (Fig. 45) or, less frequently, may be single.[95] When the lesions are stroked, the skin urticates due to the release of histamine. Various syndromes other than the purely cutaneous disease have been de-

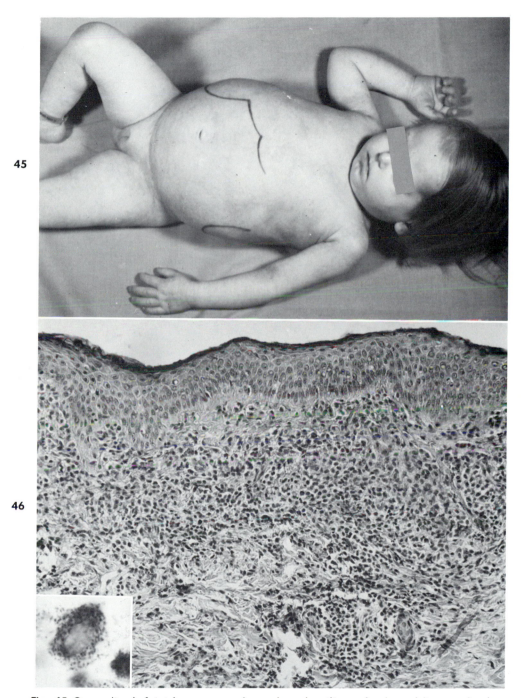

45

46

Fig. 45 Generalized, faint brown, macular rash and outlines of enlarged liver and spleen in infant with systemic mastocytosis. (WU neg. 58-1286.)
Fig. 46 Biopsy from child illustrated in Fig. 45 showing dermis heavily infiltrated with mast cells. **Inset** shows mast cell's granules stained with toluidine blue. (×120; WU neg. 62-8667; **inset,** toluidine blue; ×1,000; WU neg. 52-4400.)

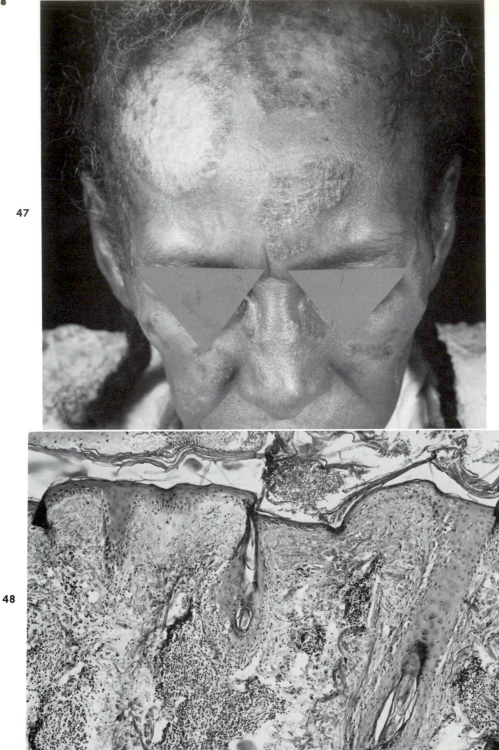

Fig. 47 Chronic discoid lupus erythematosus with involvement of cheeks, bridge of nose, forehead, and scalp. (WU neg. 60-2970.)
Fig. 48 Hyperkeratosis, follicular plugging, atrophy, liquefaction degeneration, and patchy lymphocytic infiltrate of chronic discoid lupus erythematosus. (×85; WU neg. 62-8658.)

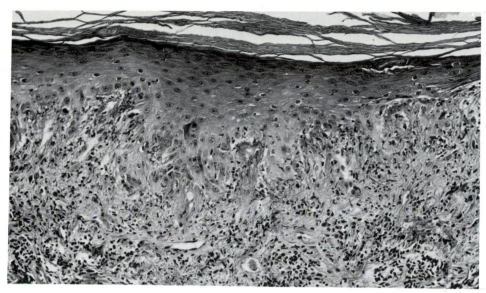

Fig. 49 Subacute lupus erythematosus in which necrosis of collagen at dermoepidermal junction and some inflammatory reactions are present. (×150; WU neg. 62-8611.)

scribed in which viscera and bone have been involved,[92, 96] and a few cases of mast cell leukemia[98] also have been described. Histologically, the lesions are easily missed unless the cytologic features of mast cells in sections stained with hematoxylin-eosin are remembered. These cells have large, pale nuclei, distinct cytoplasmic boundaries, and a faintly granular cytoplasm (Fig. 46). In sections stained with toluidine blue or Giemsa, the metachromatic granules are obvious.[93] A few eosinophilic leukocytes may be admixed with the mast cells in the dermis. Mast cell tumors of the skin are common in the dog[97] and occur in the cat and ox.[94]

Lupus erythematosus

Chronic discoid lupus erythematosus and systemic lupus erythematosus present distinct and almost uniformly separable entities. Chronic discoid lupus erythematosus is a relatively common condition with a distinct preference for women, presenting as delimited erythematous to hyperkeratotic to atrophic patches on the face, neck, scalp, and, less frequently, the arms and trunk (Fig. 47). Sunlight may cause exacerbations. Histologically, the lesions are characterized by predominantly follicular hyperkeratosis, epidermal atrophy with liquefaction degeneration of the basal layer, and a distinct, patchy, periadnexal lymphocytic infiltrate (Fig. 48). The changes seen in biopsies reflect the stage and type of lesion sampled. None of the changes is pathognomonic. Polymorphous light eruption may be difficult to differentiate from chronic discoid lupus erythematosus, perhaps because it is a variant thereof. The same may be said for lymphocytic infiltration of the skin described by Jessner and Kanof.[100] Chronic discoid lupus erythematosus very rarely progresses to the acute disease.[99, 102] Therapy with antimalarial drugs such as chloroquine is reasonably satisfactory.

Systemic lupus erythematosus is an "autoimmune" malady in which antibodies to homologous and heterologous deoxyribonucleic acid have been demonstrated. It manifests a protean symptomatology usually characterized by fatigue, fever, arthritis, various cutaneous lesions of which the erythematous bimalar "butterfly" blush is most common, signs of renal involvement, lymphadenopathy, and panserositis. The typical, but not always present, der-

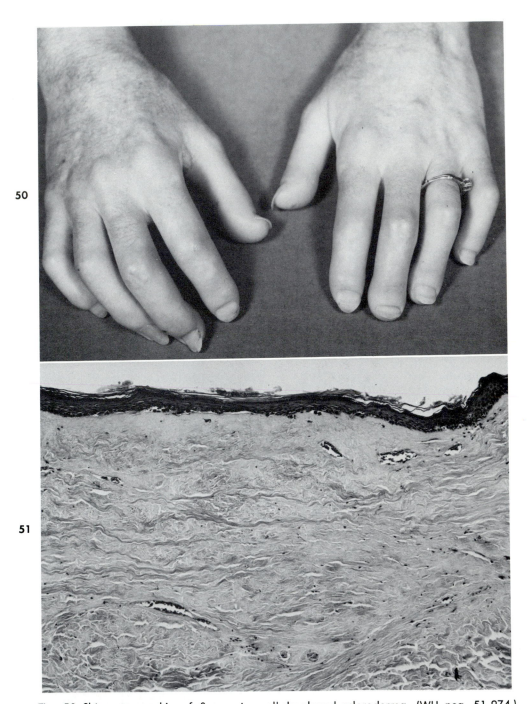

50

51

Fig. 50 Shiny, tense skin of fingers in well-developed scleroderma. (WU neg. 51-974.)
Fig. 51 Distinct increase in amount of dermal collagen, epidermal atrophy, and slight hyperkeratosis in patch of localized scleroderma (morphea). (×85; WU neg. 62-8613.)

mal histologic picture is fibrinoid necrosis at the dermoepidermal junction accompanied by atrophy and liquefaction degeneration of the epidermis (Fig. 49). The systemic lesions are often described but no better than in the original paper by Klemperer et al.[101]

Dermatomyositis

No unique morphologic features occur in the skin in dermatomyositis.[105] Biopsies of the afflicted muscles show distinct myositis with necrosis of myofibers, fragmentation, phagocytosis, and some sarcolemmal nuclear proliferation. In the later stages, fibrosis, fat infiltration, and fascicular atrophy appear.[103] Williams[106] reviewed the experience of many regarding the incidence or coincidence of adenocarcinoma with dermatomyositis. He found that 15% of the patients have neoplasms of the stomach, breast, ovary, lung, and colon. Curtis et al.[104] demonstrated an autoimmune reaction in which the patients developed antibodies specific for extracts of their own cancer. Remissions have occurred following resection of the neoplasm. Thus careful investigation of adults with dermatomyositis for undetected carcinoma is certainly worthwhile. However, in the majority none will be found, and the etiology remains obscure. Corticosteroid therapy is beneficial.

In long-standing dermatomyositis and, in fact, in lupus erythematosus, acrodermatitis atrophicans, and mycosis fungoides, a secondary change called poikiloderma atrophicans vasculare may appear. The histologic changes are generally those of the associated disease.

Scleroderma

Scleroderma is manifest in two distinct forms: localized scleroderma or morphea[107] and systemic scleroderma, in which the skin, particularly of the face, upper trunk, hands, and arms (acrosclerosis) (Fig. 50), the esophagus, the heart, and the lungs are diseased. The etiology and pathogenesis are unknown.[110] Systemic sclerosis is often classified as one of the "collagen diseases." The dominant change is an increase in the amount of collagen. This is, morphologically (by light and electron microscopy) and biochemically, normal collagen.[108, 109] Thus the histologic diagnosis depends on the evaluation of increments in the amount and distribution of collagen. The "smudging," "homogenization," and variable tinctorial changes seen in sections stained with hematoxylin-eosin do not necessarily indicate structural changes in the collagen. In fact, some care should be exercised not to confuse the changes of senile elastosis and basophilic degeneration of collagen and the normally thicker dermis of the fingers with scleroderma. The dermis, particularly the papillary portion, becomes a dense feltwork of closely woven collagen bundles (Fig. 51). The sclerosis may extend in depth to encircle the secretory coils of the eccrine sweat glands. Concomitantly, the epidermis becomes atrophic. Varying amounts of mild and nonspecific inflammatory reaction may be seen in the dermis, more so at the advancing edge of a patch of morphea. Dystrophic calcification may occur in scleroderma, and in some patients the dominant pattern is that of acrosclerosis preceded by, or associated with, Raynaud's phenomenon.

Vesiculobullous diseases

Diagnosis of the vesiculobullous dermatoses is simplified if the planes of separation and the types of cellular change are noted.[112]

Subepidermal "pressure" bullae, in which the intact epidermis is separated from the dermis, occur in *dermatitis herpetiformis*[117] (Fig. 52), in *bullous erythema multiforme,* in *bullous pemphigoid,* and in *porphyria cutanea tarda.* Histologic differentiation of these lesions is not possible, although minor differences, such as the presence or absence of an inflammatory infiltrate, its character and distribution, may be found.[115] For example, eosinophilic leukocytes are numerous in dermatitis herpetiformis (Fig. 53), but they are also present in bullous

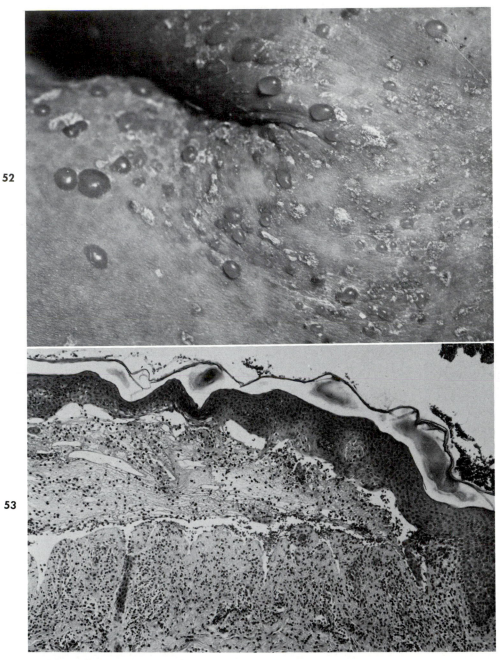

52

53

Fig. 52 Bullae of dermatitis herpetiformis on anterior portion of chest and upper arm. Previous lesions have ruptured, causing changes between intact blisters. (WU neg. 62-5916.)
Fig. 53 Subepidermal bulla from patient with dermatitis herpetiformis. Many of the inflammatory cells are eosinophilic leukocytes. Junction with intact skin is at right. (WU neg. 62-8608.)

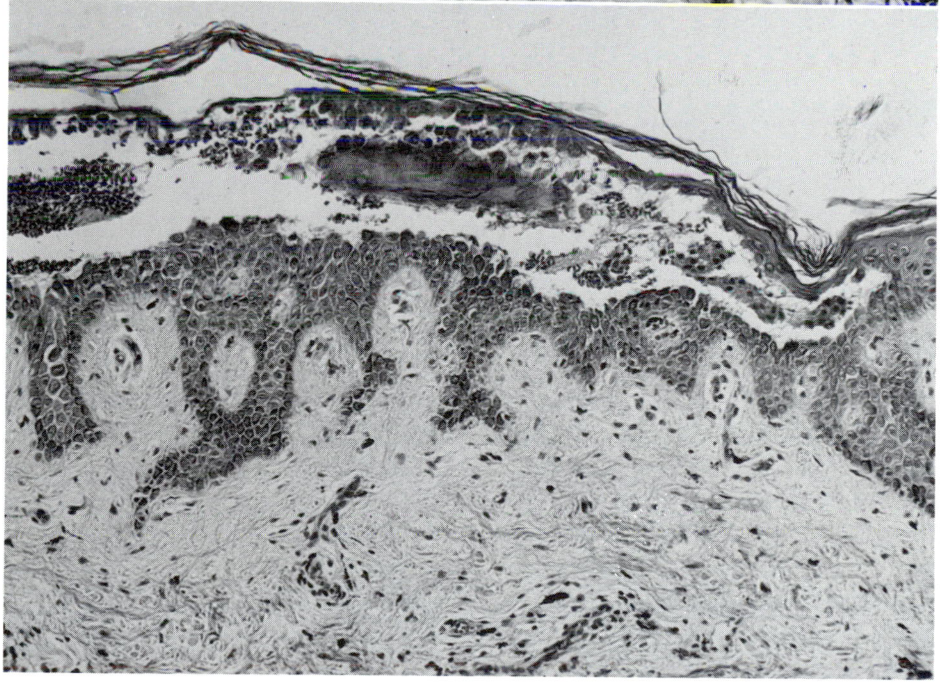

Fig. 54 Pemphigus vuglaris in which characteristic suprabasal bulla and dark acantholytic cells can be seen. (×85; WU neg. 62-8612.)
Fig. 55 Pemphigus foliaceus with its high intraepidermal cleavage plane. (×85; WU neg. 62-8659.)

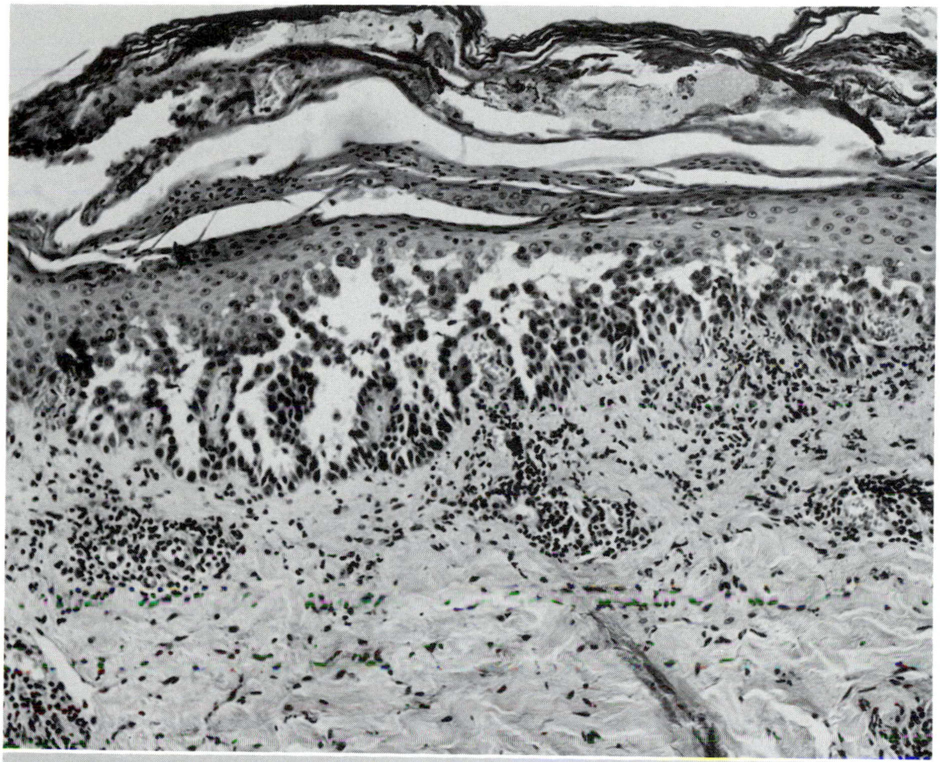

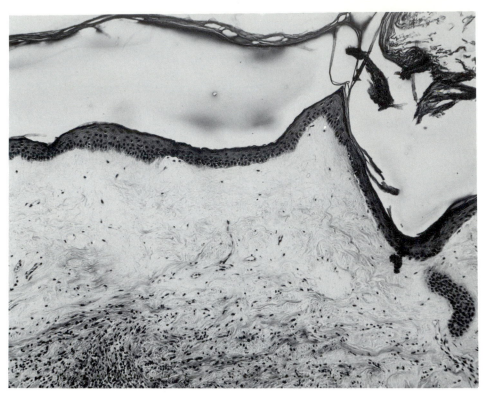

Fig. 56 Edematous hypocellular band of upper dermis, epidermal atrophy, and hyperkeratosis typical of lichen sclerosus et atrophicus. Keratin is artifactually lifted from epidermis. (×120; WU neg. 62-8660.)

pemphigoid. The clinical features such as the intense pruritus of dermatitis herpetiformis, its association with a spinelike enteropathy,[113] and its response to sulfapyridine and diazone allow accurate differentiation. The significance of the pathologist's report lies in determining that the lesion is subepidermal and that acantholysis is absent. A common trap is that the regrowth of epithelium across the base of the bulla, covering the denuded dermis, may be rapid. Thus if older lesions are biopsied, an intraepidermal bulla may be found. Large intraepidermal bullae unassociated with acantholytic changes should be suspect of being healing subepidermal bullae. Occasionally, subepidermal clefts, due to severe liquefaction of the basal layer, appear in chronic discoid lupus erythematosus and lichen planus.

Among the intraepidermal bullous dermatoses are *pemphigus vulgaris* and a var-

iant thereof, *pemphigus vegetans*. In these diseases, the cleavage plane is just above the basal layer and is due to acantholysis (Fig. 54). Indirect immunofluorescent stains demonstrate antiepithelial antibodies in the sera of patients with pemphigus.[111] In contrast, the separation in *pemphigus foliaceus*[114] is in or just below the granular layer (Fig. 55). In *subcorneal pustular dermatosis*,[116] the vesicles are just beneath the keratin layer, as they are in *impetigo contagiosa*.

Another subcorneal vesicular lesion we have seen mistaken for junctional nevus is the blood blister, in which the erythrocytes are trapped beneath the thick stratum corneum of the toes or fingers.

Degenerative and miscellaneous diseases
Lichen sclerosus et atrophicus

Lichen sclerosus et atrophicus occurs most often on the upper trunk and neck.[120]

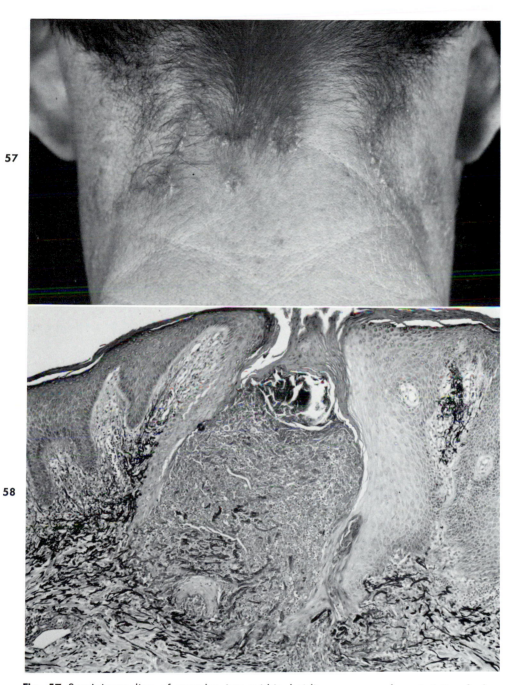

Fig. 57 Serpiginous line of papules just within hairline on nape characteristic of elastosis perforans. (WU neg. 62-5920.)
Fig. 58 Skeins of abnormally coarse elastica in papillae can be seen on right. Penetrating strands can be seen entering follicle that is plugged with necrotic debris. (Verhoeff–van Gieson; ×85; WU neg. 62-8665.)

It may be seen limited to the vulva and perineum.[118] In the past, the same lesion on the glans penis was called balanitis xerotica obliterans. Atrophy and hyperkeratosis of the epidermis are associated with complete obliteration of the structure of the upper dermis. It is replaced by an edematous, hypocellular, faintly staining band beneath which a moderate chronic inflammatory infiltrate appears (Fig. 56). In older lesions, some hyalinization and angiectasia occur in this band. This lesion has no relation to leukoplakia of the vulva and should not be mistaken for it. Simple vulvectomies have been done because of such errors. The "precancerous" lesions of the vulvar skin are well described and discussed by Jeff-coate and Woodcock[119] and Taylor.[121]

Elastosis perforans

In elastosis perforans, clumps and strands of abnormally coarse elastic fibers penetrate the epidermis and produce a focal epidermal hyperplasia.[122, 123] The common site is the back of the neck in adolescent boys (Fig. 57). The altered elastica in the

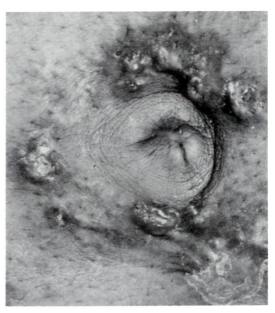

Fig. 59 Nodules and plaques about umbilicus in patient with pseudoxanthoma elasticum. (WU neg. 51-2732.)

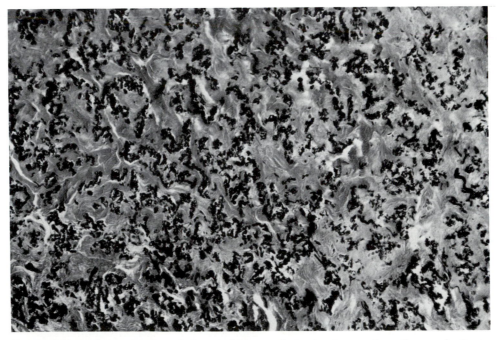

Fig. 60 Coarse, fragmented, and clustered pieces of elastica in pseudoxanthoma elasticum. (Verhoeff's elastic tissue stain; ×150; WU neg. 62-8940.)

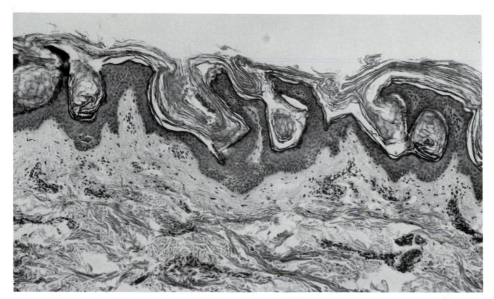

Fig. 61 Biopsy from axilla showing papillomatosis and hyperkeratosis of acanthosis nigricans. (×80; WU neg. 62-8662.)

papillary dermis is easily missed, and recognition usually requires elastic tissue stains. These changes are illustrated in Fig. 58.

Pseudoxanthoma elasticum

The dermal changes in pseudoxanthoma elasticum are manifestations of a generalized disorder of connective tissue.[125] Angioid streaks in the retina and degenerative changes in arteries leading to occlusion or rupture are described. Yellow streaks and plaques of the skin, particularly in areas of creases such as the neck, axillae, and groin, account for the name pseudoxanthoma (Fig. 59). Histologically, the mid and lower dermis contain clumps and strands of altered, faintly basophilic connective tissue that stain intensely with aldehyde fuchsin and Verhoeff's elastic tissue stain (Fig. 60). This tinctorial reaction suggests, as do other findings described by Graham Smith et al.,[124] that the abnormality is, in fact, one of the elastic fibers. The exact nature of the defect remains unknown.

Pretibial myxedema

Pretibial myxedema is characterized by nodular lesions that occur on the legs of patients who are or have been thyrotoxic.[127] They may become quite large. The accumulation of mucopolysaccharides in the dermis is similar to that in the orbital tissues due to excess TSH secretion by the pituitary gland.[126] Histologically, the dermal collagen is separated by aggregates of faintly basophilic material that stains with mucicarmine and with Hale's colloidal iron reaction for acid mucopolysaccharides and that is PAS positive and diastase resistant.

Acanthosis nigricans

Acanthosis nigricans is a misnomer, for the changes are those of papillomatosis and hyperkeratosis (Fig. 61). This change in the skin may be seen in patients with carcinomas of the gastrointestinal tract or other sites[129] and in obese individuals, some of whom have endocrine disorders, and in some instances it is a familial disorder.[128]

Darier's disease

The keratotic and papular lesions of Darier's disease are characterized histologically by suprabasal clefts in which acantholytic cells called grains are found.

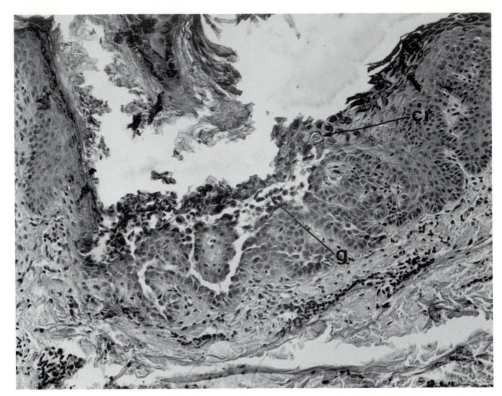

Fig. 62 Suprabasal cleft with villous projections and acantholytic and individually dyskeratotic cells of Darier's disease. Corp ronds, **cr.** Grains, **g.** (×150; WU neg. 62-8941.)

The dermal papillae covered by a layer of basal cells form small villi at the base of the lesion. In addition, within the epidermis large individually dyskeratotic cells called *corps ronds* are found (Fig. 62). When the lesions are closely spaced, the skin assumes a verrucous appearance. The oral mucosa and hairless skin may be involved, showing that the disease is not limited to the hair follicle as suggested by the name keratosis follicularis. An isolated follicular lesion, although histologically similar, is not a part of Darier's disease (p. 101).

Xanthoma

Various types of xanthomatous lesions occur[130, 131] (Fig. 63). The common lesion seen in our laboratory is the *xanthelasma*. These lesions, composed of neutral fat-laden histiocytes in the dermis of the eyelids (Fig. 64), are often excised for cosmetic reasons. Only a few of the individuals with xanthelasmas have systemic hypercholesterolosis.

Juvenile xanthogranuloma (nevoxanthoendothelioma)

The name nevoxanthoendothelioma is descriptive in that the lesion occurs in infants and thus is a nevus in the sense of congenital mark. It contains fat-laden histiocytes and Touton giant cells and thus is xanthomatous. Proliferation of small vessels may be seen (Fig. 65). A preferable name is juvenile xanthogranuloma. Most of the lesions occur in infants and are limited to the skin. However, extradermal involvement occurs, as described by Helwig and Hackney[133] and Nödl.[134] Occasionally, glaucoma and amblyopia, due to involvement of the iris and the ciliary body, are the presenting complaint.[132, 135] We studied the disease in an 11-month-old white male infant with lesions of the thigh, axilla, and right retro-orbital tissues (Fig.

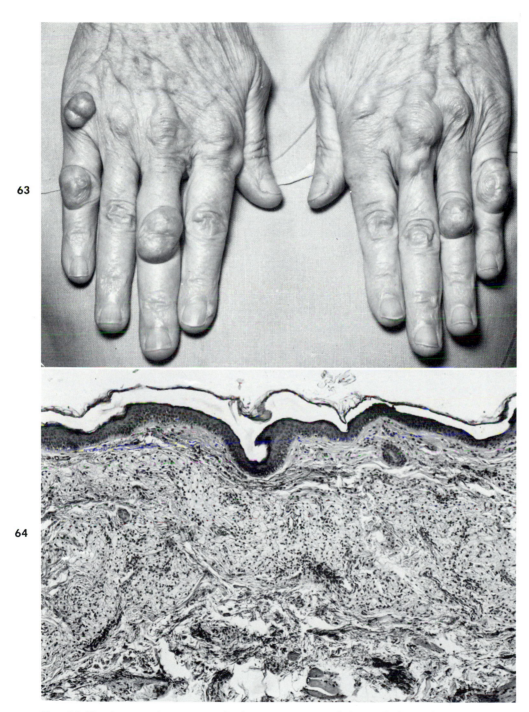

Fig. 63 Xanthoma tuberosum multiplex in patient with hypercholesterolemia. (WU neg. 62-5917.)

Fig. 64 Clusters and sheets of foamy histiocytes within dermis from xanthelasma. (×87; WU neg. 62-8936.)

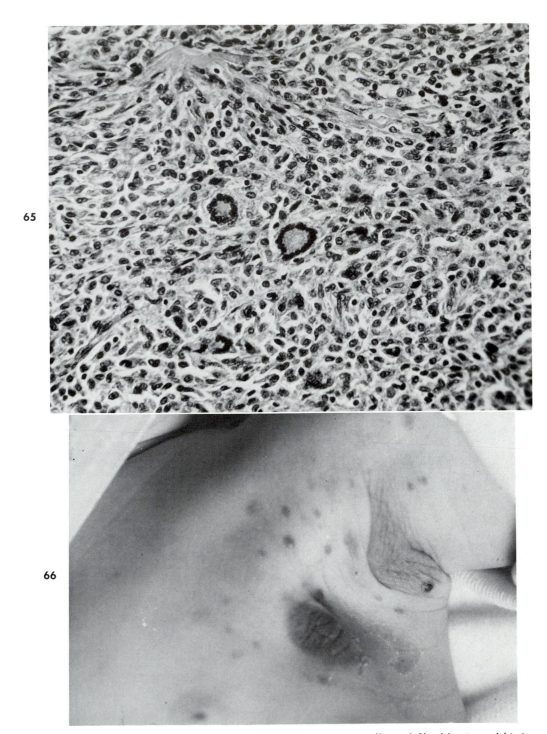

Fig. 65 Juvenile xanthogranuloma showing Touton giant cells and fibroblastic and histio-cytic proliferation. (×350; WU neg. 53-4624A.)
Fig. 66 Plaques and nodules of juvenile xanthogranuloma of axillary skin and chest wall in 11-month-old infant. (WU neg. 62-3018.)

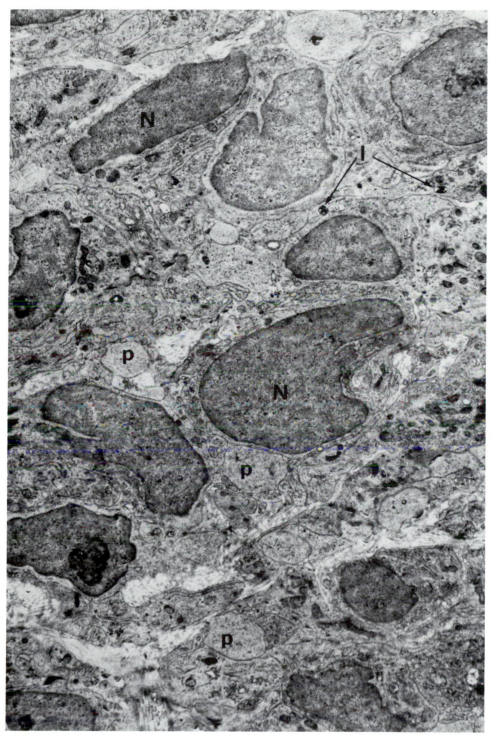

Fig. 67 Juvenile xanthogranuloma showing complex intermingling of cytoplasmic process, **p.** Cells have large nuclei, **N,** but lack specific ultrastructural characteristics. Small aggregates of lipid are labeled **I.** (Uranyl acetate–lead citrate; ×6,000.)

66). Ultrastructural studies have shown a complex tissue with two dominant cell types. One is histiocytic, and the cells contain fat in areas of regression. The other cell is probably fibrocytic (Fig. 67). The uncommon visceral involvement does not allow, in our opinion, classification of this lesion in the "lipoidoses" nor consideration of it as a *forme fruste* of Hand-Schüller-Christian syndrome.

REFERENCES

Introduction to dermatopathology

1 Allen, A. C.: The skin; a clinicopathologic treatise, ed. 2, New York, 1967, Grune & Stratton, Inc.
2 Burckhardt, W., and Epstein, S.: Atlas and manual of dermatology and venerology, ed. 2, Baltimore, 1963, The Williams & Wilkins Co.
3 Fitzpatrick, T. B., Arndt, K. A., Clark, W. H., Eisen, A. Z., van Scott, E. J., and Vaughan, J. H.: Dermatology in general medicine, New York, 1971, McGraw-Hill Book Co.
4 Gans, O.: Histologie der Hautkrankheiten, Berlin, 1928, Julius Springer, vols. I and II.
5 Kimming, J., and Jannes, M.: Color atlas of dermatology, Philadelphia, 1966, W. B. Saunders Co.
6 Lever, W. F.: Histopathology of the skin, ed. 4, Philadelphia, 1967, J. B. Lippincott Co.
7 Montagna, W., and Lobitz, W. C., Jr.: The epidermis, New York, 1964, Academic Press, Inc.
8 Montgomery, H.: Dermatopathology, New York, 1967, Hoeber Medical Division, Harper & Row, Publishers, vols. I and II.
9 Rook, A., Wilkinson, D. S., and Ebling, F. J. G.: Textbook of dermatology, ed. 2, Philadelphia, 1972, F. A. Davis Co.
10 Unna, P. G.: The histopathology of the diseases of the skin, Edinburgh, 1896, William F. Clay.

Skin
Epidermis

11 Clark, W. H., Watson, M. C., and Watson, B. E. M.: Two kinds of "clear" cells in the human epidermis, Am. J. Pathol. 39:333-344, 1961.
12 Horstman, E.: Die Haut. In Möllendorff, W. V., editor: Handbuch der microskopischen Anatomie des Menschen, vol. 3, part 3, Berlin, 1957, pp. 1-488.
13 Masson, P.: Pigment cells in man, In Miner, R. W., editor: The biology of melanoma,

New York, 1948, The New York Academy of Sciences, pp. 15-51.
14 Moore, K. L., and Barr, M. L.: Nuclear morphology, according to sex, in human tissues, Acta Anat. (Basel) 21:197-208, 1954.
15 Moorhead, P. S., Nowell, P. C., Mellman, W. J., Battips, D. M., and Hungerford, D. A.: Chromosome preparations of leukocytes cultured from human peripheral blood, Exp. Cell Res. 20:613-616, 1960.
16 Pansegrau, D. G., and Peterson, R. E.: Improved staining of sex chromatin, Am. J. Clin. Pathol. 41:266-272, 1964.

Dermis

17 Dobson, R. L., and Abele, D. C.: Cytologic changes in the eccrine sweat gland in hypothyroidism; a preliminary report, J. Invest. Dermatol. 37:457-458, 1961.
18 Gersh, I., and Catchpole, H. R.: The nature of ground substance of connective tissue, Perspect. Biol. Med. 3:282-319, 1960.
19 Horstman, E.: Die Haut. In Möllendorff, W. V., editor: Handbuch der microskopichen Anatomie des Menschen, vol. 3, part 3, Berlin, 1957, pp. 1-488.
20 Loewenthal, L. J. A.: The pathogenesis of miliaria, Arch. Dermatol. 84:2-17, 1961.
21 Lund, H. Z., and Sommerville, R. L.: Basophilic degeneration of the cutis, Am. J. Clin. Pathol. 27:183-190, 1957.
22 Montagna, W., Bentley, J. P., and Dobson, R. L.: The dermis, New York, 1968, Appleton-Century-Crofts.
23 Sams, W. M., Jr., and Smith, J. G., Jr.: The histochemistry of chronically sun-damaged skin, J. Invest. Dermatol. 37:447-453, 1961.
24 Winkelmann, R. K.: Cutaneous vascular patterns. In Advances in biology of the skin. Vol. II. The blood vessels and circulation of blood in the skin (Montagna, W., and Ellis, R. A., editors), New York, 1961, Pergamon Press, Inc.

Inflammatory diseases of known cause
Viral diseases

25 Almeida, J. D., Howatson, A. F., and Williams, M. G.: Electron microscope study of human warts; sites of virus production and nature of the inclusion bodies, J. Invest. Dermatol. 38:337-345, 1962
26 Ebert, M. H., and Otsuka, M.: Virus diseases of skin, with special reference to elementary and inclusion bodies, Arch. Dermatol. 48:635-649, 1943.
27 Goodpasture, E. W., and King, H.: A cytologic study of molluscum contagiosum, Am. J. Pathol. 3:385-394, 1927.
28 Merselis, J. G., Kaye, D., and Hook, E. W.:

Disseminated herpes zoster: report of 17 cases, Arch. Intern. Med. 113:679-686, 1964.

29 Molin, L.: Aspects of the natural history of herpes zoster, Acta Derm. Venereol. 48:569-583, 1969.

30 Rowson, K. E. K., and Mahy, B. W. J.: Human papova (wart) virus, Bacterial Rev. 31: 110-131, 1967.

31 Sutton, J. S., and Burnett, J. W.: Ultrastructural changes in dermal and epidermal cells of skin infected with molluscum contagiosum virus, J. Ultrastruct. Res. 26:177-196, 1969.

32 Wile, U. J., and Kingery, L. B.: The etiology of common warts, J.A.M.A. 73:970-973, 1919.

33 Williams, M. G., Almeida, J. D., and Howatson, A. F.: Electron microscope studies on viral skin lesions, Arch. Dermatol. 86:290-297, 1962.

Bacterial diseases

34 Binford, C. H.: Leprosy as a diagnostic problem in surgical pathology, South. Med. J. 51: 200-207, 1958.

35 Brunsting, H. A.: Hidradenitis suppurativa: abscess of the apocrine sweat glands; a study of the clinical and pathologic features with a report of 23 cases and a review of the literature, Arch. Dermatol. 39:108-119, 1939.

36 Dillon, J. S., and Spjut, H. J.: Acne aggregata seu conglobata, Ann. Surg. 195:451-455, 1964.

37 Mansfield, R. E.: Histoid leprosy, Arch. Pathol. 87:580-585, 1969.

38 Masson, J. K.: Surgical treatment for hidradenitis suppurativa, Surg. Clin. North Am. 49: 1043-1052, 1969.

39 Montgomery, H.: Histopathology of various types of cutaneous tuberculosis, Arch. Dermatol. 35:698-715, 1937.

40 Russell, B.: Tuberculosis of the skin, Practitioner 180:553-563, 1958.

41 Shelley, W. B., and Cahn, M. M.: The pathogenesis of hidradenitis suppurativa in man, Arch. Dermatol. 72:562-569, 1955.

Fungal diseases

42 Azulay, R. D., and Serruya, J.: Hematogenous dissemination in chromoblastomycosis, Arch. Dermatol. 95:57-60, 1966.

43 Baker, R. D.: Tissue reaction in human blastomycosis, Am. J. Pathol. 18:479-497, 1942.

44 French, A. J., and Russell, S. R.: Chromoblastomycosis, Arch. Dermatol. 67:129-134, 1953.

45 Graham, J. H., Johnson, W. C., Burgoon, C. F., and Helwig, E. B.: Tinea capitis, Arch. Dermatol. 89:528-543, 1964.

46 Harrell, E. R., and Curtis, A. C.: North American blastomycosis, Am. J. Med. 27:750-766, 1959.

47 Kempson, R. L., and Sternberg, W. H.: Chronic subcutaneous abscesses caused by pigmented fungi, a lesion distinguishable from cutaneous chromoblastomycosis, Am. J. Clin. Pathol. 39:598-606, 1963.

48 Moore, M., Cooper, Z. K., and Weiss, R. S.: Chromomycosis (chromoblastomycosis), J.A. M.A. 122:1237-1243, 1943.

Miscellaneous diseases
Sarcoid

49 Cronin, E.: Skin changes in sarcoidosis, Postgrad. Med. J. 46:507-509, 1970.

50 Hurley, H. J., and Shelley, W. B.: Sarcoid granulomas with intradermal tuberculin in normal human skin, Arch. Dermatol. 82:65-72, 1960.

51 Israel, H. L., and Goldstein, R. A.: Relations of Kveim-antigen reaction to lymphadenopathy, N. Engl. J. Med. 284:345-349, 1971.

52 Maycock, R. L., Bertrand, P., Morrison, C. E., and Scott, J. H.: Manifestations of sarcoidosis, Am. J. Med. 35:67-89, 1963.

53 Siltzbach, L. E.: The Kveim test in sarcoidosis, J.A.M.A. 178:476-482, 1961.

Foreign body reaction

54 Allen, A. C.: Persistent "insect bites" (dermal eosinophilic granulomas) simulating lymphoblastomas, histiocytoses, and squamous cell carcinomas, Am. J. Pathol. 24:367-387, 1948.

55 Epstein, E.: Silica granuloma of the skin, Arch. Dermatol. 71:24-35, 1955.

56 Helwig, E. B.: Chemical (beryllium) granulomas of the skin, Milit. Surg. 109:540-558, 1951.

57 Newcomer, V. D., Graham, J. H., Schaffert, R. R., and Kaplan, L.: Sclerosing lipogranuloma resulting from exogenous lipids, Arch. Dermatol. 73:361-371, 1956.

58 Shelley, W. B., and Hurley, H. J.: The allergic origin of zirconium deodorant granulomas, Br. J. Dermatol. 70:75-101, 1958.

59 Shelley, W. B., and Hurley, H. J.: The pathogenesis of silica granulomas in man: a nonallergic colloidal phenomenon, J. Invest. Dermatol. 34:107-123, 1960.

Inflammatory diseases of unknown cause
Psoriasis

60 Albert J., and Crone, R. I.: Keratosis blenorrhagica (Reiter's disease?) and its treatment, Arch. Dermatol. 79:581-586, 1959.

61 Farber, E. M., and McClintock, R. P.: A current review of psoriasis, Calif. Med. 108: 440-457, 1968.

62 Helwig, E. B.: Pathology of psoriasis, Ann. N. Y. Acad. Sci. 73:924-935, 1958.

63 Weinstein, G. D., and van Scott, E. J.: An-

toradiographic analysis of turnover times of normal and psoriatic epidermis, J. Invest. Dermatol. **45**:257-262, 1965.

Exfoliative dermatitis and erythroderma

64 Abrahams, I., McCarthy, J. T., and Sanders, S. L.: One hundred and one cases of exfoliative dermatitis, Arch. Dermatol. **87**:96-101, 1963.
65 Tombridge, T. L.: Personal communication.

Lichen planus

66 Andreasen, J. O.: Oral lichen planus; a histologic evaluation of 97 cases, Oral Surg. Oral Med. Oral Path. **25**:158-166, 1968.
67 Altman, J., and Perry, H. O.: The variations and course of lichen planus, Arch. Dermatol. **84**:179-191, 1961.
68 Lumpkin, L. R., and Helwig, E. B.: Solitary lichen planus, Arch. Dermatol. **93**:54-55, 1966.
69 Wilson, H. T. H., and Bett, D. C. G.: Miliary lesions in lichen planus, Arch. Dermatol. **83**:920-923, 1961.

Chondrodermatitis helicis

70 Barker, L. P., Young, A. W., and Sachs, W.: Chondrodermatitis of the ears; a differential study of nodules of the helix and anthelix, Arch. Dermatol. **81**:15-25, 1960.
71 Calnan, J., and Rossatti, B.: On the histopathology of chondrodermatitis nodularis helicis chronica, J. Clin. Pathol. **12**:179-182, 1959.
72 Zimmerman, M. C.: Chondrodermatitis nodularis chronica helicis. In Epstein, E., editor: Skin surgery, Springfield, Ill., 1970, Charles C Thomas, Publisher, pp. 641-643.

Granuloma faciale

73 Allen, A. C.: Persistent "insect bites" (dermal eosinophilic granulomas) simulating lymphoblastomas, histiocytoses, and squamous cell carcinomas, Am. J. Pathol. **24**:367-387, 1948.
74 Gottlieb, B., and Winkelmann, R. K.: Lymphocytic infiltration of the skin, Arch. Dermatol. **86**:626-633, 1962.
75 Johnson, W. C., Higdon, R. S., and Helwig, E. B.: Granuloma faciale, Arch. Dermatol. **79**:42-52, 1959.
76 Pedace, F. J., and Perry, H. O.: Granuloma faciale, Arch. Dermatol. **94**:387-395, 1966.

Erythema nodosum

77 Irgang, S.: Nodular vasculitis, Arch. Dermatol. **74**:245-249, 1956.
78 Perry, H. O., and Winkelmann, R. K.: Subacute nodular migratory panniculitis, Arch. Dermatol. **89**:170-179, 1964.

79 Vesey, C. M. R., and Wilkinson, D. S.: Erythema nodosum; a study of 70 cases, Br. J. Dermatol. **71**:139-155, 1959.

Granuloma annulare

80 Arner, S., and Aspegren, N.: Familial granuloma annulare, Acta Derm. Venereol. **48**:253-254, 1968.
81 Beatty, E. C.: Rheumatic-like nodules occurring in nonrheumatic children, Arch. Pathol. **68**:154-159, 1959.
82 Mesara, B. W., Brody, G. L., and Oberman, H. A.: "Pseudorheumatoid" subcutaneous nodules, Am. J. Clin. Pathol. **45**:684-691, 1966.
83 Rubin, M., and Lynch, F. W.: Subcutaneous granuloma annulare; comment on familial granuloma annulare, Arch. Dermatol. **93**:416-429, 1966.
84 Wells, R. S., and Smith, M. A.: The natural history of granuloma annulare, Br. J. Dermatol. **75**:199-205, 1963.
85 Wood, M. G., and Beerman, H.: Necrobiosis lipoidica, granuloma annulare and rheumatoid nodule, J. Invest. Dermatol. **34**:139-147, 1960.

Necrobiosis lipoidica

86 Bauer, M., and Levan, N. E.: Diabetic dermangiopathy; a spectrum including pigmented pretibial patches and necrobiosis lipoidica diabeticorum, Br. J. Dermatol. **83**:528-535, 1970.
87 Fisher, E. R., and Danowski, T. S.: Histologic, histochemical, and electron microscopic features of the shin spots of diabetes mellitus, Am. J. Clin. Pathol. **50**:547-554, 1968.
88 Muller, S. A., and Winkelmann, R. K.: Necrobiosis lipoidica diabeticorum; histopathologic study of 98 cases, Arch. Dermatol. **94**:1-10, 1966.

Weber-Christian disease

89 Christian, H. A.: Relapsing febrile nodular nonsuppurative panniculitis, Arch. Intern. Med. **42**:338-341, 1928.
90 Laymon, C. W., and Peterson, W. C., Jr.: Lipogranulomatosis subcutanea (Rothmann-Makai); an appraisal, Arch. Dermatol. **90**:288-292, 1964.
91 Lever, W. F.: Nodular nonsuppurative panniculitis (Weber-Christian disease), Arch. Dermatol. **59**:31-35, 1949.

Urticaria pigmentosa

92 Berlin, C.: Urticaria pigmentosa as a systemic disease, Arch. Dermatol. **71**:703-712, 1955.
93 Drennan, J. M.: The mast cells in urticaria pigmentosa, J. Pathol. Bacteriol. **63**:513-520, 1951.

94 Head, K. W.: Cutaneous mast cell tumors in the dog, cat, and ox, Br. J. Dermatol. **70:** 390-408, 1958.

95 Johnson, W. C., and Helwig, E. B.: Solitary mastocytosis (urticaria pigmentosa), Arch. Dermatol. **84:**806-815, 1961.

96 Nickel, W. R.: Urticaria pigmentosa, Arch. Dermatol. **76:**476-498, 1957.

97 Nielsen, S. W., and Cole, C. R.: Canine mastocytoma: a report of one hundred cases, Am. J. Vet. Res. **19:**417-432, 1958.

98 Waters, W. J., and Lacson, P. S.: Mast cell leukemia presenting as urticaria pigmentosa, Pediatrics **19:**1033-1042, 1947.

Lupus erythematosus

99 Harvey, A. M., Schulman, L. E., Tumulty, P. A., Conley, C. L., and Schoenrich, E. H.: Systemic lupus erythematosus: review of the literature and clinical analysis of 138 cases, Medicine (Baltimore) **33:**291-437, 1954.

100 Jessner, M., and Kanof, N. B.: Lymphocytic infiltration of the skin, Arch. Dermatol. **68:** 447-449, 1953.

101 Klemperer, P., Pollack, A. D., and Baehr, G.: Pathology of disseminated lupus erythematosus, Arch. Pathol. **32:**569-631, 1941.

102 Shrank, A. B., and Doniach, D.: Discoid lupus erythematosus; correlation of clinical features with serum auto-antibody pattern, Arch. Dermatol. **87:**677-685, 1963.

Dermatomyositis

103 Adams, R. D., Denny-Brown, D., Pearson, C. M.: Diseases of muscle, ed. 2, New York, 1962, Harper & Row, Publishers, pp. 414-436.

104 Curtis, A. C., Heckaman, J. H., and Wheeler, A. H.: Study of the autoimmune reaction in dermatomyositis, J.A.M.A. **178:**571-573, 1961.

105 Janis, J. F., and Winkelmann, R. K.: Histopathology of the skin in dermatomyositis, Arch. Dermatol. **97:**640-649, 1968.

106 Williams, R. C., Jr.: Dermatomyositis and malignancy: a review of the literature, Ann. Intern. Med. **50:**1174-1181, 1959.

Scleroderma

107 Christianson, H. B., Dorsey, C. S., O'Leary, P. A., and Kierland, R. R.: Localized scleroderma; a clinical study of 235 cases, Arch. Dermatol. **74:**629-639, 1956.

108 Fisher, E. R., and Rodnan, G. P.: Pathological observations concerning the cutaneous lesion of progressive systemic sclerosis: an electron microscopic histochemical and immunohistochemical study, Arthritis Rheum. **3:**536-545, 1960.

109 Fleischmajer, R.: The collagen in scleroderma, Arch. Dermatol. **89:**437-441, 1964.

110 Winkelmann, R. K.: Classification and pathogenesis of scleroderma, Mayo Clin. Proc. **46:** 83-91, 1971.

Vesiculobullous diseases

111 Beutner, E. H., Chorzelski, T. P., and Jordan, R. E.: Autosensitization in pemphigus and bullous pemphigoid, Springfield, Ill., 1971, Charles C Thomas, Publisher.

112 Lever, W. F.: Pemphigus and pemphigoid, Springfield, Ill., 1965, Charles C Thomas, Publisher.

113 Lyell, A.: Dermatitis herpetiformis enteropathy, Br. J. Dermatol. **81:**228-229- 1968.

114 Perry, H. O., and Brunsting, L. A.: Pemphigus foliaceus; further observations, Arch. Dermatol. **91:**10-23, 1965.

115 Piérard, J., and Whimster, I.: The histological diagnosis of dermatitis herpetiformis, bullous pemphigoid and erythema multiforme, Br. J. Dermatol. **73:**253-266, 1961.

116 Sneddon, I. B., and Wilkinson, D. S.: Subcorneal pustular dermatosis, Br. J. Dermatol. **68:**835-894.

117 Tollman, M. M.: Dermatitis herpetiformis, Arch. Dermatol. **77:**462-465, 1968.

Degenerative and miscellaneous diseases
Lichen sclerosus et atrophicus

118 Barker, L. P., and Gross, P.: Lichen sclerosus et atrophicus of the female genitalia, Arch. Dermatol. **85:**362-373, 1962.

119 Jeffcoate, T. N. A., and Woodcock, A. S.: Premalignant conditions of the vulva, with particular reference to chronic epithelial dystrophies, Br. Med. J. **5245:**127-134, 1961.

120 Montgomery, H., and Hill, W. R.: Lichen sclerosus et atrophicus, Arch. Dermatol. **42:** 755-779, 1940.

121 Taylor, C. W.: Dermatology of the vulva, J. Obstet. Gynaec. Br. Emp. **69:**881-887, 1962.

Elastosis perforans

122 Hitch, J. M., and Lund, H. Z.: Elastosis perforans serpiginosa, Arch. Dermatol. **79:**407-421, 1959.

123 Mehregan, A. H.: Elastosis perforans serpiginosa, Arch. Dermatol. **97:**381-393, 1968.

Pseudoxanthoma elasticum

124 Graham Smith, J., Jr., Davidson, E. A., and Clark, R. D.: Dermal elastica in actinic elastosis and pseudoxanthoma elastica, Nature (London) **195:**716-717, 1962.

125 Robertson, M. G., and Schroder, J. S.: Pseudoxanthoma elasticum; a systemic disorder, Am. J. Med. **27:**433-442, 1959.

Pretibial myxedema

126 Beierwaltes, W. H., and Bollet, A. J.: Muco-polysaccharide content of skin in patients with pretibial myxedema, J. Clin. Invest. **38:** 945-948, 1959.

127 Gabrilove, J. L., and Ludwig, A. W.: The histogenesis of myxedema, J. Clin. Endocr. **17:**925-932, 1957.

Acanthosis nigricans

128 Brown, J., and Winkelmann, R. K.: Acanthosis nigricans; a study of 90 cases, Medicine (Baltimore) **47:**33-51, 1968.

129 Curth, H. O.: Cancer associated with acanthosis nigricans, Arch. Surg. **47:**517-522, 1943.

Xanthoma

130 Altman, J., and Winkelman, R. I.: Xanthoma disseminatum, Arch. Dermatol. **86:**582-596, 1962.

131 Fredrickson, D. S.: Plasma lipid abnormalities and cutaneous xanthomas. In Fitzpatrick, T. B., Arndt, K. A., Clark, W. H., Jr., Eisen, A. Z., Van Scott, E. J., and Vaughan, J. H., editors: Dermatology in general medicine, New York, 1971, McGraw-Hill Book Co., pp. 1173-1193.

Juvenile xanthogranuloma
(nevoxanthoendothelioma)

132 Blank, H., Eglick, P. G., and Beerman, H.: Nevoxantho-endothelioma with ocular involvement, Pediatrics **4:**349-354, 1949.

133 Helwig, E. B., and Hackney, V. C.: Juvenile xanthogranuloma (nevoxanthoendothelioma), Am. J. Pathol. **30:**625-626, 1949.

134 Nödl, F.: Systematisierte grossknotige Nevoxanthoendothelioma, Arch. Klin. Exp. Dermatol. **208:**601-615, 1959.

135 Sanders, T. E.: Personal communication.

Tumors

Malcolm H. McGavran, M.D.

Introduction

The skin is, contrary to the ubiquitous simplistic concept, a remarkably heterogeneous organ. The tumors (hamartomatous, reactive, and neoplastic) that occur in the skin are more numerous than those produced by any other organ. For example, the eccrine sweat gland alone gives rise to six histologically distinct adenomas. This diversity, combined with a body of descriptive data (clinical, histologic, histochemical, and ultrastructural) amassed over the past century and dispersed in varying literatures, produces confusion, chiefly in the area of nomenclature. Within the limits inherent in this book, it is impossible to pursue finite segmentation, interesting and accurate as it may be. The more common lesions will be discussed in some detail and pertinent references provided for the rare lesions. Several excellent texts dealing in detail with tumors of the skin are available.[1-6]

Epidermis

Actinic keratosis

In that portion of the epidermis exposed to sunlight, chiefly that of the near ultraviolet spectrum, there develops a sequence of atrophic, atypical, dysplastic, and eventually hyperplastic changes known as actinic or solar keratosis (Fig. 68). The term "senile" keratosis often is inappropriate. Histologically, actinic keratoses involve the interfollicular epidermis, sparing the follicular apparatus and the intraepidermal portion of the sweat duct.[7] The stratum corneum is replaced by a parakeratotic scale. Excessive production and accumulation of this scale lead to the formation of cutaneous horns. The granular layer

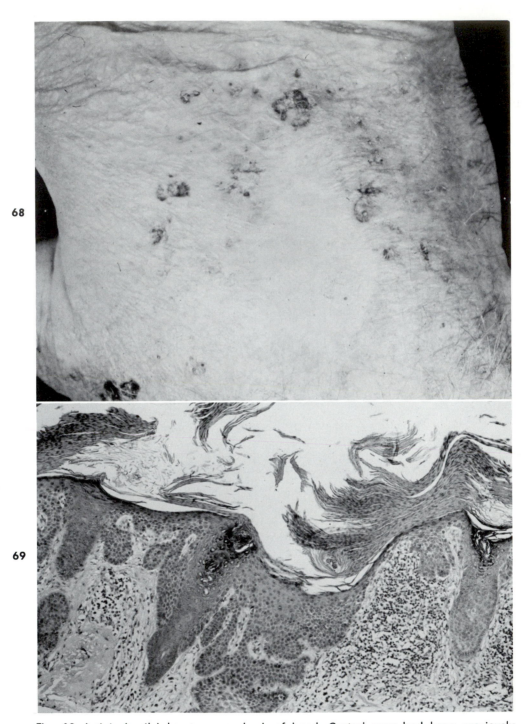

Fig. 68 Actinic (senile) keratoses on back of hand. Central area had been previously excised and grafted. (WU neg. 49-1887.)

Fig. 69 Atrophic interfollicular epidermis covered by parakeratotic scale. Follicular orifices maintain their granular layer and orthokeratosis. Slight atypia is evident in areas of acanthotic hyperplasia in this actinic keratosis. (×90; WU neg. 67-4140.)

is generally absent except at and about the follicular orifices. The stratum spinosum shows disorderly maturation as well as individually dysplastic and dyskeratotic cells (Fig. 69). On occasion, suprabasal acantholysis produces vesicles reminiscent of those seen in pemphigus vulgaris. The papillary dermis is often chronically inflamed, and basophilic degenerative changes are prominent in the collagen. In florid keratosis, the atypical epithelial proliferation produces irregularly elongated acanthotic ridges, and this process extends down the external root sheaths of the hair follicles.

Actinic keratoses may be treated by a variety of methods—freezing, superficial curettage, application of antineoplastic chemotherapeutic agents, and surgical excision.[8] Excision is, in fact, unnecessarily radical therapy except for the more florid and infiltrative types and those not responding to topical 5-fluorouracil.

Carcinoma in situ

Along the sequence of neoplastic progression in the epidermis damaged by sun appears a histologic picture identified as intraepithelial carcinoma or carcinoma in situ. The lesions show full-thickness involvement of the epidermis by neoplastic squamous cells. In contrast to this entity as found on mucosal surfaces, some surface maturation and keratinization may be found overlying carcinoma in situ of the epidermis. The lesion previously known as intraepithelial epithelioma is probably composed of a heterogeneous group of lesions as Mehregan and Pinkus[11] have described. A distinct intraepithelial tumor, composed of clear, glycogen-filled keratinocytes, is known as Degos' acanthoma or clear cell acanthoma.[9, 10]

Bowen's disease

The terms carcinoma in situ and Bowen's disease are almost inextricably confused and inappropriately used as synonyms. In point of fact, Bowen[12] described (and the condition has been repeatedly observed) a syndrome of indolent, scaly, erythematous plaques occurring predominantly on skin unexposed to sunlight (Fig. 70). Histologically, the lesions show a variety of atypical epithelial changes culminating in the pattern of frank carcinoma in situ (Fig. 71). Bowen's disease cannot be diagnosed on histologic appearance alone. Its diagnosis is made only upon the basis of the characteristic course, distribution, and morphologic pattern of the lesions. Graham and Helwig[13] found an increase in the incidence of visceral cancer in a group of patients with Bowen's disease. Searches for carcinogens, such as arsenic, in Bowen's disease have proved inconclusive. Arsenic is capable of inducing carcinoma of the skin that eventuates on a protracted hyperplastic and dysplastic prodroma.

Epidermoid (squamous) carcinoma

The incidence of epidermoid (squamous) carcinoma can be correlated directly with the amount of exposure to the sun and the lack of pigmentation of the skin. Blond, blue-eyed, fair-skinned persons living in Texas have a higher incidence of skin cancer than do their counterparts in Minnesota. Epidermoid carcinoma in black people is a rare disease. In urban populations, frankly invasive squamous carcinoma is uncommon, whereas in rural populations it is common.[19] Other factors operate in the production of epidermoid carcinoma arising from the skin. Chronic osteomyelitic sinuses, acne aggregata seu conglobata, and old burn scars, either thermal or due to x-rays, constitute one set of predispositional phenomena.[15, 18] Chemicals, including arsenic, coal tars, and soot and a variety of oils and distillation products, form another group of epidermal carcinogens. The diminished capacity of DNA repair following ultraviolet light irradiation of the cells of most, but not all, persons with xeroderma pigmentosa provides a "molecular" explanation for this tragic condition.[14]

A considerable variance of opinion exists as to what represents invasion of the der-

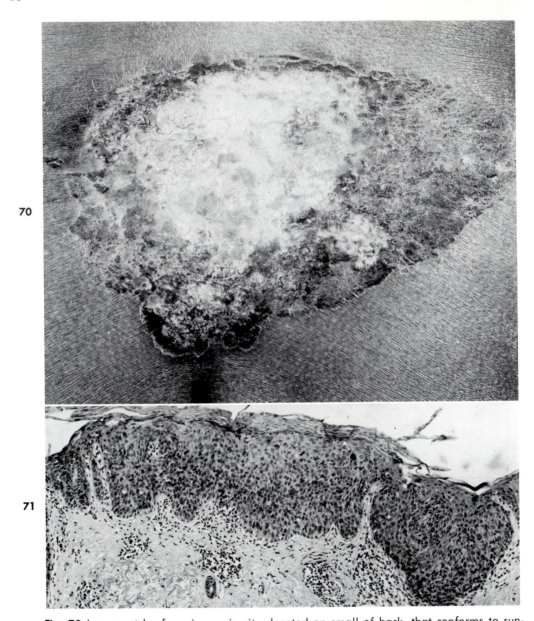

Fig. 70 Large patch of carcinoma in situ, located on small of back, that conforms to syndrome described by Bowen.[12] (WU neg. 49-5915.)

Fig. 71 Parakeratotic scale overlies dysplastic and atypical keratinocytes that involve full thickness of epidermis. This is carcinoma in situ. (×90; WU neg. 67-4141.)

mis. Thus what is considered florid actinic keratosis by some may be called superficially invasive carcinoma by others. Pragmatically, the significant fact is that metastases are rare, if they occur at all, from small (less than 1.5 cm in diameter), superficially invasive cancers of the skin.[17] Even in lesions larger than 2 cm, with unequivocal invasion into the reticular dermis, the incidence of regional lymph node metastases is low, less than 5%. The majority (80% to 90%) of epidermoid carcinomas are well to moderately differentiated (i.e., the keratinocytes maintain their ability to form keratin) (Fig. 72). A small fraction are poorly differentiated and re-

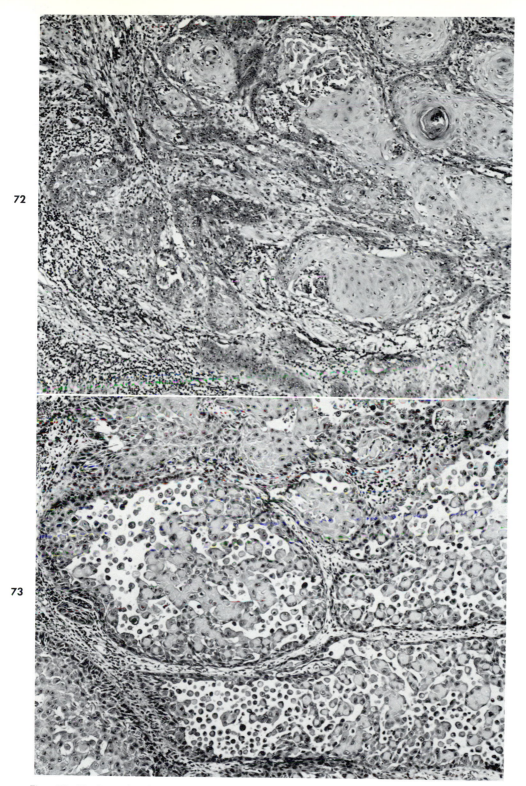

72

73

Fig. 72 Moderately differentiated to well-differentiated invasive epidermoid carcinoma that arose on forehead of 77-year-old man. (×90; WU neg. 67-4409.)
Fig. 73 False glands caused by acantholysis produce adenoid variant of epidermoid carcinoma. (×90; WU neg. 67-4144.)

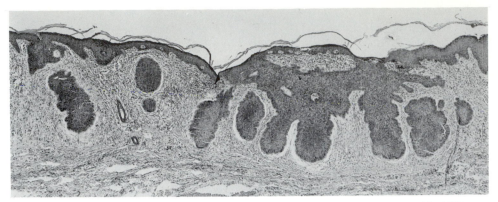

Fig. 74 Example of superficial multicentric type of basal cell carcinoma. (×35; WU neg. 67-4149.)

tain minimal evidence of their keratinocytic heritage. Many of the so-called "Grade IV" or "spindle cell" epidermoid carcinomas of the skin are, in point of fact, likely atypical fibroxanthomas (p. 104) or amelanotic melanomas. Acantholysis (the loss of cohesiveness caused by desmosomal degeneration) produces a type of epidermoid carcinoma called adenoid squamous cell carcinoma.[16] The pseudoglandular pattern of these cancers should not be mistaken for adenocarcinoma (Fig. 73).

Complete excision is requisite for cure of epidermoid carcinoma. Careful pathologic examination, including marking of the surgical margins with India ink or silver nitrate, allows identification of those cases in which tumor has been transected.

Pseudoepitheliomatous hyperplasia

At sites of trauma and chronic irritation and around ulcers, the reparative hyperplasia of the epidermis may produce seemingly invasive tongues of epithelial cells. These are generally associated with a dermal fibrocytic and angiomatous reaction and a definite acute to subacute inflammatory infiltrate. Clear separation of pseudoepitheliomatous hyperplasia from cancer is not always easy. The absence of atypical epithelial cells and the presence of the inflammatory reaction, as well as the history, are helpful in distinguishing these false cancers from the real ones. Conservatism is generally warranted.

Basal cell carcinoma

Basal cell carcinomas derive their name from their cytologic similarity to the basal cells of the epidermis and the follicle. They are the most frequent form of skin cancer and occur predominantly on the sun-exposed skin in direct proportion to the number of pilosebaceous units present therein.[24] Fair-skinned, blue-eyed persons engaged in outdoor occupations suffer a higher incidence of these tumors.[21] Metastases are vanishingly rare.[27] When allowed to grow through the skull, into the nares, into the orbit, or into the temporal bone via the auditory canal, basal cell carcinoma can kill. Most often death is the result of meningitis.

The clinical appearances of basal cell carcinoma are as variable as are its histologic patterns. Nodular, ulcerative, superficial, erythematous, multicentric, and sclerosing or morphea-like forms occur. Growth is slow and progress indolent. Excision, curettage and desiccation, irradiation, and caustic pastes used appropriately cure almost all these tumors. In instances wherein basal cell carcinoma extends to the margin of surgical excision, an occurrence of approximately 5% in large series, only one-third show evidence of recrudescence over the ensuing two to five years.[22] Thus immediate reexcision is not indicated. Careful follow-up is sufficient.

Histologically, basal cell carcinomas are seen to arise from the basal layer of the

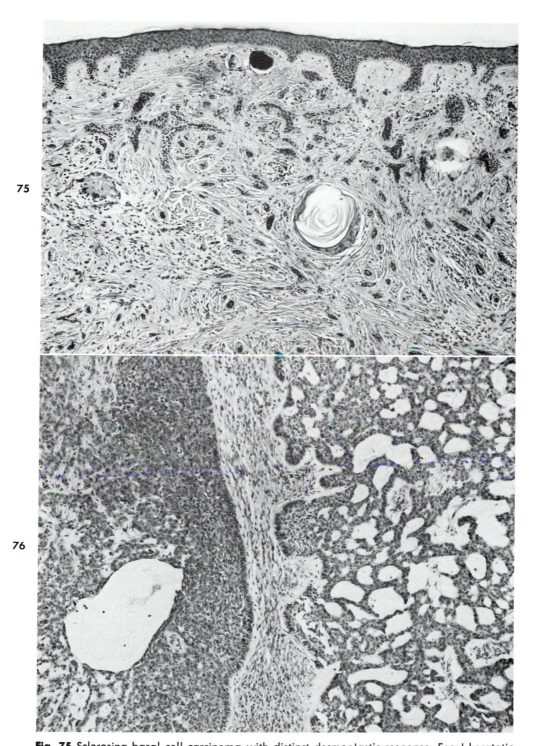

75

76

Fig. 75 Sclerosing basal cell carcinoma with distinct desmoplastic response. Focal keratotic differentiation forms nests of squamous debris. (×90; WU neg. 67-4060A.)
Fig. 76 Basal cell carcinoma with both solid (left) and adenoid (right) cystic areas. (×90; WU neg. 67-4145.)

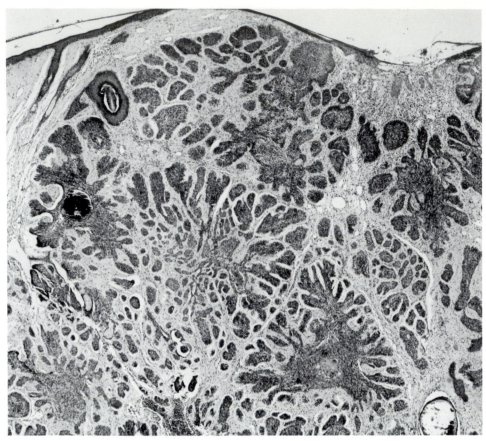

Fig. 77 Stromal component and segmentation of epithelium in basal cell tumor of tricho-epitheliomatous type. (×40; WU neg. 67-4403.)

epidermis as well as from the pilosebaceous adnexa.[25] They may have solid, cystic, adenoid, sclerosing, and keratotic patterns (Figs. 74 to 76). The presence of keratinocytic differentiation provokes much verbiage and hybrid terms such as "basosquamous carcinoma." Biologically, basal cell tumors having areas of squamous differention behave no differently than pure basal cell carcinoma. They are not an intermediate step toward epidermoid carcinoma.

A syndrome of multiple nevoid basal cell carcinomas, keratinous cysts of the jaws, skeletal anomalies, and occasional central nervous system, mesenteric, and endocrinologic abnormalities has been established in the past decade.[23] Pathologically, these basal cell carcinomas cannot be distinguished from those occurring in individuals without the syndrome. The syndrome should be suspected when basal cell cancers are seen in young persons who have multiple tumors, many of which are of the superficial multicentric type and in which osteoid is an occasional finding.[26]

Trichoepitheliomas are basal cell tumors of long standing. They may be multiple, do not ulcerate, and histologically have a prominent stromal component surrounding abortive pilar differentiation (Fig. 77). The fibroepithelial tumor of Pinkus is a polypoid lesion, often occurring on the back, in which stroma predominates[20] (Fig. 78).

Seborrheic verruca

Seborrheic verruca are common, benign, pigmented, basal and keratinocytic pro-

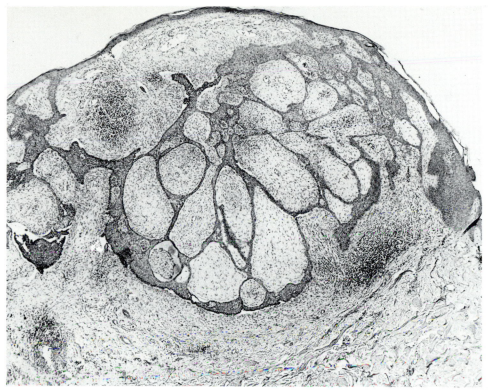

Fig. 78 Fibroepithelial tumor of Pinkus. This is a variant of basal cell carcinoma. (×40; WU neg. 67-4121.)

liferations occurring chiefly on the trunk of adults. They may be single or multiple. The lesions protrude above the surface of the skin, are soft, and vary in color from tan to black. The single, heavily pigmented seborrheic verruca may be confused clinically with malignant melanoma (Fig. 79).

The characteristic histologic features are shown in Fig. 80. Other patterns occur, and in irritated seborrheic verruca, squamous metaplasia is pronounced. Atypical seborrheic verrucae may be misdiagnosed as basosquamous carcinomas. The multiple, small, seborrheic verrucae are readily treated by superficial curettage or freezing.[28]

Extramammary (anogenital) Paget's disease

Invasion of the epidermis by cells from adenocarcinoma originating in sweat glands, the rectum, and the urethra produces the entity of extramammary Paget's disease. In perhaps one-half of the patients the underlying adenocarcinoma is not detected or may be at a site so distant that intraepidermal metastasis has to be invoked in hypothetical explanation.[30] The labia majora, scrotum, and perineum are the most frequent sites, with adjacent areas following. The lesions are grossly circinate, annular, erythematous, and eczematoid plaques. Histologically, large, pale, vacuolated cells, containing acidic mucopolysaccharides,[29] are seen concentrated just above the basal layer (Fig. 81). They may form nests and extend into the stratum spinosum. Electron microscopic examination shows that Paget's cells are not altered keratinocytes or melanocytes[31] (Fig. 82). Adequate surgical excision is the treatment of choice. The differential diagnosis of extramammary Paget's disease includes carci-

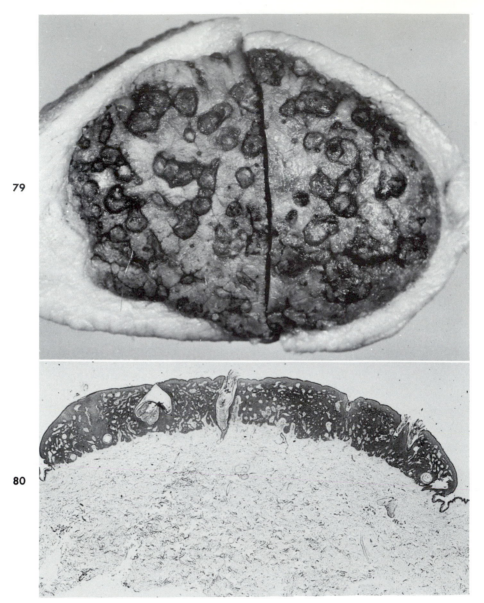

79

80

Fig. 79 Large, deeply pigmented, sharply circumscribed, elevated, seborrheic keratosis. (WU neg. 49-6197.)
Fig. 80 Seborrheic verruca projecting above level of epidermis. Cysts represent sections of hyperkeratotic follicles. (×12; WU neg. 49-5195.)

noma in situ, junctional nevi, and malignant melanoma.

Adnexa

All of the adnexa are derived from the same primitive ectodermal cell as the epidermis and thus it is not surprising that adnexal tumors have certain similar histologic appearances and cytologic features.

Readily recognizable homogeneous groups can be identified and separated and their structure and cytochemistry correlated with those of the analogous adnexa or even with a subdivision thereof.

Eccrine sweat gland

The normal anatomy and segments of the eccrine gland and the idealized gross

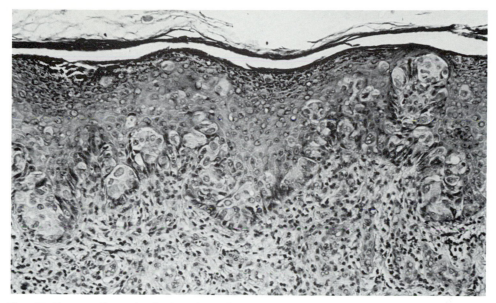

Fig. 81 Paget cells, individual and in clusters, are present just above basal layer and farther up in epidermis in this lesion from scrotum. No primary cancer, sweat gland or other, was found. Patient has had no recrudescence in nine years following surgical excision. (×150; WU neg. 67-4146A.)

appearance of its adenomas are shown in Fig. 83.

Poroma

The eccrine poroma, first described by Pinkus et al.,[45] occurs chiefly on the palms and soles. Occurrence elsewhere, however, has been reported.[44] Poromas often show a moat and hillock pattern and histologically are characterized by a sharp junction between the proliferating, nonpigmented, basal type of keratinocytes and the adjacent epidermis (Fig. 84). Within these cords and nests, ducts and ductlike structures may be formed. Ultrastructural studies show that the predominant cell has features similar to those of the acrosyringium, and histochemical similarities exist as well.[34] The dermis beneath often shows a distinct proliferation of reactive vessels and some inflammation. These lesions are to be differentiated from basal cell tumors and seborrheic verrucae.

Acrospiroma

An adenoma, also called solid-cystic hidradenoma by Winkelmann and Wolff,[48] acrospiroma arises from the distal excretory duct. It forms nodules with occasional cystic foci high in the dermis (Fig. 85). The proliferating cell is cytologically similar to that of the poroma. The acrospiroma differs from the poroma in that epidermal involvement is not found. Johnson and Helwig[39] ably discuss the differential diagnosis of this lesion.

Syringoma

Syringomas are generally multiple, yellowish, papulonodular lesions that occur chiefly on the neck and face of women. They are formed by clusters of small ducts lined by two-cell-thick epithelium, occasionally with comma-shaped extensions (Fig. 86). The ultrastructural[35] and histochemical[47] findings indicate that these lesions are eccrine and not apocrine derivatives.

Chondroid syringoma (mixed tumor)

Chondroid syringomas are benign, nodular, nonulcerated tumors that occur predominantly on the face, head, and neck but also on the extremities and trunk.[46]

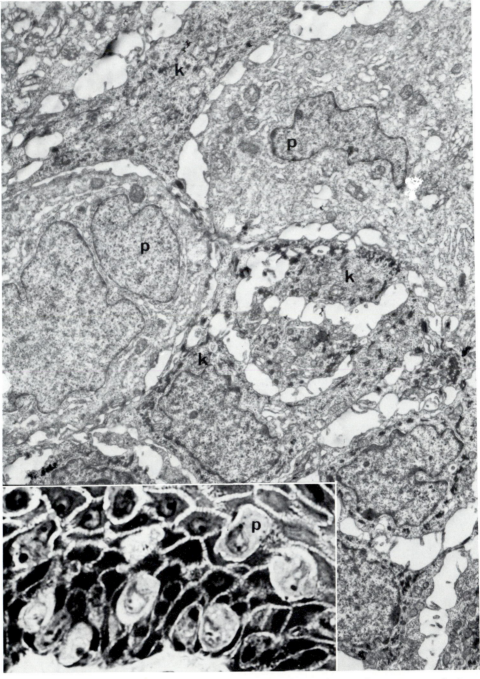

Fig. 82 Ultrastructure of Paget cells, **p,** as contrasted to adjacent keratinocytes, **k. Inset** shows large, pale Paget cells, **p,** in light micrograft from lμ thick, Epon-embedded section of epidermis. (Uranyl acetate–lead citrate; ×4,000; **inset,** ×800.)

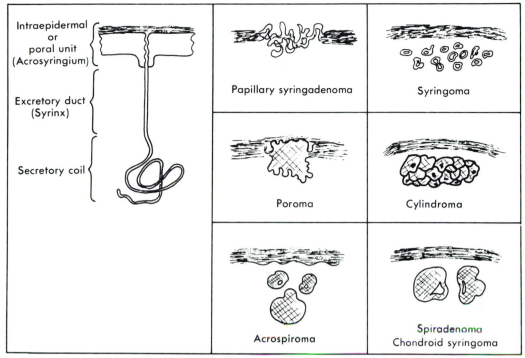

	Papillary syringadenoma	Syringoma
Intraepidermal or poral unit (Acrosyringium) Excretory duct (Syrinx) Secretory coil	Poroma	Cylindroma
	Acrospiroma	Spiradenoma Chondroid syringoma

Fig. 83 Eccrine sweat gland and adenomas.

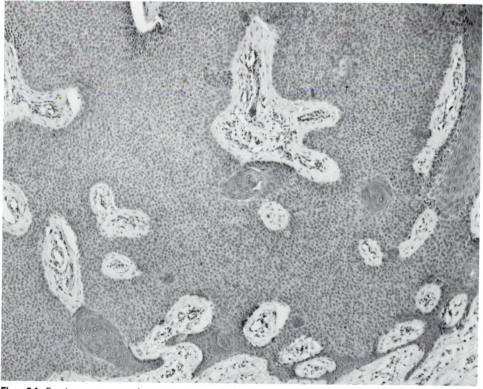

Fig. 84 Eccrine poroma showing most of the features described in text. (×90; WU neg. 67-4111A.)

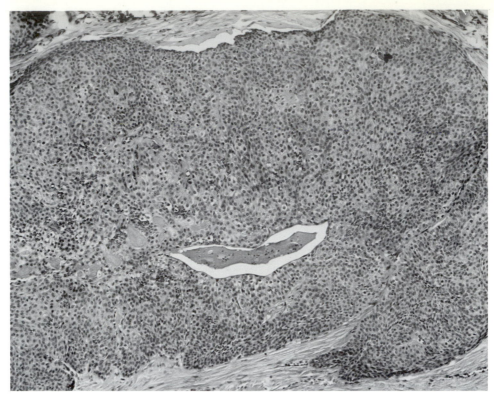

Fig. 85 Nodular eccrine adenoma showing histologic features of subgroup called acrospiroma. (×90; WU neg. 67-4113A.)

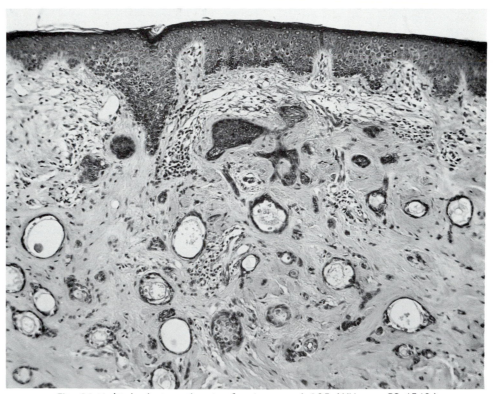

Fig. 86 Multiple ducts and cysts of syringoma. (×135; WU neg. 52-4548.)

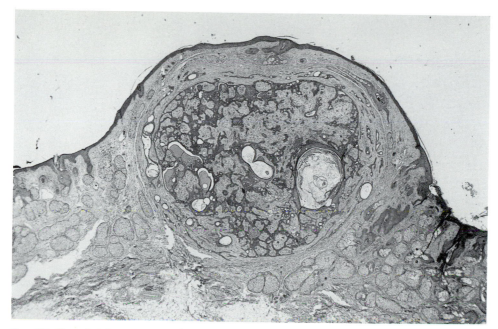

Fig. 87 Chondroid syringoma that arose on cheek of 77-year-old man. (×15; WU neg. 67-4108A.)

Histologically, their appearance is comparable to that of mixed tumors of salivary gland origin[38] (Fig. 87).

Dermal eccrine cylindroma

The past emphasis on multiplicity, enormous size, and scalp involvement of dermal eccrine cylindromas obscures the fact that the majority of these slowly growing adenomas are solitary and small and that approximately 10% occur on sites other than the head and neck.[32] The characteristic histologic and ultrastructural appearances are illustrated in Figs. 88 and 89. The heavy basement membranes surrounding the nests of cells are obvious. Intralobular accumulation of similar material also occurs.

Eccrine spiradenoma

Eccrine spiradenomas are sharply delimited, lobular, and cellular adenomas that occur almost anywhere on the body. They were first segregated by Kersting and Helwig,[40] and subsequent studies by Munger et al.[43] and Hashimoto et al.[36] have documented their relation to the lower portion of eccrine duct. Histologically,

these tumors are very cellular (Fig. 90). The scanty cytoplasm and prominent nuclei may lead the unwary to an erroneous diagnosis of malignancy.

Papillary syringadenoma

Papillary syringadenomas are verrucous, moist tumors that occur chiefly on the scalp, neck and face but are found elsewhere on the skin. They are seen from childhood to senescence, and often there is a history of slow growth or of a recent change in a "birthmark." The histologic appearance is shown in Fig. 91. Juxtaposed nevus sebaceus was found in one-third and basal cell carcinoma in one-tenth of the patients reported by Helwig and Hackney.[37]

Sweat gland cancer

Identification of adenocarcinomas arising from eccrine glands is difficult unless the lesions have obviously invasive characteristics or have metastasized when first seen.[33] These are rare tumors and comprise a minute fraction of sweat gland neoplasms even in large and collected series[42]

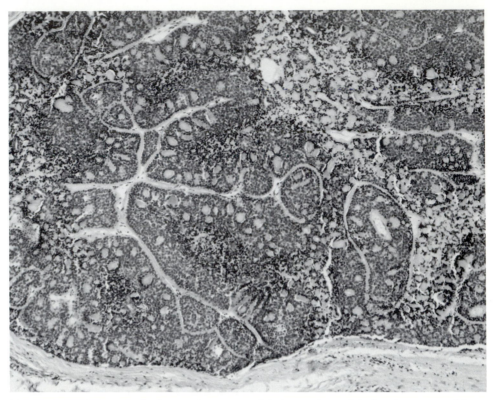

Fig. 88 Dermal eccrine cylindroma showing perilobular and intralobular deposition of basement membrane material. (×90; WU neg. 67-4059.)

(Fig. 92). A select variant, mucinous (adenocystic) carcinoma, is described by Mendoza and Helwig.[41] The presumption that two-cell-thick epithelial structure connotes benignity is not justified and, contrariwise, loss of differentiation does not always imply malignancy.

Apocrine sweat gland

Although apocrine sweat glands are concentrated in the axillae, groin, and perineum, they occur in small numbers on the face and elsewhere. Three characteristic adenomas arise from apocrine glands: papillary hidradenoma, cystadenoma, and "ceruminous" adenoma. Landry and Winkelmann[52] describe an uncommon variant.

Papillary hidradenoma

Papillary hidradenomas occur on the labia and perineum of postpubertal women.[56] These nodular and cystic lesions are distinct and differ from the papillary syringadenoma previously discussed and from the apocrine cystadenoma. The histologic appearance of the papillary hidradenoma is illustrated in the discussion on the vulva (Fig. 763, A).

The findings of Meeker et al.[53] that the lesion is limited to white women is not absolute, for we have seen a case in our material from a black woman.

Cystadenoma

Cystadenomas, also known as hydrocystomas, are cystic, nodular hyperplasias of apocrine glands, generally limited to the face. Holder et al.[50] report a case on the trunk. The lesions are often pigmented and may be confused clinically with nevi, blue nevi, and pigmented basal cell tumors.[54]

"Ceruminous" adenoma

The apocrine glands in the external auditory canal are called ceruminous

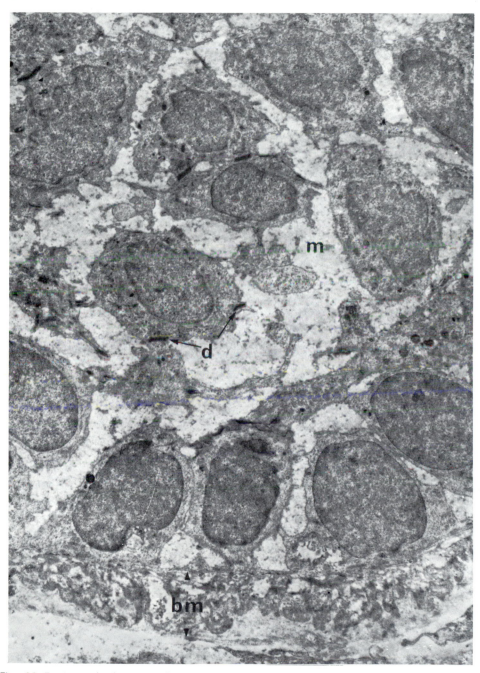

Fig. 89 Eccrine cylindroma (turban tumor) illustrating thick basement membrane, **bm,** at periphery of lobule, desmosomal attachments of cells, **d,** and mucopolysaccharide matrix, **m.** These cells are similar to eccrine duct cells. (Uranyl acetate–lead citrate; ×5,000; courtesy Dr. B. L. Munger, Hershey, Pa.)

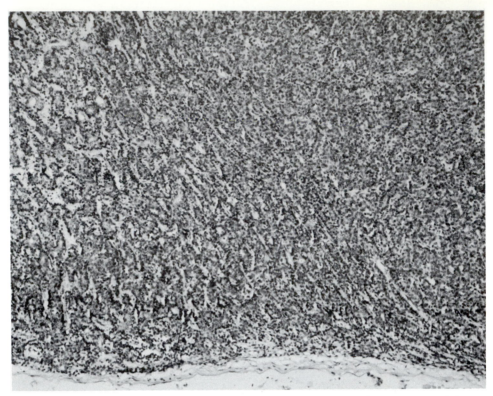

Fig. 90 Eccrine spiradenoma showing closely packed glandular and seemingly solid components. (×90; WU neg. 67-4408.)

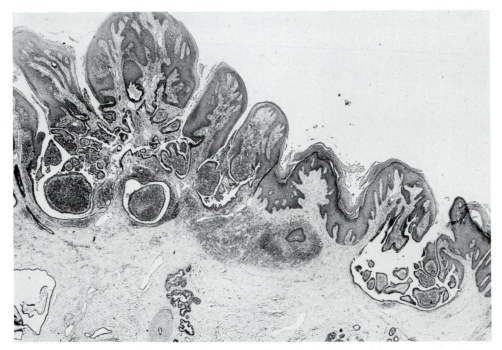

Fig. 91 At bases of epidermal papillae are clefts and glands lined by eccrine epithelium. Chronic, lymphocytic, and plasmocellular inflammatory infiltrate is not uncommon in papillary syringadenomas. (×15; WU neg. 67-4109A.)

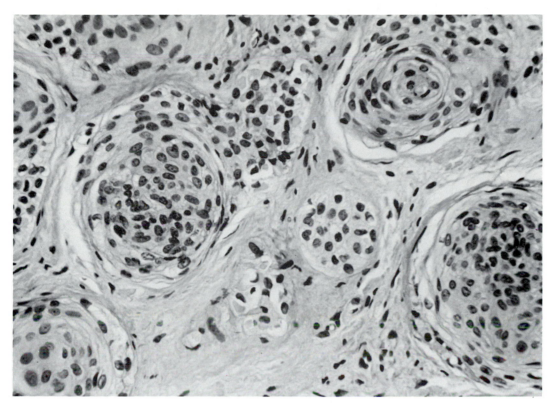

Fig. 92 Sweat gland carcinoma of skin upper lip in 28-year-old woman. (×350; WU neg. 71-6391.)

glands. They do not produce cerumin. Cerumin is the product of the sebaceous glands and not the apocrine glands. Thus continued use of the term ceruminous adenoma is not justified, as Johnstone et al.[51] aptly point out.

"Ceruminous" adenomas are rare.[55] Their initial removal is often incomplete, and recrudescences are common. Histologically, two major divisions may be made: those adenomas having characteristic two-layered epithelium set in varying amounts of stroma and a second smaller group with a poorly differentiated epithelial pattern that, on occasion, has a cylindromatous appearance.[49] Mixed tumors appearing in the ear canal may originate from sweat glands or be extensions from parotid tumors. Adequate excision is requisite for eradication of these lesions. Procrastination leads to death when the temporal bone is involved.

Sebaceous gland
Senile sebaceous hyperplasia

The most common tumor of the sebaceous glands is due to hyperplasia occurring chiefly on the nose and cheeks of elderly persons, hence the name senile sebaceous nevus or, preferably, senile sebaceous hyperplasia (Fig. 93). Bona fide adenomas occur,[57] but the lines of distinction between adenoma and adenomatous hyperplasia are indistinct. The "sebaceous adenoma" occurring in tuberous sclerosis is a fibrovascular hamartoma with little sebaceous hyperplasia.

Nevus sebaceus of Jadassohn

Nevus sebaceus of Jadassohn is a hamartomatous conglomerate of large sebaceous glands associated with heterotopic apocrine glands and defective hair follicles. The lesions occur on the scalp and face, are

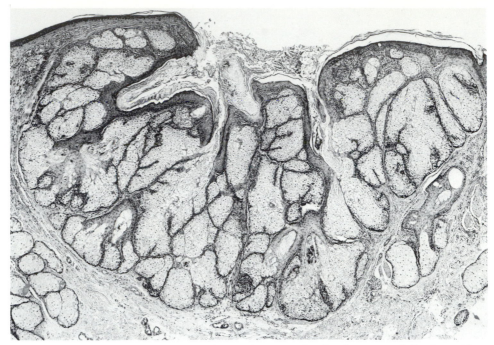

Fig. 93 Example of senile sebaceous hyperplasia in glands about two follicular orifices. (×35; WU neg. 67-4063A.)

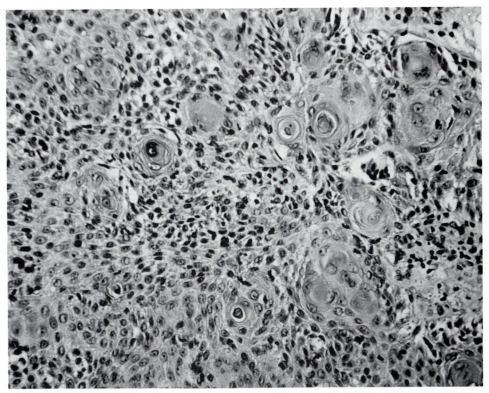

Fig. 94 Characteristic "squamous eddies" found within basal epithelium of follicular keratosis. (×260; WU neg. 67-4413.)

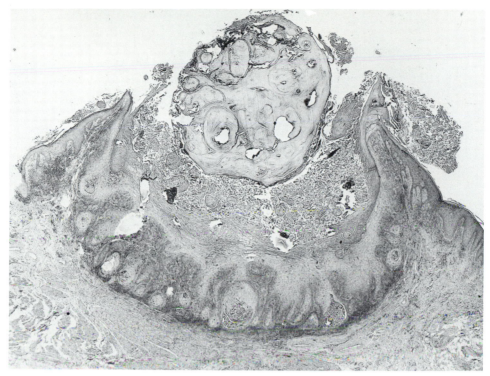

Fig. 95 Crater filled with plug of keratin surrounded by proliferating squamous epithelium characteristic of keratoacanthoma. (×18; WU neg. 67-4132.)

present from infancy, and gradually enlarge.

Other lesions

Unequivocal sebaceous carcinoma is vanishingly rare.[57] Sebaceous metaplasia, seen as focal areas of characteristic foamy lipid-laden cells, is not infrequent in basal cell carcinomas and even in squamous carcinomas.[58]

Hair follicle
Inverted follicular keratosis

The hyperplastic follicular lesions of inverted follicular keratosis are identified by the presence of squamous eddies (Fig. 94). They usually have a papillomatous as well as an acanthotic inverted component. Mehregan[74] draws an analogy between inverted follicular keratosis and the eccrine poroma, since both are derived from infundibular parts of their respective adnexa.

Trichofolliculoma

Trichofolliculomas are solitary, nodular, hamartomatous lesions that should be distinguished from trichoepitheliomas and epithelioma adenoides cysticum.[64, 65] Their characteristic dilated central follicle is surrounded by proliferating epithelium showing various stages of pilar formation.

Keratoacanthoma

Keratoacanthomas arise not from the interfollicular epidermis but from the wall of the upper portion of the hair follicle. They were historically and are currently occasionally confused with epidermoid carcinoma. Keratoacanthomas occur in males three or four times more frequently than in females and in somewhat younger persons in a similar but not identical distribution to that of epidermoid carcinoma.[77] The distinctive features of keratoacanthomas, as contrasted to squamous carcinoma, are as follows.

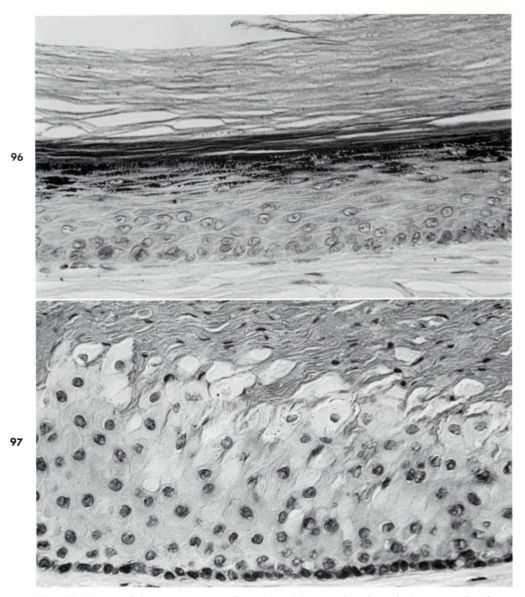

Fig. 96 Lining of keratinous cyst of epidermoid type that has distinct granular layer. (×350; WU neg. 67-4117A.)
Fig. 97 Lining of keratinous cyst of trichilemmal type which cornifies without granular layer. Pallor of cells just beneath keratin is not due to fat. (×350; WU neg. 67-4148.)

1 They arise from previously undiseased skin, whereas most cancers evolve upon antecedent actinic keratosis.
2 They have a rapid (four to six weeks) growth, producing a characteristic, dome-shaped volcano with a central crater filled by a keratotic plug. Cancer has a far more protracted course.

3 They undergo spontaneous regression over an ensuing four to six weeks and leave a slightly depressed, annular scar.[78]

Histologically, cross sections of keratoacanthomas are diagnostic (Fig. 95). Biopsies, on the other hand, may be difficult, if not impossible, to distinguish from well-

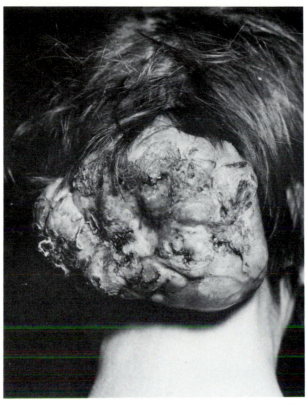

Fig. 98 Proliferating keratinous cyst of five years' duration in scalp of 52-year-old woman. It recurred following local removal, but re-excision was apparently curative. Patient has been followed for six years. (From Dabska, M.: Giant hair matrix tumor, Cancer **28**:701-706, 1971.)

differentiated epidermoid carcinoma.[60] The pattern and form of the proliferating epithelium are useful in diagnosing keratoacanthoma. Cytologic criteria commonly thought of as diagnostic of cancer are of no particular use. We have seen, though rarely, keratoacanthomas invade the sheaths of dermal nerves and extend superficially into skeletal muscle. In most instances, the rim of epithelium is surrounded by a chronic inflammatory infiltrate. This increases during the period of regression. The etiology of keratoacanthomas is unknown. In rabbits, Ghadially et al.[62] have produced similar tumors by the application of dimethylbenzanthracene. Growth and regression of keratoacanthomas, perhaps more accurately called *folliculoacanthomas*, correlate with the cyclic responses of the pilofollicular apparatus.

Keratinous cyst

The tumors of the skin most frequently misdiagnosed, both clinically and pathologically, are the cysts of the hair follicle. Sebaceous cysts are a myth, born of casual gross description and perpetuated by uncritical repetition.[69]

Two types of keratinous cyst occur. The more frequent, 90%, is lined by epithelium that cornifies, with a distinct granular layer, as does the interfollicular epidermis and the upper third of the external root sheath. Such cysts are of the *epidermoid* type (Fig. 96). Traumatic inoculation may produce such cysts on the fingers and hands. In the infrequent type of keratinous cyst, occurring almost exclusively on the scalp, cornification occurs in the absence of a granular layer. These are keratinous cysts of the *trichilemmal* (pilar) type (Fig.

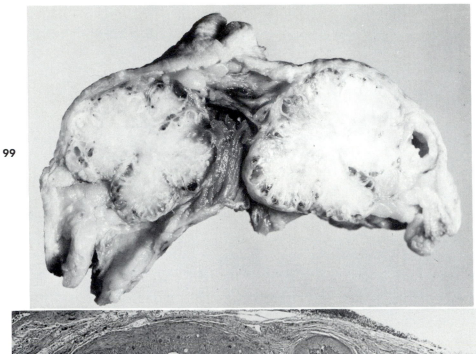

99

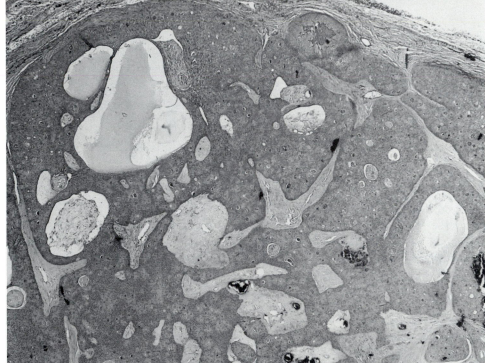

100

Fig. 99 Transected proliferating keratinous cyst. This is not epidermoid carcinoma arising in keratinous cyst. (WU neg. 53-1806.)
Fig. 100 Interlacing proliferating epithelium in proliferating keratinous cyst with microscopic features that characterize it as follicular in type. (×30; WU neg. 67-4478.)

97). These cysts do not occur on hairless skin.[72, 75] Amino acid analyses of the cornified content of these two types of cysts show (1) that the epidermoid cysts differ from stratum corneum in a reduction of cystine and the presence of citrulline and (2) that the trichilemmal cyst content is low in sulfur-containing amino acids and thus distinct from hair cortex.[73]

The majority of the reports in the literature purporting to document carcinoma arising in keratinous "sebaceous" cysts are nonsense upon critical review. It is not inconceivable that such should occur, but if it does, it is vanishingly rare. We have never seen such a case in our material nor known of one in the experience of our dermatologically sophisticated colleagues. Many of the lesions thought to be cancers are, in fact, proliferating keratinous cysts (Figs. 98 to 100) of the trichilemmal type.[59, 67, 68, 76]

Dermoid cyst

Keratinous cysts, into which adnexa open, occurring on the face of children along lines of embryonic closure are known as dermoid cysts. These are distinct from histologically comparable cysts occurring in multiples on the trunk in individuals with a strong familial incidence. This latter condition is known as steatocystoma multiplex.[70]

Isolated follicular dyskeratosis (warty dyskeratoma)

Relatively infrequently small papulonodular lesions show a peculiar follicular acantholysis and dyskeratosis identical to that seen in Darier's disease (Fig. 101). Gra-

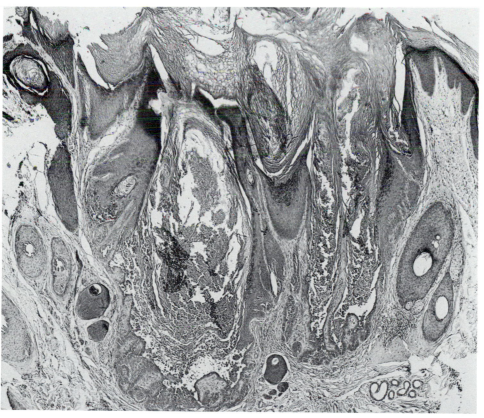

Fig. 101 Dysplastic and acantholytic process involving lower part of follicle, which, when cut appropriately, produces diagnostic picture of isolated follicular dyskeratosis. (×35; WU neg. 67-4134.)

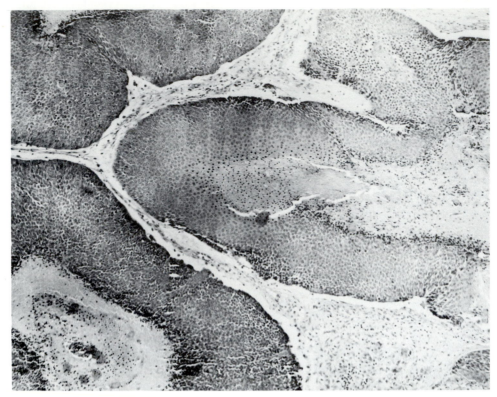

Fig. 102 In this pilomatrixoma, basal cells keratinize, as does cortex of hair without granular layer, and produce ghost cells (see Fig. 103). (×150.)

ham and Helwig[63] have shown that these are not isolated manifestations of Darier's disease.

Pilomatrixoma

Pilomatrixomas are nodular, histologically characteristic (Figs. 102 and 103), subepidermal, benign tumors that occur predominantly, but not exclusively, in children and young adults.[61] Their old name was a characteristic dermatologic eponym —calcifying epithelioma of Malherbe. The evidence derived from electron microscopic and histochemical studies documents their origin from the pilary root.[66, 71]

Dermis

Many of the mesenchymal tumors involving the dermis are discussed in the chapter on soft tissues. Only those peculiar to the skin are included here.

Keloid and scar

Reparative process in the dermis may become hyperplastic and produce keloids, particularly in black persons. These lesions can be separated on morphologic grounds from hyperplastic scars on the basis of their hypercellularity and coarse collagen bundles[82] (Fig. 104). This distinction is useful in estimating the probability of recrudescence, which is high for keloids.

Nodular subepidermal fibrosis

Under the descriptive term nodular subepidermal fibrosis is included a spectrum of firm, nodular, nonencapsulated, often pigmented lesions that occur chiefly on the extremities. Clinically, they are called nevi when pigmented and many other names when not pigmented.[81] On transection, they are yellow to tan (Fig. 105). Microscopically, the cellular, fibrocytic pro-

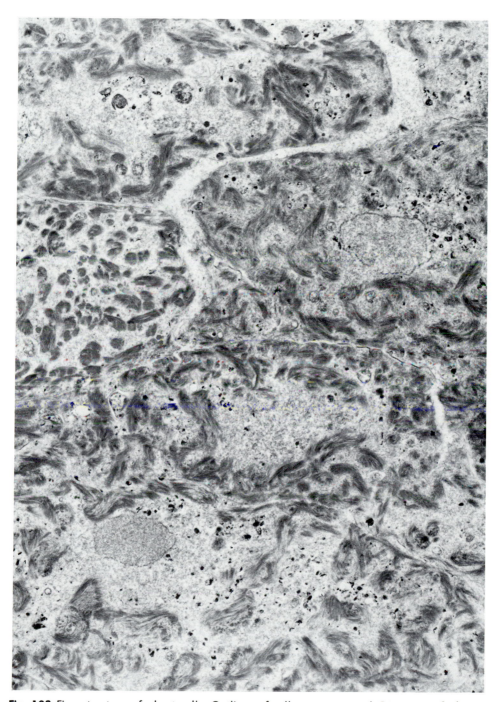

Fig. 103 Fine structure of ghost cells. Outlines of cells are preserved. Remnants of plasma membranes are visible, as are ghosts of nuclei. Sheaves of keratin form interwoven bundles, and calcification begins in mitochondria. (Uranyl acetate-lead citrate; ×4,000.)

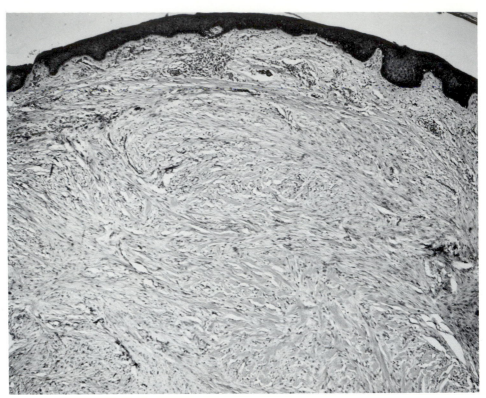

Fig. 104 Coarse collagen bundles are set in hypocellular stroma in this keloid. (×40; WU neg. 67-4404.)

liferation with admixed lipid and occasionally hemosiderin-filled histiocytes is set in a fine vascular network (Fig. 106). The lipid contents of the histiocytes is underestimated unless fat stains are done. The lesions blend imperceptibly into the adjacent dermis. The resulting variegated appearance has given rise to many diagnostic terms. The common synonyms are dermatofibroma, histiocytoma, and sclerosing hemangioma. These lesions are not small dermatofibrosarcomas for they usually lack the characteristic storiform or cartwheel swirls. The overlying epidermis may become hyperplastic and acanthotic and contribute to the clinical confusion.[107]

Atypical fibroxanthoma

Atypical fibroxanthomas are nodular ulcerative tumors that occur on the sunexposed skin of elderly persons and are clinically considered cancer[92a] (Figs. 107

and 108). Microscopically, they evoke a spectrum of malignant diagnoses varying from rhabdomyosarcoma to malignant melanoma and "grade IV" squamous carcinoma.[96] They are, nonetheless, benign reactive lesions. Histologically, the bizarre histiocytic cells are admixed with a fibrocytic stroma with varying amounts of inflammation (Fig. 109). These lesions represent one of the increasing group wherein supposedly secure cytologic criteria of neoplasia fail to correlate with biologic behavior.[97] Similar lesions have been reported at sites of irradiation damage.[84, 102]

Dermatofibrosarcoma

Dermatofibrosarcomas are slowly growing nodular, protuberant neoplasms that are peculiar to the dermis[89, 95] (Fig. 110). Local recrudescence is reported as a common phenomenon following enucleation or limited excisions.[109] This is because

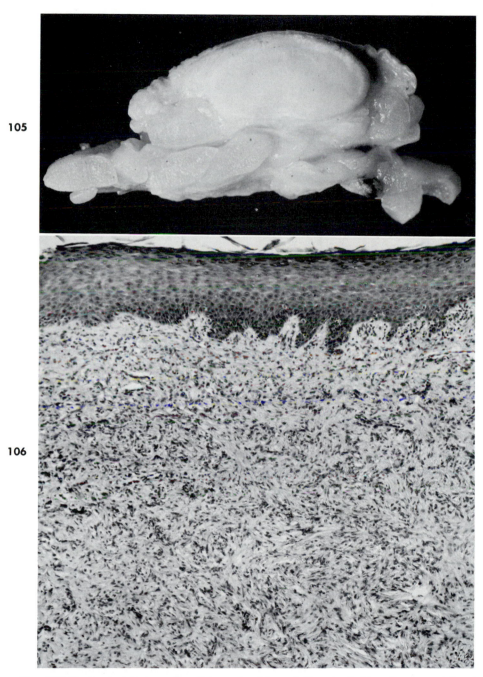

Fig. 105 Transected lesion of nodular subepidermal fibrosis. Epidermis was not involved, and lesion was bright yellow. (W.U. neg. 52-1597.)
Fig. 106 Fibrocytic proliferation of nodular subepidermal fibrosis in which histiocytic component is obscured. (×90; WU neg. 67-4406.)

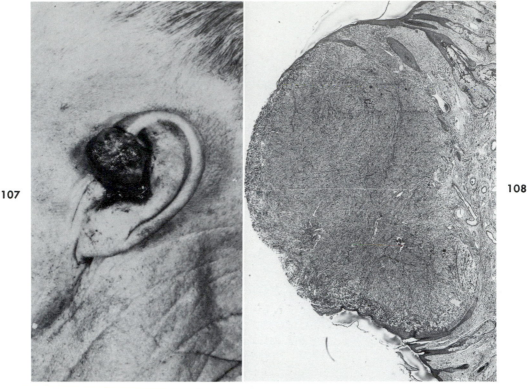

107   108

Fig. 107 Atypical fibroxanthoma arising on ear. (WU neg. 64-2738; from Kempson, R. L., and McGavran, M. H.: Atypical fibroxanthomas of the skin, Cancer **17:**1463-1471, 1964.)
Fig. 108 Low-power view of atypical fibroxanthoma showing its delimitation and cellularity. (×8; WU neg. 64-678A; from Kempson, R. L., and McGavran, M. H.: Atypical fibroxanthomas of the skin, Cancer **17:**1463-1471, 1964.)

the tumor is not encapsulated, even though grossly it may seem to be. The histologic appearance of radial whorls of fibrocytes producing the storiform or cartwheel pattern is characteristic and diagnostic (Fig. 111). Histiocytes and hemosiderin are not present except in areas of necrosis. Rarely, these tumors metastasize to regional nodes and/or the viscera.[80]

Leiomyoma

Leiomyomas rank high on the list of painful skin tumors. Two groups of leiomyomas of the skin are distinguished: (1) the "nevoid" or hamartomatous proliferation of erector pili muscles that gives rise to multiple cutaneous leiomyomas. (Figs. 112 to 114) and (2) the solitary cutaneous leiomyoma. The latter lesion is more deeply situated, at the junction of the

subcutis and dermis, and probably arises from vascular smooth muscle.[101] Primary leiomyosarcoma does occur in the skin.[105]

Metastatic carcinoma

Metastases to the skin occur chiefly on the chest and abdomen, with the scalp, face, and other sites being less common. Most of the metastases are multiple and form firm nonulcerated dermal nodules. The breast is the most common source of the primary lesion, with the gastrointestinal tract (stomach, colon, and pancreas) and the lung tied for second place.[104] In Brownstein and Helwig's study,[85] melanoma follows. Solitary skin nodules may appear from an asymptomatic primary renal cancer. On such nodules an erroneous diagnosis of clear cell sweat gland tumor may be rendered by the unwary.[87] The possibility

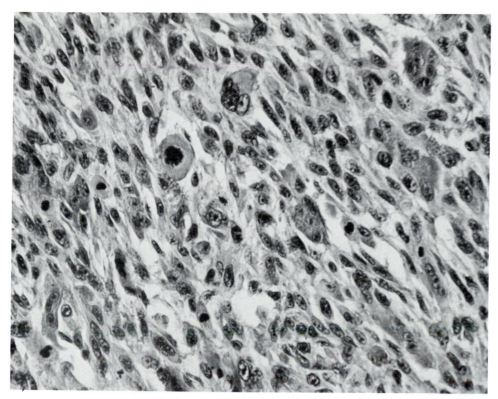

Fig. 109 Atypical and frankly bizarre cells are chiefly histiocytic, although fibrocytes have prominent nucleoli as well in atypical fibroxanthomas. (×500; WU neg. 64-3845; from Kempson, R. L., and McGavran, M. H.: Atypical fibroxanthomas of the skin, Cancer **17:** 1463-1471, 1964.)

of metastatic carcinoma must be kept in mind in the differential diagnosis of epithelial dermal nodules if errors are to be avoided. Prognostically, metastases to the skin are a sign of rapidly impending demise from disseminated disease except in patients with carcinoma of the breast.

Endometriosis

In postmenarchal and premenopausal women, endometriosis of the skin occurs in the umbilicus and groin without antecedent surgery as well as in scars from abdominal operations. It is diagnosed by the presence of endometrial glands associated with focal areas of endometrial stroma. Steck and Helwig[108] discuss the peculiarities of this entity well.

Cutaneous lymphoid hyperplasia

Cutaneous lymphoplasia, characterized by reactive nonneoplastic lymphoid nodules occurring predominantly on the face of women, is likely a response to trauma, insect bites, and other undetermined stimuli. The older diagnostic terms "lymphadenoma," "lymphocytoma benigna cutis," and "Spiegler-Fendt sarcoid" now appear unjustified. The lesions are livid nodules or plaques and histologically show admixtures of lymphocytes, histiocytes, and plasma cells (Fig. 115). Mach and Wilgram[99] subdivide their 115 cases into five groups on the basis of predominant cell type. No particular clinical correlation results, but it is helpful to recognize that these variations in appearance exist. Among the patients studied by Mach and Wilgram,[100] the lesions in eight showed a pattern of "giant" follicles. These are not nodular lymphomas involving the skin. Many of the reticulum cells in the reactive centers contain polychrome bodies (Flemming bodies). In none of these patients was systemic malignant

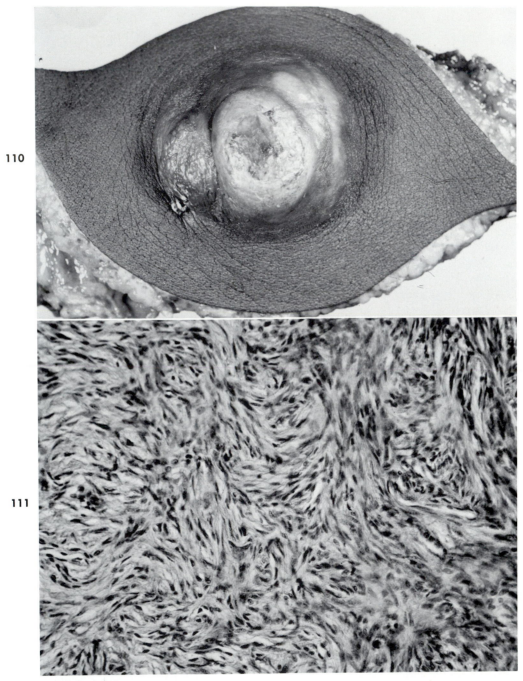

Fig. 110 Multinodular dermatofibrosarcoma from buttock. (WU neg. 57-5211.)
Fig. 111 Storiform or cartwheel pattern of dermatofibrosarcoma. (×270; WU neg. 62-7609A.)

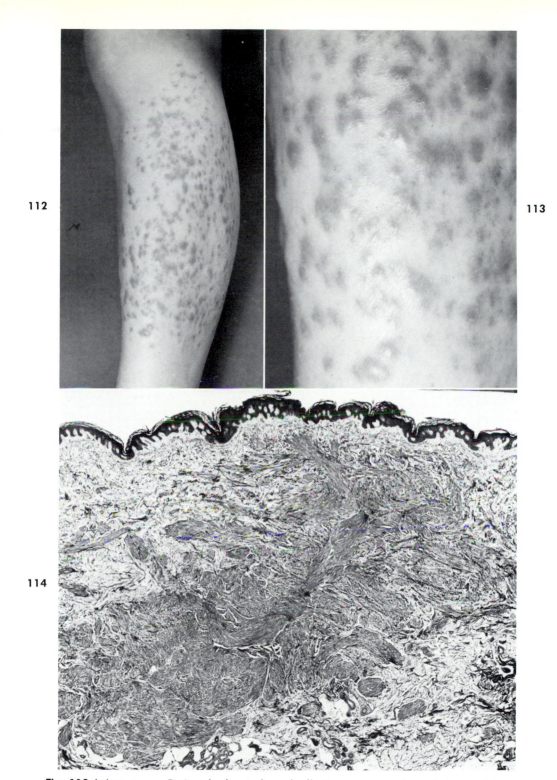

Fig. 112 Leiomyomas. Patient had noted gradually increasing number of pink nodules on one leg over period of twenty years. (WU neg. 64-1284.)

Fig. 113 Closer view of lesions illustrated in Fig. 112 showing single and confluent dermal nodules which, when pressed, caused severe pain. (WU neg. 64-1285.)

Fig. 114 Biopsy from lesions illustrated in Figs. 112 and 113 showing unencapsulated nodules of hyperplastic smooth muscle. (Masson trichrome; ×35; WU neg. 65-8446.)

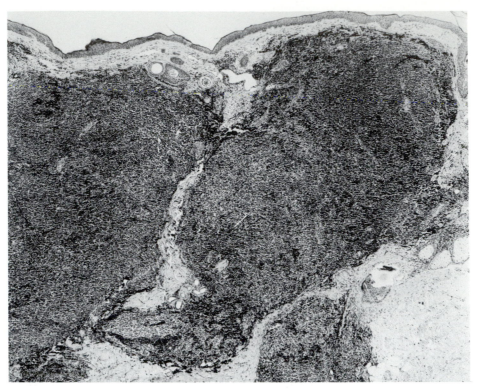

Fig. 115 Cutaneous lymphoid hyperplasia showing large aggregates of lymphoid cells in dermis. This is not malignant lymphoma of skin. (×35; WU neg. 67-4120.)

lymphoma found concomitantly or subsequently. The lesions respond to penicillin or low doses of x-ray therapy.

Malignant lymphoma

Lymphomatous neoplasms arising primarily in the skin are infrequent. Secondary involvement in patients with leukemia or widely disseminated lymphoma poses no problem so long as clinicopathologic correlation is not neglected. It is well to remember that a large portion of the skin lesions occurring in such patients are histologically nonspecific inflammatory reactions and are not due to infiltration by neoplastic cells. Of the malignant lymphomas arising primarily in the skin, with no evidence of involvement elsewhere, mycosis fungoides comes first, followed by histiocytic lymphoma. Involvement of the skin by lymphocytic or Hodgkin's lymphoma is a sign of far-advanced disease.

Mycosis fungoides

Mycosis fungoides has various manners of presentation and progression, most identified by eponymic names.[83] The simplest classification is in three stages: premycotic, mycotic, and tumorous (Fig. 116). In the premycotic stage, the skin is erythematous, scaly, and pruritic. Histologically, a chronic nonspecific dermatitis is seen associated with psoriasiform changes in the epidermis. In the mycotic stage, infiltrative plaques appear, and biopsies show a polymorphous inflammatory infiltrate in the dermis that contains small numbers of frankly atypical histiocytic cells. These cells may invade the epidermis to form Pautrier microabscesses (Fig. 117). In the tumorous stage, infiltrates of atypical histiocytic cells predominate.

The course may be protracted over a period of years, and the histologic diagnosis may be difficult or impossible until fairly

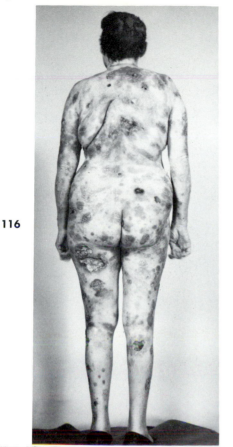

116

late in the disease. Reed and Cummings[103] have shown a definite correlation between the histologic findings and the course. Initially, patients with mycosis fungoides have no evidence of specific hematologic disorders. Sézary cells, atypical monocytes, with PAS-positive cytoplasmic granules, may be present in the blood of approximately 20% of the patients.[86] The nonspecificity of Sézary and mycosis cells has been well documented.[91, 92] Dermatopathic lymphadenitis may occur in patients with protracted exfoliative dermatitis. The terminal course of patients with mycosis fungoides demonstrates the conversion to or coincidence of distinct malignant lymphoma in approximately one-third of the

Fig. 116 Mycosis fungoides showing both infiltrative plaques and nodules, some ulcerated, over virtually entire body. (WU neg. 67-3000.)
Fig. 117 Dermal infiltrate of atypical histiocytic cells extending focally into epidermis, forming Pautrier abscess. (×200; WU neg. 67-4412.)

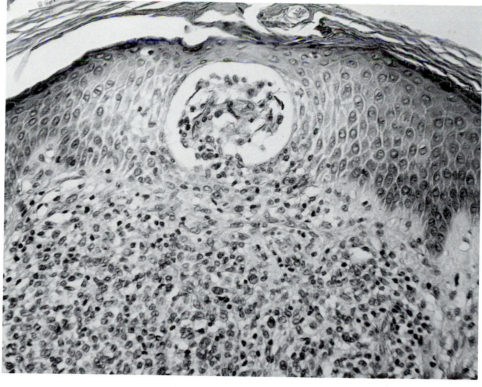

117

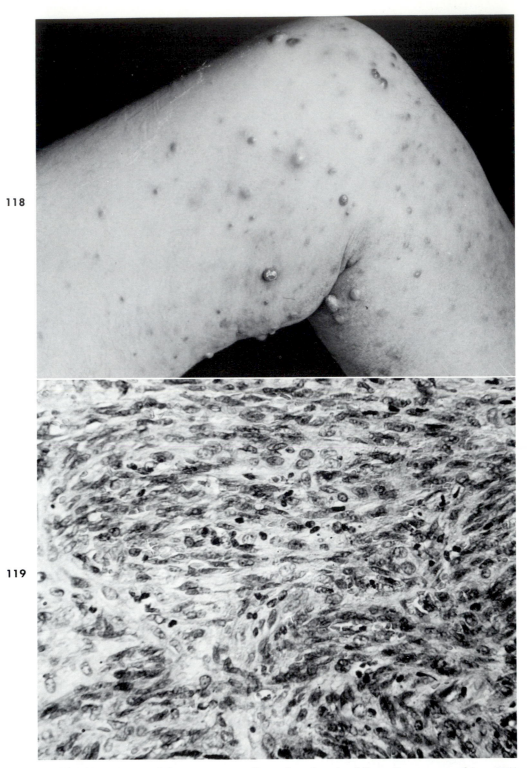

Fig. 118 Numerous nodules, some virtually pedunculated, of Kaposi's sarcoma of leg. (WU neg. 48-4296.)
Fig. 119 Sarcomatous stroma of Kaposi's sarcoma within which erythrocytes are enmeshed. (×300; WU neg. 67-3848.)

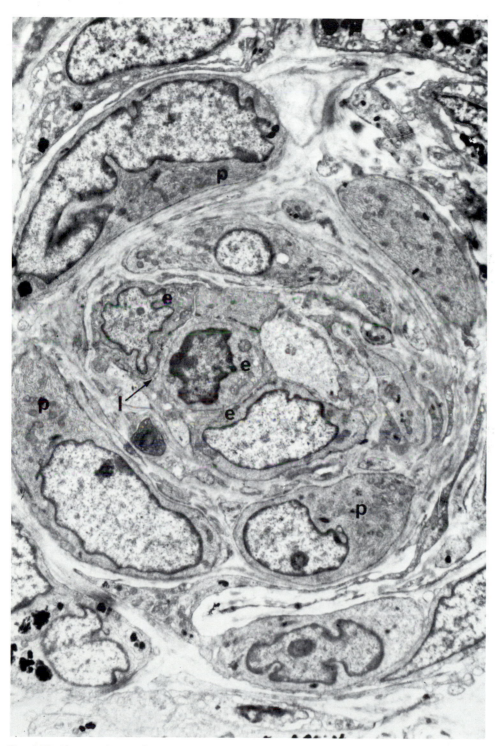

Fig. 120 Abnormal vessel in Kaposi's sarcoma. Endothelial cells, **e**, are markedly hyperplastic and have reduced lumen **l**, to fine slit. Perithelial cells, **p**, are prominent. Pigmented macrophages surround vessel. (Uranyl acetate–lead citrate; ×4,200.)

cases. Histiocytic lymphoma and monocytic leukemia, lymphocytic lymphoma and lymphoblastic leukemia, and Hodgkin's disease account for all these.[88] In the remaining patients, polymorphic infiltrates of mycosis fungoides may be found in nodes, lung, and spleen and even in the brain.[106] Sepsis is a frequent terminal complication. The most satisfactory form of palliative therapy is total body surface irradiation by the electron beam.[93] Chemotherapy may also produce temporary remissions.[90, 111]

Histiocytic lymphoma

Most of the patients presenting with dermal histiocytic lymphoma (reticulum cell sarcoma) give a history of rapid appearance of multiple pink dermal nodules. Biopsies show pure histiocytic lymphoma and the usual studies (radiographs, bone marrow aspirates, etc.) fail to demonstrate disease elsewhere. Though histiocytic lymphoma is among the neoplasms of man in which documented spontaneous remission may occur,[98] the majority of the patients eventually manifest disseminated disease and run the usual course.

Kaposi's sarcoma

Although infrequent in the United States, Kaposi's sarcoma comprises 10% of all malignant neoplasms in parts of Africa.[79] Clinically, it is usually manifest by multiple blue dermal plaques or nodules starting on the feet and legs (Fig. 118). These nodules progress up the extremity and occasionally assume the pedunculated appearance of pyogenic granulomas. By angiographic techniques, clinically inapparent subcutaneous nodules can be identified. Temporary control is effected by irradiation, chemotherapy, or, if sharply delimited, excision. The course of Kaposi's sarcoma is variable although usually prolonged. Some elderly persons die of intercurrent disease. In patients in whom the disease runs its full course, widespread visceral involvement may be found. Four clinical types of Kaposi's sarcoma have been delineated by Taylor et al.[110]

Histologically, these angiomatous lesions have characteristic areas of spindle cells within which erythrocytes are enmeshed (Fig. 119). Admixed in these lesions are hemosiderin-laden, phagocytic cells. Histochemical and ultrastructural studies (Fig. 120) show that this tumor is derived from vasoformative mesenchyme. Cutaneous angiosarcoma should and can be differentiated from Kaposi's sarcoma.[94]

REFERENCES
Introduction

1 Allen, A. C.: The skin; a clinicopathologic treatise, ed. 2, New York, 1967, Grune & Stratton, Inc.
2 Hashimoto, K., and Lever, W. F.: Appendage tumors of the skin, Springfield, Ill., 1968, Charles C Thomas, Publisher.
3 Lever, W. F.: Histopathology of the skin, ed. 4, Philadelphia, 1967, J. B. Lippincott Co.
4 Lund, H. Z.: Tumors of the skin. In Atlas of tumor pathology, Sect. I, Fasc. 2, Washington, D. C., 1957, Armed Forces Institute of Pathology.
5 Montgomery, H.: Dermatopathology, New York, 1967, Hoeber Medical Division, Harper & Row, Publishers, vols. I and II.
6 Pinkus, H., and Mehregan, A. H.: A guide to dermatohistopathology, New York, 1967, Appleton-Century-Crofts.

Epidermis
Actinic keratosis

7 Pinkus, H.: Keratosis senilis: a biologic concept of its pathogenesis and diagnosis based on the study of normal epidermis and 1730 seborrheic and senile keratoses, Am. J. Clin. Pathol. **29**:193-207, 1958.
8 Spira, M., Freeman, R., Arfai, P., Gerow, F. J., and Hardy, S. B.: Clinical comparison of chemical peeling, dermabrasion and 5-FU for senile keratoses, Plast. Reconstr. Surg. **46**:61-66, 1970.

Carcinoma in situ

9 Brownstein, M. H., Fernando, S., and Shapiro, L.: Clear cell acanthoma; clinicopathologic analysis of 37 new cases, Am. J. Clin. Pathol. **59**:306-311, 1973.
10 Landry, M., and Winkelmann, R. K.: Multiple clear-cell acanthoma and ichthyosis, Arch. Dermatol. **105**:371-383, 1972.
11 Mehregan, A. H., and Pinkus, H.: Intraepidermal epithelioma: a critical study, Cancer **17**:609-636, 1964.

Bowen's disease

12 Bowen, J. T.: Precancerous dermatoses: a study of two cases of chronic atypical epithelial proliferation, J. Cutan. Dis. **30**:241-255, 1912.

13 Graham, J. H., and Helwig, E. B.: Bowen's disease and its relationship to systemic cancer, Arch. Dermatol. **80**:133-159, 1959.

Epidermoid (squamous) carcinoma

14 Cleaver, J. E.: Xeroderma pigmentosa: variants with normal DNA repair and normal sensitivity to ultraviolet light, J. Invest. Dermatol. **58**:124-128, 1972.

15 Johnson, L. L., and Kempson, R. L.: Epidermoid carcinoma in chronic osteomyelitis: diagnostic problems and management, J. Bone Joint Surg. **47-A**:133-145, 1965.

16 Johnson, W. C., and Helwig, E. B.: Adenoid squamous cell carcinoma (adenoacanthoma), Cancer **19**:1639-1650, 1966.

17 Lund, H. Z.: How often does squamous cell carcinoma metastasize? Arch. Dermatol. **92**:635-637, 1965.

18 Martin, H., Strong, E., and Spiro, R. H.: Radiation-induced skin cancer of the head and neck, Cancer **25**:61-71, 1970.

19 Urbach, F.: Geographic pathology of skin cancer. In Urbach, F., editor: International conference on the biologic effects of ultraviolet radiation (with emphasis on the skin), New York, 1969, Pergamon Press, Inc., pp. 635-650.

Basal cell carcinoma

20 Gellin, G. E., and Bender, B.: Giant premalignant fibroepithelioma, Arch. Dermatol. **94**:70-73, 1966.

21 Gellin, G. E., Kopf, A. W., and Garfinkel, L.: Basal cell epithelioma: a controlled study of associated factors, Arch. Dermatol. **91**:38-45, 1965.

22 Gooding, C. A., White, G., and Yatsuhashi, M.: Significance of marginal extension in excised basal cell carcinoma, N. Engl. J. Med. **273**:923-924, 1965.

23 Gorlin, R. J., Vickers, R. A., Kelln, E., and Williamson, J. J.: The multiple basal-cell nevi syndrome: an analysis of a syndrome consisting of multiple nevoid basal cell carcinoma, jaw cysts, skeletal anomalies, medulloblastoma, and hyporesponsiveness to parathormone, Cancer **18**:89-104, 1965.

24 Graham, P. G., and McGavran, M. H.: Basal-cell carcinomas and sebaceous glands, Cancer **17**:803-806, 1964.

25 Kint, A.: Histogenetic study of the basal cell epithelioma, Curr. Probl. Dermatol. **3**:82-123, 1970.

26 Mason, J. K., Helwig, E. B., and Graham, J. H.: Pathology of the nevoid basal cell carcinoma syndrome, Arch. Pathol. **79**:401-408, 1965.

27 Wermuth, B. M., and Fajardo, L. F.: Metastatic basal cell carcinoma; a review, Arch. Pathol. **90**:458-462, 1970.

Seborrheic verruca

28 Scully, J. P.: Treatment of seborrheic keratosis, J.A.M.A. **213**:1498, 1970.

Extramammary (anogenital) Paget's disease

29 Fisher, E. R., and Beyer, F., Jr.: Differentiation of neoplastic lesions characterized by large vacuolated intraepidermal (pagetoid) cells, Arch. Pathol. **67**:140-145, 1959.

30 Helwig, E. B., and Graham, J. H.: Anogenital (extramammary) Paget's disease: a clinicopathological study, Cancer **16**:387-403, 1963.

31 Koss, L. G., and Brockunier, A., Jr.: Ultrastructural aspects of Paget's disease of the vulva, Arch. Pathol. **87**:592-600, 1969.

Adnexa
Eccrine sweat gland

32 Crain, R. C., and Helwig, E. B.: Dermal cylindroma (dermal eccrine cylindroma), Am. J. Clin. Pathol. **35**:504-515, 1961.

33 Futrell, J. W., Krueger, G. R., Chretien, P. B., and Ketchan, A. S.: Multiple primary sweat gland carcinomas, Cancer **28**:686-691, 1971.

34 Hashimoto, K., and Lever, W. F.: Eccrine poroma; histochemical and electron microscopic studies, J. Invest. Dermatol. **43**:237-247, 1964.

35 Hashimoto, K., Gross, B. G., and Lever, W. F.: Syringoma: histochemical and electron microscopic studies, J. Invest. Dermatol. **46**:150-166, 1966.

36 Hashimoto, K., Gross, B. G., Nelson, R. G., and Lever, W. F.: Eccrine spiradenoma; histochemical and electron microscopic studies, J. Invest. Dermatol. **46**:347-365, 1966.

37 Helwig, E. B., and Hackney, V. C.: Syringadenoma papilliferum, Arch. Dermatol. **71**:361-372, 1955.

38 Hirsch, P., and Helwig, E. B.: Chondroid syringoma, Arch. Dermatol. **84**:835-847, 1961.

39 Johnson, B. L., Jr., and Helwig, E. B.: Eccrine acrospiroma, Cancer **23**:641-657, 1969.

40 Kersting, D. W., and Helwig, E. B.: Eccrine spiradenoma, Arch. Dermatol. **73**:199-227, 1956.

41 Mendoza, S., and Helwig, E. B.: Mucinous (adenocystic) carcinoma of the skin, Arch. Dermatol. **103**:68-78, 1971.

42 Miller, W. L.: Sweat gland carcinoma, Am. J. Clin. Pathol. 47:767-780, 1967.

43 Munger, B. L., Berghorn, B. M., and Helwig, E. B.: A light and electron microscopic study of a case of multiple eccrine spiradenoma, J. Invest. Dermatol. 38:289-297, 1962.

44 Okun, M. R., and Ansell, H. B.: Eccrine poroma; report of three cases, two with an unusual location, Arch. Dermatol. 88:561-566, 1963.

45 Pinkus, H., Rogin, J. R., and Goldman, F.: Eccrine poroma; tumors exhibiting features of the epidermal sweat duct unit, Arch. Dermatol. 74:511-521, 1956.

46 Stout, A. P., and Gorman, J. G.: Mixed tumors of the skin of the salivary gland type, Cancer 12:537-543, 1959.

47 Winkelmann, R. K., and Gottlieb, B. F.: Syringoma: an enzymatic study, Cancer 16:665-669, 1963.

48 Winkelmann, R. K., and Wolff, K.: Solid-cystic hidradenoma of the skin, Arch. Dermatol. 97:651-661, 1968.

Apocrine sweat gland

49 Cankar, V., and Crowley, H.: Tumors of the ceruminous glands: a clinicopathological study of seven cases, Cancer 17:67-75, 1964.

50 Holder, W. R., Smith, J. D., and Mocega, E. E.: Giant apocrine hidrocystoma, Arch. Dermatol. 104:522-523, 1971.

51 Johnstone, J. M., Lennox, B., and Watson, A. J.: Five cases of hidradenoma of the exterior auditory canal: so-called ceruminoma, J. Pathol. Bacteriol. 73:421-427, 1957.

52 Landry, M., and Winkelmann, R. K.: An unusual tubular apocrine adenoma, Arch. Dermatol. 105:869-879, 1972.

53 Meeker, J. H., Neubecker, R. D., and Helwig, E. B.: Hidradenoma papilliferum, Am. J. Clin. Pathol. 37:182-195, 1962.

54 Mehregan, A. H.: Apocrine cystadenoma; a clinicopathologic study with special reference to the pigmented variety, Arch. Dermatol. 90:274-279, 1964.

55 Wetli, C. V., Pardo, V., Millard, M., and Gerston, K.: Tumors of ceruminous glands, Cancer 29:1169-1178, 1972.

56 Woodworth, H., Jr., Dockerty, M. B., Wilson, R. B., and Pratt, J. H.: Papillary hidradenoma of the vulva: a clinicopathologic study of 69 cases, Am. J. Obstet. Gynecol. 110:501-508, 1971.

Sebaceous glands

57 Rulon, D. B., and Helwig, E. B.: Cutaneous sebaceous neoplasms, Cancer (in press).

58 Urban, F. H., and Winkelmann, R. K.: Sebaceous malignancy, Arch. Dermatol. 84:63-72, 1961.

Hair follicle

59 Dabska, M.: Giant hair matrix tumor, Cancer 28:701-706, 1971.

60 Fisher, E. R., McCoy, M. M., and Wechsler, H. L.: Analysis of histopathologic and electron microscopic determinants of keratoacanthoma and squamous cell carcinoma, Cancer 29:1387-1397, 1972.

61 Forbis, R. J., and Helwig, E. B.: Pilomatrixoma, Arch. Dermatol. 83:606-618, 1961.

62 Ghadially, F. M., Barton, B. W., and Kerridge, D. F.: The etiology of keratoacanthoma, Cancer 16:603-611, 1963.

63 Graham, J. H., and Helwig, E. B.: Isolated follicular dyskeratosis, Arch. Dermatol. 77:377-389, 1958.

64 Gray, H. R., and Helwig, E. B.: Trichofolliculoma, Arch. Dermatol. 86:619-625, 1962.

65 Gray, H. R., and Helwig, E. B.: Epithelioma adenoides cysticum and solitary trichoepithelioma, Arch. Dermatol. 87:102-114, 1963.

66 Hashimoto, K., Nelson, R. G., and Lever, W. F.: Calcifying epithelioma of Malherbe; histochemical and electron microscopic studies, J. Invest. Dermatol. 46:391-408, 1966.

67 Holmes, E. J.: Tumors of the lower hair sheath, Cancer 21:234-248, 1968.

68 Jones, E. W.: Proliferating epidermoid cysts, Arch. Dermatol. 94:11-19, 1966.

69 Kligman, A. M.: The myth of the sebaceous cyst, Arch. Dermatol. 89:253-256, 1964.

70 Kligman, A. M., and Kirschbaum, J. D.: Steatocystoma multiplex: a dermoid tumor, J. Invest. Dermatol. 42:383-387, 1964.

71 McGavran, M. H.: Ultrastructure of pilomatrixoma (calcifying epithelioma), Cancer 18:1445-1456, 1965.

72 McGavran, M. H., and Binnington, B.: Keratinous cysts of the skin, Arch. Dermatol. 94:499-508, 1966.

73 McGavran, M. H., and Orman, S. K.: Unpublished data.

74 Mehregan, A. H.: Inverted follicular keratosis, Arch. Dermatol. 89:229-235, 1964.

75 Pinkus, H.: "Sebaceous cysts" are trichilemmal cysts, Arch. Dermatol. 99:544-553, 1969.

76 Reed, R. J., and Lamar, L. M.: Invasive hair matrix tumors of the scalp; invasive pilomatrixoma, Arch. Dermatol. 94:310-316, 1966.

77 Rook, A., and Champion, R. H.: Keratoacanthoma, Natl. Cancer Inst. Monogr. 10:257-274, 1963.

78 Rossman, R. E., Freeman, R. G., and Knox, J. M.: Multiple keratoacanthoma, Arch. Dermatol. 89:374-381, 1964.

Dermis

79 Ackerman, L. V., and Murray, J. F., editors: Symposium on Kaposi's sarcoma, Acta Un. Int. Cancr. 18:312-511, 1962.

80 Adams, J. T., and Saltzstein, S. L.: Metastasizing dermatofibrosarcoma protuberans: report of two cases, Am. Surg. **29**:879-886, 1963.

81 Black, W. C., III, McGavran, M. H., and Graham, P.: Nodular subepidermal fibrosis, Arch. Surg. **98**:296-300, 1969.

82 Blackburn, W. R., and Cosman, B.: Histologic basis of keloid and hypertrophic scar differentiation; clinicopathologic correlation, Arch. Pathol. **82**:65-71, 1966.

83 Block, J. B., Edgcomb, J., Eisen, A., and Van Scott, E. J.: Mycosis fungoides; natural history and aspects of its relationship to other malignant lymphomas, Am. J. Med. **34**:228-235, 1963.

84 Bourne, R. G.: Paradoxical fibrosarcoma of skin (pseudosarcoma): a review of 13 cases, Med. J. Aust. **1**:504-510, 1963.

85 Brownstein, M. H., and Helwig, E. B.: Metastatic tumors of the skin, Cancer **29**:1298-1307, 1972.

86 Clendenning, W. E., Brecher, G., and Van Scott, E. J.: Mycosis fungoides; relationship to malignant cutaneous reticulosis and the Sezary syndrome, Arch. Dermatol. **89**:785-791, 1964.

87 Conner, D. H., Taylor, H. B., and Helwig, E. B.: Cutaneous metastasis of renal cell carcinoma, Arch. Pathol. **76**:339-346, 1963.

88 Cyr, D. P., Geokas, M. C., and Worsley, G. H.: Mycosis fungoides: hematologic findings and terminal course, Arch. Dermatol. **94**:558-573, 1966.

89 Darier, J.: Dermatofibromes progressifs et récidivants ou fibrosarcomes de la peau, Ann. Derm. Syph. (Paris) **5**:545-562, 1924.

90 Epstein, E. H., Jr., Levin, D. L., Croft, J. D., Jr., and Lutzner, M. A.: Mycosis fungoides; survival, prognostic features, response to therapy, and autopsy findings, Medicine (Baltimore) **15**:61-72, 1972.

91 Fisher, E. R., Horvat, B. C., and Wechsler, H. L.: Ultrastructural features of mycosis fungoides, Am. J. Clin. Pathol. **58**:99-110, 1972.

92 Flaxman, B. A., Zelasny, G., and Van Scott, E. J.: Nonspecificity of characteristic cells in mycosis fungoides, Arch. Dermatol. **104**:141-147, 1971.

92a Fretzin, D. F., and Helwig, E. B.: Atypical fibroxanthoma of the skin; a clinicopathologic study of 140 cases, Cancer **31**:1541-1552, 1973.

93 Fuks, Z., and Bagshaw, M. A.: Total skin electron treatment of mycosis fungoides, Radiology **100**:145-150, 1971.

94 Girard, C., Johnson, W., and Graham, J.: Cutaneous angiosarcoma, Cancer **26**:868-883, 1970.

95 Hoffman, E.: Über das knollentreibende Fibrosarkom der Haut (Dermatofibrosarkoma protuberans), Dermatol. Z. **43**:1-28, 1925.

96 Hudson, A. W., and Winkelmann, R. K.: Atypical fibroxanthoma of the skin: a reappraisal of 19 cases in which the original diagnosis was spindle-cell squamous carcinoma, Cancer **29**:413-422, 1972.

97 Kempson, R. L., and McGavran, M. H.: Atypical fibroxanthomas of the skin, Cancer **17**:1463-1471, 1964.

98 Kim, R., Winkelmann, R. K., and Dockerty, M.: Reticulum cell sarcoma of the skin, Cancer **16**:646-655, 1963.

99 Mach, K. W., and Wilgram, G. F.: Characteristic histopathology of cutaneous lymphoplasia (lymphocytoma), Arch. Dermatol. **94**:26-34, 1966.

100 Mach, K. W., and Wilgram, G. F.: Cutaneous lymphoplasia with giant follicles, Arch. Dermatol. **94**:749-756, 1966.

101 Montgomery, H., and Winkelmann, R. K.: Smooth muscle tumors of the skin, Arch. Dermatol. **79**:32-41, 1959.

102 Rachmaninoff, N., McDonald, J. R., and Cook, J. C.: Sarcoma-like tumors of the skin following irradiation, Am. J. Clin. Pathol. **36**:427-437, 1961.

103 Reed, R. J., and Cummings, C. E.: Malignant reticulosis and related conditions of the skin; a reconsideration of mycosis fungoides, Cancer **19**:1231-1247, 1966.

104 Reingold, I. M.: Cutaneous metastases from internal carcinoma, Cancer **19**:162-168, 1966.

105 Rising, J. A., and Booth, E.: Primary leiomyosarcoma of the skin with lymphatic spread, Arch. Pathol. **81**:94-96, 1966.

106 Rosai, J., and Spiro, J.: Central nervous system involvement by mycosis fungoides, Acta Derm. Venereol. (Stockh.)**48**:482-488, 1968.

107 Schoenfield, R. J.: Epidermal proliferations overlying histiocytomas, Arch. Dermatol. **90**:266-270, 1964.

108 Steck, W. D., and Helwig, E. B.: Cutaneous endometriosis, J.A.M.A. **191**:167-170, 1965.

109 Taylor, H. B., and Helwig, E. B.: Dermatofibrosarcoma protuberans, Cancer **15**:717-725, 1962.

110 Taylor, J. F., Templeton, A. C., Vogel, C. L., Ziegler, J. L., and Kyalwazi, S. K.: Kaposi's sarcoma in Uganda; a clinico-pathological study, Int. J. Cancer **8**:122-135, 1971.

111 Van Scott, E. J., and Kalmanson, J. D.: Complete remissions of mycosis fungoides lymphoma induced by topical nitrogen mustard (HN2); control of delayed hypersensitivity to HN2 by desensitization and by induction of specific immunologic tolerance, Cancer **32**:18-30, 1973.

Nevi and malignant melanoma

Introduction

The word *nevus* (L. *naevus,* birthmark) can be properly applied to any circumscribed new growth of the skin of congenital origin. However, is is usually used as a synonym for *mole* (L. *moles,* a shapeless mass) to designate a developmental malformation of the melanocytic system, usually arising between the second and sixth year of life. The adjectives melanocytic (which we prefer), nevocellular, and pigmented refer specifically to this type of nevus.

The pathologic problems in the diagnosis of moles and melanoma include incorrect diagnosis of a cellular mole as malignant melanoma, incorrect diagnosis of a superficial malignant melanoma, failure to appreciate the potentialities of the juvenile melanoma, improper evaluation of a Hutchinson's melanotic freckle, failure to recognize nonpigmented forms of malignant melanoma, and muddy thinking regarding the origin of the mole.

Nevi
Origin and distribution

Masson's concept[50, 54] of dual origin of moles from intraepidermal melanoblasts and dermal Schwann cells is supported by many studies. The common mole has been demonstrated to have neuroectodermal origin by careful histologic study, and particularly through special staining of neurites with silver techniques.[11, 39, 50] Clark et al.[15] showed by electron microscopy that many of the clear cells seen in the basal layer of the epidermis in hematoxylin-eosin sections correspond to dendritic cells or melanocytes. Phylogenetic evidence strongly supports neural crest origin of melanoblasts.[24, 39, 63, 82]

Every person has a variable number of moles. Their distribution is not the same as malignant melanoma. They are much more common in the skin of the head, neck, and trunk, whereas a high percentage of malignant melanomas occur in the lower extremities.

Nevi of every conceivable size, shape, and degree of pigmentation occur, and they may be more or less hairy. Nevi have been variously classified, but it is most logical to divide them according to the location of the melanocytes inasmuch as their position bears a definite relationship to the likelihood of malignant transformation.

The terminology of pigment cells associated with the formation of melanin pigment as used in biology and medicine has been confusing.[9, 52] The recommended terminology[27] is given in Table 3.

Table 3 Recommended terminology of pigment cells*

Type of cell	Recommended terminology
Mature melanin-forming cell	Melanocyte
Immature melanin-forming cell	Melanoblast
Cell with phagocytized melanin	Macrophage (or melanophage)
"Contractile" cell	Melanophore

*From Fitzpatrick, T. B., and Lerner, A. B.: Terminology of pigment cells, Science 117:640, 1953.

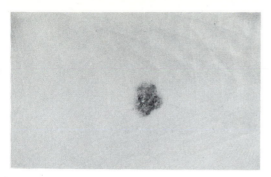

Fig. 121 Junctional nevus, nonhairy and fawn colored, on plantar surface of foot. (WU neg. 49-1492.)

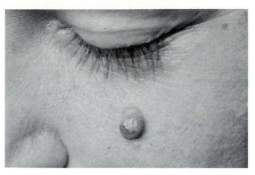

Fig. 123 Typical intradermal nevus of skin of cheek. (WU neg. 49-169.)

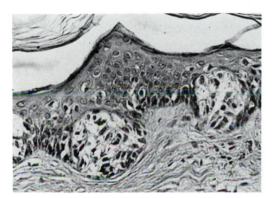

Fig. 122 Typical junctional nevus in adult. Note location of cells at dermoepidermal junction. (High power; WU neg. 51-464.)

Junctional, compound, and intradermal nevi

A *junctional nevus* is one in which the melanocytes are present at the dermoepidermal junction. Grossly, it is flat or slightly elevated, nonhairy, and fawn colored (Fig. 121). Microscopically, it is characterized by the presence of melanocytic nests in the dermoepidermal junction (Fig. 122). This is the lesion from which malignant melanomas may arise. In the *intradermal nevus,* all the melanocytes are in the dermis. This is the common adult type of nevus. It may be papillary, pedunculated, or flat (Fig. 123). Usually it is hairy, and invariably multiple. Its degree of pigmentation varies widely. Malignant melanomas practically

never arise from this type of nevus. Microscopically, small nests or bundles of melanocytes are seen in the dermis, with no evidence of circumscription (Fig. 124). Pseudoacini and giant cells may be present. Their occasional extreme cellularity may result in an incorrect diagnosis of malignant melanoma (Fig. 125). The melanosomes are well demonstrated by electron microscopy (Fig. 126). The *compound nevus* combines the features of the junctional and intradermal types.

The percentage of nevi with junctional changes decreases as the age of the patient increases.[44] Stegmaier and Montgomery[73] demonstrated junctional activity in 100 consecutive moles in children under the age of 10 years. A personal review of 156 moles from children under 15 years of age showed 110 (64%) to be junctional, whereas only fifty-four (17%) moles from adults showed junctional change. With increasing age, there is an increase of neuroid bundles and nervelike elements.[11] These findings support Masson's concept[50, 54] of the gradual migration of the epidermal melanoblasts away from the epidermis, coupled with continuous proliferation of Schwann cells in the dermis.

For some unexplained reason, in adult life junctional nevi tend either to persist or to appear in greater proportion in the lower extremity. Although in adults only a small percentage of all nevi occur below the knee, practically all of them are junc-

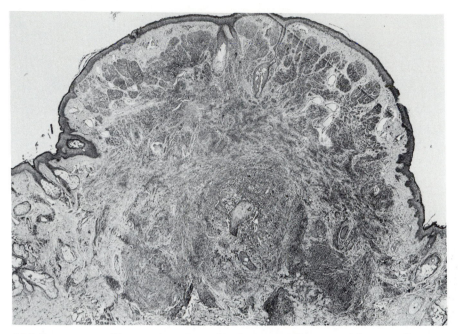

Fig. 124 Same nevus illustrated in Fig. 123 showing cells arranged in small nests and bundles lying entirely within dermis. (Low power; WU neg. 49-2024.)

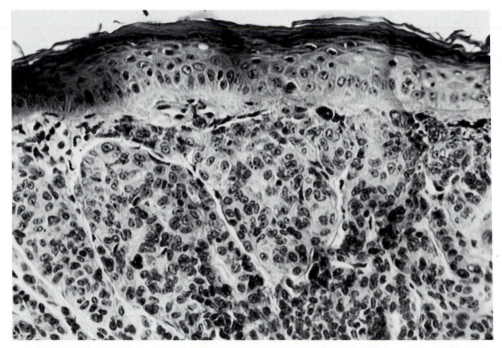

Fig. 125 Excessively cellular intradermal nevus with occasional large cells. This is the type that can be incorrectly diagnosed as malignant. (High power; WU neg. 48-6693.)

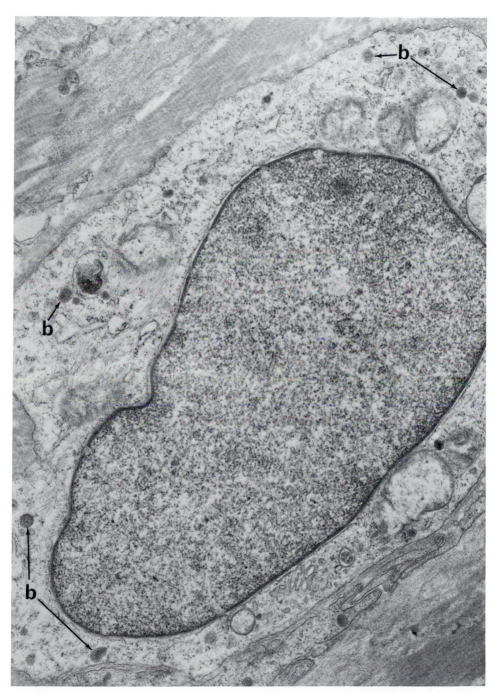

Fig. 126 Cell from intradermal nevus showing melanosomes, **b,** within thin rim of cytoplasm about large nucleus. (Uranyl acetate–lead citrate; ×15,000; courtesy Dr. H. Rodriguez, Mexico City, Mexico.)

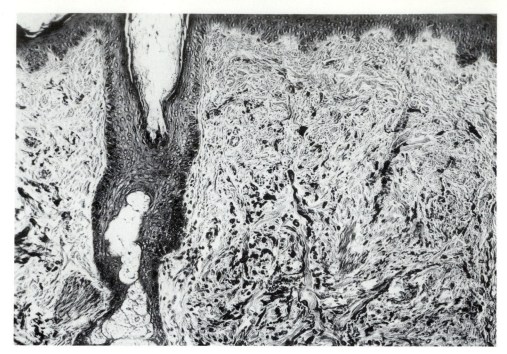

Fig. 127 Blue nevus. Note fusiform cells in dermis containing melanin pigment. (Low power.)

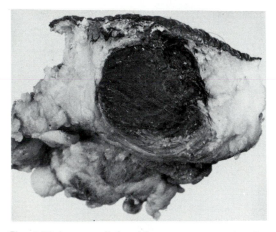

Fig. 128 Large cellular blue nevus occurring in buttock of young woman. Note lack of involvement of epidermis and well-delimited pushing borders. (WU neg. 53-5790.)

tional in character. Nevi also are common on both male and female genitalia. However, a survey of fourteen nevi of the vulva showed only two to be junctional.

We have seen perineural and lymph vessel invasion in perfectly benign nevi. Johnson and Helwig[35] reported six cases in which clusters of benign-appearing nevus cells were found in the capsule of a lymph node, usually located in the axillary region. The lymph node itself did not contain similar cells.

Nevi almost invariably arise from skin, but we have seen them in the oral cavity, tonsillar area, esophagus, larynx, and vagina.

Blue and cellular blue nevi

The *blue nevus* is characterized microscopically by an ill-defined dermal proliferation of elongated dermal melanocytes. Melanin pigment is usually abundant (Fig. 127). There is a clear space between the lesion and the epidermis, with absence of junctional component.[58] Blue nevi are sometimes misinterpreted as nodular subepidermal fibrosis. They are usually small and often located in the head, neck, or upper extremity. Combined blue and intradermal nevi occur.[41] Blue nevi have been reported in the hard palate,[31] breast,[3] cervix,[29] and prostate.[33]

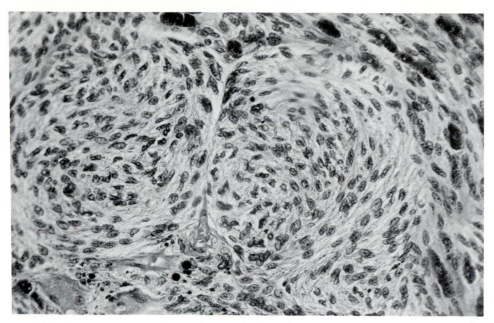

Fig. 129 Large cellular blue nevus of buttock with whorllike areas and fusiform cells producing melanin pigment. (×380; WU neg. 52-141.)

The *cellular blue nevus* is a distinctive variety, often suspected of being malignant because of its size and rather intense pigmentation[53, 65] (Fig. 128). Of the forty-five cases we have examined, twenty-three were located in the buttock or sacrococcygeal area; the scalp, face, and dorsa of the foot and hand were involved less frequently. In only one case was there local recurrence; no metastases were encountered. The regional lymph nodes draining a cellular blue nevus may be intensely pigmented, but this is not evidence of metastases since free melanin pigment alone may be carried from the nevus to the nodes by the draining lymphatics. Helwig[32] collected 192 cellular blue nevi. There were metastases to regional lymph nodes in four instances. After excision of the primary lesion and involved nodes, no further metastases developed, and all four patients were living and well at the time of his report. Three had been followed over five years.

Cellular blue nevi differ microscopically from malignant melanomas by the absence of junctional activity, epidermal invasion, peripheral inflammation, and necrosis; the presence of pushing margins, biphasic pattern, fasciculation, and neuroid structures; and the relative lack of atypia and mitotic figures (Fig. 129).

Spindle and epithelioid cell nevi

Spindle and epithelioid nevi, two variants of melanocytic nevi, were well described by Spitz[72] in 1948 under the name of *juvenile melanoma*. The majority occur in children, in whom they often present as a small (2 cm or less in diameter), raised, pink or red nodule in the skin of the face.[37] We have seen twenty-six similar lesions in adults.[25] All of them had a benign course.

Microscopically, most of these nevi are of the compound type. The spindle cell variant is characterized by cigar-shaped cells with large nuclei and prominent nucleoli (Fig. 130). The cells of the epithelioid type have similar nuclei and a large, polygonal cytoplasm with distinct borders (Fig. 131). A variant of the latter is a multinucleated giant melanocyte containing up to ten or twenty nuclei. Mitoses can

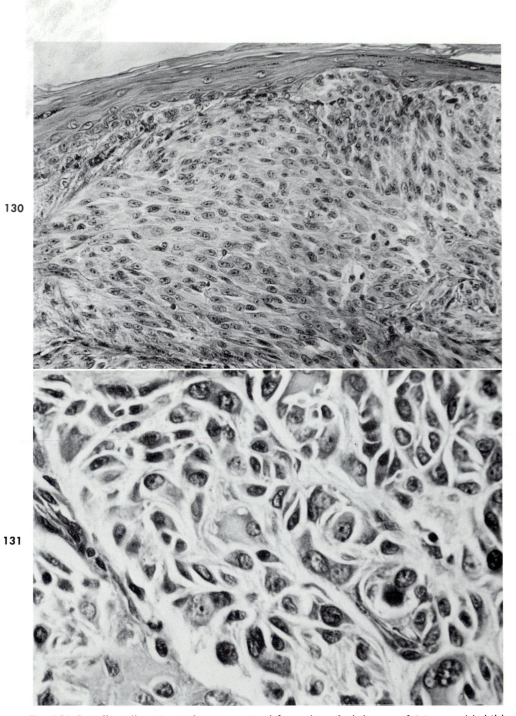

Fig. 130 Spindle cell variant of nevus excised from skin of abdomen of 14-year-old child. Cells are spindle shaped and have numerous mitotic figures, abundant cytoplasm, and uniform nuclei. (×300; WU neg. 58-125.)

Fig. 131 Epithelioid cell nevus occurring in 5-year-old child. This is the variant with typical giant cells and can be distinguished from malignant melanoma in adult. (×600; WU neg. 52-4082.)

be numerous, but atypical mitoses are exceptional. A mixture of spindle and epithelioid cells can occur. We have not yet seen a pure epithelioid cell nevus in an adult. Features that favor a diagnosis of spindle or epithelioid cell nevus over one of malignant melanoma are pushing margins, compact packing of the cells, nesting, multinucleated giant cells, telangiectasia, fibrosis, and lack of ulceration.

Other nevi

The term *halo nevus* (leukoderma acquisitum centrifugum) is used to describe a melanocytic nevus surrounded by a zone of depigmented skin[38] (Fig. 132). It is most commonly found on the trunk of young whites.[79] Microscopically, it is characterized by a heavy infiltration of the nevus by lymphocytes and histiocytes. The lesion can be confused with melanoma, lymphoma, and dermatitis. It should be mentioned that malignant melanoma may also be surrounded by a halo of depigmented skin.

Balloon nevus is another unusual variety of nevus, identified by the presence of large melanocytes with foamy cytoplasm, perhaps the result of a biochemical alteration in melanin synthesis.[68] Balloon cells also can occur in blue nevi and malignant melanomas[28] (Figs. 133 and 134).

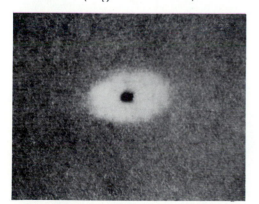

Fig. 132 Typical clinical appearance of halo nevus. Heavily pigmented center is surrounded by sharply defined oval area of depigmentation. Pigmented nevus may be situated in center, as here, or be excentric. (WU neg. 73-1207; courtesy Dr. A. W. Kopf, New York, N. Y.)

Congenital nevi differ from the more common acquired variety because of their larger size (Fig. 136), tendency to involve the reticular dermis and subcutaneous tissue, single cell permeation of dermal collagen bundles, and involvement of skin adnexae, nerves, and vessels.[49] Neuroid differentiation, such as formation of Wagner-Meissner-like corpuscles, is common (Fig. 135). The term *neuronevus* has been applied in the past to congenital (and some acquired) nevi in which this feature was particularly prominent.[51]

Giant pigmented (hairy) nevus is a variant of congenital nevus characterized by its extensive size, its surface area being by definition 144 sq cm or larger. It has a tendency to distribute along a dermatome and often has a "bathing trunk" or "garment" configuration. It may involve a whole extremity, the entire scalp, most of the trunk, and even extend into the placenta.[23] It is sometimes associated with meningeal or cerebral melanosis.[69] It may give rise to malignant melanoma of the skin or central nervous system and to related malignant neuroectodermal tumors[64] (Fig. 137). Whether the smaller congenital nevi are also subject to an increased risk of malignant transformation has not yet been established.[49]

Clinicopathologic correlation

Nevi often are removed for cosmetic purposes; obviously, all nevi cannot be removed because every adult has some ten or twenty. However, if a nevus is chronically irritated by a belt, collar, strap, or shoe, it should be removed. The signs of possible malignant change in a nevus include deepening of pigmentation, spread of the pigment beyond the gross confines of the lesion, ulceration, rapid growth, appearance of flat areas of depigmentation in a black mole, a red inflamed zone around a nevus, satellite nodules, and the presence of itching, oozing of serum, or bleeding with trivial trauma.[21]

In approximately 50% of malignant mel-

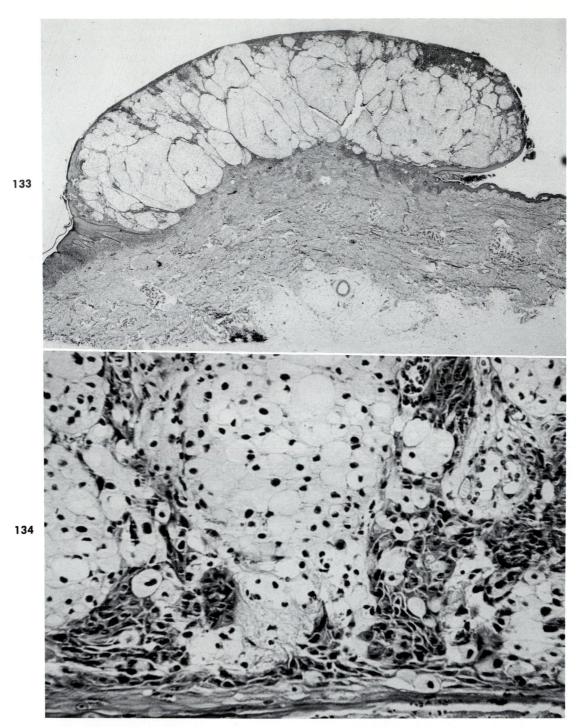

Fig. 133 Balloon cell melanoma involving skin of right shoulder of 50-year-old man. Low-power view showing polypoid tumor with only superficial dermal invasion. (×3; WU neg. 70-7159; slide contributed by Dr. W. A. Gardner, Jr., Durham, N. C.)

Fig. 134 High-power view of lesion illustrated in Fig. 133 showing tumor cells with abundant clear cytoplasm and well-defined cell membranes. (×300; WU neg. 70-7157; slide contributed by Dr. W. A. Gardner, Jr., Durham, N. C.)

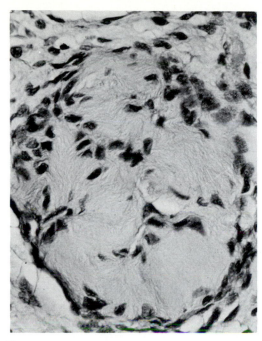

Fig. 135 Wagner-Meissner corpuscle in large congenital nevus of posterior wall of chest of infant. (×600; WU neg. 52-243.)

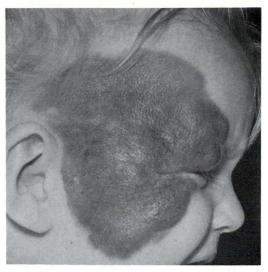

Fig. 136 Congenital nevus on skin of face of child. Lesion is elevated, well circumscribed, and uniformly brown. (WU neg. 47-5464.)

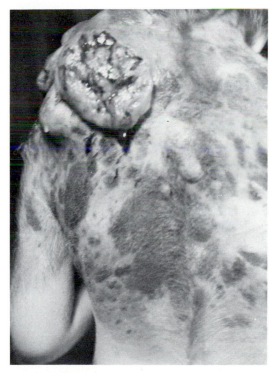

Fig. 137 Malignant ulcerating neurogenous tumor arising in giant pigmented (hairy) nevus in child. (WU neg. 53-2798.)

anomas, there is a history of preexisting nevi.[1] In practically all instances, these nevi are junctional in nature.[5, 76] However, junctional activity is, to a great extent, a function of age and development.

The appearance or enlargement of a junctional nevus in adults is probably indication for its removal. Although most plantar and palmar nevi are junctional in nature, the chances of malignant change are too low (less than 1%) to warrant routine removal.[83] Mundth et al.[58a] examined 10,000 healthy men for pigmented nevi of the palms, soles, and genitalia. Of this group, 14.9% had at least one pigmented nevus in these areas.

If a nevus is removed, a cold knife must be used.[80] Incomplete removal may result in local recrudescence but not in malignant change.[67] The recurrent lesion often shows junctional activity, even if that was not present in the original excision.[19] This, plus the nuclear enlargement and nucleolar prominence that often accompanies these recurrences, has sometimes resulted in a mistaken diagnosis of malignant melanoma. Even the most observant and astute surgeon cannot be certain that the nevus he

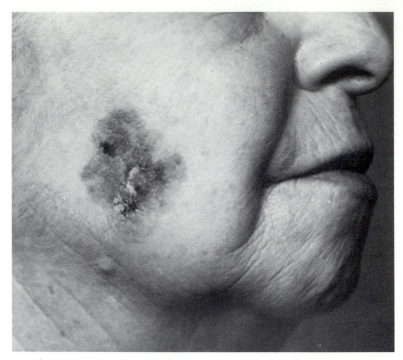

Fig. 138 Hutchinson's freckle that had been present for many years in 67-year-old woman. Raised area in center represents invasive melanoma. (WU neg. 68-3972.)

is removing is not already a melanoma. All nevi require histologic study.

Although the cautery will not cause a perfectly benign intradermal nevus to become malignant, the steam of cautery used on a malignant melanoma possibly drives cancer cells into open small venules and lymphatics, leading to the development of satellite skin nodules.[6] Furthermore, some consideration should be given to the poor pathologist. He has enough difficulty in the interpretation of borderline nevi without adding distortion of the tissue and peculiar staining reactions due to cautery. Histologic interpretation of a cauterized specimen is extremely difficult, if not impossible.

Malignant melanoma
Classification

The long-held impression that malignant melanoma can be subdivided according to certain clinical and pathologic features has recently been crystallized into three distinct clinicopathologic forms largely through the work of Clark et al.[16, 57] in the United States and McGovern[46] in Australia. These are melanoma arising in Hutchinson's freckle, superficial spreading melanoma, and nodular melanoma. A certain degree of accuracy in the differential diagnosis is possible on the basis of location and gross appearance, but the distinction is made fundamentally by microscopic evaluation of the lateral intraepidermal component when present.

Hutchinson's freckle typically occurs in the sun-exposed areas of elderly white persons (Fig. 138), most commonly on the cheek. It is a flat, slowly growing lesion, its color varying from tan to black.[17] Microscopically, it is characterized by a proliferation of atypical melanocytes in the basal layer, distributed individually as well in nests (Fig. 139). Retraction of the cytoplasm and pleomorphism are prominent. Of eighty-five cases studied by Wayte and Helwig,[78] forty-five had an invasive malignant melanoma in the center of the lesion at the time of excision. Only three patients died of the tumor; a fourth developed

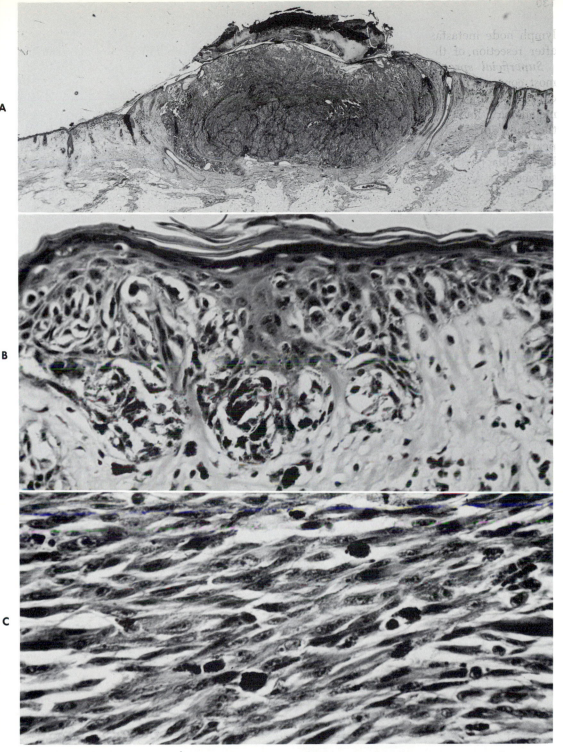

Fig. 139 Hutchinson's freckle with invasive melanoma developed in its center. **A,** Panoramic view, showing large central nodule of invasive tumor. **B,** High-power view of Hutchinson's freckle. Atypical melanocytes, isolated or forming *theques,* are present along basal layer. Numerous melanin-containing macrophages can be seen in dermis. **C,** High-power view of invasive melanoma. Tumor cells are spindle shaped and contain abundant melanin, as is often case with melanomas arising in Hutchinson's freckle. (**A,** ×60; WU neg. 71-8660; B, ×300; WU neg. 72-6048; **C,** ×350; WU neg. 72-6049.)

lymph node metastases but remained well after resection of the involved nodes.

Superficial spreading melanoma is the most common form of melanoma. It is also called premalignant melanosis or pagetoid melanoma[46] and can occur anywhere on the body surface. It has a variegated appearance, the colors including hues of tan, brown, black, blue, pink, and white. The surface is elevated and the margins palpable (Fig. 140). Microscopically, the noninvasive areas are composed of uniform atypical melanocytes with nest formation and pagetoid appearance (Fig. 141). In the series reported by Clark et al.,[16] thirty-six out of 114 patients (31.5%) died as a result of tumor spread.

Nodular melanoma can present as a smooth nodule covered by normal epidermis, as an elevated blue black plaque, or as a polypoid, frequently ulcerated mass (Fig. 142). We have seen it resembling a pyogenic granuloma. A lateral flat component is not seen clinically or microscopically. It affects all body surfaces, is usually of short duration, and occurs in a younger age group than either of the foregoing two categories. The mortality is the highest of all three forms: 56.1% in the series reported by Clark et al.[16]

Distribution

Malignant melanomas as a group occur most frequently in the head and neck area and on the lower extremities[1, 2, 4] (Table 4).

An ulcerating neoplasm on the plantar surface of the foot is almost certainly a malignant melanoma, although it may exactly resemble a callus[22] (Fig. 143). The subungual malignant melanoma is a well-recognized type.[60] If a pigmented area occurs beneath the nail, this diagnosis must be considered seriously. In time, of course, the lesion ulcerates and destroys the digit.

Huge metastases may arise from a primary melanoma no more than a few millimeters in diameter.

Biopsy

Repeated statements are made that the biopsy of a malignant melanoma causes spread. We have seen cauterization of a malignant melanoma followed by the rapid appearance of satellite skin nodules, but we know of no such instance following clean incisional biopsy with a cold knife. A comparison of patients on whom incisional biopsy was done and those who had excision without biopsy showed no differences in survival rate.[26] Primary adequate excision should be done if the lesion is located in an area in which no deformity will result. However, if the lesion is of such size and in such a location that radical

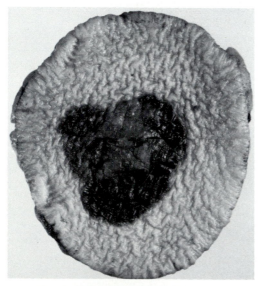

Fig. 140 Superficial spreading malignant melanoma with invasive focus in center. (WU neg. 67-2927.)

Table 4 History of preexisting mole in malignant melanoma*

Location of melanoma	Number	%	Number with history of previous mole
Lower extremities	68	37	31
Head	62	33	30
Chest	25	14	15
Upper extremities	24	13	13
Trunk	6	3	3
Total	185	100	92 (50%)

*From Ackerman, L. V.: Malignant melanoma of skin, Tex. Med. **45**:735-744, 1949.

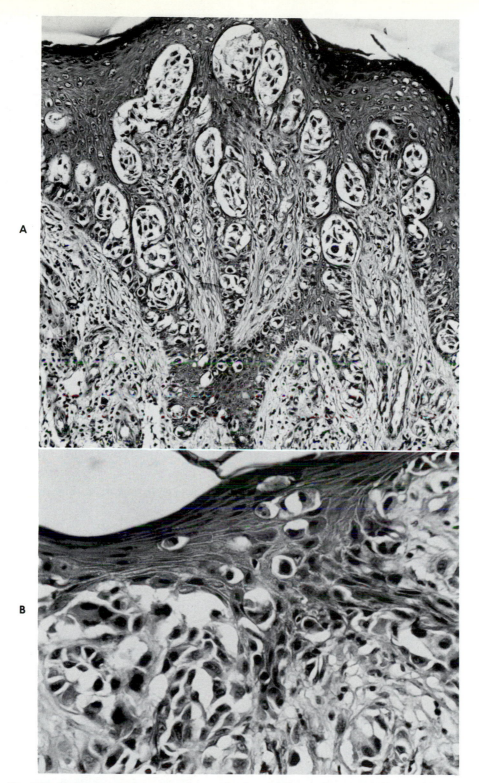

Fig. 141 Malignant melanoma of superficial spreading type. **A,** Marked proliferation of clear cells in well-defined nests resembles appearance of Paget's disease. **B,** Tumor cells have epithelioid appearance and permeate malpighian layers throughout. (**A,** ×150; WU neg. 71-6393; **B,** ×350; WU neg. 71-7653.)

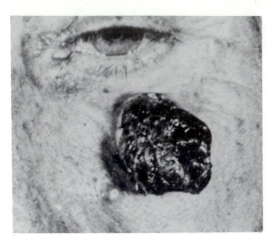

Fig. 142 Typical elevated black malignant melanoma of skin of cheek. (WU neg. 52-4098.)

excision implies disfigurement or disability, then careful incisional biopsy is indicated.

There are numerous lesions that may or may not contain melanin pigment and that can be confused clinically with malignant melanoma—nodular subepidermal fibrosis, infected hemangioma, seborrheic keratosis, and pigmented basal cell carcinoma.[75] Frequently, malignant melanomas are not recognized clinically. Becker[10] reported 151 cases that were verified microscopically, but only 115 were diagnosed clinically. Furthermore, he described 169 patients with lesions clinically thought to be malignant melanoma, but only eighty-two proved to be this lesion.

Microscopic recognition

The obvious malignant melanoma is easily identified microscopically by junctional activity, prominent melanin pigmentation, deep invasion of the surrounding tissue, and many abnormal mitotic figures. It is the interpretation of borderline lesions that taxes the ability and experience of the pathologist. In order to make a diagnosis of malignant melanoma in an adult, the following criteria are helpful:

1 There is loss of cohesiveness of the melanocytes, prominence of their nuclei and nucleoli, and a disproportionate increase of the nuclear cytoplasmic ratio.

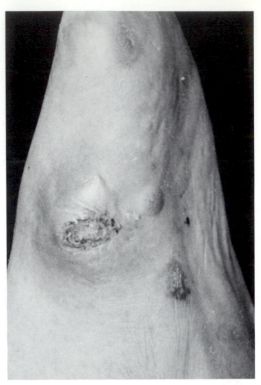

Fig. 143 Malignant melanoma of foot, relatively nonpigmented. Such lesions can be treated for long periods as benign process.

2 Melanocytes may extend throughout the epidermis to the most superficial layer, but this is not necessarily evidence that the lesion is a malignant melanoma.

3 The most important finding is the presence of atypical melanocytes growing in an infiltrative fashion into the dermis.

4 Normal mitotic figures may be found in small numbers in actively growing nevi, and sometimes in large numbers in spindle cell and epithelioid cell nevi. On the other hand, the presence of atypical mitoses is almost always indicative of melanoma and is invariably accompanied by other evidence that the lesion is malignant.

5 The early malignant melanoma is usually associated with a dermal infiltrate of chronic inflammatory cells, often with a bandlike distribution.

6 Amelanotic melanomas can often be

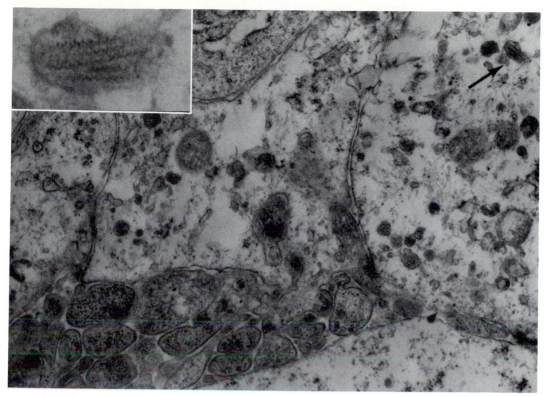

Fig. 144 Electron micrograph of formalin-fixed material from soft tissue malignant tumor involving right thigh of 30-year-old man. Tumor did not contain melanin. Possibilities considered by light microscopy were alveolar soft part sarcoma, metastatic carcinoid tumor, and malignant melanoma. Electron microscopy showed cells containing cytoplasmic prolongations with numerous ribosomes and also scattered melanosomes (arrow). **Inset,** High-power view in which typical striated configuration of melanosome can be clearly seen. (Uranyl acetate–lead citrate; ×27,800; **inset,** uranyl acetate–lead citrate; ×108,000.)

identified ultrastructurally by the presence of melanosomes (Fig. 144).

Children rather frequently have pigmented tumors. McWhorter and Woolner[48] reported 172, of which 149 were pigmented nevi, 7 were blue nevi, 11 were juvenile melanomas, and 5 were malignant melanomas. Malignant melanomas occurring in children have the same microscopic pattern as those in adults and therefore can be differentiated on morphologic grounds from spindle and epithelioid cell nevi. Of the five patients reported by McWhorter and Woolner,[48] four died. Twelve cases, all with documented metastatic disease, have been reported by Lerman et al.[42]

Junctional activity is associated with the majority of early malignant melanomas.

We have seen only one malignant melanoma unconnected with the overlying epidermis that spread and metastasized in a conventional fashion. Bimes[12] reported two instances of malignant melanomas arising from an intradermal nevus. It has been pointed out by Darier,[20] Miescher,[56] and Allen and Spitz[5] that a malignant melanoma lying entirely within the dermis is practically always metastatic.

Malignant melanomas are noted for their bizarre clinical course and great microscopic variability. Sections may be presented to a pathologist that show an unusual nonpigmented malignant tumor. He must keep constantly running through his mind a record that repeats, "Could this peculiar malignant tumor possibly be a malig-

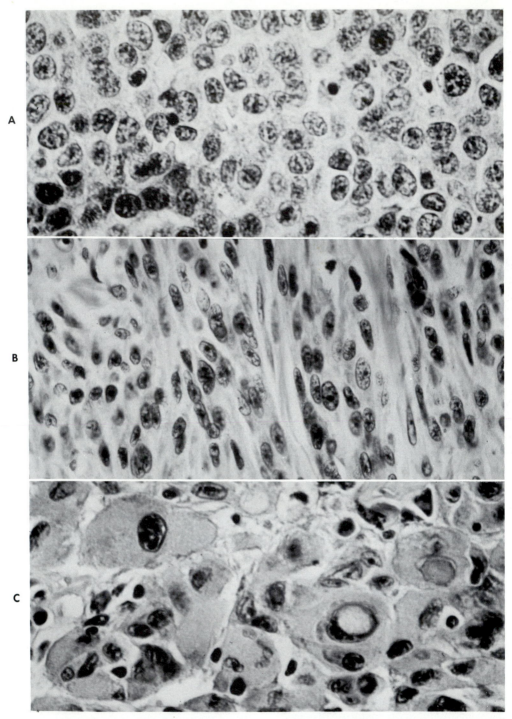

Fig. 145 Different malignant melanomas at same magnification demonstrating possible microscopic variations. Tumor shown in **A** resembles malignant lymphoma. Fusiform cells of the tumor shown in **B** resemble those of fibrosarcoma. Great variation of tumor cells and giant forms shown in **C** suggest liposarcoma. (**A** to **C**, High power.)

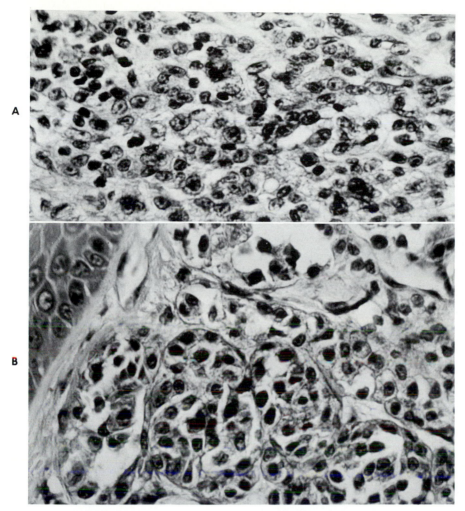

Fig. 146 **A,** Undifferentiated nonpigmented malignant melanoma metastatic to scalp in 17-year-old girl. **B,** Primary tumor contained areas similar to those shown in **A.** Its true character is indicated by nevoid pattern seen in this section taken near surface.

nant melanoma?" The pattern of this tumor can resemble a malignant lymphoma, a fibrosarcoma, or an epidermoid carcinoma (Fig. 145). A case illustrates this point. A 17-year-old girl presented with a tumor of the scalp that had destroyed underlying bone. Sections were made, and various pathologists made diagnoses of osteogenic sarcoma, reticulum cell sarcoma, and Hodgkin's disease, but none considered malignant melanoma (Fig. 146, *A*). Complete physical examination of the patient demonstrated a slightly ulcerated primary lesion 1 cm in diameter on the posterior wall of the chest (Fig. 146, *B*).

Spread

Malignant melanoma has been called the black death because of the appalling speed of its metastases and because it grows readily and luxuriantly in almost any organ. It spreads quickly by the lymphatics to regional lymph nodes, and it also spreads through the bloodstream.

The liver, lungs, and brain are commonly involved. At autopsy, metastases to the heart are found in one-half the patients. Occasionally, osteolytic metastases occur within bone. On several occasions material submitted has been from a metastasis. The primary tumor has been small,

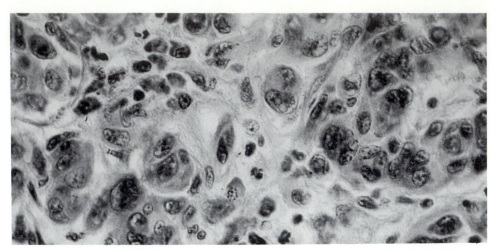

Fig. 147 Heavily irradiated malignant melanoma. Note absence of any detectable irradiation effect. (High power.)

not detectable, or previously removed. The first manifestation even may be intestinal obstruction due to metastases in the small bowel.

Clinicopathologic correlation

The treatment of malignant melanoma is wide excision of the primary lesion. A margin of 2 cm to 3 cm is sufficient for the average-sized tumor. Removal of the underlying fascia, once considered a must, has fallen in discredit in recent years.[74] Distal lymph stasis can be a serious consequence of the procedure, especially in lesions located below the knee. Furthermore, Olsen[59] observed an increased incidence of metastases to regional lymph nodes when the fascia had been removed. If the regional lymph nodes are clinically considered to be involved, a radical lymph node dissection should be performed. If metastatic disease is confirmed microscopically, the prognosis is poor. Of forty-six patients having therapeutic inguinal lymph node dissection, only five were alive and well after five years.[14] In the rare case in which melanoma is in close proximity to a lymph node group, excision of the tumor with in-continuity lymphadenectomy is indicated regardless of the clinical appearance of the nodes.[62] However, this can be applied only to a very small percentage

of melanomas. Routine removal of clinically negative lymph nodes is a very controversial subject. We do not believe that the efficacy of prophylactic node dissection has been proved. McNeer[47] is in favor of the procedure based on the finding of microscopic foci of malignant melanoma in 23% of clinically negative nodes. However, most series fail to show an improvement of survival in the patients so treated.[13, 34, 66]

The two most important microscopic features that correlate with prognosis are the type of melanoma and depth of invasion.[16] Small lesions (under 2 cm in diameter) and superficial lesions have the best prognosis.[30, 40, 45, 55] The degree of pigmentation and cytologic features of the invasive component do not influence the prognosis.[18] The five-year survival of properly treated patients is between 25% and 35%. Women treated for melanoma have a higher survival rate than men. It must be remembered, however, that recurrence is possible ten to fifteen years after treatment. Melanomas are nearly always radioresistant (Fig. 147). Pregnancy does not have an adverse effect in a woman with malignant melanoma.[61, 81]

Malignant melanoma at times acts in a very unpredictable manner. For instance, spontaneous regression of primary lesions before and with the appearance of regional node metastases has been documented.[70] Melanoma can be associated with generalized melanosis[71] and with lesions resembling vitiligo.[8] Melanin, dopa, and a variety of metabolites can be detected in the urine.[77] Hereditary and multiple forms of malignant melanoma have been described.[7, 36] Recent evidence suggests that immunologic factors are important in the evolution of malignant melanoma.[43]

REFERENCES

1 Ackerman, L. V.: Malignant melanoma of skin; clinical and pathologic analyses of 75 cases, Am. J. Clin. Pathol. **18**:602-624, 1948.

2 Ackerman, L. V.: Malignant melanoma of the skin, Tex. Med. **45**:735-744, 1949.

3 Ackerman, L. V., and Taylor, H. B.: Case 3: Blue nevus. Proceedings of the 35th Seminar of the American Society of Clinical Pathology, 1970, pp. 10-12.

4 Affleck, D. H.: Melanomas, Am. J. Cancer **27**:120-138, 1936.

5 Allen, A. C., and Spitz, S.: Malignant melanoma; a clinicopathological analysis of the criteria for diagnosis and prognosis, Cancer **6**:1-45, 1953.

6 Amadon, P. D.: Electrocoagulation of melanoma and its dangers, Surg. Gynecol. Obstet. **56**:943-946, 1933.

7 Anderson, D. E., Smith, J. L., Jr., and McBride, C. M.: Hereditary aspects of malignant melanoma, J.A.M.A. **200**:741-746, 1967.

8 Balasanov, K., Andreev, V. C., and Tchernozemski, I.: Malignant melanoma and vitiligo, Dermatologica **139**:211-219, 1969.

9 Becker, S. W.: Dermatological investigation of melanin pigmentation. In Biology of melanomas (special publication), New York Academy of Sciences **4**:82-101, 1948.

10 Becker, S. W.: Pitfalls in the diagnosis and treatment of melanoma, Arch. Dermatol. **69**:11-30, 1954.

11 Berkheiser, S. W., and Rappoport, A. E.: The comparative morphogenesis of the dermo-epidermal nevi and malignant melanoma, Am. J. Pathol. **28**:477-495, 1952.

12 Bimes, C.: Histopathologie des naevo-carcinomes, Bull. Cancer (Paris) **40**:481-528, 1953.

13 Block, G. E., and Hartwell, S. W., Jr.: Malignant melanoma: a study of 217 cases, Ann. Surg. **154**:74-101, 1961.

14 Booher, R. J., and Pack, G. T.: Malignant melanoma of the feet and hands, Surgery **42**:1084-1121, 1957.

15 Clark, W. H., Jr., Watson, M. C., and Watson, B. E. M.: Two kinds of "clear" cells in the human epidermis; with a report of a modified DOPA reaction for electron microscopy, Am. J. Pathol. Bacteriol. **39**:333-344, 1961.

16 Clark, W. H., Jr., From, L., Bernardino, E. A., and Mihm, M. C.: The histogenesis and biologic behavior of primary human malignant melanomas of the skin, Cancer Res. **29**:705-726, 1969.

17 Clark, W. H., Jr., and Mihm, M. C., Jr.: Lentigo maligna and lentigo-maligna melanoma, Am. J. Pathol. **55**:39-67, 1969.

18 Cochran, A. J.: Histology and prognosis in malignant melanoma, J. Pathol. **97**:459-468, 1969.

19 Cox, A. J., and Walton, R. G.: The induction of junctional changes in pigmented nevi, Arch. Pathol. **79**:428-434, 1965.

20 Darier, J.: Des naevocarcinomes, Bull. Cancer (Paris), Seance du Nov. 21, 1913.

21 Davis, N. C., Herron, J., and McLeon, G. R.: The macroscopic appearance of malignant melanoma of the skin, Med. J. Aust. **2**:883-886, 1966.

22 Decker, A. M., and Chamness, J. T.: Melanocarcinoma of the plantar surface of the foot, Surgery **29**:731-742, 1951.

23 Demian, S., Donnelley, W., and Monif, G. R. G.: Placental involvement in giant pigmented nevi, Am. J. Pathol. **71**:14a, 1973 (abstract).

24 DuShane, G.: Embryology of vertebrate pigment cells. I. Amphibia, Q. Rev. Biol. **18**:109-127, 1943.

25 Echevarria, R., and Ackerman, L. V.: Spindle and epithelioid cell nevi in the adult; a clinicopathologic report of 26 cases, Cancer **20**:175-189, 1967.

26 Epstein, E., Bragg, K., and Linden, G.: Biopsy and prognosis of malignant melanoma, J.A.M.A. **208**:1369-1371, 1969.

27 Fitzpatrick, T. B., and Lerner, A. B.: Terminology of pigment cells, Science **117**:640, 1953.

28 Gardner, W. A., Jr., and Vazquez, M. D.: Balloon cell melanoma, Arch. Pathol. **89**:470-472, 1970.

29 Goldman, R. L., and Friedman, N. B.: Blue nevus of the uterine cervix, Cancer **20**:210-214, 1967.

30 Handley, W. S.: The pathology of melanotic growths in relation to their operative treatment, Lancet **1**:927-996, 1907.

31 Harper, J. C., and Waldron, Ch. A.: Blue nevus of palate, Oral Surg. Oral Med. Oral Path. **20**:145-149, 1965.

32 Helwig, E. B.: Personal communication, 1958.

33 Jao, W., Fretzin, D. F., Christ, M. L., and Prinz, L. M.: Blue nevus of the prostate gland, Arch. Pathol. **91**:187-192, 1971.

34 Johnson, R. E.: Occult lymphatic metastases in malignant melanoma of the skin, Ann. Surg. **146**:931-936, 1957.

35 Johnson, W. T., and Helwig, E. B.: Benign nevus cells in the capsule of lymph nodes, Cancer 23:747-753, 1969.

36 Kahn, L. B., and Donaldson, R. C.: Multiple primary melanoma; case report and study of tumor growth in vitro, Cancer 25:1162-1169, 1970.

37 Kernen, J. A., and Ackerman, L. V.: Spindle cell nevi and epithelioid cell nevi (so-called juvenile melanomas) in children and adults; a clinicopathologic study of 27 cases, Cancer 13:612-625, 1960.

38 Kopf, A. W., Morrill, S. D., and Silberberg, I.: Broad spectrum of leukoderma acquisitum centrifugum, Arch. Dermatol. 92:14-35, 1965.

39 Laidlaw, G. F., and Murray, M. F.: Melanoma studies: theory of pigmented moles. Their relation to evolution of hair follicles, Am. J. Pathol. 9:827-838, 1933. Addendum: Theory of pigmented moles, Am. J. Pathol. 10:319-320, 1934.

40 Lane, N., Lattes, R., and Malm, J.: Clinicopathological correlations in a series of 117 malignant melanomas of the skin of adults, Cancer 11:1025-1043, 1958.

41 Leopold, J. G., and Richards, D. B.: The interrelationship of blue and common naevi, J. Pathol. Bacteriol. 95:37-46, 1968.

42 Lerman, R. I., Murray, D., O'Hara, J. M., Booher, R. H., and Foote, F. W., Jr.: Malignant melanoma of childhood; a clinicopathologic study and a report of 12 cases, Cancer 25:436-449, 1970.

43 Lewis, M. G., Ikonopisov, R. L., Nairn, R. C., Philips, T. M., Fairley, G. H., Bodenham, D. C., and Alexander, P.: Tumour-specific antibodies in human malignant melanoma and their relationship to the extent of the disease, Br. Med. J. 3:547-552, 1969.

44 Lund, H. Z., and Stobbe, G. D.: The natural history of the pigmented nevus; factors of age and anatomic location, Am. J. Pathol. 25:1117-1155, 1949.

45 Lund, R. H., and Ihnen, M.: Malignant melanoma; clinical and pathologic analysis of 93 cases; is prophylactic lymph nodes dissection indicated? Surgery 38:652-659, 1955.

46 McGovern, V. J.: The classification of melanoma and its relationship with prognosis, Pathology 2:85-98, 1970.

47 McNeer, G.: Malignant melanoma, Surg. Gynecol. Obstet. 120:343-344, 1965.

48 McWhorter, H. E., and Woolner, L. B.: Pigmented nevi, juvenile melanomas, and malignant melanomas in children, Cancer 7:564-585, 1955.

49 Mark, G. J., Mihm, M. C., Jr., Liteplo, M. G., Reed, R. J., and Clark, W. H., Jr.: Congenital melanocytic nevi of the small and garment type:

50 Masson, P.: Les naevi pigmentaires, tumeurs nerveuses, Ann. Anat. Pathol. (Paris) 3:417-453, 657-696, 1926.

51 Masson, P.: Giant neuro-naevus of the hairy scalp, Ann. Surg. 93:218-222, 1931.

52 Masson, P.: Pigment cells in man. In Biology of melanomas (special publication), New York Academy of Sciences 4:15-51, 1948.

53 Masson, P.: Neuro-nevi "bleu," Arch. De Vecchi Anat. Patol. 14:1-28, 1950.

54 Masson, P.: My conception of cellular nevi, Cancer 4:9-38, 1951.

55 Mehnert, J. H., and Heard, J. L.: Staging of malignant melanomas by depth of invasion: proposed index to prognosis, Am. J. Surg. 110:168-176, 1965.

56 Meischer, G.: Die Entstehung der bösartigen Melanome der Haut, Virchow Arch. Pathol. Anat. 264:86-142, 1927.

57 Mihm, M. C., Jr., Clark, W. H., Jr., and From, L.: The clinical diagnosis, classification and histogenetic concepts of the early stages of cutaneous malignant melanomas, N. Engl. J. Med. 284:1078-1082, 1971.

58 Montgomery, H., and Kahler, J. E.: The blue nevus (Jadassohn-Tièche): its distinction from ordinary moles and malignant melanomas, Am. J. Cancer 36:527-539, 1939.

58a Mundth, E. D., Guralnick, E. A., and Raker, J. W.: Malignant melanoma, a clinical study of 427 cases, Ann. Surg. 162:15-28, 1965.

59 Olsen, G.: Removal of fascia—cause of more frequent metastases of malignant melanomas of the skin to regional lymph nodes? Cancer 17:1159-1164, 1964.

60 Pack, G. T., and Oropeza, R.: Subungual melanoma, Surg. Gynecol. Obstet. 124:571-582, 1967.

61 Pack, G. T., and Scharnagel, I. M.: The prognosis for malignant melanoma in the pregnant woman, Cancer 4:324-334, 1951.

62 Pack, G. T., Scharnagel, I., and Morfit, M.: Principle of excision and dissection in continuity for primary and metastatic melanoma of skin, Surgery 17:849-866, 1945.

63 Rawles, M. E.: Development of melanophores from embryonic mouse tissues grown in coelom of chick embryos, Proc. Natl. Acad. Sci. U.S.A. 26:673-680, 1940.

64 Reed, W. B., Becker, S. W., Becker, S. W., Jr., and Nickel, W. R.: Giant pigmented nevi, melanoma, and leptomeningeal melanocytosis; a clinical and histopathological study, Arch. Dermatol. 91:100-119, 1965.

65 Rodriguez, H., and Ackerman, L. V.: Cellular blue nevus, Cancer 21:393-405, 1968.

66 Sandeman, T. F.: The radical treatment of enlarged lymph nodes in malignant melanoma,

clinical, histologic and ultrastructural study, Hum. Pathol. 4:395-418, 1973.

Am. J. Roentgenol. Radium Ther. Nucl. Med. **97**:969-979, 1966.

67 Schoenfeld, R. J., and Pinkus, H.: Recurrence of nevi after incomplete removal, Arch. Dermatol. **78**:30-35, 1958.

68 Schrader, W. A., and Helwig, E. B.: Balloon cell nevi, Cancer **20**:1502-1514, 1967.

69 Slaughter, J. C., Hordman, J. M., Kempe, L. G., and Earle, K. M.: Neurocutaneous melanosis and leptomeningeal melanomatosis in children, Arch. Pathol. **88**:298-304, 1969.

70 Smith, J. L., Jr., and Stehlin, J. S., Jr.: Spontaneous regression of primary malignant melanomas with regional metastases, Cancer **18**:1399-1415, 1965.

71 Sohn, N., Gang, H., Gumport, S. L., Goldstein, M., and Deppisch, L. M.: Generalized melanosis secondary to malignant melanoma, report of a case with serum and tissue tyrosinase studies, Cancer **24**:893-903, 1969.

72 Spitz, S.: Melanomas of childhood, Am. J. Pathol. **24**:591-609, 1948.

73 Stegmaier, O. C., and Montgomery, H.: Histopathologic studies of pigmented nevi in children, J. Invest. Dermatol. **20**:51-64, 1953.

74 Stehlin, J. S., Jr.: Malignant melanoma: an appraisal, Surgery **64**:1149-1157, 1968.

75 Stewart, M. J., and Bonser, G. M.: Melanin-forming epidermal tumours of skin; study of

57 personally observed cases, J. Pathol. Bacteriol. **60**:21-33, 1948.

76 Traub, E. F., and Keil, H.: "Common mole"; its clinicopathologic relations and question of malignant degeneration, Arch. Dermatol. **41**:214-252, 1940.

77 Voorhess, M. L.: Urinary excretion of DOPA and metabolites by patients with melanoma, Cancer **26**:146-149, 1970.

78 Wayte, D. M., and Helwig, E. B.: Melanotic freckle of Hutchinson, Cancer **21**:893-911, 1968.

79 Wayte, D. M., and Helwig, E. B.: Halo nevi, Cancer **22**:69-90, 1968.

80 Webster, J. P., Stevenson, T. W., and Stout, A. P.: Symposium on reparative surgery; surgical treatment of malignant melanomas of skin, Surg. Clin. North Am. **24**:319-339, 1944.

81 White, L. P., Linden, G., Breslow, L., and Harzfeld, L.: Studies on melanoma; the effect of pregnancy on survival in human melanoma, J.A.M.A. **177**:235-238, 1961.

82 Willier, B. H., and Rawles, M. E.: Control of feather control pattern by melanophores grafted from one embryo to another of different breed of fowl, Physiol. Zoöl. **13**:177-199, 1940.

83 Wilson, F. C., Jr., and Andersonk, P. C.: A dissenting view on the prophylactic removal of plantar and palmar nevi, Cancer **14**:102-104, 1961.

4 Oral cavity and pharynx

Introduction

The oral cavity is the site of numerous diseases, both congenital and acquired, affecting a large variety of tissues and systems. Only those that occur commonly enough to be of interest to the surgical pathologist are discussed here. For a thorough discussion of these and the rarer diseases, the reader is referred to the excellent treatise edited by Gorlin and Goldman.[1] Several of the dermatoses discussed in Chapter 3 can be accompanied by oral lesions, their microscopic appearance being roughly equivalent to that of the cutaneous component.

Biopsy and cytology

Dentists have the best opportunity to discover early lesions of the oral cavity. It is their responsibility to examine the oral cavity carefully for evidence of systemic disease and benign or malignant tumors.[2] Patients with a suspicious lesion should be referred for proper study and biopsy.

Lesions within the oral cavity often are not biopsied properly. An adequate biopsy may be difficult to obtain from certain intraoral lesions such as deep-lying tumors at the base of the tongue. It is imperative that a deep biopsy be taken rather than a small superficial one. In experienced hands, the accuracy of intraoral biopsy approaches 100%.[3] Cytologic examination of oral lesions is of no great practical value. In a series of 158 epidermoid carcinomas studied by Shklar et al.,[4] there was a false negative incidence of 13.9%. Furthermore, there was not a single case with positive cytology in which the biopsy had failed to reveal the tumor.

Congenital abnormalities

Dermoid cysts are seen in the midline of the floor of the mouth. Although present at birth, they may become evident later on when secondarily inflamed. They are lined by squamous epithelium and contain skin adnexa.[7] *Cysts lined by gastric or intestinal epithelium* have been reported in the tongue and floor of the mouth.[6] Minute *cysts of odontogenic origin* are commonly seen in the alveolar and palatal mucosa of newborn and older infants.[5] They need not be biopsied. Nodules of *heterotopic nerve tissue* in the palate mainly composed of glial elements and ependymal-lined clefts have been reported by Zarem et al.[9] *White sponge nevus,* an autosomal dominantly inherited disease, is characterized by large white plaques in the oral mucosa. Microscopically, there is striking intracellular edema throughout the malpighian layer.[8] *Fordyce's disease* refers to the presence of normal sebaceous glands inside the oral cavity, a very common occurrence. The entity *lingual thyroid* is discussed in the chapter on the thyroid gland.

Reactive processes

Chronic inflammatory lesions are produced in the oral cavity by ill-fitting dentures, ragged, sharp teeth, and poor dental hygiene (Fig. 148). Removal of the offending agent allows the pathologic process to subside.[13] Bhaskar et al.[12] described 341

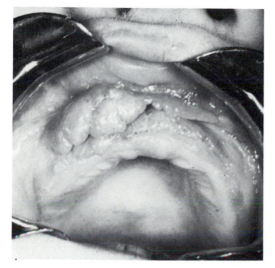

Fig. 148 Localized nonneoplastic overgrowth of upper alveolus produced by ill-fitting denture. (WU neg. 52-4100; courtesy Dr. C. A. Waldron, Atlanta, Ga.)

cases of inflammatory papillary hyperplasia of the oral mucosa associated with the use of dentures; 82.7% of the lesions were located in the palate. Localized overgrowth of the epithelium with or without ulceration is frequent, and it is not rare to see large pseudotumors made up of fibrous tissue and chronic inflammatory cells, among which plasma cells may be prominent[11] (Figs. 149 and 150). The inflammation distorts the epithelial pegs and may produce areas in which squamous cells are isolated from the overlying epithelium[10] (Fig. 151). If the pathologist pays attention to the inflammatory process and notes that the squamous cells are well differentiated and that inflammatory cells are present between them, he will diagnose the lesion correctly.

On rare occasions, the epithelial distortion is so intense that a diagnosis of cancer may be made even by the experienced pathologist. We have seen four patients exhibiting marked epithelial abnormalities and destruction of the mandible who were treated by irradiation and/or radical resection and neck dissection. Needless to say, the lymph nodes contained no tumor. Dilantin therapy can cause tremendous hypertrophy of the mucosa of

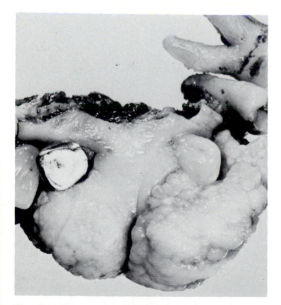

Fig. 149 Resected pseudotumor of alveolar process made up of fibrous tissue and chronic inflammatory cells. (WU neg. 52-3842.)

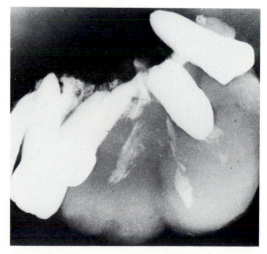

Fig. 150 Alveolar process from which pseudotumor shown in Fig. 149 was resected, showing extent of soft tissue mass.

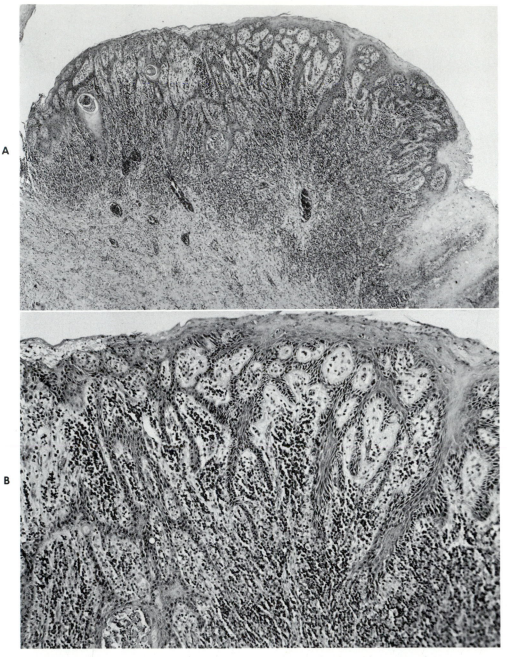

Fig. 151 Extreme pseudoepitheliomatous hyperplasia of inflamed gingiva that was incorrectly diagnosed as carcinoma by several experienced pathologists. Long, thin strands of distorted, well-differentiated squamous cells infiltrated by inflammatory cells are present. (**A,** ×40; WU neg. 57-4783; **B,** ×115; WU neg. 57-4784.)

the gums necessitating surgical removal (Fig. 152).

A reactive process of altogether different microscopic appearance is the *oral sub-*

mucous fibrosis seen in Indians and Pakistanians.[18] It is thought to be the result of hypersensitivity to chillies. The overlying epithelium is usually atrophic. A re-

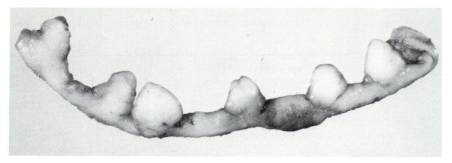

Fig. 152 Surgically removed tremendously hypertrophied gingival mucosa caused by Dilantin therapy in 13-year-old girl. (WU neg. 62-6348.)

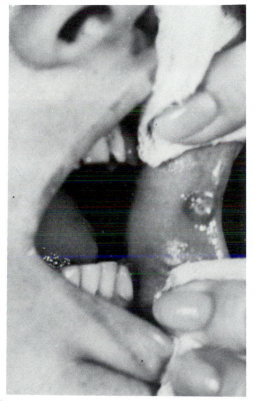

Fig. 153 Sharply circumscribed and elevated pyogenic granuloma of buccal mucosa. (EFSCH 13461.)

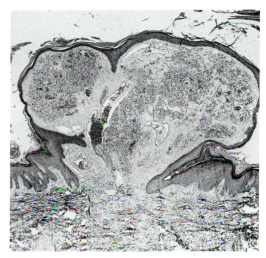

Fig. 154 Typical low-power pattern of pyogenic granuloma. Note elevation above lining epithelium and its narrowing at base. (WU neg. 51-1069.)

lationship with oral carcinoma has been suggested but not yet established with certainty.

The term ***mucous cyst (mucocele)*** when applied to a lesion of the oral cavity refers to a well-localized focus of stromal reaction to spillage of mucus from a minor salivary gland. The lower lip is the classical location. The most common microscopic pattern is that of granulation tissue surrounding one or more spaces containing mucin.[16]

Pyogenic granuloma is an exaggerated response to minor trauma. It appears in the oral cavity as an elevated, dark red lesion that may or may not be ulcerated (Fig. 153). Large masses of proliferating endothelial cells are separated by an edematous stroma containing inflammatory cells. Characteristically, the covering epithelium almost meets at the base of the lesion (Fig. 154). It heals as a residual fibrous mass or fibroepithelial papilloma.[15] An identical lesion occurring during pregnancy is often incorrectly diagnosed as an infected hemangioma.[17]

The so-called *peripheral giant cell granu-loma (giant cell epulis)* is seen in all age groups and is more common in females.[14] Maxilla and mandible are equally affected. A soft to firm mass forms that pushes the teeth aside and may erode the mandible. Microscopically, the lesion shows numerous giant cells, an active vascular stroma, and, at times, small amounts of bone production.

Specific infections

Tuberculosis is a rare lesion within the oral cavity. It is usually seen on the tongue as a painful ulcer, but it also may occur on the buccal mucosa.[21] It nearly always is associated with advanced pulmonary disease. Microscopically, there are typical tubercles.

Syphilis may produce a gumma in the tongue or palate appearing as a painless indurated mass. Microscopically, there is a granuloma with giant cells, numerous plasma cells, and prominent vascular changes. There seems to be a relationship between syphilis and tongue cancer, although the percentage of patients with such association is no longer as high as old reports would indicate. A study of 243 patients with cancer of the tongue revealed that only fifteen (6.1%) had a history of syphilis.[20]

Histoplasmosis can occur anywhere in the oral cavity and can closely simulate epidermoid carcinoma on clinical examination. Indurated ulcers (Fig. 155), nodular lesions, or verrucous masses can be present. The microscopic appearance is that of a granuloma, although sometimes only a nonspecific inflammatory reaction is seen (Fig. 156). Special stains (Gomori's, methenamine-silver, or PAS-Gridley) are necessary for the identification of the fungi (Fig. 156, *inset*).[19]

Tumors
Tumors of surface epithelium

Leukoplakia is a clinical term. It has been defined by Pindborg[32] as a white patch or plaque, not less than 5 mm in diameter, which cannot be removed by rubbing and which cannot be classified as any other diagnosable disease (Fig. 157). As suggested by King,[29] it is more appropriate to diagnose this lesion microscopically as epithelial atrophy or hyperplasia, grading the atypicality (if any) as mild, moderate, or severe. The commonest location of leukoplakia is the buccal gingival gutter.[33] Pindborg[32] divides this lesion into two types: speckled and homogeneous. Over 60% of the former have superimposed infection by *Candida albicans.*[34] Cases of leukoplakia with atypical epithelial changes are morphologically quite similar to actinic keratosis of the skin. Warty dyskeratoma, a skin condition, considered by some a variant of actinic keratosis, also has been reported in the oral cavity.[27] Pindborg et al.[32] followed 248 patients with oral leukoplakia for one to ten years: 4.4% developed epidermoid carcinoma. Most of the cases were of the speckled type. In Einhorn's series[26]

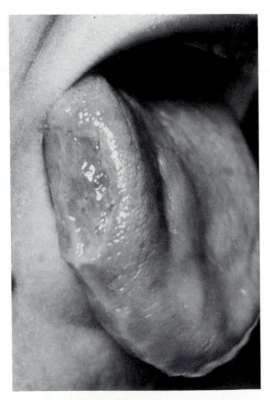

Fig. 155 Oral histoplasmosis presenting as indurated ulcer of tongue. (WU neg. 57-6589.)

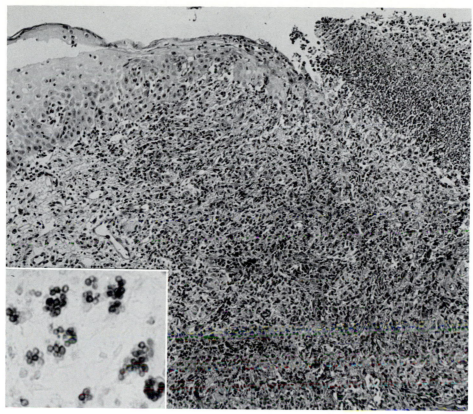

Fig. 156 Histoplasmosis of oral cavity. Ulcer shows histiocytic and chronic inflammatory reaction without granulomas. **Inset,** Numerous fungi can be seen with PAS stain. (×140; WU neg. 66-12081; **inset,** periodic acid–Schiff; ×720; WU neg. 66-12085.)

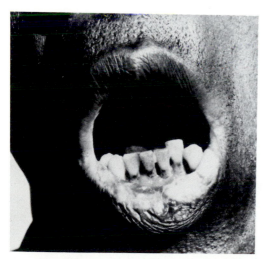

Fig. 157 Marked leukoplakia of lower lip in Bantu. (Courtesy Dr. A. Schamaman, Johannesburg, South Africa.)

of 782 patients with a mean follow-up of 11.7 years, the incidence of carcinoma was 2.4% after ten years and 4% after twenty years.

Epidermoid carcinoma in situ can be a precursor of invasive oral cancer (Fig. 158). How often this occurs is not known. Neither is the speed of its evolution.

We have seen a 60-year-old man with a small, slightly elevated, pinkish gray area on the floor of the mouth that was excised and found to be epidermoid carcinoma in situ. Three months later, invasive carcinoma was present at the site of excision and in the underlying mandible. Another patient had epidermoid carcinoma in situ with multiple foci of origin over a wide area of the oral mucosa. This lesion was present for five years before invasive carci-

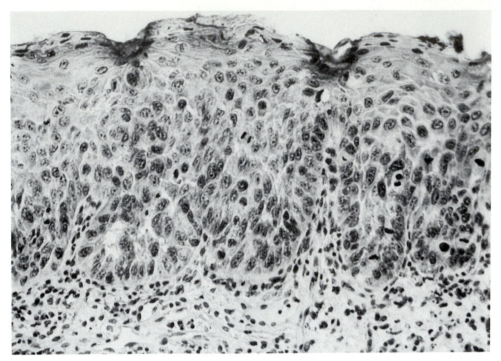

Fig. 158 Epidermoid carcinoma in situ of floor of mouth. Note intact basement membrane, complete disorganization of epithelium throughout all layers, and many mitotic figures. (×270; WU neg. 51-4661.)

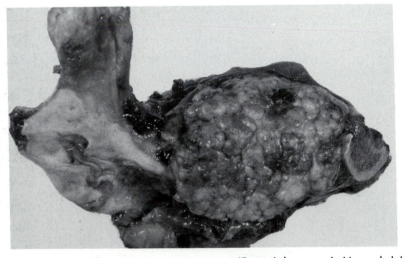

Fig. 159 Extensive papillary verrucous carcinoma. (From Ackerman, L. V., and del Regato, J. A.: Cancer, ed. 4, St. Louis, 1970, The C. V. Mosby Co.)

noma appeared and caused the death of the patient.

Epidermoid carcinoma in situ also may exist at the periphery of an obvious car-

cinoma. Therefore, it is necessary to encompass the invasive carcinoma, whether treatment be by irradiation therapy or by excision. As more and more carcinomas of

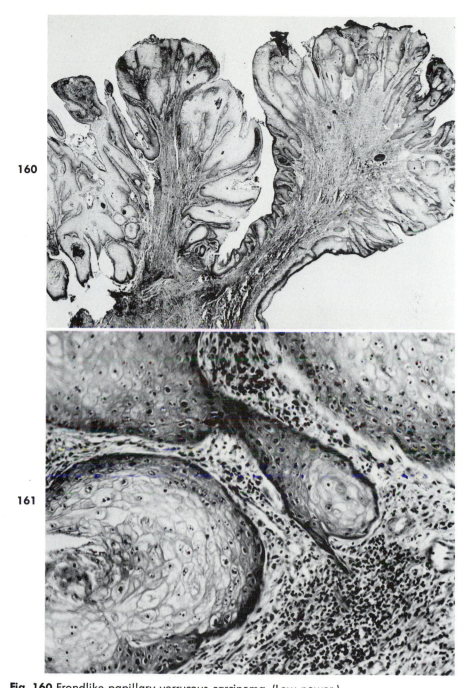

Fig. 160 Frondlike papillary verrucous carcinoma. (Low power.)
Fig. 161 Detailed view of swollen rete ridges of deeply invasive verrucous carcinoma with intact basement membrane.

the oral cavity are cured, it is becoming apparent that the entire mucosa of the oral cavity is susceptible to the development of carcinoma. If a patient has one carcinoma of the oral cavity, the chances of that patient developing another are increased.[25, 35] Among 206 patients with carcinoma of the oral cavity seen at the Ellis Fischel State

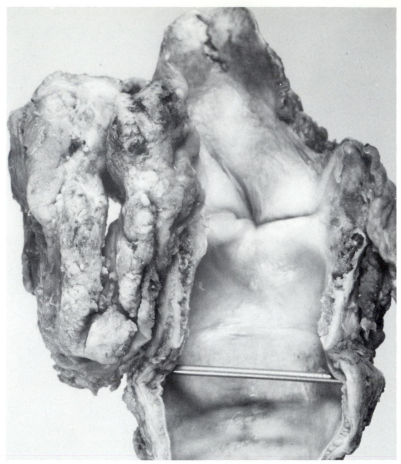

Fig. 162 Large ulcerating primary carcinoma of piriform sinus occurring in 69-year-old man. (WU neg. 62-6529.)

Cancer Hospital, two patients had two independent carcinomas on admission and eight developed second "primary" carcinomas after treatment of the initial tumor.[23]

Table 5 Intraoral distribution of verrucous carcinoma*

Location	Patients
Oral cavity	77
Buccal mucosa	50
Gingiva	21
Tongue	3
Anterior tonsillar pillar	1
Hard palate	2
Larynx	12
Nasal fossa	4
Total	93

*From Kraus, F. T., and Perez-Mesa, C.: Verrucous carcinoma, Cancer 19:26-38, 1966.

Verrucous carcinoma is a form of epidermoid carcinoma with a distinctive morphologic pattern and clinical evolution. The intraoral distribution of this lesion is shown in Table 5.

Verrucous carcinoma occurs most frequently on the buccal mucosa and lower gingiva and is almost invariably associated with leukoplakia. It occurs predominantly in men who chew tobacco. In time, this lesion may produce a large, fungating, soft papillary growth (Fig. 159). It tends to become infected and slowly to invade contiguous structures. We have seen it destroy the mandible, grow through the soft tissues of the cheek, and invade the maxilla. Metastases from this tumor are exceedingly rare.

The microscopic diagnosis of verrucous carcinoma may be difficult because of its well-differentiated character. Sections of an adequate biopsy show swollen and voluminous rete pegs that extend into the deeper tissues, where their pattern becomes quite complex. Once the pattern has been seen, it can be recognized easily (Figs. 160 and 161). Resection is the treatment of choice. If surgery is inadequate, the tumor will recur.[22] Radiation therapy should not be employed, since it may alter the nature of the tumor to a highly malignant, rapidly metastasizing, poorly differentiated epidermoid carcinoma.[30]

Epidermoid carcinoma is the most frequent malignant tumor of the oral cavity and pharynx (Fig. 162). In the oral cavity,

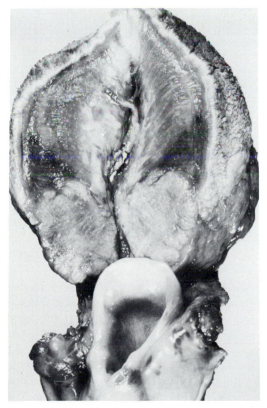

Fig. 163 Poorly differentiated squamous carcinoma in base of tongue. Patient had cervical node metastases. Primary lesion shown was not discovered clinically because of lack of proper palpation. Lesion was found after death. (WU neg. 50-371.)

the lesion may arise in areas of leukoplakia or carcinoma in situ. It gradually forms an ulcer with firm, indurated borders. Epidermoid carcinomas within the oral cavity are often only moderately well differentiated. In the base of the tongue or the nasopharynx, they frequently are undifferentiated (Fig. 163). They quickly invade the lingual muscles and spread widely into surrounding structures. Squamous carcinoma of the nasopharynx invades the base of the skull and often involves nerves. Both differentiated and undifferentiated squamous carcinomas metastasize primarily by lymphatics. The distribution of lymph node involvement depends on the anatomy of lymphatic drainage. For instance, the more anterior the lesion, the lower will be the position of the node metastases in the neck. Carcinoma of the lips is associated with sunlight, smoking, and chronic mechanical irritation.[24] The lower lip is involved in the large majority of cases (over 90%). In rare instances, the tumor has a spindle cell configuration simulating sarcoma[28] (Fig. 164). Carcinoma of the tongue tends to produce multiple small metastases that may not be palpable. Carcinomas of the base of the tongue and the nasopharynx metastasize to the deep retropharyngeal lymph nodes (Fig. 165).

Treatment of lesions in the anterior two-thirds of the tongue usually combines irradiation and neck dissection. Interstitial radium is placed in the tongue, and a radical neck dissection is done on the homolateral side. About 25% of the tongue lesions are cured by this procedure. Relatively few of the squamous carcinomas of the nasopharynx and the base of the tongue are cured, the reasons for failure being the inability to sterilize the primary lesion locally by irradiation and the frequency of widespread metastases.

Lymphoepithelioma is a poor name for a type of pharyngeal poorly differentiated carcinoma diffusely infiltrated by lymphocytes.[36] The lymphocytes are not true components of the tumor. By electron microscopy, we have demonstrated

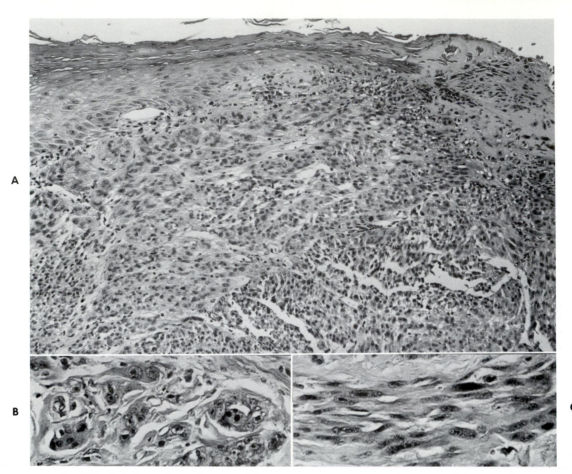

Fig. 164 Spindle cell carcinoma of lip. **A,** Panoramic view, showing cellular neoplasm growing beneath attenuated and partially ulcerated epidermis. **B,** In this area, tumor cells have clear-cut epithelial appearance. **C,** In other foci, cellular shape and pattern of growth closely simulate sarcoma. This peculiar variety of squamous cell carcinoma, which has strong predilection for involvement of lip, should be clearly separated from atypical fibroxanthoma of skin and from "pseudosarcoma" of upper respiratory and digestive tracts. (**A,** ×150; WU neg. 73-2666; **B,** ×300; WU neg. 73-2690; **C,** ×300; WU neg. 73-2691.)

tonofilaments and desmosomes, clear evidence that this tumor is of epithelial origin (Fig. 3). According to Lin et al.,[31] the tumor cells resemble those of transional cell carcinoma and probably arise from the cells of the basal layers of pseudostratified and stratified epithelia. Undifferentiated carcinoma of the nasopharynx metastatic to lymph nodes closely simulates histiocytic lymphoma. The focal (predominantly sinusal) nature of the involvement and the large vesicular nuclei with a single prominent nucleolus seen in metastatic car-

cinoma are useful features in the differential diagnosis. We have also seen several cases in which the metastatic tumor was accompanied by a marked infiltration by eosinophils, thus resulting in a mistaken diagnosis of Hodgkin's disease. This type of carcinoma occurs frequently in the Chinese. About 25% of the lesions are cured by irradiation.[37]

Epidermoid carcinoma of the oral cavity and larynx associated with polypoid sarcoma-like masses ("pseudosarcoma") is discussed in Chapter 6.

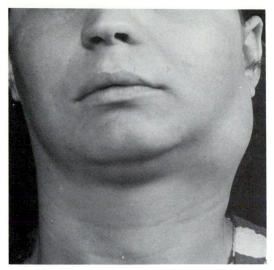

Fig. 165 Clinical photograph of nodal metastasis from nasopharyngeal carcinoma. This is typical location of involved nodes. (WU neg. 48-4426.)

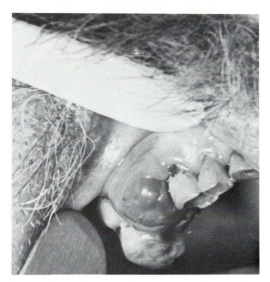

Fig. 166 Malignant lymphoma arising from upper alveolus.

Tumors of minor salivary glands

Minor salivary glands, present in practically all structures within the oral cavity, participate in many of the diseases affecting their major counterparts, a feature of diagnostic value. Thus, biopsy of the lower lip has shown involvement of the minor salivary glands in cases of mucoviscidosis[41] and Sjögren's syndrome.[39] The glands also can be the site of benign and malignant tumors. Microscopically, the tumors do not differ from those located in the major glands (Chapter 17). However, they differ from the latter in their relative incidence rate and natural history.[38] The hard palate is the most common location, but the tumors also occur in the gingiva, floor of the mouth, tongue, and lip (usually the upper). Benign mixed tumors, which constitute 78% of all parotid neoplasms, make up only 56% of the salivary gland tumors of the palate.[40] Adenoid cystic carcinoma and mucoepidermoid carcinoma comprise 85% of all intraoral malignant salivary gland tumors, whereas there is an even distribution of several tumor types in the parotid gland. The prognosis of adenoid cystic carcinoma is better when the tumor is located in the palate than when present in the parotid or submaxillary gland.[40] We have seen tumors of the deep lobe of the parotid gland presenting as primary intraoral masses. They present a difficult therapeutic problem.

Tumors of lymphoid tissue

Benign nodules made of well-differentiated lymphocytes, with or without an admixture of histiocytes, are not uncommon in the oral cavity. They may represent enlarged buccal lymph nodes or hypertrophic buccal tonsils or may be associated with cystic glandular structures (so-called lymphoepithelial cysts).[43] The most prominent of these benign lymphoid proliferations are designated **lymphoid polyps** or **pseudolymphomas.** Saltzstein[45] has reviewed the microscopic criteria for the differential diagnosis with malignant lymphomas.

Malignant lymphoma most commonly occurs in the tonsil and in Waldeyer's ring of lymphoid tissue within the pharynx. It forms bulky masses that are very soft and cellular. We have seen it arising from the base of the tongue and the upper and lower gingivae (Fig. 166). The lesion

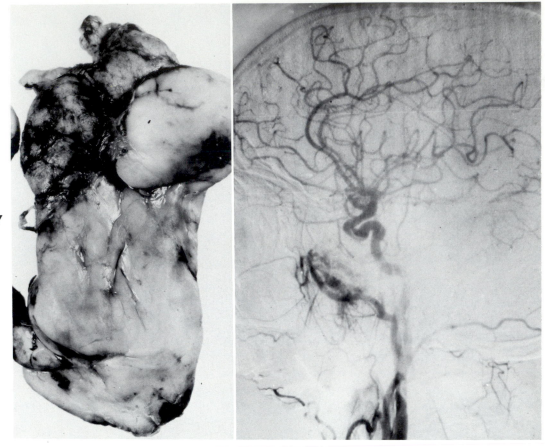

Fig. 167 Large nasopharyngeal angiofibroma in 12-year-old boy. (WU neg. 71-9827.)
Fig. 168 Nasopharyngeal angiofibroma in 13-year-old boy well demonstrated by subtraction arteriography. (WU neg. 67-9774.)

shows the microscopic patterns that are seen in malignant lymphomas elsewhere. Both lymphocytic and histiocytic types are common. Conversely, Hodgkin's disease presenting primarily as an oral cavity tumor is exceptional. In about two-thirds of the oral lymphomas, there is cervical lymph node involvement. In a series of 225 patients reported by Banfi et al.,[42] lymphangiography revealed retroperitoneal lymph node involvement in one-third. Irradiation therapy is capable of sterilizing both the intraoral tumor and the involved cervical lymph nodes.

Plasmacytomas can occur in the soft tissues of the oral cavity, although not so commonly as in the upper air passages.[44] It is important to differentiate them from the much more common plasma cell granulomas of reactive nature. The latter are composed of mature plasma cells, have an admixture of other inflammatory cells, and are associated with fibrosis.

Tumors of melanocytic system

Both *ephelis* and *lentigo* can present as solitary lesions of the lip. They are characterized by hyperpigmentation of the basal layer, associated in the latter with elongation of the rete ridges. If multiple, the possibility of gastrointestinal polyposis (Peutz-Jeghers syndrome) should be investigated.

All varieties of *melanocytic nevi* occur. Trodahl et al.[48] collected three junctional, thirty compound, thirty-two intramucosal

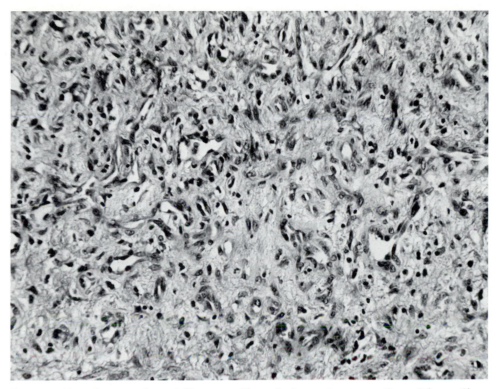

Fig. 169 Nasopharyngeal angiofibroma with typical prominent vessels and loose fibro-blastic stroma. (×250; WU neg. 62-3620.)

(the equivalent of the cutaneous intra-dermal), and six blue nevi. The lips are the most common site of involvement. On the other hand, malignant melanoma pre-fers the palate and gingiva. Both pig-mented and amelanotic varieties occur.[46] An intramucosal lesion microscopically in-distinguishable from Hutchinson's freckle of the skin has been discussed by Robin-son and Hukill.[47]

Nasopharyngeal angiofibroma

The nasopharyngeal angiofibroma occurs almost exclusively in males between 10 and 25 years of age.[49a] It arises from the wall of the nasopharyngeal cavity or posterior nasal space. It can grow to occlude the involved nares completely (Fig. 167). It may protrude below the free edge of the soft palate, extend into the antrum, and grow to the external orifice of the nares, posteriorly into the nasopharynx, or even into the orbit and cranial cavity.[49] McGav-

ran et al.[50] studied thirty cases. A total of thirty-eight recurrences were seen in seventeen patients. Of these, thirty-five were manifested within twelve months, and none occurred after two years. Selective carotid arteriograms are helpful in deter-mining the gross confines of the tumor (Fig. 168).

Nasopharyngeal angiofibromas contain abnormal irregular vessels sometimes hav-ing smooth muscle in their wall. The larg-est vessels are located at the base of the lesion (Fig. 169). There may be a con-siderable number of mast cells. Electron microscopy shows peculiar intranuclear dense bodies in stromal cells (Fig. 170). There is no doubt that some large lesions spontaneously regress after puberty. The tumors tend to bleed severely on manipu-lation and biopsy. Since they occur almost exclusively in young males, they are prob-ably influenced by some unknown endo-crine factor.[51]

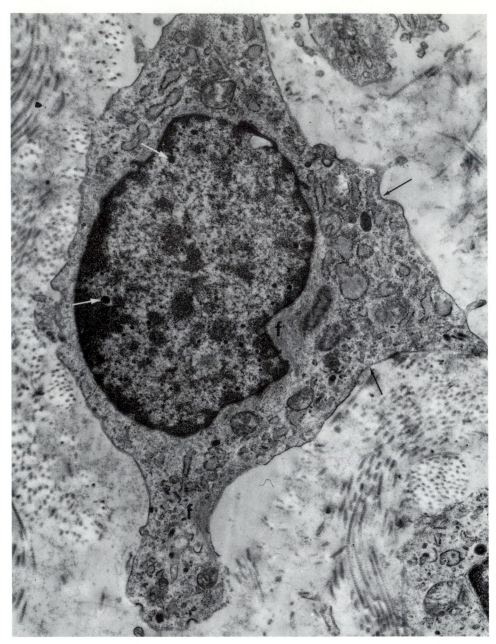

Fig. 170 Stromal cells in nasopharyngeal angiofibromas have peculiar multiple nuclear dense bodies (white arrows), nature of which is unknown. Their cytoplasm is fibrocytic in type, with fine filaments, **f,** and pinocytic vesicles along plasma membrane (black arrows). (Uranyl acetate–lead citrate; ×9,000.)

Other tumors

Hemangioma and lymphangioma are vascular malformations that frequently occur on the tongue or gingiva in children or young adults. We have seen such lesions on the tongue form soft cystic masses so large that they interfered with speech and mastication. Microscopically, they show endothelial-lined spaces, some of which contain blood. Treatment by excision or sodium morrhuate injection depends upon size and location.

Smooth muscle tumors of the oral cavity were reviewed by MacDonald.[55] Most leiomyomas are located in the tongue, whereas leiomyosarcomas prefer the cheek region.

Rhabdomyomas have a special predilection for the oral cavity and neck. Both solitary and multiple forms have been observed.[52]

We have seen two **neurilemomas** involving the tongue and several **neurofibromas** beneath the epithelium of the pharynx.[56] Multiple mucosal neuromas, microscopically resembling traumatic neuromas, occur in the lips, tongue, conjunctiva, and nasal and laryngeal mucosa as part of a familial syndrome whose other components are pheochromocytoma and medullary carcinoma of the thyroid gland.[53]

Granular cell tumor, a lesion of disputed histogenesis, may arise within the tongue and cause prominent epithelial alterations that may be confused with cancer (p. 193). A lesion that is indistinguishable from granular cell tumor by light and electron microscopy is seen occasionally in the gingiva of newborn infants and is designated **congenital epulis.**[54]

Metastatic tumors may present as primary intraoral masses. The gingiva is the classical location, with or without bony involvement. We have seen metastatic renal cell carcinoma masquerading clinically and microscopically as a pyogenic granuloma.

REFERENCES
Introduction

1 Gorlin, R. J., and Goldman, H. M.: Thoma's Oral pathology, St. Louis, 1970, The C. V. Mosby Co., vols. I and II.

Biopsy and cytology

2 Bhaskar, S. N.: Oral pathology in the dental office: survey of 20,575 biopsy specimens, J. Am. Dent. Assoc. **76:**761-766, 1968.
3 Giunta, J., Meyer, I., and Shklar, G.: The accuracy of the oral biopsy in the diagnosis of cancer, Oral Surg. Oral Med. Oral Path. **28:**552-556, 1969.
4 Shklar, G., Cataldo, E., and Meyer, I.: Reliability of cytologic smear in diagnosis of oral cancer; a controlled study, Arch. Otolaryngol. **91:**158-160, 1970.

Congenital abnormalities

5 Cataldo, E., and Berkman, M. D.: Cysts of the oral mucosa in newborns, Am. J. Dis. Child. **116:**44-48, 1968.
6 Gorlin, R. J., and Jirasek, J. E.: Oral cysts containing gastric or intestinal mucosa; an unusual embryological accident or heterotopia, Arch. Otolaryngol. **91:**594-597, 1970.
7 Meyer, I.: Dermoid cysts (dermoids) of the floor of the mouth, Oral Surg. Oral Med. Oral Path. **8:**1149-1164, 1955.
8 Simpson, H. E.: White sponge nevus, J. Oral Surg. **24:**463-466, 1966.
9 Zarem, H. A., Gray, G. F., Jr., and Morehead, D.: Heterotopic brain in the nasopharynx and soft palate, Surgery **61:**483-486, 1967.

Reactive processes

10 Ackerman, L. V., and McGavran, M. H.: Proliferating benign and malignant epithelial lesions of the oral cavity, J. Oral Surg. **16:**400-413, 1958.
11 Barker, D. S., and Lucas, R. B.: Localized fibrous overgrowths of the oral mucosa, Br. J. Oral Surg. **5:**86-92, 1967.
12 Bhaskar, S. N., Beasley, J. D., and Cutright, D. E.: Inflammatory papillary hyperplasia of the oral mucosa: report of 341 cases, J. Am. Dent. Assoc. **81:**949-952, 1970.
13 Bodine, R. L.: Oral lesions caused by ill-fitting dentures, J. Prosthet. Dent. **21:**580-588, 1969.
14 Giansanti, J. S., and Waldron, C. A.: Peripheral giant cell granuloma: review of 720 cases, J. Oral Surg. **27:**787-791, 1969.
15 Kerr, D. A.: Granuloma pyogenicum, Oral Surg. **4:**158-176, 1951.
16 Lattanand, A., Johnson, W. C., and Graham, J. H.: Mucous cyst (mucocele); a clinicopathologic and histochemical study, Arch. Dermatol. **101:**673-678, 1970.
17 MacVicar, J., and Dunn, M. F.: Pregnancy tumour of the gums, J. Obstet. Gynaecol. Br. Commonw. **76:**260-263, 1969.
18 Pindborg, J. J., Poulsen, H. E., and Zachariah, J.: Oral epithelial changes in thirty Indians with oral cancer and submucous fibrosis, Cancer **20:**1141-1146, 1967.

Specific infections

19 Bennett, D. E.: Histoplasmosis of the oral cavity and larynx; a clinicopathologic study, Arch. Intern. Med. **120:**417-427, 1967.
20 Meyer, I., and Abbey, L. M.: Relationship of syphilis to primary carcinoma of tongue, Oral Surg. Oral Med. Oral Path. **30:**678-681, 1970.

21 Oppenheim, H., Livingston, C. S., Nixon, J. W., and Miller, C. D.: Streptomycin therapy in oral tuberculosis, Oral Surg. Oral Med. Oral Path. 4:1389-1405, 1951.

Tumors

Tumors of surface epithelium

22 Ackerman, L. V.: Verrucous carcinoma of the oral cavity, Surgery 23:670-678, 1948.

23 Ackerman, L. V., and Johnson, R.: Present-day concepts of intraoral histopathology, Proc. Second Natl. Cancer Conf. 1:403-414, 1952.

24 Anderson, D. L.: Cause and prevention of lip cancer, J. Can. Dent. Assoc. 37:138-142, 1971.

25 Byars, L. T., and Anderson, R.: Multiple cancers of the oral cavity, Am. Surg. 18:386-391, 1952.

26 Einhorn, J., and Wersäll, J.: Incidence of oral carcinoma in patients with leukoplakia of the oral mucosa, Cancer 20:2189-2193, 1967.

27 Gorlin, R. J., and Peterson, W. C., Jr.: Warty dyskeratoma; a note concerning its occurrence on the oral mucosa, Arch. Dermatol. 95:292-293, 1967.

28 Green, G. W., Jr., and Bernier, J.: Spindle cell squamous carcinoma of the lip; report of four cases, Oral Surg. Oral Med. Oral Path. 12:1008-1016, 1959.

29 King, O. H.: Intraoral leukoplakia? Cancer 17:131-136, 1964.

30 Kraus, F. T., and Perez-Mesa, C.: Verrucous carcinoma; clinical and pathologic study of 105 cases involving oral cavity, larynx and genitalia, Cancer 19:26-38, 1966.

31 Lin, H.-S., Lin, C.-S., Yeh, S., and Tu, S.-M.: Fine structure of nasopharyngeal carcinoma with special reference to the anaplastic type, Cancer 23:390-405, 1969.

32 Pindborg, J. J., Jølst, O., Renstrup, G., and Roed-Petersen, B.: Studies in oral leukoplakia: a preliminary report on the period prevalence of malignant transformation in leukoplakia based on a follow-up study of 248 patients, J. Am. Dent. Assoc. 76:767-771, 1968.

33 Renstrup, G.: Leukoplakia of the oral cavity; a clinical and histopathologic study, Acta Odontol. Scand. 16:99-111, 1958.

34 Renstrup, G.: Occurrence of Candida in oral leukoplakias, Acta Pathol. Microbiol. Scand. [B] 78:421-424, 1970.

35 Slaughter, D. P.: Multicentric origin of intra-oral carcinoma, Surgery 20:113-146, 1946.

36 Teoh, T. B.: Epidermoid carcinoma of the nasopharynx among Chinese: a study of 31 necropsies, J. Pathol. Bacteriol. 73:451-465, 1957.

37 Vaeth, J. M.: Nasopharyngeal malignant tumors: 82 consecutive patients treated in a period of twenty-two years, Radiology 74:364-372, 1960.

Tumors of minor salivary glands

38 Chaudhry, A. P., Vickers, R. A., and Gorlin, R. J.: Intraoral minor salivary gland tumors; an analysis of 1414 cases, Oral Surg. Oral Med. Oral Path. 14:1194-1226, 1961.

39 Chisholm, D. M., and Mason, D. K.: Labial salivary gland biopsy in Sjögren's disease, J. Clin. Pathol. 21:656-660, 1968.

40 Eneroth, C.-M.: Incidence and prognosis of salivary-gland tumors at different sites; a study of parotid, submandibular and palatal tumors in 2632 patients, Acta Otolaryngol. (Stockholm) 263:174-178, 1970.

41 Warwick, W. J., Bernard, B., and Meskin, L. H.: The involvement of the labial mucous salivary gland in patients with cystic fibrosis, Pediatrics 34:621-628, 1964.

Tumors of lymphoid tissue

42 Banfi, A., Bonadonna, G., Carnevali, G., Molinari, R., Monfardini, R., and Salvini, E.: Lymphoreticular sarcomas with primary involvement of Waldeyer's ring; clinical evaluation of 225 cases, Cancer 26:341-351, 1970.

43 Bernier, J. L., and Bhaskar, S. N.: Lymphoepithelial lesions of salivary glands; histogenesis and classification based on 186 cases, Cancer 11:1156-1179, 1958.

44 Ewing, M. R., and Foote, F. W., Jr.: Plasma-cell tumors of the mouth and upper air passages, Cancer 5:499-513, 1952.

45 Saltzstein, S. L.: Extranodal malignant lymphomas and pseudolymphomas. In Sommers, S. C., editor: Pathology Annual, vol. 4, New York, 1969, Appleton-Century-Crofts, pp. 159-184.

Tumors of melanocytic system

46 Chaudhry, A. P., Hampel, A., and Gorlin, R. J.: Primary malignant melanoma of the oral cavity: a review of 105 cases, Cancer 11:923-928, 1958.

47 Robinson, L., and Hukill, P.: Hutchinson's melanotic freckle in oral mucous membrane, Cancer 26:297-302, 1970.

48 Trodahl, J. N., and Sprague, W. G.: Benign and malignant melanocytic lesions of the oral mucosa; an analysis of 135 cases, Cancer 25:812-823, 1970.

Nasopharyngeal angiofibroma

49 Harma, R. A.: Nasopharyngeal angiofibroma, Acta Otolaryngol. (Stockholm) 146(suppl.):1-74, 1958.

49a Hicks, J. L., and Nelson, J. F.: Juvenile nasopharyngeal angiofibroma, Oral Surg. Oral Med. Oral Path. 35:807-817, 1973.

50 McGavran, M. G., Sessions, D. G., Dorfman, R. D., Davis, D. O., and Ogura, J. H.: Naso-

pharyngeal angiofibroma, Arch. Otolaryngol. 90:94-104, 1969.

51 Sternberg, S. S.: Pathology of juvenile naso-pharyngeal angiofibroma—a lesion of adolescent males, Cancer 7:15-28, 1954.

Other tumors

52 Assor, D., and Thomas, J. R.: Multifocal rhabdomyoma; report of a case, Arch. Otolaryngol. 90:489-491, 1969.

53 Gorlin, R. J., Sedano, H. O., Vickers, R. A., and Červenka, J.: Multiple mucosal neuromas, pheochromocytoma and medullary carcinoma of the thyroid—a syndrome, Cancer 22:293-299, 1968.

54 Kay, S., Elzay, R. P., and Wilson, M. A.: Ultrastructural observations on a gingival granular cell tumor (congenital epulis), Cancer 27:674-680, 1971.

55 MacDonald, D. G.: Smooth muscle tumours of the mouth, Br. J. Oral Surg. 6:207-214, 1969.

56 Oberman, H. A., and Sullenger, G.: Neurogenous tumors of the head and neck, Cancer 20:1992-2001, 1967.

5 Mandible and maxilla

Introduction

The mandible and the maxilla are discussed here because of the specialized nature of the lesions that occur within them and the intimate relationship of the lesions within the oral cavity to these bony structures. Salivary gland tumors and squamous carcinoma within the oral cavity may secondarily involve the maxilla or the mandible, producing destruction of bone.

Osteomyelitis

Acute and chronic forms of osteomyelitis occur. The focal chronic variety involves the alveolus and usually is secondary to a dental infection.[1] It can be erroneously diagnosed clinically, radiographically, and microscopically as fibrous dysplasia or ossifying fibroma.

Simple bone cyst

Simple bone cyst usually occurs in young patients. We prefer the designation *simple bone cyst* to that of traumatic bone cyst or hemorrhagic bone cyst because there is a history of previous trauma in only one-half of the patients and the content of the cyst is hemorrhagic in only a small proportion of cases.[2] Jaffe[3] believes it represents the counterpart in the jaw of the lesion of long bones designated as solitary (or unicameral) bone cyst. It should be differentiated from the so-called "latent bone cavity," a symptomless open cavity situated below and behind the inferior dental canal near the angle of the mandible and often containing salivary gland tissue.[2]

We know of an 11-year-old girl who, following a tooth extraction, developed swelling of the mandible over a ten-day interval. Roentgenographic examination demonstrated a large area of radiolucent destruction of the mandible (Fig. 171). Unfortunately, hemiresection of the mandible was done because of an erroneous clinical and radiographic diagnosis of ameloblastoma. Grossly, the cystic space was filled with brownish yellow material and brown fluid. Microscopic examination showed a shell of the cortex of the mandible. The periosteum adjacent to the dead bone showed prominent intramembranous

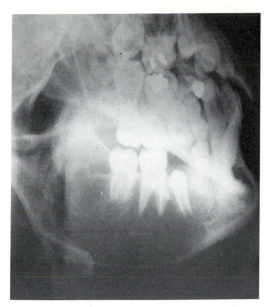

Fig. 171 Traumatic cyst of mandible in 11-year-old girl. Note thin shell of remaining mandible. (WU neg. 52-3857.)

new bone formation (see Fig. 984). Cure could have been effected by unroofing the lesion and evacuating the blood.

Giant cell lesions

True giant cell tumors of the mandible and maxilla are exceptional.[5] Pathogenetically, giant cell lesions of these bones are heterogeneous. The most common type has been referred to as giant cell reparative granuloma of the jaw by Jaffe[6] (Fig. 172). This disease affects children, mainly girls, and occurs almost twice as frequently in the mandible as in the maxilla.[7, 9] It produces a cystic lesion of the bone which, microscopically, shows large numbers of giant cells, rather cellular vascular stroma, and often new bone formation (Fig. 173). The osteoclast-like giant cells have a patchy distribution usually associated with areas of hemorrhage.

Tombridge[8] presented good evidence that the bilateral familial lesion occurring in children and young adults and causing usually bilateral smooth mandibular enlargement represented giant cell reparative granuloma. This lesion is often called "cherubism" because of the clinical appearance of the patient.

Giant cell reparative granuloma cannot be differentiated on morphologic grounds from the "brown tumor" of hyperparathyroidism. Therefore, the presence of a giant cell lesion of the mandibular and maxillary region requires that hyperparathyroidism be ruled out.[4] In our experience, the recurrence rate for giant cell reparative granuloma treated by curettage has been 69%.[4a]

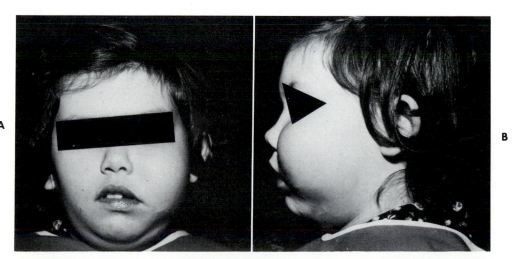

Fig. 172 **A,** Young girl with extensive giant cell reparative granuloma almost completely replacing maxilla. **B,** Four years after operation, patient is without deformity. (**A,** WU neg. 58-268; **B,** WU neg. 58-267; **A** and **B,** courtesy Dr. A. J. Murphy, Pittsburgh, Pa.)

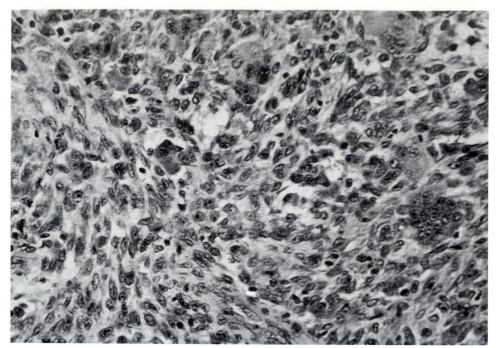

Fig. 173 Giant cell reparative granuloma with highly cellular fibrous tissue and collections of giant cells. Lesion occurred in maxilla of 10½-year-old white girl. (×30; WU neg. 62-1005.)

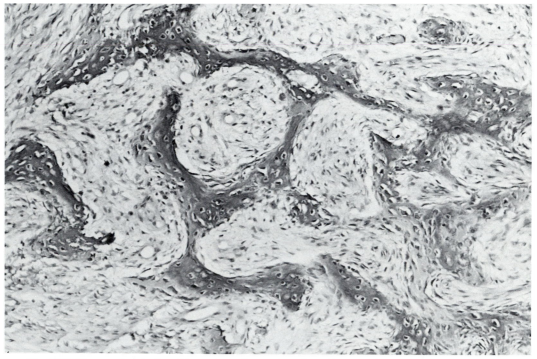

Fig. 174 Fibrous dysplasia of jaw. Irregular trabeculae of woven bone can be seen arising directly from fibrous stroma. Note absence of osteoblastic rimming. (×120; slide contributed by Dr. A. Schmaman, Johannesburg, South Africa.)

Fibro-osseous lesions

Benign jaw lesions composed of an admixture of fibrous and osseous tissue can be divided into three main types: fibrous dysplasia, ossifying fibroma (fibrous osteoma), and cementifying fibroma. There is still considerable controversy about the relationship among these three conditions.[13] Many authors believe that ossifying fibroma is simply a variant of fibrous dysplasia, a view with which we disagree. On the other hand, we have seen some cases with features of both ossifying fibroma and cementifying fibroma.[14, 18] Be as it may, we think there are enough differences among these three conditions to justify their separation.

Fibrous dysplasia represents maturation arrest of bone at the woven bone stage. Trabeculae of bone do not show rimming by osteoblasts, and they show no evidence of lamellar transformation[15, 17] (Fig. 174).

Ossifying fibroma occurs in young persons, causing diffuse enlargement of the mandible or maxilla. Radiographically, there is an increased density if considerable bone formation is present (Fig. 175). Decreased density results if the lesion is predominantly fibrous.[11] Microscopically, bone trabeculae rimmed by orderly rows of osteoblasts and many immature trabeculae bordered by lamellar osteoid are seen. The picture varies from many spicules of new bone with a cellular vascular stroma to very dense bone.[10] The more cellular types may be incorrectly diagnosed as osteosarcoma. In the past, Phemister and Grimson[16] recognized fibrous osteoma as benign and treated it conservatively. Smith and Zavaleta[19] demonstrated good correlation between the age of the patient and the maturation of the lesion. We have seen a patient with a long time interval between surgical excisions. The first lesion was highly cellular and very active and could easily have been diagnosed as a malignant tumor. The second lesion showed mature, thick bone trabeculae in a relatively avascular stroma.

Cementifying fibroma forms a large well-defined radiolucent mass that gradually becomes radiopaque. It may involve the maxilla as well as the mandible, but the commonest location is the mandibular premolar or molar region. It should be separated from the benign cementoblastoma (true cementoma), which usually involves

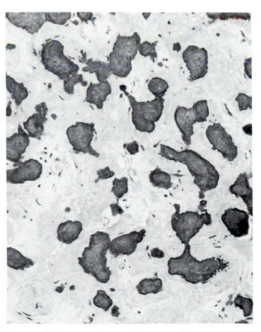

Fig. 176 Cementifying fibroma showing innumerable foci of cementum regularly scattered in background of fibrohyaline stroma. (×120; slide contributed by Dr. A. Schmaman, Johannesburg, South Africa.)

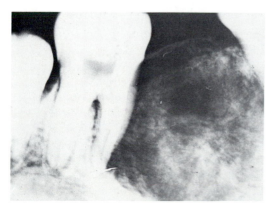

Fig. 175 Ossifying fibroma in 17-year-old black girl. Note sharp border of lesion. (Courtesy Dr. C. A. Waldron, Atlanta, Ga.)

the periapical region of anterior mandibular teeth and which is discussed under odontogenic tumor below. Microscopically, cementifying fibroma does not show osteoblastic rimming. Lacunae are not present (Fig. 176). The distinguishing feature is the presence of PAS-positive droplet cementum. A probably related lesion of similar microscopic appearance and most commonly located in the mandibular incisor region of middle-aged women is sometimes referred to as *periapical cemental dysplasia* or *periapical fibrous dysplasia*.[12]

Epithelial cysts

Epithelial-lined cysts of the maxilla and mandible may arise as a result of a developmental defect or, more commonly, secondary to inflammation of the dental pulp.[30, 31, 35] The former may arise either as a result of a malformation of the tooth-developing apparatus or from entrapment of primitive epithelium when the several processes of the face fuse.[25, 28, 36] We use the following classification, adopted by the World Health Organization.[32]

A Developmental
  1 Odontogenic
    a Primordial cyst (keratocyst)
    b Gingival cyst
    c Eruption cyst
    d Dentigerous (follicular) cyst
  2 Nonodontogenic
    a Nasopalatine duct (incisive canal) cyst
    b Globulomaxillary cyst
    c Nasolabial (nasoalveolar) cyst
B Inflammatory
  1 Radicular cyst

In the evaluation of these lesions, it is essential to be familiar with the clinical and radiographic findings. The microscopic appearance alone is practically never diagnostic.

Primordial cyst (keratocyst)

The primordial cyst usually has no special relationship with a tooth, although in some cases it may be present in an area of a missing tooth. It has been reported in patients from 8 to 83 years of age, with a mean age of 32 years. The most common location is the posterior body and ramus of the mandible.[34] Clinically, there is swelling in about one-half of the cases. Occasionally, pain and limitation of function are also present. Radiographically, it presents as a unilocular or multilocular radiolucent lesion with a distinct radiopaque boundary.[23] The cystic spaces may have a scalloped border. Microscopically, the cyst is lined by stratified squamous epithelium with no rete processes and surrounded by a thin fibrous capsule sometimes containing islands of odontogenic epithelium and accessory cysts. The lumen is filled with desquamated keratinocytes. Secondary inflammation may be present.

Multiple primordial cysts are a component of the *multiple nevoid basal cell carcinoma syndrome,* which is inherited as an autosomal dominant trait and is characterized by multiple basal cell nevi of skin, jaw cysts, skeletal anomalies (particularly bifid ribs), a characteristic facies, and hyporesponsiveness to parathormone.[29] Medulloblastoma has been a complication in some of these cases.

The so-called *developmental lateral periodontal cyst* is considered a specific type of primordial cyst.[37] It is seen most frequently in the cuspid-premolar area of the mandible but can occur as far anteriorly as the lateral incisor and as far posteriorly as the first molar. It also has been reported in the maxilla. It typically occurs in relation to the lateral margin of a vital tooth.

Primordial cysts are treated by curettage or enucleation. The recurrence rate is high, in the range of 25%.

Gingival cyst

The gingival cyst is primarily a soft tissue lesion that arises from extraalveolar remnants of the dental lamina.[21] It occurs in early to middle adulthood and presents as a smooth-surfaced hard elevation of the gingivae. The radiographs are usually negative, but on occasion a cup-shaped depression of the alveolar ridge may be evident. Microscopically, the cyst is lined by stratified squamous epithelium, often keratinized. The lumen contains a proteinaceous fluid. Inflammation is usually absent. The gingival cyst is easily enucleated, and recurrence is rare.

A similar lesion, sometimes designated as *dental lamina cyst* or *Epstein's pearl,* is often seen in the soft tissues overlying the tooth-bearing areas in newborn infants. The maxillary alveolar ridge is most commonly affected. The process is self-limited, disappears within the first few months of life, and requires no therapy.

Eruption cyst

The eruption cyst presents as a dome-shaped bluish swelling in the alveolus, in an area where a tooth will erupt. Microscopically, it is lined by stratified squamous epithelium. It may be regarded as a type of dentigerous cyst.

Dentigerous (follicular) cyst

The dentigerous cyst is the most common developmental odontogenic cyst. It arises

in the enamel organ of an unerupted tooth. It is usually discovered during the second and third decades and is asymptomatic unless secondarily infected. If left untreated, it can attain large size. The most common locations are the mandibular third molars, maxillary cuspids, maxillary third molars, and mandibular second premolars. Radiographically, it appears as a well-defined radiolucency around the crown of an unerupted tooth (Fig. 177). The larger cysts are rarely multilocular. The lining stratified squamous epithelium is thicker than in the primordial cyst, but rete processes are unusual in the absence of inflammation. Mucus-producing cells and ciliated cells are sometimes present. Islands of odontogenic epithelium are often seen around the main cyst. The treatment is curettage. Recurrence is unusual. Dentigerous cysts have the potentiality, only rarely expressed, to develop into ameloblastoma and epidermoid carcinoma.[24, 26, 38]

Nasopalatine duct (incisive canal) cyst

The nasopalatine duct cyst is the most common nonodontogenic epithelial cyst of the jaws.[20] It is rarely observed before the third decade. It is found in the midline of the maxilla, immediately behind the central incisors and superior to the incisive papilla. It presents radiographically as a well-defined, round, ovoid, or heart-shaped radiolucency as large as 4 cm in diameter. It may be present as a lump in the palate but is most often discovered during a routine radiographic investigation. The lining may be of stratified squamous epithelium, pseudostratified ciliated columnar epithelium, or a mixture of both. The fibrous capsule characteristically contains large nerves and vessels and sometimes even mucous glands and adipose tissue. Enucleation is curative.

Globulomaxillary cyst

The globulomaxillary cyst has been reported in all age groups from the second to the fifth decades.[22] It is located beneath the maxillary lateral incisor and cuspid and is symptomatic only if secondarily

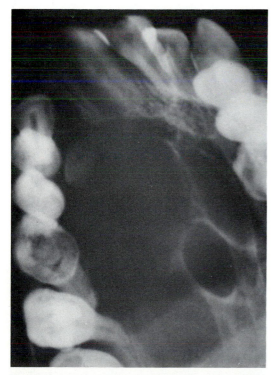

Fig. 177 Large dentigerous cyst in maxilla that arose from enamel organ of small supernumerary tooth seen in anterior portion of cystic cavity. (WU neg. 62-8761.)

infected. Radiographically, it presents as an inverted, pear-shaped radiolucency with distinct margins. Microscopically, it may be lined by stratified squamous cuboidal or ciliated columnar epithelium, with or without rete peg formation. Odontogenic epithelial islands may be present within the cyst wall. Treatment is by enucleation.[27]

Nasolabial (nasoalveolar) cyst

The nasolabial cyst is situated on the alveolar process near the base of the nostril.[33] It is primarily a soft tissue lesion but may result in erosion of the maxilla. The epithelial lining may be squamous, pseudostratified, ciliated columnar, or a mixture.

Radicular cyst

The radicular cyst, also designated as apical periodontal, is the most common of all of the epithelial cysts of the jaws.[30] It arises as a result of inflammation and eventually necrosis of the dental pulp. Most frequently, it represents a sequel of dental caries, although it may result also from trauma. It can occur in all age groups but is more frequent during the third and fourth decades. The most common location is the maxilla, particularly in connection with both central and lateral incisors. Radiographically, it presents as a well-circumscribed radiolucency at the apex of the affected tooth (Fig. 178).

Microscopically, it is lined by stratified squamous epithelium, the thickness of which varies according to the degree of inflammation present. Rete peg formation is frequently seen. Mucous or ciliated cells may be present. Peculiar double-contoured hyaline bodies of uncertain nature are sometimes seen embedded in the epithelium. The inflammatory infiltrate in the wall may be acute or chronic. Aggregates of cholesterol crystals, foamy macrophages, multinucleated giant cells, and plasma cells are common. The cyst usually is shelled out easily from the surrounding bone, and recurrences are rare. When the affected tooth is extracted, the cyst is often re-

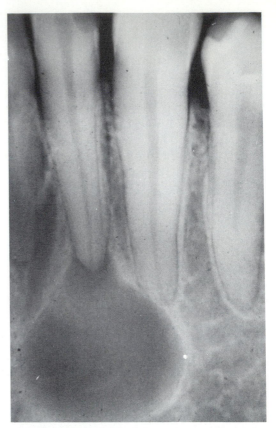

Fig. 178 Radicular periodontal cyst demonstrating continuity with pulp canal of nonvital tooth. (WU neg. 62-8855.)

moved with the root. Neoplastic transformation into epidermoid carcinoma has been reported, although this is exceptional.

Radicular cysts left within the substance of the jaw after the offending tooth has been extracted are sometimes designated as *residual cysts*.

Odontogenic tumors

Some of the lesions included in the category of odontogenic tumors are probably hamartomas rather than true neoplasms. In some, the odontogenic origin is disputed. They are considered together in this chapter because they present similar clinical and/or pathologic features. Odontogenic tumors vary markedly in appearance from case to case, largely as a result of different degrees of induction exerted by the odontogenic epithelium. The tumor

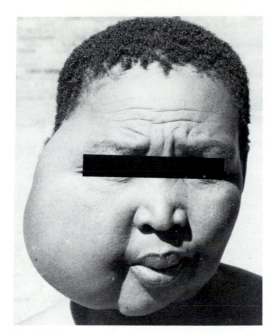

Fig. 179 Recurrent ameloblastoma following limited surgical excision. (Courtesy Dr. A. Schmaman, Johannesburg, South Africa.)

types described below represent the better defined categories, atlhough it should be recognized that cases with intermediate features are often encountered, suggesting the existence of a continuous morphologic spectrum.[51, 59]

Ameloblastoma

The ameloblastoma is a true neoplasm of the odontogenic epithelium that mimics the morphology of the developing tooth. It occurs in a wide age range of patients but most often during the fourth and fifth decades. It shows a slight predilection for males and is usually found in the molar area of the mandible. The clinical duration may range from a few weeks to fifty years, 5.8 years being the average period.[70, 76] Clinically, it begins as a painless swelling that may ulcerate and produce limitation of function in later stages (Fig. 179). Radiographically, this lesion may manifest as a unilocular or multilocular radiolucency usually having well-defined margins[74] (Fig. 180). An embedded tooth may be present.

Microscopically, the ameloblastoma is composed of epithelial strands or islands of varying size. On the periphery of these islands are tall, columnar, ameloblast-like cells with their nuclei polarized toward the basement membrane. Also present are central cells of a spinous appearance that resemble stellate reticulum. These central cells may degenerate, leaving cystic spaces, may cornify to the level of forming acanthomatous islands, or may alter till they form granular cells. These various histologic manifestations can be given little prognostic significance, since they can all sometimes be seen in a single example of the disease. Pindborg and Kramer[68] described the different patterns of growth as follicular, plexiform, acanthomatous, basal cell, and granular cell types (Figs. 181 to 183). Variations also are prominent at an electron microscopic level.[61] The granular cell type closely resembles the appearance of the granular cell tumor, except for the peripheral lining of clearly identifiable ameloblasts.[45] The epithelial nature of the granular cells was demonstrated ultrastructurally by Navarrete and Smith.[62] It is likely that the so-called *congenital epulis of infancy* also represents a granular degeneration of odontogenic epithelium.[48, 58]

The early stages in the development of ameloblastoma were described by Vickers and Gorlin.[79] Ameloblastoma is a locally aggressive disease that is resistant to therapy and prone to recurrence.[54] The usual therapy is curettage, resection, or hemisection. Recurrences have been reported in about one-third of the surgically treated patients. Radiotherapy is ineffective. There have been isolated reports of ameloblastoma extending to distant sites, such as the lung. For the most part, these "metastases" have been interpreted as the result of aspiration of tumor to the lung, but in a very few instances metastases have been found in the regional lymph nodes.[55, 56, 71] The latter need to be differentiated from intraosseous epidermoid carcinoma, carcinomas of salivary gland origin, and metastatic carcinoma (Fig. 184).

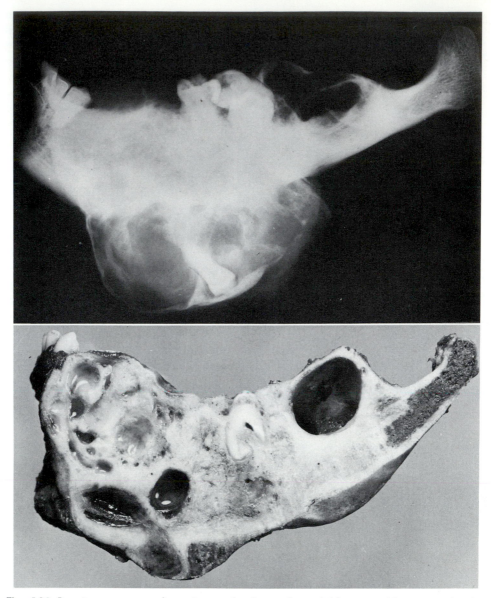

Fig. 180 Roentgenogram and specimen of advanced ameloblastoma. Note extensive involvement of mandible with characteristic multiloculation. (WU negs. 52-4760 and 52-4635.)

Calcifying epithelial odontogenic tumor

The calcifying epithelial odontogenic tumor has a growth potential and biology similar to the ameloblastoma. The initial series of cases was limited to males, but later reports have indicated no sex predilection. This disease occurs in the same age group as the ameloblastoma and is most prevalent in the molar area of the mandible. It is often associated with the coronal aspect of an unerupted tooth. Radiographically, it appears as a well or poorly defined radiolucency with a varying degree of radiodensity (Fig. 185).

Microscopically, the lesion is composed of sheets or islands of polyhedral, often densely eosinophilic, epithelial cells. Intercellular bridges are prominent. Often these epithelial cells demonstrate considerable pleomorphism and hyperchromasia.[66, 67, 78] Scat-

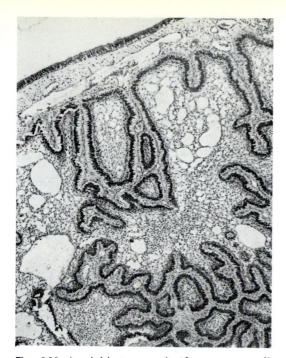

Fig. 181 Ameloblastoma, plexiform type, well differentiated. Similarity to odontogenic epithelium in normal enamel organ is well demonstrated. Early degeneration of stellate reticulum with microcyst formation is apparent. Respiratory epithelium lining maxillary sinus can be seen at upper left. (WU neg. 62-448.)

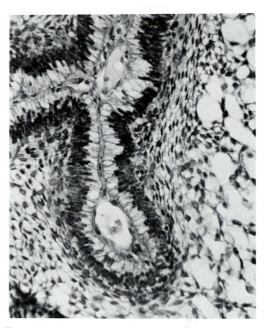

Fig. 182 Same ameloblastoma shown in Fig. 181 under higher power, demonstrating polarized columnar cells resembling ameloblasts that lie adjacent to sparse, mature, fibrous tissue stroma. (WU neg. 62-449.)

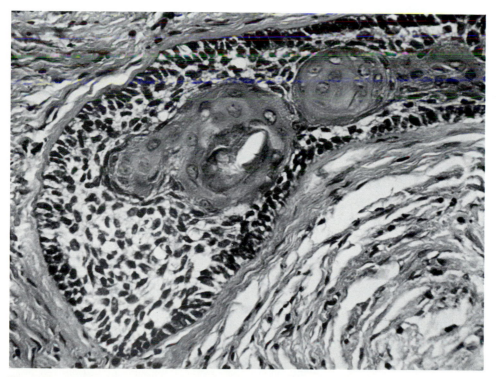

Fig. 183 Acanthomatous type of ameloblastoma. Squamous metaplasia within stellate reticulum must not be mistaken for squamous cell carcinoma. (×400; WU neg. 62-6842.)

tered throughout the tumor are varying numbers of spherical calcified bodies exhibiting Liesegang's phenomenon (Fig. 186). The staining reactions of the material are similar to those of amyloid,[69] but the ultrastructural features are not.[46] This substance probably represents a fibrillar protein secreted by the tumor cells. This tumor is treated by curettage or resection. Recurrence was noted in less than one-fourth of the reported cases.

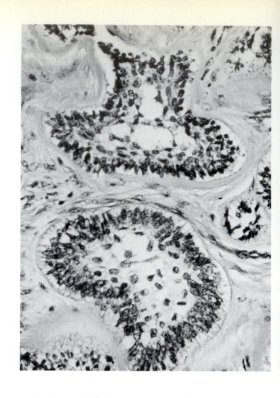

Fig. 184 Metastasizing ameloblastoma reported by Schweitzer and Barnfield,[71] representing one of the surgical excisions, which shows distinctive pattern of usual ameloblastoma with central areas suggesting stellate reticulum and tall peripheral palisaded cells. There is no microscopic evidence of malignancy. (×360; WU neg. 52-4086.)

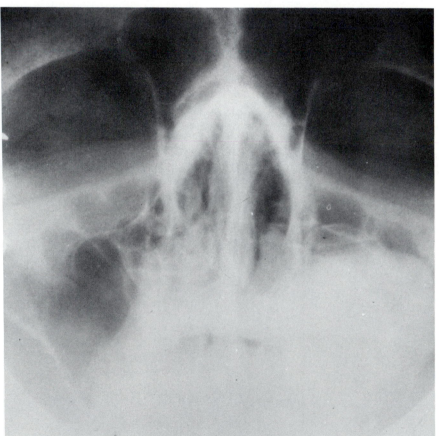

Fig. 185 Calcifying epithelial odontogenic tumor involving maxilla in 58-year-old man. (WU neg. 61-8229.)

Ameloblastic fibroma

The ameloblastic fibroma is a slow-growing, usually asymptomatic, expansile lesion of the jaws composed of both the epithelial and mesenchymal portions of the odontogenic apparatus. This disease occurs primarily in young individuals. It does not exhibit any sexual preference, and the premolar-molar region of the mandible is affected most often. Radiographically, the lesion appears as a well-delineated, often spherical radiolucency.

Microscopically, the ameloblastic fibroma presents as an encapsulated mass composed of cords, strands, and occasionally islands of cuboidal odontogenic epithelium. The connective tissue element is composed of plump, immature, spindle-shaped fibroblasts with an associated fibrillar framework of collagen[72] (Fig. 187). A granular cell variant has been described, as in the ameloblastoma.[49] This lesion is treated by curettage. Recurrence is very unusual even if treatment is incomplete. Exceptionally, the mesenchymal component of an ameloblastic fibroma exhibits malignant cytologic features. This neoplasm is designated as *ameloblastic fibrosarcoma* if pure and as *ameloblastic odontosarcoma* if some dysplastic dentin and enamel also are present.[47, 68]

Adenomatoid odontogenic tumor (adenoameloblastoma)

The adenomatoid odontogenic tumor has been reported in patients ranging in age from 5 to 48 years, most cases occurring in the second decade. The usual site of

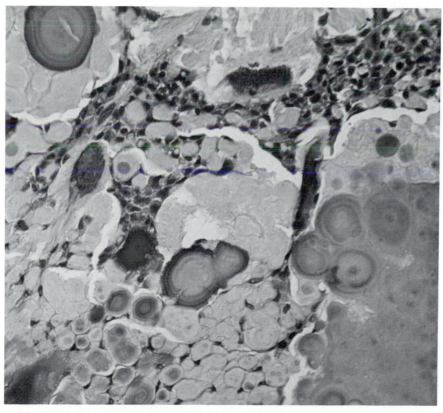

Fig. 186 Features characteristic of calcifying epithelial odontogenic tumor: small cells with hyperchromatic nuclei (upper right), large cells with faint eosinophilic cytoplasm and pyknotic nuclei pressed against cell membrane, and calcifying spherules developing within eosinophilic cytoplasm in various stages (exhibiting Liesegang's phenomenon) coalescing to form large calcific masses (lower right). (×340; WU neg. 63-273.)

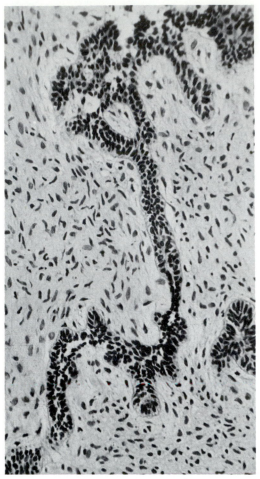

Fig. 187 Ameloblastic fibroma showing narrow strands of odontogenic epithelium within abundance of uniform, immature, fibrous tissue. This type of tumor does not metastasize and only rarely recurs. (Low power; WU neg. 62-7249A.)

occurrence is the anterior portion of the maxilla, especially the cuspid region, but sporadic cases have been reported in other sites.[50, 77] The disease is usually discovered on routine examination. Radiographically, it presents as a well-defined radiolucency often associated with an impacted tooth. Within this radiolucency, a soft tissue outline is occasionally observed, sometimes with small specks of radiodensity. This tumor can also present as an extraosseous soft tissue lesion.

Histologically, the tumor is an encapsulated lesion with a cystic lumen and an attached intraluminal mass composed of ductlike structures made up of columnar or cuboidal epithelial cells, often containing eosinophilic material. Surrounding these ductlike structures and making up the bulk of the lesion are spindle-shaped epithelial cells[40] (Fig. 188). Scattered throughout the epithelium are varying numbers of round and irregularly shaped calcified bodies. The ameloblastic adenomatoid tumor is a slow-growing expansile lesion which, when treated by simple curettage, rarely recurs.[44, 64]

Calcifying odontogenic cyst

The calcifying odontogenic cyst is best considered with the odontogenic tumors rather than with the odontogenic cysts, since its morphology and behavior is more similar to the former.[39, 52] This lesion has been reported to occur in patients ranging from 8 to 71 years of age, the mean age being 24 years. There is no demonstrable sex predilection. The reported cases have been nearly evenly distributed in both jaws, in both anterior and posterior segments. Some cases have occurred as soft tissue lesions with little or no bony involvement. Radiographically, the lesion presents as a well-defined radiolucency, occasionally with flecks of radiodensity.

Microscopically, there is an outer layer of columnar-shaped epithelial cells reminiscent of stellate reticulum. Within these central cells are eosinophilic masses (sometimes called ghost cells) that represent individual cell keratinization. They closely resemble the appearance seen in pilomatrixoma of the skin. In areas in which the integrity of the basal epithelial layer has been interrupted, the masses of keratin frequently elicit a foreign body reaction. In these same areas, a calcified material reminiscent of bone or dentin may be demonstrated. This was designated as dentinoid by Gorlin et al.[52] The calcifying epithelial cyst is treated by curettage. Recurrence is unusual. Generally, this lesion behaves in a benign fashion, but in isolated cases it has demonstrated a growth potential similar to that of ameloblastoma.

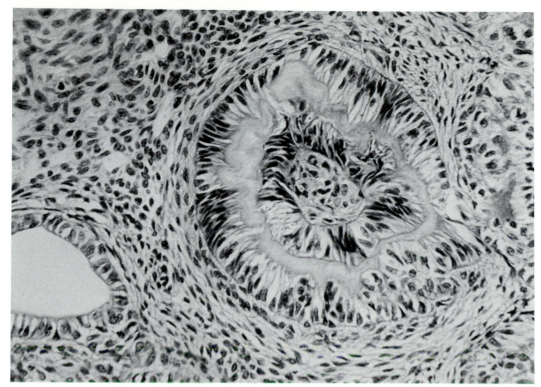

Fig. 188 Adenomatoid odontogenic tumor (adenoameloblastoma). Odontogenic epithelium with ductlike structures and cellular connective tissue stroma are demonstrated. (×300; WU neg. 72-11210; slide contributed by Dr. J. Segura, San José, Costa Rica.)

Dentinoma

Dentinoma is one of the rarest odontogenic neoplasms. It appears on x-ray films as a well-defined radiolucent lesion often containing radiopaque foci.[41] Microscopically, odontogenic epithelium is present in the form of thin irregular strands, surrounded by immature connective tissue, resembling that of the dental papilla.[60] The characteristic feature of this lesion is the presence of a poorly mineralized, dysplastic dentin.[65]

Ameloblastic fibro-odontoma

The ameloblastic fibro-odontoma is basically an odontoma with an associated ameloblastic fibroma. This disease has been reported to occur in patients ranging in age from 6 months to 40 years, 11 years being the mean. There is a slight predilection for the mandible over the maxilla, the pre-molar-molar area being the commonest site. No sex predilection seems to exist.

This disease often presents as a painless swelling, although mild pain, altered occlusion, and delayed eruption are reported in patients with the larger lesions. Radiographically, the lesion appears as a well-defined radiolucency with varied amounts of included radiopaque material. Histologically, it is composed of an odontoma with areas of actively growing ameloblastic fibroma. It is a slow-growing expansile lesion which is nonetheless capable of local destruction and the attainment of huge size. This disease is treated by curettage or other conservative techniques, and recurrence is unusual.

Odontoameloblastoma

Odontoameloblastoma occurs particularly in childhood and is characterized by the presence of enamel, dentin, and an odontogenic epithelium with an appearance similar to that of ameloblastoma.[63] Radiographically, it appears as a well-defined focus of mineralization.[53, 57]

Odontoma

The odontoma is a malformation which is most often diagnosed in the second decade of life and is reported to be twice as common in females as males. Most of the lesions occur in the premolar-molar areas, with a slight preference for the mandible. They are usually asymptomatic, and expansion of the jaws is very unusual. On radiographic examination, the odontoma is found to be a radiolucent lesion with varying levels of radiodensity.

Histologically, the lesion is composed

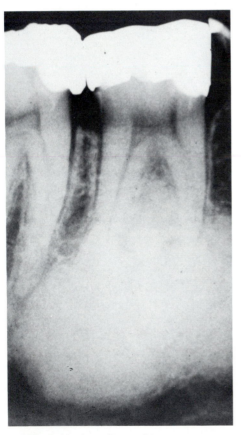

Fig. 189 Typical radiographic appearance of cementoblastoma. Dense, homogeneous mass is seen in continuity with tooth root. (Courtesy Dr. C. A. Waldron, Atlanta, Ga.)

of all of the elements of tooth formation—viz., enamel, dentin, cementum, and dental pulp. When these tissues exist in a random arrangement, the lesion is called a *complex odontoma;* when they are arranged in normal tooth patterns, the designation of *compound odontoma* is used. These lesions are treated by simple curettage, and recurrence is very rare.

Fibroma (odontogenic fibroma)

This lesion is mainly composed of mature fibrous tissue in which islands of odontogenic epithelium are included. In the absence of the epithelial component, the differentiation from other fibroblastic lesions of the jaw becomes difficult.

Myxoma (myxofibroma)

This neoplasm often presents radiographically with a characteristic "soap-bubble" appearance. It is locally invasive and often extends into the soft tissues.[81] This is the reason for its high incidence of local recurrence. Distant metastases do not occur. Microscopically, it consists of rounded and stellate cells floating in an abundant mucoid matrix.[42] Atypical nuclei may be present, but mitoses are exceptional.

Cementoma

Cementoma is a generic term for lesions of the jaw containing cementum-like tissue.[68] Cementifying fibroma and periapical cemental dysplasia have been discussed under fibro-osseous lesions.

Benign cementoblastoma (true cementoma) is a distinctive neoplasm almost always found around the root of a premolar or molar, sometimes fused to it.[43, 80] The mandible is involved more commonly than the maxilla. Radiographically, a central radiopaque mass is seen surrounded by a uniform radiolucent shell (Fig. 189). Microscopically, cementum-like material is deposited throughout. The appearance of this lesion may resemble that of Paget's disease, osteosarcoma, and osteoid osteoma.

Gigantiform cementoma (familial multiple cementoma) presents radiographically

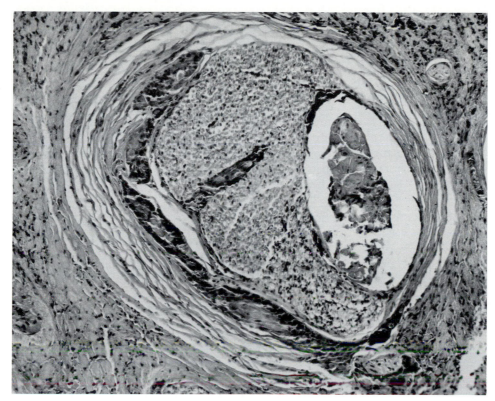

Fig. 190 Epidermoid carcinoma invading nerve of dental foramen. (×150; WU neg. 58-237.)

as multiple, dense, lobulated masses, often symmetrically involving the jaws. Microscopically, the cementum-like material present is dense, highly calcified, almost acellular.

Primary intraosseous epidermoid carcinoma

A rare tumor, primary intraosseous epidermoid carcinoma, arises within the jaw. Only those cases having no connection with the oral mucosa can be accepted with certainty. It is probable that it represents an heterogeneous group, some cases representing squamous metaplasia of ameloblastoma and others a malignant change in an odontogenic cyst. Carcinoma of salivary gland origin (particularly mucoepidermoid carcinoma) should be considered in the differential diagnosis.[75] It also should be remembered that most epidermoid carcinomas found within the jaws represent direct extensions from tumors of the tongue, floor of the mouth, or gingivae.[73]

Metastatic tumors

Secondary involvement of the mandible by invasion is common from squamous carcinomas of the alveolar ridge, the buccal mucosa, and the floor of the mouth.[82] The tumor destroys the periosteum, infiltrates beneath it, extends into the dental foramina, and finally destroys the mandible (Fig. 190). Squamous carcinoma metastatic to submaxillary lymph nodes can invade the mandible secondarily. We have seen similar encroachment by primary malignant tumors of the submaxillary gland.

Metastatic carcinoma may involve the mandible as a part of a disseminated process.[83] We have seen such involvement by tumors from the breast, thyroid gland, and prostate. McDaniel et al.[84] reviewed thirty-two cases of metastatic tumors in the jaw. In nine cases, the jaw metastasis was the first symptom of the disease. The breast and the lung were the most common sites for the primary tumor (nine cases each), followed by the thyroid gland (four cases).

In children, metastatic rhabdomyosarcoma, adrenal neuroblastoma, Wilms' tumor, and leukemia may all present clinically as jaw tumors.[83a]

Other tumors and tumorlike conditions

The bony structures of the jaw rarely may be involved by many other benign and malignant conditions. Some of these may contain a large number of multinucleated giant cells, a point to be remembered in the differential diagnosis of the giant cell lesions previously mentioned. Among the benign lesions, we have seen aneurysmal bone cyst,[86] osteoblastoma, neurofibroma, desmoplastic fibroma,[94] and hemangioma.[96] Paget's disease of the mandible and maxilla can occur as a dominant clinical expression of a generalized process.[85] Eosinophilic granuloma causes a localized ragged zone of destruction, more often in the mandible than in the maxilla.[93]

Among the primary malignant bone tumors, *osteosarcoma* is the most common. Of the fifty-six cases reported by Garrington et al.,[90] thirty-eight involved the mandible. The worst prognosis was for those involving the maxillary antrum, whereas the best outcome was seen in lesions of the mandibular symphysis. Cases of parosteal osteosarcoma have been reported.[95] *Chondrosarcoma* of the jaw shows a striking predilection for the maxilla.[88] Conversely, of the twelve cases of jaw *fibrosarcoma* tabulated by Dahlin,[89] ten were located in the mandible. *Plasma cell myeloma* can present in the jaw, either as part of a generalized process or as the prime manifestation of the disease.[91] We have seen *malignant lymphomas* (usually of histiocytic type) presenting as primary mandibular lesions. They were incorrectly diagnosed radiographically as chronic osteomyelitis. The predilection of *Burkitt's lymphoma* for these structures is well known. We have also seen a case of *Ewing's sarcoma* arising in the maxilla.

Pigmented neuroectodermal tumor of infancy (melanotic progonoma; retinal anlage tumor) is a rare benign neoplasm of neuroectodermal derivation previously thought to arise from odontogenic epithelium.[92] The maxilla is the most common location. However, we have seen it also in the mandible, skull, shoulder, epididymis, and soft tissues of the extremities. Borello and Gorlin[87] reported a case in which there was production of vanilmandelic acid, further supporting a neural origin.

REFERENCES
Osteomyelitis

1 Titterington, W. P.: Osteomyelitis and osteoradionecrosis of the jaws, J. Oral Med. **26**:7-16, 1971.

Simple bone cyst

2 Howe, G. L.: "Haemorrhagic cysts" of the mandible, Br. J. Oral Surg. **3**:55-76, 77-91, 1965.
3 Jaffe, H. L.: Giant-cell reparative granuloma, traumatic bone cyst, and fibrous (fibro-osseous) dysplasia of the jawbones, Oral Surg. Oral Med. Oral Path. **6**:159-175, 1953.

Giant cell lesions

4 Black, B. K., and Ackerman, L. V.: Tumors of the parathyroid; a review of twenty-three cases, Cancer **3**:415-444, 1950 (extensive bibliography).
4a Dehner, L. P.: Tumors of the mandible and maxilla in children. I. Clinicopathologic study of 46 histologically benign lesions, Cancer **31**:364-384, 1973.
5 Hamlin, W. B., and Lund, P. K.: "Giant cell tumors" of the mandible and facial bones, Arch. Otolaryngol. **86**:658-665, 1967.
6 Jaffe, H. L.: Giant cell reparative granuloma, traumatic bone cyst, and fibrous (fibro-osseous) dysplasia of the jawbones, Oral Surg. Oral Med. Oral Path. **6**:159-175, 1953.
7 Radcliffe, A., and Friedmann, I.: Reparative giant-cell granuloma of the jaw, Br. J. Surg. **45**:50-54, 1957.
8 Tombridge, T. L.: Familial giant cell reparative granuloma of the mandible ("cherubism"), Am. J. Clin. Pathol. **37**:196-203, 1962.
9 Waldron, C. A., and Shafer, W. G.: The central giant cell reparative granuloma of the jaws; an analysis of 38 cases, Am. J. Clin. Pathol. **45**:437-447, 1966.

Fibro-osseous lesions

10 Billing, L., and Ringertz, N.: Fibro-osteoma; a pathologico-anatomical and roentgenological study, Acta Radiol. **27**:129-152, 1946.

11 Cahn, L. R.: Bone pathology as it relates to some phases of oral surgery, Oral Surg. Oral Med. Oral Path. **1**:917-933, 1948.

12 Chaudhry, A. P., Spink, J. H., and Gorlin, R. J.: Periapical fibrous dysplasia (cementoma), J. Oral Surg. **22**:218-226, 1964.

13 Dehner, L. P.: Tumors of the mandible and maxilla in children. I. Clinicopathologic study of 46 histologically benign lesions, Cancer **31**: 364-384, 1973.

14 Hamner, J. E., III, Scofield, H. H., and Cornyn, J.: Benign fibro-osseous jaw lesions of periodontal membrane origin; an analysis of 249 cases, Cancer **22**:861-878, 1968.

15 Harris, W. H., Dudley, H. R., and Barry, R. J.: The natural history of fibrous dysplasia, J. Bone Joint Surg. **44-A**:207-233, 1962.

16 Phemister, D. B., and Grimson, K. S.: Fibrous osteoma of the jaws, Ann. Surg. **105**:564-583, 1937.

17 Reed, R. J.: Fibrous dysplasia of bone, Arch. Pathol. **75**:480-495, 1963.

18 Schmaman, A., Smith, I., and Ackerman, L. V.: Benign fibro-osseous lesions of the mandible and maxilla; a review of 35 cases, Cancer **26**:303-312, 1970.

19 Smith, A. G., and Zavaleta, A.: Osteoma, ossifying fibroma, and fibrous dysplasia of facial and cranial bones, Arch. Pathol. **54**:507-527, 1952.

Epithelial cysts

20 Abrams, A. M., Howell, F. V., and Bullock, W. K.: Nasopalatine cysts, Oral Surg. Oral Med. Oral Path. **16**:306-332, 1963.

21 Bhaskar, S. N., Loskin, D. M.: Gingival cysts, Oral Surg. Oral Med. Oral Path. **8**:803-807, 1955.

22 Brown, P. R. H.: An unusual case of globulomaxillary cyst, Oral Surg. Oral Med. Oral Path. **24**:719-725, 1967.

23 Browne, R. M.: The odontogenic keratocyst, Br. Dent. J. **128**:225-231, 1970.

24 Browne, R. M., and Gough, N. G.: Malignant changes in the epithelium lining odontogenic cysts, Cancer **29**:1199-1207, 1972.

25 Cabrini, R. L., Barras, R. E., and Albano, H.: Cysts of the jaws: a statistical analysis, J. Oral Surg. **28**:485-489, 1970.

26 Chretien, P. B., Carpenter, D. F., White, N. S., Harrah, J. D., and Lightbody, P. M.: Squamous carcinoma arising in a dentigerous cyst; presentation of a fatal case and review of four previously reported cases, Oral Surg. Oral Med. Oral Path. **30**:809-816, 1970.

27 Christ, T. F.: The globulomaxillary cyst: an embryologic misconception, Oral Surg. Oral Med. Oral Path. **30**:515-526, 1970.

28 Gorlin, R. J.: Potentialities of oral epithelium manifest by mandibular dentigerous cysts, Oral Surg. Oral Med. Oral Path. **10**:271-284, 1957.

29 Gorlin, R. J., Vickers, R. A., Kelly, E., and Williamson, J. J.: The multiple basal cell nevi syndrome, Cancer **18**:89-104, 1965.

30 Killey H. C., and Kay, L. W.: Benign cystic lesions of the jaws, Edinburgh, 1966, E. S. Livingstone Ltd., pp. 86-93.

31 Killey, H. C., and Kay, L. W.: An analysis of 471 benign cystic lesions of the jaws, Int. Surg. **46**:540-545, 1966.

32 Pindborg, J. J., and Kramer, I. R. H.: Histologic typing of odontogenic tumours, jaw cysts, and allied lesions. In International Histological Classification of Tumours, vol. 5, Geneva, 1971, World Health Organization.

33 Roed-Petersen, B.: Nasolabial cysts; a presentation of five patients with a review of the literature, Br. J. Oral Surg. **7**:84-95, 1969.

34 Shear, M.: Primordial cysts, J. Dent. Ass. S. Afr. **15**:211-217, 1960.

35 Sonesson, A.: Odontogenic cysts and cystic tumors of the jaws, Acta Radiol. **81**(suppl.): 1-159, 1950 (extensive bibliography).

36 Soskolne, W. A., and Shear, M.: Observations of the pathogenesis of primordial cysts, Br. Dent. J. **123**:321-326, 1967.

37 Standish, S. M., and Shafer, W. G.: The lateral periodontal cyst, J. Periodontol. **29**: 27-33, 1958.

38 Stanley, H. R.: Ameloblastoma potential of follicular cysts, Oral Surg. Oral Med. Oral Path. **20**:260-268, 1965.

Odontogenic tumors

39 Abrams, A. M., and Howell, F. V.: The calcifying odontogenic cyst; report of four cases, Oral Surg. Oral Med. Oral Path. **25**:594-606, 1968.

40 Abrams, A. M., Melrose, R. J., and Howell, F. V.: Adenoameloblastoma, Cancer **22**:175-185, 1968.

41 Azaz, B., Ulmansky, M., and Lewin-Epstein, J.: Dentinoma; report of a case, Oral Surg. Oral Med. Oral Path. **24**:659-663, 1967.

42 Barros, R. E., Dominguez, F. V., and Cabrini, R. L.: Myxoma of the jaws, Oral Surg. Oral Med. Oral Path. **27**:225-236, 1969.

43 Bernier, J. L., and Thompson, H. C.: The histogenesis of the cementoma; report of 15 cases, Am. J. Orthod. (Oral Surg. Sect.) **32**: 543-555, 1946.

44 Bhaskar, S. N.: Adenoameloblastoma: its histogenesis and report of 15 new cases, J. Oral Surg. **22**:218-226, 1964.

45 Campbell, J. A. H.: Adamantinoma containing tissue resembling granular-cell myoblastoma, J. Pathol. Bacteriol. **71**:45-49, 1956.

46 Chaudhry, A. P., Hanks, C. T., Leifer, C., and Gargiulo, E. A.: Calcifying epithelial odontogenic tumor; a histochemical and ultrastructural study, Cancer **30**:1036-1045, 1972.

47 Cina, M. T., Dahlin, D. C., and Gores, R. J.:

Ameloblastic sarcoma; report of two cases, Oral Surg. Oral Med. Oral Path. **15**:696-700, 1962.

48 Costas, J. B., and DiPiramo, S.: Congenital epulis (congenital granular cell myoblastoma); report of 2 cases, Oral Surg. Oral Med. Oral Path. **26**:497-504, 1968.

49 Couch, R. D., Morris, E. E., and Vellios, F.: Granular cell ameloblastic fibroma; report of 2 cases in adults, with observations of its similarity to congenital epulis, Am. J. Clin. Pathol. **37**:398-404, 1962.

50 Giansanti, J. S., Someren, A., and Waldron, C. A.: Odontogenic adenomatoid tumor (adenoameloblastoma); survey of 111 cases, Oral Surg. Oral Med. Oral Path. **30**:69-88, 1970.

51 Gorlin, R. J., Chaudhry, A. P., and Pindborg, J. J.: Odontogenic tumors; classification, histopathology, and clinical behavior in man and domesticated animals, Cancer **14**:73-101, 1961.

52 Gorlin, R. J., Pindborg, J. J., Clausen, F. P., and Vickers, R. A.: The calcifying odontogenic cyst: a possible analogue of the cutaneous calcifying epithelioma of Malherbe; an analysis of fifteen cases, Oral Surg. Oral Med. Oral Path. **15**:1235-1243, 1962.

53 Hamner, J. E., and Pizer, M. E.: Ameloblastic odontoma, Am. J. Dis. Child. **115**:332-336, 1968.

54 Hoffman, P. J., Baden, E., Rankow, R. M., and Potter, G. D.: Fate of uncontrolled ameloblastoma, Oral Surg. Oral Med. Oral Path. **26**:419-426, 1968.

55 Hoke, H. F., Jr., and Harrelson, A. B.: Granular cell ameloblastomas with metastases to cervical vertebrae, Cancer **20**:991-999, 1967.

56 Ikemura, K., Tashiro, H., Fujino, H., Ohbu, D., and Nakajima, K.: Ameloblastoma of the mandible with metastasis to the lungs and lymph nodes, Cancer **29**:930-940, 1972.

57 Jacobsohn, P. H., and Quinn, J. H.: Ameloblastic odontomas; report of three cases, Oral Surg. Oral Med. Oral Path. **26**:829-836, 1968.

58 Kay, S., Elzay, R. P., and Willson, M. A.: Ultrastructural observations on a gingival granular cell tumor (congenital epulis), Cancer **27**:674-680, 1971.

59 Lucas, R. B.: Pathology of tumours of the oral tissues, ed. 2, Edinburgh and London, 1972, Churchill Livingstone.

60 Manning, G. L., and Browne, R. M.: Dentinoma, Br. Dent. J. **128**:178-181, 1970.

61 Mincer, H. H., and McGinnis, J. P.: Ultrastructure of three histologic variants of the ameloblastoma, Cancer **30**:1036-1045, 1972.

62 Navarrete, A. R., and Smith, M.: Ultrastructure of granular cell ameloblastoma, Cancer **27**:948-955, 1971.

63 Olech, E., and Alvares, O.: Ameloblastic

odontoma, Oral Surg. Oral Med. Oral Path. **23**:487-492, 1967.

64 Philipsen, H. P., and Birn, H.: The adenomatoid odontogenic tumour; ameloblastic adenomatoid tumour or adeno-ameloblastoma, Acta Pathol. Microbiol. Scand. **75**:375-398, 1969.

65 Pindborg, J. J.: Dissertations in honorem svenonis petri; on dentinomas with report of a case, Acta Pathol. Microbiol. Scand. Suppl. **105**:135-144, 1955.

66 Pindborg, J. J.: A calcifying epithelial odontogenic tumor, Cancer **11**:838-843, 1958.

67 Pindborg, J. J.: The calcifying epithelial odontogenic tumor: review of the literature and report of an extraosseous case, Acta Odontol. Scand. **24**:419-430, 1966.

68 Pindborg, J. J., and Kramer, I. R. H.: Histologic typing of odontogenic tumours, jaw cysts, and allied lesions, In International Histological Classification of Tumours, vol. 5, Geneva, 1971, World Health Organization.

69 Ranlov, P., and Pindborg, J. J.: The amyloid nature of the homogeneous substance in the calcifying epithelial odontogenic tumour, Acta Pathol. Microbiol. Scand. **68**:169-174, 1966.

70 Robinson, H. B. G.: Ameloblastoma; survey of 379 cases from literature, Arch. Pathol. **23**:831-843, 1937.

71 Schweitzer, F. C., and Barnfield, W. F.: Ameloblastoma of the mandible with metastasis to the lungs, J. Oral Surg. **1**:287-295, 1943.

72 Shafer, W. G.: Ameloblastic fibroma, J. Oral Surg. **13**:317-321, 1955.

73 Shear, M.: Primary intra-alveolar epidermoid carcinoma of the jaw, J. Pathol. **97**:645-651, 1969.

74 Sherman, R. S.: Resume of the roentgen diagnosis of tumors of the jawbones, Oral Surg. Oral Med. Oral Path. **4**:1427-1443, 1951.

75 Silvergrade, L. B., Alvares, O. F., and Olech, E.: Central mucoepidermoid tumors of the jaws; review of the literature and case report, Cancer **22**:650-653, 1968.

76 Small, I. A., and Waldron, C. A.: Ameloblastomas of the jaws, Oral Surg. Oral Med. Oral Path. **8**:281-297, 1955.

77 Spouge, J. D.: The adenoameloblastoma, Oral Surg. Oral Med. Oral Path. **23**:470-482, 1967.

78 Vap, D. R., Dahlin, D. C., and Turlington, E. G.: Pindborg tumor: the so-called calcifying epithelial odontogenic tumor, Cancer **25**:629-636, 1970.

79 Vickers, R. A., and Gorlin, R. J.: Ameloblastoma: delineation of early histopathologic features of neoplasia, Cancer **26**:699-710, 1970.

80 Zegarelli, E. V., and Ziskin, D. E.: Cementomas; a report of 50 cases, Am. J. Orthod. (Oral Surg. Sect.) **29**:285-292, 1943.

81 Zimmerman, D. C., and Dahlin, D. C.: Myxomatous tumors of jaws, Oral Surg. Oral Med. Oral Path. **11**:1069-1080, 1958.

Metastatic tumors

82 Buirge, R. E.: Secondary carcinoma of the mandible, Surgery 15:553-564, 1944.

83 Byars, L. T., and Sarnat, B. G.: Mandibular tumors, Surg. Gynecol. Obstet. 83:355-363, 1946.

83a Dehner, L. P.: Tumors of the mandible and maxilla in children. II. A study of 14 primary and secondary malignant tumors, Cancer 32: 112-120, 1973.

84 McDaniel, R. K., Luna, M. A., and Stimson, P. G.: Metastatic tumors in the jaws, Oral Surg. Oral Med. Oral Path. 31:380-386, 1971.

Other tumors and tumorlike conditions

85 Ash, J. E., and Raum, M.: An atlas of otolaryngic pathology, 1956, The American Academy of Ophthalmology and Otolaryngology, The American Registry of Pathology, and The Armed Forces Institute of Pathology.

86 Bhaskar, S. N., Bernier, J. L., and Godby, F.: Aneurysmal bone cyst and other giant cell lesions of the jaws: report of 104 cases, J. Oral Surg. 17:30-41, 1959.

87 Borello, E. D., and Gorlin, R. J.: Melanotic neuroectodermal tumor of infancy—a neoplasm of neural crest origin, Cancer 19:196-206, 1966.

88 Chaudhry, A. P., Rabinovitch, M. R., Mitchell, D. F., and Vickers, R. A.: Chondrogenic tumors of the jaws, Am. J. Surg. 102:403-411, 1961.

89 Dahlin, D. C.: Bone tumors; general aspects and data on 3,987 cases, ed. 2, Springfield, Ill., 1967, Charles C Thomas, Publisher.

90 Garrington, G. E., Scofield, H. H., Cornyn, J., and Hooker, S. P.: Osteosarcoma of the jaws; analysis of 56 cases, Cancer 20:377-391, 1967.

91 Henderson, D., and Rowe, N. L.: Myelomatosis affecting the jaws, Br. J. Oral Surg. 6: 161-172, 1969.

92 Lurie, H. I.: Congenital melanocarcinoma, melanotic adamantinoma, retinal anlage tumor, progonoma, and pigmented epulis of infancy; summary and review of the literature and report of the first case in an adult, Cancer 14:1090-1108, 1961.

93 McGavran, M. H., and Spady, H. A.: Eosinophilic granuloma of bone; a study of twenty-eight cases, J. Bone Joint Surg. 42-A:979-992, 1960.

94 Rabhan, W. N., and Rosai, J.: Desmoplastic fibroma; report of ten cases and review of the literature, J. Bone Joint Surg. 50-A:487-502, 1968.

95 Roca, A. N., Smith, J. L., Jr., and Jing, B.-S.: Osteosarcoma and parosteal osteogenic sarcoma of the maxilla and mandible; study of 20 cases, Am. J. Clin. Pathol. 54:625-636, 1970.

96 Taylor, B. G., and Etheredge, S. N.: Hemangiomas of mandible and maxilla presenting as surgical emergencies, Am. J. Surg. 108:574-577, 1964.

6 Respiratory tract

Nose and paranasal sinuses
Larynx and trachea
Lung

Nose and paranasal sinuses

Inflammatory ("allergic") polyp
Tumors
    Papilloma
    Carcinoma
    Neurogenous and related tumors
    Malignant melanoma
    Plasma cell tumor
Other lesions

Inflammatory ("allergic") polyp

Nasal polyps are not true neoplasms. Their formation is associated with either infection or allergy. These soft polypoid lesions tend to be bilateral. Microscopically, they are composed of a loose mucoid stroma and mucous glands and are covered by respiratory epithelium. They are infiltrated by lymphocytes, plasma cells, and eosinophils.

Prominent thickening of the basement membrane is a common finding. The surface epithelium often exhibits foci of squamous metaplasia. If proper attention is placed on the stromal changes, confusion with true papillomas is unlikely to occur. The polyps presumably associated with an allergy have, at times, a marked eosinophilic leukocytic infiltrate. They tend to recur after removal.

From 6% to 10% of patients with mucoviscidosis (cystic fibrosis) develop polyps in the nasal cavity and paranasal sinuses. Therefore, children with nasal polyps should be investigated for this condition. Microscopically, the polyps differ from the ordinary variety only by the presence of large cystic glands with inspissated secretion in their lumina.[1]

Tumors
Papilloma

Nasal and paranasal papillomas are benign neoplasms of the respiratory mucosa (Fig. 191). Many adjectives have been attached to them, such as inverted, cylindric cell, transitional, squamous, and schneiderian. Excluded from this group are the papillary tumors arising from the stratified squamous epithelium lining the nasal vestibule, which are analogous to tumors occurring elsewhere in the skin. Nasal papillomas are not related to inflammatory polyps. The latter are bilateral in a high proportion of cases, but this was true only in six out of 315 papillomas reviewed by Hyams.[2] Microscopically, the tumors are composed of proliferating columnar or squamous epi-

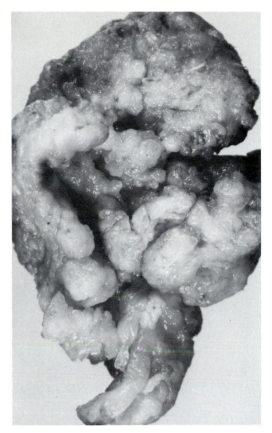

Fig. 191 Nasal papilloma, inverted type, in 57-year-old man. (WU neg. 62-6743.)

thelial cells, with an admixture of mucin-containing cells.[3] Those arising in the nasal septum are usually exophytic, mushroom shaped, with a thin central core of connective tissue (Fig. 192). Those located in the lateral wall (middle meatus or middle or inferior turbinate) are of the inverted type, with inward growth of the epithelium into the stroma. This last feature can be misinterpreted as invasion and the lesion incorrectly diagnosed as carcinoma.

Nasal papillomas have a marked tendency to recur.[3a] It is stated that they may become malignant. Although we have seen a few unquestionable cases of invasive squamous cell carcinoma *in* a papilloma, most of the cases supposed to show this transformation were carcinomas from their inception and had been originally misinter-preted as papillomas because of their well-differentiated nature.

Carcinoma

Squamous cell carcinoma is by far the most common type of cancer in the nose and paranasal sinuses.[4, 7] In most instances, the microscopic diagnosis is obvious because of the atypicality and stromal infiltration. There are, however, two varieties that can be erroneously diagnosed as benign: one is the type having a growth pattern quite similar to that of a papilloma (Fig. 193). It often shows no obvious stromal invasion, and the differential diagnosis with papilloma has to be made on the basis of cellular abnormalities such as loss of polarity and atypical nuclear changes.[5] It should be remembered that mitoses and some degree of nuclear hyperchromasia can be present in benign lesions. The second type is *verrucous carcinoma,* of which we have seen four examples in the nasal cavity (p. 148).

Tumors of salivary gland origin occur in the nose as well as in the sinuses. The maxillary sinus is the most common location. Of thirty-seven cases reviewed by Rafla,[6] twenty-one were in the antrum, nine in the ethmoid, five in the nasal fossa, and two in the sphenoid. They are almost always malignant. Adenoid cystic carcinoma is the most common variety.

Adenocarcinomas of the nasal cavity with a microscopic appearance resembling that of colonic carcinomas have been studied by Sanchez-Casis et al.[8] These are locally aggressive tumors with a propensity for recurrence (Fig. 194).

Neurogenous and related tumors

Encephaloceles and ***glial heterotopias*** (commonly called nasal gliomas) are related malformational "tumors" usually affecting newborn and older infants. They may present as subcutaneous masses at the base of the nose or as intranasal polyps. Associated bony defects are the rule with the encephaloceles, but they are unusual with the glial heterotopias, a feature to be

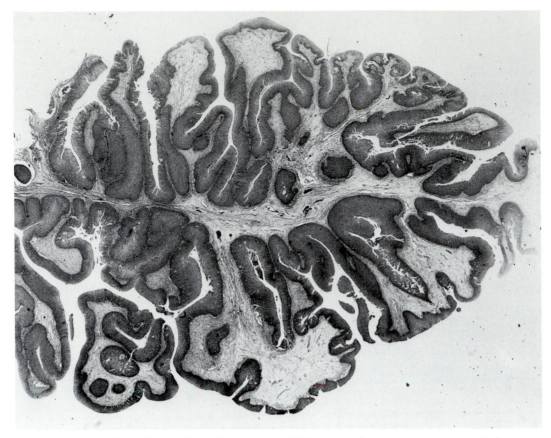

Fig. 192 Nasal papilloma of exophytic variety. Thick layer of mature squamous epithelium invaginates about central fibrovascular core. (×10; WU neg. 72-6555.)

evaluated at the time of removal. *Neuri-lemomas* and *neurofibromas* are extremely rare. Intracranial *meningiomas* may invade the sphenoid or frontal sinuses secondarily. We also have seen them presenting as primary intranasal masses.[12]

Olfactory neuroblastomas are low-grade malignant neoplasms arising from neuroepithelial elements in the olfactory membrane. They are often incorrectly diagnosed as undifferentiated carcinoma or malignant lymphoma (Fig. 195). Electron microscopic examination may be of considerable help in the diagnosis. The tumors spread frequently to surrounding structures and sometimes metastasize to cervical lymph nodes.[9, 10]

Invasion of the nasal cavity by *pituitary adenomas* has been observed.[11] A case of intranasal *paraganglioma* was reported by Parisier and Sinclair.[13]

Malignant melanoma

Primary malignant melanomas of the nasal cavity and paranasal sinuses usually present as solid polypoid growths. Holdcraft and Gallagher[14] collected thirty-nine cases. Of these, twenty-one were located in the nasal cavity, four in the antrum, two in the ethmoid, and one in both frontal and ethmoid sinuses. Of thirty-one patients in whom follow-up was available, twenty-six died as a result of metastatic disease.

Plasma cell tumor

Plasma cell tumors arising in the nasopharynx may present primarily in the nose as a soft bleeding mass.[16] Microscopic ex-

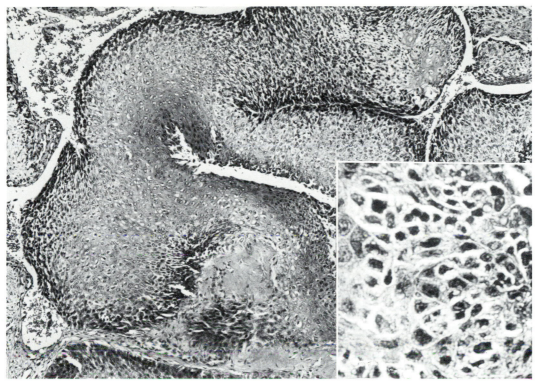

Fig. 193 Squamous cell carcinoma of nasal cavity. The well-differentiated nature of tumor and papillomatous pattern of growth often result in mistaken diagnosis of papilloma. **Inset,** High-power view shows, however, that tumor cells have malignant cytologic features. (×90; WU neg. 72-6399; **inset,** WU neg. 72-11215.)

amination shows a monomorphic infiltration by immature plasma cells.[15, 17] In our experience, all patients with apparently solitary plasma cell tumors of the upper air passages in whom there was adequate follow-up developed disseminated myeloma. In some, this process took ten or more years to become manifest.

Other lesions

Dermoid cysts are dorsal developmental defects located in the midline. They may be associated with bony defects and sinus

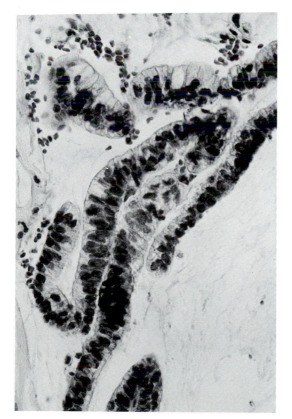

Fig. 194 Well-differentiated adenocarcinoma of nares in 70-year-old man. This tumor was first incorrectly diagnosed as benign polyp but since then stubbornly recurred over four-year period. (×210; WU neg. 52-593.)

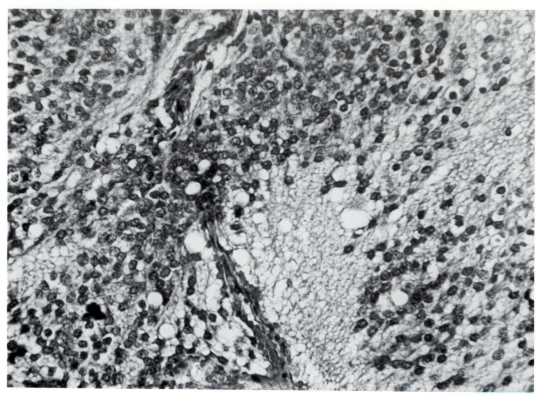

Fig. 195 Typical microscopic appearance of olfactory neuroblastoma. Compact nests of small round cells alternate with reticular areas formed by tangles of neurites emanating from tumor cells. (×350; WU neg. 72-6550.)

tracts. *Teratomas* have been reported in the sinuses and nasopharynx of infants and children. The large majority are benign.[19] *Mucoceles* of the maxilla may expand gradually and cause destruction of contiguous bones and thus be mistaken for a malignant neoplasm. *Wegener's granulomatosis* is a rapidly progressive, usually fatal condition in which nasal involvement is accompanied by pulmonary and renal disease. Microscopically, a necrotizing vasculitis with secondary granulomatous reaction and epithelial ulceration are seen. Multiple, deep biopsies may be necessary to find the diagnostic areas. Elastic tissue stains are helpful in identifying remnants of badly damaged vessels. *Lethal midline granuloma* is an ill-defined clinical syndrome that encompasses a variety of pathologic conditions.[20] *Malignant lymphomas,*[18] *leiomyosarcomas,*[21] and *embryonal rhabdomyosarcomas,*[22] can present as primary neo-

plasms of the paranasal sinuses. We have seen a *glomus tumor* presenting as a polypoid intranasal mass.

REFERENCES
Inflammatory ("allergic") polyp

1 Schwachman, H., Kulczycki, L. L., Mueller, H. L., and Flake, C. G.: Nasal polyposis in patients with cystic fibrosis, Pediatrics 30:389-401, 1962.

Tumors
Papilloma

2 Hyams, V. J.: Papillomas of the nasal cavity and paranasal sinuses; a clinicopathologic study of 315 cases, Ann. Otol. Rhinol. Laryngol. 80:192-206, 1971.
3 Oberman, H. A.: Papillomas of the nose and paranasal sinuses, Am. J. Clin. Pathol. 42:245-258, 1964.
3a Snyder, R. N., and Perzin, K. H.: Papillomatosis of nasal cavity and paranasal sinuses (inverted papilloma, squamous papilloma); a clinicopathologic study, Cancer 30:668-690, 1972.

Carcinoma

4 Frazell, E. L., and Lewis, J. S.: Cancer of the nasal cavity and accessory sinuses, Cancer **16:**1293-1301, 1963.

5 Osborn, D. A.: Nature and behavior of transitional tumors in the upper respiratory tract, Cancer **25:**50-60, 1970.

6 Rafla, S.: Mucous gland tumors of paranasal sinuses, Cancer **24:**683-691, 1969.

7 Ringertz, N.: Pathology of malignant tumors arising in the nasal and paranasal cavities and maxilla, Acta Otolaryngol. [Suppl.] (Stockh.) **27:**1-405, 1938.

8 Sanchez-Casis, G., Devine, K. D., and Weiland, L. H.: Nasal adenocarcinomas that closely simulate colonic carcinomas, Cancer **28:**714-720, 1971.

Neurogenous and related tumors

9 Gerard-Marchant, R., and Micheau, C.: Microscopical diagnosis of olfactory esthesioneuromas; general review and report of five cases, J. Natl. Cancer Inst. **35:**75-82, 1965.

10 Hutter, R. V. P., Lewis, J. S., Foote, F. W., Jr., and Tollefsen, H. R.: Esthesioneuroblastoma, Am. J. Surg. **106:**748-753, 1963.

11 Kay, S., Lees, J. K., and Stout, A. P.: Pituitary chromophobe tumors of the nasal cavity, Cancer **3:**695-704, 1950.

12 McGavran, M. H., Biller, H., and Ogura, J. H.: Primary intranasal meningioma, Arch. Otolaryngol. **93:**95-97, 1971.

13 Parisier, S. C., and Sinclair, G. M.: Glomus tumor of the nasal cavity, Laryngoscope **78:**2013-2024, 1968.

Malignant melanoma

14 Holdcraft, J., and Gallagher, J. C.: Malignant melanomas of the nasal and paranasal sinus mucosa, Ann. Otol. Rhinol. Laryngol. **78:**5-20, 1969.

Plasma cell tumor

15 Ewing, M. R., and Foote, F. W., Jr.: Plasma-cell tumors of the mouth and upper air passages, Cancer **5:**499-513, 1952.

16 Kotner, L. M., and Wang, C. C.: Plasmacytoma of the upper air and food passages, Cancer **30:**414-418, 1972.

17 Webb, H. E., Harrison, E. G., Masson, J. K., and ReMine, W. H.: Solitary extramedullary myeloma (plasmacytoma) of the upper part of the respiratory tract and oropharynx, Cancer **15:**1142-1155, 1962.

Other lesions

18 Birt, B. D.: Reticulum cell sarcoma of the nose and paranasal sinuses, J. Laryngol. Otol. **84:**615-630, 1970.

19 Boies, L. R., Jr., and Harris, D.: Nasopharyngeal dermoid of the newborn, Laryngoscope **75:**763-767, 1965.

20 Kassel, S. H., Echevarria, R. A., and Guzzo, F. P.: Midline malignant reticulosis (so-called lethal midline granuloma), Cancer **23:**920-935, 1969.

21 Kawabe, Y., Kondo, T., and Hosoda, S.: Two cases of leiomyosarcoma of the maxillary sinuses, Arch. Otolaryngol. **90:**492-495, 1969.

22 Manon, J. K., and Soule, E. H.: Embryonal rhabdomyosarcoma of the head and neck; report on eighty-eight cases, Am. J. Surg. **110:**585-591, 1965.

Larynx and trachea

LARYNX
Cysts

Cysts of the larynx have been divided by DeSanto et al.[1] according to their mechanism of formation into *saccular* (24%) and *ductal* (75%). The former arise from cystic distention of the laryngeal saccule. They are large and deep and are often found inside the ventricle. Ductal cysts, which are the result of dilatation of mucous glands, are small and superficial and are usually located in the true cord or epiglottis. Both types can be lined by either squamous or respiratory epithelium or a combination of both.

Rarely, laryngeal cysts are lined partially or completely by oncocytes. Papillary infoldings are usually present. Gallagher and Puzon,[2] who collected eighteen examples, considered them the result of epithelial hyperplasia and metaplasia rather than true neoplasms.

The term *laryngocele* refers to an air-containing saccular dilatation of the appendix of the ventricle of Morgagni, communicating with the lumen of the ventricle by a narrow stalk.[3] The internal variety presents with hoarseness, dyspnea, or reflex cough, whereas the external type appears as a soft mass in the lateral aspect of the neck. Combined forms occur.

Infection

Chronic *nonspecific laryngitis* can be the result of infection, overuse of the voice, exposure to chemical or physical agents, or irritation by tobacco and alcohol. Microscopically, a lymphocytic infiltrate is seen beneath the mucosa with an inconstant admixture of plasma cells and histiocytes.

The most frequent infection involving the larynx is *tuberculosis.* This process begins with interarytenoid edema, followed by involvement of the true cord. It may spread throughout the larynx. Roentgenographic examination of the chest invariably shows active advanced tuberculosis. Laryngeal biopsy shows typical granulomas.

Other specific laryngitides are *syphilitic, lepromatous,* and *fungal.* We have diagnosed several cases of histoplasmosis and one of blastomycosis. In histoplasmosis, the early lesions are frequently located in the vocal cords and epiglottis[5] (Figs. 196 and 197). A granulomatous lesion involving *only* the anterior portions of the larynx (especially the epiglottis) or having associated oral lesions is more likely to be histoplasmosis than tuberculosis. Laryngeal *granulomas* due to endotracheal trauma caused by intubation can occur and be mistaken for a neoplasm.[4] *Arthritis* of the cricoarytenoid joint is commonly associated with generalized arthritis of a rheumatoid nature.[6]

Fig. 196 Laryngogram demonstrating mass interpreted radiographically as carcinoma on free surface of epiglottis. (WU negs. 66-13136 and 66-13137.)

Fig. 197 Section of lesion shown in Fig. 196 illustrating granulomas due to histoplasmosis. (WU neg. 66-11898A.)

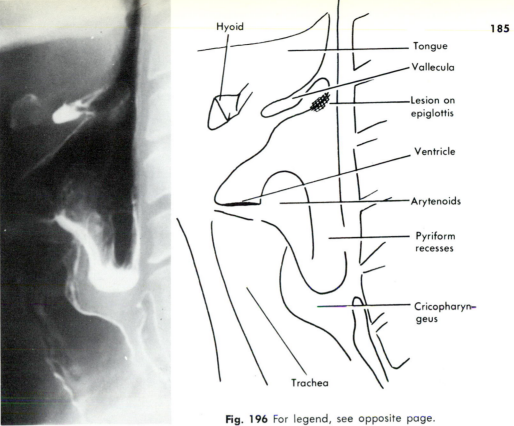

Hyoid

Tongue

Vallecula

Lesion on
epiglottis

Ventricle

Arytenoids

Pyriform
recesses

Cricopharyn-
geus

Trachea

Fig. 196 For legend, see opposite page.

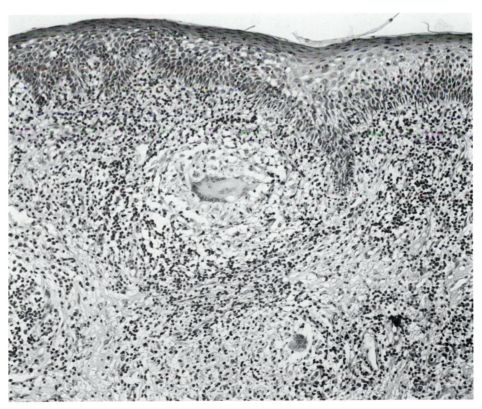

Fig. 197 For legend, see opposite page.

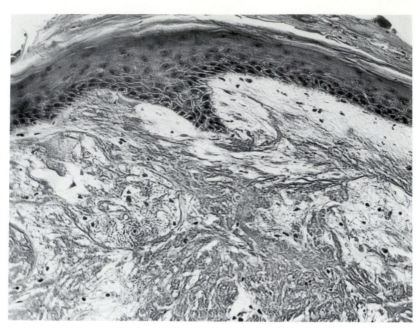

Fig. 198 Laryngeal nodule. Note amorphous, poorly stained material beneath intact epithelium. (Low power; WU neg. 50-479.)

Laryngeal nodule

Laryngeal nodules represent a peculiar noninflammatory reaction to injury causing hoarseness and appear in people who misuse their voices. They occur chiefly on the anterior third of the vocal cords and have been variously called singers' nodes, amyloid tumors, polyps, and varices.

Microscopically, these nodules have varying patterns, depending on their stage of evolution.[7] In the early stages, they show edema and proliferation of young fibroblasts. Later, dilated blood vessels and hyalinization of the stroma appear. Cases with a prominent vascular component are frequently mistaken for hemangioma. The hyaline stage is the one previously designated "amyloid tumor" (Fig. 198). This is a misnomer. True localized amyloid deposits do occur in the tracheobronchial tree.[8]

Tumors
Papillomatosis

Papillomatosis of the larynx is a disease probably viral in origin,[11] usually of childhood and adolescence, in which multi-

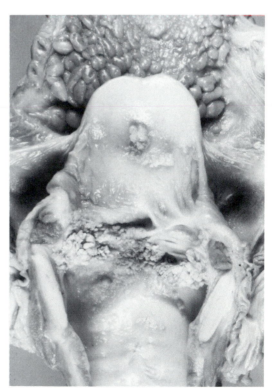

Fig. 199 Extensive papillomatosis in 18-year-old boy. Patient had had almost fifty resections of this process, beginning at 7 years of age, and finally died of suffocation. (WU neg. 66-8331.)

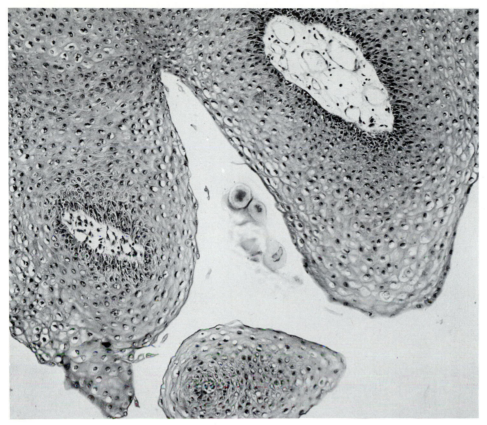

Fig. 200 Papillomatosis of larynx in child. Note papillary character and excellent differentiation of epithelium. (×120; WU neg. 58-235.)

ple papillary tumors occur on the true cord and may involve also the false cord and subglottic area.[10] When extensive, papillomatosis may cause extreme respiratory embarrassment and even death[9] (Fig. 199). Moore and Lattes[12] reported a case in which recurrent laryngeal papillomatosis was followed by extensive bronchial papillomatosis. Microscopic examination shows a papillary growth of well-differentiated squamous cells with an orderly maturation pattern (Fig. 200).

These tumors tend to recur over a long period of time but invariably maintain their orderly character. Rarely, invasive squamous carcinoma develops in association with laryngeal papillomatosis. Rabbett[13] has pointed out that in all the reported cases of juvenile laryngeal papillomatosis that had undergone malignant transformation, irradiation therapy previously had been given to the diseased area. This was also true in the two cases we have observed.

Keratosis

Keratosis of the larynx involves the true cords and interarytenoid area. This lesion often occurs in persons who smoke, in singers, and in those who use their voices excessively. Examination shows a thickening of the vocal cord. Biopsy reveals hyperkeratotic epithelium, often with a granular layer, with downgrowth of the underlying squamous cells (Fig. 201).

Cellular atypia, when present, is graded as mild, moderate, or severe. The chances of development of a squamous cell carcinoma, although always small, are higher for the lesions with increasing degrees of atypia.

Of eighty-four patients with laryngeal

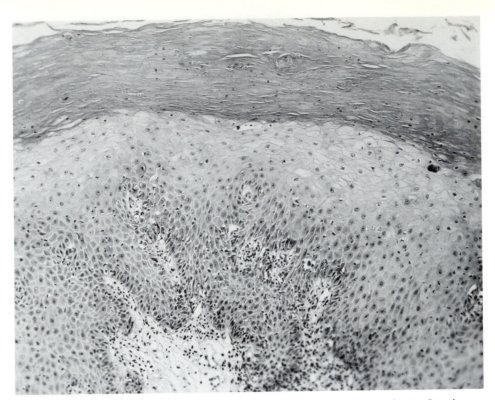

Fig. 201 Keratosis of larynx with hyperkeratotic epithelium and acanthosis. Basal membrane is intact. (×115; WU neg. 51-1320.)

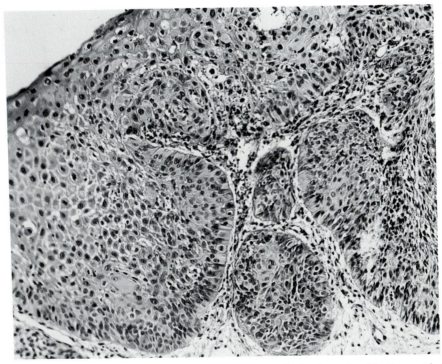

Fig. 202 Epidermoid carcinoma in situ of larynx. Note thickening of epithelium with intact basement membrane and complete disorganization of all layers. (×200; WU neg. 50-960.)

keratosis followed for a minimum of five and a maximum of fifteen years, only three developed laryngeal carcinomas. These occurred nine months, six years, and eight years, respectively, after the diagnosis of keratosis. One of the patients died of laryngeal carcinoma.[14] We believe, therefore, that conservative therapy is indicated, even for the lesions with severe atypia, if proper periodic examinations are carried out. We have seen a patient in whom forty-six biopsies of the cord, taken over a ten-year period, showed various degrees of keratosis without evidence of cancer.

Carcinoma in situ

Epidermoid carcinoma in situ is now recognized as a definite entity. It may occur at the peripheral margin of an invasive cancer or be present without invasion. The former situation is definitely the most common. Patients with this entity have hoarseness and may show slight reddening of the true cord. The microscopic criteria for diagnosis are the same as for its more common counterpart in the uterine cervix; i.e., the presence of atypical changes

throughout the epithelium without evidence of surface maturation (Fig. 202).

Such a lesion may be cured by biopsy, local excision, laryngeal fissure, stripping, or irradiation therapy. In certain instances, it may appear later on the opposite cord. We suspect that if carcinoma in situ is not treated, it will progress in time to invasive carcinoma, but the length of this interval is unknown.[15] We know of several patients who have had carcinoma in situ for five to eight years without developing invasive cancer. We also know that a significant proportion (75%) of invasive car-

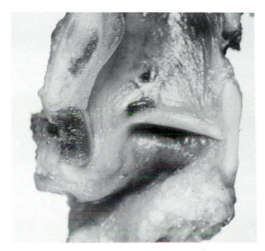

Fig. 204 Sagittal section of gross specimen of larynx showing small area of involvement of true cord. (WU neg. 49-6450.)

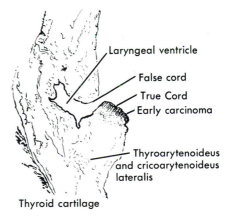

Fig. 205 Schematic representation and anatomy of lesion shown in Fig. 206. (WU neg. 52-4745.)

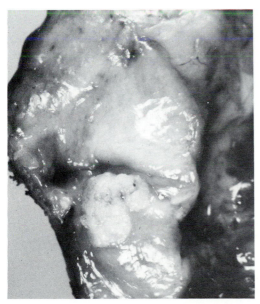

Fig. 203 Well-differentiated squamous cancer of true cord, without involvement of vocal muscle. Margins were free of tumor. (WU neg. 67-7099.)

cinomas *are associated with* in situ cancer.[16] Careful examination of the patients, including critical histologic appraisal, judicious therapy, and adequate follow-up, should clarify the status of epidermoid carcinoma in situ of the larynx.

Invasive epidermoid carcinoma

Invasive epidermoid carcinoma occurs most often in men of the older age group and comprises almost 99% of all malignant laryngeal neoplasms. It is divided, according to its location, into four types[18] as follows, in order of frequency.

1 *Glottic.* These are tumors limited to the true vocal cords (Fig. 203). They may be confined to the membranous portion of one cord (T1) or may extend to the anterior commissure, arytenoid, opposite cord, or up to 1 cm subglottically (T2). The glot-

tis is the most common location of laryngeal cancers. They are usually well differentiated and tend to remain localized because of the surrounding cartilaginous wall and the paucity of lymphatics (Figs. 204 to 206). Ipsilateral lymph node metastases were not found in any of forty-one T1 lesions and in only 7.3% of T2 tumors.[25] Therefore, prophylactic lymph node dissection is not indicated. Early cases can be treated by irradiation therapy with excellent results[24, 26] (Fig. 207). If irradiation fails, surgery will still save most of the patients. Actually, some small, superficially invasive epidermoid carcinomas of the true cord can be cured by endoscopic biopsy removal alone.[27] T2 glottic cancers are best treated by hemilaryngectomy.[19]

2 *Supraglottic.* These tumors involve the false cord and/or the laryngeal surface of

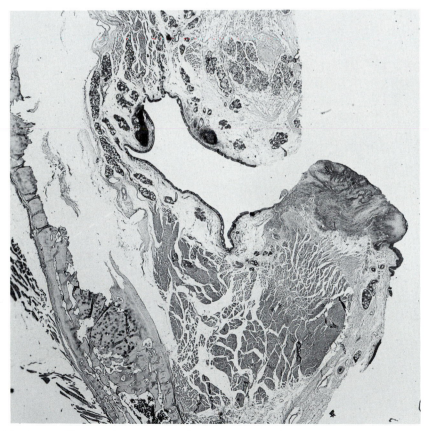

Fig. 206 Lesion illustrated in Fig. 204 showing topography of larynx and superficial character of carcinoma. Lesion could have been cured as well by good irradiation therapy as by laryngectomy. (Low power; WU neg. 51-147.)

the epiglottis. One-third of the supraglottic cancers arise from the latter structure. The incidence of lymph node metastases is 33%. However, the frequency of clinically undetected metastases is quite low (one out of twenty-five cases in the series reported by McGavran et al.[23]). In our institution, supraglottic tumors are treated with irradiation followed by partial laryngectomy.

3 Transglottic. This term is applied to cancers that cross the laryngeal ventricle. They have the highest incidence of lymph node involvement (52%). Of sixteen transglottic cancers examined by McGavran et al.,[23] five (31%) had clinically undetected node metastases. This figure indicates that elective lymph node dissection should be performed for tumors in this location, in addition to laryngectomy.

4 Infraglottic. Under this category are included cancers involving the true cord with a subglottic extension of more than 1 cm (Fig. 208) as well as tumors entirely confined to the subglottic area. The latter are unusual in our experience (Fig. 209). Of the infraglottic cancers studied by McGavran et al.,[23] 19% were associated with lymph node metastases, all of them clinically undetected. This speaks again of the advisability of elective node dissection for this group of neoplasms.

Tumors situated on the glossal surface of the epiglottis, pyriform sinus, or postcricoid areas are considered of pharyngeal origin and discussed in Chapter 4.

Verrucous carcinoma is a rare variant of laryngeal carcinoma that behaves like verrucous carcinoma in other locations (Fig. 210). Extensive local invasion may occur, but regional lymph node metastases prac-

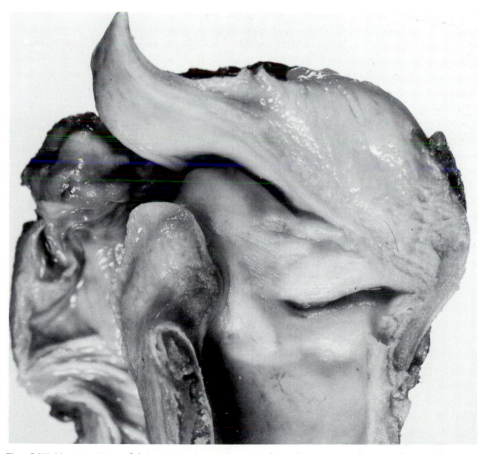

Fig. 207 Hemisection of larynx at autopsy more than five years after irradiation for carcinoma of true cord. Note perfectly normal true and false cords. Patient died of cardiovascular disease. (WU neg. 61-1715.)

tically never develop. Of twelve patients with laryngeal verrucous carcinoma reviewed by Kraus and Perez-Mesa,[21] none had metastases.

Epidermoid carcinoma with sarcoma-like stroma ("pseudosarcoma") is a peculiar neoplasm restricted to the upper respiratory and digestive tracts.[17, 20, 22] We have

have seen no examples in the larynx. Lymph node metastases are composed of either the carcinomatous component alone or of both elements. However, we now have a case in which a metastatic lymph node, serially sectioned, contained only the sarcoma-like growth. This finding proves that this component is also malignant. If

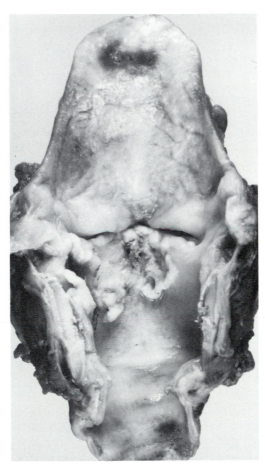

Fig. 208 Laryngeal carcinoma involving both true cords and extending into subglottic area for distance of 1.7 cm. This type is classified as subglottic carcinoma. (WU neg. 69-16.)

examined eleven cases, five of them located in the larynx. They all had a polypoid configuration (Fig. 211). Microscopically, they have an element of epidermoid carcinoma (often inconspicuous and frequently in situ) and a pleomorphic sarcoma-like component, which makes the bulk of the lesion. It is microscopically distinct from carcinosarcoma, of which we

it is a true sarcoma or a carcinoma in disguise is still a matter of controversy.

Other tumors

The *subglottic hemangioma* characteristically occurs in infants. It presents as a sessile, poorly circumscribed mass immediately below the true cord. Symptoms of upper respiratory tract obstruction may be

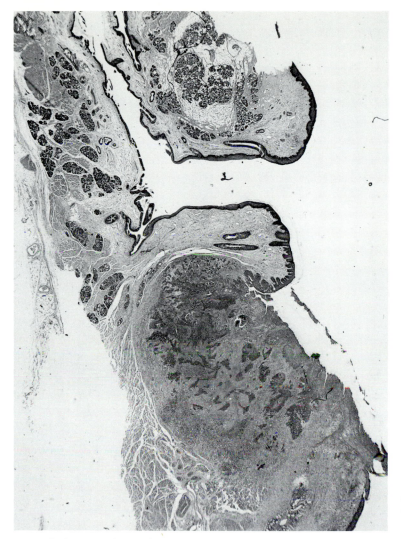

Fig. 209 True subglottic epidermoid carcinoma in 42-year-old man. Hemilaryngectomy was performed. All margins were free. This was third proved subglottic carcinoma out of 600 laryngectomies. (Low power; WU neg. 62-7389.)

severe. One-half of the patients have associated hemangiomas in the skin, an important diagnostic sign. Biopsy can precipitate massive bleeding. The treatment of choice is radiation therapy, sometimes preceded by tracheotomy.[34]

Granular cell tumor may involve the true cord. We have seen two cases mistaken microscopically for epidermoid carcinoma because of the secondary pseudoepitheliomatous hyperplasia present in conjunction with the lesions.[30]

Rhabdomyoma has a predilection for the head and neck area, including the larynx.

Cross striations are often found in addition to peculiar crystal-like intracytoplasmic particles.[29]

Other benign tumors we have encountered in the larynx include *paraganglioma, neurilemoma,* and a single instance of *inflammatory pseudotumor (pseudolymphoma).*

Cady et al.[31] found thirty-one nonepidermoid primary malignant tumors in a review of 2,500 laryngeal cancers (an incidence of 1.25%). These included seventeen adenocarcinomas, four malignant melanomas, three malignant lymphomas, three

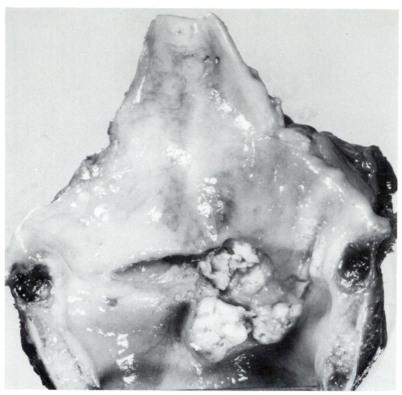

Fig. 210 Verrucous carcinoma of larynx with obliteration of right vocal cord and extension into subglottis. (WU neg. 59-941; from Kraus, F. T., and Perez-Mesa, C.: Verrucous carcinoma; clinical and pathologic study of 105 cases involving oral cavity, larynx, and genitalia, Cancer **19**:26-28, 1966.)

rhabdomyosarcomas, two chondrosarcomas, and one plasmacytoma. Three of the seventeen *adenocarcinomas* were of the adenoid cystic type (Fig. 212). The *rhabdomyosarcomas* are invariably of the embryonal variety.[28] *Plasmacytomas,* although initially appearing localized in the larynx, always become disseminated.[32]

Cartilaginous tumors of the larynx often arise from the cricoid cartilage and appear posteriorly in the subglottic region. Goeth-

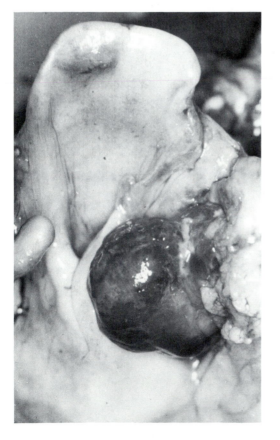

Fig. 211 Epidermoid carcinoma with sarcoma-like stroma ("pseudosarcoma") involving pharyngeal wall. Note typical polypoid configuration. (From Cornes, J. S., and Lewis, M. S.: Polypoid carcinomas of the pharynx with sarcomatous or pseudosarcomatous stroma, Br. J. Surg. **53**:340-344, 1966.)

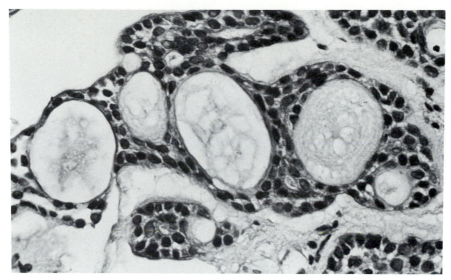

Fig. 212 Adenoid cystic carcinoma arising from mucous glands of larynx. Extensive lymph node and pulmonary metastases were present at time of this biopsy. (×500; WU neg. 52-4079.)

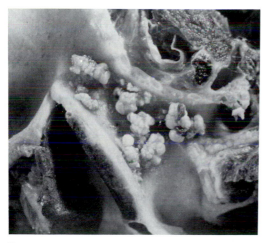

Fig. 213 Extensive papillomatosis of trachea and bronchi. (AFIP 289980.)

als et al.[33] classified four of their twenty-two cases as benign and all of the others as chondrosarcomas by applying the same microscopic criteria used for the skeletal tumors. However, none of the tumors metastasized, and only six recurred locally. These findings indicate that surgery should be as conservative as possible for cartilaginous neoplasms occurring in this location.

We have also seen examples of *fibrosarcoma, carcinoid tumor,* and an instance of *metastatic renal cell carcinoma* first presenting with laryngeal symptoms.

TRACHEA

Papilloma and *papillomatosis* of the trachea are similar to the lesions seen in the larynx[37] (Fig. 213).

In *tracheopathia osteoplastica,* multiple small submucosal nodules composed of mature bone and cartilage are found beneath the mucosa.[36] The etiology is unknown. Most *malignant tumors* involving the trachea represent direct extension from a bronchial or esophageal carcinoma. Of fifty-three primary treacheal carcinomas collected by Houston et al.,[39] twenty-four were squamous cell carcinomas and nineteen were adenoid cystic carcinomas (Fig. 214). The prognosis is poor for both tumor types, but the clinical course is quite different. Squamous cell carcinoma in most cases causes rapid death, whereas adenoid cystic carcinoma follows a protracted (up to thirty years) but relentless clinical course.[40] The majority of squamous cell carcinomas arise in the lower one-third of the trachea, whereas most adenoid cystic cancers and mucus-secreting adenocarcinomas occur in the upper one-third.[38]

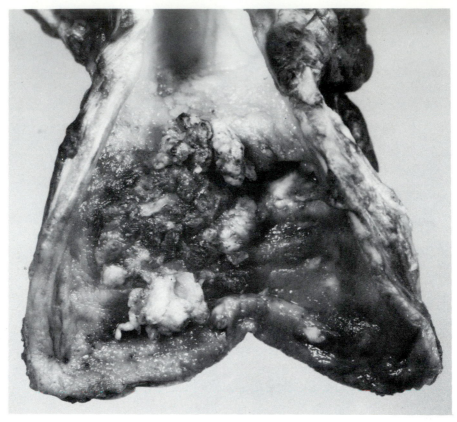

Fig. 214 Epidermoid carcinoma of trachea, excised following course of radiation therapy (6,000 R). Patient is alive and without evidence of disease four years later. (WU neg. 67-8073.)

REFERENCES

LARYNX

Cysts

1 DeSanto, L. W., Devine, K. D., and Weiland, L. H.: Cysts of the larynx—classification, Laryngoscope **80**:145-176, 1970.
2 Gallagher, J. C., and Puzon, B. Q.: Oncocytic lesions of the larynx, Ann. Otol. Rhinol. Laryngol. **78**:307-318, 1969.
3 Giovaniello, J., Grieco, R. V., and Bartone, N. F.: Laryngocele, Am. J. Roentgenol. Radium Ther. Nucl. Med. **108**:825-829, 1970.

Infection

4 Barton, R. T.: Observation on the pathogenesis of laryngeal granuloma due to endotracheal anesthesia, N. Engl. J. Med. **248**:1097-1099, 1953.
5 Bennett, D. E.: Histoplasmosis of the oral cavity and larynx; a clinicopathologic study, Arch. Intern. Med. **120**:417-427, 1967.
6 Bienestock, H., Ehrlich, G. E., and Freyberg, R. H.: Rheumatoid arthritis of the cricoarytenoid joint; a clinicopathologic study, Arthritis Rheum. **6**:48-63, 1963.

Laryngeal nodule

7 Ash, J. E., and Schwartz, L.: The laryngeal (vocal cord) node, Trans. Am. Acad. Ophthalmol. Otolaryngol. **48**:323-332, 1944.
8 Kamberg, S., Loitman, B. S., and Holtz, S.: Amyloidosis of the tracheobronchial tree, N. Engl. J. Med. **266**:587-591, 1962.

Tumors

Papillomatosis

9 Björk, H., and Weber, C.: Papilloma of the larynx, Acta Otolaryngol. (Stockh.) **46**:499, 1956.
10 Holinger, P. H., Schild, J. A., and Maurizi, D. G.: Laryngeal papilloma; review of etiology and therapy, Laryngoscope **78**:1462-1474, 1968.
11 Meesen, J., and Schultz, H.: Electron microscope demonstration of a virus in human laryngeal papilloma, Klin. Wochenschr. **35**:771-773, 1957.
12 Moore, R. L., and Lattes, R.: Papillomatosis of the larynx and bronchi, Cancer **12**:117-126, 1959.
13 Rabbett, W. F.: Juvenile laryngeal papillomatosis; relation of irradiation to malignant de-

generation in this disease, Ann. Otol. Rhinol. Laryngol. **74**:1149-1163, 1965.

Keratosis

14 McGavran, M. H., Bauer, W. C., and Ogura, J. H.: Isolated laryngeal keratosis; its relation to carcinoma of the larynx based on a clinico-pathologic study of 87 consecutive cases with long-term follow-up, Laryngoscope **70**:932-951, 1960.

Carcinoma in situ

15 Altman, F., Ginsberg, I., and Stout, A. P.: Intraepithelial carcinoma (cancer in situ) of the larynx, Arch. Otolaryngol. **56**:121-133, 1952.
16 Bauer, W. C., and McGavran, M. H.: Carcinoma-in-situ and evaluation of epithelial changes in laryngo-pharyngeal biopsies, J.A.M.A. **221**:72-75, 1972.

Invasive epidermoid carcinoma

17 Appelman, H. D., and Oberman, H. A.: Squamous cell carcinoma of the larynx with sarcoma-like stroma; a clinicopathologic assessment of spindle cell carcinoma and "pseudosarcoma", Am. J. Clin. Pathol. **44**:135-145, 1965.
18 Bauer, W. C., Edwards, D. L., and McGavran, M. H.: A critical analysis of laryngectomy in the treatment of epidermoid carcinoma of the larynx, Cancer **15**:263-270, 1962.
19 Biller, H. F., Ogura, J. H., and Pratt, L. L.: Hemilaryngectomy for T2 glottic cancers, Arch. Otolaryngol. **93**:238-243, 1971.
20 Goellner, J. R., Devine, K. D., and Weiland, L. H.: Pseudosarcoma of the larynx, Am. J. Clin. Pathol. **59**:312-326, 1973.
21 Kraus, F. T., and Perez-Mesa, C.: Verrucous carcinoma; clinical and pathologic study of 105 cases involving oral cavity, larynx, and genitalia, Cancer **19**:26-28, 1966.
22 Lane, N.: Pseudosarcoma (polypoid sarcoma-like masses) associated with squamous-cell carcinoma of the mouth, fauces and larynx; report of ten cases, Cancer **10**:19-41, 1957.
23 McGavran, M. H., Bauer, W. C., and Ogura, J. H.: The incidence of cervical lymph node metastases from epidermoid carcinoma of the larynx and their relationship to certain characteristics of the primary tumor; a study based on the clinical and pathological findings for 96 patients treated by primary en bloc laryngectomy and radical neck dissection, Cancer **14**:55-65, 1961.
24 Marks, R. D., Jr., Fitz-Hugh, G. S., and Constable, W. C.: Fourteen years' experience with cobalt-60 radiation therapy in the treatment of early cancer of the true vocal cords, Cancer **28**:571-576, 1971.

25 Ogura, J. H., and Biller, H. F.: Neck dissection for carcinoma of the larynx and hypopharynx, Proceedings of the Sixth National Cancer Conference, Philadelphia, 1970, J. B. Lippincott Co., pp. 671-675.
26 Perez, C. A., Holtz, S., Ogura, J. H., Dedo, H. H., and Powers, W. E.: Radiation therapy of early carcinoma of the true vocal cords, Cancer **21**:764-771, 1968.
27 Stutsman, A. C., and McGavran, M. H.: Ultra-conservative management of superficially invasive epidermoid carcinoma of the true vocal cord, Ann. Otol. Rhinol. Laryngol. **80**:507-512, 1971.

Other tumors

28 Batsakis, J. G., and Fox, J. E.: Rhabdomyosarcoma of the larynx, Arch. Otolaryngol. **91**:136-140, 1970.
29 Batsakis, J. G., and Fox, J. E.: Supporting tissue neoplasms of the larynx, Surg. Gynecol. Obstet. **131**:989-997, 1970.
30 Booth, J. B., and Osborn, D. A.: Granular cell myoblastoma of the larynx, Acta Otolaryngol. (Stockh.) **70**:279-293, 1970.
31 Cady, B., Rippey, J. H., and Frazell, E. L.: Non-epidermoid cancer of the larynx, Ann. Surg. **167**:116-120, 1968.
32 Costen, J. B.: Plasmacytoma; a case with original lesion of the epiglottis and metastasis to the tibia, Laryngoscope **61**:266-270, 1951.
33 Goethals, P. L., Dahlin, D. C., and Devine, K. D.: Cartilaginous tumors of the larynx, Surg. Gynecol. Obstet. **117**:77-82, 1963.
34 Tefft, M.: The radiotherapeutic management of subglottic hemangioma in children, Radiology **85**:207-214, 1966.
35 Vetters, J. M., and Toner, P. G.: Chemodectoma of the larynx, J. Pathol. **101**:259-265, 1970.

TRACHEA

36 Ashley, D. J.: Bony metaplasia in trachea and bronchi, J. Pathol. **102**:186-188, 1970.
37 Buffmire, D. K., Clagett, O. T., and McDonald, J. R.: Papillomas of the larynx, trachea and bronchi; report of a case, Mayo Clin. Proc. **25**:595-600, 1950.
38 Hajdu, S. I., Huvos, A. G., Goodner, J. T., Foote, F. W., Jr., and Beattie, E. J., Jr.: Carcinoma of the trachea; clinicopathologic study of 41 cases, Cancer **25**:1448-1456, 1970.
39 Houston, H. E., Payne, W. S., Harrison, E. G., Jr., and Olsen, A. M.: Primary cancers of the trachea, Arch. Surg. **99**:132-140, 1969.
40 Markel, S. F., and Abell, M. R.: Adenocystic basal cell carcinoma of the trachea, J. Thorac. Cardiovasc. Surg. **48**:211-225, 1964.

Lung

Introduction

Since 1933, when the first lung was successfully resected for bronchogenic carcinoma, advances in thoracic surgery have been extremely rapid. As a result, exploratory thoracotomy has become so safe that debatable lesions of the lung or bronchus are explored without hesitation. Only those lesions pertaining particularly to surgical pathology are described in this section.

The most frequent specimens submitted by an active thoracic surgery service are from segmental resections, lobectomies, and pneumonectomies. Unfortunately, some pathologists are content to make a simple diagnosis of tuberculosis, bronchiectasis, or cancer. To extend the knowledge of pulmonary pathology and to give the surgeon more information than a mere diagnosis, it is necessary to have a well-organized method for studying the specimens, which may differ according to the pathologic change present.

In most cases, we inject the specimen with formalin through the bronchial tree and, after it is fixed, dissect it with careful regard to its anatomy. Using the nomenclature of Brock[1] and Jackson and Huber,[3] we have devised stamps in order to identify the site of pathologic change (Fig. 215). In this fashion, the pathologist quickly gains a concept of the areas in the various lobes that are most commonly involved in different pathologic processes. If the lesion is carcinoma, sections must be taken at the bronchial line of resection, and all lymph nodes must be studied. In cases of metastatic carcinoma, Hodgkin's disease, or other potentially multifocal diseases, we study the lung after fixation by cutting thin (2 mm to 3 mm) slices with an electrically driven commercial meat slicer and carefully examining each cut surface.

It is imperative to have thorough bacteriologic study for the identification of various inflammatory and granulomatous processes. Fixed sections often hinder the identification of the tubercle bacillus, *Histoplasma capsulatum, Brucella,* and other organisms.

Weed et al.[5] stressed that many granulomatous lesions that have similar microscopic patterns may be caused by a variety of agents. It has been our experience that tuberculosis occasionally has an unusual pattern that makes its true nature unsuspected.[4] Therefore, material from any specimen containing pathology not yet diagnosed should be cultured prior to fixation. Furthermore, by using fluorescent antibody techniques, granulomatous-producing lesions caused by tularemia[6] and *Histoplasma capsulatum*[2, 7] may be identified. In cases of suspected pneumoconiosis or other occupational diseases, a portion of lung should be saved in formalin for possible physical or chemical determinations.

PLEURA
Biopsy and cytology

Needle biopsy of the parietal pleura is very useful for the differential diagnosis between inflammatory disease and malignancy.[11] Aaron et al.[8] combined pleural biopsy with biopsy of the lung parenchyma and hilar lymph nodes in the study of eighty-nine patients with diffuse pulmonary disease and/or hilar adenopathy and persistent pleural effusion. A definite diagnosis was reached in sixty-two cases. If tuberculosis is suspected, part of the pleural biopsy should be cultured. Levine et al.[10] found that culture of a single specimen from pleural biopsy was positive with greater frequency than multiple cultures of pleural fluid.

Whenever the possibility of malignancy is considered in the presence of pleural effusion, a cytologic examination of the pleural fluid should always be performed, regardless of its gross appearance.

In patients with long-standing pleural effusion, bloody fluid used to be considered indicative of cancer and serous effusion suggestive of tuberculosis. In a series of such patients who had exploratory thoracotomy, biopsy, and often decortication, the diagnosis was found to have little correlation with the type of fluid. A high percentage of the patients had nonspecific fibrosis and chronic inflammation, and the mere presence of bloody fluid did not indicate a malignant neoplasm.[9]

Obliterative pleuritis

Inflammatory disease of the lung may involve the pleura. The pulmonary lesion may completely resolve, leaving a pleural symphysis secondary to prominent fibrous thickening (up to several centimeters) of the pleura. These changes were seen frequently during World War II following penetrating injury to the chest. The underlying lung parenchyma may be perfectly normal. Its expansion is prevented by the surrounding rigid and contracted "thickened pleura." In many instances, this "thickened pleura" can be peeled away, with marked improvement of the underlying pulmonary function.

During World War II, an organizing hematoma often formed following a penetrating wound of the thorax. If this hematoma were allowed to remain for a long time, decortication was extremely difficult. If the chest were entered too early before cleavage planes could be established, decortication was impossible. A three-week to five-week interval was found to be ideal.[12] It should be emphasized that the material obtained by decortication represents an organized hematoma made up of fibrous tissue *without elastic tissue*, which, in itself, is proof that the underlying pleura is not involved. Infection may cause more rapid organization of the hematoma.

Mesothelioma

A highly controversial group of neoplasms, mesotheliomas, have gained wide recognition in recent years, largely as a result of their increasing frequency and the discovery of their relationship with exposure to asbestos. Wagner et al.[21] reported a marked increase in the incidence of diffuse pleural mesotheliomas in workers of large asbestos mining areas in South Africa. Proof of the widespread use of this material is the findings of asbestos bodies in lung smears (particularly from the lower lobes) in approximately 40% of persons autopsied in the United States.[14] It should be noted that the asbestos bodies are more commonly found in the lung than within the mesothelioma. The chemistry and morphology of asbestos bodies have been well reviewed by Gaensler and Addington.[16] Peculiar cytoplasmic hyaline masses were found by Kuhn and Kuo[17] in the alveolar cells of the lung in asbestosis.

Pleural mesotheliomas can be divided into four reasonably distinct clinico-pathologic varieties: benign fibrous, benign epithelial, malignant fibrous, and malignant epithelial.

Benign fibrous mesothelioma is always well circumscribed or encapsulated. It is usually asymptomatic, although on occasion patients present with prominent pulmonary osteoarthropathy that rapidly re-

gresses when the tumor is removed.[13] Grossly, the lesion is firm, lobulated, and gray-white to yellow-white, with frequent whorling and fasciculation. Unlike the neurilemoma, it does not undergo cystic degeneration (Fig. 216). It may be found attached to the parietal pleura or visceral pleura or within an interlobar fissure.

Microscopically, the tumor forms a tangled network of fibrous tissue with abundant reticulin and foci of dense collagenous material. The degree of cellularity varies a great deal from case to case. The

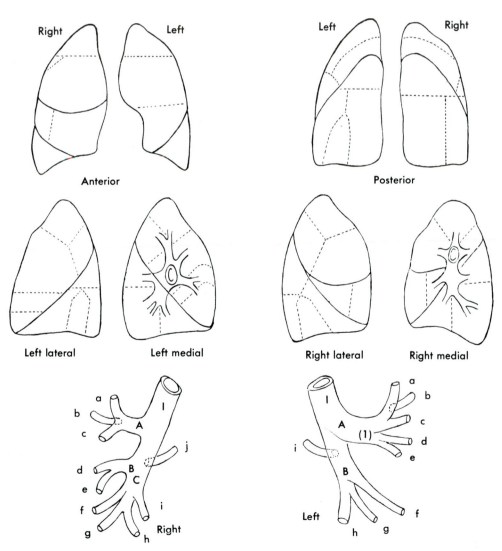

Fig. 215 Diagrammatic sketch of main branches of bronchi of lungs, using nomenclature of Brock[1] and Jackson and Huber.[3] (For key, see opposite page.)

most cellular types are sometimes misdiagnosed as fibrosarcoma or neurofibrosarcoma (Fig. 217). If proper attention is paid to the lack of nuclear aberrations and the rarity or absence of mitoses, confusion is unlikely to occur. In some instances, foci of epithelial cells forming papillae, tubules, or solid nests are found in the periphery of predominantly fibrous tumors. It is not clear if they are a constituent of the neoplasm or merely entrapped mesothelium or pulmonary epithelium.[15, 19] The theory of the mesothelial origin of this neoplasm, not too obvious by light or electron microscopic examination, is largely based on tissue culture studies published by Stout and Murray in 1942.[20] We agree with Ratzer et al.[19] that confirmation of this work with modern tissue culture techniques is needed. The large majority of these neoplasms are permanently cured by local excision. However, we have now seen two patients in whom repeated local recurrences developed, with eventual tumor invasion of the chest wall.

Benign epithelial mesothelioma, which makes a good percentage of peritoneal mesotheliomas, is exceptional in the pleura. We have seen only three cases.[15] Grossly, it is a soft friable mass, mottled pink, gray, and yellow. Microscopically, papillary processes lined by one or several layers of cuboidal mesothelial cells are seen. The differentiation with the malignant epithelial mesothelioma is made on the basis of the lack of significant atypia and the well-circumscribed, solitary nature of the lesion.

Malignant fibrous mesothelioma often presents with chest pain and/or dyspnea. Association with hypoglycemia has been reported, with disappearance of the symptom on removal of the tumor.[18] Pleural effusion was found in twelve of the fifteen cases reported by Ratzer et al.[19] Grossly, this tumor is relatively well circumscribed but not encapsulated. Hemorrhage, necrosis, and cystic changes are common. Microscopically, the tumor is highly cellular, formed by interwoven bundles of spindle cells. Nuclear atypia is present, and mi-

Brock's nomenclature	Jackson-Huber's nomenclature

Right bronchial tree (I, main bronchus; **A**, upper lobe bronchus; **B**, middle lobe bronchus; **C**, lower lobe bronchus)

Brock's nomenclature	Jackson-Huber's nomenclature
a. Apical bronchus, upper lobe	a. Apical bronchus, upper lobe
b. Subapical bronchus, upper lobe	b. Anterior bronchus, upper lobe
c. Pectoral bronchus, upper lobe	c. Posterior bronchus, upper lobe
d. Medial division, middle lobe	d. Medial division, middle lobe
e. Lateral division, middle lobe	e. Lateral division, middle lobe
f. Anterior basal bronchus, lower lobe	f. Anterior basal bronchus, lower lobe
g. Middle basal bronchus, lower lobe	g. Lateral basal bronchus, lower lobe
h. Posterior basal bronchus, lower lobe	h. Posterior basal bronchus, lower lobe
i. Cardiac bronchus, lower lobe	i. Medial basal bronchus, lower lobe
j. Apical bronchus, lower lobe	j. Superior bronchus, lower lobe

Left bronchial tree (I, main bronchus; **A**, upper lobe bronchus; **B**, lower lobe bronchus; (1), lingular bronchus)

Brock's nomenclature	Jackson-Huber's nomenclature
a. Apical bronchus, upper lobe	a. Superior division, upper lobe
b. Subapical bronchus, upper lobe	b. Apical posterior, upper lobe
c. Pectoral bronchus, upper lobe	c. Anterior bronchus, upper lobe
d. Upper division, lingular, upper lobe	d. Superior lingular, inferior division, upper lobe
e. Lower division, lingular, upper lobe	e. Inferior lingular, inferior division, upper lobe
f. Anterior basal bronchus, lower lobe	f. Anterior-medial basal, lower lobe
g. Middle basal bronchus, lower lobe	g. Lateral basal, lower lobe
h. Posterior basal bronchus, lower lobe	h. Posterior basal, lower lobe
i. Apical bronchus, lower lobe	i. Superior bronchus, lower lobe

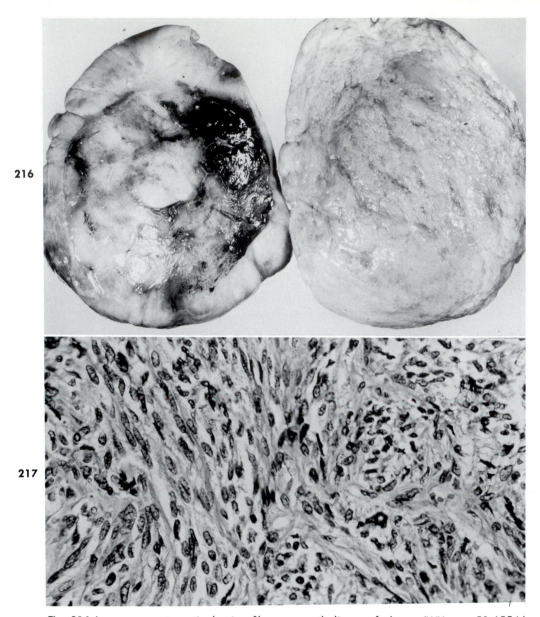

Fig. 216 Large, asymptomatic, benign fibrous mesothelioma of pleura. (WU neg. 50-6554.)
Fig. 217 Highly cellular fibrous mesothelioma. Changes shown may cause incorrect diagnosis of sarcoma. (×460; WU neg. 52-3455.)

totic figures are common. The prognosis is extremely poor. The histogenetic considerations given for the benign fibrous mesothelioma also apply to this malignant counterpart.

Malignant epithelial mesothelioma is a diffuse neoplasm that often involves the lower half of a hemithorax but may spread to the entire pleural space, both pleurae, or even to the peritoneum. Distant metastases occur late in the course of the disease. Grossly, multiple gray or white ill-defined nodules are seen in a diffusely thickened pleura. Pleural effusion is almost always present. Microscopically, the epithelial formations may form papillae or

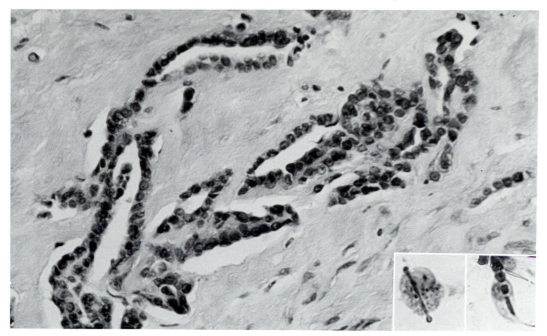

Fig. 218 Malignant diffuse mesothelioma of epithelial variety. Glandlike spaces grow in dense fibrous stroma. **Insets,** Asbestos bodies found in patient's sputum. (×350; WU neg. 72-6055; **insets,** Papanicolaou; ×720; WU negs. 72-1093 and 72-1094.)

pseudoacini or grow as solid nests (Fig. 218). The cytoplasm is abundant and acidophilic. Spindle tumor cells are sometimes observed, and the appearance of the tumor may be reminiscent of synovial sarcoma. Early cases must be differentiated from reactive mesothelial hyperplasia and obviously malignant tumors from metastatic carcinoma. The prognosis is uniformly poor. Fifteen of sixteen patients reported by Ratzer et al.[19] died from eleven to fifty-eight months following onset of symptoms.

Other lesions

Pleural hyaline plaques are sometimes found by the surgeon incidentally during the course of a thoracotomy. They are located on the parietal and diaphragmatic surfaces, are usually multiple, and tend to follow the course of the ribs.[25] Calcification may develop focally, and this can be detected by radiographic examination. Asbestos fibers have been implicated as the etiologic agent.[22]

Rheumatoid disease occasionally involves the lung and pleura. It may produce pneumonitis, diffuse interstitial fibrosis, discrete rheumatoid nodules (with or without cavitation) or diffuse pleural reaction with effusion.[24] The microscopic appearance of the pleural biopsy is often nonspecific. In some instances, however, the presence of palisaded spindle histiocytes underlying a layer of fibrin and arranged perpendicularly to the pleural surface should make the pathologist suspect a rheumatoid etiology.[23]

Endometriosis of the pleura and diaphragm has been reported. Most of the cases have occurred in the right side and have been associated with widespread intra-abdominal endometriosis.[26]

PULMONARY PARENCHYMA AND BRONCHI
Abscess

Lung abscesses are most often located in the right lower lobe (Fig. 219), right upper lobe, and left lower lobe according to a series reported from Barnes Hospital.[27] The right side and the lower lobes were

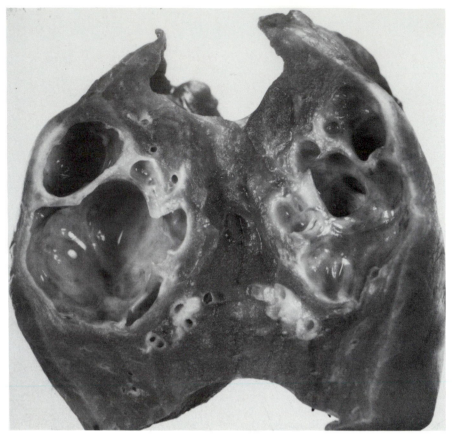

Fig. 219 Chronic abscess of right lower lobe of lung in child following two-week history of pneumonia. Abscess is well delimited with smooth walls. (WU neg. 67-299.)

more frequently involved than the left side and the upper lobes.[27]

In Brock's series[29] of fifty cases, the right upper lobe was involved in twenty, the right lower lobe in twelve, the left upper lobe in seven, and the left lower lobe in eight. Brock emphasized that the apical segments of the upper lobes are only rarely the site of an abscess. The subapical segment is the most frequent site in the right upper lobe, and the axillary branch of the pectoral segment is the most common site in the left upper lobe. The anterior position of the bronchus of the middle lobe is responsible for the infrequent occurrence of abscess in this lobe.

The apical segment of the lower lobes is particularly vulnerable in patients who must assume a supine position. The basal bronchi of the lower lobes are about equal-

ly susceptible. Brock[28, 29] pointed out that involvement of the basal segment by atelectasis and infection is frequent following abdominal operations because of their dependency, limited movement of the diaphragm and abdominal muscles, tight bandaging, excessive sedation, and dehydration.

The causes and treatment of lung abscess have changed considerably with the advent of antibiotics. In the past, lung abscesses often followed tonsillectomies and operations in the throat, but today this complication is relatively infrequent. Lung abscess most frequently follows the aspiration of infected or foreign material (Fig. 220). Embolism from a distant source does not cause unilocular abscess. The number of chronic abscesses removed on our thoracic surgery service has lessened. If emboli of

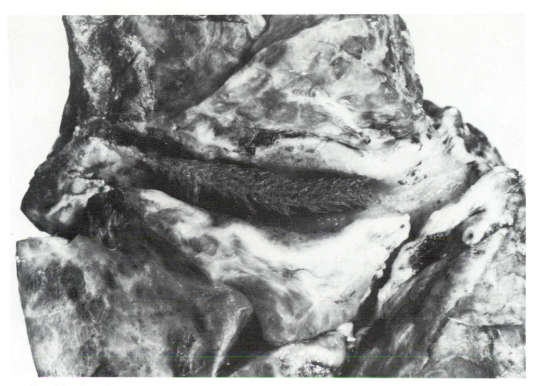

Fig. 220 Bronchopneumonia with abscess formation in 2-year-old boy secondary to aspiration of foreign body (Timothy grass inflorescence). (From Kissane, J. M., and Smith, M. G.: Pathology of infancy and childhood, St. Louis, 1967, The C. V. Mosby Co.)
First recorded case of this condition seems to be that recorded in book entitled *Some account of Lord Boringdon's accident on July 21st, 1817, and its consequences* as follows: "In 1662, Armand de Boutree, son of the Compte de Nogent, was seized with a violent fever, accompanied by a great difficulty in breathing, a dry cough, afterwards spotting of blood, sleeplessless, and great pain in the right side. A tumor at length appeared on that side, and a surgeon extracted from it an ear of barley almost entire which was quite green and had undergone no change."

infected material reach the lung, bilateral sepsis usually follows. Lung abscesses and other long-standing pulmonary cavities may be complicated by the growth of fungi, particularly *Mucor* and *Aspergillus* (Fig. 221).

It must be remembered that lung abscess may be secondary to a carcinoma. Brock[29] reported fifty-six patients with abscesses, fifty-three of whom were past 45 years of age. Of the latter patients, 30% had abscesses secondary to cancer. In about one-half of the patients, the cause was unknown. Frequently, patients are seen first and treated by an internist. Often, the abscess clears, particularly when it is small. Chronic abscesses are best treated surgically. Today, drainage by resection of a

rib is seldom done. In small unilocular abscesses, partial resection of the lobe may be curative.[32] However, Burford[30] believes that lobectomy is preferable because complications such as bronchopleural fistula and empyema are much less frequent. The larger, more complicated abscess is invariably associated with fibrosis and bronchiectasis of the lung. In these cases, lobectomy and occasionally pneumonectomy are necessary.

Grossly and microscopically, chronic abscesses have thick fibrotic walls and are surrounded by areas of organizing pneumonia. The bronchi communicating with them show prominent bronchiectasis. The clinical result of abscess resection is ex-

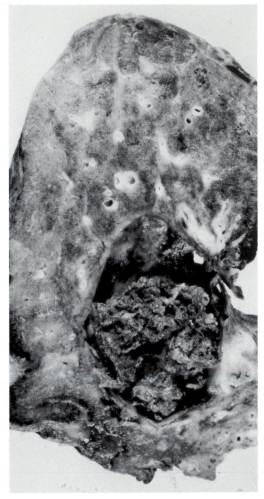

Fig. 221 Chronic pulmonary abscess complicated by growth of "fungus ball." Organism was identified as *Mucor*. (WU neg. 72-2862.)

cellent. The mortality rate in the patients treated by Harter[31] was under 5%.

Complications of untreated lung abscesses include brain abscesses, empyema, exsanguinating hemorrhage, overwhelming illness, and spread of the process. The newer methods of treatment have greatly reduced the frequency of these complications.

Tuberculosis

The use of the new antimicrobial agents and isoniazid has modified both the natural history and the pathology of *tuberculosis.* However, there is still an appreciable number of patients who, because of inadequate response to drug therapy, become candidates for surgery. Most of the surgical procedures done at the present time for tuberculosis are resectional—wedge excision, subsegmental resections, lobectomy, and pneumonectomy. Strieder et al.[41] summarized the indications for pulmonary resection as follows:

1 Open cavity (with or without positive sputum) after a suitable period (four to six months) on a satisfactory drug regimen
2 Residual caseous or fibrocaseous disease, with or without positive sputum
3 Irreversible destructive lesions, such as bronchostenosis, and bronchiectasis[39]
4 Recurrent or persistent hemorrhage, usually arising in a cavity or bronchiectasis
5 Thoracoplasty failure
6 Unexpandable lobe or lung, with associated chronic encapsulated tuberculous empyema
7 Suspected neoplasm

In most reported series of surgically treated tuberculous patients, 80% to 85% have inactive disease two to five years after surgery. Most complications of surgery, such as bronchopleural fistula, occur in patients with positive sputum preoperatively.[37]

Grossly, the lung or lobe surgically resected for tuberculosis usually consists of nonfunctioning pulmonary parenchyma. When tuberculosis predominantly involves the bronchi, causing stricture formation, the more peripheral lung becomes nonfunctioning. The pathologic process is a combination of tuberculosis and a superimposed infection. The strictures may be in major bronchi or, rarely, may involve smaller ramifications of the bronchial tree (Figs. 222 and 223). Usually, bronchiectasis in the upper lobes is nonspecific in nature because of good drainage. However, in the lower lobes, it is more often complicated by extensive active tuberculosis.

It is probable that the histogenesis of

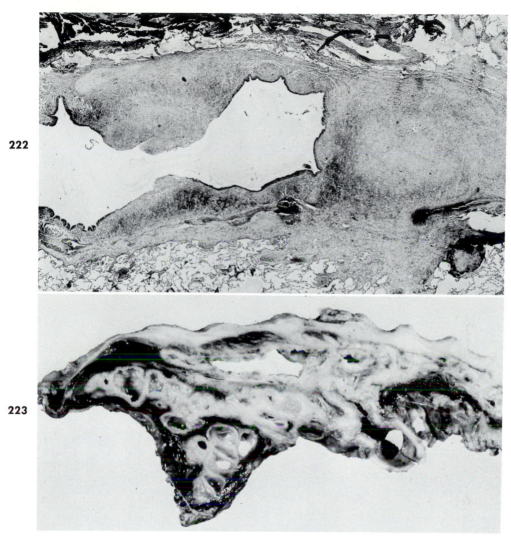

Fig. 222 Tuberculosis involving small bronchus, with narrowing of lumen, ulceration, and peribronchial involvement. (Low power; WU neg. 49-5636.)
Fig. 223 Extensive tuberculosis involving entire left lung with prominent bonchiectasis, cavitation, and thickened pleura. It is obvious that compression therapy cannot cure such lesions. (WU neg. 50-5257.)

tuberculosis of the bronchi is due to the retrograde spread of tubercle bacilli down the ducts of the mucous glands, direct implantation of these bacilli on the bronchial mucosa, and spread through the lymphatics to involve adjacent bronchi. Peribronchial tuberculous lymph nodes may infect the mucous glands of bronchi by direct extension. As Meissner[38] said, "Many of the lymphatics drain down the wall of the bronchus; the submucosa of the bronchus is also rich in lymphatics. Thus, the entire course of the bronchus . . . which leads from a parenchymal lesion is potentially subject to tuberculosis if tubercle bacilli will but lodge in its walls".*

Sweany and Seiler[43] reported their observations on thirty-four specimens in patients

*From Meissner, W. A.: Surgical pathology of endobronchial tuberculosis, Dis. Chest. **11:**18-25, 1945.

who had received rest and prolonged anti-microbial therapy. They demonstrated that about 25% of the advanced lesions showed healing by approximation of the walls of the cavities with granulation tissue, followed by fibrosis and stellate scars. There was also a group of patients with advanced disease in whom the lesions stabilized as chronic open cavities. Potential danger exists when a cavity with a communicating bronchus heals by inpissation of caseous material.[34] With the newer drugs, cavities can completely or almost completely heal, leaving a thin, fibrous wall with a smooth surface. The inner lining of the cavity has no epithelium except at the point at which

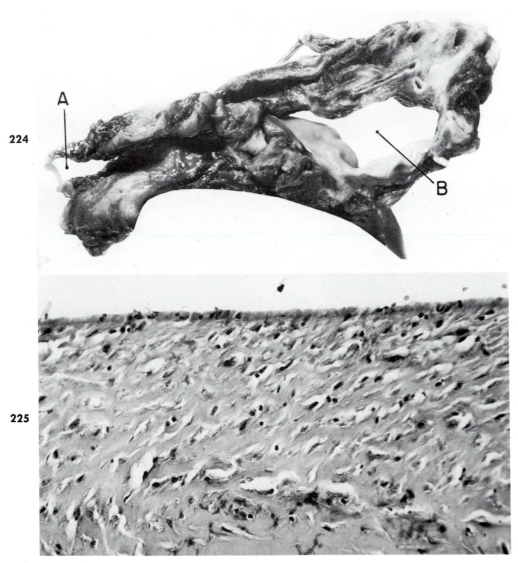

224

225

Fig. 224 Two apparently healed cavities, **A** and **B**, of right middle lobe. (From Auerbach, O., and Small, M. J.: The syndrome of persistent cavitation and noninfectious sputum during chemotherapy and its relation to the open healing of cavities, Am. Rev. Tuberc. **75**:242-258, 1957.)

Fig. 225 Lining of healed cavity shown in Fig. 224. There is no epithelium and no evidence of activity of process. (×260; WU neg. 58-128A; slide contributed by Dr. O. Auerbach, East Orange, N. J.)

the bronchus enters the cavity (Figs. 224 and 225). In this zone, it is squamous in nature. Examination for acid-fast organisms is invariably negative.[42] Such healing is relatively rare.[33, 44]

Tuberculomas are relatively infrequent lesions. Of 887 resected solitary pulmonary nodules collected by Steele,[40] there were 474 granulomas, 316 malignant tumors, 65 hamartomas, 23 miscellaneous lesions, and

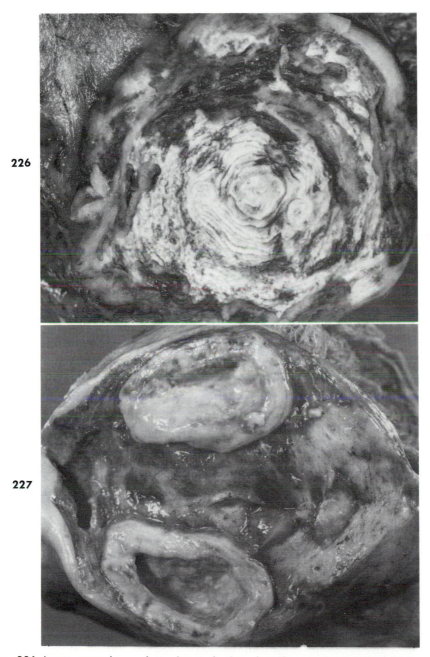

226

227

Fig. 226 Large granuloma that elevated pleural surface and presented laminated appearance. These laminated lesions often are caused by histoplasmosis. (WU neg. 48-5592.)
Fig. 227 Tuberculoma with central cavitation. These lesions may rupture and cause widespread pulmonary tuberculosis. (WU neg. 48-5009.)

9 pleural or chest wall tumors. Of these granulomas, 121 were due to tuberculosis. In only 17 (14%) of these was there a history of previous tuberculosis. In eighteen patients with such lesions seen at Barnes Hospital, eleven were past 40 years of age.[35] Tuberculomas are located immediately beneath the pleura and form discrete, firm, round masses. The pleura overlying the lesion is white or slightly yellow in color. There are usually no pleural adhesions. On section, the lesions may show concentric laminations of calcification (Fig. 226). Infrequently, they show areas of central cavitation (Fig. 227).

Evidence suggests that the tuberculoma is a reinfection rather than a primary Ghon focus. The large size, subpleural location, thick capsule, presence of separate satellite nodules, absence of bone, and evidence in some cases of separate Ranke's complexes support this viewpoint. Microscopically, we have invariably found areas of *persistent caseation*. Elastic and connective tissue stains outline the shadows of persistent alveoli, demonstrating that this process is the end stage of a caseous lobular tuberculous pneumonia. There is also prominent subpleural fibrous thickening. In a few instances, we have demonstrated communication of the process with a bronchus. Small active tubercles may be present in the immediate vicinity of the main lesion. Lesions of an identical gross pattern may be caused by organisms other than the tubercle bacilli, particularly by *Histoplasma* and other fungi. In thirty-five surgically resected, discrete pulmonary granulomas, Zimmerman[45] identified tubercle bacilli in six lesions, *Coccidioides* in three, and *Histoplasma* in nineteen. No organisms were found in the remaining seven.

An apparently increasing number of granulomatous infections of the lung is due to "atypical" or "unclassified" acid-fast mycobacteriae. We know of no way to differentiate them pathologically from tuberculosis, short of culture of the organism. The surgical approach follows the same general rules as in tuberculosis.[36]

Radiologically, it may be impossible to differentiate tuberculomas from primary or secondary neoplasms. The presence of concentric or focal areas of calcification strongly supports a diagnosis of granuloma. However, we have seen two carcinomas of the lung with focal calcification, both incorrectly diagnosed radiographically as tuberculomas. Because these lesions contain persistent areas of caseation and cannot be differentiated from a neoplasm, they must be resected. Gross examination at operation is almost always diagnostic, but the diagnosis should be confirmed by frozen section.

Other granulomatous diseases

There are many granulomatous processes which become focal and chronic within the lung and which are usually resected because of the difficulty in differentiating them from neoplasms. Frequently, all that can be said after studying these lesions is that the process is a chronic granulomatous one.

We have come to realize that various bacteria and fungi can give similar microscopic patterns. For this reason, we have made it our custom in all debatable lesions of the lung to put small pieces of tissue in the refrigerator so that they may be thoroughly studied bacteriologically if the permanent sections are not diagnostic. As a result of this procedure, we have found unexpected tuberculosis, atypical myobacteriosis, histoplasmosis, blastomycosis, and other diseases. The recognition particularly of fungi is aided by the use of Schiff and Gridley stains. The Schiff stain selectively outlines the capsule of the organism. Diffuse noncaseating granulomas also can be seen in sarcoidosis and, as an expression of hypersensitivity, in farmer's lung, maplebark stripper's lung, pigeon-breeder's lung, budgerigar-fancier's lung, mushroom-picker's lung, Wegener's granulomatosis, eosinophilic pneumonia, and bronchial chondromalacia.[46] Silo-filler's disease should be clearly separated from the aforementioned group, since it is a form of chemical pneumonitis secondary to nitrogen dioxide inhalation and is not characterized by the presence of granulomas.

Interstitial pneumonia

Following the routine use of open lung biopsy in the presence of a persistent unexplained pulmonary infiltrate, valuable information on the group of diseases usually grouped under the term "interstitial pneumonia" has been obtained. If the course of the disease is rapid, with death within a matter of months, the eponymic designation of Hamman-Rich syndrome is usually employed. Most of the cases, however, follow a protracted clinical course. They are characterized microscopically by irregular fibrosis, smooth muscle proliferation, mononuclear infiltrate, and variable proliferation of alveolar cells. Necrosis, hyaline membranes, and fibrin are present in the early stages. In some instances, there is, in addition, damage to the bronchioles, as evidenced by "bronchiolitis obliterans" and distal endogenous lipoid pneumonia. Some of the interstitial pneumonias are the result of viral, mycoplasmal, or chemical pneumonia, whereas others represent the residue of a diffuse granulomatous process. Still others are associated with one of the so-called collagen diseases (such as rheumatoid arthritis or scleroderma) or to obstruction of the pulmonary veins.[47] Several instances of familial incidence have been reported.[48] Liebow[52] has tentatively separated from this group three types with distinctive morphologic features: desquamative interstitial pneumonia, lymphoid interstitial pneumonia, and giant cell interstitial pneumonia. The remaining cases, which represent the large majority, constitute the "usual" or "classical" type of interstitial pneumonia. Desquamative interstitial pneumonia is characterized by a filling of the alveolar spaces by large mononuclear cells, associated with relatively minor interstitial changes.[50, 53] In the cases examined electron microscopically in our institution, the desquamated cells had the features of macrophages rather than of granular pneumocytes, although hyperplasia of the latter was seen in the alveolar wall.[51] Necrosis, hyaline membranes, and fibrin are absent. Radiographically, a ground-glass type of opacification is seen bilaterally in the periphery of the lung bases. Good response to steroids was noted by Liebow et al[53] in their original series of eighteen patients. Lymphoid interstitial pneumonia can be regarded as the diffuse variant of pulmonary pseudolymphoma. A lymphocytic infiltrate, often admixed with histiocytes and plasma cells, occupies the lung interstitium. Response to steroids is poor. Differentiation with malignant lymphoma may be difficult.

Scadding et al.[54] use the pathogenetically more satisfactory term *diffuse fibrosing alveolitis* to designate this group of conditions. They consider Liebow's "usual interstitial pneumonia" and "desquamative interstitial pneumonia," which they call the "mural type" and the "desquamative type" of diffuse fibrosing alveolitis, respectively, as the opposite ends of a continuous spectrum rather than as two separate entities. We agree with this viewpoint. Several cases of carcinoma arising in lungs with diffuse interstitial fibrosis have been reported.[49]

Broncholith

Broncholiths occur rather infrequently. They are usually produced by erosion of partially calcified tuberculous lymph nodes into the bronchial lumen. In bronchiectasis, bronchial cartilage may undergo ossification and ulcerate into the lumen[55] (Fig. 228).

Lipoid pneumonia

Lipoid pneumonia is often a complication of debilitating disease or an incidental postmortem finding.[56] However, the local expressions of this process are often confused particularly with malignant neoplasms and consequently have become a surgical problem. Lipoid pneumonia can be divided into two types: exogenous and endogenous.

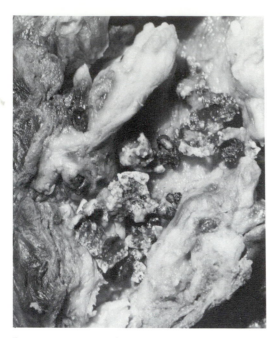

Fig. 228 Extensive broncholiths associated with advanced bronchiectasis. (WU neg. 48-4214.)

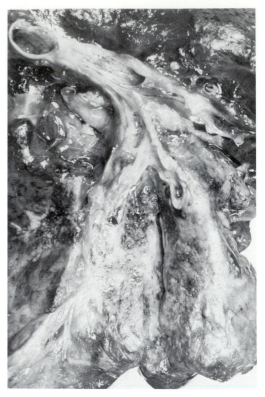

Fig. 229 Exogenous lipoid pneumonia producing firm, indurated area that, grossly, was considered to be carcinoma. (WU neg. 48-5291.)

In the *exogenous* type, lipoid reaches the lungs in various ways (oily nasal sprays, cod-liver oil, and mineral oil). We have seen one instance of partial esophageal obstruction that facilitated aspiration of oily medication. The patient's symptoms may warrant radiographic examination, which may show either a well-defined or a diffuse pulmonary process.[59] Examination of the sputum for the presence of fat particles is not diagnostic. Peculiar-appearing macrophages may be seen in the sputum and may be confused cytologically with carcinoma. At the time of exploration, a localized lesion of lipoid pneumonia may be extremely firm (Fig. 229). The lymphatics over the surface of the lung are often prominent, suggesting lymphatic permeation by carcinoma. The surgeon may see fat droplets if he cuts across one of these lesions.

The microscopic pattern shows fibrous tissue and sudanophilic material filling large spaces (Fig. 230). Frozen section may be difficult to interpret in the rare instance in which there is proliferation of alveolar cells. This change is similar to that described by Pinkerton[57, 58] in experimental animals. He has described methods of recognition of the various types of oils within the lung.

Endogenous lipoid pneumonia is characterized by the presence of yellow areas representing large amounts of lipid in the lung. These lesions we designate as endogenous because they are usually associated with some degree of bronchial block and represent the accumulation of fat of endogenous origin. The pathologist should be aware of this possibility, for such localized areas of lipoid pneumonia may be present peripheral to a blocked bronchus due to a carcinoma.

Organizing pneumonia

Pneumonia is not usually considered a surgical problem. However, if the disease,

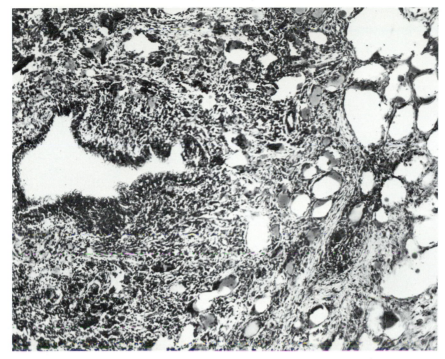

Fig. 230 Exogenous lipoid pneumonia demonstrating fibrosis and empty spaces that contained sudanophilic material. (Low power; WU neg. 48-3873.)

instead of resolving, organizes, shadows occur in the lung that may be mistaken for tumor (Fig. 231). We have seen fifteen patients with persistent lesions in various areas of the lung (often in the upper lobe) who had cough, hemoptysis, and weight loss justifying a clinical diagnosis of carcinoma.[60] Radiographically, the diagnosis was often carcinoma. Cytologic studies in these patients were negative. At the time of exploration, the involved area was extremely firm, and a diagnosis of organizing pneumonia was made only after frozen section.

Grossly, the lobes contain yellow areas and are very firm, but the pattern of the lung persists. The process extends to the pleura, which is invariably thickened. Microscopically, the exudate is organized. The cellularity of the connective tissue depends on the duration of the process. Necrotizing lesions of small-sized and moderate-sized bronchi are present. Bacteriologic study has not been rewarding.

Bronchiectasis

Bronchiectasis is a disease usually contracted in the first two decades of life (69% of a large group studied by Perry and King[71]). In a series of children with bronchiectasis reported by Field,[64-66] there was a history of pneumonia in 35% and of pertussis in 30%. Bronchiectasis involves the left side more often than the right, possibly because the right side is better drained. It is thought that the pulmonary artery constricts the left bronchus. The combination of sinusitis, complete situs inversus, and bronchiectasis is designated Kartagener's syndrome.[69] Sinusitis often has been incriminated as the cause of bronchiectasis, but this concept lacks proof since sinusitis follows just as often as it precedes bronchiectasis.

The pathogenesis of bronchiectasis appears to be a combination of blockage of a bronchus and infection. In the presence of pneumonitis there may be atelectasis, but without infection bronchiectasis does

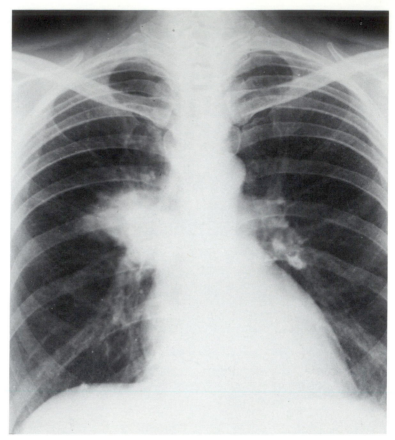

Fig. 231 Hilar mass that was considered radiographically to be bronchogenic cancer but proved pathologically to be organizing pneumonia. (WU neg. 52-7380.)

not occur.[62] Probably the sequence of infection, pneumonitis, atelectasis, and bronchiectasis is most frequent. With atelectasis, intrapleural pressure becomes more negative. This negative pressure is transmitted through the solid nonexpanded pulmonary tissue to the elastic and expansible bronchial walls.[61] This sequence may be initiated by foreign bodies or by any process partially occluding the bronchial tree.

With infection, the regional lymph nodes often are greatly enlarged.[70] Infection without atelectasis or pneumonitis is rarely a factor in the development of bronchiectasis.[69] The lower lobes are most frequently involved. When the left lower lobe is the site of bronchiectasis, the lingual division of the left upper lobe also is almost always afflicted. Lander and Davidson[67] pointed out that with collapse of the left lower lobe

the lingular bronchus is displaced and that with collapse of the right lower lobe drainage of the right middle lobe and pectoral branch of the right upper lobe is affected. When bronchiectasis has been long established in an area of the lung, it usually remains confined to that area. *Spread rarely takes place* unless there is additional pulmonary infection and atelectasis.

Grossly, the pleura frequently is thickened and the lung is heavier than normal. Bronchiectasis is broadly classified as saccular, cystic, or cylindrical (Fig. 232). The walls of the bronchi are thickened and dilated and at times widen to include abscesses, and infrequently pleural perforation and empyema occur. The intervening lung parenchyma shows variable degrees of inflammation and fibrosis.

Microscopically, bronchiectasis is usu-

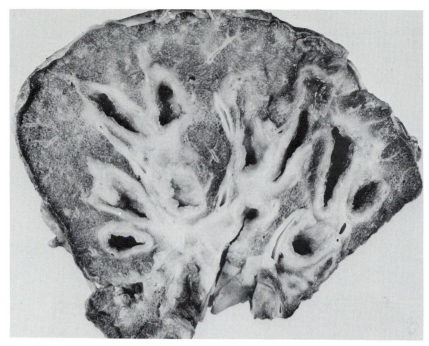

Fig. 232 Extensive bronchiectasis involving entire right lower lobe with diffuse parenchymal involvement. (WU neg. 49-5677.)

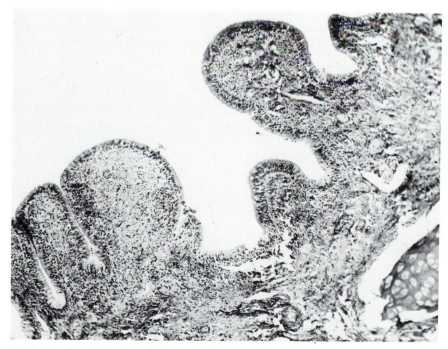

Fig. 233 Bronchiectasis, in which epithelium is still present, showing diffuse chronic inflammation, absence of muscularis mucosae, and fragmented bronchial cartilage. (Low power; WU neg. 48-4907.)

ally well delimited. The bronchial epithelium may be ulcerated, but squamous epithelial metaplasia is infrequent. The persistent epithelium is normal and ciliated. With advanced bronchiectasis, the submucosa contains granulation tissue, the cartilage is fragmented or destroyed, and the muscularis mucosae is erased or focally hyperplastic. Excess lymphoid tissue around the bronchi, often containing germinal follicles, occurs particularly in the younger patients (Fig. 233). The mucous glands are not changed. Communications are common between the bronchial and pulmonary arteries, the bronchial arteries often being greatly enlarged, tortuous, and thick walled.[68] Anastomoses of the bronchial artery and pulmonary artery are found along the branches of the bronchi of the fourth order. The changes in the lung parenchyma vary from none to advanced organizing pneumonia and fibrosis.

Clinicopathologic correlation

Patients with bronchiectasis have foul, fetid, abundant sputum. In the past, the only really effective treatment was surgical resection. Before the use of antimicrobial drugs, the majority of patients who contracted the disease before the age of 10 years and were not treated surgically died before 40 years of age.

The complications of bronchiectasis such as brain abscess and bronchopleural fistula with empyema are infrequent today. Burford[63] believes that surgical resection is indicated in patients with predominant unilateral disease and in those with hemorrhage and repeated pulmonary infections. In most instances, however, conservative treatment with the newer drugs is sufficient to control the disease. It is important to realize that the process is focal and that the extent of the disease is entirely dependent upon the primary insult. For instance, in 114 patients reported by Perry and King,[71] only six developed a spread of disease. All six had had intercurrent pneumonia. Bronchiectasis is only rarely associated with amyloid disease.

Cystic diseases

Blebs are formed by rupture of an alveolus directly beneath the pleura, with escape of air into the areolar layer of the pleura, which results in interstitial emphysema. A bleb may rupture into the free pleural space, causing pneumothorax. Emphysematous bullae result from rupture of an alveolus into adjoining alveoli. A large air space may be formed from the continued accumulation of air that is covered by a stretched, thin pleura. The symptoms of such bullae depend upon compression of residual nondiseased lung or result from hemorrhage and infection.

Large bullae can be treated by simple excision of the walls with closure of bronchiolar fistulas and obliteration of the pleural space.[72, 74] Obstructive focal emphysema can occur in young children on the basis of many causes, including mucosal folds, plugs of mucus, and deficiencies in the bronchial cartilages. This abnormality occurs only in the upper lobes and right middle lobe. Lobectomy is curative.

Congenital cystic disease often is diagnosed incorrectly. It certainly exists, for such lesions have been found at birth. However, it is extremely rare, and the criteria for its recognition are poorly defined. The absence of coal pigment in cystic areas is not absolutely diagnostic. The presence of other abnormalities of the bronchi are helpful but are not certain indications of the congenital nature of the lesion. It must be remembered that a chronic lung abscess may completely heal, leaving a large unilocular cyst with smooth lining.

Honeycombing is a gross descriptive term applied to a localized or diffuse area of coarsening of the lung parenchyma with increased porosity, distinguishable from emphysema by virtue of the fibrosis present and representing the end result of an interstitial pneumonia, regardless of what the etiologic agent of the latter might have been. The term *bronchiolar emphysema* has been used inappropriately for this condition in the past. There is no evidence that honeycombing is ever of congenital origin. The superior portions of the upper and lower lobes are the most common sites of involvement. Atypical foci of acinar and squamous proliferation are often seen in late stages of honeycombing. Meyer and Liebow[75] consider this a precancerous change, in view of its frequent association with malignant tumors, particularly adenocarcinomas. Another kind of atypical epithelial proliferation, which should be clearly separated from the ones just described, is the type variously called spindle-celled proliferation, Witwell's tumourlet, or carcinoid-like proliferation. Most of the cases have been found in association with saccular bronchiectasis.[73] We interpret the three cases reported by Womack and Graham[76] as belonging to this category. These proliferations are small, solid, often multiple, and composed of uniform spindle cells. Their striking microscopic similarity with bronchial carcinoid tumors suggests that they represent nodular proliferations of Kulchitsky's (enterochromaffin) cells. There is no evidence that they are related to bronchial carcinoma.

Bronchopulmonary sequestration

Bronchopulmonary sequestration is a definite clinicopathologic entity. There is partial or complete separation of a portion of a lobe of the lung, with no connection to the bronchial tree.

In the *extralobar* variety, the tissue is enveloped by its own pleural covering and exists as a nodule apart from the lung, at any level from the thoracic inlet to the diaphragm, or even within the abdominal cavity. About 90% of the cases occur in the left side. Other congenital malformations, especially diaphragmatic hernia, occur in approximately 20% of the patients.[77] The arterial supply is usually by one or several small arteries from the aorta or one of its branches. The venous drainage is into the azygos system.

The *intralobar* variety is characteristically located within the lower lobe, especially in the posterior basal segment. About 60%

of the cases occur on the left side. The segment is supplied by a *large* artery arising from the aorta or one of its branches, arising above the diaphragm in 75% of the patients and below the diaphragm in the remainder. Failure of the surgeon to appreciate this fact may result in death from hemorrhage. Despite its origin, the artery is always of the elastic pulmonary type. Shunts between the anomalous arteries and intrapulmonary vessels have been demonstrated.[78] The venous blood flows into the pulmonary venous system. Grossly, the sequestered portion may present as a single cyst, as a multicystic area, or as a solid mass. Microscopically, there is usually chronic inflammation and fibrosis. Obliterative changes of blood vessels are prominent. The pathogenesis of this condition is not clear. Pryce et al.[79] believe that the persistence of the systemic arterial supply is the primary cause of this anomaly. Smith,[80] on the other hand, attributes it to a defect in the pulmonary arterial development.

Arteriovenous fistula

Arteriovenous fistulas are radiographically discernible, are frequently multiple, and occur often in the right lower and middle lobes of the lungs (Figs. 234 and 235). These probably congenital lesions are made up of large vascular channels with arteriovenous communications.[82]

Microscopically, the vessels are abnormal, often showing deficiencies and excesses of muscle, which make it impossible to differentiate artery from vein.[81] Because of the shunt, there are bruit, cyanosis, polycythemia, and low oxygen content of arterial blood. Excision is curative.

Miscellaneous lesions

Solitary *infarcts* may present on radiographic examination as masses suggestive of carcinoma. We have seen a case located in the upper lobe that was interpreted radiographically as possibly malignant and was therefore resected (Fig. 236).

Eosinophilic granuloma can be circum-

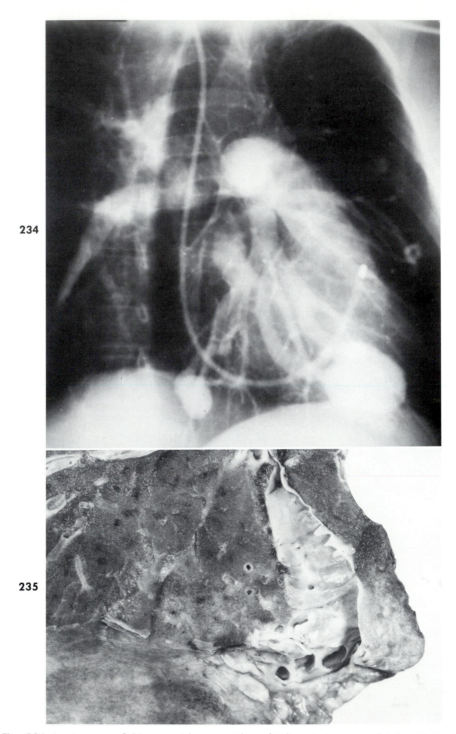

234

235

Fig. 234 Angiogram of 28-year-old man with multiple arteriovenous fistulas. Patient had Rendu-Osler-Weber syndrome. After left lower lobectomy, oxygen saturation went from 86% to 95%. (WU neg. 63-9767.)

Fig. 235 Dilated vessel with smooth wall in large arteriovenous shunt in 24-year-old woman. (WU neg. 67-3921.)

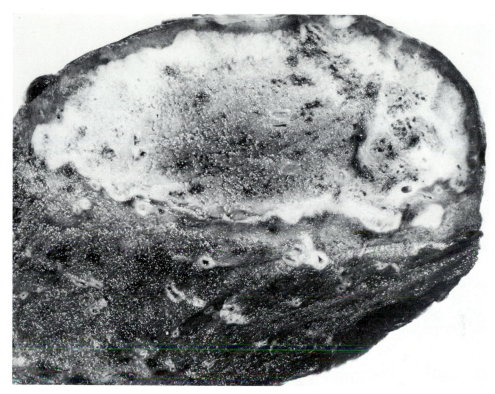

Fig. 236 Well-delimited infected infarct in 51-year-old man that was thought possibly to be primary carcinoma. (WU neg. 61-1036.)

scribed or diffuse. It predominates in the upper lobes and can produce nodular as well as cavitary lesions. In approximately 20% of the patients, there is associated extrapulmonary involvement, usually in bones or the pituitary region. Spontaneous pneumothorax is a common complication. Microscopically, there is a compact interstitial infiltrate, often subpleural, composed of mature histiocytes, numerous eosinophils, and reactive mesothelial cells. Hemosiderin deposition and necrosis are common.[86]

Liebow and Carrington[87] group under the term *eosinophilic pneumonia* all pulmonary infiltrations associated with eosinophilia, as well as infiltrations of the lung by eosinophils with or without peripheral eosinophilia. The acute form, characterized by flitting pulmonary infiltrates accompanied by eosinophilia and lasting no more than a month, is commonly referred as Löffler's syndrome. Most cases of eosinophilic pneumonia are of a chronic nature.

Response to steroids is unpredictable. Helminths, drugs, *Aspergillus, Filaria,* and *Dirofilaria* have been identified as the etiologic agents in some of the cases.[89] If the changes of eosinophilic pneumonia are accompanied by necrotizing vasculitis, there is a good probability of extrapulmonary involvement.

In classical **Wegener's granulomatosis,** necrotic and granulomatous changes in the lungs are accompanied by similar upper respiratory and renal lesions, the disease running an accelerated clinical course.[90] Carrington and Liebow[83] have described a "limited" form confined to the lungs and having a more prolonged clinical course. Grossly, there are multiple, bilateral round nodules, frequently located in the lower lobes (Fig. 237). Microscopically, the disease is indistinguishable from the classical variety. A requisite for the diagnosis is the presence of vasculitis *away* from the areas of necrosis. A further varia-

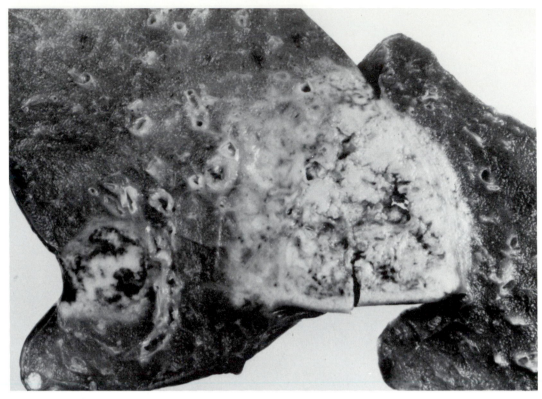

Fig. 237 Limited form of Wegener's granulomatosis in 69-year-old woman. Several necrotic granulomatous foci are evident. Largest has infarctlike shape, a feature of diagnostic significance. (WU neg. 71-10985.)

tion in the theme is lymphomatoid granulomatous as described by Liebow et al.[86a, 88] In it, the typical changes of Wegener's disease are obscured by an intense round cell infiltrate, predominantly lymphocytic but also containing histiocytes and plasmocytoid cells. This disease can be easily confused with malignant lymphoma. In autopsied patients with this condition, similar nodular changes are often found in the kidneys.

Alveolar proteinosis is perihilar in distribution, resembling radiographically the picture of pulmonary edema. Microscopically, the striking abnormality is the accumulation of a lipoproteinaceous material in the alveolar lumina, associated with some proliferation and desquamation of granular pneumocytes and small lymphoid accumulations in the interstitium.[91] The disease seems to be the result of a failure in removing the products of cell necrosis.

Focal changes of alveolar proteinosis have been described in otherwise typical cases of pulmonary tuberculosis.[93]

Patients with **idiopathic hemosiderosis** classically present with hemoptysis and refractory anemia. Roentgenograms of the lung often show a granular perihilar infiltrate. Microscopically, large accumulations of hemosiderin-laden macrophages in the alveolar lumina are accompanied by proliferation of alveolar lining cells. Necrosis and lymphoid follicles do not occur.

Round pulmonary masses, radiographically resembling neoplasms, can be the result of nodular **amyloidosis**[85] or intrapulmonary **hematoma,**[84] the latter occurring as a complication of blunt trauma to the thorax.

Tumors
Hamartoma (chondroma)

The hamartoma (often called chondroma) is a relatively rare tumor that usually

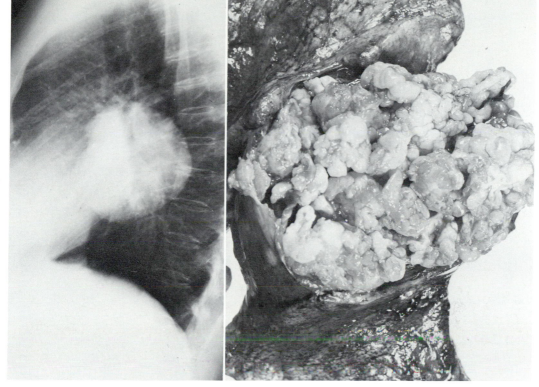

238

239

Fig. 238 Large well-delineated hamartoma of lung. (WU neg. 49-2120.)
Fig. 239 Same lesion shown in Fig. 238 demonstrating typical glistening nodules of carti-lage on cross section. (WU neg. 49-1756.)

occurs in adults.[96] The most common va-riety is located in the lung parenchyma just beneath the pleura and varies in size from a small lesion to a mass occupying the entire lobe. It is sharply delineated and lobulated. On cross section, its ap-pearance is characterized by glistening nodules of cartilage (Figs. 238 and 239). The second and less common type presents as a polypoid mass inside a large bron-chus.[95] We have seen one large hamartoma growing in the hilum. Fragments of this lesion were obtained through the broncho-scope. The patient finally died of infection secondary to the tumor.

Microscopically, the tumor contains is-lands of cartilage with definite perichon-dria that often show calcification and rare-ly ossification. Anthracotic coal pigment is absent. This lesion has been designated as a hamartoma because it conforms to

the definition of this term by Albrecht[94]: "Hamartomata are tumor-like malforma-tions in which occur only abnormal mixing of the normal components of the organ. The abnormalities may take the form of a change in quantity, arrangement, or de-gree, or may comprise all three."*

The hamartoma is made up of normal cartilage arranged in islands, fat, smooth muscle, and clefts lined by respiratory epithelium. At times, this epithelium may be ciliated. These elements are intermin-gled throughout the tumor. The cartilage often shows calcification and rarely ossi-fication. Anthracotic coal pigment is ab-sent. This lesion is often discovered as a clear-cut shadow in roentgenograms of the chest. It is diagnosed easily by its

---

*From Albrecht, E.: Ueber Hamartome, Verh. Dtsch. Pathol. Ges. **7**:153-157, 1904.

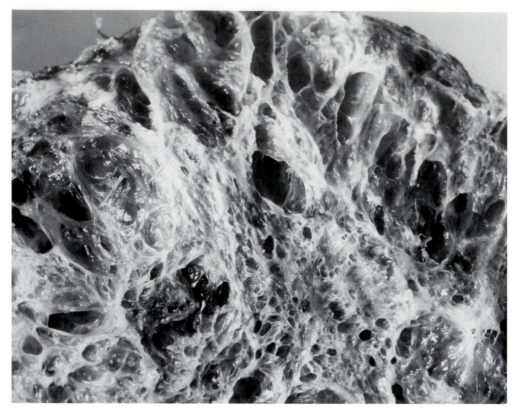

Fig. 240 Extensive honeycombing of right upper lobe in 63-year-old woman who had associated adenocarcinoma. Regional lymph nodes were negative. (WU neg. 66-12771.)

gross appearance and should be treated by local resection.

Fibroxanthoma

There is a group of pulmonary lesions presenting as more or less circumscribed nodules, having as a common feature the proliferation of histiocytic cells. Wide variations on this basic theme occur from case to case or even within the same case and are responsible for the many names and histogenetic interpretations that this group of lesions has received. These variations include vascular proliferation, fibrosis and hyalinization, fat accumulation with formation of xanthoma cells, hemosiderin deposition, and presence of other inflammatory cells, such as lymphocytes and plasma cells.[99]

We believe that many of the lesions diagnosed as sclerosing hemangioma and inflammatory pseudotumor belong to this category.[97, 98] Whether fibroxanthoma is a true neoplasm or merely a reactive proliferation is still debated. Most cases present as small peripheral nodules, yellow and firm, covered by an intact pleura. The large majority of the patients are asymptomatic. We have seen the lesions confused with hemangiopericytoma, carcinoid tumor, and metastatic carcinoma. Excision is curative.

Carcinoma

Carcinoma of the lung has become increasingly frequent during the past thirty years. This is due not only to increased recognition and better radiologic and bronchoscopic diagnoses but also to a steep rise in incidence. In some institutions, such as veterans' hospitals and those in which thoracic surgery is a prominent specialty, carcinoma of the lung is the most frequent neoplasm. This increase is almost entirely in male patients with epidermoid and oat cell carcinomas of the bronchus.

There has been much speculation as to the cause of this increase. Many factors previously considered of etiologic importance can now be eliminated (tuberculosis, tarring of roads, the influenza epidemic of 1918, anthracosis, and anthracosilicosis). There appears to be little doubt that exposure to chromates,[105] asbestos,[101, 104] and radioactivity in certain mines[108] accounts for a small fraction of this increase. Cigarette smoking has been strongly associated with carcinoma of the lung. In a series of male patients with squamous carcinoma and oat cell carcinoma that we recently reviewed, practically 100% smoked excessively. In female patients with squamous cancer, only one-third of those we reviewed did not smoke.[109] Male smokers living in an urban area have a higher incidence of lung cancer than those living in a rural area.[107] This suggests that air pollution potentiates the carcinogenic action of tobacco in susceptible male individuals.

The meticulous histologic observations of Auerbach et al.[100] on the tracheobronchial trees of 117 patients seen at autopsy support a relationship of heavy cigarette smoking to cancer of the bronchus. "Although definite carcinoma-in-situ was present in all groups, with a parallel rise in proportion to increasing cigarette consumption, there was an almost similar distribution of this change in those who smoked more than one package a day (6.0%) and in the cases of bronchogenic carcinoma (6.3%)."*

Excessive cigarette smoking is also associated with pulmonary emphysema, frequently a crippling disease.

Meyer and Liebow[106] reported that 22% of 153 consecutively resected pulmonary tumors were associated with honeycomb-

---

*From Auerbach, O., Gere, J. B., Forman, J. B., Petrick, T. G., Smilin, H. J., Muehsam, G. E., Kassouny, D. Y., and Stout, A. P.: Changes in the bronchial epithelium in relation to smoking and cancer of the lung, N. Engl. J. Med. **256:** 97-104, 1957.

ing and atypical epithelial proliferation (Fig. 240). Most of the neoplasms associated with such atypical epithelial proliferation occurred in the upper lobe, and 31% were adenocarcinomas. Similarly, the majority of cancers arising in connection with localized scars are of either adenocarcinomatous or adenosquamous type.[103]

Most lung cancers are of considerable size when first detected. Rarely, however, and mainly as a result of cytologic examination, in situ or early invasive bronchogenic carcinomas are discovered. Woolner et al.[110] collected twenty-eight such cases seen at the Mayo Clinic in a twenty-three-year-period. The prognosis in their series was good: only three patients died of the cancer, in two of whom there was evidence of multicentricity.

Multiple invasive bronchogenic carcinomas are rare. LeGal and Bauer[102] found that 6.4% of sixty-three patients who had survived at least thirty months following surgical excision of a bronchogenic carcinoma developed a second primary lung cancer.

Microscopic types

Many different microscopic classifications of lung carcinoma exist. The one we use has been slightly modified from the classifications of Kreyberg[123] and the World Health Organization[124] and include the following categories:

1 Squamous cell carcinoma
  a Well differentiated (keratinized)
  b Poorly differentiated (nonkeratinized)
2 Adenocarcinoma and related tumors, latter group including:
  a Clear cell carcinoma
  b Giant cell carcinoma
  c Bronchiolar ("alveolar cell") carcinoma
3 Adenosquamous (mixed) carcinoma
4 Oat cell (small cell) carcinoma
5 Undifferentiated carcinoma
6 Mucous gland carcinomas
  a Adenoid cystic carcinoma
  b Mucoepidermoid carcinoma

About 96% of the *squamous cell carcinomas* occur in males. Most cases arise from the mucosa of major bronchi (Fig.

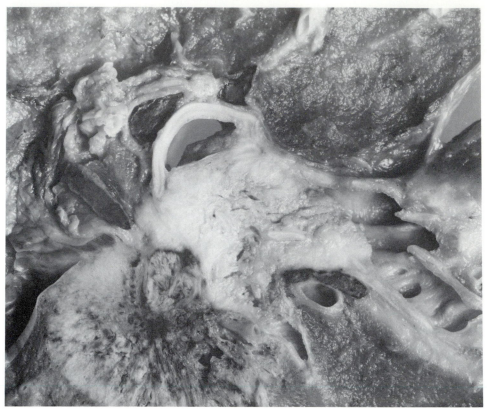

Fig. 241 Bronchial carcinoma arising in major bronchus. Tumor replaces portion of bronchial wall and extends into surrounding parenchyma. Organizing pneumonia can be seen peripherally. (WU neg. 71-7169.)

241) and therefore present as hilar or perihilar masses in chest roentgenograms. As a group, they are larger than the other types at the time of the diagnosis.[113] Signs of bronchial obstruction, such as obstructive pneumonitis or atelectasis, are found in approximately one-half of the patients. The tumors have a special tendency to undergo central necrosis with cavitation. Thus, of forty-four tumors with radiographically demonstrable cavitation examined by Strang and Simpson,[133] thirty-six were of squamous cell type. On the other hand, calcification is extremely unusual. Rarely, squamous cell carcinomas present as intrabronchial polypoid masses, with only minor extrabronchial spread. Microscopically, the presence of keratin is the single most important criterion for the diagnosis. This may be apparent in isolated cells or, more commonly,

in the form of "keratin pearls." In doubtful cases, Kreyberg's stain[123] can be of help in differentiating keratin from necrotic debris. In the absence of keratin, the diagnosis is based on the presence of intercellular bridges, whorl formation, or definite stratification of the tumor cells. The bronchial mucosa adjacent to the tumor usually shows squamous metaplasia and sometimes carcinoma in situ.[117] We have seen instances in which carcinoma in situ spread along the bronchus several centimeters from the primary tumor. We have also seen a patient who developed a contralateral primary lung cancer six years after a pneumonectomy for cancer had shown carcinoma in situ at the line of resection.

Adenocarcinomas and related tumor types comprise 49% of all lung cancers in females, whereas the corresponding fig-

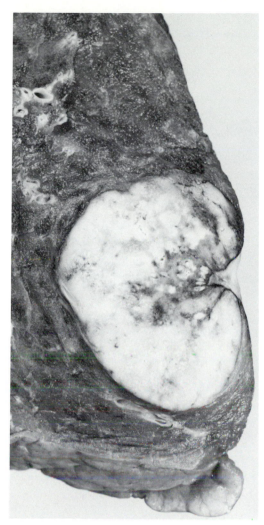

Fig. 242 Large peripheral carcinoma with marked pleural retraction. Latter finding is seen much more commonly in primary rather than in metastatic tumors. (WU neg. 60-5571.)

eycombing and may show foci of atypical acinar proliferation in the neighboring air spaces.[129] Microscopically, the diagnosis of adenocarcinoma is based on the identification of definite glandular or papillary structures and/or the presence of mucin secretion. Lining of tumor cells along alveolar walls, a pattern of growth that any tumor type may exibit, can simulate gland formation. Blood vessel invasion was identified by Bennett et al.[115] in 86% of the 100 adenocarcinomas they examined. In the same series, metastases to peribronchial or hilar lymph nodes were found in one-half of the patients. The resectability rate was 71%, about twice the overall rates for bronchogenic carcinoma. However, the overall five-year survival rate was only 9%.

Most observers regard *clear cell carcinoma*[130] and *giant cell carcinoma*[131] as variants of adenocarcinoma due to the fact that in a certain percentage of cases, foci of glandular differentiation and/or mucin production have been identified.[121] Both tumors have a peripheral location and are associated with a grave prognosis.

Bronchiolar cell carcinoma has two distinct gross patterns: well-delimited nodules, usually multiple, and a single poorly defined mass within a lobe. Because there is no lesion in the major bronchi, the process may suggest an organizing pneumonia (Figs. 243 and 244). The mass may have a mucoid surface. Usually the surgeon is not aware that the lesion is a neoplasm. Microscopically, the tumor forms well-differentiated papillary masses of tall columnar cells that contain epithelial mucin[134] (Fig. 245). Tumor nodules have a topographic association with bronchioles and not with bronchi. Continuity between tumor cells lining alveoli and the epithelium of respiratory bronchioles or alveolar ducts can be demonstrated.[126] Inflammatory cells and fat-filled macrophages are frequently associated with the tumor. Psammoma bodies are present in 13% of the cases.[114] The histogenesis of this neoplasm has been debated for many

ure in males is only 9%.[115] In absolute numbers, however, they are more common in males than in females. Grossly, they usually present as poorly circumscribed gray yellowish lesions. If they secrete mucin, they have a mucoid, glairy appearance. About 65% of the cases are located peripherally, and 77% have involvement of the visceral pleura at the time of excision (Fig. 242). Cavitation is very unusual. A large percentage of adenocarcinomas arise in association with a peripheral scar or hon-

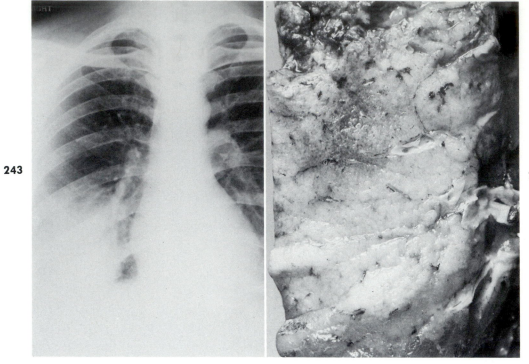

243

244

Fig. 243 Typical roentgenogram of bronchiolar (alveolar cell) carcinoma. Note poorly defined shadow in right lower lung field. (WU neg. 48-4750.)
Fig. 244 Typical gross appearance of bronchiolar (alveolar cell) carcinoma: mucoid surface, appearance somewhat like organizing pneumonia, and poorly defined borders. (WU neg. 50-3577.)

years. Electron microscopic studies[125] have given support to the theory that the tumor arises from terminal bronchiolar epithelium rather than from alveolar cells and is therefore a morphologic variant of adenocarcinoma.[120] Bennett and Sasser[114] compared thirty cases of bronchiolar carcinoma with 100 cases of ordinary lung adenocarcinoma and found frequent overlapping of patterns. The main differences encountered were a higher incidence of multiplicity and a slightly better survival rate in the patients with bronchiolar carcinoma.

We use the term *adenosquamous carcinoma* for lung tumors arising from bronchial surface epithelium in which unquestionable evidence of squamous and glandular differentiation is found in the same neoplasm in a roughly equivalent amount. (Figs. 246 and 247). Squamous cell carcinomas having occasional mucin-producing cells or adenocarcinomas with minute foci

of squamous differentiation are named according to their predominant component. Thus defined, adenosquamous carcinomas comprises less than 10% of lung cancers. Most of the cases are located peripherally and often are associated with a scar, suggesting a closer relationship with adenocarcinoma than with squamous cell carcinoma.

Oat cell carcinoma should be viewed as a highly distinctive tumor type rather than as an undifferentiated form of lung cancer. The microscopic pathology has been well described by Azzopardi.[112] Small cells, varying in shape from nearly round to fine spindle, are the main constituents of the neoplasm (Fig. 248). "Spindling" artifact is quite common in biopsy material and can render the diagnosis impossible. Azzopardi[112] has described the presence of hematoxyphilic areas in the wall of blood vessels in areas of necrosis. They are Feul-

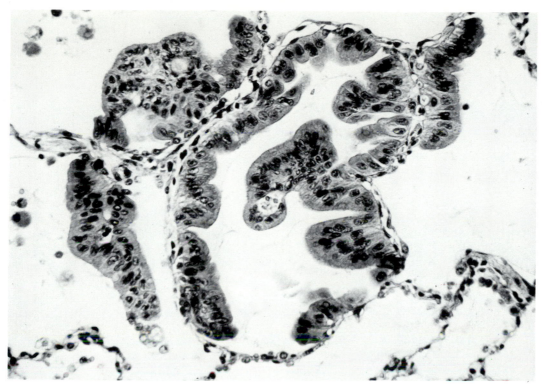

Fig. 245 Typical well-differentiated bronchiolar (alveolar cell) carcinoma. Tumor cells line wall of terminal air spaces. (×250; WU neg. 63-9076.)

gen positive and probably represent deposition of DNA from degenerated tumor cells. The presence of ribbons and rosettes, the identification of dense-core secretory granules by electron microscopy,[116] the finding of serotonin in the tumor extracts,[119] and the well-known association with a variety of endocrine syndromes all suggest an origin from Kulschitsky's type neuroendocrine cells. A further point favoring this interpretation is the existence of cases with a microscopic appearance intermediate between oat cell carcinoma and bronchial carcinoid, as we have observed in several instances.[111] Oat cell carcinoma comprises 10% of all lung cancers. Approximately 95% of the patients are males, and 85% are smokers.[122] It is typically a lesion of the central portions of the lung. Bronchoscopic biopsy is often positive, even if no gross abnormalities are seen. The prognosis is extremely poor. Only two of 138 patients treated in our institution were alive and free of tumor seven years following resection.[122]

Undifferentiated carcinomas are pleomorphic epithelial tumors without any evidence of squamous or glandular differentiation. The tumor cells are often large, although they can be medium sized or even small. Since the lesions often present as peripheral tumors, it has been suggested that most cases represent anaplastic varieties of adenocarcinoma.[118]

There are two major types of carcinomas arising from bronchial mucous glands: adenoid cystic carcinoma and mucoepidermoid carcinoma. Their microscopic appearance and natural history are essentially the same as those of the homologous tumors occurring in the salivary glands (Fig. 249). Both tumor types have been included in the past in the heterogeneous group of bronchial adenoma.

Adenoid cystic carcinoma arises in the major bronchi and often involves the trachea.[127] Metastases to regional lymph nodes and lung parenchyma are frequent (Fig. 250). If this tumor is diagnosed by broncho-

scopic biopsy, pneumonectomy is indicated. Irradiation therapy may be helpful. The total duration of the disease is long, but the ultimate prognosis is very poor.[128]

Mucoepidermoid carcinomas can be di-

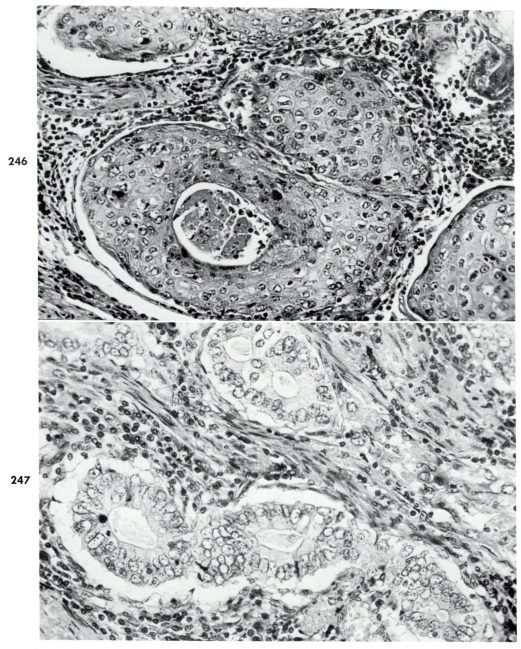

Fig. 246 Carcinoma of lung showing squamous differentiation. (×300; WU neg. 50-5216.)
Fig. 247 Same tumor shown in Fig. 246 demonstrating adenocarcinoma in adjacent zone. (×300; WU neg. 50-5215.)

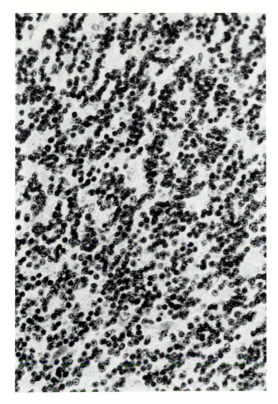

vided, as in the salivary gland, in a low-grade and a high-grade variety. The former has a low malignant potential, characterized mainly by local invasion.[132] The high-grade variety carries an extremely poor prognosis. All twelve patients with this tumor type reviewed by Turnbull et al.[135] were dead of the disease regardless of treatment within eighteen months of the onset of their first symptom.

Lung neoplasms are sometimes associated with extrapulmonary manifestations not related with the presence of metastatic disease. Although exceptions occur, there is a fairly good correlation between some morphologic parameters and the systemic effect produced. These are summarized in Table 6.

Fig. 248 Oat cell carcinoma of round cell type. This type of bronchogenic carcinoma is practically never curable. (×300; WU neg. 48-6218.)

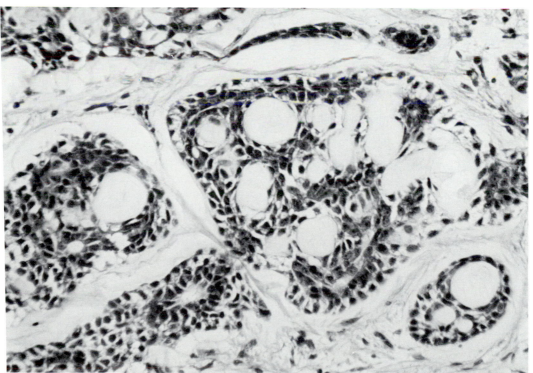

Fig. 249 Adenoid cystic carcinoma arising in major bronchus. Microscopic appearance is identical to homologous salivary gland neoplasm. (×100; WU neg. 63-9077.)

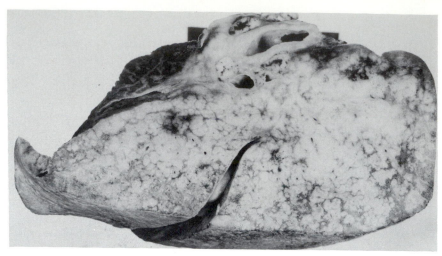

Fig. 250 Extensive involvement of lung, bronchi, and regional lymph nodes by adenoid cystic carcinoma. (WU neg. 48-5015.)

Table 6 Systemic effects of lung cancer and their relationship with tumor type

Systemic effect	Tumor type
Cushing syndrome	Oat cell carcinoma
	Bronchial carcinoid
Carcinoid syndrome	Bronchial carcinoid
	Oat cell carcinoma
Hyponatremia due to inappropriate secretion of ADH	Oat cell carcinoma
Hyperparathyroidism	Squamous cell carcinoma
Gynecomastia due to gonadotropin secretion	All tumor types
Clubbing of fingers and hypertrophic pulmonary osteoarthopathy	Unrelated to tumor type; mainly dependent on proximity to pleural surface
Mental syndromes (i.e., toxic confusional psychosis)	Oat cell carcinoma
Cortical cerebellar degeneration	All tumor types
Encephalomyelitis	Oat cell carcinoma
Sensory neuropathy	Oat cell carcinoma
Myopathic-myastenic syndrome	Oat cell carcinoma

Cytology

Michael Kyriakos, M.D.

Exfoliative cytology has reached a high level of accuracy since Wandall's classical monograph.[152] By examination of the sputum and/or bronchial secretions, it is now possible to make a diagnosis in 80% to 90% of the patients with cancer, whereas bronchoscopic biopsy in operable carcinoma of the lung is positive in only one-third of the patients.[143, 149] Tumor invasion of the pleura is readily detected by pleural fluid examination.[150]

In patients with primary bronchogenic carcinoma, a single bronchial washing will be positive in 35% to 40%. In those who yield positive cytology, a bronchial washing is positive in approximately two-thirds. A single sputum specimen has been reported to be positive in 42% to 61% of the patients, but the ease with which sputum can be obtained raises the detection rate to 80% when three and to over 90% when five sputum specimens are submitted.[139] In about one-third of the patients, cytology provides the only microscopic diagnosis before thoracic surgery.[140] The development of the bronchial brushing technique under fluroscopic control has expanded the role of pulmonary cytology.[138, 142] Peripheral carcinomas, which yield positive cytology in only about one-half the cases, can now be diagnosed in 70% to 80% of the patients.

In patients who have either a negative or no bronchial biopsy, cytology is of

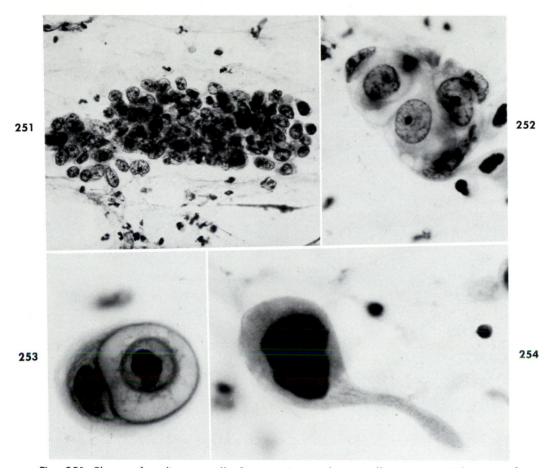

Fig. 251 Clump of malignant cells from patient with oat cell carcinoma. Piling up of cells and their grouping in strands are characteristic of this tumor type.

Fig. 252 Clump of reactive macrophages mistaken for malignant tumor. Resection of lobe demonstrated only lipoid pneumonia. (×1,080; WU neg. 48-4588.)

Fig. 253 Apparent "cannibalism" of one tumor cell by another. In actuality, one cell overrides other. This is more frequently seen in epidermoid carcinoma but may be found in other tumor types as well.

Fig. 254 Tadpole-shaped cell in patient with epidermoid cell carcinoma. Large "ink dot" type of nucleus is common in epidermoid carcinoma of lung.

Table 7 Cytology and biopsy in patients with operable cancer*

Biopsy	Positive cytology	Negative or suspicious cytology
Positive bronchial biopsy	35 (17.7%)	25 (12.6%)
Negative bronchial biopsy	18 (9.1%)	20 (10.1%)
No bronchial biopsy	41 (20.3%)	59 (30.2%)

*From Spjut, H. J., Fier, D. J., and Ackerman, L. V.: Exfoliative cytology and pulmonary cancer, J. Thorac. Surg. **30:**90-107, 1955.

great value (Table 7). In fifty-nine such patients, thirteen frozen sections were requested, eleven of which demonstrated cancer. Thus, forty-eight patients having pulmonary resections had a positive cytology as the only preoperative tissue diagnosis. Cancer was present in every instance.[147, 149]

In most instances, tumor cells are easily recognized because they occur in clumps or as numerous single bizarre cells (Figs. 251, 253, and 254). Recognition becomes more difficult in the oat cell carcinoma in which individual cells may suggest lymphocytes rather than tumor.

The diagnosis of exfoliative material should be on a conservative basis. Our reports are made as follows:

1 "Unsatisfactory (saliva only)" when no macrophages are present in the smear
2 "Negative" when no abnormal cells are observed in a technically satisfactory smear
3 "Benign atypia" when epithelial bronchial cells with hyperplastic and metaplastic changes secondary to inflammation are identified
4 "Suspicious but not diagnostic" (This report is an indication for repeat examination.)
5 "Positive for cancer cells" (In 87% of these cases that we have examined, there was agreement between the cytologic and microscopic diagnosis in regard to the cell type.)

False positive diagnoses have been made in patients with infarct, bronchiectasis, fungal disease, viral pneumonia, irradiation changes, or lipoid pneumonia (Fig. 252). Usually, the cells that are misinterpreted as cancer are either macrophages or altered alveolar lining cells.

Pearson et al.[146] have reported patients with positive cytology and negative roentgenograms of the chest. It is important to emphasize that blind exploratory thoracotomy is not indicated for these patients. Lesions of the oral cavity, pharynx, larynx, and esophagus can all yield positive "respiratory" cytology. We had a 70-year-old male patient with positive cytology for epidermoid carcinoma. Tumor cells were obtained at the time of bronchoscopy and at the time of esophagoscopy. The tumor was in reality in the piriform fossa.

Bronchoscopic biopsy

Tissue obtained at the time of bronchoscopy may be insignificant in amount because of the timidity of the bronchoscopist or the inaccessibility of the lesion. A biopsy should be fairly generous. In spite of the fact that we have at times seen pulmonary parenchyma and even mediastinal pleura in bronchoscopic biopsies, no untoward effects resulted except when small blood vessels were severed.

The fragments obtained should be quickly put in fixative. The tissue should be sectioned at various levels, for frequently tumor will be found at one level and not at another. Still more rarely, the biopsy may be taken from the edge of the tumor, and epidermoid carcinoma in situ may be observed. If longitudinal furrows have become obliterated or if there is thickening, granularity, or a nodular appearance of the mucosa, this may indicate carcinoma in situ.[153]

On several occasions, we also have seen clumps of neoplastic cells apart from the bronchoscopic biopsy, and on these we have been able to make a cytologic diagnosis of carcinoma (Fig. 255). The presence of squamous metaplasia in a biopsy specimen merely means that some form of inflammatory process is present that may or may not be combined with carcinoma (Fig. 256).

Frozen section

Frozen section is an important procedure in debatable lesions of the lung and has its greatest value in peripheral lesions. If a patient has a resectable cancer of the lung, the bronchoscopic biopsy will be positive in only 30% of the instances. Cytologic examination will raise this percentage to 80% only if an adequate number of specimens (three) are studied. This means that a number of patients with cancer will undergo surgery without a definite preoperative diagnosis.

It is our policy to excise debatable lesions with a margin of normal lung. This excision may imply lobectomy. Frozen section is then done. Frequently, the lesion proves to be a benign process such as tuberculoma, hamartoma, or organizing pneumonia. If it is cancer, the thoracic surgeon decides the extent of resection.

It is much more important that the pathologist make a definite diagnosis in lesions of the lung than in lesions of the breast, for a second thoracotomy carries

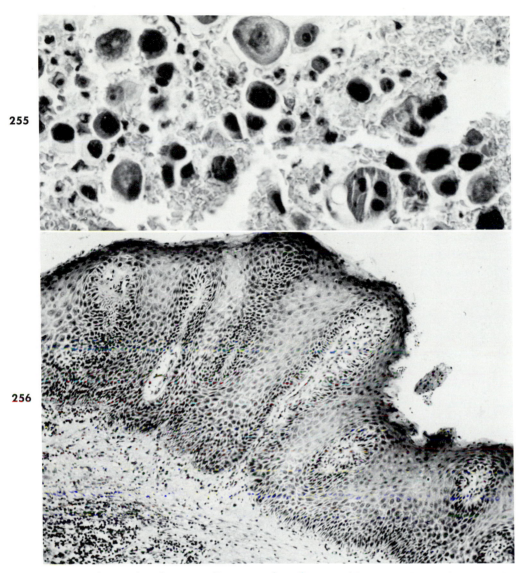

Fig. 255 Clump of malignant cells seen in bronchoscopic biopsy specimen. Note variation in cell size and atypical nuclei. (×600; WU neg. 52-3604.)
Fig. 256 Prominent squamous metaplasia of bronchus. (Low power; WU neg. 48-4908.)

with it considerable morbidity and additional risk. He must not be misled into making a diagnosis of carcinoma in highly cellular inflammatory lesions, in organizing pneumonia, or especially in lipoid pneumonia. Conversely, some of the poorly differentiated neoplasms of the lung may have a considerable inflammatory infiltrate and be incorrectly diagnosed as nonneoplastic.

Biopsy of lymph nodes and lung parenchyma

Aspiration biopsy of lesions of the lung are infrequently done by most thoracic surgeons because of possible morbidity and the risk of implantation of tumor. However, it is rare to have complications, and implantation, in our experience, practically never occurs. This method should probably be used much more frequently, particularly in peripheral masses of uncertain nature.[151]

There have been numerous procedures devised to diagnose bronchogenic cancer from lymph nodes outside the thoracic cage. If these nodes contain cancer, then thoracotomy may be avoided. Daniels[137] devised a procedure for exploration of the lymph nodes in the prescalene fat pad. Paulson[144] has explored the cervical region and the superior portion of the mediastinum through limited incisions in the neck and in the second intercostal space. Positive nodes were found in eighty-two of 182 patients. The positive nodes were found in 60% of the patients with negative x-ray films of the mediastinum. If such an exploration is negative, there is a 90% correlation between the findings by mediastinal exploration and subsequent resectability. Scalene nodes biopsy is being replaced in most medical centers by mediastinoscopy, which can be done with practically no risk. If a mediastinal node is involved by cancer, the patient is inoperable in practically every instance.[145]

In patients with bilateral disseminated pulmonary disease of unknown etiology, thoracotomy with lung biopsy is indicated. By this method not only can the pathologic diagnosis be made, but also bacterial studies and chemical analyses can be carried out.[136] The site of the incision is planned according to the distribution of the lesions.

Grant and Trivedi[141] believe that if the scalene nodes are not palpable, thoracotomy should be done without delay. A diagnosis nearly always can be made. These diagnoses include such diverse lesions as pneumoconioses, fungal diseases, sarcoidosis, primary and metastatic carcinomas, and Hodgkin's disease.

Clinicopathologic correlation

The early symptoms and signs of bronchogenic carcinoma are related to partial or complete block of a bronchus. The symptoms produced are usually those of an inflammatory condition. The radio-graphic picture changes with variation in the degree of bronchial block.

Unfortunately, the symptoms and roentgenographic findings may be erroneously interpreted as a viral pneumonia, tuberculosis, or some other inflammatory process. In the periphery of the lung, the lesion is silent until it reaches a sufficient size to ulcerate into a bronchus or to involve the pleural surface.

Of every 100 patients who come to the Thoracic Surgery Clinic at Barnes Hospital, only about fifty can be explored, and only twenty-five have a pneumonectomy with hope of cure. Routine chest surveys of asymptomatic individuals occasionally show lesions that are carcinoma. Hood et al.[157] reported 156 solitary circumscribed lesions of the lung. One out of three lesions proved to be malignant tumor. Calcification was not present in a single malignant lesion, and 42% of the noncalcified lesions were malignant. Early exploratory thoracotomy will increase the number of tumors suitable for resection. If the lesion has extended to involve a rib, the recurrent laryngeal nerve, or the pericardium or has extensively implicated hilar lymph nodes, cure is practically impossible even by the most aggressive surgical procedure.

Epidermoid carcinoma has the best prognosis.[158] Collier et al.[155] stressed the prognostic value of true vein invasion. Blood vessel invasion and lymph node metastases appear to be of equal prognostic significance, and their effect upon survival is additive.[159] The oat cell carcinomas are seldom resectable and practically never curable.

Exploratory thoracotomy at the present time has practically no operative mortality. Pneumonectomy by experienced thoracic surgeons has a mortality of 5% or less. Gibbon et al.[156] reported 532 consecutive cases of cancer of the lung. Of the patients having pneumonectomy or lobectomy, 22% survived five years (9% of the entire group). Our results have been comparable. Between Jan. 1, 1948, and Dec. 31, 1955, 1,008 patients with carcinoma of

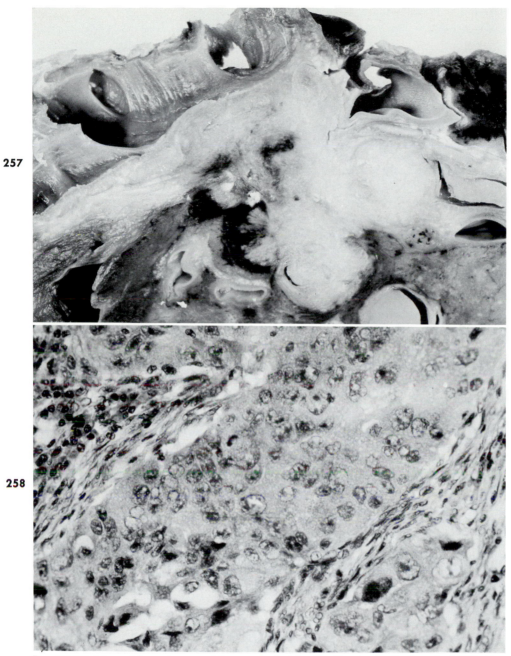

Fig. 257 Epidermoid carcinoma of lung resected by Dr. Evarts A. Graham in 1933. Note extension into surrounding lung and involvement of two regional lymph nodes. Patient died in 1962 without evidence of cancer. (WU neg. 48-5900.)
Fig. 258 Poorly differentiated squamous carcinoma shown in Fig. 257. (High power; WU neg. 48-6220.)

the lung were seen on the Thoracic Surgery Service at Barnes Hospital. Of these, 390 were inoperable and fifteen refused operation. Of 603 exploratory thoracoto-mies, the tumor was resected in 356. There were 280 pneumonectomies, seventy-four lobectomies, and two segmental resections.

Five-year follow-up was possible in 482

patients. Of these, thirty-eight were cured, an overall salvage of 8%, or 21.3% of the resected cases.[154]

The first successful lung resection for epidermoid carcinoma was performed by Dr. Evarts A. Graham in 1933. The patient, a physician, died thirty years later of an unrelated disease (Figs. 257 and 258).

Bronchial carcinoid

The term *bronchial adenoma* should be discarded, since it embraces three unrelated lung neoplasms of differing degrees of malignancy: bronchial carcinoid, adenoid cystic carcinoma, and mucoepidermoid tumor.[175] Bronchial carcinoid, which comprises the largest percentage of these lesions has been a much-debated neoplasm.[168, 169] It is a relatively infrequent tumor, making up less than 5% of all neoplasms of the bronchi. It is an important neoplasm, however, for it is resectable and curable in most instances. In Moersch and McDonald's series,[177] there were forty-five men (average age, 42 years) and forty-one women (average age, 38 years).

Carcinoid tumors most frequently arise in the main stem bronchi but may be found in the smaller ramifications of the bronchopulmonary tree. They are seldom entirely intrabronchial (Figs. 259 and 260). In our group of fifty-three patients, the most superficial tumor was firmly fixed below the level of the cartilaginous rings. In a few instances, about half the tumor was within and the other half outside the bronchus. In most instances, however, the bronchial component microscopically was only a small fraction of the entire neoplasm. Usually, the bronchial epithelium is not ulcerated. However, with increased growth, with biopsy, and with infection, superficial ulceration may occur. The lack of ulceration is the reason tumor cells from bronchial carcinoid are not recognized in the sputum or in the bronchial secretions. We have found such cells in two patients in whom ulceration of the lesion occurred. Biopsy is usually positive in these patients (seventy-five of seventy-eight reported by Moersch and McDonald[177]).

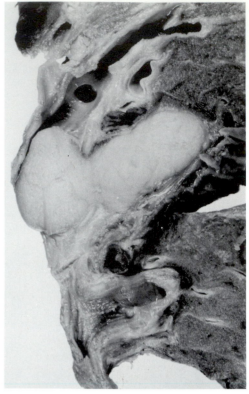

Fig. 259 Bronchial carcinoid with prominent intrabronchial and extrabronchial component. (WU neg. 49-1827.)

These tumors grow slowly but may become so large that they extend all the way to the pleura.[174] Frequently, they invade and destroy bronchial cartilage, and rarely they directly invade or metastasize to regional lymph nodes. Local invasion of surrounding structures can occur. We have seen the myocardium invaded in one instance.[163]

On section, the tumor is extremely vascular, often has a grayish yellow color, and at times contains many fibrous septa. The vascularity may lead to excessive hemorrhage on biopsy. Credit should be given to Graham and Womack[172] for insisting that this tumor has invasive characteristics and the capacity to metastasize locally and at times distantly.

The microscopic pattern varies in different sections and, at times, from field to field.[173] Most tumor cells are small and uniform, with round central nuclei (Fig.

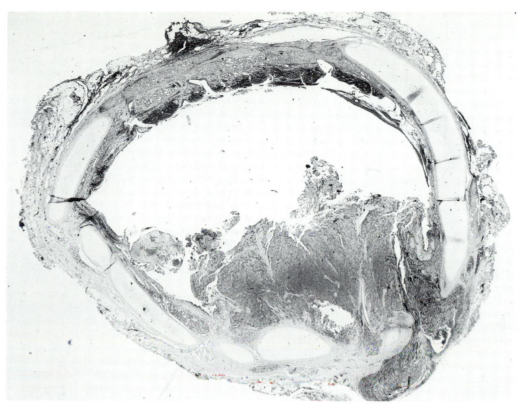

Fig. 260 Typical growth pattern of bronchial carcinoid. Most of tumor is endobronchial and polypoid, but a portion is infiltrating wall and invading peribronchial soft tissues. (×5; WU neg. 72-6547.)

261). Mitoses are rare or absent. Spindle metaplasia is often seen, especially in the peripherally situated tumors[167] Ribbons and festoons are common, whereas rosettes are only rarely present. Solid growth of cells is a less common pattern of growth. In rare cases, some or all of the tumor cells are large, with abundant acidophilic cytoplasm, therefore resembling oncocytes[165] (Fig. 262). Argentaffin cells (defined here as cells containing silver granules after Masson-Hamperl stain in formalin-fixed, paraffin-embedded material) are rare in bronchial carcinoid, whereas argyrophilic cells are the rule. We use routinely the Sevier-Munger technique to demonstrate the latter. The histochemical features of bronchial carcinoid thus resemble those of carcinoid tumors arising from other foregut derivatives, such as stomach and duodenum, and differ from the more common carcinoid tumors of the appendix and distal small bowel.[164, 183] By electron microscopy, the cells contain "neurosecretory" granules of uniform size, sometimes aligned along the cell membrane[162] (Fig. 263). The origin of these neoplasms is from cells of Kulchitzky's type normally present in the bronchial and bronchiolar epithelium.[171, 179a]

Most bronchial carcinoids are "nonfunctioning" tumors. However, cases with typical carcinoid syndrome and elevated 5-HIAA in the urine have been documented.[179, 181, 185] In some instances, the tumor has been found to secrete 5-hydroxytryptophan instead of serotonin, another feature associated with foregut-derived carcinoid tumors.[178]

When this tumor invades bronchial cartilage, fragments of the cartilage may undergo metaplasia to bone. Islands of cartilage and bone may become separated

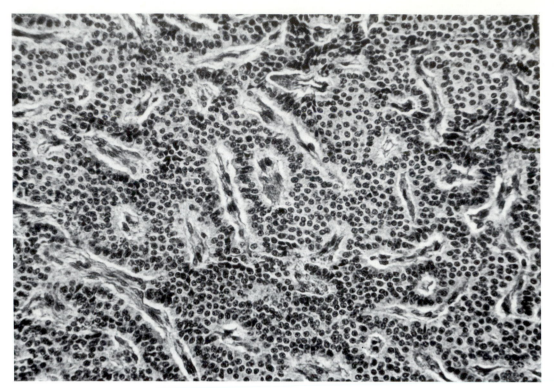

Fig. 261 Bronchial carcinoid. Note uniformity of tumor cells and peculiar relationship with blood vessels. (×100; WU neg. 69-9552.)

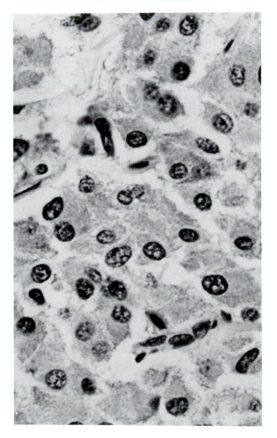

and appear within the tumor, but these islands are not an integral part of the tumor. Intermediate forms between bronchial carcinoid and oat cell carcinoma have been described.[161]

Clinicopathologic correlation

Carcinoid tumors (so-called bronchial adenomas) occur in major bronchi and, because of their vascularity, frequently cause hemoptysis. With either partial or complete blockage of the bronchi, pulmonary infection dominates the clinical picture. Owing to their polypoid endobronchial type of growth, bronchoscopy and bronchoscopic biopsy are usually positive. Of seventy-six patients who underwent bronchoscopy in

Fig. 262 Bronchial carcinoid of oncocytic variety with large cells, eosinophilic cytoplasm, small nucleus, and no mitotic figures. (×400; WU neg. 48-5779.)

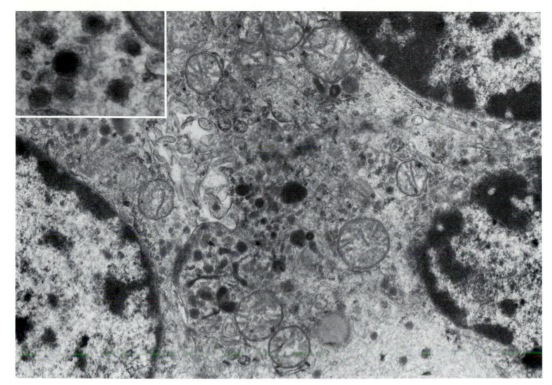

Fig. 263 Electron micrograph of bronchial carcinoid. Numerous neurosecretory granules are arranged in clusters beneath plasma membrane. Perinuclear cytoplasm contains numerous microfilaments, a common finding in endocrine neoplasms. **Inset,** Higher magnification of secretory granules. They contain homogeneous dense core surrounded by membrane, thin clear space existing in between. (Uranyl acetate–lead citrate; ×18,300; **inset,** uranyl acetate–lead citrate; ×55,300.)

the series reported by Wilkins et al.,[182] in only four was the tumor not visible. Care should be exercised in the diagnosis of bronchial carcinoid in a small bronchial biopsy. Confusion with oat cell carcinoma is particularly common.

These tumors cannot be removed completely by morselization through the bronchoscope. If the tumor is so located that lobectomy is possible, this should be done. If complete removal is impossible by lobectomy or if secondary inflammatory changes have destroyed the rest of the lung, then pneumonectomy is indicated.

Wilkins et al.[182] reviewed the results of surgical therapy in eighty-two patients with bronchial carcinoid. The overall ten-year cumulative survival was 70%; for resected cases only, it was 82%, whereas of eleven patients treated by bronchoscopic methods,

only one was alive. Distant metastases from these tumors are rare but have been reported by numerous observers.[160, 170, 176] Bone metastases are characteristically of the osteoblastic type.[180]

Bronchial carcinoid has been reported in association with Cushing's syndrome[166] and multiple endocrine adenomatosis.[184]

Carcinosarcoma and blastoma

Carcinosarcoma of the lung is a rare neoplasm that often presents as an endobronchial polypoid mass. Microscopically, an intermingling of carcinomatous and spindle, sarcoma-like cells is present. The epithelial component is usually of squamous type. Bronchoscopic biopsy may show one or both elements. Distant metastases were present in nine of the twenty-four cases analyzed by Stackhouse et al.[188] The

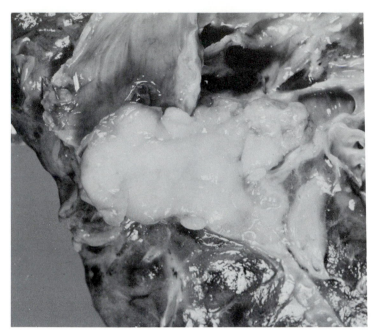

Fig. 264 Polypoid carcinosarcoma of bronchus. Patient has now survived over five years. (WU neg. 49-1939.)

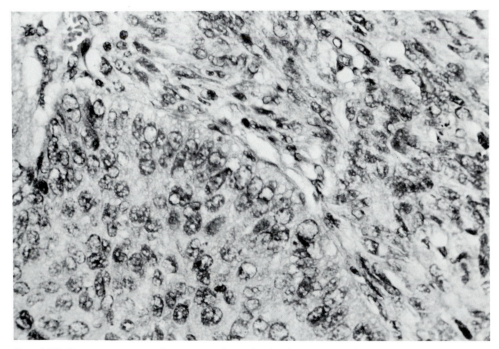

Fig. 265 Carcinosarcoma showing rather sharp demarcation between squamous carcinoma and sarcoma. (×460; WU neg. 50-5417.)

prognosis is rather unpredictable although as a group better than for bronchial carcinoma. We have had two patients with carcinosarcoma who have now survived over five years following pneumonectomy[186] (Figs. 264 and 265).

Pulmonary blastoma, also known as embryoma, is characterized by the presence of well-differentiated glands in a cellular stroma composed of undifferentiated spindle cells. The microscopic appearance is reminiscent of Wilms' tumor.[187] Metastases were present in five of twelve cases reviewed by Stackhouse et al.[188]

Both pulmonary blastoma and carcinosarcoma are malignant mixed tumors of adult individuals. However, they differ in several respects: in pulmonary blastoma, the epithelial component is always glandular, whereas in carcinosarcoma it is usually squamous; pulmonary blastoma is often peripheral, whereas carcinosarcoma is central, associated with a large bronchus; finally, pulmonary blastoma seems to have a better prognosis than carcinosarcoma.

Malignant lymphoma and pseudolymphoma

Primary pulmonary **malignant lymphomas** can be of histiocytic, lymphocytic, or, exceptionally, of Hodgkin's disease type (Fig. 266). Not included in this group are the cases of pulmonary spread from hilar lymph nodes, as it often occurs in Hodgkin's disease. Lymphocytic lymphoma must be differentiated from **pseudolymphoma,** a condition of probable inflammatory nature in which mature lymphocytes infiltrate the lung parenchyma and produce an ill-defined tumor mass (Fig. 267). Features favoring the diagnosis of pseudolymphoma include absence of hilar lymph node involvement, presence of germinal centers, and presence of other inflammatory cells.[189]

Metastatic tumors

Metastatic tumors of all types grow freely in the lung parenchyma. These metastases may be single or be restricted to a single lobe of the lung and thereby

be curable by resection. Habein et al.[192] reported pulmonary resection for metastatic malignant lesions in ninety-six patients. Sixteen were living without evidence of recurrence three or more years after the operation. The most common carcinomas of the total group (seventy-three) were carcinomas of the large bowel and breast, and the most common sarcomas (twenty) were osteosarcomas and fibrosarcomas.

No conclusions can be drawn concerning survival from the type of neoplasm. Generally, the neoplasms most favorable for resection are well-differentiated sarcomas (Fig. 268). We have resected well-differentiated fibrosarcomas and leiomyosarcomas.[191] The resectable tumors do not usually cause any pulmonary symptoms and are discovered on roentgenograms of the chest taken at properly spaced intervals. The most important prognostic sign is the interval between the primary operation and the appearance of a metastasis. This was found directly proportional to survival time thereafter in the series of Edlich et al.[190] when the group was considered as a whole. Bad prognostic signs are multiplicity of metastases and presence of lymph node involvement.

Infrequently, metastatic cancer involves hilar lymph nodes or lung and extends secondarily into the bronchus. We have seen this occur in testicular tumors, carcinoma of the kidney, and carcinoma of the rectum (Fig. 269). Certain neoplasms grow so rapidly and produce such diffuse pulmonary involvement that attempted resection is not indicated. Among these are carcinoma of the stomach and testis, malignant bone neoplasms, and carcinomas of the breast.

Other tumors

The so-called **granular cell tumor** can present as a polypoid intrabronchial mass and produce signs of bronchial obstruction.[197] Multicentric lesions have been described. We have seen an instance of a polypoid **inflammatory polyp** completely blocking a bronchus. We have also seen

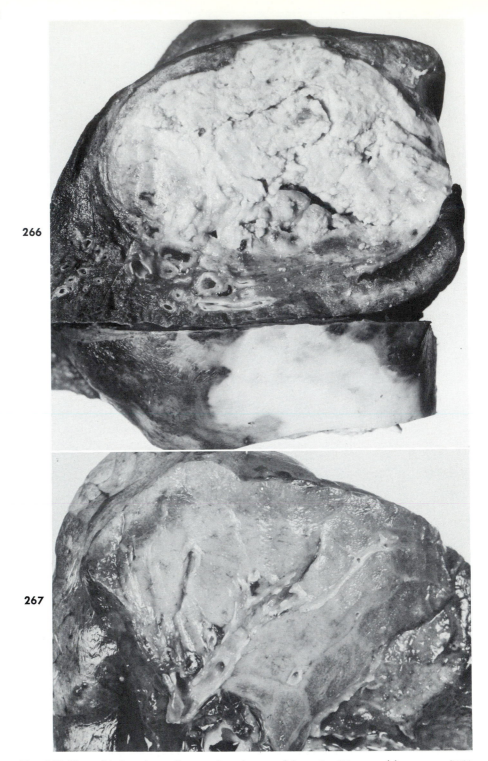

Fig. 266 Huge histiocytic malignant lymphoma of lung in 45-year-old woman. (WU neg. 55-3939.)

Fig. 267 Homogeneous localized pseudolymphoma occurring in left upper lobe in 74-year-old woman. Regional lymph nodes were hyperplastic. Pneumonectomy was done by Dr. Evarts A. Graham. Patient died five years later without evidence of cancer. (WU neg. 48-7010.)

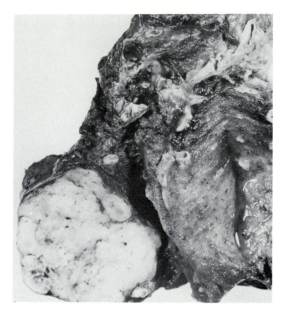

Fig. 268 Well-defined chondrosarcoma metastatic to lung in patient who had had this type of tumor in tibia several years before. (WU neg. 49-1757.)

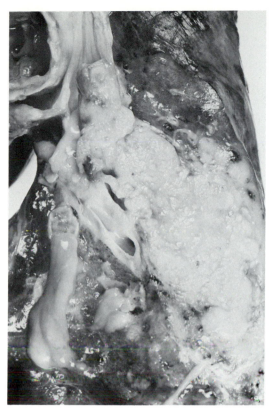

Fig. 269 Metastatic carcinoma of rectum forming polypoid mass in bronchus—a rare occurrence. (WU neg. 51-857.)

an intrapulmonary *thymoma,*[206] a *neurofibroma* growing between the pulmonary fissures, several bonafide *hemangiomas* of the lung parenchyma, two *leiomyomas* occurring beneath the pleural surface,[205] and a large bronchial *lipoma*[195] (Fig. 270). *Papillomas* of the trachea and large bronchi can occur alone or, more commonly, associated with laryngeal involvement.[202] Cases of *mucous gland adenoma* have been reviewed by Kroe and Pitcock.[200] An authentic pulmonary *oncocytoma,* unrelated to bronchial carcinoid, has been studied by Fechner and Bentinck.[196a]

Liebow and Castleman[201] have reported twelve cases of a neoplasm they designate as *benign clear cell ("sugar") tumor.* Grossly, it presents as a round or ovoid mass of small size, usually located in the peripheral lung. Microscopically, it is made up of large cells with clear cytoplasm crowded with glycogen granules. Fat is absent. Mitoses and areas of necrosis are not seen. These are the main features that differentiate this neoplasm from primary "clear cell carcinoma" and metastatic

renal cell carcinoma. Becker and Soifer[193] examined one of these neoplasms by electron microscopy and made the interesting observation that most of the glycogen is membrane-bound in lysosome-like organelles, in a pattern reminiscent of glycogenosis II.

Heppleston[198] reported an instance of an intrapulmonary *paraganglioma.* Multiple microscopic foci interpreted as chemoreceptor cells proliferation can be rarely seen as an incidental finding in surgically excised lungs. Their relationship with blood vessels distinguishes them from "tumourlets."[199]

We have examined an intrabronchial polypoid *fibrosarcoma* treated by pneumonectomy, in which the patient was free of symptoms five years later, only to have local recurrence that caused death by invasion of the pericardium.[194] Primary *leio-*

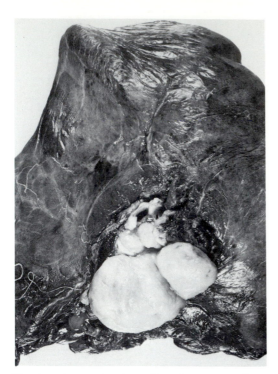

Fig. 270 Large, bright yellow lipoma involving bronchus. (WU neg. 51-1695.)

myosarcomas, chondrosarcomas,[196] *osteosarcomas,*[204] and *malignant melanomas*[203] have been described in the lung. However, in the presence of any of these tumors, all efforts should be made to rule out the possibility of a primary tumor elsewhere.

REFERENCES

Introduction

1 Brock, R. C.: The anatomy of the bronchial tree, with special reference to the surgery of lung abscess, ed. 2, London, 1954, Oxford University Press.

2 Hodgson, C. H., Weed, L. A., and Clagett, O. T.: Pulmonary histoplasmosis; summary of data on reported cases and a report on two patients treated by lobectomy, J.A.M.A. **145:**807-810, 1951.

3 Jackson, C. L., and Huber, J. F.: Correlated applied anatomy of the bronchial tree and lungs with a system of nomenclature, Dis. Chest. **9:**319-326, 1943.

4 McDonald, J. R., and Weed, L. A.: Histopathologic examination for tuberculosis, Mayo Clin. Proc. **25:**417-434, 1950.

5 Weed, L. A., Dahlin, D. C., Pugh, D. G., and Ivins, J. C.: Brucella in tissues removed at surgery, Am. J. Clin. Pathol. **22:**10-21, 1952.

6 White, J. D., and McGavran, M. H.: Identifi-

cation of Pasteurella tularensis by immunofluorescence, J.A.M.A. **194:**294-296, 1965.

7 Yamaguchi, B. T., Adriano, S., and Braunstein, H.: Histoplasma capsulatum in the pulmonary primary complex: immunohistochemical demonstration, Am. J. Pathol. **43:**713-719, 1963.

PLEURA

Biopsy and cytology

8 Aaron, B. L., Bellinger, S. B., Shepard, B. M., and Doohen, D. J.: Open lung biopsy; a strong stand, Chest **59:**18-22, 1971.

9 Ferguson, T. B., and Burford, T. H.: The role of surgery in the management of unilateral pleural effusion, Ann. Intern. Med. **50:**981-998, 1959.

10 Levine, H., Metzger, W., Lacera, D., and Kay, L.: Diagnosis of tuberculous pleurisy by culture of pleural biopsy specimen, Arch. Intern. Med. **126:**269-271, 1970.

11 Rao, V., Jones, P. O., Greenberg, S. D., Bahar, D., Daysog, A. O., Jr., Schweppe, H. I., Jr., and Jenkins, D. E.: Needle biopsy of parietal pleura in 124 cases, Arch. Intern. Med. **115:**34-51, 1965.

Obliterative pleuritis

12 Samson, P. C., and Burford, T. H.: Total pulmonary decortication, J. Thorac. Surg. **16:**127-145, 1947.

Mesothelioma

13 Benoit, H. W., Jr., and Ackerman, L. V.: Solitary pleural mesotheliomas, J. Thorac. Surg. **25:**346-357, 1953.

14 Cauna, D., Totten, R. S., and Gross, P.: Asbestos bodies in human lungs at autopsy, J.A.M.A. **192:**371-373, 1965.

15 Foster, E. A., and Ackerman, L. V.: Localized mesotheliomas of the pleura; the pathologic evaluation of 18 cases, Am. J. Clin. Pathol. **34:**349-364, 1960.

16 Gaensler, E. A., and Addington, W. W.: Asbestos or ferruginous bodies, N. Engl. J. Med. **280:**288-292, 1969.

17 Kuhn, C., III, and Kuo, T. T.: Cytoplasmic hyalin in asbestosis, Arch. Pathol. **95:**190-194, 1973.

18 McPeak, C. J., and Papaiannou, A. N.: Nonpancreatic tumors associated with hypoglycemia, Arch. Surg. **93:**1019-1024, 1966.

19 Ratzer, E. R., Pool, J. L., and Melamed, M. R.: Pleural mesotheliomas; clinical experiences with thirty-seven patients, Am. J. Roentgenol. Radium Ther. Nucl. Med. **99:**863-880, 1967.

20 Stout, A. P., and Murray, M. R.: Localized pleural mesothelioma; investigation of its characteristics and histogenesis by the method

of tissue culture, Arch. Pathol. 34:50-64, 1951.

21 Wagner, J. C., Sleggs, C. A., and Marchand, P.: Diffuse pleural mesothelioma and asbestos exposure in the North Western Cape Province, Br. J. Int. Med. 17:260-271, 1960.

Other lesions

22 Hourihane, D. O'B., Lessof, L., and Richardson, P. C.: Hyaline and calcified pleural plaques as an index of exposure to asbestos; a study of radiological and pathological features of 100 cases with a consideration of epidemiology, Br. Med. J. 1:1069-1074, 1966.

23 Martel, W., Abell, M. R., Mikkelsen, W. M., and Whitehouse, W. M.: Pulmonary and pleural lesions in rheumatoid disease, Radiology 90:641-653, 1968.

24 Petty, T. L., and Wilkins, M.: The five manifestations of rheumatoid lung, Dis. Chest 49:75-82, 1966.

25 Rous, V., and Studeny, J.: Aetiology of pleural plaques, Thorax 25:270-284, 1970.

26 Yeh, T. J.: Endometriosis within the thorax: metaplasia, implantation, or metastasis? J. Thorac. Cardiovasc. Surg. 53:201-205, 1967.

PULMONARY PARENCHYMA AND BRONCHI
Abscess

27 Bosher, L. H., Jr.: A review of surgically treated lung abscess, J. Thorac. Surg. 21:370-376, 1951.

28 Brock, R. C.: The anatomy of the bronchial tree, with special reference to the surgery of lung abscess, ed. 2, London, 1954, Oxford University Press.

29 Brock, R. C.: Studies in lung abscess, Guys Hosp. Rep. 97-98:196-229, 1948-1949.

30 Burford, T.: Personal communication, 1962.

31 Harter, J. S.: Treatment of the lung abscess, South. Surg. 16:191-195, 1950.

32 Myers, R. T., and Bradshaw, H. H.: Conservative resection of chronic lung abscess, Ann. Surg. 131:985-993, 1950.

Tuberculosis

33 Auerbach, O., and Small, M. J.: The syndrome of persistent cavitation and noninfectious sputum during chemotherapy and its relation to the open healing of cavities, Am. Rev. Tuberc. 75:242-258, 1957.

34 Auerbach, O., Hobby, G. L., Small, M. J., Lenert, T. F., and Comer, J. V.: The clinicopathologic significance of the demonstration of viable tubercle bacilli in resected lesions, J. Thorac. Surg. 29:109-132, 1955.

35 Black, H., and Ackerman, L. V.: The clinical and pathologic aspects of tuberculoma of the lung; an analysis of 18 cases, Surg. Clin. North Am. 30:1279-1297, 1950 (extensive bibliography).

36 Hattler, B. G., Jr., Young, W. G., Jr., Sealy, W. C., Gentry, W. H., and Cox, C. B.: Surgical management of pulmonary tuberculosis due to atypical mycobacteria, J. Thorac. Cardiovasc. Surg. 59:366-371, 1970.

37 Malave, G., Foster, E. D., Wilson, J. A., and Munro, D. D.: Bronchopleural fistula—present-day study of an old problem; a review of 52 cases, Ann. Thorac. Surg. 11:1-10, 1971.

38 Meissner, W. A.: Surgical pathology of endobronchial tuberculosis, Dis. Chest. 11:18-25, 1945.

39 Parker, E. F., Brailsford, L. E., and Gregg, D. B.: Tuberculous bronchiectasis, Am. Rev. Respir. Dis. 98:240-249, 1968.

40 Steele, J. D.: The solitary pulmonary nodule; with a foreword by Leo J. Rigler (The John Alexander monograph series on various phases of thoracic surgery, no. 6), Springfield, Ill., 1964, Charles C Thomas, Publisher.

41 Strieder, J. W., Laforet, E. G., and Lynch, J. P.: The surgery of pulmonary tuberculosis, N. Engl. J. Med. 276:960-965, 1967.

42 Sutinen, S.: Evaluation of activity in tuberculous cavities of the lung; a histopathologic and bacteriologic study of resected specimens with clinical and roentgenographic correlations, Scand. J. Respir. Dis. (suppl.) 67:5-78, 1968.

43 Sweany, H. C., and Seiler, H. H.: The pathology and bacteriology of resected lesions in pulmonary tuberculosis, Dis. Chest 29:119-152, 1956.

44 Thompson, J. R.: "Open healing" of tuberculous cavities, Am. Rev. Tuberc. 72:601-612, 1955.

45 Zimmerman, L. E.: Demonstration of histoplasma and coccidioides in so-called tuberculomas of lung, Arch. Intern. Med. 94:690-699, 1954.

Other granulomatous diseases

46 Nicholson, D. P.: Extrinsic allergic pneumonias, Am. J. Med. 53:131-136, 1972.

Interstitial pneumonia

47 Andrews, E. C., Jr.: Five cases of an undescribed form of pulmonary interstitial fibrosis caused by obstruction of the pulmonary veins, Bull. Johns Hopkins Hosp. 100:28-42, 1957.

48 Bonanni, P. P., Frymoyer, J. W., and Jacox, R. F.: A family study of idiopathic pulmonary fibrosis, Am. J. Med. 39:411-421, 1965.

49 Fraire, A. E., and Greenberg, S. D.: Carcinoma and diffuse interstitial fibrosis of lung, Cancer 31:1078-1086, 1973.

50 Gaensler, E. A., Goff, A. M., and Prowse, C. M.: Desquamative interstitial pneumonia, N. Engl. J. Med. 274:113-128, 1966.

51 Kuhn, C., III: Personal communication, 1973.
52 Liebow, A. A.: New concepts and entities in pulmonary disease. In Liebow, A. A., and Smith, D. E., editors: The lung (Monograph of the International Academy of Pathology), Baltimore, 1968, The Williams & Wilkins Co., pp. 332-365.
53 Liebow, A. A., Steer, A., and Billingsley, J. G.: Desquamative interstitial pneumonia, Am. J. Med. 39:369-404, 1965.
54 Scadding, J. G., and Hinson, K. F. W.: Diffuse fibrosing alveolitis (diffuse interstitial fibrosis of the lungs); correlation of histology at biopsy with prognosis, Thorax 22:291-304, 1967.

Broncholith

55 Schmidt, H. W., Clagett, O. T., and McDonald, J. R.: Broncholithiasis, J. Thorac. Surg. 19:226-245, 1950 (extensive bibliography).

Lipoid pneumonia

56 Berg, R., Jr., and Burford, T. H.: Pulmonary paraffinoma (lipoid pneumonia), J. Thorac. Surg. 20:418-428, 1950.
57 Pinkerton, H.: Oils and fats in the lung, Am. J. Dis. Child. 33:259-285, 1927.
58 Pinkerton, H.: The reaction to oils and fats in the lung, Arch. Pathol. 5:380-401, 1928.
59 Robbins, L. L., and Sniffen, R. C.: Correlation between the roentgenologic and pathologic findings in chronic pneumonitis of cholesterol type, Radiology 53:187-202, 1949.

Organizing pneumonia

60 Ackerman, L. V., Elliott, G. V., and Alanis, M.: Localized organizing pneumonia: its resemblance to carcinoma; review of its clinical, roentgenographic and pathologic features, Am. J. Roentgenol. Radium Ther. Nucl. Med. 71:988-996, 1954.

Bronchiectasis

61 Andrus, P. M.: Bronchiectasis; an analysis of its causes, Am. Rev. Tuberc. 36:46-81, 1937.
62 Anspach, W. E.: Atelectasis and bronchiectasis in children; a study of fifty cases presenting a triangular shadow at the base of the lung, Am. J. Dis. Child. 47:1011-1050, 1934.
63 Burford, T. H.: Personal communication, 1958.
64 Field, C. E.: Bronchiectasis in childhood. I. Clinical survey of 160 cases, Pediatrics 4:21-45, 1949.
65 Field, C. E.: Bronchiectasis in childhood. II. Aetiology and pathogenesis, including a survey of 272 cases of doubtful irreversible bronchiectasis, Pediatrics 4:231-248, 1949.
66 Field, C. E.: Bronchiectasis in childhood. III. Prophylaxis, treatment and progress with a follow-up study of 202 cases of established bronchiectasis, Pediatrics 4:355-372, 1949.
67 Lander, F. P. L., and Davidson, M.: Aetiology of bronchiectasis, Br. J. Radiol. 11:65-89, 1938.
68 Liebow, A. A., Hales, M. R., and Lindskog, G. E.: Enlargement of the bronchial arteries and their anastomoses with the pulmonary arteries in bronchiectasis, Am. J. Pathol. 25:211-232, 1949.
69 Mallory, T. B.: The pathogenesis of bronchiectasis, bronchial infection and atelectasis, N. Engl. J. Med. 237:795-798, 1947.
70 Ogilvie, A. G.: Natural history of bronchiectasis; clinical, roentgenologic and pathologic study, Arch. Intern. Med. 68:395-465, 1941.
71 Perry, K. M. A., and King, D. S.: Bronchiectasis; study of prognosis based on follow-up of 400 patients, Am. Rev. Tuberc. 41:531-548, 1940.

Cystic diseases

72 Allbritten, F. F., Jr., and Templeton, J. Y.: Treatment of giant cysts of the lung, J. Thorac. Surg. 20:749-760, 1950.
73 Cunningham, G. J., Nassau, E., and Walter, J. B.: The frequency of tumour-like formations in bronchiectatic lungs, Thorax 13:64-68, 1958.
74 Jewsbury, P.: Surgical treatment of cystic disease and emphysema in young children, Br. J. Surg. 42:601, 1955.
75 Meyer, E. C., and Liebow, A. A.: Relationship of interstitial pneumonia, honeycombing and atypical epithelial proliferation to cancer of the lung, Cancer 18:322-351, 1965.
76 Womack, N. A., and Graham, E. A.: Epithelial metaplasia in congenital cystic disease of the lung, Am. J. Pathol. 17:645-654, 1941.

Bronchopulmonary sequestration

77 Bruwer, A., Clagett, O. T., and McDonald, J. R.: Intralobar bronchopulmonary sequestration, Med. Clin. North Am. 38:1081-1090, 1954.
78 Johnston, D. G.: Inflammatory and vascular lesions of bronchopulmonary sequestration, Am. J. Clin. Pathol. 26:636-644, 1956.
79 Pryce, D. M., Sellors, T. H., and Blair, L. G.: Intralobar sequestration of lung associated with an abnormal pulmonary artery, Br. J. Surg. 35:18-29, 1947.
80 Smith, R. A.: Some controversial aspects of intralobar sequestration of the lung, Surg. Gynecol. Obstet. 114:57-68, 1962.

Arteriovenous fistula

81 Liebow, A. A.: Tumors of the lower respiratory tract. In Atlas of tumor pathology, Sect. V, Fasc. 17, Washington, D. C., 1952, Armed Forces Institute of Pathology.

82 Lingskog, G. E., Liebow, A. A., Kausel, H., and Janzen, A.: Pulmonary arteriovenous aneurysm, Ann. Surg. **132**:591-606, 1950.

Miscellaneous lesions

83 Carrington, C. B., and Liebow, A. A.: Limited forms of angiitis and granulomatosis of Wegener's type, Am. J. Med. **41**:497-527, 1966.

84 Errion, A. R., Hauk, V. N., and Kettering, D. L.: Pulmonary hematoma due to blunt nonpenetrating thoracic trauma, Am. Rev. Respir. Dis. **88**:384-392, 1963.

85 Fors, B., and Ryden, L.: Tumoral amyloidosis of the lung, Acta Pathol. Microbiol. Scand. **61**:1-12, 1964.

86 Lewis, J. G.: Eosinophilic granuloma and its variants with special reference to lung involvement, Q. J. Med. **33**:337-359, 1964.

86a Liebow, A. A.: Pulmonary angiitis and granulomatosis (the J. Burns Amberson lecture), Am. Rev. Respir. Dis. **108**:1-18, 1973.

87 Liebow, A. A., and Carrington, C. B.: The eosinophilic pneumonias, Medicine (Baltimore) **48**:251-285, 1969.

88 Liebow, A. A., Carrington, C. R. B., and Friedman, P. J.: Lymphomatoid granulomatosis, Hum. Pathol. **3**:457-558, 1972.

89 Neafie, R. C., and Piggott, J.: Human pulmonary dirofilariasis, Arch. Pathol. **92**:342-349, 1971.

90 Nielsen, K., Christiansen, I., and Jensen, E.: Wegener's granulomatosis; a survey and three cases, Acta Med. Scand. **181**:577-582, 1967.

91 Rosen, S. H., Castleman, B., and Liebow, A. A.: Pulmonary alveolar proteinosis, New Engl. J. Med. **258**:1123-1142, 1958.

92 Soergel, K. H., and Sommers, S. C.: Idiopathic pulmonary hemosiderosis and related syndromes, Am. J. Med. **32**:499-511, 1962.

93 Steer, A.: Focal pulmonary alveolar proteinosis in pulmonary tuberculosis, Arch. Pathol. **87**:347-352, 1969.

Tumors

Hamartoma (chondroma)

94 Albrecht, E.: Ueber Hamartome, Verh. Dtsch. Pathol. Ges. **7**:153-157, 1904.

95 Butler, C., and Kleinerman, J.: Pulmonary hamartoma, Arch. Pathol. **88**:584-592, 1969.

96 McDonald, J. R., Harrington, S. W., and Clagett, O. T.: Hamartoma (often called chondroma) of the lung, J. Thorac. Surg. **14**:128-143, 1945.

Fibroxanthoma

97 Liebow, A. A., and Hubbel, D. S.: Sclerosing hemangioma (histiocytoma, xanthoma) of lung, Cancer **9**:53-75, 1956.

98 Titus, J. L., Harrison, E. G., Clagett, O. T., Anderson, M. W., and Knaff, L. J.: Xanthomatous and inflammatory pseudotumors of the lung, Cancer **15**:522-538, 1962.

99 Wentworth, P., Lynch, M. J., Fallis, J. C., Turner, J. A. P., Lowden, J. A., and Conen, P. E.: Xanthomatous pseudotumor of lung; a case report with electron microscope and lipid studies, Cancer **22**:345-355, 1968.

Carcinoma

100 Auerbach, O., Gere, J. B., Forman, J. B., Petrick, T. G., Smolin, H. J., Muehsam, G. E., Kassouny, D. Y., and Stout, A. P.: Changes in the bronchial epithelium in relation to smoking and cancer of the lung, N. Engl. J. Med. **256**:97-104, 1957.

101 Kannerstein, M., and Churg, J.: Pathology of carcinoma of the lung associated with asbestos exposure, Cancer **30**:14-21, 1972.

102 LeGal, Y., and Bauer, W. G.: Second primary bronchogenic carcinoma, J. Thorac. Cardiovasc. Surg. **41**:114-124, 1961.

103 Limas, C., Japaze, H., and Garcia-Bunuel, R.: "Scar" carcinoma of the lung, Chest **59**:219-222, 1971.

104 Lynch, K. M., and Smith, W. A.: Pulmonary asbestosis; a report of bronchial carcinoma and epithelial metaplasia, Am. J. Cancer **36**:567-573, 1939.

105 Machle, W., and Gregorius, F.: Cancer of the respiratory system in United States chromate-producing industry, Public Health Rep. **63**:1114-1127, 1948.

106 Meyer, E. C., and Liebow, A. A.: Relationship of interstitial pneumonia honeycombing and atypical epithelial proliferation to cancer of the lung, Cancer **18**:322-351, 1965.

107 Mills, C. A., and Porter, M. M.: Tobacco smoking, motor exhaust fumes, and general air pollution in relation to lung cancer incidence, Cancer Res. **17**:981-990, 1957.

108 Sikl, H.: The present status of knowledge about the Jachymov disease (cancer of the lungs in the miners of the radium mines), Acta Un. Int. Cancr. **6**(6):1366-1375, 1950.

109 Vincent, T. N., Satterfield, J. V., and Ackerman, L. V.: Carcinoma of the lung in women, Cancer **18**:559-570, 1965.

110 Woolner, L. B., David, E., Fontana, R. S., Andersen, H. A., and Bernatz, P. E.: In situ and early invasive bronchogenic carcinoma; report of 28 cases with postoperative survival data, J. Thorac. Cardiovasc. Surg. **60**:275-290, 1970.

Microscopic types

111 Arrigoni, M. G., Woolner, L. B., and Beruatz, P. E.: Atypical carcinoid tumors of the lung, J. Thorac. Cardiovasc. Surg. **64**:413-421, 1972.

112 Azzopardi, J. G.: Oat cell carcinoma of the bronchus, J. Pathol. Bacteriol. **78**:513-519, 1959.

113 Bateson, E. M.: The solitary circumscribed bronchogenic carcinoma; a radiological study of 100 cases, Br. J. Radiol. 37:598-607, 1964.

114 Bennett, D. E., and Sasser, W. F.: Bronchiolar carcinoma; a valid clinicopathologic entity? A study of 30 cases, Cancer 24:876-887, 1969.

115 Bennett, D. E., Sasser, W. F., and Ferguson, T.: Adenocarcinoma of the lung in men; a clinicopathologic study of 100 cases, Cancer 23:431-439, 1969.

116 Bensch, K. G., Corrin, B., Pariente, R., and Spencer, H.: Oat-cell carcinoma of the lung; its origin and relationship to bronchial carcinoid, Cancer 22:1163-1172, 1968.

117 Black, H., and Ackerman, L. V.: The importance of epidermoid carcinoma in situ in the histogenesis of carcinoma of the lung, Ann. Surg. 136:44-55, 1952.

118 Byrd, R. B., Miller, W. E., Carr, D. T., Payne, W. S., and Woolner, L. B.: The roentgenographic appearance of large cell carcinoma of the bronchus, Mayo Clin. Proc. 43:333-336, 1968.

119 Hattori, S., Matsuda, M., Tateishi, R., Nishihara, H., and Horai, T.: Oat-cell carcinoma of the lung; clinical and morphological studies in relation to its histogenesis, Cancer 30:1014-1024, 1972.

120 Herbut, P. A.: "Alveolar cell tumor" of the lung, Arch. Pathol. 41:175-184, 1946.

121 Herman, D. L., Bullock, W. K., and Waken, J. K.: Giant cell adenocarcinoma of the lung, Cancer 19:1337-1346, 1966.

122 Kato, Y., Ferguson, T. B., Bennett, D. E., and Burford, T. H.: Oat cell carcinoma of the lung; a review of 138 cases, Cancer 23:517-524, 1969.

123 Kreyberg, L.: Main histological types of primary epithelial lung tumours, Br. J. Cancer 15:206-210, 1961.

124 Kreyberg, L., Liebow, A. A., and Uehlinger, E. A.: Histological typing of lung tumours, vol. 1 of International histological classification of tumours, Geneva, 1967, World Health Organization.

125 Kuhn, C., III: Fine structure of bronchioloalveolar cell carcinoma, Cancer 30:1107-1118, 1972.

126 Laipply, T. C., Sherrick, J. C., and Cape, W. E.: Bronchiolar (alveolar cell) tumors, Arch. Pathol. 59:35-50, 1955.

127 McDonald, J. R., Moersch, J. H., and Tinney, W. S.: Cylindroma of the bronchus, J. Thorac. Surg. 14:445-453, 1945.

128 Markel, S. F., Abell, M. R., Haight, C., and French, A. J.: Neoplasms of bronchus commonly designated as adenomas, Cancer 17:590-608, 1964.

129 Meyer, E. C., and Liebow, A. A.: Relationship of interstitial pneumonia honeycombing and atypical epithelial proliferation to cancer of the lung, Cancer 18:322-351, 1965.

130 Morgan, A. D., and Mackenzie, D. H.: Clear-cell carcinoma of the lung, J. Pathol. Bacteriol. 87:25-27, 1964.

131 Nash, A. D., and Stout, A. P.: Giant cell carcinoma of the lung, Cancer 11:369-376, 1958.

132 Reichle, F. A., and Rosemond, G. P.: Mucoepidermoid tumors of the bronchus, J. Thorac. Cardiovasc. Surg. 51:443-448, 1966.

133 Strang, C., and Simpson, J. A.: Carcinomatous abscess of the lung, Thorax 8:11-28, 1953.

134 Swan, L. L.: Pulmonary adenomatosis of man, Arch. Pathol. 47:517-544, 1949.

135 Turnbull, A. D., Huvos, A. G., Goodner, J. T., and Foote, F. W., Jr.: Mucoepidermoid tumors of bronchial glands, Cancer 28:539-544, 1971.

Cytology/Biopsy/Frozen section

136 Andrews, N. C., and Klassen, K. P.: Eight years' experience with pulmonary biopsy, J.A.M.A. 164:1061-1065, 1957.

137 Daniels, A. C.: Method of biopsy useful in diagnosing certain intrathoracic diseases, Dis. Chest 16:360-366, 1949.

138 Fennessy, J. J., Fry, W. A., Manalo-Estrella, P., and Hidvegi, D. V. S. F.: The bronchial brushing technique for obtaining cytologic specimens from peripheral lung lesions, Acta Cytol. (Baltimore) 14:25-30, 1970.

139 Fontana, R. S., Carr, D. T., Woolner, L. B., and Miller, F. K.: An evaluation of methods of inducing sputum production in patients with suspected cancer of the lung, Mayo Clin. Proc. 37:113-121, 1962.

140 Frenzel, H., and Papageorgiou, A.: Malignant cells in the sputum in coin lesions of the lung, Ger. Med. Mon. 9:1-10, 1964.

141 Grant, L. J., and Trivedi, S. A.: Open lung biopsy for diffuse pulmonary lesions, Br. Med. J. 1:17-21, 1960.

142 Hattori, S., Matsuda, M., Sugiyama, T., and Matsoda, H.: Cytologic diagnosis of early lung cancer: brushing method under x-ray television fluoroscopy, Dis. Chest 45:129-142, 1964.

143 Koss, L. G., Melamed, M. R., and Goodner, J. T.: Pulmonary cytology—a brief survey of diagnostic results from July 1st, 1952 until December 31st, 1960, Acta Cytol. (Baltimore) 8:104-113, 1964.

144 Paulson, D. L.: A philosophy of treatment for bronchogenic carcinoma, Ann. Thorac. Surg. 5:289-299, 1968.

145 Pearson, F. G., Nelems, J. M., Henderson, R. D., and Delarue, N. C.: The role of mediastinoscopy in the selection of treatment for bronchial carcinoma with involvement of su-

perior mediastinal lymph nodes, J. Thorac. Cardiovasc. Surg. **64**:382-390, 1972.

146 Pearson, F. G., Thompson, D. W., and Delarue, N. C.: Experience with the cytologic detection, localization, and treatment of radiographically undemonstrable bronchial carcinoma, J. Thorac. Cardiovasc. Surg. **54**:371-382, 1967.

147 Russell, W. O., Neidhardt, H. W., Mountain, C. E., Griffith, K. M., and Chang, J. P.: Cytodiagnosis of lung cancer, Acta Cytol. (Baltimore) **7**:1-44, 1963 (extensive bibliography).

148 Sison, B. S., and Weiss, W.: Needle biopsy of the parietal pleura in patients with pleural effusion, Br. Med. J. **1**:298-300, 1962.

149 Spjut, H. J., Fier, D. J., and Ackerman, L. V.: Exfoliative cytology and pulmonary cancer, J. Thorac. Surg. **30**:90-107, 1955.

150 Spjut, H. J., Hendrix, V. J., Ramirez, G. A., and Roper, C. L.: Carcinoma cells in pleural cavity washings, Cancer **11**:1222-1225, 1958.

151 Stevens, G. M., Weigen, J. F., and Lillington, G. A.: Needle aspiration biopsy of localized pulmonary lesions with amplified fluoroscopic guidance, Am. J. Roentgenol. Radium Ther. Nucl. Med. **103**:561-571, 1968.

152 Wandall, H. H.: A study of neoplastic cells in sputum as a contribution to the diagnosis of primary lung cancer. Acta Chir. Scand. **91** (suppl. 93):1-143, 1944.

153 Wierman, W. H., McDonald, J. R., and Clagett, O. T.: Occult carcinoma of the major bronchi, Surgery **35**:335-345, 1934.

Clinicopathologic correlation

154 Burford, T. H., Ferguson, T. B., and Spjut, H. J.: Results in the treatment of bronchogenic carcinoma, J. Thorac. Surg. **36**:316-328, 1958.

155 Collier, F. C., Blakemore, W. S., Kyle, R. H., Enterline, H. T., Kirby, C. K., and Johnson, J.: Carcinoma of the lung; factors which influence five-year-survival with special reference to blood vessel invasion, Ann. Surg. **146**:417-423, 1957.

156 Gibbon, J. H., Jr., Allbritten, F. F., Jr., Templeton, J. Y., III, and Nealon, T. F., Jr.: Cancer of the lung—an analysis of 532 consecutive cases. Ann. Surg. **138**:489-501, 1953.

157 Hood, R. T., Jr., Good, C. A., Clagett, O. T., and McDonald, J. R.: Solitary circumscribed lesions of the lung, J.A.M.A. **152**:1185-1191, 1953.

158 Overholt, R. H., and Schmidt, I. C.: Survival in primary carcinoma of the lung, N. Engl. J. Med. **240**:491-497, 1949.

159 Spjut, H. J., Roper, C. L., and Butcher, H. R., Jr.: Pulmonary cancer and its prognosis; a study of the relationship of certain factors to survival of patients treated by pulmonary resection, Cancer **14**:1251-1258, 1961.

Bronchial carcinoid

160 Anderson, W M.: Bronchial adenoma with metastasis to the liver, J. Thorac. Surg. **12**:351-360, 1943.

161 Arrigoni, M. G., Woolner, L. B., and Beruatz, P. E.: Atypical carcinoid tumors of the lung, J. Thorac. Cardiovasc. Surg. **64**:413-421, 1972.

162 Bensch, K. G., Gordon, G. B., and Miller, L. R.: Electron microscopic and biochemical studies on the bronchial carcinoid tumor, Cancer **18**:592-602, 1965.

163 Black, B.: Personal communication, 1951.

164 Black, W. C., III: Enterochromaffin cell types and corresponding carcinoid tumors, Lab. Invest. **19**:473-486, 1968.

165 Black, W. C., III: Pulmonary oncocytoma, Cancer **23**:1347-1357, 1969.

166 Cohen, R. B., Toll, G. D., and Castleman, B.: Bronchial adenomas in Cushing's syndrome; their relation to thymomas and oat cell carcinomas associated with hyperadrenocorticism, Cancer **13**:812-817, 1960.

167 Felton, W. L., II: Liebow, A. A., and Lindskog, G. E.: Peripheral and multiple bronchial adenomas, Cancer **6**:555-567, 1953.

168 Feyrter, F.: Über das Bronchuscarcinoid, Virchows Arch. Pathol. Anat. **332**:25-43, 1959.

169 Foster-Carter, A. F.: Bronchial adenoma, Q. J. Med. **10**:139-174, 1941.

170 Geever, E. F., Williams, W. S., and McWilliams, J. E.: Bronchial adenoma with cancerous transformation, Am. J. Clin. Pathol. **19**:836-839, 1949.

171 Gmelich, J. T., Bensch, K. G., and Liebow, A. A.: Cells of Kultschitzky type in bronchioles and their relation to the origin of peripheral carcinoid tumor, Lab. Invest. **17**:88-98, 1967.

172 Graham, E. A., and Womack, N. A.: The problem of the so-called bronchial adenoma, J. Thorac. Surg. **14**:106-127, 1945.

173 Holley, S. W.: Bronchial adenomas, Milit. Surg. **99**:528-554, 1946.

174 Maier, H. C., and Fischer, W. W.: Adenomas arising from small bronchi not visible bronchoscopically, J. Thorac. Surg. **16**:392-398, 1947.

175 Markel, S. F., Abell, M. R., Haight, C., and French, A. J.: Neoplasms of bronchus commonly designated as adenomas, Cancer **17**:590-608, 1964.

176 Meissner, W. A.: The pathology of so-called bronchial adenomas, Proceedings of the Second National Cancer Conference, New York, 1952, American Cancer Society, Inc.

177 Moersch, H. J., and McDonald, J. R.: Bron-

chial adenoma, J.A.M.A. **142**:299-303, 1950.

178 Sandler, M., Scheuer, P. J., and Watt, P. J.: 5-hydroxytroptophan-secreting bronchial carcinoid tumour, Lancet **2**:1067-1069, 1961.

179 Stanford, W. R., Davis, J. E., Gunter, J. U., and Hobart, S. G., Jr.: Bronchial adenoma (carcinoid type) with solitary metastasis and associated functioning carcinoid syndrome, South. Med. J. **51**:449-454, 1958.

179a Tateishi, R.: Distribution of argyrophil cells in adult human lungs, Arch. Pathol. **96**:198-202, 1973.

180 Thomas, B. M.: Three unusual carcinoid tumours, with particular reference to osteoblastic bone metastases, Clin. Radiol. **19**:221-225, 1968.

181 Warner, R. R. P., Kirschner, P. A., and Warner, G. M.: Serotonin production by bronchial adenomas without the carcinoid syndrome, J.A.M.A. **178**:1175-1179, 1961.

182 Wilkins, E. W., Jr., Darling, R. C., Soutter, L., and Sniffen, R. C.: A continuing clinical survey of adenomas of the trachea and bronchus in a general hospital, J. Thorac. Cardiovasc. Surg. **46**:279-291, 1963.

183 Williams, E. D.: The classification of carcinoid tumours, Lancet **1**:238-239, 1963.

184 Williams, E. D., and Celestin, L. R.: The association of bronchial carcinoid and pluriglandular adenomatosis, Thorax **17**:120-127, 1962.

185 Williams, E. D., and Azzopardi, J. G.: Tumors of lung and carcinoid syndrome, Thorax **15**:30-36, 1960.

Carcinosarcoma and blastoma

186 Bergmann, M., Ackerman, L. V., and Kemler, R. L.: Carcinosarcoma of the lung; review of the literature and report of two cases treated by pneumonectomy, Cancer **4**:919-929, 1951.

187 Minken, S. L., Craver, W. L., and Adams, J. T.: Pulmonary blastoma, Arch. Pathol. **86**:442-446, 1968.

188 Stackhouse, E. M., Harrison, E. G., Jr., and Ellis, F. H.: Primary mixed malignancies of lung; carcinosarcoma and blastoma, J. Thorac. Cardiovasc. Surg. **57**:385-399, 1969.

Malignant lymphoma and pseudolymphoma

189 Saltzstein, S. L.: Pulmonary malignant lymphomas and pseudolymphomas; classification, therapy, and prognosis, Cancer **16**:928-955, 1963.

Metastatic tumors

190 Edlich, R. F., Shea, M. A., Foker, J. E., Grondin, C., Castaneda, A. R., and Varco, R. L.: A review of 26 years' experience with pulmonary resection for metastatic cancer, Dis. Chest **49**:587-594, 1966.

191 Feldman, P. S., and Kyriakos, M.: Pulmonary resection for metastatic sarcoma, J. Thorac. Cardiovasc. Surg. **64**:784-799, 1972.

192 Habein, H. C., Jr., Clagett, O. T., and McDonald, J. R.: Pulmonary resection for metastatic tumors, Arch. Surg. **78**:716-723, 1959.

Other tumors

193 Becker, N. H., and Soifer, L.: Benign clear cell tumor ("sugar tumor") of the lung, Cancer **27**:712-719, 1971.

194 Black, H.: Fibrosarcoma of the bronchus, J. Thorac. Surg. **19**:123-134, 1950.

195 Crutcher, R. R., Waltuck, T. L., and Ghosh, A. K.: Bronchial lipoma, J. Thorac. Cardiovasc. Surg. **55**:422-425, 1968.

196 Daniels, A. C., Conner, G. H., and Straus, F. H.: Primary chondrosarcoma of the tracheobronchial tree; report of a unique case and brief review, Arch. Pathol. **84**:615-624, 1967.

196a Fechner, R. E., and Bentinck, B. R.: Ultrastructure of bronchial oncocytoma, Cancer **31**:1451-1457, 1973.

197 Gallivan, G. J., Dolan, C. T., Stam, R. E., Eggerston, B. S., Jr., and Tovey, J. D.: Granular cell myoblastoma of the bronchus, J. Thorac. Cardiovasc. Surg. **52**:875-881, 1966.

198 Heppleston, A. G.: A carotid-body-like tumour in the lung, J. Pathol. Bacteriol. **75**:461-464, 1958.

199 Korn, D., Bensch, K., Liebow, A. A., and Castleman, B.: Multiple minute pulmonary tumors resembling chemodectomas, Am. J. Pathol. **37**:641-672, 1960.

200 Kroe, D. J., and Pitcock, J. A.: Benign mucous gland adenoma of the bronchus, Arch. Pathol. **84**:539-542, 1967.

201 Liebow, A. A., and Castleman, B.: Benign clear cell ("sugar") tumors of the lung, Yale J. Biol. Med. **43**:213-222, 1971.

202 Moore, R. L., and Lattes, R.: Papillomatosis of larynx and bronchi, Cancer **12**:117-126, 1959.

203 Reid, J. D., and Mehta, V. T.: Melanoma of the lower respiratory tract, Cancer **19**:627-631, 1966.

204 Reingold, L. M., and Amromin, G. D.: Extraosseous osteosarcoma of the lung, Cancer **28**:491-498, 1971.

205 Taylor, T. L., and Miller, D. R.: Leiomyoma of the bronchus, J. Thorac. Cardiovasc. Surg. **57**:284-288, 1969.

206 Thorburn, J. D., Stephens, H. B., and Grimes, O. F.: Benign thymoma in the hilus of the lung, J. Thorac. Surg. **24**:540-543, 1952.

7 Mediastinum

Introduction

The mediastinum is the portion of the thoracic cavity located between the pleural cavities, extending anteroposteriorly from the sternum to the spine and sagitally from the thoracic inlet to the diaphragm. It contains many organs and structures from which various types of cysts and neoplasms may arise. At present, thoracic surgery has advanced so far in technique and safety that exploratory thoracotomy can be performed with little risk. For instance, Blades[1] reported 109 patients treated by thoracotomy at army thoracic surgery centers with no operative mortality. Therefore, the nature of these neoplasms has assumed great practical significance. The pathologist has been forced by the advances in thoracic surgery to differentiate and classify them more accurately.

If a mass is seen on roentgenographic examination, it is far better to explore the mediastinum than to give a so-called test dose of irradiation, for the lesion may be a resectable neoplasm or perhaps only a cyst. Large tumors of the anterior portion of the mediastinum, including thymomas, substernal thyroid tissue, and malignant neoplasms, have been successfully identified by needle biopsy. Because of faulty embryogenesis, thyroid tissue may be present in the mediastinum, usually in the superior or anterior portion. We have seen it just above the diaphragm in the posterior portion (Chapter 9). Parathyroid tissue also may be intramediastinal (Chapter 8).

Tumors secondarily invading the mediastinum from the esophagus, lung parenchyma, bronchus, pleura, chest wall, or vertebra may be confused with primary mediastinal neoplasms, but these will not be discussed here.

An arbitrary division of the mediastinum into *superior, anterior, middle* and *posterior* compartments has proved useful, since most cysts and neoplasms have a predilection for one compartment over the others. The most common mediastinal lesions are noted in Fig. 302 according to their frequency and most common site of occurrence.[2, 3]

Nonneoplastic cysts
Pericardial cysts (coelomic)

Pericardial cysts arise as failures in embryonic development.[8] The pericardium is formed by the fusion of multiple disconnected lacunae. Failure of one of the lacunar cavities to merge with the others may

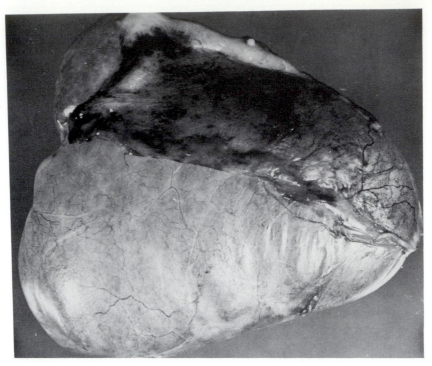

Fig. 271 Unilocular thin-walled pericardial cyst. (WU neg. 48-3399.)

result in the development of a pericardial coelomic cyst. Such cysts commonly occur in the right cardiophrenic angle.[9] They are soft and unilocular, usually loosely adherent to the pericardium and sometimes communicate with the pericardial cavity (Fig. 271). At times, multiple cysts may be present. They contain clear fluid unless infected.

These lesions may be strongly suspected but cannot be accurately diagnosed without exploration. We have seen one patient in whom the radiographic configuration suggested metastatic carcinoma. The blood supply for pericardial cysts comes from the pericardium. The inner surface of the cyst wall is covered by a thin layer of mesothelium.

Bronchial, esophageal, gastric, and enteric cysts

Laipply's explanation[7] of the development of tracheal, bronchial, esophageal, gastroenteric, and gastric cysts appears well supported. In the embryonic stage, the fusion of the lateral walls that form the tra-

cheoesophageal septum begins caudally. At this time, if a small bud or diverticulum of the foregut is pinched off, this bud might be carried into the mediastinum by the downward growth of lungs. The diverticulum would contain entoderm and mesoderm that were destined to become part of the trachea, bronchi, esophagus, stomach, or intestine.

Bronchial cysts occur along the tracheobronchial tree most commonly immediately posterior to the carina. Rarely, they occur just above the diaphragm.[10] Communication with the lumen of the tracheobronchial tree is exceptional. In children, these cysts can be missed on plain films but cause severe respiratory distress because of airway compression. Barium-swallow studies are very helpful in diagnosis.[6] These cysts contain clear or gelatinous fluid and do not reach a large size (Fig. 272). Microscopic examination reveals that they usually are lined by ciliated columnar epithelium (Fig. 273). The wall may contain hyaline cartilage, smooth muscle, and

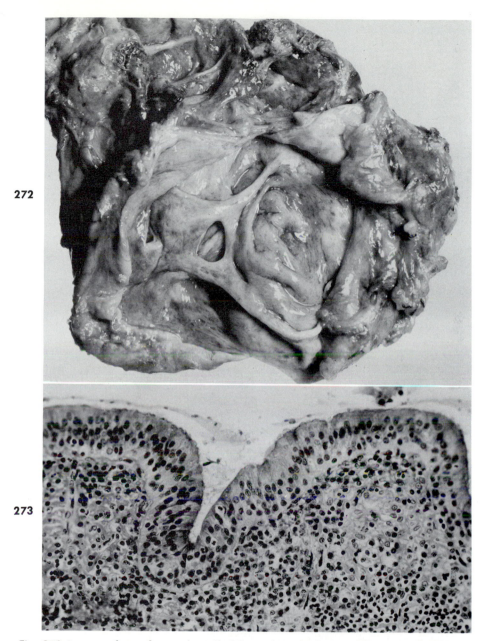

Fig. 272 Inner surface of smooth-walled large bronchial cyst. (WU neg. 48-6734.)
Fig. 273 Lining of cyst shown in Fig. 272. Surface epithelium is ciliated and columnar.
(×240; WU neg. 49-344.)

nerve trunks. Because of variation in location, they may cause symptoms or be an entirely incidental finding.

Esophageal cysts are usually not reported as such but as portions of mixed cysts consisting of bronchial and esophageal elements or of gastric and esophageal elements. The latter are seen in adults in the lower half of the esophagus and can be lined by pseudostratified ciliated epithelium, squamous epithelium, or a mixture of both.

Gastric and *enteric cysts* are usually located paravertebrally in the posterior por-

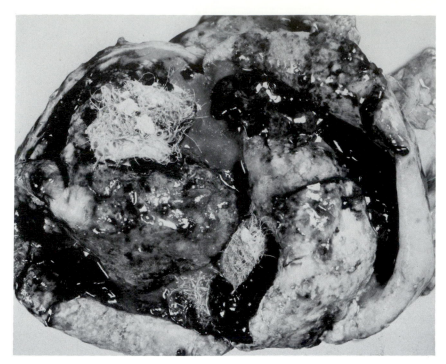

Fig. 274 Large benign cystic teratoma of anterior portion of mediastinum in which hair is clearly visible. (WU neg. 48-899.)

tion of the mediastinum attached to the wall of the esophagus or even embedded within the muscular layer of this organ. The gastric variety is made up of the same coats as the stomach, whereas the enteric type simulates the wall of normal intestine. Combined forms occur and are designated as **gastroenteric cysts.** Nerve fibers and ganglia are often present.[4]

These congenital cysts only exceptionally communicate with the tracheobronchial tree or the esophagus. They are not neoplasms, and malignant change does not take place within them. Symptoms from these cysts are related to pressure phenomena and consist of cough, dysphagia, recurrent pulmonary infection, dyspnea, pain, and rarely hemoptysis. The gastric variety can be life threatening because of the occurrence of gastric secretion and the resulting hemorrhage, peptic ulcer, or perforation.[5]

Inflammatory diseases

Acute mediastinitis is usually the result of traumatic perforation of the esophagus.[13]

Chronic mediastinitis can produce compression of the vena cava and simulate a malignant process. The typical location is the anterior mediastinum, in front of the tracheal bifurcation. Microscopically, one may find granulomas, fibrosis, or a combination of both.[15] In some of these cases, a fungal (histoplasmosis) or tuberculous etiology can be documented.[14] In most instances, a specific etiology cannot be demonstrated.[11] The predominantly fibrous cases may be associated with similar changes in the retroperitoneum.[12]

Tumors
Germinal tumors

Teratomas represent the most common variety of mediastinal germinal neoplasms. They usually become clinically apparent in early adult life. They grow to a large size and often have a distinct, sharply delineated wall that may become calcified. The cystic tumor may become adherent to surrounding structures.[18] Calcification may be present within the neoplasm.

These tumors sometimes perforate into

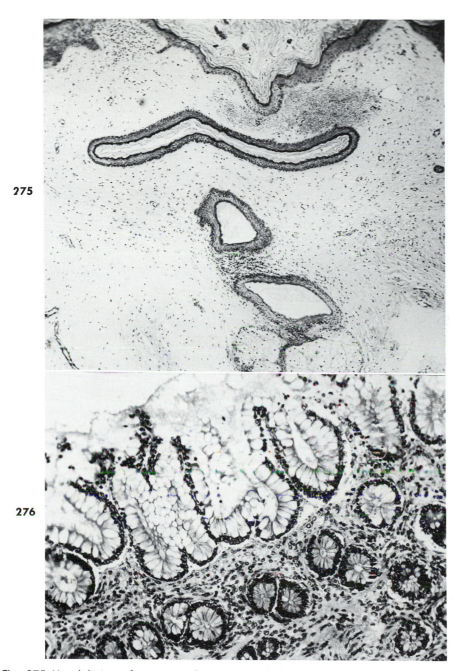

Fig. 275 Usual lining of teratoma showing stratified squamous epithelium and abundant sebaceous glands. (Low power; WU neg. 49-256.)
Fig. 276 Epithelium suggesting large bowel in benign teratoma. (×200; WU neg. 49-253.)

the tracheobronchial tree, and the patient may cough up sebaceous oily material and hair (Fig. 274). If the sebaceous material within them escapes, a prominent inflammatory reaction results.

Microscopically, the benign adult terato-

mas resemble those of the ovary. They are lined by stratified squamous epithelium and contain abundant sebaceous glands (Fig. 275). Hair is invariably present. The more tissue sections made, the more types of tissue revealed. It is common to find

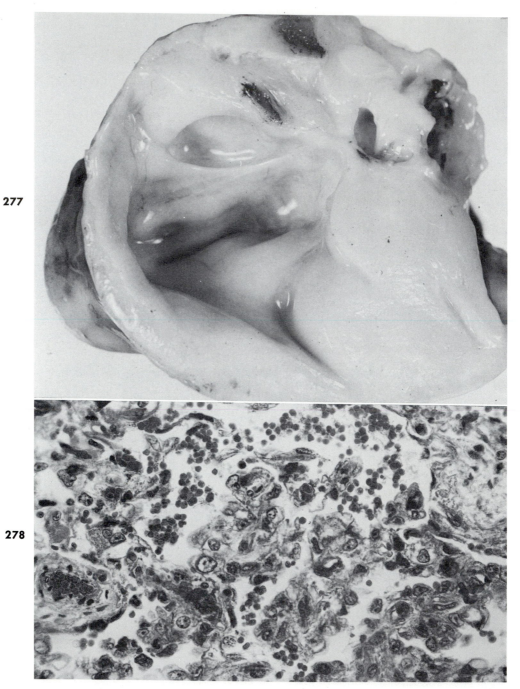

277

278

Fig. 277 Malignant teratoma of mediastinum that was highly cellular but still encapsulated. (WU neg. 48-5292.)
Fig. 278 Malignant teratoma in which tumor cells are poorly differentiated. (High power; WU neg. 49-588A.)

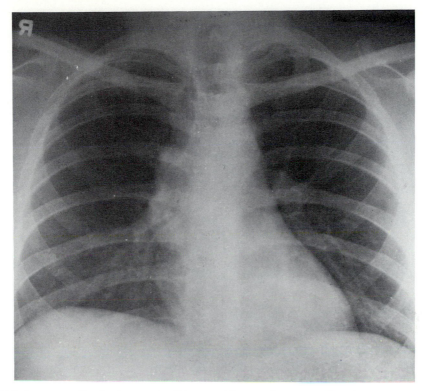

Fig. 279 Large mediastinal mass in 24-year-old man that proved to be seminoma. Patient was treated by irradiation and has survived over ten years. (WU neg. 66-770.)

tissues from skin, intestine (Fig. 276), bronchus, bone, cartilage, and nerve. Pancreatic tissue, strangely enough, is also quite frequent.[19]

Malignant teratomas make up only a small fraction (less than 5%) of all mediastinal teratomas. Although they grow more rapidly, some malignant teratomas cannot be distinguished from their benign counterparts at the time of roentgenographic or gross examination. In others, rapid infiltrative growth and local and distant metastases make their malignant nature evident.

Grossly, areas of hemorrhage and necrosis are present (Fig. 277). Microscopically, a malignant component (usually epidermoid or undifferentiated carcinoma) is seen in addition to mature foci similar to those seen in the benign counterpart (Fig. 278).

Primary *choriocarcinomas* of the mediastinum are rare.[20, 22] All but one of the fifteen reported cases have occurred in males. They are often associated with gynecomastia and positive pregnancy tests. The prognosis is extremely poor. Before accepting a diagnosis of primary mediastinal choriocarcinoma, the possibility of a metastasis from an occult testicular tumor should always be investigated. That choriocarcinoma can occur as a primary lesion in the mediastinum has been demonstrated rather convincingly by serially sectioning both testes and finding no abnormalities in them.[16] Some observers even believe that a small scar found in a testis may be evidence of a previously existing choriocarcinoma.[20]

Primary *seminoma (germinoma)* of the mediastinum also occurs and may be cured by irradiation therapy[17] (Figs. 279 and 289). The majority occur in young males and have a microscopic appearance identical to that of their testicular counterpart. Glycogen is almost always present in the

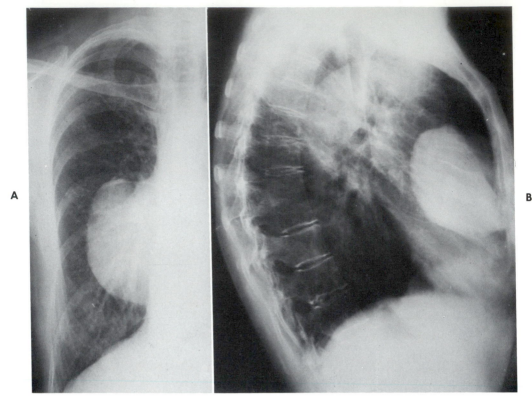

Fig. 280 Lobulated large benign thymoma located in anterior portion of mediastinum. (**A**, WU neg. 49-3479; **B**, WU neg. 49-3480.)

cytoplasm, a useful feature for their differentiation from malignant lymphomas.

Embryonal carcinoma and *endodermal sinus tumor* also have been reported as primary mediastinal neoplasms.[21] Both have an ominous prognosis. The microscopic appearance again is indistinguishable from that of the analogous gonadal neoplasms.

Thymic cysts and tumors

Thymic cysts, derived from a remnant of the third bronchial pouch, can occur in the neck or in the mediastinum.[25] The former can be seen anywhere along a line extending from the angle of the mandible to the manubrium sterni.[40] The only distinguishing feature is the presence of thymic tissue in the wall. The epithelial lining may be squamous or columnar. Degenerative changes are common, with prominent cholesterol granulomas. A large proportion of "nonspecific cysts" of the antero-

superior portion of the mediastinum are probably of thymic origin. Care should always be exercised in excluding the possibility of thymoma with cystic degeneration, a not uncommon occurrence.[27]

Thymolipomas are encapsulated benign neoplasms that can attain large size but nearly always remain asymptomatic. Microscopically, they are composed of an admixture of mature adipose tissue and normal thymic tissue.[46]

Thymoma is a generic term for the mysterious group of tumors made of thymic epithelial cells and almost always accompanied by a variable admixture of lymphocytes. The latter elements are probably nonneoplastic. The usual location is the anterosuperior portion of the mediastinum. However, they also can occur in other portions of the mediastinum or in the neck.[41] Radiographically, they produce a characteristic lobulated shadow (Fig. 280). Grossly,

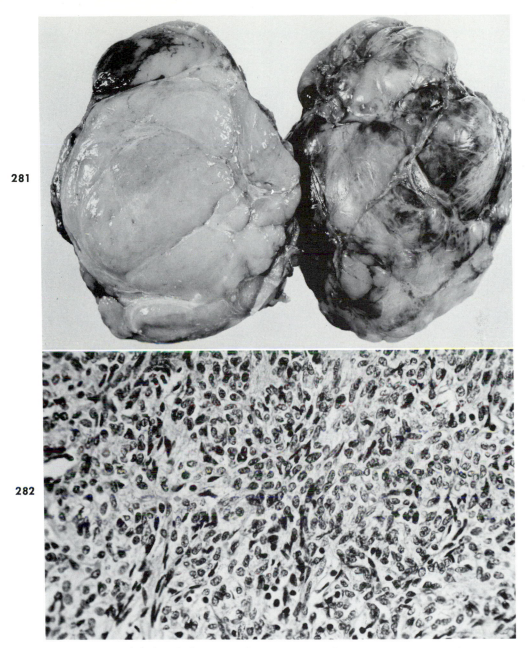

Fig. 281 Large lobulated thymoma showing encapsulation, no necrosis, and connective tissue trabeculae. (WU neg. 49-3096.)
Fig. 282 Same tumor illustrated in Fig. 281 showing spindle-shaped epithelial elements. These changes usually indicate that patient does not have myasthenia gravis. (×400; WU neg. 50-3949.)

they are often large, gray yellowish, and separated in lobules by connective tissue septa (Fig. 281). In approximately 80% of the cases, the tumor is well encapsulated and can be removed with ease. In the remaining 20%, infiltration of surrounding structures is noted at surgery.

Microscopically, the large majority of

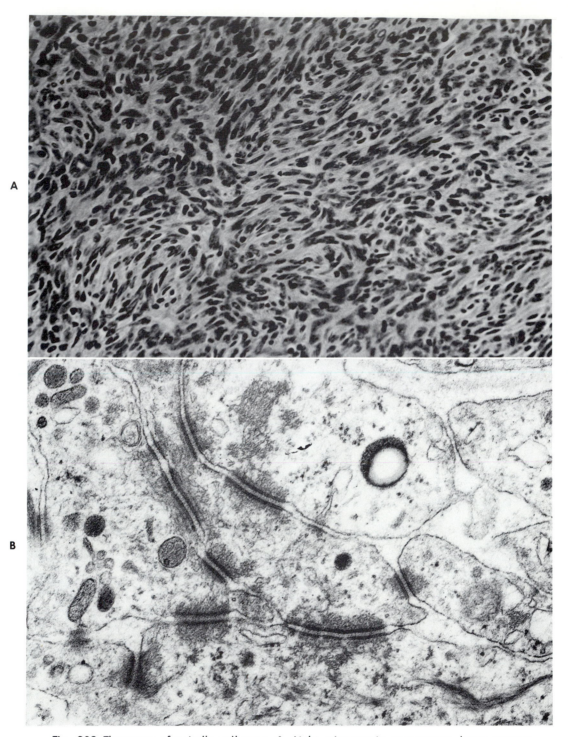

Fig. 283 Thymoma of spindle cell type. **A,** Light microscopic appearance. Large masses of spindle tumor cells alternate with collections of lymphocytes. **B,** Numerous desmosomes and tonofibrils in tumor cells indicate its epithelial origin. (**A,** ×350; WU neg. 72-11212; courtesy Dr. G. D. Levine, Stanford, Calif.; **B,** uranyl acetate–lead citrate; ×54,500; from Levine, G. D., and Bensch, K. G.: Epithelial nature of spindle-cell thymoma; an ultra-structural study, Cancer **30:**500-511, 1972.)

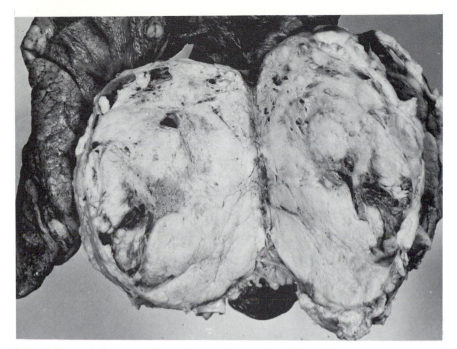

Fig. 284 Malignant thymoma found in anterior portion of mediastinum at autopsy. There was invasion of surrounding structures but no distant metastases. (WU neg. 51-4318.)

thymomas are composed of an admixture of lymphocytes and epithelial cells (Fig. 282). Predominantly lymphocytic thymomas can be confused with malignant lymphoma, whereas purely epithelial thymomas can simulate carcinoma or hemangiopericytoma. Features that we have found helpful in the diagnosis of thymoma include presence of two cell types; a thick fibrous (sometimes calcified) capsule; fibrous septa between tumor nodules; perivascular spaces occupied by proteinaceous fluid, lymphocytes, old blood cells, foamy cells, or fibrous tissue; foci of medullary differentiation; and pseudoglandular formations in the capsule and within the tumor. The epithelial tumor cells may have a round, oval, or spindle shape. Occasionally, they are arranged in whorls, but well-defined Hassall's corpuscles are rare. By electron microscopy, they exhibit tonofibrils and desmosomes, further proof of their epithelial derivation[36, 48] (Fig. 283).

The large majority of encapsulated thymomas are cured by surgical excision. On rare occasions, they may recur, either as a solitary mediastinal mass or as multiple small mediastinal and pleural implants.[29] The grossly infiltrative variety, which cannot be excised completely, often kills the patient by impinging upon vital structures (Fig. 284). This variety is designated malignant thymoma on the basis of the gross features, inasmuch as the microscopy hardly differs from that of the encapsulated type[34] (Fig. 285). It should be emphasized, however, that in some clinically aggressive thymomas the cytologic features are clearly those of a malignant neoplasm.[38] Distant metastases are exceptional, although unquestionable cases have been reported.[31]

Thymomas can be associated with a variety of syndromes, of which myasthenia gravis is the most important. In a series of 658 patients with myasthenia gravis seen at Massachusetts General Hospital, fifty-six (8.5%) had thymoma.[49] A few of the remainder had a microscopically normal thymus, whereas the large majority had thymic hyperplasia. The latter is defined as the presence of lymphoid follicles in the thymus and is independent of the size of the gland. Thymic hyperplasia also can

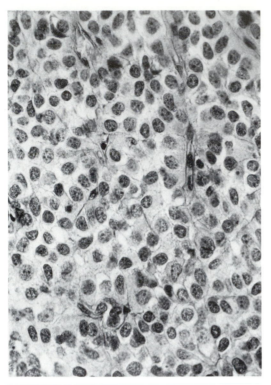

Fig. 285 Malignant thymoma. Tumor appears well differentiated, yet tumor implants and blood vessel invasion were present. (×200; WU neg. 52-112.)

be seen in hyperthyroidism, Addison's disease, lupus erythematosus, and other autoimmune diseases.[39] Rarely, myasthenia gravis develops months or years after the excision of a thymoma.[24] Thymomas associated with myasthenia gravis almost always have epithelial cells of plump shape (although the reverse is not necessarily true) (Fig. 286). The relative proportion of epithelial cells and lymphocytes is not important. The best way to predict the presence of myasthenia gravis is to find lymphoid follicles in the adjacent thymic tissue or, exceptionally, even in the thymoma itself.[23] In a large series reported by Wilkins et al.[49] the ten-year cumulative survival rate for patients with thymoma without myasthenia gravis was 67%, and in those with thymoma with myasthenia gravis, it was 32%. Most of the deaths in the latter group were due to myasthenic crisis. The ten-year survival rate for patients with encapsulated thymomas without myasthenia gravis approached 100%, and for those with invasive thymomas with myasthenia gravis, it was zero.

Thymomas also have been found associ-

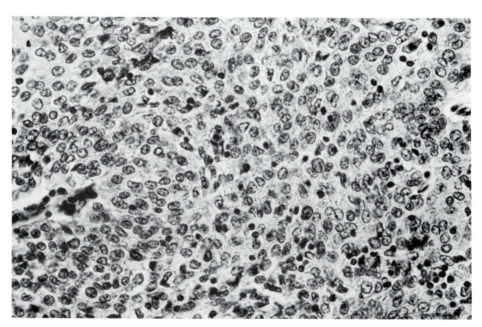

Fig. 286 Thymoma in patient with myasthenia gravis. Note plump appearance of epithelial cells. Approximately 8.5% of patients with myasthenia gravis have associated thymoma. (×400; WU neg. 52-3449.)

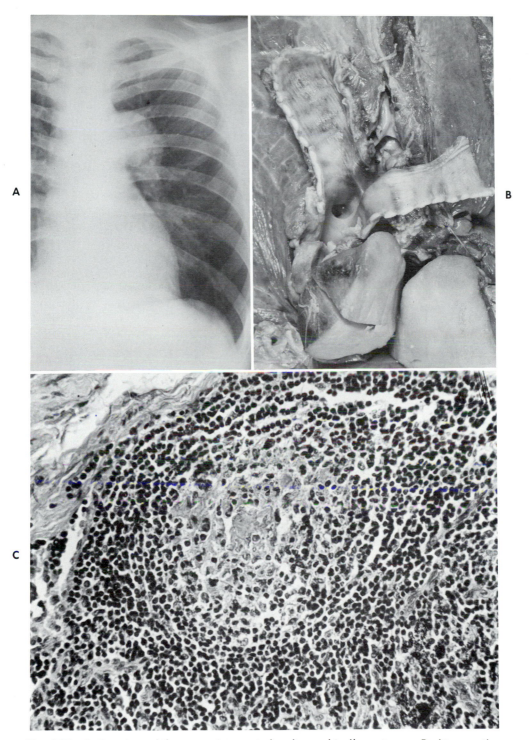

Fig. 287   A, Prominent hilar mass interpreted radiographically as tumor. **B,** At operation, firm mass intimately associated with bronchus was thought to represent neoplasm. **C,** Microscopically, mass proved to be hyperplastic fused lymph nodes with prominent hyalinized germinal centers. (**A,** WU neg. 56-3604; **B,** WU neg. 55-1278; **C,** ×600; WU neg. 58-127.)

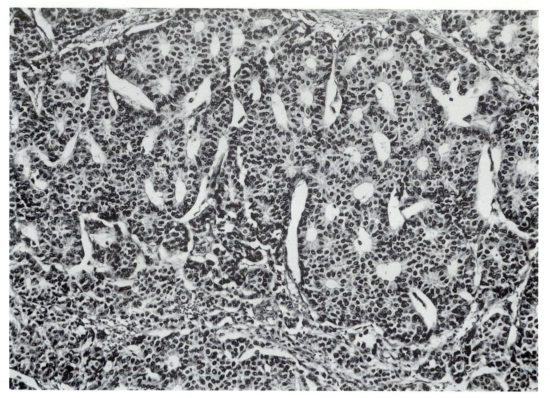

Fig. 288 Carcinoid tumor of thymus. Tumor cells of uniform appearance and predominantly solid pattern of growth form regularly distributed rosettes. (×150; WU neg. 73-7010; slide contributed by Dr. H. C. Taylor, St. Louis, Mo.)

ated with hypogammaglobulinemia (12% of the cases), erythroid hypoplasia (5%), and more rarely with myositis, myocarditis, dermatomyositis, lupus erythematosus, rheumatoid arthritis, scleroderma, Sjögren's disease, multiple myeloma, bullous dermatitis, hyperglobulinemic purpura, and an increased incidence of carcinoma.[30, 32, 45]

There are several tumors and tumorlike conditions often diagnosed as thymoma that we believe should be clearly separated from the latter. One is the condition designated by Castleman et al.[26] as *localized mediastinal lymph node hyperplasia*. It is made up of very large masses of lymph nodes, sometimes reaching 12 cm in diameter and 100 gm in weight. The germinal centers, which are prominent, hyalinized, and with thick-walled blood vessels, are often misinterpreted as Hassall's corpuscles (Fig. 287). Similar lesions have been found in the neck, axilla, and retroperitoneum.[47]

We believe they represent hyperplasia of lymph nodes rather than hamartomas of lymphoid tissue.

We have seen many examples of the so-called *granulomatous thymoma*.[37] We believe they represent Hodgkin's disease of the nodular sclerosing type involving the thymus gland and eliciting a peculiar response of the thymic epithelium.[28, 33]

We have collected eleven examples of a mediastinal endocrine tumor with features akin to those of carcinoid tumors[42] (Fig. 288). Three of the patients had, in addition, the typical manifestations of the multiple endocrine adenoma syndrome.[43] We believe these tumors arise not from thymic lymphocytic or epithelial elements but from enterochromaffin cells, which are probably located within the thymus gland itself. It is likely that the reported cases of thymoma associated with Cushing's syndrome belong to the same category.[44]

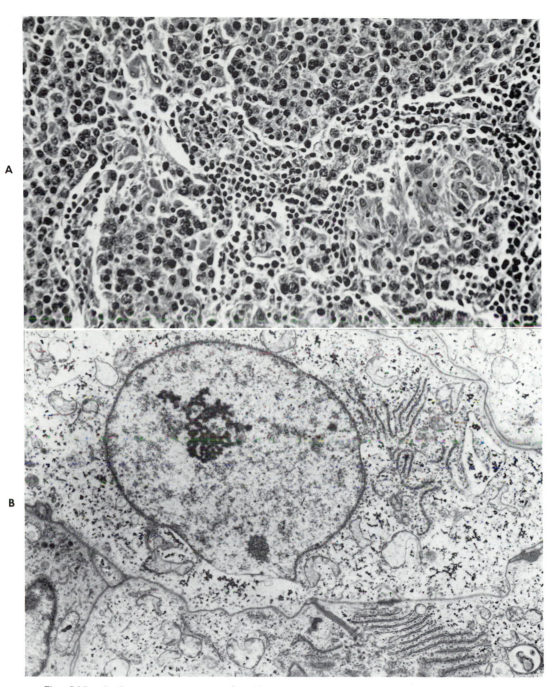

Fig. 289 **A,** Primary seminoma of mediastinum arising within thymic gland. Collections of large undifferentiated cells are separated by fibrous strands containing numerous lymphocytes and epithelioid cell granulomas. **B,** Ultrastructural appearance of tumor cells. Similarity to testicular seminoma is striking (compare with Fig. 712). (**A,** ×350; WU neg. 72-6552; courtesy Dr. G. D. Levine, Stanford, Calif.; **B,** uranyl acetate–lead citrate; ×8,800; from Levine, G. D.: Primary thymic seminoma—a neoplasm ultrastructurally similar to testicular seminoma and distinct from epithelial thymoma, Cancer **31:**729-741, 1973.)

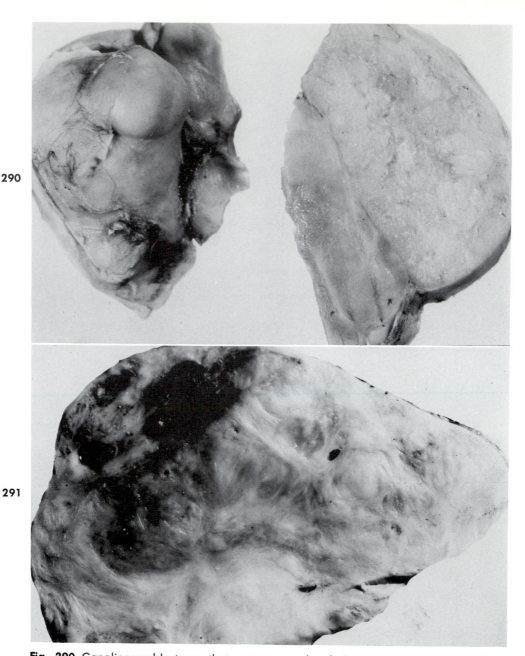

Fig. 290 Ganglioneuroblastoma that was encapsulated. Patient has remained well for over decade. (WU neg. 49-7106; from Ackerman, L. V., and Taylor, F. H.: Neurogenous tumors within the thorax; a clinical pathologic evaluation of forty-eight cases, Cancer **4:** 669-691, 1951.)

Fig. 291 Large ganglioneuroma removed from posterior portion of mediastinum. (From Ackerman, L. V., and Taylor, F. H.: Neurogenous tumors within the thorax; a clinical pathologic evaluation of forty-eight cases, Cancer **4:**669-691, 1951.)

Seminomas of the thymus should also be separated from bonafide thymomas, although on occasion the microscopic dif-ferentiation may be difficult. They represent primary mediastinal germinal tumors rather than thymic neoplasms[35] (Fig. 289).

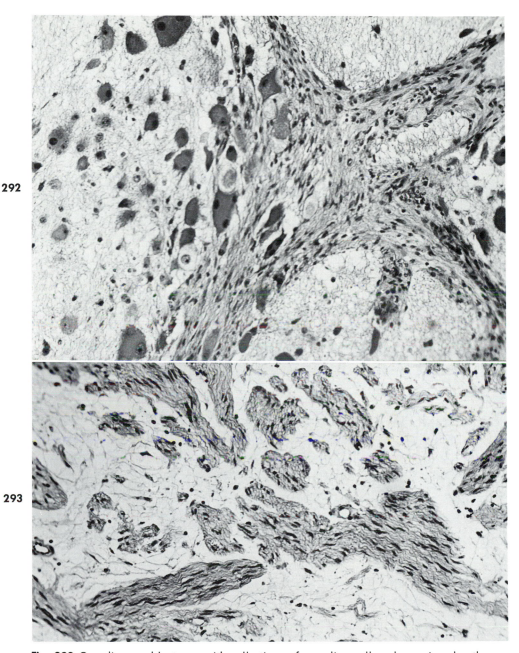

Fig. 292 Ganglioneuroblastoma with collections of ganglion cells, schwannian sheath proliferation, and cobwebby material. (×200; WU neg. 50-554; from Ackerman, L. V., and
Taylor, F. H.: Neurogenous tumors within the thorax; a clinical pathologic evaluation of
forty-eight cases, Cancer **4**:669-691, 1951.)
Fig. 293 Another area in same tumor illustrated in Fig. 292 showing prominent schwannian sheath proliferation. (×200; WU neg. 50-553; from Ackerman, L. V., and Taylor, F.
H.: Neurogenous tumors within the thorax; a clinical pathologic evaluation of forty-eight
cases, Cancer **4**:669-691, 1951.)

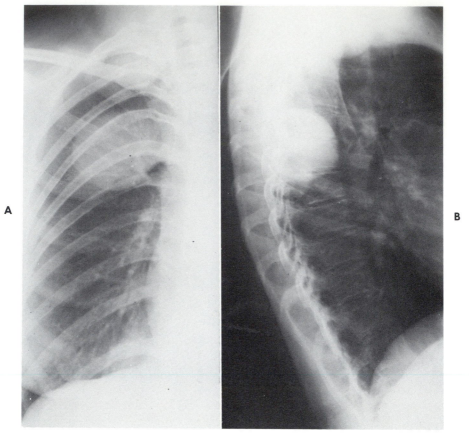

Fig. 294 Sharply delimited neurilemoma occurring in posterior portion of mediastinum. (**A**, WU neg. 48-5735; **B**, WU neg. 48-5734.)

We also have seen several instances of metastatic oat cell carcinoma of the lung and mediastinal malignant lymphoma mistakenly interpreted as thymomas.

Neurogenic tumors

The neurogenic tumors of the mediastinum can be classified as follows:

A Tumors of sympathetic nervous system
   1 Neuroblastoma
   2 Ganglioneuroblastoma
   3 Ganglioneuroma
B Tumors of nerve sheath origin
   1 Neurilemoma (including "ancient neurilemoma")
   2 Neurofibroma
   3 Malignant schwannoma (neurofibrosarcoma)
C Tumors of paraganglia

Tumors of sympathetic nervous system

The tumors of the sympathetic nervous system show variable cellular differentia-
tion. A sharp division into the different types cannot be made because one type often blends into another. Different degrees of differentiation may occur in the same tumor. It is, therefore, important to make multiple sections of these tumors.

Neuroblastoma occurs with higher frequency in children.[51] It appears high in the mediastinum, is usually unencapsulated, and infiltrates surrounding tissue. Microscopically, the tumor cells are slightly larger than lymphocytes, stain deeply, and may show rosette formation and small focal areas of calcification (Chapter 15).

Ganglioneuroblastoma shows an intermediate degree of differentiation. Grossly, encapsulation takes place and the tumor acquires a lobulated appearance (Fig. 290). Areas of calcification possibly secondary to regressive changes are common. Microscopically, the tumor cells are larger than

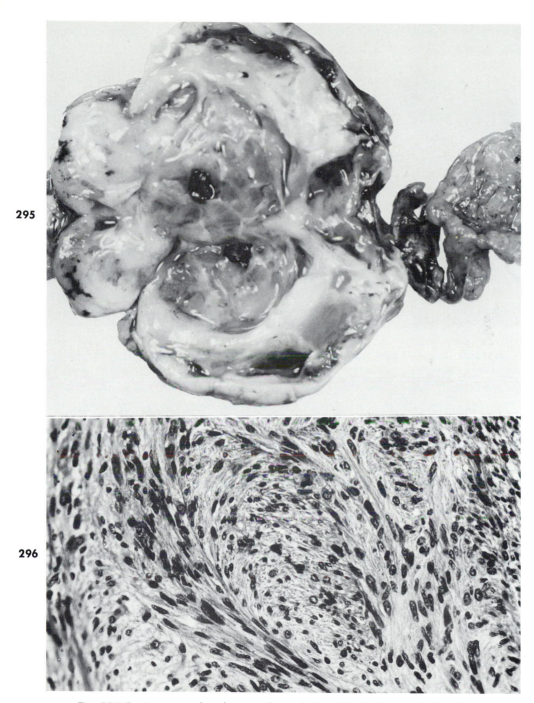

Fig. 295 Cystic encapsulated tumor shown in Fig. 294. (WU neg. 48-5199.)
Fig. 296 Cellular area in neurilemoma with palisading. (×350; WU neg. 49-248.)

those of ganglioneuroma, the nuclei do not stain so heavily, and a cytoplasmic cobweblike material appears that represents the formation of dendritelike specializations by the tumor cells. The presence of this

material between tumor cells is an important diagnostic sign.

Ganglioneuroma occurs in older persons and is the most common of the three tumors. Grossly, it forms a smooth, well-

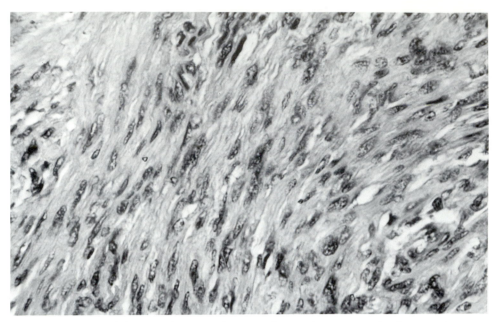

Fig. 297 Highly cellular neurilemoma that was benign but incorrectly diagnosed as malignant because of cellularity. (×600; WU neg. 50-1594; from Ackerman, L. V., and Taylor, F. H.: Neurogenous tumors within the thorax; a clinical pathologic evaluation of forty-eight cases, Cancer **4:**669-691, 1951.)

encapsulated mass, usually in the posterior mediastinum, and on section is often fibrous and yellowish gray (Fig. 291). It may contain cystic areas and fatty degeneration. Necrosis is infrequent. Microscopically, islands of ganglion cells, often twenty or thirty at a time, are observed (Fig. 292). These ganglion cells may have several nuclei. Often associated with these cells are large masses of nonmyelinated sheaths, which are more numerous than might be expected from the number of ganglion cells present[57] (Fig. 293). Focal collections of lymphocytes are often present. They should not be confused with the immature cells of ganglioneuroblastomas.[56]

The survival rate in patients with tumors of the sympathetic nervous system is directly related to the differentiation of the tumor. Adequate excision effects cure in all patients with ganglioneuromas. The prognosis in patients with ganglioneuroblastomas that contain both elements is somewhat unpredictable, but cure is not rare. Even patients with neuroblastoma with liver metastases can be cured. In our series of thirty-six children with tumors of the sympathetic nervous system, a crude survival rate of 50% for five years was obtained. Mediastinal neuroblastoma in two patients and adrenal neuroblastoma in one patient showed histologic evidence of maturation to a ganglioneuroma several years after radiation therapy.[55]

Tumors of the sympathetic nervous system can be multiple and can occur in different locations with different degrees of differentiation.[59]

Tumors of nerve sheath origin

Stout[58] divided the tumors of nerve sheath origin into two distinct types: neurofibroma and neurilemoma.

Neurofibroma is nonencapsulated, having a tangled network showing schwannian sheath proliferation. Special stains show large numbers of neurites. Mast cells are often present in large numbers. This type of tumor may undergo malignant change.[53]

Neurilemoma, on the other hand, is encapsulated and is made up of Antoni type

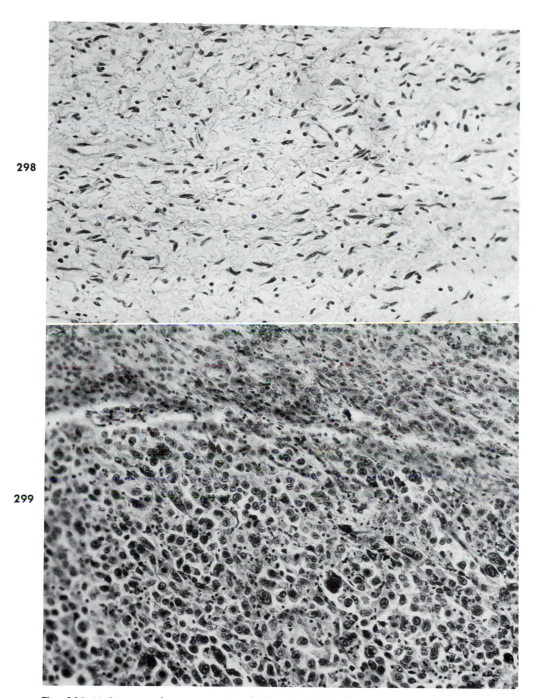

Fig. 298 Malignant schwannoma in which individual cells are quite uniform. From such single microscopic field, it would be difficult, if not impossible, to tell that tumor was malignant. (×200; WU neg. 50-549; from Ackerman, L. V., and Taylor, F. H.: Neurogenous tumors within the thorax; a clinical pathologic evaluation of forty-eight cases, Cancer **4:** 669-691, 1951.)

Fig. 299 Same tumor shown in Fig. 298 at later time period showing highly undifferentiated area with numerous tumor giant cells. (×200; WU neg. 50-5511.)

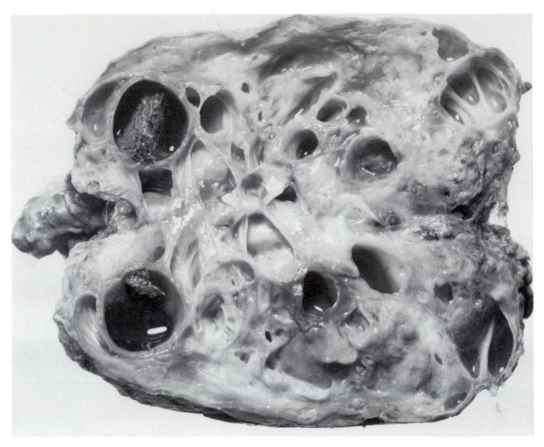

Fig. 300 Large cystic hygroma (17 cm × 15 cm × 7 cm) in neck of 18-month-old male infant extending into superior portion of mediastinum. (WU neg. 61-1668.)

A and type B tissue. Antoni type A tissue is composed of bands of cells with their nuclei arranged in parallel order. Antoni type B tissue is made up of cystic spaces containing gelatinous-like material. Collections of foamy macrophages are often seen. Neurites are seen only in the compressed capsule. This tumor is nonmalignant. Apparently the worst it ever does is to recur locally.

The sharp differentiation described by Stout[58] may not be apparent in tumors of nerve sheath origin in the posterior portion of the mediastinum (Fig. 294). In fact, practically all tumors of nerve sheath origin in this region are encapsulated tumors. These tumors grow rather slowly and are often discovered on routine roentgenographic examination. Regressive change within them, such as fatty degeneration, hemorrhage, and cystic formation, is common (Figs. 295 and 296).

We have seen several neurilemomas that were completely cystic. Such regressive changes with overgrowth of fibrous tissue make recognition difficult. We have designated them as *ancient neurilemomas*.[50] Other neurilemomas can be very cellular and be confused with sarcoma (Fig. 297). A point to remember is that despite their marked cellularity, they have practically no mitotic activity.

In our series, four patients had ***malignant schwannomas*** apparently arising from preexisting neurofibromas. Three of these patients had florid Recklinghausen's disease.[50] When these tumors become malignant, the change may be hardly perceptible microscopically, the only suggestion being some slight increase in cellularity.

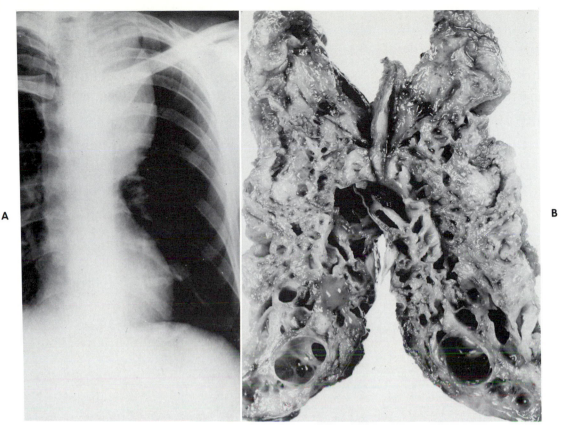

Fig. 301   A, Lymphangioma of anterior portion of mediastinum. **B,** Lymphangioma demonstrating large, cystic, smooth-walled spaces. (**A,** WU neg. 49-5186; **B,** WU neg. 49-5163.)

With outspoken malignant change, the tumor cells individually may become bizarre, and it then may be impossible to recognize the malignant tumor as originating from a preexisting neurofibroma (Figs. 298 and 299). In these instances, the presence of Recklinghausen's disease, previous biopsy, or the presence of other neurofibromas may suggest the diagnosis.

The prognosis in patients with tumors of nerve sheath origin is excellent with the exception of those with malignant schwannomas. We had ten patients with neurilemomas, eleven with ancient neurilemomas, and ten with neurofibromas. Twenty-eight of these patients are still living and well without evidence of disease. Of four patients with malignant schwannoma, three are dead, and the other is living without evidence of tumor.

Tumors of paraganglia

Most mediastinal paragangliomas occur in association with the aortic chemoreceptor bodies and therefore occur in the anterosuperior mediastinum close to the base of the heart.[54] Their histologic appearance is identical to that of carotid body tumors. They are almost always nonfunctioning and benign.

Functioning paragangliomas, often referred to as extra-adrenal pheochromocytomas, rarely occur in the mediastinum. The large majority are benign.[52]

Malignant lymphoma

Malignant lymphoma can present as an anterior, superior, or middle mediastinal mass, in this order of frequency.[61] It represents the most common neoplasm of the middle portion of the mediastinum. It may

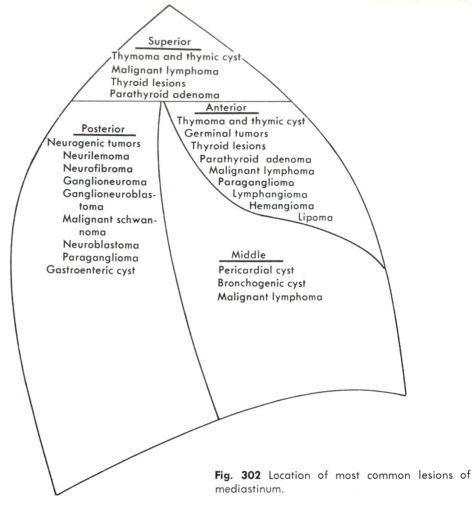

Fig. 302 Location of most common lesions of mediastinum.

appear in this area as a manifestation of a disseminated process, or it may present as a primary mediastinal disease. Van Heerden et al.[61] collected ninety-seven examples of the latter. Fifty-seven patients had Hodgkin's disease, and 61.3% of these survived five years. The majority were of the nodular sclerosing type.[60] Forty patients had lymphocytic and/or histiocytic lymphomas, and only 15% of these survived five years. The diagnosis of mediastinal malignant lymphoma may be suggested by the radiographic appearance, but it cannot be made with certainty without exploratory thoracotomy. Radiation therapy is the treatment of choice. However, there is some evidence suggesting that in nodular sclerosing Hodgkin's disease, in which the

lesion is often sharply circumscribed, a combination of surgery and radiation therapy is the most effective therapy.[60, 61]

We have encountered a plasma cell granuloma in the mediastinum associated with amyloid formation and secondarily involving the lung parenchyma.

Mesenchymal tumors

Lipomas and **lymphangiomas** are the two most common benign mesenchymal neoplasms of the mediastinum (Figs. 300 and 301). The lipomas are often very large, are located just above the diaphragm, and can extend into both sides of the pleural cavity, making complete removal difficult.[62, 63]

Hemangiomas,   hemangiopericytomas,

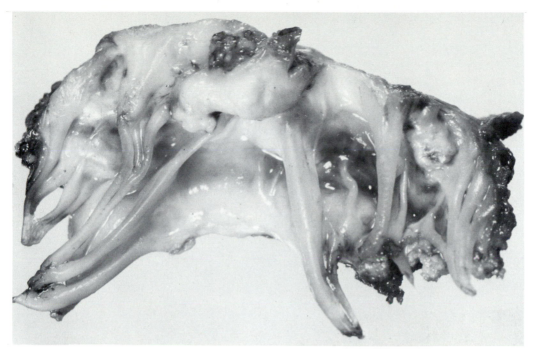

Fig. 303 Surgical specimen of mitral valve distorted by rheumatic heart disease in 40-year-old man who had disease for over ten years. Valve was resected and replaced by prosthesis. Unfortunately, it failed. (WU neg. 62-1352.)

leiomyomas, and *benign mesenchymomas* also occur.[64] Svane et al.[65] collected thirty-two cases of cavernous hemangioma and indicated that even when the tumors were incompletely removed, usually no further trouble resulted. Microscopically, these tumors consist of thin spaces separated by fine septa lined by endothelium. Smooth muscle, lymphoid tissue, and cholesterol crystals may be present.

Among the malignant mesenchymal tumors, *liposarcomas* and *fibrosarcomas* predominate. We have seen mediastinal liposarcoma occurring in conjunction with liposarcoma of the thigh. We also have seen a few *embryonal rhabdomyosarcomas* of the superior portion of the mediastinum in children in close proximity to the thymus gland.

Metastatic tumors

Metastatic malignant tumors are cited only because of their clinical similarity to primary malignant mediastinal tumors. Confusion occurs most often when there are metastases to the mediastinum from bronchogenic carcinoma. However, many other types of malignant tumors can metastasize to the mediastinum and simulate a primary tumor of this area.

We have seen inconspicuous primary carcinomas of the breast and esophagus produce secondary voluminous metastatic masses that mimic a primary mediastinal tumor. Testicular tumors are particularly prone to develop mediastinal metastatic masses. Carcinoma of the lung and various types of lymphomas are the most common cause of superior vena cava syndrome.

Clinicopathologic correlation

It is apparent from this short résumé of the more common lesions that the mediastinum is a veritable Pandora's box. Congenital remnants, benign tumors, and primary and metastatic neoplasms occur in it.

The location of lesions in the mediastinum (Fig. 302), together with their configuration, may give some hint as to the correct diagnosis, but many, both benign and malignant, give similar radiographic shadows. Exploration is mandatory for all of them. Its risk is practically zero.

Cure is effected by excision of the congenital cysts and benign neoplasms. A few patients with malignant tumors may be cured by resection of the tumor.

Heart and aorta

The heart and aorta used to be considered outside the province of the surgeon, but during the past twenty-five years ad-

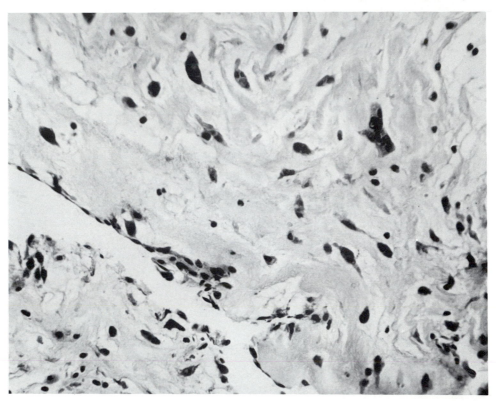

Fig. 304 Patient (33-year-old woman), who was thought to have rheumatic heart disease, developed signs of embolism to one of large arteries of leg. Artery was opened and peculiar jellylike clot found. It was thought by surgeon to be extremely atypical. Microscopically, it showed cells with bizarre nuclei against mucoid background. This pattern was thought to be typical of myxoma, and it was predicted that patient had myxoma of left side of heart. Appropriate studies were made, and thoracic surgeon removed myxoma found in left atrium. Patient had uneventful postoperative recovery. She did not have rheumatic heart disease. (×275; WU neg. 62-7388.)

Fig. 305 A, Patient, 28-year-old man, complained of dyspnea on exertion. Roentgenogram of chest revealed multiple small nodular densities in both lung fields. Open lung biopsy revealed tumor emboli filling branches of pumonary artery. **Inset,** Thin rows of small regular tumor cells can be seen in abundant myxoid matrix. Pathologic diagnosis was "metastatic carcinoma, primary site undetermined." **B,** Nature of disease became obvious only nine years later, when large cardiac myxoma was removed from right atrium. Pulmonary nodules obviously represent emboli from tumor. **Inset,** Tumor cells, although larger and slightly more atypical, have same configuration and stromal background as those in lungs. (**A,** ×30; WU neg. 73-1360; **inset,** ×350; WU neg. 73-1358; **B,** ×40; WU neg. 73-1359; **inset,** ×350; WU neg. 73-1359; **A, B,** and **insets,** courtesy Dr. Y. LeGal, Strasbourg, France.)

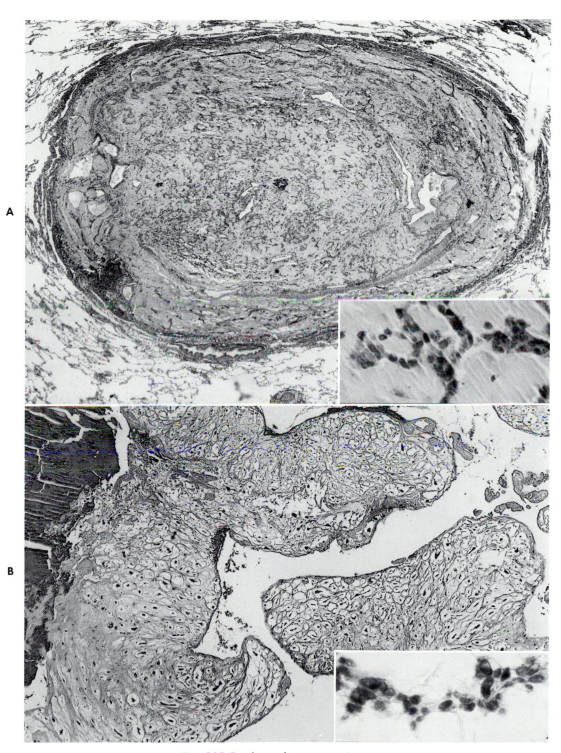

Fig. 305 For legend, see opposite page.

vances in thoracic surgery have followed better understanding of the physiology of the heart and refinement of new procedures in diagnosis and treatment (cardiac catheterization, angiocardiography, hypothermia, and extracorporeal circulation). Entire books have been written about congenital heart disease.[75] Most operations for congenital cardiovascular malformations are directed toward improvement in the flow of oxygenated blood by such procedures as ligation or division of a patent ductus or the Blalock operation, the closure of interatrial and interventricular septal defects. Methods have been devised to relieve pulmonary, aortic, and mitral valvular stenosis. In these procedures, the surgical pathologist rarely receives tissue. If the operation fails, the cause of failure becomes the concern of the general pathologist. Therefore, the various cardiac abnormalities and their methods of treatment will not be presented in detail.

Cardiac valves

Operations to correct major defects of the valves by resection and prosthetic replacement are being successfully performed (Fig. 303). Roberts and Morrow[79] emphasize that the most precise diagnosis will be made from the gross appearance of the valve and that usually the microscopic examination is of little help. Photographic and radiographic examination of the specimen is also well indicated. Careful examination of the gross specimen with knowledge of the clinical history often allows a distinction between a rheumatic or a congenital origin for a chronic valvulopathy to be made. Microscopically, both show fibrosis, calcification, and occasional inflammatory cells. Distinct mucinous changes were seen in twenty-one of 140 cardiac valves examined by Frable.[69] These were found to be nonspecific, inasmuch as seven of the patients suffered from congenital heart disease, four from rheumatic heart disease, and three from subacute bacterial endocarditis. In seven cases, all occurring in the aorta of adults, no specific etiology

could be ascertained. These were considered examples of the "floppy valve syndrome,"[77] although the existence of such an entity is still debated.

Left atrium in mitral stenosis

Mitral valvulotomy for patients with mitral stenosis may be accompanied by biopsy of the atrial appendage. These appendages are always abnormal, showing hypertrophy of the muscle and various other alterations. About one-half of them show actual Aschoff nodules.[66] We have not been able to correlate the presence of

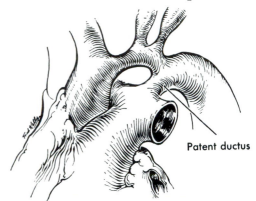

Fig. 306 Infantile (diffuse) type of coarctation of aorta. (From Burford, T. H.: Symposium on clinical surgery; coarctation of aorta and its treatment, Surg. Clin. North Am. **30:**1249-1258, 1950.)

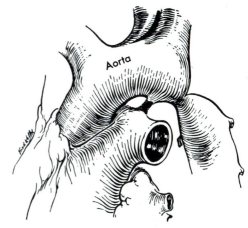

Fig. 307 Adult (localized) type of coarctation of aorta. (From Burford, T. H.: Symposium on clinical surgery; coarctation of aorta and its treatment, Surg. Clin. North Am. **30:**1249-1258, 1950.)

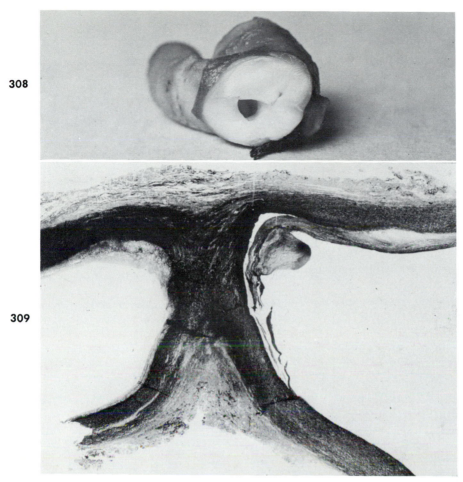

308

309

Fig. 308 Coarctation of aorta, adult type, showing greatly narrowed lumen. (WU neg. 48-5295.)
Fig. 309 Coarctation of aorta at point of constriction showing subintimal thickening and medial distortion. (Low power; WU neg. 48-6704.)

these nodules with the postoperative course nor with clinical evidence of activity of the rheumatic process.

Cardiac tumors

Myxomas constitute approximately 50% of primary tumors of the heart. The large majority are located in the left atrium.[70] They may present with signs of mitral stenosis, or insufficiency, multiple emboli (Figs. 304 and 305), or with symptoms secondary to hypergammaglobulinemia.[74, 81] Grossly, they are soft polypoid masses often attached by a stalk to the septum near the foramen ovale. Microscopically, round or polygonal cells are seen surrounded by abundant loose stroma rich in acid mucopolysaccharides.[68] Surgical excision is often curative.

Other primary heart tumors, all extremely rare, include several types of sarcomas, hemangiomas, and so-called rhabdomyomas.[76] Involvement of the heart by metastatic carcinoma or by malignant lymphoma is a commoner event but rarely seen as a surgical specimen.[72, 80]

Coarctation of aorta

Coarctation of the aorta is usually divided into infantile and adult types, but it is probably better to call them diffuse or localized[73] (Figs. 306 and 307).

In the diffuse type, the coarctated segment lies proximal to the ductus arteriosus. This type was incompatible with life, but Gross and Hufnagel[71] used homografts to repair the defect. In the localized type, the short, narrowed segment of the aorta is at the level of the aortic insertion of the ductus or just distal to it. If resection is not done, about 60% of the patients die before 40 years of age[78] of aortic rupture, endocarditis, hypertension, or congestive failure (Fig. 308).

Grossly, the vessel is narrowed at the point of insertion of the ligamentum arteriosum. On opening the aorta, a diaphragm-like structure lies across the lumen, through which there is an aperture usually 1 mm or less in diameter.[67] Often there is localized subintimal thickening, and beneath this the media is distorted and thickened (Fig. 309).

Operations for coarctation of the aorta are often difficult in older patients because of advanced arteriosclerotic changes in the aorta.

REFERENCES

Introduction

1 Blades, B.: Mediastinal tumors; report of cases treated at army thoracic surgery centers in the United States, Ann. Surg. **123**:749-765, 1946.
2 Oldham, H. N., Jr., and Sabiston, D. C., Jr.: Primary tumors and cysts of the mediastinum, Monogr. Surg. Sci. **4**:243-279, 1967.
3 Ringertz, N., and Lidholm, S. O.: Mediastinal tumors and cysts, J. Thorac. Surg. **31**:458-487, 1956.

Nonneoplastic cysts

4 Abell, M. R.: Mediastinal cysts, Arch. Pathol. **61**:360-379, 1956.
5 Chitale, A. R.: Gastric cyst of the mediastinum; a distinct clinicopathological entity, J. Pediatr. **75**:104-110, 1969.
6 Eraklis, A. J., Griscom, N. T., and McGovern, J. B.: Bronchogenic cysts of the mediastinum in infancy, N. Engl. J. Med. **281**:1150-1155, 1969.
7 Laipply, T. C.: Cysts and cystic tumors of the mediastinum, Arch. Pathol. **39**:153-161, 1945 (extensive bibliography).
8 Lambert, A. V. S.: Etiology of thin-walled thoracic cysts, J. Thorac. Surg. **10**:1-7, 1940.

9 Lillie, W. I., McDonald, J. R., and Clagett, O. T.: Pericardial celomic cysts and pericardial diverticula; a concept of etiology and report of cases, J. Thorac. Surg. **20**:494-504, 1950.
10 Maier, H. C.: Bronchiogenic cysts of the mediastinum, Ann. Surg. **127**:476-502, 1948.

Inflammatory diseases

11 Kunkel, W. M., Jr., Clagett, O. T., and McDonald, J. R.: Mediastinal granulomas, J. Thorac. Surg. **27**:565-574, 1954.
12 Mitchinson, M. J.: The pathology of idiopathic retroperitoneal fibrosis, J. Clin. Pathol. **23**:681-689, 1970.
13 Payne, W. S., and Larson, R. H.: Acute mediastinitis, Surg. Clin. North Am. **49**:999-1009, 1969.
14 Salyer, J. M., Harrison, H. N., Winn, D. F., Jr., and Taylor, R. R.: Chronic fibrous mediastinitis and superior vena caval obstruction due to histoplasmosis, Dis. Chest. **35**:364-377, 1959.
15 Schowengerdt, C. G., Suyemoto, R., and Main, F. B.: Granulomatous and fibrous mediastinitis; a review and analysis of 180 cases, J. Thorac. Cardiovasc. Surg. **57**:365-379, 1969.

Tumors
Germinal tumors

16 Laipply, T. C., and Shipley, R. A.: Extragenital choriocarcinoma in the male, Am. J. Pathol. **21**:921-933, 1945.
17 Oberman, H. A., and Libcke, J. H.: Malignant germinal neoplasms of the mediastinum, Cancer **17**:498-507, 1964.
18 Rusby, N. L.: Dermoid cysts and teratomata of the mediastinum; a review, J. Thorac. Surg. **13**:169-222, 1944.
19 Schlumberger, H. G.: Teratoma of the anterior mediastinum in the group of military age; a study of sixteen cases, and a review of theories of genesis, Arch. Pathol. **41**:398-444, 1946.
20 Symeonidis, A.: Zur Frage der extragenitalen teratogenen Chorionepitheliome und der chorionepitheliomähnlichen Geschwülste, Zentralbl. Allg. Pathol. **62**:177-186, 1935.
21 Teilmann, I., Kassis, H., and Pietra, G.: Primary germ cell tumor of the anterior mediastinum with features of endodermal sinus tumor (mesoblastoma vitellinum), Acta Pathol. Microbiol. Scand. **70**:267-278, 1967.
22 Wenger, M. E., Dines, D. E., Ahmann, D. L., and Good, C. A.: Primary mediastinal choriocarcinoma, Mayo Clin. Proc. **43**:570-575, 1968.

Thymic cysts and tumors

23 Alpert, L. I., Papatestas, A., Kark, A., Osserman, R. S., and Osserman, K.: A histologic reappraisal of the thymus in myasthenia gravis; a correlative study of thymic pathology and

response to thymectomy, Arch. Pathol. **91:** 55-61, 1971.

24 Azer, M. S., Zikria, E., and Ford, W. B.: Myasthenia gravis appearing after removal of a thymoma; report of a case and review of the literature, Am. Surg. 37:109-113, 1971.

25 Bleger, R. C., and McAdams, A. J.: Thymic cysts, Arch. Pathol. 82:535-541, 1966.

26 Castleman, B., Iverson, L., and Menendez, V. P.: Localized mediastinal lymph-node hyperplasia resembling thymoma, Cancer 9:822-830, 1956.

27 Dyer, N. H.: Cystic thymomas and thymic cysts; a review, Thorax 22:408-421, 1967.

28 Fechner, R. E.: Hodgkin's disease of the thymus, Cancer 23:16-23, 1969.

29 Fechner, R. E.: Recurrence of noninvasive thymomas; report of four cases and review of the literature, Cancer 23:1423-1427, 1969.

30 Goldstein, G., and Mackay, I. R.: The human thymus, St. Louis, 1969, Warren H. Green, Inc. (extensive bibliography).

31 Guillan, R. A., Zelman, S., Smalley, R. L., and Iglesias, P. A.: Malignant thymoma associated with myasthenia gravis, and evidence of extrathoracic metastases; an analysis of published cases and report of a case, Cancer 27: 823-830, 1971.

32 Hirst, E., and Robertson, T. I.: The syndrome of thymoma and erythroblastopenic anemia; a review of 56 cases including 3 case reports, Medicine (Baltimore) 46:225-264, 1967.

33 Katz, A., and Lattes, R.: Granulomatous thymoma or Hodgkin's disease of thymus? A clinical and histologic study and a re-evaluation, Cancer 23:1-15, 1969.

34 Lattes, R.: Thymoma and other tumors of the thymus; an analysis of 107 cases, Cancer 15: 1224-1260, 1962.

35 Levine, G. D.: Primary thymic seminoma—a neoplasm ultrastructurally similar to testicular seminoma and distinct from epithelial thymoma, Cancer 31:729-741, 1973.

36 Levine, G. D., and Bensch, K. G.: Epithelial nature of spindle-cell thymoma; an ultrastructural study, Cancer 30:500-511, 1972.

37 Lowenhaupt, E., and Brown, R.: Carcinoma of the thymus of granulomatous type, Cancer 4:1193-1209, 1951.

38 Minkowitz, S., Solomon, L., and Nicastri, A. D.: Cytologically malignant thymoma with distant metastasis, Cancer 21:426-433, 1968.

39 Okabe, H.: Thymic lymph follicles; a histopathological study of 1,356 autopsy cases, Acta Pathol. Jap. 16:109-130, 1966.

40 Ratnesar, P.: Unilateral cervical thymic cyst, J. Laryngol. Otol. 85:293-298, 1971.

41 Ridenhour, C. E., Henzel, J. H., DeWeese, M. S., and Kerr, S. E.: Thymoma arising from undescended cervical thymus, Surgery 67: 614-619, 1970.

42 Rosai, J., and Higa, E.: Mediastinal endocrine neoplasm, of probable thymic origin, related to carcinoid tumor; clinicopathologic study of 8 cases, Cancer 29:1061-1074, 1972.

43 Rosai, J., Higa, E., and Davie, J. M.: Mediastinal endocrine neoplasm in patients with multiple endocrine adenomatosis; a previously unrecognized association, Cancer 29:1075-1083, 1972.

44 Scholz, D. A., and Bahn, R. C.: Thymic tumors associated with Cushing's syndrome; review of 3 cases, Mayo Clin. Proc. 34:433-441, 1959.

45 Souadjian, J. V., Silverstein, M. N., and Titus, J. L.: Thymoma and cancer, Cancer 22:1221-1225, 1968.

46 Trites, A. E. W.: Thyrolipoma, thymolipoma and pharyngeal lipoma; a syndrome, Can. Med. Assoc. J. 95:1254-1259, 1966.

47 Tung, K. S. K., and McCormack, L. J.: Angiomatous lymphoid hamartoma, Cancer 20: 525-536, 1967.

48 Watanabe, H.: A pathological study of thymomas, Acta. Pathol. Jap. 16:323-358, 1966.

49 Wilkins, E. W., Jr., Edmunds, L. H., Jr., and Castleman, B.: Cases of thymoma at the Massachusetts General Hospital, J. Thorac. Cardiovasc. Surg. 52:322-330, 1966.

Neurogenic tumors

50 Ackerman, L. V., and Taylor, F. H.: Neurogenous tumors within the thorax; a clinical pathologic evaluation of forty-eight cases, Cancer 4:669-691, 1951. (Extensive bibliography.)

51 Blacklock, J. W. S.: Neurogenic tumors of the sympathetic system in children, J. Pathol. Bacteriol. 39:27-48, 1934.

52 Edmunds, L. H.: Mediastinal pheochromocytoma, Ann. Thorac. Surg. 2:742-751, 1966.

53 Oberman, H. A., and Abell, M. R.: Neurogenous neoplasms of the mediastinum, Cancer 13:882-898, 1960.

54 Pachter, M. R.: Mediastinal nonchromaffin paraganglioma; a clinicopathological study based on eight cases, J. Thorac. Cardiovasc. Surg. 45: 152-160, 1963.

55 Perez, C. A., Vietti, T., Ackerman, L. V., Eagleton, M. D., and Powers, W. E.: Tumors of the sympathetic nervous system in children; an appraisal of treatment and results, Radiology 88:750-760, 1967.

56 Schweisguth, O., Mathey, J., Renault, P., and Binet, J. P.: Intrathoracic neurogenic tumors in infants and children; a study of forty cases, Am. Surg. 150:29-41, 1959.

57 Stout, A. P.: Ganglioneuroma of the sympathetic nervous system, Surg. Gynecol. Obstet. 84:101-110, 1947.

58 Stout, A. P.: Tumors of the peripheral nervous system. In Atlas of tumor pathology, Sect. II,

Fasc. 6, Washington, D. C., 1949, Armed Forces Institute of Pathology.

59 Wahl, H. R., and Craig, P. E.: Multiple tumors of the sympathetic nervous system, Am. J. Pathol. **14**:797-808, 1938.

Malignant lymphoma

60 Burke, W. A., Burford, T. H., and Dorfman, R. F.: Hodgkin's disease in the mediastinum, J. Thorac. Cardiovasc. Surg. **3**:287-296, 1967.

61 Van Heerden, J. A., Harrison, E. G., Jr., Bernatz, P. E., and Kiely, J. M.: Mediastinal malignant lymphoma, Chest **57**:518-529, 1970.

Mesenchymal tumors

62 Gremmel, H., Rotthoff, F., and Willmann, K. H.: Intrathorakale lipome, Thoraxchirurgie **6**: 75-85, 1958.

63 McCorkle, R. G., Koerth, C. J., and Donaldson, J. M., Jr.: Thoracic lipomas, J. Thorac. Surg. **9**:568-582, 1940.

64 Pachter, M. R., and Lattes, R.: Mesenchymal tumors of the mediastinum, Cancer **16**:74-94, 95-107, and 108-117, 1963.

65 Svane, H., and Ottosen, P.: Cavernous haemangioma of the mediastinum; a rare tumour form, Acta Chir. Scand. **118**:405-408, 1960.

Heart and aorta

66 Clark, R. M., and Anderson, W.: Rheumatic activity in auricular appendages removed at mitral valvoplasty, Am. J. Pathol. **31**:809-819, 1955.

67 Edwards, J. E., Christensen, N. A., Clagett, O. T., and McDonald, J. R.: Pathologic considerations in coarctation of the aorta, Mayo Clin. Proc. **23**:324-332, 1948.

68 Fine, G., Morales, A., and Horn, R. C., Jr.: Cardiac myxoma; a morphologic and histogenetic appraisal, Cancer **22**:1156-1162, 1968.

69 Frable, W. J.: Mucinous degeneration of the cardiac valves, J. Thorac. Cardiovasc. Surg. **58**:62-70, 1969.

70 Goodwin, J. F.: Diagnosis of left atrial myxoma, Lancet **1**:464-468, 1963.

71 Gross, R. E., and Hufnagel, C.: Coarctation of the aorta, N. Engl. J. Med. **233**:287-293, 1945.

72 Hanfling, S. M.: Metastatic cancer to the heart, Circulation **22**:474-483, 1960.

73 Hanlon, C. R.: Present status of cardiovascular surgery, J.A.M.A. **149**:1-7, 1952.

74 Heath, D.: Pathology of cardiac tumors, Am. J. Cardiol. **21**:315-327, 1968.

75 Kjellberg, S. R., Mannheim, E., Rudhe, U., and Jonsson, B.: Diagnosis of congenital heart disease, ed. 2, Chicago, 1959, Year Book Medical Publishers, Inc.

76 Prichard, R. W.: Tumors of the heart; review of the subject and report of one hundred and fifty cases, Arch. Pathol. **51**:98-128, 1951.

77 Read, R. C., Thal, A. P., and Wendt, V. E.: Symptomatic valvular myxomatous transformation (the floppy valve syndrome); a possible forme fruste of the Marfan syndrome, Circulation **32**:897-910, 1965.

78 Reifenstein, G. H., Levine, S. A., and Gross, R. E.: Coarctation of the aorta; a review of 104 autopsied cases of the "adult type" 2 years of age or older, Am. Heart J. **33**:146, 168, 1947.

79 Roberts, W. C., and Morrow, A. G.: Cardiac valves and the surgical pathologist, Arch. Pathol. **82**:309-313, 1966.

80 Roberts, W. C., Glancy, D. L., and DeVita, V. T., Jr.: Heart in malignant lymphoma (Hodgkin's disease, lymphosarcoma, reticulum cell sarcoma and mycosis fungoides); study of 196 autopsy cases, Am. J. Cardiol. **22**:85-107, 1968.

81 Silverman, J., Olwin, J. S., and Graettinger, J. S.: Cardiac myxomas with systemic embolization; review of the literature and report of a case, Circulation **26**:99-103, 1962.

8 Parathyroid glands

Anatomy

Normally, there are four oval, resilient parathyroid glands, each averaging 4 mm × 3 mm × 1.5 mm. Exceptionally, more than four glands are present. Thus, in a study of 527 autopsy cases, Gilmour and Martin[5] found two instances in which there were six glands and thirty-one in which there were five. Variations in the size and weight of the normal glands were studied by Gilmour and Martin,[5] who found that in 189 cases the mean weight was 117.6 mg ± 4 mg in men and 131.3 ± 5.8 mg in women. The color may vary from reddish brown to light tan, depending upon fat content, which, in turn, depends on age, nutrition, and activity of the individual.

Parathyroid glands are arranged in two pairs, the upper pair usually located on the middle third of the posterolateral border of the thyroid gland and the lower pair at, just behind, or slightly below the lower pole of the thyroid gland, in close proximity to the inferior thyroid artery.

The upper pair of glands arises from the fourth branchial cleft and descends into the neck with the thyroid gland during embryonic life. The lower pair arises from the third branchial cleft and descends with the thymus to the level of the lower pole of the thyroid gland. Faulty migrations of the glands during embryonic life result in anomalous positions. The upper glands may be found inside the carotid sheath or behind the cervical or thoracic esophagus. The lower glands may continue their descent with the thymus into the anterior portion of the mediastinum. They also may be located inside the thyroid gland or in the pharynx.[6]

There has been a rather rigid division of various types of cells in the parathyroid glands, and each of these types has been given numerous synonyms. There is evidence that the *chief cell* is the basic cell type and that the others represent functional modifications of the former, with differences in morphology and metabolic activity (Fig. 310).

The chief cell measures 6μ to 8μ in diameter and has ill-defined scanty cytoplasm. Minor changes in cell size and cytoplasmic clarity have been correlated with more striking ultrastructural variation and with functional activity by Roth and Raisz.[9] The *oxyphil cell*, small clusters of which are normally present in the parathyroid glands of adults, is larger than the chief cell and has eosinophilic granular cytoplasm. Ultrastructurally, oxyphils contain many large mitochondria and have a rich content of oxidative enzymes, when compared with the chief cell. Secretion droplets (presumably parathormone) are variably prominent in chief cells, depend-

283

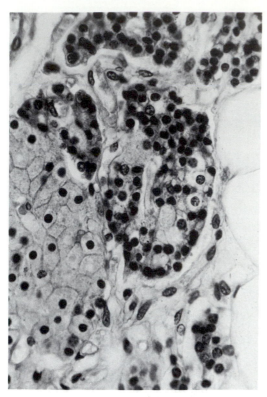

Fig. 310 Normal parathyroid gland. Note lack of encapsulation and persistence of fat. Cells with deep-staining nuclei are chief cells, and those with prominent cytoplasm are oxyphil cells. (×500; WU neg. 49-814.)

ing upon the stage of function of the cell, but are rarely seen in oxyphils[9] (Fig. 311).

Cells intermediate in appearance between the chief and the oxyphil cells and designated as *transitional oxyphil cells* may be seen, particularly in adenomas or chief cell hyperplasia. Normally, an inverse relationship between cellular content of glycogen and secretion is seen, but in cells from adenomas or hyperplastic glands, large quantities of both often are present.

The *water-clear cell* is characterized by abundant poorly stained cytoplasm and better defined cell membranes. Forms intermediate between the normal chief cell and and water-clear cell *(transitional water-clear cells)* are common in adenomas and forms of hyperplasia. Biochemical and physiologic explanations for these morphologic observations are not yet available.

The frequency distribution of the different cells varies with the age of the patient. Until puberty, the gland is composed wholly of chief cells with slight tendency to vacuolization. These cells contain a fair amount of glycogen but no fat. Fat appears soon after puberty as very fine droplets. At puberty, or soon afterward, pale oxyphils gradually appear, at first singly and then in pairs, frequently forming large islands after 40 to 50 years of age. These islands of oxyphil cells are sharply circumscribed but not encapsulated. Often, continuous cords of parenchymal cells can be traced across the margin of the island into the surrounding gland.

Following puberty, large fat cells appear in the stroma and increase in number until about 40 years of age. The fat tissue remains fairly constant during middle and old age. It is interesting to note that when an adult gland is smaller than normal, the decreased size is due to the absence or marked diminution of fat cells, whereas the parenchymal cell volume is about the same as in a normal-sized, fat-containing gland. This has been proved by actual measurement by Gilmour.[4]

Cysts of varying sizes are observed in about one-half of the patients beyond puberty. These cysts are sometimes filled with granular and cellular debris or with a dark blue-staining, finely granular material that has been designated incorrectly as colloid.

There are times when it is difficult to make the histologic differentiation between parathyroid and thyroid tissue. Colloidlike material in parathyroid tumors and within the thyroid gland appears to be the same. In the normal parathyroid gland and in parathyroid tumors, there is considerable glycogen. In the normal thyroid gland, there is practically no glycogen. Thyroid nodules and thyroid cancer contain small amounts of glycogen. Thus, the presence and the amount of glycogen observed may be helpful in making a distinction between parathyroid tissue and thyroid tissue.[7]

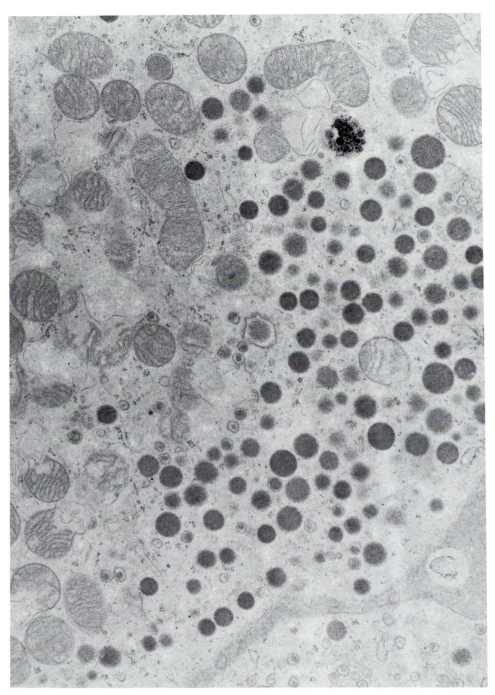

Fig. 311 Membrane-limited secretory granules are far more numerous in this cell from parathyroid adenoma than in normal chief cells. Granules vary in size depending on their stages of maturity. (Uranyl acetate; approximately ×12,000.)

Physiology

The parathyroid glands mediate their endocrine function through the production of parathormone.[1] The chief cells are most critically sensitive to calcium concentrations in vivo and in vitro. Roth and Raisz[9] have shown convincing ultrastructural changes corresponding to enhanced production of secretion (parathormone) when calcium concentration is reduced. These active cells contain abundant secretion granules, a prominent Golgi apparatus, and very little glycogen. Under conditions of elevated calcium concentration, the cells are nearly devoid of secretion, have an inconspicuous Golgi apparatus, and contain abundant glycogen. This critical experiment provides objective proof of the role of iodized serum calcium in regulating chief cell function and parathormone production.

Osteoclastic resorption of bone with elevation of serum calcium is the most important function physiologically. Depression of tubular resorption of phosphorus with subsequent increased urinary phosphate is a secondary aspect of parathormone activity. A single hormone is probably responsible for both renal and osseous effects and appears to stimulate tubular resorption and intestinal absorption of calcium as well. An influence in magnesium metabolism may occur, and low serum levels have been reported in hyperparathyroidism.[8] Recent studies suggest that the mechanism of action of parathormone in the receptor tissues is a rapid stimulation of adenyl-cyclase, a membrane-bound enzyme, with a resulting increase in the intracellular concentration of cyclic 3',5' AMP.[3] Chang[2] demonstrated that if autogenous and homogenous transplantations of parathyroid gland were made to the subperiosteal area in the parietal bone in young rats and mice, prominent resorption of parietal bone and minimal new bone deposition occurred. These changes strongly suggested a direct local effect. Similar transplants of many other organs, such as urinary bladder mucosa, testis, pancreas, compact bone, etc., caused no changes.

Primary hyperparathyroidism

The designation *primary hyperparathyroidism* is applied to a group of parathyroid lesions characterized by the production of increased levels of parathormone, in which there is no evidence of previous parathyroid stimulation by hypocalcemia resulting from chronic renal, osseous, or intestinal disease.

With a pathologically increased secretion of parathormone, the following sequence of events occurs. Serum calcium levels rise secondary to calcium release from bone. The increased calcium-ion concentration in the bloodstream exceeds the kidney threshold for calcium ions, and increased quantities of calcium may be excreted—hypercalciuria. The decreased reabsorption of inorganic phosphate results in increased excretion of phosphorus in the urine—hyperphosphaturia. Hypophosphatemia accompanies the hyperphosphaturia. Therefore, the results of increased parathormone secretion are hypercalcemia, hypophosphatemia, and hyperphosphaturia and, less predictably, hypercalciuria. Another associated chemical finding is an inconstant elevation of the serum alkaline phosphatase level.

According to the clinical presentation, patients with primary hyperparathyroidism

Table 8 Clues to diagnosis of hyperparathyroidism in 343 patients (Massachusetts General Hospital series, 1930-1965)*

Clue	Number of patients
Bone disease	80
Renal stones	195
Peptic ulcer	27
Pancreatitis	9
Fatigue	10
Hypertension	6
Mental disturbance	3
Central nervous system signs	7
No symptoms	2
Multiple endocrine abnormalities	3
Lump in neck	1

*From Cope, O.: The story of hyperparathyroidism at the Massachusetts General Hospital, N. Engl. J. Med. **274:**1174-1182, 1966.

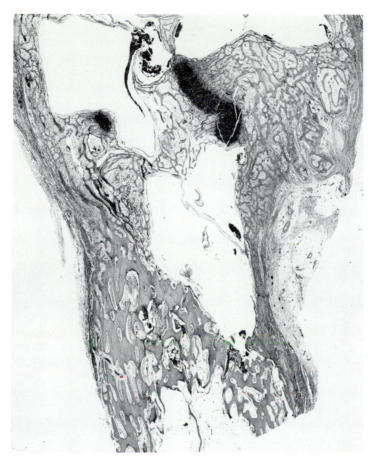

Fig. 312 Osteitis fibrosa cystica. Note bone production and destruction with cyst formation. Dark areas represent hemorrhage and giant cell formation (brown tumor). (Low power; WU neg. 49-4562.)

may be classified into the following types: (1) those with osseous manifestations, (2) those with renal manifestations, and (3) those with neither of the foregoing (Table 8). With the routine use of the serum autoanalyzer in most hospital centers, there has been a sharp increase in the incidence of the latter group.[15] Practically all patients with primary hyperparathyroidism have hypercalcemia and increased levels or circulating parathormone, as measured by radioimmunoassay.[18] However, well-documented instances of normocalcemic primary hyperparathyroidism have been reported.[22]

Bone changes in hyperparathyroidism depend on many factors, including the calcium intake, the renal function, and the level at which the parathyroid lesion is functioning. With minimal changes, the x-ray film may show simply generalized diminished bone density. With advanced changes, cyst formation occurs. It must be emphasized that such changes are generalized, and if a given bone is examined roentgenologically, it will show involvement of the entire bone rather than a localized lesion surrounded by normal bone, such as in fibrous dysplasia.

Frequently, the first sign is a cystic lesion of the maxilla or the mandible. Biopsy of this lesion or other cystic lesions may lead to an erroneous diagnosis of primary giant cell tumor. In any such instance, parathyroid lesions must be excluded. Unfortunately, we have not been able to distinguish microscopically between lesions of the mandible secondary to hyperparathyroidism and those lesions that are independent and solitary (so-called giant cell reparative granulomas).

In patients with hyperparathyroidism and bone changes, hypercalcemia and hypophosphatemia are usually marked. These alterations are associated with an elevated serum alkaline phosphatase level and a reduced renal tubular reabsorption of phosphate. It is rare to see a functioning parathyroid tumor with radiographic evidence of bone changes without an elevated alkaline phosphatase level. In the past, bone changes often became extensive, with deformity, formation of many cysts, and even fractures (Fig. 312).

Microscopically, bone biopsy of such a lesion demonstrates bone destruction, new bone formation, cysts, and so-called brown tumors. These brown tumors show areas of hemorrhage and giant cells. This combination of microscopic findings should make the pathologist suspect a functioning parathyroid adenoma[12] (Figs. 313 and 314). Removal of the parathyroid adenoma is followed by a rapid reversal to normal (Figs. 315 and 316). We have seen such a reversal take place within a two-month period even with advanced alterations. Repair of some cystic lesions does not take place, and for this reason small cysts may persist (Fig. 317).

The renal changes of primary hyperparathyroidism include renal stones, nephrocalcinosis, polyuria and polydipsia, and impairment of renal function. It is now recognized that renal calculus is the most common clinical manifestation of hyperparathyroidism.[19] If the renal lesions are

severe at the time of the removal of the parathyroid lesion, they often progress, are frequently associated with hypertension, and are the most important cause of death.

Other manifestations of hyperparathyroidism include hypertension, peptic ulcer, acute and chronic pancreatitis, and mental disturbances. Duodenal ulcer occurred in twelve of fifty patients in Hellström and

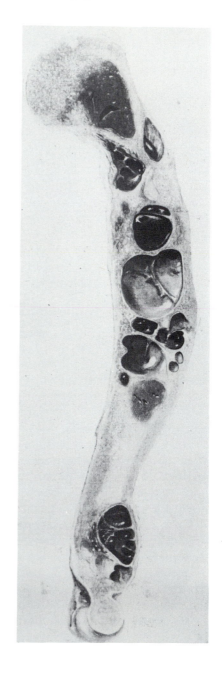

Fig. 313 Extreme osteitis fibrosa cystica. Note deformity of bone with numerous cysts and brown tumors. (WU neg. 49-4586; from Hunter, D., and Turnbull, H. N.: Hyperparathyroidism: generalized osteitis fibrosa, with observations upon bones, parathyroid tumours, and normal parathyroid glands, Br. J. Surg. **19**:203-284, 1931.)

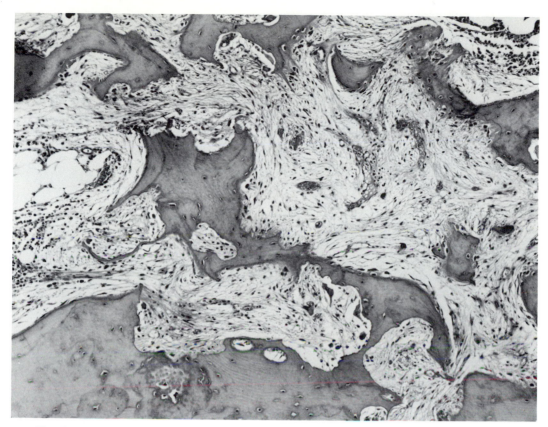

Fig. 314 Bone changes in hyperparathyroidism: marrow fibrosis, extreme osteoclastic resorption, and some bone production. Patient had extensive bone disease with normal renal function. (×90; WU neg. 72-5961.)

Ivemark's series.[16] The incidence of duodenal ulcer was highest in men. It is interesting that Schiffrin[20] demonstrated that parathyroid extract injected into dogs causes an increase in the volume, acidity, and pepsin content of gastric secretion. With removal of the adenoma, the ulcer usually heals. Dent et al.[14] found elevated levels of plasma gastrin in ten of twenty patients with hyperparathyroidism without achlorhydria. These levels fell after removal of the diseased parathyroid, together with the serum calcium and the parathyroid hormone concentration. Rarely, acute gastrointestinal, cardiovascular, or central nervous system symptoms develop because of very high serum calcium levels. This condition, designated as *parathyroid crisis*, is fatal unless the offending gland or glands are rapidly excised.[17]

Familial hyperparathyroidism may occur. We have studied a family in which eleven members were affected.[13] Hyperparathyroidism and Zollinger-Ellison syndrome constitute the two most prominent manifestations of multiple endocrine adenomatosis.[10] Association with sarcoidosis also has been documented.[23]

Primary hyperparathyroidism may be caused by adenoma (single or multiple), chief cell hyperplasia, water-clear cell hyperplasia, or carcinoma. Classically, a single adenoma has been regarded as the responsible cause in the large majority of cases. (Table 9). However, follow-up studies of patients so diagnosed, as well as studies of asymptomatic (presumably early) cases, have shown an increased incidence of chief cell hyperplasia as a cause of primary hyperparathyroidism.[15, 21] Thus,

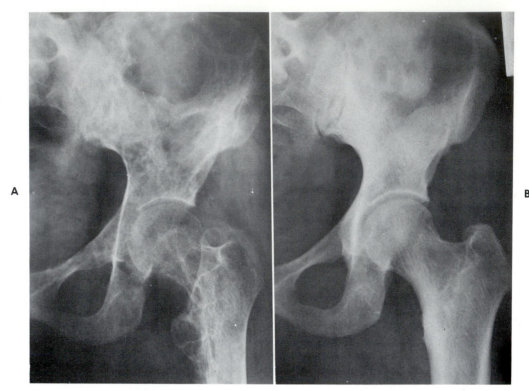

Fig. 315 A, Extensive changes in bones of pelvis and femur caused by functioning parathyroid adenoma. **B,** Same pelvis and femur eight years following removal of adenoma.
Note complete reversion to normal. (**A,** WU neg. 49-3694; **B,** WU neg. 49-3695; **A** and
B, from Black, B. K., and Ackerman, L. V.: Tumors of the parathyroid; a review of twenty-
three cases, Cancer **3:**415-444, 1950.)

Table 9 Causes of hyperparathyroidism in 343
patients (Massachusetts General Hospital series,
1930-1965)*

Cause	Number of patients
Neoplasia	
Single adenoma	263
Double adenoma	13
Carcinoma	15
Primary hyperplasia	
Clear cell	15
Chief cell	37

*From Cope, O.: The story of hyperparathyroidism at
the Massachusetts General Hospital, N. Engl. J. Med.
274:1174-1182, 1966.

in a series of forty-seven patients operated
at Barnes Hospital in a thirty-month period,
nineteen harbored an adenoma, whereas
twenty-three were found to have chief
cell hyperplasia.[15] These studies also have

cast doubts on the validity of the rigid
distinction classically applied between adenoma and hyperplasia. It may well be,
as Black and Utley[11] have suggested, that
they merely represent different morphologic
manifestations of the same process. However, we think they should be separated
whenever possible because of the differences in therapeutic approach.

Adenoma

Parathyroid adenoma should ideally be
confined to one gland, have a definite rim
of normal parathyroid separated by a fibrous band, and be accompanied by other
glands with normal (or atrophic) microscopic appearance. Double and even triple
adenomas have been reported,[25, 26] but we
would interpret most of them as instances
of chief cell hyperplasia. The rim of nor-

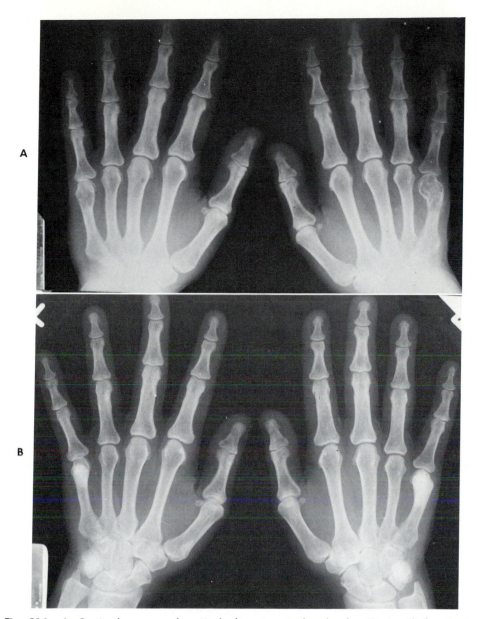

Fig. 316   A, Cystic changes and cortical alterations in hands of patient with functioning parathyroid adenoma. **B,** Dramatic change evident nine months after removal of adenoma. (**A,** WU neg. 57-6267; **B,** WU neg. 57-6268.)

mal parathyroid may be absent, or it may be missed on the plane of section. We could identify it in 58% of our adenomas. It may be simulated by compressed, less hyperplastic tissue in chief cell hyperplasia. The presence of a *microscopically normal* second gland is the best guarantee that a given lesion is an adenoma.

Adenomas occur in women and men in a ratio of 3:1. They can occur at almost any age, but most occur in patients in the fourth decade. A few cases have been reported in children.[24] Adenomas vary in weight from 0.4 gm to 120 gm. The mean weight of such tumors reported prior to 1947 was approximately 7 gm. An adenoma of this weight measures about 3 cm × 2 cm × 1.5 cm. Adenomas are usually oval,

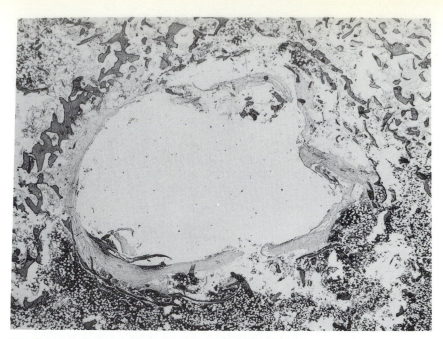

Fig. 317 Failure of repair of cystic lesions of bone in hyperparathyroidism. Section was made twenty-three months after removal of functioning parathyroid adenoma. This man, who died of renal insufficiency, was the first patient in whom a functioning adenoma of parathyroid gland was successfully diagnosed and surgically treated (1928) (reported by Barr, D. P., and Bulger, H. A.: Clinical syndrome of hyperparathyroidism, Am. J. Med. Sci. **179**:449-476, 1930). (Low power; WU neg. 49-5193.)

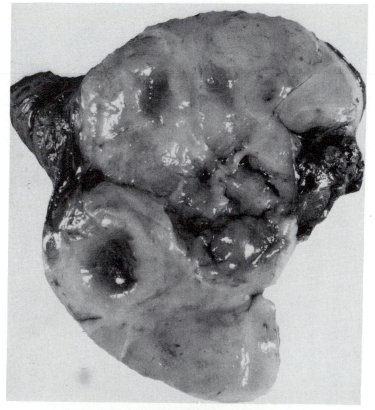

Fig. 318 Functioning parathyroid adenoma. Note encapsulation and cystic change. (WU neg. 46-8635; from Black, B. K., and Ackerman, L. V.: Tumors of the parathyroid; a review of twenty-three cases, Cancer **3**:415-444, 1950.)

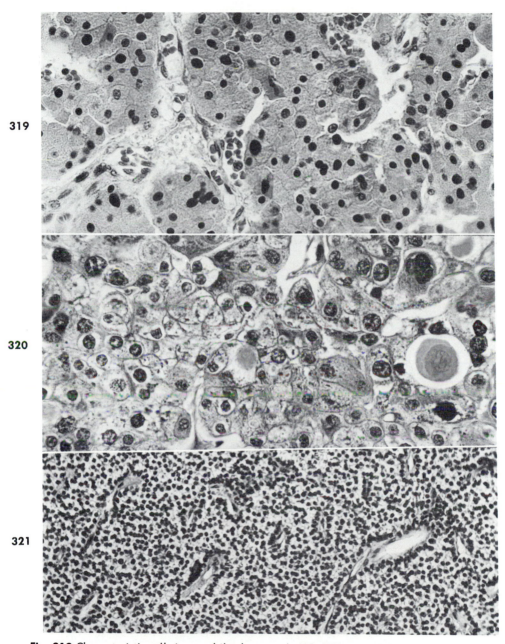

Fig. 319 Characteristic cells in oxyphil adenoma. (×400; WU neg. 49-3701.)
Fig. 320 Functioning parathyroid adenoma with extreme variation in nuclear size. Patient has survived eighteen years following operation. (×500; WU neg. 49-816; from Black, B. K., and Ackerman, L. V.: Tumors of the parathyroid; a review of twenty-three cases, Cancer **3:**415-444, 1950.)
Fig. 321 Functioning parathyroid adenoma. Note difference in microscopic pattern from adenoma shown in Fig. 320. Patient has survived eleven years. (×185; WU neg. 49-3700.)

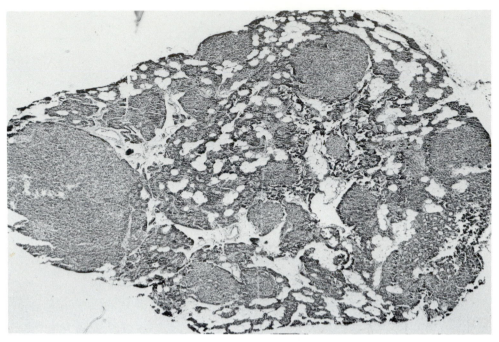

Fig. 322 Nodular chief cell hyperplasia in normal-sized parathyroid gland. Some fat is still present. This illustration demonstrates that parathyroid gland may not be enlarged but still, because of its cellular population, be hyperplastic. (×45; WU neg. 67-4472.)

may show slight lobulation, and usually have a thin connective tissue capsule. On section, they are usually grayish brown (Fig. 318). Foci of hemorrhage and even calcification may occur. Parathyroid adenomas may not be large enough to be felt but may produce pressure deformities recognized radiographically in the esophagus or the trachea. Wyman and Robbins localized twenty of thirty-four lesions.[27]

Microscopically, parathyroid adenomas are made up of any one of various cell types (Fig. 319). Frequently, the tumors harbor cysts containing a varying amount of colloidlike material. Often variation in cellular and nuclear size is conspicuous (Figs. 320 and 321). Mitotic figures are rare or absent. We believe that the chief cell, the transitional water-clear cell, the water-clear cell, and rarely the oxyphil cell can all produce parathormone.

Chief cell hyperplasia

Primary chief cell hyperplasia is an entity described by Cope et al.[30] in which there is evidence of increased production of parathormone. It occurs without previous impairment of renal function and is frequently seen in patients with multiple endocrine changes. In this entity, all parathyroid glands are enlarged and tend to be reddish brown in color.[28] The predominant cell is the chief cell, but other cells are present. The superior glands are larger than the inferior ones, although the difference is not so striking as in the case of water-clear cell hyperplasia. The microscopic distinction with adenoma may be exceedingly difficult.[29] Size, shape, color, consistency, and cell types present and their relative frequency are of no help in this regard. Presence of a rim of normal parenchyma and the identification of at least a normal parathyroid gland are the only definite criteria by which a diagnosis of adenoma can be made over that of chief cell hyperplasia. Black and Haff[29] examined thirty-nine patients with chief cell hyperplasia. In thirteen, all parathyroid glands were obviously enlarged and,

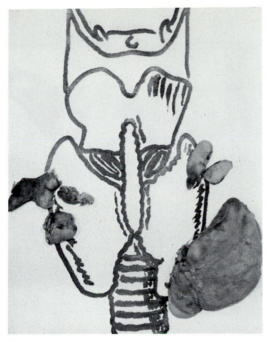

Fig. 323 Distribution of parathyroid tissue in water-clear cell hyperplasia in 48-year-old woman. Total weight of tissue removed was 125 gm. Patient died thirty-five months after first operation, and equal amount of parathyroid tissue was again found. There were generalized diminished bone density and only mild hyperparathyroidism.

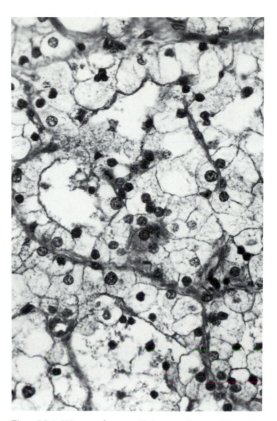

Fig. 324 Water-clear cell hyperplasia. Note increase in size and number of water-clear cells. (High power; WU neg. 49-3060.)

therefore, conformed to the classic description. In twelve patients, only one gland was large and nodular, whereas the others were nearly normal in size, the picture therefore simulating that of an adenoma. In the remaining fourteen patients, all four parathyroid glands seemed normal in size and appearance to the surgeon, and only minimal microscopic evidence of hyperplasia could be detected in them.

Another exceedingly difficult differential diagnosis is that between primary and secondary chief cell hyperplasia. As a rule, in primary hyperplasia the glands are more nodular, traversed by fibrous septa, and have more acinar formations and giant cells than in the secondary form[28] (Fig. 322). However, in many cases the distinction can be made only on the basis of a detailed clinical history.

Water-clear cell hyperplasia

A rare condition, water-clear cell hyperplasia is characterized by extreme enlargement of all parathyroid tissue so that the total weight of the glands may exceed 65 gm. We have seen a case in which the tissue removed weighed 125 gm (Fig. 323). The enlargement is due to a combination of hyperplasia and hypertrophy of water-clear cells (Fig. 324). Rogers et al.[32] showed that even though the hypertrophy may exceed sixty times the normal volume, this alone could not be responsible for the size of the gland, and therefore hyperplasia must be a contributing factor.

A distinct correlation may be made between the weight of the parathyroid tissue and the degree of hyperparathyroidism, a correlation that can also be made with adenomas.[31] Whatever the mechanism in-

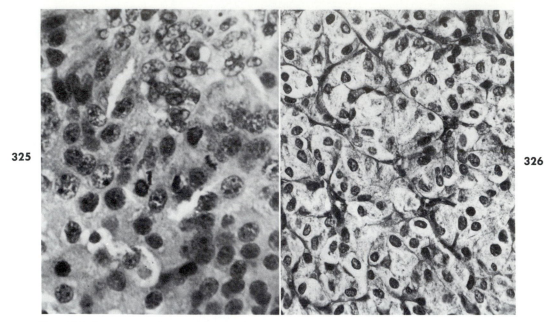

325   326

Fig. 325 Carcinoma of parathyroid gland in which nerve invasion, tumor thrombi, and numerous mitotic figures occurred. Mitotic figures are absent in parathyroid adenomas. (×600; WU neg. 52-138.)

Fig. 326 Carcinoma of parathyroid gland. Note trabecular pattern. Lesion recurred after operation and finally invaded mediastinum widely. (×400; WU neg. 49-3966.)

volved, the glands apparently respond to the stimulus by an all-or-none reaction.

Grossly, the superior glands are usually larger than the inferior, but this may be due to the differences in their original size. Moreover, glands may coalesce so that two glands appear as one. They are soft and have a typical chocolate brown color. Cysts and hemorrhages have been observed. Another gross characteristic is the formation of pseudopods that may extend a considerable distance from the main mass of the gland.

Microscopically, the most constant feature is the presence of very large, clear cells, the diameters of which may range from 10μ to 40μ (Fig. 324). These cells may vary markedly in size, however, so that in some regions they do not appear much larger than the water-clear cells found in small numbers in normal parathyroid tissue. In most regions, the cytoplasm of the cell is water clear, but in some cells small eosinophilic granules are

present. High-power examination of thin sections reveals that the clarity of the cytoplasm is the result of a conglomerate of spherical clear vacuoles that are surrounded by thin portions of eosinophilic cytoplasmic material.

The nucleus averages from 6μ to 7μ. The size may vary, but no giant nuclei are seen. Basal orientation of the nuclei is one of the most striking features. The most frequent pattern is an alveolar one. There may be areas of pseudoglandular formation, however, and in other places a compact arrangement of the cells. The connective tissue is delicate and sparse for the most part, but in some areas it may be dense. Chief cells are rarely found.

Carcinoma

Erroneous diagnoses of carcinoma of the parathyroid gland have been made too frequently in the past, the error usually occurring when a malignant tumor in the region of the gland has metastasized. Since

such tumors do not produce parathormone, they cannot be proved to be of
parathyroid origin.

The often exceedingly variable microscopic pattern of parathyroid adenomas
was used incorrectly by Alexander et al.[33]
as an indication of malignant change. We
also do not believe that nests of cells of
an adenoma trapped in the capsule or lying
free within the lumina of veins are evidences of malignant change. In order for
tumor in a vein to be of any significance,
it must be a true tumor thrombus attached
firmly to the wall. The only valid evidence
of malignant change in a parathyroid
adenoma is the presence of invasion of
contiguous structures at the time of first
operation or the presence of local lymph
node or distant metastases.

Holmes et al.[34] have reviewed the forty-
six cases of functioning parathyroid carcinomas using strict criteria as defined in the
literature. Skeletal disease was present in
73% of the patients and renal disease in
32%. Metastases to the cervical lymph
nodes occurred in 32% and to the lung
in 26%. Features suggestive of carcinoma
in a hyperparathyroid patient include very
high values of serum calcium, a palpable
cervical mass, vocal cord paralysis, and
recurrence of hyperparathyroidism a short
time (a few months) following surgery.
At operation, most carcinomas are hard,
are surrounded by a dense fibrous reaction,
and are often adherent to and infiltrate
adjacent structures. Microscopically, carcinomas differ from adenomas mainly by
virtue of a trabecular arrangement, spindle shape of the tumor cells, and presence
of mitotic figures (Figs. 325 and 326).

In a recent review of a large series of
parathyroid carcinomas, Schantz and
Castleman[35] found fibrous trabeculae in
90% of the cases, mitoses in 81%, capsular
invasion in 6%, and blood vessel invasion
in 12%. They emphasized that the presence
of mitotic figures in a parathyroid lesion
is strongly suggestive of carcinoma. In a
follow-up of forty-three patients reported
by Holmes et al.,[34] it was found that

thirty (65%) of the patients were dead,
five were living with persistent tumor, and
eight were living without evidence of recurrent disease. Of thirty-nine patients
studied by Schantz and Castleman,[35] 41%
were alive and well, 13% were alive with
disease, and 46% were dead of carcinoma.
Local recurrence within the first two years
after surgery was found to be an ominous
prognostic sign.

Secondary hyperparathyroidism

Secondary hyperplasia of the parathyroid
gland occurs with chronic renal disease
such as renal rickets, chronic pyelonephritis, multiple myeloma, diffuse metastatic
carcinoma, and osteomalacia. Enlargement
usually develops because of renal insufficiency, elevation of the serum phosphatase
level, and reciprocal decrease of serum
calcium concentrations, with the resulting
stimulation of the parathyroid glands. Vitamin D resistance is a characteristic of advanced renal disease and may also play
a factor by contributing to a reduction
in serum calcium concentrations.[36] Radioimmunoassay determinations of parathormone have shown this to be roughly proportional to the severity of renal failure.
It was also found that levels of circulating
parathormone were higher in renal failure
than in any form of primary hyperparathyroidism.[38]

All of the glands usually become enlarged, measuring as much as 2 cm × 1
cm × 1 cm, but usually they do not reach
the size of an adenoma. They are creamy
gray rather than orange-brown because
the fat is replaced by cells. Because of
the replacement of fat by cells, there is
not necessarily any enlargement of the
glands. In 200 cases studied by Roth and
Marshall,[39] the parathyroid weights ranged
from 120 mg to 6 gm and showed an inverse correlation with the mean serum
calcium level.

Microscopically, the glands show little
fat, but usually the intercellular fat tissue
is not completely absent. Chief cells of
normal size dominate. Frequently, there are

increased numbers of oxyphil and transitional oxyphil cells that form hyperplastic nodular collections.

The bone changes in secondary hyperparathyroidism are similar to those in primary hyperparathyroidism but are usually much milder in degree. Rarely, severe bone changes occur with cyst formation.[37] The bony trabeculae are usually calcified. This calcification is helpful in the differential diagnosis, since it does not occur in Fanconi's syndrome or rickets.

"Tertiary" hyperparathyroidism

The term *"tertiary" hyperparathyroidism* is applied to patients with hyperparathyroidism secondary to chronic renal disease or intestinal malabsorption in whom one or more of the stimulated parathyroid glands seem to become autonomous.[41] Most cases have been detected after correction of the renal disease by hemodialysis or homotransplantation.[43] The existence of such an entity is still debated. Follow-up studies seem to indicate that if enough time is given, the parathyroid glands will revert to a normal state in the large majority of cases.[42] The microscopic appearance of these supposedly autonomous parathyroid glands is not different from that seen in the usual "suppressible" secondary hyperparathyroidism.[40]

Electron microscopy

The hyperactive parathyroid chief cell has a typical fine structural appearance, which is the same for adenoma, primary chief cell hyperplasia, and secondary hyperplasia. It is characterized by prominent Golgi apparatus, abundant cisternae of granular endoplasmic reticulum, and numerous ribosomes.[45] Electron microscopic study can confirm the hyperplastic nature of a gland that is debatable by light microscopy.[44] The cells of water-clear cell hyperplasia contain characteristic large, membrane-bound vacuoles, measuring 0.2μ to 2μ in diameter. Roth[46] has suggested that these vacuoles derive from the Golgi apparatus. Oxyphil cells are characterized

by a cytoplasm packed by mitochondria. Some of them may contain, in addition, typical secretory granules.[47]

Hyperparathyroidism secondary to nonparathyroidism tumors

Typical symptoms and signs of hyperparathyroidism may sometimes be the result of malignant tumors of nonparathyroid origin in the absence of significant osseous metastases. Omenn et al.[49] have reviewed seventy-three cases of this condition. Renal cell carcinoma and epidermoid carcinoma of lung account for 60% of the cases.[48] The parathyroid glands, when examined at autopsy, have been found to be normal or atrophic. Immunoassay of the patient's serum and tumor extracts have demonstrated the presence of a substance immunologically indistinguishable from parathormone.

Nonfunctioning lesions

Parathyroid cysts usually arise from the inferior glands. In most cases, they cause no symptoms other than those related to pressure.[50] They are lined by cuboidal or low columnar epithelial cells and often contain parathyroid tissue in their wall.[51] The few reported cases of cysts associated with hyperparathyroidism most likely represent adenomas with cystic degeneration.[53]

Oxyphil adenomas are almost always asymptomatic. Those associated with hyperparathyroidism often have an admixture of chief cells. Selzman and Fechner[54] have reported a hyperfunctioning oxyphil adenoma in which electron microscopy showed evidence of secretion by the oxyphil cells.

Carcinomas may theoretically be nonfunctioning, and a few convincing cases have been reported.[52, 55]

Exploratory operation and treatment

Both Walton[67] and Cope[58] strongly emphasized the information a surgeon must have when he prepares to operate upon a patient suspected of having a parathyroid adenoma. In the first place, he must have a thorough knowledge of parathyroid physiology and, in the second, a complete knowledge of the appearance and possible location of the parathyroid glands in the neck and mediastinum. Cope[58] pointed out that the parathyroid glands usually have a symmetrical distribution—when one superior parathyroid gland is located in one place, the opposite parathyroid gland will be in a similar area.

The statistical location of 197 tumors as reported by Norris[63] in 1947 may aid the surgeon in his approach to an adenoma that cannot be palpated. Norris[63] found that of those located in the neck, 43% were in the area of the right inferior gland, 41% in the area of the left inferior gland, 9% near the right superior gland, and 7% near the left superior gland. In his series, 10% were found in abnormal positions: approximately two-thirds in the mediastinum, 30% within the thyroid gland, and the remainder in the area behind the esophagus. In our series, five of twenty-three were located in abnormal areas, with three in the anterior portion of the mediastinum and two behind the esophagus.

Operation must be as bloodless as possible so that the parathyroid glands can be identified. The necessity of making every effort to visualize all four glands at each operation for parathyroid disease cannot be overstressed. In the past, obvious clinical and laboratory findings often were found in patients with a functioning parathyroid adenoma, and at operation usually a single, well-defined parathyroid adenoma was present. Under such circumstances, we used to say that if an atrophic parathyroid gland was found, this was an indication that a functioning parathyroid adenoma was present. We are rather doubtful that such a finding ever existed which could be recognized by either the surgeon or the pathologist.

The parathyroid glands are reddish brown after puberty. With increase in fat, they become yellow. If this fatty tissue is replaced with cells, the parathyroid tissue will again become brown in color. The vascular supply of the lower parathyroid glands comes from branches of the inferior thyroid arteries. This supply is usually independent, a circumstance that may be helpful in locating abnormally placed parathyroid adenomas. If one of these arteries is ligated, infarction of the parathyroid gland may result.[67]

If a thorough exploration of the neck reveals only three normal parathyroid glands, there is some justification for terminating the operation with a hemithyroidectomy on the side of the missing gland, since 2% of all adenomas are found in this location.[60] If this also proves negative, sternotomy and mediastinal exploration should be considered two or three weeks later. The majority of the mediastinal parathyroid adenomas can be removed from the neck, through a low collar thyroid incision. Of eighty-four cases reviewed by Nathaniels et al.,[62] mediastinotomy was necessary in only nineteen.

In patients with apparent parathyroid disease, the pathologist must know the details of the clinical history and the results of the laboratory tests, and these must include the renal function studies. He should also have the opportunity of reviewing the films. The pathologist can use frozen section to determine whether a given nodule is, in reality, parathyroid tissue. Nodules of thyroid gland, small lymph nodes, aberrant thymic tissue, and even fat may be mistaken grossly for parathyroid tissue.

The pathologist can recognize primary water-clear cell hyperplasia because of uniform enlargement of all parathyroid glands and because of the characteristically large clear cells. Carcinoma of the parathyroid gland, when it has invaded local tissues and has spindle cells with mitotic figures, also can be identified. If there is a large gland with a definite capsule and the other three glands are small, the microscopic diagnosis of an adenoma is usually not difficult. In patients with profound renal damage, the differentiation between chief cell hyperplasia and secondary hyperplasia is impossible.[65, 66] If renal function is normal, all glands are enlarged, and there is separation of parathyroid tissue into fibrous nodules, chief cell hyperplasia can be diagnosed. Bone biopsy, preferably of the iliac crest, is recommended when a patient is explored for a parathyroid lesion.

Adenomas are adequately treated by local excision of the tumor. It is imperative *to excise or biopsy at least one other parathyroid gland* in order to rule out the possibility of chief cell hyperplasia.

Primary water-clear cell and chief cell hyperplasia are conventionally treated by total excision of three glands and partial excision of the fourth. Parathyroid carcinoma is best treated by excision of the tumor and surrounding soft tissues, removal of the ipsilateral thyroid lobe, and ipsilateral lymph node dissection.[61]

The large majority of patients with secondary and "tertiary" hyperparathyroidism respond well to medical treatment.[56, 59] However, if bone lesions are severe and if the hypercalcemia is excessive, subtotal parathyroidectomy may become necessary.[57]

It is not yet known if asymptomatic individuals who are found to have mild hypercalcemia on routine screening should be operated upon. A group of such patients is now being followed to determine their outcome. So far, and after a thirty-month period, only 13.8% have required operation.[64]

REFERENCES

Anatomy/Physiology

1 Albright, F., and Reifenstein, E. C., Jr.: The parathyroid glands in metabolic bone disease; selected studies, Baltimore, 1948, The Williams & Wilkins Co.

2 Chang, H.: Grafts of parathyroid and other tissues to bone, Anat. Rec. 111:23-39, 1951.

3 Chase, L. R., and Aurbach, G. D.: Parathyroid function and the renal excretion of 3'5'-adenylic acid, Proc. Natl. Acad. Sci. USA 58:518-525, 1967.

4 Gilmour, J. R.: The parathyroid glands and skeleton in renal diseases, London, 1947, Oxford University Press.

5 Gilmour, J. R., and Martin, W. J.: The weight of the parathyroid glands, J. Pathol. Bacteriol. 44:431-462, 1937.

6 Herrold, K. M., Rabson, A. S., and Ketcham, A. S.: Aberrant parathyroid gland in pharyngeal submucosa, Arch. Pathol. 73:60-62, 1962.

7 Klinck, G. H.: Unpublished observations.

8 Pyrah, L. N., Hodgkinson, A., and Anderson, C. K.: Critical review: primary hyperparathyroidism, Br. J. Surg. 53:245-316, 1966 (excellent review and extensive bibliography).

9 Roth, S. I., and Raisz, L. G.: The course and reversibility of the calcium effect on the ultrastructure of the rat parathyroid gland in organ culture, Lab. Invest. 15:1187-1211, 1966.

Primary hyperparathyroidism

10 Ballard, H. S., Frame, B., and Hartsock, R. J.: Familial multiple endocrine adenoma–peptic ulcer complex, Medicine (Baltimore) 43:481-516, 1964.

11 Black, W. C., III, and Utley, J. R.: The differential diagnosis of parathyroid adenoma and chief cell hyperplasia, Am. J. Clin. Pathol. 49:761-775, 1968.

12 Byers, P. D., and Smith, R.: Quantitative histology of bone in hyperparathyroidism; its relation to clinical features, x-ray, and biochemistry, Q. J. Med. 40:471-486, 1971.

13 Cutler, R. E., Reiss, E., and Ackerman, L. V.: Familial hyperparathyroidism; a kindred involving eleven cases with a discussion of primary chief cell hyperplasia, N. Engl. J. Med. 270:859-865, 1964.

14 Dent, R. I., James, H. J., Wang, C., Deftos, L. J., Talamo, R., and Fischer, J. E.: Hyperparathyroidism; gastric acid secretion and gastrin, Ann. Surg. 176:360-369, 1972.

15 Haff, R. C., Black, W. C., and Ballinger, W. F., II: Primary hyperparathyroidism: changing clinical, surgical and pathological aspects, Ann. Surg. 171:85-92, 1970.

16 Hellström, J., and Ivemark, B. I.: Primary hyperparathyroidism; clinical and structural findings in 138 cases, Acta Chir. Scand. (suppl.) 294:1-113, 1962.

17 MacLeod, W. A. J., and Holloway, C. K.: Hyperparathyroid crisis; a collective review, Ann. Surg. 166:1012-1015, 1967.

18 Potts, J. T., Jr., Murray, T. M., Peacock, M., Niall, H. D., Tregear, G. W., Keutmann, H. T., Powell, D., and Deftos, L. J.: Parathyroid hormone: sequence, synthesis, immunoassay studies, Am. J. Med. 50:639-649, 1971.

19 Pyrah, L. N., Hodgkinson, A., and Anderson, C. K.: Critical review; primary hyperparathyroidism. Br. J. Surg. 53:245-316, 1966 (excellent review and extensive bibliography).

20 Schiffrin, M. J.: Relationship between the parathyroid and the gastric glands in the dog, Am. J. Physiol. 135:660-669, 1942.

21 Utley, J. R., and Black, W. C.: Hyperparathyroidism; a clinicopathologic evaluation, Am. J. Surg. 114:788-795, 1967.

22 Wills, M. R.: Normocalcaemic primary hyper-parathyroidism, Lancet **1**:849-853, 1971.

23 Winnacker, J. L., Becker, K. L., Friedlander, M., Higgins, G. A., Jr., and Moore, C. F.: Sarcoidosis and hyperparathyroidism, Am. J. Med. **46**:305-312, 1969.

Adenoma

24 Nolan, R. B., Hayles, A. B., and Woolner, L. B.: Adenoma of the parathyroid gland in children; report of case and brief review of the litera-ture, Am. J. Dis. Child. **99**:622-627, 1960.

25 Norris, E. H.: Collective review; parathyroid adenoma; study of 322 cases. Int. Abstr. Surg. **84**:1-41, 1947; in Surg. Gynecol. Obstet., Jan. 1947.

26 Woolner, L. B., Keating, F. R., Jr., and Black, B. M.: Tumors and hyperplasia of the parathy-roid glands; a review of the pathological find-ings in 140 cases of primary hyperparathy-roidism, Cancer **5**:1069-1088, 1952.

27 Wyman, S. M., and Robbins, L. L.: Roentgen recognition of parathyroid adenoma, Am. J. Roentgenol., Radium Ther. Nucl. Med. **71**: 5, 777-784, 1954.

Chief cell hyperplasia

28 Adams, P. H., Chalmers, T. M., Peters, N., Rack, J. H., and Truscott, B. McN.: Primary chief cell hyperplasia of the parathyroid glands, Ann. Intern. Med. **63**:454-467, 1965.

29 Black, W. C., and Haff, R. C.: The surgical pathology of parathyroid chief cell hyperplasia, Am. J. Clin. Pathol. **53**:565-579, 1970.

30 Cope, O., Keynes, W. M., Roth, S. I., and Castleman, B.: Primary chief-cell hyperplasia of the parathyroid glands: a new entity in the surgery of hyperparathyroidism, Ann. Surg. **148**:375-388, 1958.

Water-clear cell hyperplasia

31 Albright, F., Sulkowitch, H. W., and Bloom-berg, E.: Hyperparathyroidism due to idio-pathic hypertrophy (hyperplasia?) of parathy-roid tissue; follow-up report of 6 cases, Arch. Intern. Med. **62**:199-215, 1938.

32 Rogers, H. M., Keating, F. R., Jr., Morlock, C. G., and Baker, N. W.: Primary hyper-trophy and hyperplasia of the parathyroid gland associated with duodenal ulcer (report of additional case with special reference to metabolic, gastrointestinal and vascular mani-festations), Arch. Intern. Med. **79**:307-321, 1947.

Carcinoma

33 Alexander, H. B., Pemberton, J. D., Kepler, E. J., and Broders, A. C.: Functional parathy-roid tumors and hyperparathyroidism, Am. J. Surg. **65**:157-188, 1944.

34 Holmes, E. C., Morton, D. L., and Ketcham, A. S.: Parathyroid carcinoma: a collective re-view, Ann. Surg. **169**:631-640, 1969.

35 Schantz, A., and Castleman, B.: Parathyroid carcinoma, Cancer **31**:600-605, 1973.

Secondary hyperparathyroidism

36 Bricker, N. S., Slatopolsky, E., Reiss, E., and Avioli, L. V.: Calcium phosphorus, and bone in renal disease and transplantation, Arch. In-tern. Med. **123**:543-553, 1969.

37 Morgan, A. D., and Maclagan, N. F.: Renal disease in hyperparathyroidism, Am. J. Pathol. **30**:1141-1168, 1954.

38 Reiss, E., Canterbury, J. M., and Egdahl, R. H.: Experience with radioimmunoassay of PTH in human sera, Trans. Assoc. Am. Physi-cians **81**:104-115, 1968.

39 Roth, S. I., and Marshall, R. B.: Pathology and ultrastructure of the human parathyroid glands in chronic renal failure, Arch. Intern. Med. **124**:397-407, 1969.

"Tertiary" hyperparathyroidism

40 Black, W. C., Slatopolsky, E., Elkan, I., and Hoffsten, P.: Parathyroid morphology in sup-pressible and nonsuppressible renal hyperpara-thyroidism, Lab. Invest. **23**:497-509, 1970.

41 Davies, D. R., Dent, C. E., and Watson, L.: Tertiary hyperparathyroidism, Br. Med. J. **3**: 395-399, 1968.

42 Johnson, J. W., Hattner, R. S., Hampers, C. L., Bernstein, D. S., Merrill, J. P., and Sher-wood, L. M.: Secondary hyperparathyroidism in chronic renal failure; effects of renal homo-transplantaion, J.A.M.A. **215**:478-480, 1971.

43 McIntosh, D. A., Peterson, E. W., and Mc-Phaul, J. J., Jr.: Autonomy of parathyroid function after renal homotransplantation, Ann. Intern. Med. **65**:900-907, 1966.

Electron microscopy

44 Black W. C., III: Correlative light and elec-tron microscopy in primary hyperparathy-roidism, Arch. Pathol. **88**:225-241, 1969.

45 Faccini, J. M.: The ultrastructure of parathy-roid glands removed from patients with pri-mary hyperparathyroidism: a report of 40 cases, including four carcinomata, J. Pathol. **102**:189-199, 1970.

46 Roth, S. I.: The ultrastructure of primary water-clear cell hyperplasia of the parathyroid glands, Am. J. Pathol. **61**:233-240, 1970.

47 Selzman, H. M., and Fechner, R. E.: Oxyphil adenoma and primary hyperparathyroidism; clinical and ultrastructural observations, J.A.M.A. **199**:359-361, 1967.

**Hyperparathyroidism secondary to
nonparathyroid tumors**

48 Lafferty, F. W.: Pseudohyperparathyroidism, Medicine (Baltimore) **45**:247-260, 1966.
49 Omenn, G. S., Roth, S. I., and Baker, W. H.: Hyperparathyroidism associated with malignant tumors of nonparathyroid origin, Cancer **24**: 1004-1012, 1969.

Nonfunctioning lesions

50 Gordon, A., and Harcourt-Webster, J. N.: Parathyroid cysts: a report of two cases, J. Pathol. Bacteriol. **89**:374-377, 1965.
51 Maxwell, D. B., Horn, R. C., Jr., and Rhoads, J. E.: Cysts of the parathyroid: report of three cases clinically simulating nodular goiter, Arch. Surg. **64**:208-213, 1952.
52 Pachter, M. R., and Lattes, R.: Uncommon mediastinal tumors; report of two parathyroid adenomas, one nonfunctional parathyroid carcinoma and one "bronchial-type-adenoma," Dis. Chest **43**:519-528, 1963.
53 Rogers, L. A., Fetter, B. F., and Peete, W. P. J.: Parathyroid cyst and cystic degeneration of parathyroid adenoma, Arch. Pathol. **88**: 476-479, 1969.
54 Selzman, H. M., and Fechner, R. E.: Oxyphil adenoma and primary hyperparathyroidism; clinical and ultrastructural observations, J.A. M.A. **199**:359-361, 1967.
55 Sieracki, J. C., and Horn, R. C., Jr.: Nonfunctional carcinoma of the parathyroid, Cancer **13**:502-506, 1960.

Exploratory operation and treatment

56 Bricker, N. S., Slatopolsky, E., Reiss, E., and Avioli, L. V.: Calcium, phosphorus, and bone in renal disease and transplantation, Arch. Intern. Med. **123**:543-553, 1969.
57 Buck, B. A., and Robertson, R. D.: Indications for parathyroidectomy in advanced renal disease, Surg. Gynecol. Obstet. **133**:218-224, 1971.
58 Cope, O.: Surgery of hyperparathyroidism: the occurrence of parathyroids in the anterior mediastinum and the division of the operation into two stages, Ann. Surg. **114**:706-733, 1941.
59 Goldsmith, R. S., Furszyfer, J., Johnson, W. J., Fournier, A. E., and Arnaud, C. D.: Control of secondary hyperparathyroidism during longterm hemodialysis, Am. J. Med. **50**:692-699, 1971.
60 Goodman, M. L., Egdahl, R. H., Kemp, A., and Carey, L. C.: Hyperparathyroidism from intrathyroid parathyroid adenomas, Arch. Pathol. **87**:418-422, 1969.
61 Holmes, E. C., Morton, D. L., and Ketcham, A. S.: Parathyroid carcinoma: a collective review, Ann. Surg. **169**:631-640, 1969.
62 Nathaniels, E. K., Nathaniels, A. M., and Wang, C.-A.: Mediastinal parathyroid tumors: a clinical and pathological study of 84 cases, Ann. Surg. **171**:165-170, 1970.
63 Norris, E. H.: Collective review; parathyroid adenoma; study of 322 cases, Int. Abstr. Surg. **84**:1-41, 1947; in Surg. Gynecol. Obstet., Jan. 1947.
64 Purnell, D. C., Smith, L. H., Scholz, D. A., Elvebach, L. R., and Arnaud, C. D.: Primary hyperparathyroidism: a prospective clinical study, Am. J. Med. **50**:670-678, 1971.
65 Roth, S. I.: Pathology of the parathyroids in hyperparathyroidism, Arch. Pathol. **73**:495-510, 1962 (extensive bibliography).
66 Roth, S. I., and Munger, B. L.: The cytology of the adenomatous, atrophic, and hyperplastic parathyroid glands of man; a light- and electron-microscopic study, Virchows Arch. Pathol. Anat. **335**:389-410, 1962.
67 Walton, A. J.: The surgical treatment of parathyroid tumours, Br. J. Surg. **19**:285-291, 1931.

9 Thyroid gland

Introduction

The pathology of the thyroid gland is confusing chiefly because of the wide variations in the gross and microscopic patterns. Since these changes have been in-fluenced by the presence or absence of adequate iodine intake, the pathology varies in different areas of the world. In the United States, such differences have been erased at least in part because of the availability of iodized salt. Classification of thyroid disease has also been in a chaotic state, particularly from the viewpoint of neoplasms.

The thyroid parenchyma is not arranged in lobules, for in reconstruction models, follicles or vesicles are closed cavities not communicating with each other.[3] These vesicles vary in size from 20μ to 100μ, are lined with epithelium, and are filled with a stainable substance called colloid. The epithelial lining has a basement membrane and rests on fine connective tissue in which there are capillary blood vessels, lymphatics, and nerves. Between the follicles there are collections of endocrine cells believed to secrete calcitonin and therefore designated as C cells by Pearse.[2] They are difficult to identify in normal human thyroid glands, but recent electron microscopic studies have documented their presence[4] (Fig. 327). Klinck et al.[1] have described the electron microscopic features of the normal human thyroid gland in detail.

Thyroglossal duct cyst, branchial cleft cyst, and heterotopic thyroid tissue

"The thyroid anlage appears in the 2.0 to 2.5 mm. embryo as a midline structure, projecting downward from the pharynx between the first and second branchial arches. This point of origin corresponds to the

303

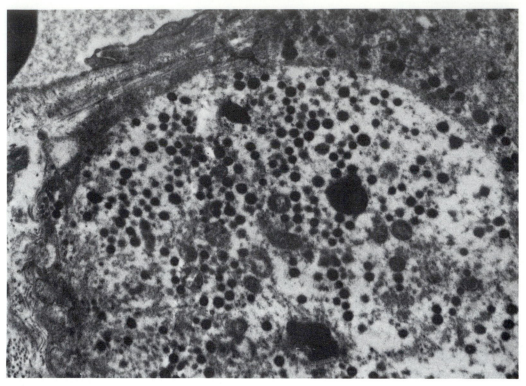

Fig. 327 Group of parafollicular cells in normal human thyroid gland. Cytoplasm contains numerous ''neurosecretory'' granules. (Courtesy Dr. S. Teitelbaum, St. Louis, Mo.)

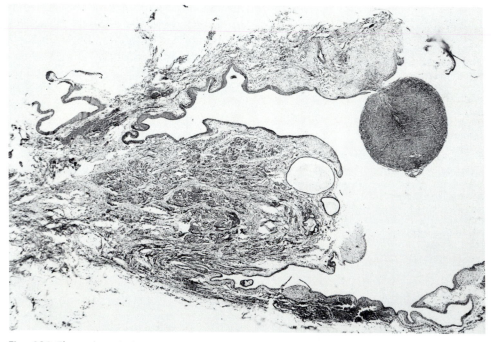

Fig. 328 Thyroglossal duct cyst. Note lymphoid tissue, epithelial lining, and cystic spaces. (Low power; WU neg. 50-2837.)

foramen cecum in adult life. The midline thyroid anlage then descends in the course of development to its position in the anterior neck. In the normal course of events, any connection between the cervical thyroid and its point of origin at the base of the tongue is obliterated and disappears. However, in certain instances, remnants of the strand of tissue connecting these points may remain, along with portions of the epithelial lining of the mouth cavity which have been dragged downward as the thyroid descends, to persist as definite structures and form cysts, sinuses, and fistulae found in later life."*

The hyoid bone formed from the second arch appears in the embryo following the descent of the thyroid gland. This bone divides the thyroglossal remnant into an infrahyoid and a suprahyoid portion. The tract passes anteriorly, posteriorly, or through the bone. The *cyst and sinuses of thyroglossal origin* are lined by pseudostratified and ciliated columnar cells. A squamous lining and mucous glands may be present[8] (Fig. 328). An inflammatory process is common.

The most frequent abnormality is a midline cyst usually in the region of the hyoid bone[16] (Fig. 329). The sinuses may develop from the suprasternal notch to the region of the hyoid bone. In order to treat this lesion adequately, it is essential that the tract be completely removed from the foramen cecum with resection of the central portion of the hyoid bone. A cyst may develop because there is secretion from the cells lining the tract. If the foramen cecum remains open, the tract may become directly infected. Cutaneous sinuses may develop.[13] These cysts are most common in childhood but may assume clinical significance even after the age of 50 years.[7] Cancer can rarely arise in thyroglossal duct remnants. Jaques et al.[9] reviewed thirty-

seven published cases and added eighteen of their own. The large majority were papillary carcinomas.

Branchial cleft cysts and sinuses may appear in the anterior lateral portion of the neck from the preauricular region to the clavicle. A cyst or sinus appearing in the preauricular area or beneath the posterior half of the mandible usually is derived from the first branchial cleft and may be connected to the external auditory canal. These lesions are rare. Lesions appearing just anterior to the sternocleidomastoid muscle in the lower half of the neck probably are remnants of the second branchial cleft. These may have an open squamous-lined tract that communicates with the pharynx near the superior fold of the tonsil. These cleft defects may consist of patent pharyngocutaneous fistulas, simple sinuses, and blind cysts (Fig. 330). Cysts also occasionally communicate with the pharynx but not with the skin.[10]

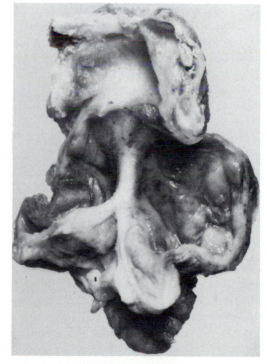

Fig. 329 Thyroglossal duct cyst from 62-year-old man. Cyst measured 6 cm × 6 cm. (WU neg. 66-7878.)

*From Stahl, W. M., Jr., and Lyall, D.: Cervical cysts and fistulae of thyroglossal tract origin, Ann. Surg. **139**:123-128, 1954.

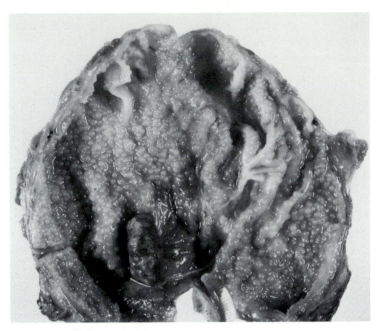

Fig. 330 Branchial cleft cyst measuring 4.5 cm × 3 cm × 1.5 cm removed from 18-year-old youth. It has been opened to expose inner surface. This is made irregular by presence of folds and innumerable hyperplastic lymphoid follicles. (WU neg. 67-1473).

The lining of these cysts and fistulous tracts is usually squamous epithelium, but columnar ciliated epithelium is common. Abundant lymphoid tissue, often with germinal centers, is observed beneath this epithelium. Mucous glands are rare. Infection may complicate the microscopic picture. We have yet to see an unquestionable case of epidermoid cancer arising in a branchial cleft cyst. Any cystic mass in the neck containing squamous cancer must be considered a lymph node metastasis with cystic degeneration.

If there is faulty descent of the thyroid gland, it may be situated anywhere along the course of the duct.[12] The most frequent location of this *heterotopic thyroid tissue* is in the region of the base of the tongue or in the pharyngeal portion of the foramen cecum. Sauk[15] examined microscopically the area of the foramen cecum in 200 consecutive autopsies and found thyroid elements in twenty cases. Very rarely, lingual thyroid tissue may be present anteriorly in the tongue[14] or within the larynx[6] (Fig. 331). Rather frequently, thy-

roid tissue also may be found free in the anterior portion of the mediastinum but rarely in the posterior portion.[17]

Grossly, the thyroid tissue found in such heterotopic nodules does not differ from that found elsewhere. When such tissue is located near the base of the tongue, there may be an imperfect capsule with nodules of thyroid tissue between muscle bundles. This may cause confusion and may result in an erroneous diagnosis of carcinoma.[19] Although aberrant thyroid tissue is usually benign, carcinomas have been reported.[5, 18]

Patients with lingual thyroid gland have some difficulty in swallowing and some degree of pharyngeal and laryngeal obstruction (Fig. 332). We have seen an infant die of respiratory insufficiency because of a large unrecognized lingual thyroid gland. Lingual thyroid glands may first present clinically during puberty and adolescence.[11]

When heterotopic thyroid tissue is present, complete absence of the thyroid gland in its normal location occurs in approximately 70% of instances. Therefore, myxedema often follows removal of hetero-

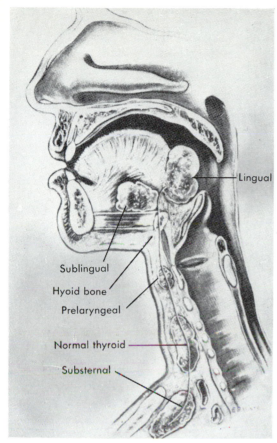

Fig. 331 Distribution of heterotopic thyroid tissue. (WU neg. 50-1570; from Lemmon, W. T., and Paschal, G. W., Jr.: Lingual thyroid, Am. J. Surg. **52**:82-85, 1941.)

topic thyroid tissue if thyroid extract is not given.

Specific infections
Syphilis

Syphilis of the thyroid gland is rare. Grossly, the lesion is asymmetrical and frequently hard and may cause fixation of the gland to the surrounding structures and even paralysis of the recurrent laryngeal nerve. This lesion is a manifestation of tertiary syphilis. We have not seen this condition.

Children may also have gummatous nodules of the thyroid gland associated with syphilitic visceral lesions. Microscopically, the lesion is a nodular gummatous process.

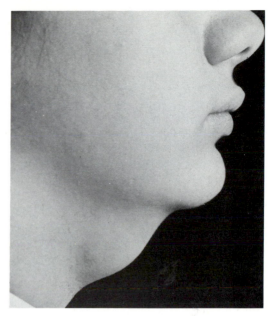

Fig. 332 Young girl with heterotopic thyroid gland. (WU neg. 49-1754.)

Clinically, it is often thought to be carcinoma.

Tuberculosis

Tuberculosis as a primary clinical manifestation within the thyroid gland is a pathologic rarity. In disseminated miliary tuberculosis, it is not rare for an occasional tubercle to occur within the gland. It is also possible for tuberculous cervical lymph nodes or tuberculous involvement of the larynx to involve the thyroid gland secondarily.

In the past, tuberculosis was frequently misdiagnosed in cases of subacute (de Quervain's) thyroiditis because of the presence of Langhans' type giant cells arranged around disintegrating follicles and forming a granuloma.

Acute infectious thyroiditis

A rare form of inflammation, acute infectious thyroiditis may be nonsuppurative or of purulent character. It is often associated with acute infections of the pharynx and upper respiratory tract. *Streptococcus hemolyticus*, *Staphylococcus aureus*, and

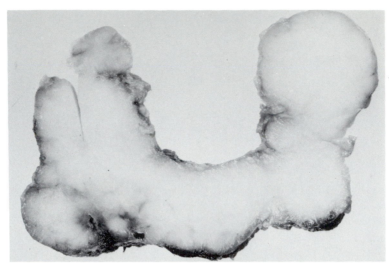

Fig. 333 Cross section of thyroid gland with chronic granulomatous thyroiditis. Note preservation of normal symmetry and presence of capsule. Patient had minimal pressure signs and symptoms. (WU neg. 49-868.)

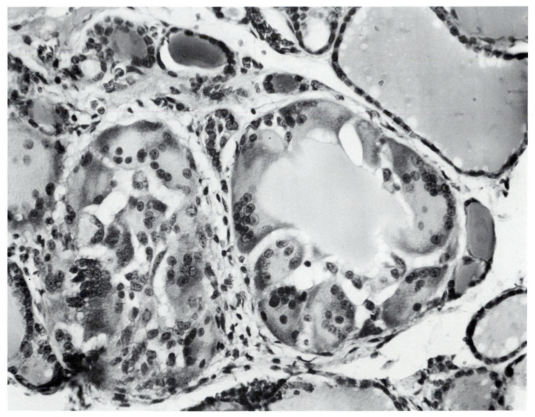

Fig. 334 Focus of granulomatous thyroiditis. Note intimate relation and formation of giant cells around colloid. (×300; WU neg. 72-5906.)

Pneumococcus are the organisms most commonly responsible.[20]

Subacute (granulomatous or de Quervain) thyroiditis

Subacute thyroiditis, a relatively common form of thyroiditis, is probably not related to infection. It may be associated with infections about the oral cavity. However, the lesion within the thyroid gland is nonbacterial in nature.[23]

Grossly, the process usually involves the entire gland, but the enlargement is often asymmetrical. The gland usually is enlarged approximately twice its normal size. In the advanced stage of the process, the involved areas are firm (Fig. 333). In contrast to Riedel's struma, there is usually little or no adherence to the surrounding structures.

The microscopic changes have been described well by de Quervain and Giordanengo.[22] Focal areas of acute inflammation and giant cells engulfing colloid are frequent (Fig. 334). Occasionally, microabscesses and granulomatous zones are present. The same thyroid tissue may show different stages of the inflammatory process.[24]

Clinicopathologic correlation

Early in the evolution of this process, the throat may be sore, deglutition may be quite painful, and the thyroid gland may be extremely tender. Patients with thyroiditis often are explored for carcinoma inasmuch as pressure symptoms, hypothyroidism, and signs suggestive of malignancy may occur after the acute process has subsided. Thyroiditis can rarely occur with papillary carcinoma and be confusing clinically and pathologically.[21] The diagnosis is usually made by frozen section at the time of surgical exploration.

The best treatment has not been defined. ACTH and cortisone have proved valuable. Irradiation therapy has not been very successful. Frequently, subtotal thyroidectomy is performed.

Riedel's struma (struma fibrosa)

Riedel's struma was described by Riedel[29] in 1896. Joll[28] reported finding an incidence of about five times as many cases of Hashimoto's disease as Riedel's struma. Although the disease predominates slightly in females, it has approximately the same incidence as other diseases of the thyroid gland in similar geographic areas. In the cases reported by Woolner et al.,[30] the patients were between 30 and 67 years of age.

The pathogenesis of invasive thyroiditis is obscure, but most authorities believe it is an independent entity bearing no relation to Hashimoto's disease. It also appears

Table 10 Gross and microscopic characteristics of subacute thyroiditis, Hashimoto's disease, and Riedel's struma

Characteristics	Subacute thyroiditis (granulomatous)	Hashimoto's disease	Riedel's struma (struma fibrosa)
Gross			
Consistency	Firm	Firm	Extremely firm
Involvement	Diffuse	Diffuse	Asymmetrical
Adherence to surrounding structures	Delicate if present	Delicate if present	Strongly adherent
Microscopic			
Microabscesses	Present	Absent	Absent
Lymphoid tissue	Minimal	Present throughout with germinal centers	Minimal
Giant cells	Common	Rare	Absent
Fibrous tissue	Increased	Slightly increased; fine, with even distribution	Extremely prominent

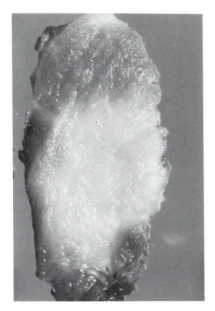

Fig. 335 Riedel's struma. Diffuse fibrotic process involves thyroid gland and surrounding tissues and obliterates anatomic boundaries. (WU neg. 60-4758.)

to bear no relation to subacute thyroiditis (Table 10).

Grossly, the process is asymmetrical and involves only localized areas of the thyroid gland (Fig. 335). The involved portion is stony hard and fixed to surrounding structures. At operation, the tissue plane about the capsule is obliterated. Dense fibrous strands extend from the capsule into adjacent muscle. The gland cuts with great resistance. On cross section, the fibrous tissue present may completely obliterate the normal architecture. Outside a poorly demarcated border, the thyroid gland usually appears quite normal.

Microscopically, fibrous tissue that is frequently extensively hyalinized completely replaces the area of the gland involved (Fig. 336). Muscle cells in the immediate area are often directly infiltrated by this connective tissue. Giant cells are absent, and no evidence of acute inflammation exists.

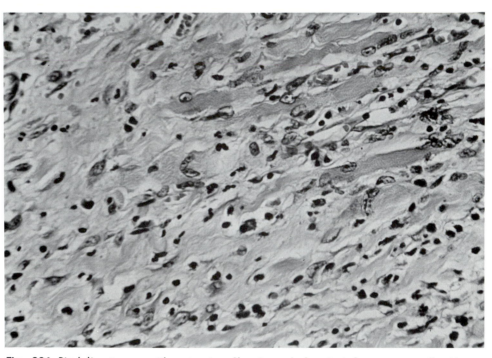

Fig. 336 Riedel's struma with extensive fibrosis and chronic inflammatory cells. No residual thyroid tissue can be identified. (×370; WU neg. 57-4809; slide contributed by Dr. L. Woolner, Rochester, Minn.)

Clinicopathologic correlation

Riedel's struma is not preceded clinically by an acute inflammatory process or by tenderness of the thyroid gland.[26, 27] It is almost impossible to differentiate it clinically from carcinoma. It binds the surrounding structures of the neck in an iron collar and may compress the trachea to a slitlike state. Patients frequently have profound dyspnea, particularly when in a recumbent position. Frozen section is diagnostic in differentiating this condition from carcinoma. If a definitive diagnosis can be made, it is wise to resect the area surgically, for this lesion is focal, and resection relieves the obstructive symptoms.

Resection is often quite difficult because no plane of cleavage exists. Large veins may be torn. Adjoining muscles frequently must be cut and partially resected in order to remove the diseased thyroid tissue. The regional lymph nodes do not become involved, a factor that may provide a clue to the diagnosis. Hypothyroidism does not usually follow resection. Riedel's struma is a rare lesion. Woolner et al.[30] were able to find only twenty cases in the Mayo Clinic files between 1920 and 1955. There was only one case per 2,000 thyroidectomies. Riedel's struma has been seen associated with mediastinal fibrosis, retroperitoneal fibrosis, sclerosing cholangitis, and pseudotumor of the orbit.[25]

Hashimoto's disease (struma lymphomatosa)

Struma lymphomatosa was first described by Hashimoto[36] in 1912, and the clinical and pathologic description of his four cases is still classical. The pathogenesis of this condition is obscure. Doniach and Roitt[34] demonstrated that the serum of patients with Hashimoto's disease contains autoantibodies against thyroglobulin. The antibody is organ specific.

Schade et al.[42] demonstrated that circulating antibody to thyroglobulin was significantly associated with lymphocytic infiltrate in patients with Graves' disease, toxic adenoma, and nontoxic nodular goiter. To complicate this picture, Balfour et al.,[31] with fluorescent antibody technique, showed autoantibodies to thyroid colloid components other than thyroglobulin in human thyroiditis. Furthermore, DeGroot et al.[33] believe that circulating autoantibodies are not the cause of Hashimoto's thyroiditis and think that this may be a reaction of a delayed hypersensitivity type. The final microscopic pattern is the result of exhaustion atrophy.

Hashimoto's disease is predominantly a disease of women over 40 years of age and bears no relation to Riedel's struma, which often occurs at an earlier age. In Marshall and Meissner's series[41] of 114 patients, 112 were women. Biopsies taken at different times usually reveal a similar histologic picture.[39] Graham and McCullagh,[35] Joll,[38] and McSwain and Moore[40] support the concept that Hashimoto's disease is a separate entity from Riedel's struma.

Grossly, the entire thyroid gland is involved by disease and is enlarged proportionately. It is asymmetrical only when the lobes of the gland are asymmetrical. It has a firm but not stony hard consistency. The fascial attachment between the thyroid gland and the tracheal wall is, at times, slightly thickened, but there is no strong fixation. On section, early lesions are quite friable. The gland is pseudolobulated and has a pale pink and yellowish white color. The cross section looks somewhat like a hyperplastic lymph node replaced by yellowish gray material (Fig. 337). Necrosis, abscess, and calcification are absent, and colloid is not clearly discernible.

Microscopically, there is diffuse infiltration by lymphoid tissue, and invariably large follicles with definite germinal centers are present (Fig. 338). This lymphoid tissue is distributed both interlobularly and intralobularly. The surrounding acini are small and invariably atrophic. The cells that form these acini are large and have acidophilic cytoplasm. Foreign body giant cells are not frequent. Connective tissue, when present, is evenly distributed and is

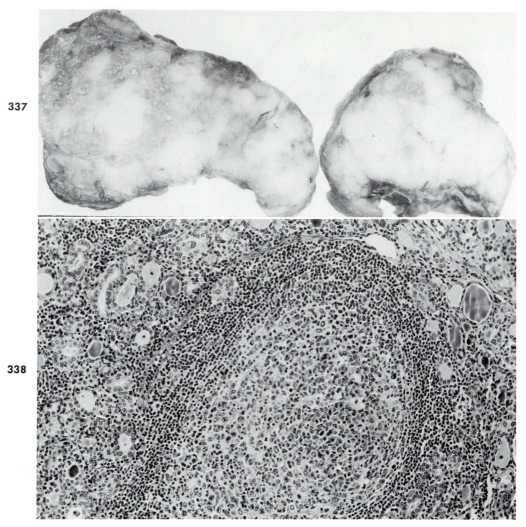

Fig. 337 Hashimoto's disease in child demonstrating homogeneous yellowish gray areas, representing increased lymphoid tissue. (WU neg. 50-1462.)
Fig. 338 Hashimoto's disease. Note increased lymphoid tissue with germinal center. Cells lining follicles are oxyphilic. (×150; WU neg. 50-683.)

seen only in the advanced stages of the disease.

The lymphoid infiltration in Hashimoto's disease must be distinguished from that seen in hyperplastic thyroid glands. The latter usually lacks germinal centers and is associated with focal or diffuse hyperplasia of the follicular cells.

Clinicopathologic correlation

Hashimoto's disease causes diffuse, firm enlargement of the thyroid gland and early signs of compression of the trachea or esophagus. At operation, the thyroid gland is usually quite easily separated from other structures. Because of the firm character of the lesion, it may be confused with carcinoma, but the diffuse involvement without fixation to the surrounding structures should be strong evidence against it. The diagnosis is usually made on frozen section, and subtotal thyroidectomy is done. The resulting hypothyroidism must be controlled with thyroid extract.

The diagnosis of Hashimoto's disease is relatively simple when it conforms to the gross and microscopic patterns described. There are numerous examples, however, in which there are focal areas of lymphoid tissue with perhaps slight evidence of follicular hyperplasia.[43] In such instances, we have dismissed the lymphoid hyperplasia as a simple accompaniment of the epithelial changes.

We do not know the pathogenesis of Hashimoto's disease. Neither do we have evidence that it ever becomes Riedel's struma or that patients with Hashimoto's disease ever had preexisting thyrotoxicosis. In twenty patients with Hashimoto's disease reported by Heptinstall and Eastcott,[37] none had thyrotoxicosis, and none had passed through a toxic phase. In a study made at our institution by Spjut et al.,[44] the minimal histologic findings for a diagnosis of Hashimoto's disease included a diffuse, or almost diffuse, oxyphilic transformation of the follicle epithelium, the presence of lymphoid follicles, and fibrosis of the stroma. In a study of thyroid specimens removed at interval operations on seventy-six patients with Graves' disease and toxic (nonexophthalmic) and nontoxic goiters, we were unable to demonstrate, convincingly, progression of thyroid hyperplasia to struma lymphomatosa, chronic thyroiditis, or Riedel's struma. Papillary carcinoma and malignant lymphoma of the thyroid gland may be associated with Hashimoto's disease.[32]

Lymphocytic thyroiditis

Lymphocytic thyroiditis is a common cause of goiter in children.[45] It can be accurately diagnosed by needle biopsy.[46] Patients with this condition usually present with asymptomatic goiter, often of short duration. Grossly, there is diffuse enlargement of the gland and increased consistency. Microscopically, there is extensive lymphocytic infiltration, germinal centers often being present. The feature distinguishing it from Hashimoto's disease is the absence or inconspicuousness of oxyphilic epithelial changes. It is likely that some of these cases represent an early stage in the evolution of Hashimoto's disease.

Diffuse hyperplasia (Graves' disease; exophthalmic goiter)

The pathogenesis of Graves' disease is not well understood. It is generally included among the autoimmune thyroid diseases, together with Hashimoto's disease and idiopathic myxedema. Long-acting thyroid stimulator (LATS), a 7S γ-globulin with thyroid-stimulating properties, is present in approximately 70% of the patients with Graves' disease and is probably the most important thyroid stimulator. There is good evidence that pituitary TSH is not involved in the pathogenesis of Graves' disease.[49] The onset may be related to psychogenic factors.

Grossly, the smooth symmetrical gland of hyperthyroidism usually is not much enlarged. The changes in the gland may be altered by preoperative therapy: Lugol's solution (5% elemental iodine and 10% potassium iodide) or related compounds tend to produce involutionary changes; propylthiouracil and its relaxed compounds block the release of thyroxine and cause rapid disappearance of symptoms. The gland itself, however, is still grossly and microscopically unchanged, and bleeding from it may be difficult to control. For this reason, propylthiouracil therapy is supplemented with Lugol's solution for approximately ten days before operation.

The gland is usually succulent and vascular and on section has the consistency of pancreatic tissue. It is uniformly brown, yellow, gray, or red, varying in vascularity, colloid content, and degree of hyperplasia (Fig. 339). Usually follicles can be found. If the disease is of long duration, the gland is often friable and dull yellow.

Microscopically, the changes that allow a diagnosis of hyperplasia rest primarily on epithelial alterations. The prominence of these epithelial changes depends on the degree of hyperplasia and the response of the gland to therapeutic measures tending to produce involution (Lugol's solution; roentgen ray therapy).

In the normal gland, the individual cells are flat cuboidal, with nuclei resting at the base. With increased activity, the epithe-

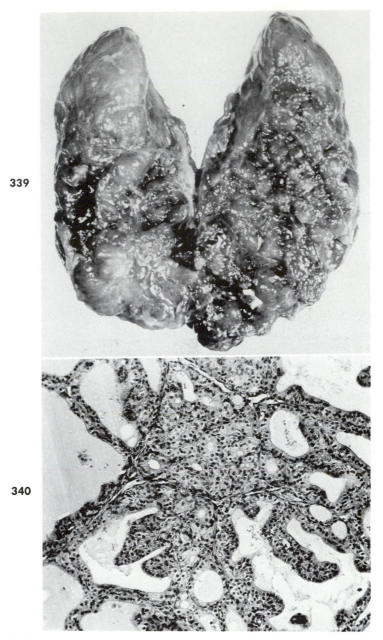

Fig. 339 Thyroid gland in diffuse hyperplasia. Gland is diffusely enlarged, hyperemic, and without nodules. (WU neg. 48-5014.)

Fig. 340 Hyperplasia of thyroid gland. Note solid masses of cells, high columnar epithelium, and papillary infolding. (High power; WU neg. 48-3404.)

lium becomes columnar and often papillary. Papillary proliferation occurs as the gland becomes increasingly vascular (Fig. 340). At times, this epithelial proliferation is so pronounced that an inexperienced pathologist may be tempted to call the changes carcinoma. In fact, it may be so extreme that papillary epithelial proliferation will extend into contiguous muscle[51] (Fig. 341). Even with pronounced involu-

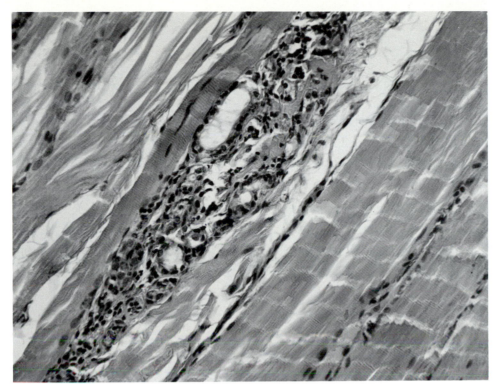

Fig. 341 Hyperplastic thyroid tissue invading muscle in 29-year-old man with Graves disease. (×275; WU neg. 62-3623; slide contributed by Dr. J. Glenn, Billings, Mont.)

tionary changes, if enough sections are cut, the pathologist can usually determine the presence of preexisting hyperplasia.

Other changes supporting the diagnosis of hyperplasia include pale, finely vacuolated colloid and aggregations of lymphoid tissue without germinal centers. This lymphoid tissue persists after involution. If the process is of long duration, the connective tissue is increased. Cells of primary hyperplasia may contain foamy cytoplasm. These cells also may be present in adenomatous goiters and rarely in tumors. In some instances, the fat and glycogen stains are positive.[51]

The thyroid glands of patients treated with I^{131} for thyrotoxicosis have been examined at autopsy at varying times after treatment.[47] The early changes are pronounced nuclear abnormalities, dissolution of some of the follicles, and specific irradiational vascular alterations. Later, there is great reduction in the size of the thyroid gland, with zones of scarring, and only scattered small follicles.

Clinicopathologic correlation

Classical Graves' disease usually appears in highly emotional patients and is accompanied by the typical eye signs, a markedly elevated basal metabolic rate, tachycardia, and often a great increase of appetite. Atrial fibrillation may occur. In patients with advanced disease, cardiac failure and liver damage may exist. Muscle weakness, weight loss, and increased resting pulse rate are important clinical manifestations. Thyroid acropachy, a late manifestation of hyperthyroidism, consists of swelling of the extremities and clubbing of the fingers and/or toes. The latter change is due to a characteristic type of periosteal new bone formation.[52] Elevation of the serum protein-bound iodine level and the increased radioactive iodine uptake are the most objective laboratory find-

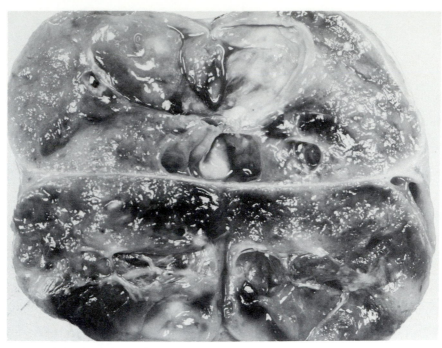

Fig. 342 Nodular hyperplasia of thyroid gland with cystic and hemorrhagic areas. (WU neg. 48-5204.)

ings supporting diagnosis of Graves' disease.

All of the clinical signs and symptoms, with the exception of exophthalmos, dramatically subside under appropriate therapy. By use of radioactive iodine, Goode et al.[48] demonstrated that even after the most radical operation, one-fifth the normal uptake could be expected within one year. Unfortunately, this is not true for other types of thyroid pathology. In Hashimoto's disease, progressive atrophy takes place. Furthermore, if a resected hyperplastic gland microscopically shows evidence of thyroid exhaustion (oxyphilia and lymphocytic infiltration), the patient has a greater chance of developing myxedema than when these changes are absent.[50]

Nodular hyperplasia with or without hyperthyroidism

The incidence of nodular hyperplasia will depend, to a great extent, on the geographic distribution of patients. Of 544,918 patients in the Boston City Hospital, the Massachusetts General Hospital, and Johns Hopkins Hospital, only 0.59% were admitted for goiter.[58] By contrast, 1.7% of 68,573 patients admitted to the Illinois Research Hospital (during 11.5 years) had nodular goiters (roughly 3.5 times the incidence on the Atlantic Seaboard).[53] In areas of endemic thyroid disease, some degree of nodular thyroid inevitably is found at postmortem examination. Of course, in endemic areas a considerable discrepancy exists between the frequency of clinical nontoxic nodular goiter and the almost 100% frequency of such disease at postmortem examination.

Grossly, the shape of a nodular thyroid gland is greatly distorted (Fig. 342). One lobe frequently is much larger than the other. The capsule of the lobe usually is intact. On cross section, multiple areas of hemorrhage and calcification are frequent. The variable individual nodules within the lobe are frequently surrounded by an incomplete fibrous tissue capsule. Occasionally, a large cystic area of degen-

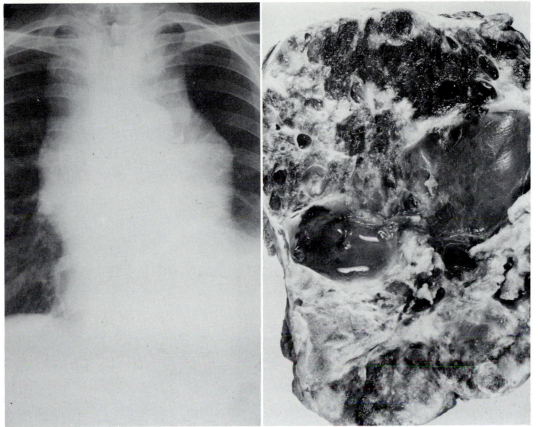

343 344

Fig. 343 Large anterior mediastinal nodular thyroid gland. (WU neg. 49-5739.)
Fig. 344 Same nodular thyroid gland shown in Fig. 343. Note nodulation, hemorrhage, and cyst formation. (WU neg. 49-6863.)

eration in which hemorrhage has occurred is removed as a dominant nodule. Because of the increased frequency of carcinoma in these thyroid glands, it is important that the gross specimen be fixed first and step sections made so that discovery of questionable areas of malignancy will be more likely seen.

These thyroid glands usually are removed because of pressure signs, cosmetic reasons, increased evidence of thyrotoxicosis in women at the menopause, and, finally, because of the increased chance of carcinoma. Such nodular glands may be located substernally (Figs. 343 and 344).

Microscopically, nodular thyroid glands are variable. The follicles differ tremendously in size. Giant follicles lined by flattened epithelium are frequent. If colloid escapes into the interstitial tissue, it provokes an interstitial reaction. Frequently there are areas of recent, as well as old, hemorrhage, often containing deposits of hemosiderin. Coarse trabeculae of fibrous tissue completely separate the lobules. Areas of calcification are frequent, but bone formation is rare. Greatly thickened vessels may occur around the periphery of the gland. Their media is often calcified.

The nodular gland always shows some evidence of hyperplasia, but it is very difficult to predict on the basis of the microscopic appearance whether or not the patient will have clinical or laboratory evidence of hyperthyroidism. Hyperplastic epithelium in an enlarged nodu-

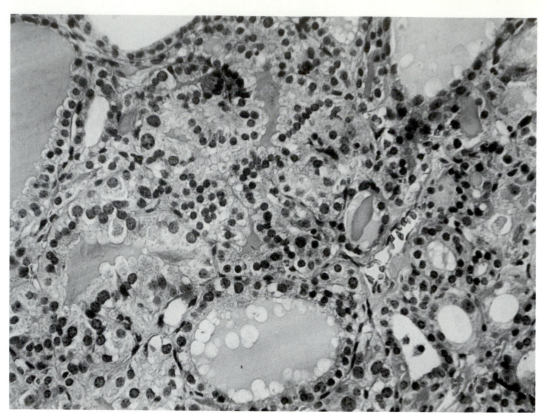

Fig. 345 Thyroid gland from 13-year-old Marshallese girl who developed nodular thyroid ten years after accidental exposure to radioactive fallout. Many nuclei are enlarged and hyperchromatic. (×340; WU neg. 67-530.)

lar gland should not be accepted as evidence of thyrotoxicosis. The prominent eye signs of Graves' disease do not occur in patients with nodular toxic goiter. The presence of thyroid cells with atypical nuclei in a multinodular gland should make the pathologist suspect previous exposure to radioactive substances (Fig. 345).

Radioautography is useful in correlating pathology of the thyroid gland with its function. "Hot" nodules of the thyroid gland are usually benign except in the rare instance in which they hide a small nonfunctioning carcinoma (two cases in our experience). It is common for a "hot" nodule to undergo cystic degeneration so that only a rim of highly functioning thyroid remains. "Cold" nodules are nondiagnostic and may represent either cancer or

a nontoxic, nonfunctioning nodular thyroid gland or a nonfunctioning adenoma.[55] Autoradiography indicates the difficulty of appraising the activity of a given follicle (Fig. 346).

Occasionally, a patient may be euthyroid and still have focal papillary areas of hyperplasia that take up radioactive iodine. Autoradiography is useful in such cases. We have seen such areas of focal hyperplasia mistaken for papillary cancer (Fig. 347).

Clinicopathologic correlation

The nodular thyroid gland, particularly the one without clinical evidence of hyperthyroidism, may manifest itself as a single, firm, dominant lump that clinically may exactly simulate a neoplasm. However, if the tumor is soft and poorly defined and

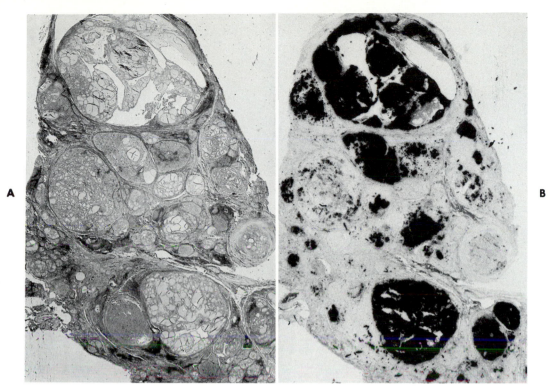

Fig. 346 Photomicrograph and autoradiograph of hyperplastic nodule. Note variation in uptake. It is impossible microscopically to make such distinctions. (**A**, WU neg. 61-1125; **B**, WU neg. 61-1126; **A** and **B**, courtesy Dr. J. S. Meyer, St. Louis, Mo.)

waxes and wanes with physiologic function, the chances are great that it is not malignant. The fully blown nodular thyroid gland may become very large, cause some degree of tracheal obstruction, and produce considerable facial disfigurement. For these reasons, it should be removed. When hyperplasia is present, there is very little chance that carcinoma is coexistent.

Any association of carcinoma and diffuse hyperplasia in the same thyroid gland is probably coincidence.[57] It is only with clinically demonstrable, nodular, nontoxic thyroid glands that the frequency of carcinoma reaches an important figure. The association between various types of thyroid disease and cancer is shown in Table 11.

Obviously, the high incidence of carcinoma associated with clinically solitary nontoxic nodular goiter reported in Table 11 is the result of patient selection. Although the data represent the incidence

of thyroid cancer in patients undergoing thyroidectomy, this rate is far in excess of that found in the total population.[59] Greene[54] and Hargreaves and Garner[56] have shown a striking correlation between the degree of lymphocytic infiltration present in the resected thyroid gland and the incidence of postoperative hypothyroidism.

Colloid and congenital goiter

Diffuse colloid goiter is an expression of iodine lack, and it is infrequent in the United States even in endemic areas because of the use of iodized salt. The thyroid glands are diffusely enlarged and simply show enlarged follicles filled with colloid. Congenital goiter in the United States also is extremely rare because of the use of iodized salt. In Switzerland before the obligatory use of iodized salt, congenital goiter was frequent. A child showing such change may have a "goiterous"

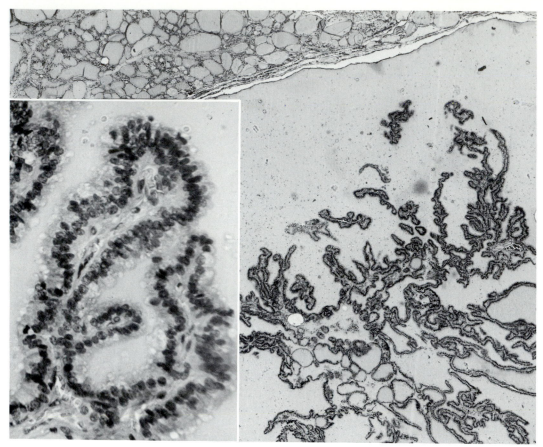

Fig. 347 Focal papillary area in thyroid gland diagnosed incorrectly as papillary cancer. It was really a "hot" zone, and this could have been demonstrated by autoradiography. **Inset** demonstrates typical pattern of hyperplastic fronds with tall columnar cells. (×34; WU Neg. 72-230; **inset,** ×300; WU neg. 72-226.)

Table 11 Incidence of carcinoma in nodular goiter as obtained from numerous reports in literature*

Author	Nodular goiter (toxic and nontoxic)		Nodular nontoxic goiter		Carcinoma in solitary nontoxic nodular goiter (%)
	Number of patients	%	Number of patients	%	
Horn et al. Philadelphia, Pa. 1947	1,135	6.3	637	9.8	
Ward San Francisco, Calif. 1947	3,539	4.8			15.6
Crile Cleveland, Ohio 1948	537	5.6	274	10.9	24.5
Cole et al. Chicago, Ill. 1948	663	8.0	285	17.1	24.4

*From Cole, W. H., Slaughter, D. P., and Majarakis, J. D.: Carcinoma of the thyroid gland, Surg. Gynecol. Obstet. **89:** 349-356, 1949; by permission of Surgery, Gynecology & Obstetrics.

mother.[61] Because such goiters regress with iodine therapy, it is rare that a surgical pathologist has the opportunity of seeing one.

There are several types of goiter due to enzyme defects in hormone synthesis[60, 63] (Figs. 348 and 349). Kennedy[62] found, in a review of thirty such cases, that in those associated with the formation of an abnormal iodoprotein, the thyroid gland had a characteristic microcystic pattern on gross examination. Microscopically, nodules were often present, formed by trabeculae and small follicles with scanty colloid. Papillary foci and a moderate degree of cellular pleomorphism were also noted. Goiters associated with defective deiodination of monoiodotyrosine and diiodotyrosine were always nodular and simulated malignancy to a striking degree because of papillary proliferation, pleomorphism, and invasion of capsule and wall of blood vessels. Goiters secondary to defective organification of iodine were also nodular and trabecular/microfollicular but showed only a moderate degree of cellular atypia.

Tumors

Classification

Following is a classification of neoplasms of the thyroid gland:

A Benign tumors
  1 Adenoma
    a Simple
    b Hürthle cell
B Malignant tumors
  1 Carcinoma
    a Papillary
    b Follicular (alveolar)
      Invasive
      Encapsulated angioinvasive
    c Hürthle cell
    d Anaplastic
      (1) Small cell
      (2) Giant cell
      (3) Spindle cell
    e Occult sclerosing
    f Epidermoid
    g Medullary
  2 Other primary tumors
    a Malignant lymphoma
    b Plasmacytoma
    c Fibrosarcoma
    d Angiosarcoma
    e Teratoma
  3 Metastatic carcinoma

Table 12 A study of 301 cancers of thyroid gland*

	Number	%
Papillary adenocarcinoma	139	46
Follicular and alveolar adenocarcinoma	22	7
Solid adenocarcinoma	56	19
Giant cell carcinoma	39	13
Hürthle cell carcinoma	27	9
Unclassified†	18	6
Total	301	100

(Lymphosarcomas and squamous carcinomas omitted)

*From Frazell, E. L., and Foote, F. W.: The natural history of thyroid cancer, J. Clin. Endocrinol. Metab. 9:1023-1030, 1949.
†Histologic material not adequate to classify.

Table 13 A study of 439 cancers of thyroid gland*

	Number	%
Group 1—Adenoma with invasion	108	24.6
(a) Blood vessel invasion	12	
(b) Capsular or lymphatic invasion	61	
(c) Capsular or lymphatic plus blood vessel invasion	35	
Group 2—Adenocarcinoma	203	46.2
(a) Papillary type	154	
(b) Alveolar type	49	
Group 3—Carcinoma simplex	108	24.6
(a) Small cell type	72	
(b) Giant cell type	36	
Miscellaneous	20	4.6
(a) Hürthle cell carcinoma	7	
(b) Fibrosarcoma	7	
(c) Lymphoma	3	
(d) Epidermoid carcinoma	2	
(e) Unclassified	1	
Total	439	100

*From Meissner, W. A., and Lahey, F. H.: Cancer of the thyroid in a thyroid clinic, J. Clin. Endocrinol. Metab. 8:749-761, 1948.

The frequency of various types of carcinoma of the thyroid gland in two large series[64, 65] is shown in Tables 12 and 13.

It must be remembered that the classifi-

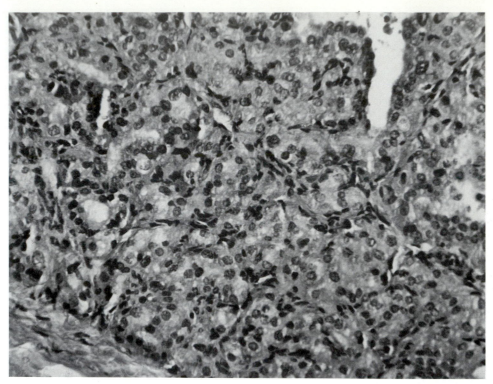

Fig. 348 Congenital goiter in 14-day-old male infant. It is a cellular lesion with practically no colloid. (×300; WU neg. 62-1003.)

cation of thyroid tumors is valuable in diagnosing and assessing clinical behavior and treatment in groups of cases. One tumor may be composed of more than one type of neoplasm. We have had the experience of seeing a great variation of types in a single case that came to post-mortem examination (Fig. 350). Such variation in microscopic pattern may have some bearing on the differences in uptake of radioactive iodine in the metastases.

Benign tumors
Simple adenoma

There have been numerous classifications of adenomas with many subdivisions, but any breakdown into individual types is probably not justified. For instance, the so-called colloid adenoma is usually not a true neoplasm but simply represents a poorly defined and partially encapsulated focus of nodular goiter. The terms fetal and embryonal adenomas are confusing because they can be interpreted as implying origin of the lesion in fetal life. They are probably variations of the same neoplasm. It is preferable to classify them simply as adenomas.

Nodules of nodular hyperplasia are still being diagnosed as adenomas or true neoplasms, so that when the question, "What percentage of adenomas become malignant?" is asked, the figure is much lower than the true incidence. However, if strict pathologic criteria are used in the diagnosis of adenomas, approximately 10% of these lesions will be malignant.[71]

The criteria for the diagnosis of adenoma should be very rigid and accurate and should include the following: the adenoma should have *complete* fibrous encapsulation, it should be dissimilar from the surrounding thyroid parenchyma, and it should compress the surrounding thyroid tissue (Fig. 351). Very frequently these adenomas show central fibrous scarring and

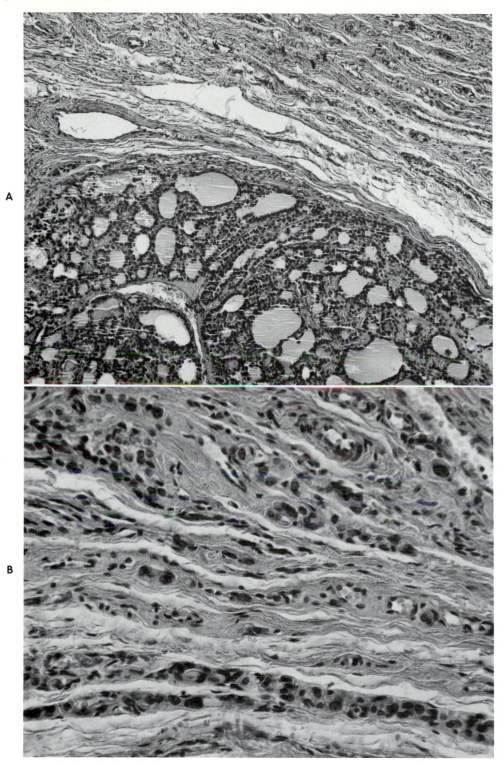

Fig. 349 Thyroid gland of cretin showing focal area of glandular proliferation associated with another zone in which follicles are atrophic and nuclei are atypical. (**A,** ×200; WU neg. 62-7613; **B,** ×350; WU neg. 62-7612; **A** and **B,** slides contributed by Dr. G. H. Moore, Denver, Colo.)

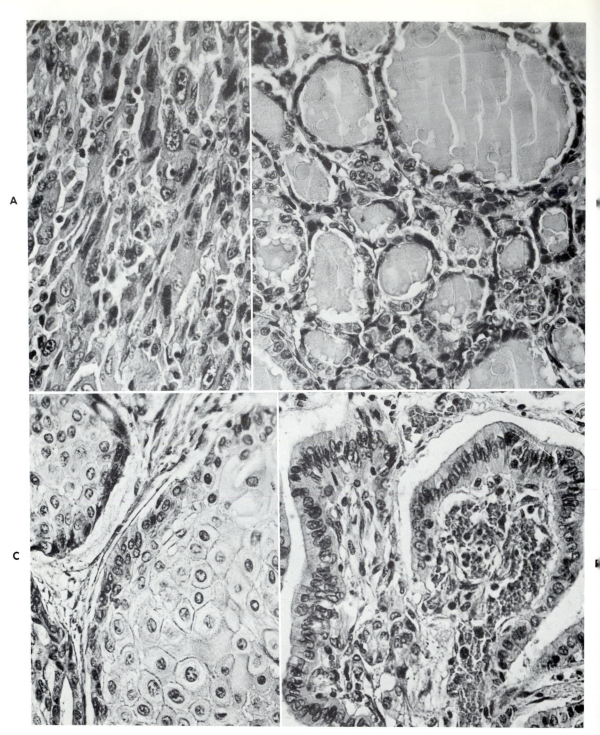

Fig. 350 Photomicrographs demonstrating variation possible in primary thyroid carcinoma and its metastases. Such variation may explain differences in uptake of radioactive iodine. **A,** Primary tumor is highly undifferentiated and could be designated as giant cell type. **B,** Metastasis to kidney. This could be called follicular type of carcinoma of thyroid gland. **C,** Metastasis to hilar lymph nodes. This could be designated as squamous carcinoma of thyroid gland. **D,** Metastasis to lung. This could be called papillary carcinoma of thyroid gland. (**A,** ×500; WU neg. 50-3342; **B,** ×400; WU neg. 50-3341; **C,** ×400; WU neg. 50-3340; **D,** ×400; WU neg. 50-3343.)

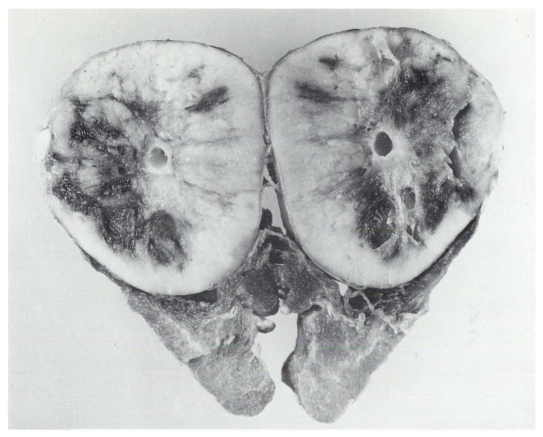

Fig. 351 Sharply circumscribed cellular adenoma of thyroid gland with central hemorrhage. Note sharp demarcation between tumor and normal thyroid gland. (WU neg. 52-2706.)

occasionally contain areas of hemorrhage. The Hürthle cell lesion is very frequently cellular and often large.

Microscopically, the simple adenoma (fetal and embryonal) is the most common of all thyroid adenomas and is usually made up of small thyroid follicles that may or may not contain small amounts of colloid (Fig. 352). Zones of fibrosis are often present in the center, and evidence of recent or old hemorrhage is common. At times, the cells have a trabecular arrangement. Considerable variation in the size and shape of the cells may be seen, but these

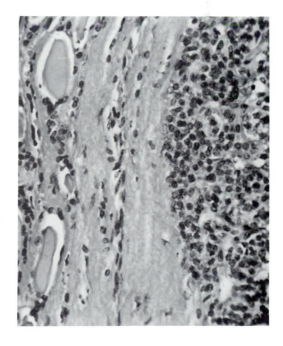

Fig. 352 Boundary between cellular adenoma and normal thyroid gland. Note difference in appearance between adenoma and thyroid gland and presence of well-defined capsule. (×300.)

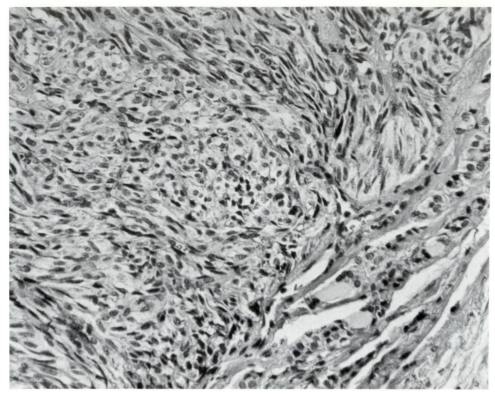

Fig. 353 Atypical adenoma of thyroid gland in 30-year-old woman. Capsule was intact, and there was no evidence of vessel invasion. (×300; WU neg. 66-9182; slide contributed by Dr. G. H. Klinck, Washington, D. C.)

changes, even when very prominent, are not necessarily an indication of malignant alteration (Fig. 353). Hazard and Kenyon[68] have coined the term *atypical adenoma* for this pseudomalignant variant.

Some correlation between the microscopic appearance of an adenoma and its activity as judged by the scan appearance is possible.[66] In general, hyperfunctioning ("hot") adenomas are more cellular and their cells have more abundant cytoplasm (and therefore a decreased nucleo-cytoplasmic ratio) than nonfunctioning ("cold") tumors.

Hürthle cell adenoma

Microscopically, the Hürthle cell adenoma, a relatively rare but distinct type of adenoma, is made up of large cells with abundant granular pink cytoplasm.[69] Nuclei are well defined, with relatively prominent nucleoli. Atypia is more common than in simple adenomas but, again is not necessarily indicative of malignant change. The cells are frequently arranged in solid masses and at times in columns. Small follicles with a small amount of central colloid may be seen. Mitotic figures are infrequent.[67, 70]

Malignant tumors
Papillary carcinoma

We believe that papillary carcinoma is cancer from its inception. We seriously doubt the existence of benign papillary cystadenoma. Papillary carcinoma metastasizes through the lymphatics in a high percentage of instances. Metastasis through the bloodstream is infrequent, but if it occurs distant metastases to lungs and bone appear.

Grossly, the primary tumor may be an extremely small, grayish white, poorly delimited area. At times it is found only on microscopic section. Our smallest primary tumor measured 4 mm. Consequently, very complete sectioning of the glands may be necessary to demonstrate the primary tumor. The larger lesions have a papillary character that can be discerned grossly (Figs. 354, 355, and 356, A).

The involved lymph nodes retain their original shape and may not be enlarged, but very frequently the architecture is completely obliterated and replaced by grayish white tumor tissue. Involved nodes may not be palpable because they are not enlarged, and their consistency does not differ from that of a normal node. This finding is well substantiated by Frazell and Foote,[74] who found that in sixty-seven patients who had no clinical evidence of disease within the lymph nodes prior to neck dissection, forty-one had involved nodes (61%) on microscopic examination.

Microscopically, the tumor in the thyroid gland and that in the nodes usually have a similar pattern, but the regularity of the architecture may vary from area to area. These tumors have a papillary character, but focal areas of follicular cancer also may be present. Mixed (papillary and follicular) carcinomas should be included with the papillary carcinomas because of their similar natural history. When cancer is present, the individual papillary zones may be multilayered and vary markedly in size and shape (Fig. 356, B and C). The nuclei of the tumor cells are characteristically large, indented, and empty-looking, even in the nonpapillary area of the tumor. At least in some instances, the latter feature is due to cytoplasmic invaginations.[75]

Fairly often, small calcific spherules (psammoma bodies) may be seen within the epithelial areas arising from the connective tissue of the stalk, evidence that tumor has been present for a long time. Their presence is usually diagnostic of papillary carcinoma, and this fact may be of great practical value in frozen section[76] (Fig. 371). These crystalline bodies stain for iron. Klinck and Winship[76] found them in 61% of papillary cancers and 26% of follicular cancers. In 21% of the glands, psammoma bodies were observed in normal thyroid tissue outside the primary tumor, as much as 1 cm distant. On the other hand, their presence in nonmalignant glands is exceptional.[78] Klinck and Winship[76] found them only once in a review of 2,153 noncancerous thyroid glands. Thus, their presence in an apparently benign gland should make the pathologist search for a carcinoma. We have seen two cases in which psammoma bodies were present in otherwise normal cervical lymph nodes. Serial sections in both cases showed the existence of a metastatic thyroid papillary carcinoma.

Psammoma bodies can sometimes be detected radiographically and can usually be distinguished from the nonspecific coarse calcium depositions seen secondarily to hemorrhage and necrosis.[77]

Both thyroid and salivary gland cancers may contain papillary areas and material that looks like colloid. This material will stain positively with ferric ferricyanide in patients with cancer of the thyroid gland but not in patients with cancer of the salivary gland.[73] Albores-Saavedra et al.[72] have described the fine structural features of this neoplasm.

Errors in the diagnosis of papillary cancer occur under the following circumstances. A patient may be euthyroid and a nodule is removed. This nodule has a papillary pattern and is called papillary cancer. In reality, it represents a zone of focal increased function, and the colloid will often be pale and finely vacuolated. By radioautography, such zones will have focal increased activity. No psammoma bodies will be present.

Follicular carcinoma

There are two distinct types of thyroid cancer that can be designated as follicular carcinoma, the *invasive type* and the so-called *encapsulated angioinvasive type* (low-grade carcinoma; carcinoma arising in

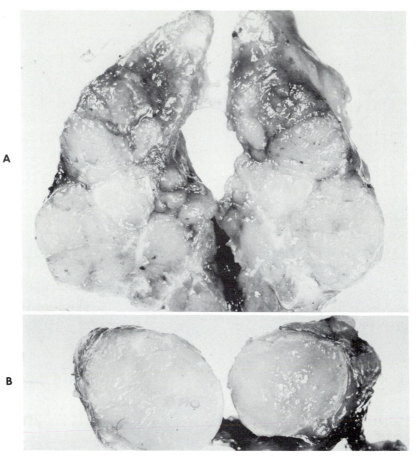

Fig. 354 **A,** Lobe of thyroid gland completely replaced by papillary carcinoma. **B,** Small mass represents complete replacement of lymph node. (**A** and **B,** WU neg. 50-504.)

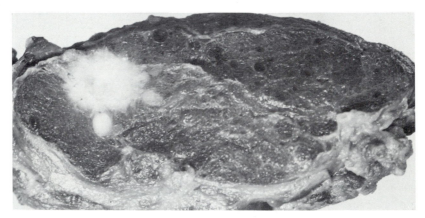

Fig. 355 Papillary carcinoma of thyroid gland measuring about 1 cm. Patient had extensive lymph node metastases. Naturally, primary tumor could not be felt. (WU neg. 52-3904.)

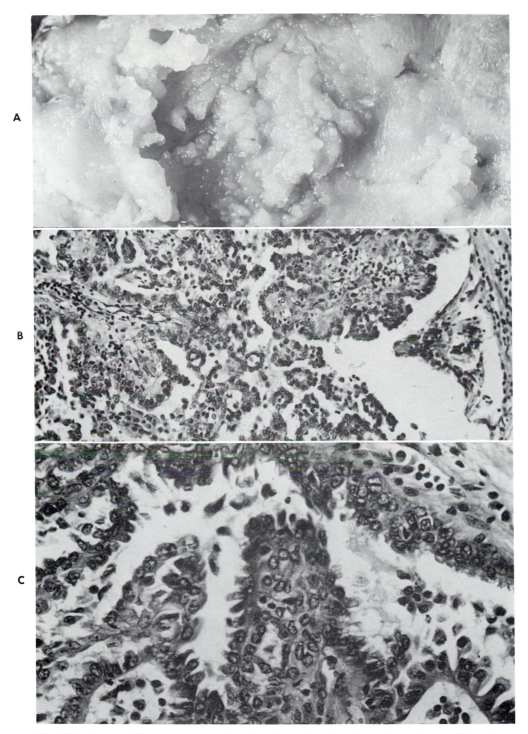

Fig. 356   A, Papillary carcinoma. This has been slightly enlarged so that papillary character of tumor can be seen. **B,** Low-power photomicrograph demonstrating papillary character of same tumor. **C,** High-power photomicrograph demonstrating layering of cells in individual papillae of same tumor. (**A,** WU neg. 51-5865; **B,** WU neg. 48-5637; **C,** WU neg. 48-5641.)

a follicular adenoma). The former rarely presents a diagnostic problem. Grossly, it presents as a single mass, nonencapsulated, of grayish white color. Microscopically, it is composed of small follicles that infiltrate the surrounding parenchyma and are associated with some fibrosis. Blood vessel invasion may or may not be present. A certain degree of atypia can be identified in most cases. However, in some instances, the cytologic features are hardly different from those of a normal gland. In these, the presence of clear-cut invasion into the thyroid parenchyma or, even better, into the surrounding perithyroid tissue, is the only evidence of a cancerous growth.

This tumor metastasizes frequently to the lungs, the bones of the shoulder girdle, sternum, skull, and large bones such as the ilium. If the primary tumor of the thyroid gland is small, the metastatic lesion may grow slowly and produce a mass that pulsates because of its vascularity. The chances are high that a metastatic pulsating lesion arises from either the kidney or the thyroid gland.

This is the type of carcinoma which shows a strong avidity for radioactive iodine. The more closely thyroid cancer resembles normal thyroid tissue, the greater the chance for an appreciable uptake. Only a small portion of the papillary carcinomas take up radioactive iodine to any degree. The undifferentiated carcinomas do not take up significant amounts. In the well-differentiated follicular type, radioactive iodine may be used as a palliative therapeutic agent when the disease has become disseminated, but sterilization of metastatic cancer practically never occurs.

The type of follicular cancer designated as encapsulated angioinvasive has gross and

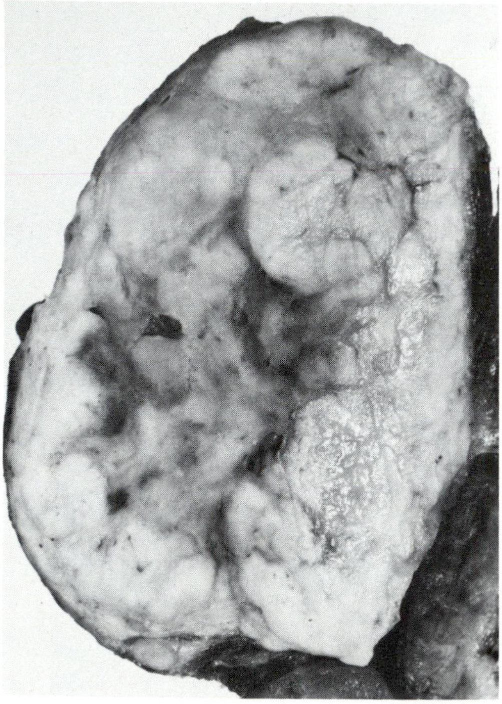

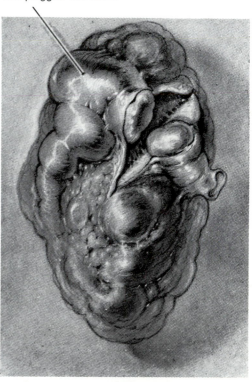

Vein plugged with tumor

Fig. 357 Follicular carcinoma of encapsulated angioinvasive type. Gross appearance is indistinguishable from that of adenoma. Microscopically, invasion of several veins by tumor cells was evident. (WU neg. 68-7713.)

Fig. 358 Large encapsulated follicular carcinoma of thyroid gland with gross evidence of vein invasion. This finding is extremely unusual in our experience.

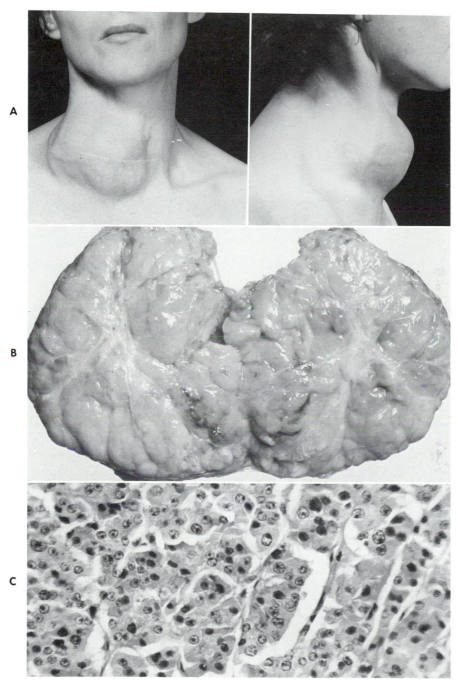

Fig. 359 Hürthle cell carcinoma of thyroid gland. **A,** Well-circumscribed thyroid nodule of two years' duration in 44-year-old woman. Scar is from operation done nine years before for hyperthyroidism. **B,** Note relative circumscription and cellularity of tumor. **C,** Note large cells with prominent cytoplasm. Tumor invaded veins. Patient died with bone and lung metastases six years after operation. (**A,** WU negs. 48-4150 and 48-4151; **B,** WU neg. 48-4259; **C,** X625; WU neg. 52-2872.)

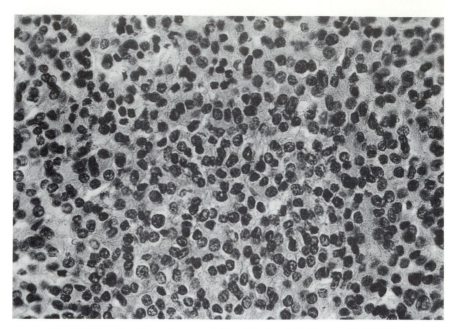

Fig. 360 Small cell carcinoma of thyroid gland (WU neg. 48-5642.)

microscopic features practically identical to those of a simple adenoma, including a well-formed capsule (Fig. 357). Its distinguishing feature is the presence of blood vessel invasion. It is therefore important that the large veins surrounding a thyroid solitary nodule be examined, because in rare instances the tumor may directly invade, block, and distend these veins (Fig. 358). On section, grayish white tumor fills their lumina. It is important that multiple sections be cut in the region of the capsule. At least five or six sections should be taken and stained not only in the conventional fashion but also with elastic tissue stain (Verhoeff's) to demonstrate the blood vessel wall and permit better assessment of the presence or absence of blood vessel invasion. Tumor cells often seen lying free within the lumina of small veins *are not evidence of cancer*. These tumor cells must be attached to the vein wall and a true tumor thrombus must be present before a diagnosis of cancer can be made.

Hürthle cell carcinoma

The Hürthle cell carcinoma is a rare malignant neoplasm that metastasizes in the same way as other malignant tumors of the thyroid gland. It reveals its identity by its microscopic pattern: large polyhedral cells with abundant eosinophilic granular cytoplasm[79, 80] (Fig. 359). Atypia cannot be relied on as a sign of malignancy, since it is often present in Hürthle cell adenomas. Instead, the presence of stromal and vascular invasion should be used as the diagnostic criteria.

Anaplastic carcinoma

Anaplastic carcinoma, a highly lethal neoplasm, can be subdivided into small cell, giant cell, and spindle cell types. *Small cell carcinoma* involves large areas of the thyroid gland and frequently invades the surrounding structures. It is made up of monotonous masses of small cells with scanty cytoplasm and homogeneously staining nucleus (Fig. 360). When this tumor grows in a diffuse fashion, the differential diagnosis with malignant lymphoma may be impossible.[85] It is only when strands and columns of tumor cells are present that the diagnosis of carcinoma can be made with certainty.[82] Small cell carcinoma of the thyroid gland is a vanishingly rare

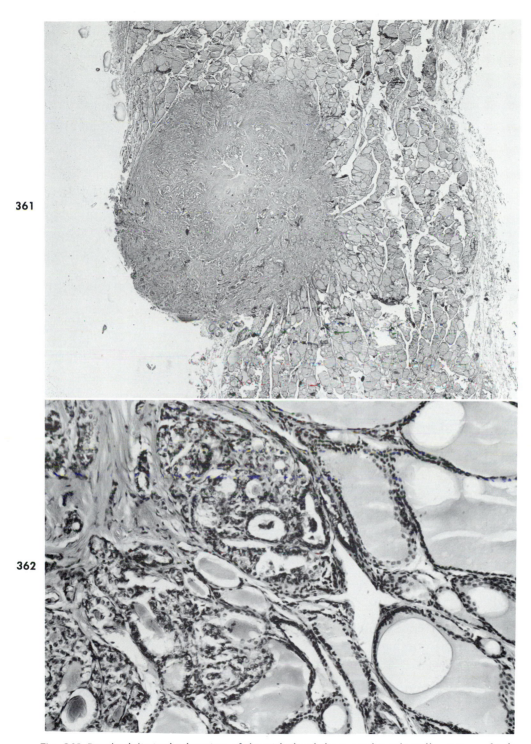

Fig. 361 Poorly delimited sclerosing of thyroid gland discovered incidentally at time of sub-total thyroidectomy for nontoxic nodular goiter. (Low power; WU neg. 55-4663.)
Fig. 362 Same lesion shown in Fig. 361. Tumor is growing as follicular carcinoma. (×130; WU neg. 55-4664.)

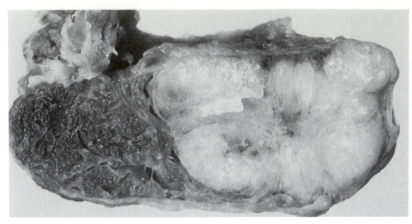

Fig. 363 Medullary carcinoma in 29-year-old man. There were lymph node metastases in neck dissection specimen. (WU neg. 59-4549.)

neoplasm. Many of the cases submitted to us with this diagnosis were in reality malignant lymphomas or medullary carcinomas. *Giant cell carcinoma* and *spindle cell carcinoma* are highly undifferentiated neoplasms that spread outside the thyroid gland and infiltrate the ribbon muscles, esophagus, trachea, and even contiguous bones. The prognosis is extremely poor.[83] Although distant metastases are common, death is usually the result of obstruction in the air passages.

There is growing evidence that many anaplastic carcinomas of the thyroid gland do not arise *de novo* but rather on the basis of a preexisting well-differentiated tumor, usually of the papillary variety.[81, 86] Fortunately, this is an extremely rare occurrence.

Giant cell carcinoma of thyroid gland should be differentiated from another rare thyroid neoplasm composed of stromal cells and osteoclast-like giant cells, with an appearance indistinguishable from that of giant cell tumor of bone.[84] We have seen only one example of this tumor type.

Occult sclerosing carcinoma

Hazard et al.[88] gave the name of nonencapsulated sclerosing tumors to minute neoplasms found incidentally in patients who had thyroidectomy for other reasons. Such lesions do not constitute a special microscopic type of thyroid cancer but simply a microscopic variant of follicular or, most commonly, papillary cancer, associated with fibrosis of the stroma.[87] They were first considered to be of little clinical significance. However, they have been found to metastasize to regional lymph nodes in at least one-third of the patients[89] (Figs. 361 and 362).

Epidermoid carcinoma

Epidermoid carcinomas may possibly arise from remnants of the thyroglossal duct or, most commonly, through squamous metaplasia of the follicular epithelium. Huang and Assor[90] found four cases among 130 consecutive malignant thyroid tumors. They occurred in elderly persons with long histories of goiter or other chronic thyroid diseases. Squamous metaplasia unrelated to carcinoma may occur in a variety of pathologic states and should not be confused with carcinoma.[91]

Medullary carcinoma

Hazard et al.[95] reported an unusual form of carcinoma which they designated as medullary. Twenty-one of 600 carcinomas of the thyroid gland were of this type. The regional lymph nodes contained metastases in ten of the twenty-one patients (Fig. 363). Fletcher[93] analyzed the clinicopathologic features of the 249 cases so far reported.

Medullary carcinoma is a remarkable neo-

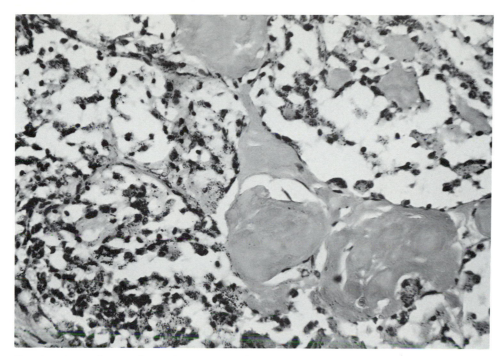

Fig. 364 Same lesion shown in Fig. 363 demonstrating large masses of amyloid. (High power; WU neg. 59-4752.)

plasm.[97] It may be associated with bilateral pheochromocytomas,[104] mucosal neuromas,[105] Cushing's disease,[103] intractable diarrhea,[102] and bilateral parathyroid hyperplasia and adenomas.[101] It arises from C cells and secretes thyrocalcitonin, as shown by electron microscopy and biochemical determinations.[92, 98, 100] It also may secrete 5-hydroxytryptamine, prostaglandins,[104a] and histaminase.[91a]

The tumor has a distinctive microscopic pattern consisting of solid masses of cells, often having a plasmacytoid appearance.[94] Amyloid is usually present in the primary tumor as well as in the metastases (Fig. 364) but is not a necessary requirement for a diagnosis of medullary carcinoma to be made. The similarities with gastrointestinal carcinoid may be striking.[96] The secretory granules in the tumor cells can be demonstrated with the Grimelius argyrophylic stain following fixation in Bouin's fluid. The tumor may have focal papillary areas, pseudofollicles, and psammoma bodies.

The amyloid in the medullary carcinoma is probably produced by the carcinoma cells. It can be demonstrated by electron microscopy[99] (Fig. 365).

Familial cases almost always show multicentric foci of involvement, whereas most sporadic cases are solitary.[97a]

Malignant lymphoma

True primary malignant lymphomas of the thyroid gland occur. They should be separated from small cell carcinomas that do not respond to irradiation and from generalized malignant lymphomas where the thyroid gland is only one more site of involvement. They may arise in a previously normal gland or be associated with Hashimoto's disease.[106] This tumor may exist both in the thyroid gland and in its regional lymph nodes and still be controlled by irradiation (Figs. 366 and 367). However, when malignant lymphoma extends beyond the capsule of the thyroid gland, the mortality is high.[107]

Plasmacytoma

Plasmacytoma of the thyroid gland has been reported by Shaw and Smith.[110] We

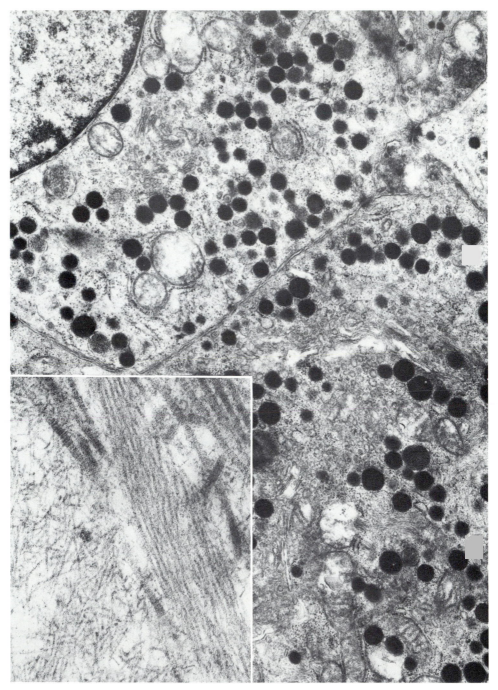

Fig. 365 Portions of two cells from medullary carcinoma of thyroid gland showing multiple dense secretory granules in cytoplasm. Each granule is surrounded by single membrane, and dense central portion is separated from it by clear zone. **Inset** shows both oriented and randomly placed amyloid filaments and may be contrasted with larger banded collagen fibers. (Courtesy Dr. J. S. Meyer, St. Louis, Mo.)

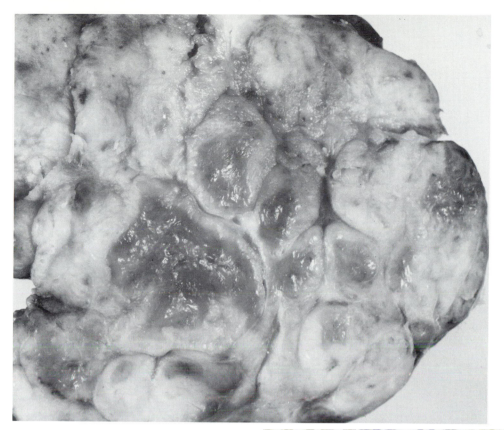

Fig. 366 Large malignant lymphoma of thyroid gland in 63-year-old man. Cervical lymph node on same side also was involved. (WU neg. 62-3130.)

have seen one diffusely involving the thyroid gland without invasion of other organs. In this case, a subtotal thyroidectomy was followed by irradiation to the remaining thyroid tissue.[109] We have also seen several instances of prominent nonneoplastic plasma cell infiltration. A 41-year-old woman had tumorlike involvement of the thyroid gland (300 gm) that was resected.[108] At the time of writing, she had no evidence of disease elsewhere, including the bones. The changes present probably were nonneoplastic. Our diag-

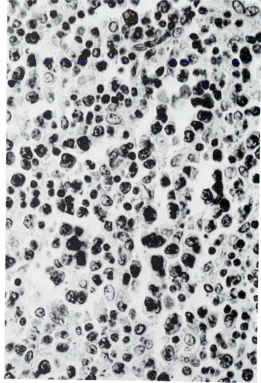

Fig. 367 Histiocytic malignant lymphoma of thyroid gland in adult treated by irradiation therapy. Tumor completely disappeared, and patient was still alive more than seven years after irradiation therapy. (WU neg. 50-694.)

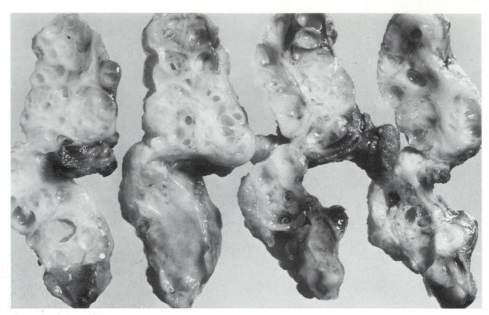

Fig. 368 Cystic teratoma of thyroid gland in 4-week-old white male infant. Clinically, lesion was considered to be congenital goiter. (WU neg. 54-1492.)

nosis, therefore, was plasma cell granuloma. Follow-up supports this opinion.

Fibrosarcoma, angiosarcoma, and teratoma

Most tumors designated as fibrosarcomas are in reality undifferentiated carcinomas with spindle cells. In a few rare instances true *fibrosarcomas* have been reported.[112] The existence of *angiosarcoma* of the thyroid gland is still controversial. Histochemical and electron microscopic studies are needed in order to determine whether this tumor is indeed of vascular origin or whether it merely represents a well-vascularized undifferentiated carcinoma. Cystic *teratomas* of the thyroid gland usually occur in children[111] (Fig. 368). Of the seventy-one published cases, only four were malignant.

Metastatic carcinoma

In widely disseminating carcinomas, invasion of the thyroid gland may occur via the bloodstream. We have seen metastases from malignant melanoma and from carcinoma of the kidney, cervix, breast, and lung. Carcinomas of the larynx sometimes invade the thyroid gland secondarily. Metastatic involvement of the thyroid gland was found by Shimaoka et al.[113] in 9.5% of 1,980 patients dying with malignant tumors. The most common primary tumors were malignant melanoma (39%) and carcinoma of the breast (21%), kidney (12%), and lung (11%).

Presence of thyroid tissue outside gland (including so-called lateral aberrant thyroid)

There are several circumstances in which normal or abnormal thyroid tissue may be found outside the confines of the thyroid gland. We have already mentioned all the sites in which aberrant thyroid tissue may be located as a result of faulty embryogenesis and the occasional occurrence of thyroid follicles in soft tissue or muscle in cases of Graves' disease. Thyroid tissue may be implanted in the soft tissues of the neck at the time of surgery and appear later as a separate mass. Suture material is usually identified microscopically in the area. Thyroid nodules may be pedunculated and connected with the gland by only a thin fibrous strand. If this connec-

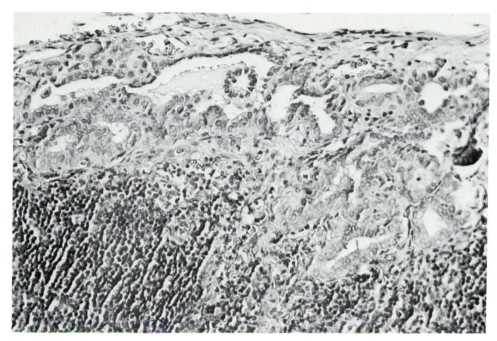

Fig. 369 Papillary carcinoma metastatic to cervical lymph node. (×230; WU neg. 51-6018.)

tion is missed by the surgeon, or if it disappears altogether, the nodule will appear as a mass independent from the thyroid gland.[121] These nodules show the same pathologic process as the main gland, such as nodular goiter or Hashimoto's disease.[117] We have seen Hashimoto's disease in such a nodule diagnosed as metastatic carcinoma.

The most difficult problem confronting the pathologist is the evaluation of thyroid tissue in cervical lymph nodes in the presence of an apparently normal thyroid gland. This phenomenon accounts for most cases of the condition formerly called lateral aberrant thyroid. It is now clear that this may be the result of two totally unrelated processes and that microscopic examination permits their separation in the majority of the instances.

Most cases represent metastases of clinically undetected thyroid carcinomas, usually of the papillary variety. King and Pemberton,[118] in 1941, analyzed fifty-four cases and found that practically all of the lesions represented metastatic extensions into deep cervical lymph nodes from primary

carcinoma of the homolateral lobe of the thyroid gland. It should be emphasized that the finding of this primary neoplasm may require extremely careful microscopic study with blocking of the entire thyroid gland and cutting of the blocks at various levels.[122] If these metastatic deposits are carefully examined, their distribution will be normal for the nodes in that area. Moreover, if they are cut at various levels, a rim of remaining compressed lymphoid tissue of the node frequently is discovered (Fig. 369). Lymphoid tissue is usually absent within the thyroid gland harboring papillary adenocarcinoma. The microscopic appearance of these metastases is not that of normal thyroid tissue, although it can closely resemble it. Papillary infoldings are often seen, and there is usually some degree of pleomorphism among the tumor cells. Their nuclei may be larger than the normal ones or may have a peculiar "empty-looking appearance.[115]

The suggestion made by Frantz[114] in 1942, that normal thyroid follicles may occasionally be found inside cervical lymph nodes is now well documented.[116, 120] Meyer

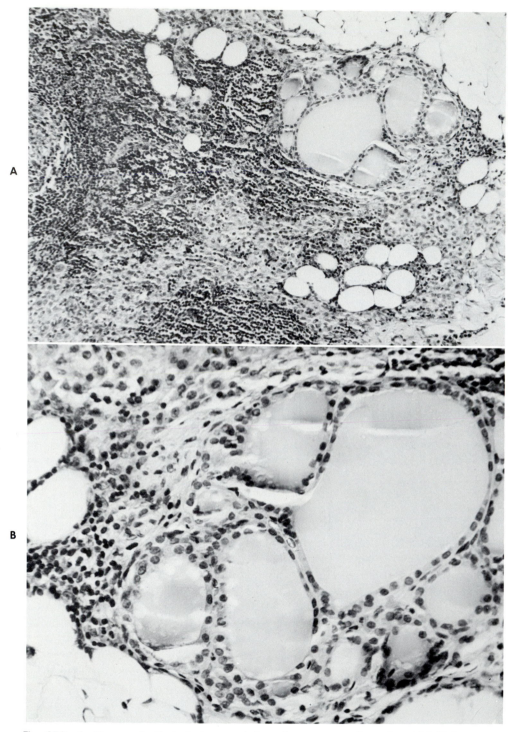

Fig. 370 A, Nonneoplastic inclusion consisting of aggregate of ten thyroid follicles at periphery of cervical lymph node. **B,** Similarity of these follicles to normal thyroid tissue is apparent. (**A,** ×80; WU neg. 64-3517; **B,** ×340; WU neg. 64-3518.)

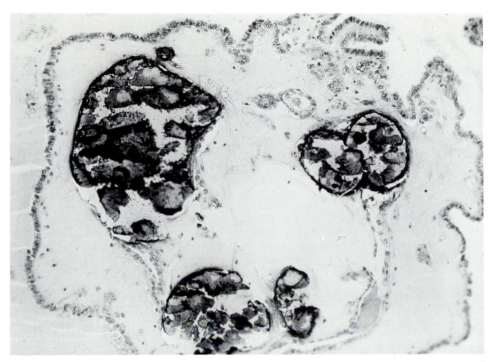

Fig. 371 Classic psammoma bodies occurring as small calcific spherules within stalk of well-differentiated papillary carcinoma. (×180; WU neg. 54-134A.)

and Steinberg[119] serially sectioned cervical lymph nodes from 106 autopsies and found thyroid tissue in five of them. Serial section of the whole thyroid gland in these cases failed to reveal carcinoma (except for a probably unrelated microscopic papillary carcinoma in the contralateral lobe of one case). Therefore, we now believe that under unusual circumstances normal thyroid tissue can travel via the lymphatics to a cervical lymph node. This should not disturb us, for we have already seen endometrium, portions of a benign nevus, and portions of an intraductal papilloma in regional lymph nodes. The typical microscopic appearance is that of a small conglomerate of follicles in the periphery of the node, *without any cell atypia or papillary foci* (Fig. 370).

Frozen section and biopsy

Since the nature of a thyroid tumor cannot be determined clinically, surgical investigation is indicated. The most common reason for exploration is the presence of a dominant, apparently single nodule in the thyroid gland in a patient without clinical signs of toxicity. At the time of exposure of the thyroid gland, multiple nodules rather than a single one are often discovered so that a diagnosis of nodular nontoxic goiter is obvious. In some instances, the patient will have a pathologic process that invades the contiguous muscle. Frozen section of this muscle usually will show invasive adenocarcinoma but rarely may show fibrous thyroiditis. In other instances, there may be enlarged lymph nodes in the region of the isthmus or in the region of the lymphatic drainage of the thyroid gland. Frozen sections of such nodes may show metastatic carcinoma. If exploration of the neck in the region of the thyroid gland is unrewarding, the surgeon must then turn his attention to the single nodule. This nodule, if small, can be removed with a margin of normal thyroid tissue, but in most instances its removal implies hemithyroidectomy. This nodule *must never be enucleated*, for if it is cancer it may be implanted throughout the tissues of the neck.

After removal of the nodule, the pathologist sections it and does a frozen section. The diagnosis will invariably be one of three things: a nodule of nodular hyperplasia, a true adenoma, or a carcinoma. The microscopic diagnosis will determine the therapy. Any pathologist with a good background in surgical pathology should have no difficulty in making a definitive diagnosis in over 90% of instances. If the patient has a pronounced hyperplasia of the thyroid gland, it may even infiltrate the surrounding muscle. If the pathologist is aware of the clinical situation, confusions will not arise.

Undifferentiated carcinoma will be an obvious diagnosis, and the diagnosis of papillary carcinoma will be probable, particularly if *psammoma bodies* are seen (Fig. 371). The greatest difficulty will occur, of course, in the recognition of the encapsulated angioinvasive form of follicular carcinoma. In some of these cases, the diagnosis will be missed because the sections examined will not contain the involved vessels. Fortunately, this does not create a therapeutic problem since the treatment for this tumor is the same as for adenomas—viz., simple lobectomy.

Needle biopsy may be useful in the diagnosis of thyroid lesions. It is particularly helpful in diffuse diseases such as struma lymphomatosa and in confirming the diagnosis of an advanced malignant neoplasm. Needle biopsy is contraindicated in all clinically solitary thyroid nodules because of danger of implantation.[123]

Clinicopathologic correlation

Carcinoma of the thyroid gland is still an infrequent neoplasm. It does not occur except coincidentally with diffuse hyperplasia. It is associated with nodular nontoxic thyroid in an appreciable number of patients, and there is a real risk of its presence in a single nontoxic nodule. The proper treatment of such single nodules is important in the cure of cancer of the thyroid gland. The indiscriminate removal of nontoxic nodules is not indicated because it is associated with measurable morbidity and mortality. We agree with Sokal[133] that skilled physicians can select the thyroid glands that should be removed. In such cases, Shimaoka et al.[132] estimated that the incidence of cancer would be one out of five.

The classification of thyroid cancer has merit, for there is a rough parallelism between the well-differentiated forms and prognosis. It is fortunate that a high percentage of thyroid carcinomas are well differentiated.[128]

It must be remembered that in the evaluation of any group of thyroid carcinomas, patients with papillary adenocarcinoma, and the well-differentiated follicular type may have an exceedingly long clinical course. For instance, in papillary cancer, it is not rare for metastases to be present in lymph nodes or even the lungs for over five years. We know of one patient who has had papillary carcinoma for twenty years. It is important for the physician to realize that thyroid cancer can occur in young persons and that it is not a rarity in children.[135, 136] Many of the thyroid cancers in children appear to be related to cervical or thymic irradiation in early life[129] (Fig. 372). Anaplastic cancer does not occur in children.[127] The only possible method of cure is by adequate surgery. Well-planned irradiation and radioactive iodine are only palliative agents.[125]

The common papillary carcinoma deserves special comment because of its many controversial aspects. The long natural history of the disease makes evaluation of any form of treatment extremely difficult. It has now been shown that this lesion has either multiple foci of origin within the thyroid gland or that it originates focally and extends widely through the gland by means of the abundant lymphatic network. In surgical specimens, the incidence of multiple areas of

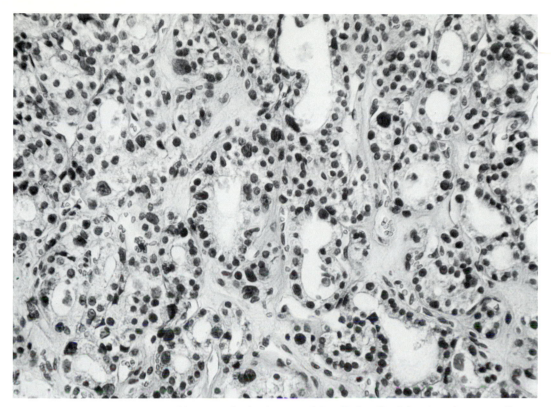

Fig. 372 Patient, 20-year-old man, who had received irradiation for "thymic enlargement" at age of 5 months, developed papillary carcinoma of thyroid gland. This photomicrograph was taken from nontumoral thyroid gland to illustrate nuclear aberrations frequently seen in patients with history of past irradiation. (WU neg. 66-7572.)

involvement in the gland is at least 80%.[131] Hemithyroidectomy, therefore, or local removal of a nodule will not remove the cancer in over one-half the patients. Furthermore, lymph node metastases are very common. If the cervical nodes are palpable, the chances of their being involved are almost 100%. If the nodes are clinically negative, they will still show microscopic metastases is at least 60% of the cases.[126]

In view of these observations, total thyroidectomy with radical neck dissection would seem the most logical operation for this neoplasm. However, the evidence for this being the case is not clear cut from the many clinical and follow-up studies that have been carried out. Recurrence in the thyroid stump can certainly occur,[130] and death from local recurrence in the neck and upper thorax has been reported.[134] However, this exceptional occurrence

should be weighed against the morbidity derived from a total thyroidectomy, such as the danger of hypothyroidism and severing of recurrent laryngeal nerves.[124] In regard to the cervical nodes, there is general agreement that they should be removed if clinically positive. On the other hand, the advisability of a lymph node dissection in the presence of clinically negative nodes is doubtful. Hutter et al.[127a] concluded that in patients who do not have elective node dissection but who later have therapeutic radical neck dissection if cervical metastases appear clinically, the prognosis is not compromised.

REFERENCES
Introduction

1 Klinck, G. H., Oertel, J. E., and Winship, T.: Ultrastructure of normal human thyroid, Lab. Invest. **22:**2-22, 1970.
2 Pearse, A. G. E.: The cytochemistry of the

C cells and their relationship to calcitonin, Proc. R. Soc. Lond. (Biol.) **164**:478-487, 1966.

3 Rienhoff, W. F.: Gross and microscopic structure of the thyroid gland in man, Arch. Surg. **19**:986-1036, 1929.

4 Teitelbaum, S. L., Moore, K. E., and Shieber, W.: Parafollicular cells in the normal human thyroid, Nature (Lond.) **230**:334-335, 1971.

Thyroglossal duct cyst, branchial cleft cyst, and heterotopic thyroid tissue

5 Ashhurst, A. P. C., and White, C. Y.: Carcinoma in an aberrant thyroid at the base of the tongue, J.A.M.A. **85**:1219-1220, 1925.

6 Beeson, H. B.: Aberrant goiter, Arch. Otolaryngol. **25**:449-454, 1937.

7 Brintnall, E. S., Davies, J. Huffman, W. C., and Lierle, D. M.: Thyroglossal ducts and cysts, Arch. Otolaryngol. **59**:282-289, 1954.

8 Dalgaard, J. B., and Witteland, P.: Thyroglossal anomalies; a follow-up study of 58 cases, Acta Chir. Scand. **111**:444-455, 1956.

9 Jaques, D. A., Chambers, R. G., and Oertel, J. E.: Thyroglossal tract carcinoma; a review of the literature and addition of eighteen cases, Am. J. Surg. **120**:439-446, 1970.

10 Lyall, D., and Stahl, W. M., Jr.: Lateral cervical cysts, sinuses, and fistulas of congenital origin, Int. Abstr. Surg. **102**:417-434, 1956 (extensive bibliography).

11 Montgomery, M. L.: Lingual thyroid, Trans. Am. Assoc. Study Goiter, pp. 145-153, 1935.

12 Ray, B. S.: Lingual thyroid, Arch. Surg. **37**:316-326, 1938.

13 Rees, C. E., and Brown, M. J.: Cysts of the thyroglossal duct, Am. J. Surg. **85**:597-599, 1953.

14 Rosedale, R. S.: Intralingual thyroid, Ann. Otol. Rhinol. Laryngol. **45**:1009-1018, 1936.

15 Sauk, J. J., Jr.: Ectopic lingual thyroid, J. Pathol. **102**:239-243, 1970.

16 Stahl, W. M., Jr., and Lyall, D.: Cervical cysts and fistulae of thyroglossal tract origin, Ann. Surg. **139**:123-128, 1954.

17 Sweet, R. H.: Intrathoracic goiter located in the posterior mediastinum, Surg. Gynecol. Obstet. **89**:57-66, 1949.

18 Tyler, A.: Carcinoma of lingual thyroid with metastases in lungs, J. Radiol. **4**:381-384, 1923.

19 Wapshaw, H.: Lingual thyroid, Br. J. Surg. **30**:160-165, 1942.

Acute infectious thyroiditis

20 Hazard, J. B.: Thyroiditis; a review, Am. J. Clin. Pathol. **25**:289-298, and 399-426, 1955.

Subacute (granulomatous or de Quervain) thyroiditis

21 Crile, G., Jr., and Fisher, E. R.: Simultaneous occurrence of thyroiditis and papillary carcinoma; report of two cases, Cancer **6**:57-62, 1953.

22 de Quervain, F., and Giordanengo, G.: Die akute und subakute nichteitrige Thyreoiditis, Mitt. Grenzgeb. Med. Chir. **44**:538-590, 1936.

23 Greene, J. N.: Subacute thyroiditis, Am. J. Surg. **51**:97-108, 1971.

24 Stein, A. A., Hernandez, I., and McClintock, J. C.: Subacute granulomatous thyroiditis, Ann. Surg. **153**:149-156, 1961.

Riedel's struma (struma fibrosa)

25 Comings, D. E., Skubi, K. B., Van Eyes, J., and Motulsky, A. G.: Familial multifocal fibrosclerosis, Ann. Intern. Med. **66**:884-892, 1967.

26 de Quervain, F.: Die akute, nicht eiterige Thyreoiditis, Mitt. Grenzgeb. Med. Chir. (Suppl. 2), pp. 1-165, 1904.

27 de Quervain, F.: Thyreoiditis simplex und toxische Reaktion der Schilddrüse, Mitt. Grenzgeb. Med. Chir. **15**:297-304, 1906.

28 Joll, C. A.: Diseases of the thyroid gland, London, 1932, William Heinemann, Ltd.

29 Riedel, H.: Die chronische, die Bildung eisenharter Tumoren führende Entzündung der Schilddrüse, Verh. Dtsch. Ges. Chir., 1896.

30 Woolner, L. B., McConaher, W. M., and Beahrs, O. H.: Invasive fibrous thyroiditis, J. Clin. Endocrinol. Metab. **17**:2, 201-220, 1957.

Hashimoto's disease (struma lymphomatosa)

31 Balfour, B. M., Doniach, D., Roitt, F., and Couchman, K. G.: Fluorescent antibody studies in human thyroiditis; autoantibodies to an antigen of the thyroid colloid distinct from thyroglobulin, Br. J. Exp. Pathol. **42**:307-316, 1961.

32 Dailey, M. E., Lindsay, S., and Skahen, R.: Relation of thyroid neoplasms to Hashimoto's disease of the thyroid gland, Arch. Surg. **70**:291-297, 1955.

33 DeGroot, L. J., Hall, R., McDermott, W. W., Jr., and Davis, A. M.: Hashimoto's thyroiditis, N. Engl. J. Med. **267**:267-273, 1962.

34 Doniach, D., and Roitt, I. M.: Auto-immunity in Hashimoto's disease and its implications, J. Clin. Endocrinol. Metab. **17**:1293-1304, 1957.

35 Graham, A., and McCullagh, E. P.: Atrophy and fibrosis associated with lymphoid tissue in the thyroid, Arch. Surg. **22**:548-567, 1931.

36 Hashimoto, H.: Zur Kenntniss der Lymphomatosen Veranderung der Schilddrüse (struma lymphomatosa), Arch. Klin. Chir. **97**:219-248, 1912.

37 Heptinstall, R. H., and Eastcott, H. H. G.: Hashimoto's disease (struma lymphomatosa), Br. J. Surg. **41**:471-477, 1954.

38 Joll, C. L.: The pathology, diagnosis and treatment of Hashimoto's disease (struma lymphomatosa), Br. J. Surg. **27**:351-389, 1939.

39 McClintock, J. C., and Wright, A. W.: Riedel's struma and struma lymphomatosa (Hashimoto), Ann. Surg. **106**:11-32, 1937.

40 McSwain, B., and Moore, S. W.: Struma lymphomatosa, Surg. Gynecol. Obstet. **76**:562-569, 1943.

41 Marshall, S. F., and Meissner, W. A.: Struma lymphomatosa (Hashimoto's disease), Ann. Surg. **141**:737-746, 1955.

42 Schade, R. O. K., Owen, S. G., Smart, G. A., and Hall, R.: The relation of thyroid autoimmunity to round-cell infiltration of the thyroid gland, J. Clin. Pathol. **13**:499-501, 1960.

43 Simmonds, M.: Über lymphatische Herde in der Schilddrüse, Virchows Arch. Pathol. Anat. **211**:73-89, 1913.

44 Spjut, H. J., Warren, W. D., and Ackerman, L. V.: A clinical-pathologic study of 76 cases of recurrent Graves' disease, toxic (non-exophthalmic) goiter, and non-toxic goiter, Am. J. Clin. Pathol. **27**:367-392, 1957.

Lymphocytic thyroiditis

45 Greenberg, A. H., Czernichow, P., Hung, W., Shelley, W., Winship, T., and Blizzard, R. M.: Juvenile chronic lymphocytic thyroiditis: clinical, laboratory and histological correlations, J. Clin. Endocrinol. Metab. **30**:293-301, 1970.

46 Weitzman, J. J., Ling, S. M., Kaplan, S. A., Reed, G. B., Costin, G., and Landing, B. H.: Percutaneous needle biopsy of goiter in childhood, J. Pediatr. Surg. **5**:251-255, 1970.

Diffuse hyperplasia (Graves' disease; exophthalmic goiter)

47 Curran, R. C., Eckert, H., and Wilson, G. M.: The thyroid gland after treatment of hyperthyroidism by partial thyroidectomy or iodine 131, J. Pathol. Bacteriol. **76**:541-560, 1958.

48 Goode, J. V., Grollman, A., and Reid, A. F.: Regeneration of human thyroid after so-called total thyroidectomy, Ann. Surg. **134**:541-545, 1951.

49 Hall, R.: Hyperthyroidism—pathogenesis and diagnosis, Br. Med. J. **1**:743-745, 1970.

50 Hargreaves, A. W., and Garner, A.: The significance of lymphocytic infiltration of the thyroid gland in thyrotoxicosis, Br. J. Surg. **55**:543-545, 1968.

51 Meissner, W.: Personal communication, 1952, 1955.

52 Nixon, D. W., and Samols, E.: Acral changes associated with thyroid diseases, J.A.M.A. **212**:1175-1181, 1970.

Nodular hyperplasia with or without hyperthyroidism

53 Cole, W. H., Slaughter, D. P., and Majarakis, J. D.: Carcinoma of the thyroid gland, Surg. Gynecol. Obstet. **89**:349-356, 1949.

53a Doniach, I.: Ætiological consideration of thyroid carcinoma. In Smithers, D., editor: Tumors of the thyroid gland, Vol. 6 of Monographs on neoplastic disease at various sites, Edinburgh and London, 1970, E. & S. Livingstone.

54 Greene, R.: Lymphadenoid change in the thyroid gland and its relation to postoperative hypothyroidism, Mem. Soc. Endocrinol. **1**:16-20, 1953.

55 Greene, R.: Discrete nodules of the thyroid gland, with special reference to carcinoma, Ann. R. Coll. Surg. Engl. **21**:73-89, 1957.

56 Hargreaves, A. W., and Garner, A.: The significance of lymphocytic infiltration of the thyroid gland in thyrotoxicosis, Br. J. Surg. **55**:543-545, 1968.

57 Pemberton, F. J.: The association of cancer of the thyroid gland and exophthalmic goiter, Surg. Clin. North Am. **28**:735-752, 1948.

58 Rogers, W. F., Asper, S. P., and Williams, R. H.: Clinical significance of malignant neoplasms of thyroid gland, N. Engl. J. Med. **237**:569-576, 1947.

59 Sokal, J. E.: Problem of malignancy in nodular goiter; recapitulation and a challenge, J.A.M.A **170**:405-412, 1959.

Colloid and congenital goiter

60 Batsakis, J. G., Nishiyama, R. H., and Schmidt, R. W.: Sporadic goiter syndrome; a clinico-pathologic analysis, Am. J. Clin. Pathol. **39**:241-251, 1963.

61 Hiilesmaa, V.: Studies of the thyroid gland of parturients and newborn infants in Southern Finland (Helsinki), Acta Obstet. Gynecol. Scand. **28**(Suppl. 1):1-100, 1948.

62 Kennedy, J. S.: The pathology of dyshormonogenetic goiter, J. Pathol. **99**:251-264, 1969.

63 Moore, G. H.: The thyroid in sporadic goitrous cretinism, Arch. Pathol. **74**:35-46, 1962.

Tumors
Classification

64 Frazell, E. L., and Foote, F. W.: The natural history of thyroid cancer, J. Clin. Endocrinol. Metab. **9**:1023-1030, 1949.

65 Meissner, W. A., and Lahey, F. H.: Cancer of the thyroid in a thyroid clinic, J. Clin. Endocrinol. Metab. **8**:749-761, 1948.

Benign tumors

66 Campbell, W. L., Santiago, H. E., Perzin, K. H., and Johnson, P. M.: The autonomous thyroid nodule: correlation of scan appearance and histopathology, Radiology **107**:133-138, 1973.

67 Gardner, L. W.: Hürthle-cell tumors of the thyroid, Arch. Pathol. **59**:372-381, 1955.

68 Hazard, J. B., and Kenyon, R.: Atypical

adenoma of the thyroid, Arch. Pathol. **58**: 554-563, 1954.

69 Heimann, P., Ljunggren, J.-G., Löwhagen, T., and Hjern, B.: Oxyphilic adenoma of the human thyroid; a morphological and biochemical study, Cancer **31**:246-254, 1973.

70 Horn, R. C., Jr.: Hürthle-cell tumors of the thyroid, Cancer **7**:234-244, 1954.

71 Meissner, W. A., and Lahey, F. H.: Cancer of the thyroid in a thyroid clinic, J. Clin. Endocrinol. Metab. **8**:749-761, 1948.

Malignant tumors
  Papillary carcinoma

72 Albores-Saavedra, J., Altamirano-Dimas, M., Alcorta-Anguizola, B., and Smith, M.: Fine structure of human papillary thyroid carcinoma, Cancer **28**:763-774, 1971.

73 Fisher, E. R., and Hellström, H. R.: Differential diagnosis of papillary carcinomas of thyroid and salivary gland origin, Am. J. Clin. Pathol. **37**:633-638, 1962.

74 Frazell, E. L., and Foote, F. W., Jr.: Papillary thyroid carcinoma; pathological findings in cases with and without clinical evidence of cervical node involvement, Cancer **8**:1165-1166, 1955.

75 Gray, A., and Doniach, I.: Morphology of the nuclei of papillary carcinoma of the thyroid, Br. J. Cancer **23**:49-51, 1969.

76 Klinck, G. H., and Winship, T.: Psammoma bodies and thyroid cancer, Cancer **12**:656-662, 1959.

77 Margolin, F. R., Winfield, J., and Steinbach, H. L.: Patterns of thyroid calcifications; roentgenologic-histologic study of excised specimens, Invest. Radiol. **2**:208-212, 1967.

78 Patchefsky, A. S., and Hoch, W. S.: Psammoma bodies in diffuse toxic goiter, Am. J. Clin. Pathol. **57**:551-556, 1972.

  Hürthle cell carcinoma

79 Frazell, E. L., and Duffy, B. J., Jr.: Hürthle-cell cancer of the thyroid; a review of forty cases, Cancer **4**:952-956, 1951.

80 Horn, R. C., Jr.: Hürthle-cell tumors of the thyroid, Cancer **7**:234-244, 1954.

  Anaplastic carcinoma

81 Hutter, R. V. P., Tollefsen, H. R., DeCosse, J. J., Foote, F. W., Jr., and Frazell, E. L.: Spindle and giant cell metaplasia in papillary carcinoma of the thyroid, Am. J. Surg. **110**: 660-668, 1965.

82 Meissner, W. A., and Phillips, M. J.: Diffuse small-cell carcinoma of the thyroid, Arch. Pathol. **74**:291-296, 1962.

83 Nishiyama, R. H., Dunn, E. L., and Thompson, N. W.: Anaplastic spindle-cell and giant-cell tumors of the thyroid gland, Cancer **30**: 113-127, 1972.

84 Silverberg, S. G., and DeGiorgi, L. S.: Osteoclastoma-like giant cell tumor of the thyroid, Cancer **31**:621-625, 1973.

85 Walt, A. J., Woolner, L. B., and Black, B. M.: Small-cell malignant lesions of the thyroid gland, J. Clin. Endocrinol. Metab. **17**: 45-60, 1957.

86 Wychulis, A. R., and Beahrs, O. R.: Papillary carcinoma with associated anaplastic carcinoma in the thyroid gland, Surg. Gynecol. Obstet. **120**:28-34, 1965.

  Occult sclerosing carcinoma

87 Hazard, J. B.: Small papillary carcinoma of the thyroid; a study with special reference to so-called nonencapsulated sclerosing tumor, Lab. Invest. **9**:86-97, 1960.

88 Hazard, J. B., Crile, G., Jr., and Dempsey, W. S.: Nonencapsulated sclerosing tumors of the thyroid, J. Clin. Endocrinol. Metab. **9**: 1216-1231, 1949.

89 Klinck, G. H., and Winship, T.: Occult sclerosing carcinoma of the thyroid, Cancer **8**:701-706, 1955.

  Epidermoid carcinoma

90 Huang, T.-Y., and Assor, D.: Primary squamous cell carcinoma of the thyroid gland: a report of four cases, Am. J. Clin. Pathol. **55**:93-98, 1971.

91 Klinck, G. H., and Menk, K. F.: Squamous cells in the human thyroid, Milit. Surg. **109**: 406-414, 1951.

  Medullary carcinoma

91a Baylin, S. B., Beaven, M. A., Buja, L. M., and Keiser, H. R.: Histaminase activity: a biochemical marker for medullary carcinoma of thyroid, Am. J. Med. **53**:723-733, 1972.

92 Cunliffe, W. J., Black, M. M., Hall, R., Johnston, I. A. D., Hudgson, P., Shuster, S., Gudmundsson, T. V., Joplin, G. F., Williams, E. D., Woodhouse, N. J. Y., Galante, L., and MacIntyre, I.: Calcitonin-secreting thyroid carcinoma, Lancet **2**:63-66, 1968.

93 Fletcher, J. R.: Medullary (solid) carcinoma of the thyroid gland; a review of 249 cases, Arch. Surg. **100**:257-262, 1970.

94 Gordon, P. R., Huvos, A. G., and Strong, E. W.: Medullary carcinoma of the thyroid gland; a clinicopathologic study of 40 cases, Cancer **31**:915-924, 1973.

95 Hazard, J. B., Hawk, W. A., and Crile, G., Jr.: Medullary (solid) carcinoma of the thyroid—a clinocopathologic entity, J. Clin. Endocrinol. Metab. **19**:152-161, 1959.

96 Horvath, E., Kovacs, K., and Ross, R. C.: Medullary cancer of the thyroid gland and

its possible relations to carcinoids; an ultrastructural study, Virchows Arch. [Pathol. Anat.] 356:281-292, 1972.

97 Ibanez, M. L., Cole, V. W., Russell, W. O., and Clarke, R. L.: Solid carcinoma of the thyroid gland; analysis of 53 cases, Cancer 20:706-723, 1967.

97a Ljungberg, O.: On medullary carcinoma of the thyroid, Acta. Pathol. Microbiol. Scand. (A), suppl. 231:1-57, 1972.

98 Melvin, K. E. W., Miller, H. H., and Tashjian, A. H., Jr.: Early diagnosis of medullary carcinoma of the thyroid gland by means of calcitonin assay, N. Engl. J. Med. 285:1115-1120, 1971.

99 Meyer, J. S.: Fine structure of two amyloid-forming medullary carcinomas of thyroid, Cancer 21:406-425, 1968.

100 Meyer, J. S., and Abdel-Bari, W.: Granules and thyrocalcitonin-like activity in medullary carcinoma of the thyroid gland, N. Engl. J. Med. 278:523-529, 1968.

101 Sapira, J. D., Altman, M., Vandyk, K., and Shapiro, A. P.: Bilateral adrenal pheochromocytoma and medullary thyroid carcinoma, N. Engl. J. Med. 273:140-143, 1965.

102 Steinfeld, C. M., Moertel, C. G., and Woolner, L. B.: Diarrhea and medullary carcinoma of the thyroid, Cancer 31:1237-1239, 1973.

103 Szijj, I., Csapó, Z., Laszló, F. A., and Kovács, K.: Medullary cancer of the thyroid gland associated with hypercorticism, Cancer 24:167-173, 1969.

104 Williams, E. D.: A review of 17 cases of carcinoma of thyroid and phaeochromocytoma, J. Clin. Pathol. 18:288-292, 1965.

104a Williams, E. D., Karim, S. M. M., and Sandler, M.: Prostaglandin secretion by medullary carcinoma of the thyroid; a possible cause of the associated diarrhœa, Lancet 1:22-23, 1968.

105 Williams, E. D., and Pollock, D. J.: Multiple mucosal neuromata with endocrine tumours; syndrome allied to von Recklinghausen's disease, J. Pathol. Bacteriol. 91:71-80, 1966.

Malignant lymphoma

106 Ranström, S.: Malignant lymphoma of the thyroid and its relation to Hashimoto's and Brill-Symmers' disease, Acta. Chir. Scand. 113:185-193, 1957.

107 Woolner, L. B., McConahey, W. M., Beahrs, O. H., and Black, B. M.: Primary malignant lymphoma of the thyroid; review of forty six cases, Am. J. Surg. 111:502-523, 1966.

Plasmacytoma

108 Heptinstall, R. H.: Personal communication, 1957.

109 Pinkerton, H.: Personal communication.

110 Shaw, R. C., and Smith, F. B.: Plasmacytoma of the thyroid gland, Arch. Surg. 40:646-657, 1940.

Fibrosarcoma, angiosarcoma, and teratoma

111 Bale, G. F.: Teratoma of the neck in the region of the thyroid gland; a review of the literature and report of four cases, Am. J. Pathol. 26:565-580, 1950.

112 Zeckwer, I. T.: Fibrosarcoma of the thyroid, Arch. Surg. 12:561-570, 1926.

Metastatic carcinoma

113 Shimaoka, K., Sokal, J. E., and Pickren, J. W.: Metastatic neoplasms in the thyroid gland; pathological and clinical findings, Cancer 15:557-565, 1962.

Presence of thyroid tissue outside gland (including so-called lateral aberrant thyroid)

114 Frantz, V. K., Forsythe, R., Hanford, J. M., and Rogers, W. M.: Lateral aberrant thyroids, Ann. Surg. 115:161-183, 1942.

115 Gray, A., and Doniach, I.: Morphology of the nuclei of papillary carcinoma of the thyroid, Br. J. Cancer 23:49-51, 1969.

116 Gricouroff, G.: Sur les tumeurs de type thyroidien d'origine extra-thyroidienne, Bull. Cancer (Paris) 50:329-331, 1963.

117 Hathaway, B. M.: Innocuous accessory thyroid nodules, Arch. Surg. 90:222-227, 1965.

118 King, W. L., and Pemberton, J. de J.: So-called lateral aberrant thyroid tumors, Trans. Am. Assoc. Study Goiter, pp. 177-195, 1941.

119 Meyer, J. S., and Steinberg, L. S.: Microscopically benign thyroid follicles in cervical lymph nodes; serial section study of lymph node inclusions and entire thyroid gland in 5 cases, Cancer 24:302-311, 1969.

120 Roth, L. M.: Inclusions of non-neoplastic thyroid tissue within cervical lymph nodes, Cancer 18:105-111, 1965.

121 Sisson, J. C., Schmidt, R. W., and Beierwaltes, W. H.: Sequestered nodular goiter, N. Engl. J. Med. 270:927-932, 1964.

122 Wozencraft, P., Foote, F. W., Jr., and Frazell, E. L.: Occult carcinomas of the thyroid: their bearing on the concept of lateral aberrant thyroid cancer, Cancer 1:574-583, 1948.

Frozen section and biopsy

123 Hawk, W. A., Crile, G., Jr., Hazard, J. B., and Barrett, D. L.: Needle biopsy of thyroid gland, Surg. Gynecol. Obstet. 122:1053-1065, 1966.

Clinicopathologic correlation

124 Crile, G., Jr.: Changing end results in patients with papillary carcinoma of the thy-

roid, Surg. Gynecol. Obstet. **132**:460-468, 1971.

125 Fitzgerald, P. J., Foote, F. W., Jr., and Hill, R. F.: Concentration of I[131] in thyroid cancer shown by radioautography, Cancer **3**: 86-105, 1950.

126 Frazell, E. L., and Foote, F. W., Jr.: Papillary thyroid carcinoma; pathological findings in cases with and without clinical evidence of cervical node involvement, Cancer **8**:1165-1166, 1955.

127 Hayles, A. B., Kennedy, R. L. J., Beahrs, O. H., and Woolner, L. B.: Carcinoma of the thyroid gland in children, Am. J. Dis. Child. **90**: 705-715, 1955.

127a Hutter, R. V. P., Frazell, E. L., and Foote, F. W., Jr.: Elective radical neck dissection: an assessment of its use in the management of papillary thyroid cancer, CA **20**:87-93, 1970.

128 Meissner, W. A., and McManus, R. G.: A comparison of the histologic pattern of benign and malignant thyroid tumors, J. Clin. Endocrinol. Metab. **12**:1474-1479, 1952.

129 Root, A. W.: Cancer of the thyroid in childhood and adolescence, Am. J. Med. Sci.

246:734-749, 1963 (extensive bibliography).

130 Rundle, F. F., and Basser, A. G.: Stump recurrence and total thyroidectomy in papillary thyroid cancer, Cancer **9**:692-697, 1956.

131 Russell, W. O., Ibanez, M. L., Clark, R. L., and White, E. C.: Thyroid carcinoma; classification, intraglandular dissemination and clinicopathological study based upon whole organ sections of 80 glands, Cancer **16**:1425-1460, 1963.

132 Shimaoka, K., Badillo, J., Sokal, J. E., and Marchetta, F. C.: Clinical differentiation between thyroid cancer and benign goiter; an evaluation, J.A.M.A. **181**:179-185, 1962.

133 Sokal, J. E.: Problem of malignancy in nodular goiter; recapitulation and challenge, J.A.M.A. **170**:405-412, 1959.

134 Tollefsen, H. R., DeCosse, J. J., and Hutter, R. V. P.: Papillary carcinoma of the thyroid, Cancer **17**:1035-1044, 1964.

135 Winship, T., and Rosvoll, R. V.: A study of thyroid cancer in children, Am. J. Surg. **102**:747-752, 1961.

136 Winship, T., and Rosvoll, R. V.: Childhood thyroid carcinoma, Cancer **14**:734-743, 1961 (extensive bibliography).

10 Gastrointestinal tract

Esophagus
Stomach
Small bowel

Appendix
Large bowel
Anus

Esophagus

Biopsy and cytology
Peptic ulcer and "reflux esophagitis"
Esophageal rings and webs
Lye strictures
Achalasia and giant muscular hypertrophy
Heterotopic gastric mucosa
Diverticula
Congenital defects
Tumors
    Smooth muscle tumors
    Epidermoid carcinoma
    Adenocarcinoma
    Other tumors

Biopsy and cytology

Exfoliative cytology in experienced hands is one of the most accurate techniques for the evaluation of esophageal lesions.[1, 3, 4] MacDonald et al.[2] reported 166 patients with pathologically proved lesions of the esophagus or cardiac portion of the stomach. In seventy-two carcinoma was present, and the cytology was positive in sixty-eight (94%). In these same patients, the radiographic diagnosis was benign or equivocal in 25%. By esophagoscopy, the lesion was interpreted as benign or equivocal in 40%. A biopsy was done at esophagoscopy in twenty-six patients, in fourteen of whom it did not contain tumor.

There were ninety-four patients with benign lesions. The cytology was reported negative in all cases, whereas the radiographic diagnosis was equivocal or called malignant in 18%. Esophagoscopy was interpreted as either cancer or equivocal in 28% of the cases.

Peptic ulcer and "reflux esophagitis"

Both peptic ulcer and "reflux esophagitis" are the result of esophageal reflux. They are always associated with a sliding hiatal hernia, although it should be stressed that it is the reflux and not the hernia that is the cause of these abnormalities. Barrett[6] clearly separated these two lesions on the basis of clinical and pathologic features. "Reflux esophagitis," a relatively common disorder, arises in esophageal epithelium and is accompanied by regurgitation, heartburn, pain, and dysphagia. Massive bleeding and perforation almost never occur. The early microscopic lesions are those of epithelial hyperplasia and infiltration by neutrophils.[10] The lesion may progress to congestion, superficial ulceration, spread of the inflammation to the wall, and circumferential fibrosis, with stricture formation and fixation to the surrounding structures.[11, 13] On the other hand, "peptic ulcer of the esophagus" has gross and micro-

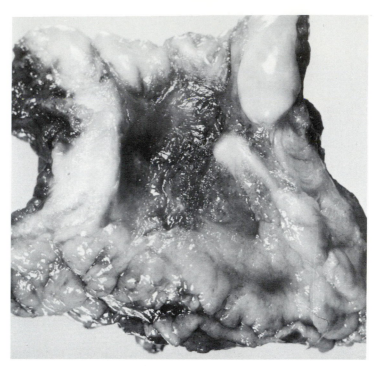

Fig. 373 Resected terminal third of esophagus demonstrating chronic peptic ulceration with deep penetration into wall. (WU neg. 49-3670.)

scopic features identical to those of a gastric ulcer. It is often large, oval, and well circumscribed, with elevated borders and deep crater (Fig. 373). It probably arises in epithelium of gastric type.[5, 7] It may result in massive bleeding or perforation, but only rarely in stricture formation. Microscopic examination of the short tubular segment distal to the ulcer, anatomically resembling esophagus, shows the segment to be lined by gastric mucosa.[12] It is still debated whether this is a congenital or acquired abnormality.[9] It is also argued what this segment should be called— *esophagus* because of its shape and motility or *stomach* because of its lining. Since there is not an agreed-upon definition on what the gastroesophageal junction is, this semantic question remains unanswerable.[8]

Esophageal rings and webs

Esophageal shadows with a configuration resembling rings and webs are often described by radiologists in patients complaining of dysphagia. Those located in the upper esophagus of women and associated with iron-deficient anemia are a component of the Plummer-Vinson or Paterson-Kelly syndrome, in which an increased incidence of carcinoma has been described. Those located in the lower esophagus are commonly referred as "Schatzki's ring" or "lower esophageal ring." The nature of the morphologic structure behind these shadows is unclear because of the lack of correlative radiographic and microscopic studies. Goyal et al.[14] partially corrected this deficiency by examining 100 autopsy specimens by these two techniques. They found two structurally different types of rings, which could be separated on radiographic examination. Nine were formed by a transverse circumferential fold of the mucosa; they were located at the squamo-columnar junction and produced a thin weblike shadow on x-ray films. Five were formed by a localized annular thickening

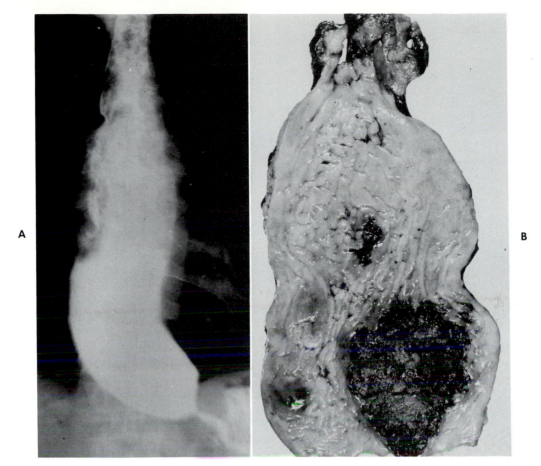

Fig. 374   A, Achalasia (megaesophagus) with superimposed ulcerating squamous carcinoma. **B,** Same lesion shown in **A.** (**A,** WU neg. 49-3478.)

of the muscle. They were proximal to the site of the mucosal ring, were covered by squamous epithelium, and produced a wide constriction when examined radiographically.

Lye strictures

Lye strictures of the esophagus are most common at the level of the bifurcation of the trachea.[18] If lye stricture is well established, the only method of cure is surgical resection.[16, 17] Carcinoma of the esophagus may develop at the site of a lye stricture.[15]

Achalasia and giant muscular hypertrophy

Achalasia (cardiospasm; megaesophagus) is related basically to emotional stress.[25] It may be due to a failure of the cardiac

mechanism to open when peristaltic waves conveying food through the esophagus reach it.[23] Supporting this theory are degenerative changes in the ganglion cells of Auerbach's (myenteric) plexus.[24] Cassella et al.[19] believe that the difficulty in achalasia of the esophagus rests centrally in the dorsal motor nuclei of the vagus and that the changes in the myenteric plexus, as well as the atrophy of the smooth muscle, are secondary changes. Misiewicz et al.[22] performed pharmacologic and histologic studies on strips of muscle removed at surgery for achalasia. They found loss of β-adrenergic activity (which mediates the relaxation of the muscle). Ganglion cells in this strip were either absent or abnormal.

In the early stages, this process is reversible. With the passage of time, how-

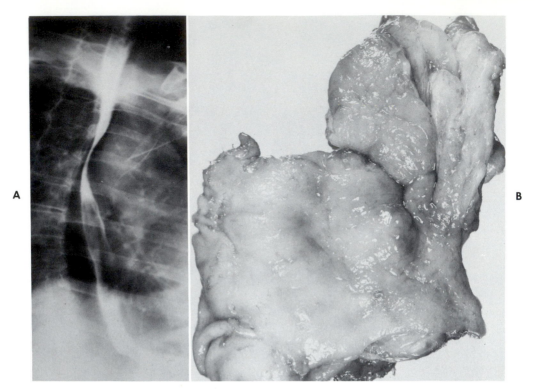

Fig. 375 **A,** Esophagogram showing smooth filling defect with compression. **B,** Resected esophagus illustrated in **A** showing smooth heterotopic gastric mucosa containing area of ulceration. (**A,** WU neg. 50-1507; **B,** WU neg. 50-727.)

ever, chronic inflammation and ulceration supervene, and fibrotic stricture results. Rarely, cancer is associated with long-standing achalasia[21] (Fig. 374). Wychulis et al.[26] observed seven cases in a group of 1,318 patients. Achalasia had been present for an average of twenty-eight years prior to the diagnosis of carcinoma. The tumors arose at all levels of the esophagus and were of epidermoid type in all but one patient.

Chagas' disease, an endemic parasitosis of South America, can be associated with alterations of Auerbach's plexus and mega-esophagus.

Giant muscular hypertrophy (diffuse spasm; corkscrew esophagus) is a motor disorder of the esophagus characterized clinically by dysphagia and pain and pathologically by focal or diffuse hypertrophy of the muscular layer, up to a thickness of 1 cm. Ferguson et al.[20] reported fourteen

cases of this disorder and pointed out that surgical therapy is not so successful as in achalasia.

Heterotopic gastric mucosa

Heterotopic gastric mucosa can occur at any point in the esophagus but appears most frequently in the postcricoid region.[29, 30] We have seen it produce a filling defect in the midportion of the esophagus[27] (Fig. 375, A). It may produce signs and symptoms suggesting a malignant neoplasm. Grossly, the surface resembles gastric mucosa (Fig. 375, B). Frequently, the lesion is sharply delineated, and the border with the normal stratified epithelium is apparent. At times, ulceration occurs.

Microscopically, this gastric mucosa is usually made up of long, typical gastric glands that are almost entirely mucin secreting (Fig. 376). The specific cells (parietal and chief) of the mucosa are rare.

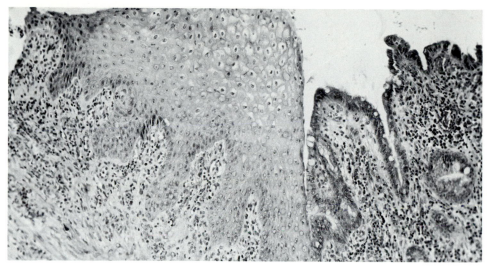

Fig. 376 Heterotopic gastric mucosa demonstrating abrupt transition between gastric and squamous epithelium. (×135; WU neg. 50-2062.)

There often is excessive inflammatory reaction which, coupled with the presence of the glands, may be erroneously diagnosed as adenocarcinoma. We have seen a single instance of carcinoma arising in heterotopic gastric mucosa in which normal lining squamous epithelium was present both proximal and distal to the lesion.[28]

Diverticula

The diverticula appearing in the upper portion of the esophagus are the result of outpouching esophageal mucosa at points of weakness in the wall of the esophagus. In the upper portion of the esophagus, the impairments are at the junction of the pharynx and the esophagus. They are more properly designated as diverticula of the hypopharynx and are classified as pulsion diverticula. They occur at this point because of the relationship between the inferior constrictor muscle and the obliquely passing fibers of the cricopharyngei as they descend upon the posterior wall of the esophagus to become longitudinal.[32]

In the lower third of the esophagus and in the region of the hilum of the lung, inflammatory lymph nodes (usually tuberculous) can become firmly attached to the esophagus and produce traction diverticula.

Just above the diaphragm, so-called epiphrenic diverticula of the pulsion variety occur rarely.[31] The outpouchings are false diverticula that contain mucosa, submucosa, and often muscularis mucosae. They are lined by squamous epithelium and may be associated with considerable inflammation. Complications may include obstruction, infection with perforation and mediastinitis, hemorrhage, and even carcinoma. Wychulis et al.[33] found three cases of carcinoma in 961 surgical cases of pharyngoesophageal diverticulum, an incidence of 0.31%. The prognosis is poor.

Congenital defects

The esophagus of a 3-week-old embryo is an annular constriction between the pharynx and the stomach. With growth of lung buds and elongation of the neck, it becomes tubular. At first, the cephalad portions of the esophagus and the trachea form a single channel. Later, a septum grows in and separates them.

Various types of defects may persist, the most frequent being esophageal atresia with fistula between the esophagus and trachea at the level of the tracheal bifurcation or at the level of the right main stem bronchus.[34-36] In this deformity, the hypertrophied dilated upper portion of the esophagus ends blindly at varying distances below the larynx. The lower portion of the esophagus usually communicates with the trachea about 0.5 cm above the bifurcation. Striated muscle is present in the upper portion of the esophagus and absent in the lower portion. Tracheal structures are often found in the fistulous end of the lower segment of the esophagus.[37]

There also can be defects of the esophagus alone, congenital narrowing or shortening of the whole esophagus, stenosis of the lower or upper end, or an occluding diaphragm of mucous membrane.

Surgery can close a tracheoesophageal fistula and establish continuity of the esophagus.[36]

Tumors
Smooth muscle tumors

Of the 200 benign tumors of the esophagus that were discussed by Totten et al.,[43] the *leiomyoma* was the most frequent. It occurs much less often than carcinoma. At times, these tumors are multiple.[42] Grossly, they form well-defined masses, which are grayish white on cross section, arising from the smooth muscle in the wall of the esophagus. If they grow intraluminally, they encroach upon the mucosa and appear as a sessile or pedunculated polyp. Ulceration of the overlying mucosa is a rare event, in contrast to its common occurrence in gastric leiomyomas.

Esophageal leiomyomas can encircle the entire esophagus in its lower third and constrict it.[39] Microscopically, they have the characteristics of a benign smooth muscle tumor. Local resection or enucleation of leiomyomatous tumors is usually successful.[40]

Leiomyosarcomas are quite unusual. Only thirty-eight reported cases were found by Athanasoulis and Aral[38] in their review. Grossly, they may be indistinguishable from leiomyoma.[41] Presence of a significant number of mitotic figures is the main criterion by which they are separated from their benign counterpart.

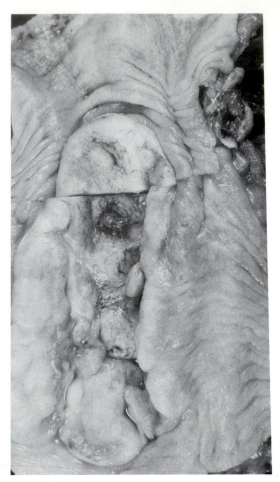

Fig. 377 Epidermoid carcinoma of terminal third of esophagus demonstrating well-delineated mass with central ulceration. (WU neg. 51-1200.)

Epidermoid carcinoma

Carcinoma of the esophagus occurs most frequently in men over 50 years of age. Rarely, it is associated with a benign stricture[44] or with achalasia,[45] but it is not related to leukoplakia of the esophagus (Fig. 374). It should be pointed out that most lesions diagnosed as "leukoplakia" in the esophagus have no microscopic resemblance to the common leukoplakia of the oral cavity. They represent, instead, focal thickening of the epithelium with increase in glycogen content.[52] In the United States, carcinoma of the esophagus is second in frequency only to carcinoma of the large

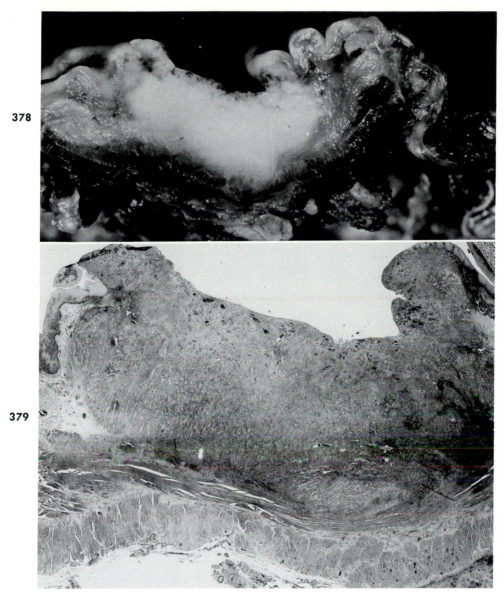

Fig. 378 Cross section of specimen of tumor shown in Fig. 377. Tumor is still confined to esophageal wall. (WU neg. 51-1199.)

Fig. 379 Tumor shown in Fig. 378. Patient died eighteen years later of unrelated disorder. (WU neg. 51-1217.)

bowel and stomach. By contrast, it is the most common malignant tumor of the alimentary tract in the African Bantus. It can occur in any portion of the esophagus, but it is most common in the middle and lower thirds.[48] It gradually obstructs the lumen of the esophagus in 90% of the patients.

Grossly, the tumor usually is circumferential and has sharply demarcated margins (Fig. 377). On cut section, grayish white tumor frequently replaces the entire wall of the esophagus and may extend into the surrounding soft tissue and trachea (Figs. 378 to 380). When tumor is present in the lower third of the esophagus, the

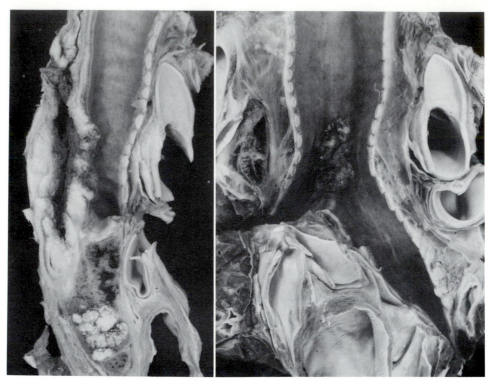

Fig. 380 Carcinoma of esophagus involving entire circumference of organ, invading trachea, and producing intratracheal polypoid mass. This may result in mistaken diagnosis of primary tracheal carcinoma. There are metastases in mediastinal lymph nodes. (Courtesy Dr. E. F. Lascano, Buenos Aires, Argentina.)

stomach is often invaded (Figs. 381 and 382).

Failure to cure carcinoma of the esophagus is the result of the growth characteristics of the neoplasm. Usually, these tumors quickly spread through the muscle to the periesophageal tissue. The esophagus is abundantly supplied with lymphatics that often transport tumor below the diaphragm or upward into the cervical lymph nodes. Unexpected extension of the tumor may be found in careful examination of surgical specimens. We subserially cut a surgical specimen of a carcinoma of the esophagus and found tumor 5 cm above and 7 cm below the gross limits of the tumor. This submucosal extension could not be seen or felt grossly. Burgess et al.[46] studied fifteen specimens of carcinoma of the esophagus microscopically and found intramural spread from 1 cm to 4 cm beyond the gross limits of the tumors.

In one of our specimens, epidermoid carcinoma in situ of the epithelium was found apart from the primary tumor, supporting the concept of multiple foci of origin.[54] In the small group of patients with resectable carcinomas, cures are infrequent because of early metastases. Guernsey and Knudsen[47] performed laparotomy with celiac lymph node biopsy in forty patients having esophageal carcinoma without evidence of metastatic disease by conventional techniques. Metastases in the celiac nodes were found in sixteen patients (40%). When operative removal of an epidermoid carcinoma of the esophagus is performed, frozen section of tissue at the levels of transection will help establish the adequacy of the resection.

Considerable palliation is achieved by well-planned irradiation, and cures have been reported by this form of treatment[49, 51] (Fig. 383). Radiation therapy is best indi-

381

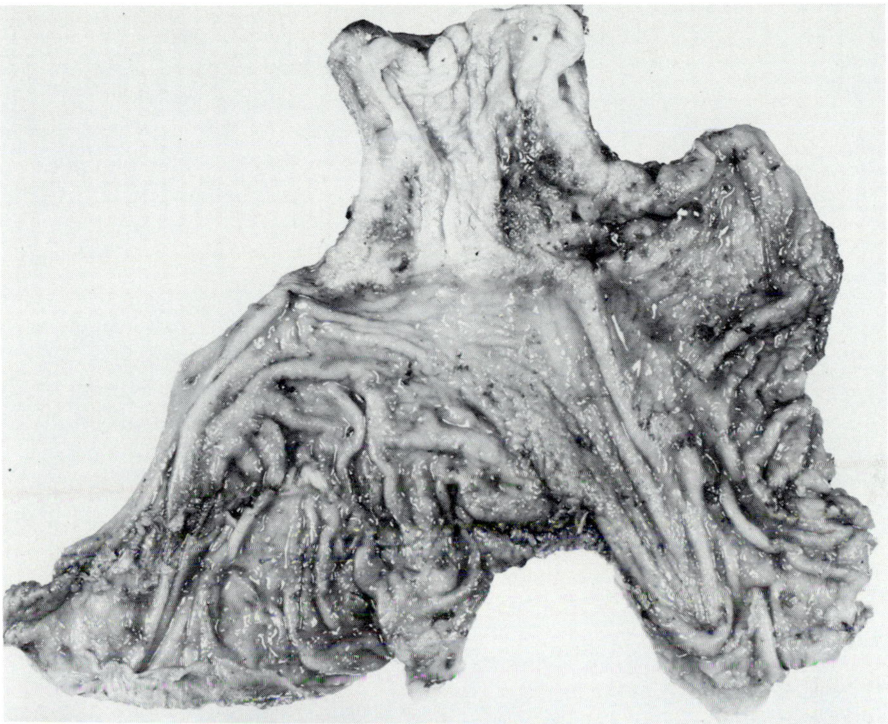

382

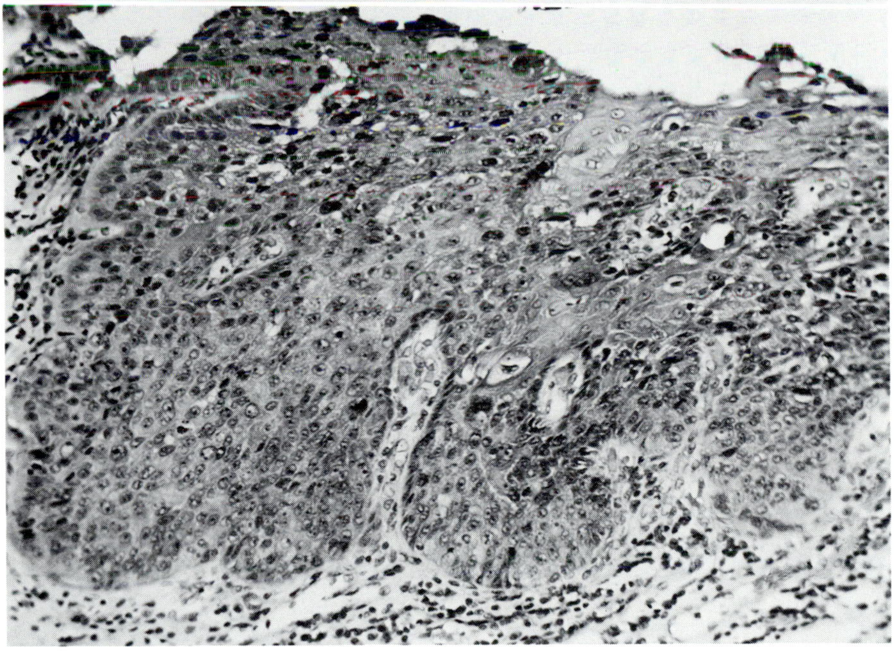

Fig. 381 Epidermoid carcinoma of lower third of esophagus invading stomach. (WU neg. 49-6554.)

Fig. 382 Peripheral margin of tumor shown in Fig. 381. This is zone of epidermoid carcinoma in situ. (×200; WU neg. 50-2976.)

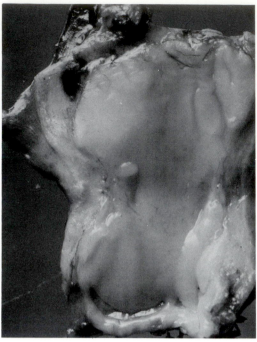

Fig. 383 Specimen illustrating effect of pre-operative irradiation. It is a resected segment of esophagus at junction of upper and middle thirds. There was previously at this point a large ulcerated carcinoma that was heavily irradiated. Ulceration disappeared and was replaced by smooth mucosa. However, after taking many sections, residual carcinoma was found in wall. There was also metastatic cancer in regional lymph nodes. (WU neg. 49-1328.)

cated for carcinoma of the upper third of the esophagus, and surgery is best indicated for carcinoma of the lower third. Cancer of the middle third responds poorly to both methods of treatment. Smithers[53] reviewed the world literature and found seventy-four five-year survivors among patients treated by surgery who had carcinoma of the lower third of the esophagus and sixty-one five-year survivors among patients treated by radiotherapy who had carcinoma of the upper third of the esophagus.

Verrucous carcinoma, an extremely well-differentiated neoplasm that invades locally but is only rarely associated with lymph node metastases, has been reported in the esophagus by Minielly et al.[50]

Adenocarcinoma

Primary adenocarcinoma of the esophagus is a very rare tumor. It may arise from normal esophageal glands or from a focus of ectopic gastric mucosa. The only unquestionable cases are those in which there is normal esophageal (squamous) eipthelium in the proximal as well as in the *distal* margin. This eliminates the large majority of cardiac tumors, in which the lower margin is continued by gastric mucosa. Although theoretically some of these tumors could be arising from esophageal glands or from "gastric-lined esophagus," the possibility of esophageal extension from a gastric carcinoma can never be ruled out. For practical purposes, it is best to consider all adenocarcinomas involving both sides of the cardioesophageal junction as primary gastric tumors with esophageal spread and all pure epidermoid carcinomas of similar location as primary esophageal cancers with secondary gastric involvement.

Other tumors

Other malignant tumors of the esophagus are a rarity. *Epidermoid carcinoma with sarcoma-like stroma ("pseudosarcoma")* usually presents as a large polypoid neoplasm[58, 63] (Fig. 384). The microscopic and histogenetic considerations are the same as for the laryngeal form of this enigmatic tumor (Chapter 6). We have also observed *metastatic carcinoma* in nodes about the esophagus that has secondarily invaded it.[64] Approximately thirty cases of *primary malignant melanoma* have been reported.[55] Presence of "junctional activity" at the periphery is required in order to rule out a metastatic neoplasm. In some cases, the melanoma has been associated with focal or diffuse melanosis.[61] The prognosis is exceedingly poor.

Heitzman et al.[59] reported an instance of *amyloidosis* with perforation and hematemesis. Rojas and Vallecillo[62] published a case of *adenoid cystic carcinoma* of the esophagus. We have seen an example in the upper third of the esophagus.

Flege and Edmonds[57] have reported a

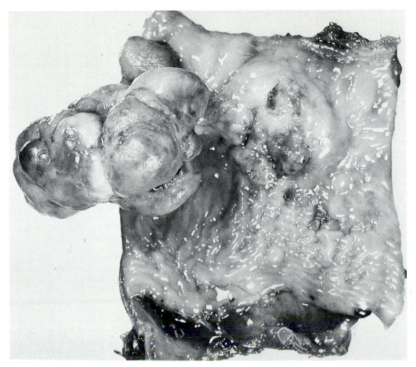

Fig. 384 Epidermoid carcinoma with sarcoma-like stroma ("pseudosarcoma") of upper third of esophagus in 66-year-old man. Note typical polypoid configuration. There were no metastases, and tumor had not extended through wall. (WU neg. 52-3827.)

granular cell tumor and Brenner et al.[56] a *carcinoid tumor.* Most of the fifty-three cases of *fibrovascular polyps* reviewed by Jang et al.[60] were pedunculated, usually solitary, occurring in adults. About 85% were located in the upper third of the esophagus. Microscopically, they are composed of fibrous tissue and numerous blood vessels, with stromal edema and occasional lymphocytic infiltration. The overlying mucosa is often ulcerated.

Paget's disease has been described in the esophagus associated with squamous cell carcinoma.[65]

REFERENCES
Biopsy and cytology

1 Johnson, W. D., Koss, L. G., Papanicolaou, G. N., and Seybolt, J. F.: Cytology of esophageal washings, Cancer **8**:951-957, 1955.
2 MacDonald, W. C., Brandburg, L. L., Taniguchi, L., and Rubin, C. E.: Esophageal exfoliative cytology, Ann. Intern. Med. **59**: 332-337, 1963.
3 Prolla, J. C., Taebel, D. W., and Kirsner, J. B.: Current status of exfoliative cytology in diagnoses of malignant neoplasms of the esophagus, Surg. Gynecol. Obstet. **121**:743-752, 1965.
4 Raskin, H. R., Kirsner, J. B., and Palmer, W. L.: Role of exfoliative cytology in the diagnosis of cancer of the digestive tract, J.A.M.A. **169**: 789-791, 1959.

Peptic ulcer and "reflux esophagitis"

5 Allison, P. R.: Peptic ulcer of the esophagus, Thorax **3**:20-42, 1948.
6 Barrett, N. R.: Chronic peptic ulcer of the oesophagus and "oesophagitis," Br. J. Surg. **38**:175-182, 1950.
7 Belsey, R.: Peptic ulcer of the oesophagus, Ann. R. Coll. Surg. Engl. **14**:303-322, 1954.
8 Harrison, C. P.: Where is the gastroesophageal junction? (letter to the editor), Can. Med. Assoc. J. **99**:867-868, 1968.
9 Heitmann, P., Csendes, A., and Strauszer, T.: Esophageal strictures and lower esophagus lined with columnar epithelium, Am. J. Dig. Dis. **16**: 307-320, 1971.
10 Ismail-Beigi, F., Horton, P. F., and Pope, C. E., II: Histological consequences of gastroesophageal reflux in man, Gastroenterology **58**: 163-174, 1970.
11 Sandry, R. J.: Pathology of reflux esophagitis.

in Skinner, D. B., Belsey, R. H. R., Hendrix, T. R., and Zuidema, G. D., editors: Gastroesophageal reflux in hiatal hernia, Boston, 1972, Little, Brown and Co.

12 Trier, J. S.: Morphology of the epithelium of the distal esophagus in patients with mid-esophageal peptic strictures, Gastroenterology **58**:444-461, 1970.

13 Yardley, J. H.: Biopsy findings in low-grade reflux esophagitis. In Skinner, D. B., Belsey, R. H. R., Hendrix, T. R., and Zuidema, G. D., editors: Gastroesophageal reflux and hiatal hernia, Boston, 1972, Little, Brown and Co.

Esophageal rings and webs

14 Goyal, R. K., Bauer, J. L., and Spiro, H. M.: The nature and location of lower esophageal ring, N. Engl. J. Med. **284**:1175-1180, 1971.

Lye strictures

15 Bigelow, N. H.: Carcinoma of the esophagus developing at the site of lye stricture, Cancer **6**:1159-1164, 1953.

16 Bosher, L. H., Jr., Burford, T. H., and Ackerman, L. V.: The pathology of experimentally produced lye burns and strictures of the esophagus, J. Thorac. Surg. **21**:483-489, 1951.

17 Burford, T., Webb, W. R., and Ackerman, L. V.: Caustic burns of the esophagus and their surgical management, Ann. Surg. **138**:453-460, 1953.

18 Kiviranta, U. K.: Corrosion of esophagus and stomach: sequels and therapy; clinical studies and follow-up examination of 379 patients, Acta Otolaryngol. (Stockh.) (Suppl. 81), pp. 1-128, 1949.

Achalasia and giant muscular hypertrophy

19 Cassella, R. R., Brown, A. L., Jr., Sayre, G. P., and Ellis, F. H., Jr.: Achalasia of the esophagus, Ann. Surg. **160**:474-487, 1964.

20 Ferguson, T. B., Woodbury, J. D., Roper, C. L., and Burford, T. H.: Giant muscular hypertrophy of the esophagus, Ann. Thorac. Surg. **8**:209-218, 1969.

21 Just-Viera, J. O., and Haight, C.: Achalasia and carcinoma of the esophagus, Surg. Gynecol. Obstet. **128**:1081-1095, 1969.

22 Misiewicz, J. J., Waller, S. L., Anthony, P. P., and Gummer, J. W. P.: Achalasia of the cardia; pharmacology and histopathology of isolated cardiac sphincteric muscle from patients with and without achalasia, Q. J. Med. **149**:17-30, 1969.

23 Puppel, I. D:. The role of esophageal motility in the surgical treatment of megaesophagus, J. Thorac. Surg. **19**:371-390, 1950.

24 Rake, G. W.: On the pathology of achalasia of the cardia, Guys Hosp. Rep. **77**:141-150, 1927.

25 Wolf, S., and Almy, T. P.: Experimental observations on cardiospasm in man, Gastroenterology **13**:401-421, 1949.

26 Wychulis, A. R., Woolam, G. L., Andersen, H. A., and Ellis, F. H., Jr.: Achalasia and carcinoma of the esophagus, J.A.M.A. **215**:1638-1641, 1971.

Heterotopic gastric mucosa

27 Bosher, L. H., Jr., and Taylor, F. H.: Heterotopic gastric mucosa in the esophagus with ulceration and stricture formation, J. Thorac. Surg. **21**:306-312, 1951.

28 Foraker, A. G.: Personal communication, 1957.

29 Rector, L. E., and Connerley, M. L.: Aberrant mucosa in the esophagus in infants and children, Arch. Pathol. **31**:285-294, 1941.

30 Schridde, H.: Über Magenschleimbaut-Inseln vom Bau der Cardialdrüsenzone und Fundusdrüsenregion und den unteren, oesophagealen Cardialdrüsen gleichende Drüsen im obersten Oesophagusabschnitt, Virchows Arch. Pathol. Anat. **175**:1-16, 1904.

Diverticula

31 Janes, R. M.: Diverticula of the lower thoracic esophagus, Ann. Surg. **124**:637-652, 1946.

32 Lahey, F. H.: Pharyngoesophageal diverticulum: its management and complications, Ann. Surg. **124**:617-652, 1946.

33 Wychulis, A. R., Gunnlaugsson, G. H., and Clagett, O. T.: Carcinoma occurring in pharyngoesophageal diverticulum; report of three cases, Surgery **66**:976-979, 1969.

Congenital defects

34 Clatworthy, H. W., Jr.: Esophageal atresia; importance of early diagnosis and adequate treatment illustrated by a series of patients, Pediatrics **16**:122-128, 1955.

35 Holden, M. P., and Wooler, G. H.: Tracheo-oesophageal fistula and oesophageal atresia: results of 30 years' experience, Thorax **25**:406-412, 1970.

36 Holder, T. M., Cloud, D. T., Lewis, J. E., Jr., and Pilling, G. P., IV: Esophageal atresia and tracheoesophageal fistula; a survey of its members by the Surgical Section of the American Academy of Pediatrics, Pediatrics **34**:542-549, 1964.

37 Rosenthal, A. H.: Congenital atresia of the esophagus with tracheo-esophageal fistula, Arch. Pathol. **12**:756-772, 1931 (extensive bibliography).

Tumors
Smooth muscle tumors

38 Athanasoulis, C. A., and Aral, I. M.: Leiomyosarcoma of the esophagus, Gastroenterology **54**:271-274, 1968.

39 Harrington, S. W.: Surgical treatment of be-

nign and secondarily malignant tumors of the esophagus, Arch. Surg. **58**:646-661, 1949.

40 Lewis, B., and Maxfield, R. G.: Leiomyoma of the esophagus; case report and review of the literature, Int. Abstr. Surg. **99**:2, 105-128, 1954.

41 Rainer, W. G., and Brus, R.: Leiomyosarcoma of the esophagus; review of the literature and report of 3 cases, Surgery **50**:343-350, 1965.

42 Rose, J. D.: Myomata of the esophagus, **Br.** J. Surg. **24**:297-308, 1936.

43 Totten, R. S., Stout, A. P., Humphreys, G. H., II, and Moore, R. L.: Benign tumors and cysts of the esophagus, J. Thorac. Surg. **25**:606-622, 1953.

Epidermoid carcinoma

44 Benedict, E. B.: Carcinoma of the esophagus developing in benign strictures, N. Engl. J. Med. **224**:408-412, 1941.

45 Bersack, S. R.: Carcinoma of the esophagus in association with achalasia of the cardia, Radiology **42**:220-223, 1944.

46 Burgess, H. M., Baggenstoss, A. H., Moersch, H. J., and Clagett, O. T.: Carcinoma of the esophagus: a clinical pathologic study, Surg. Clin. North Am. **31**:965-976, 1951.

47 Guernsey, J. M., and Knudsen, D. F.: Abdominal exploration in the evaluation of patients with carcinoma of the thoracic esophagus, J. Thorac. Cardiovasc. Surg. **59**:62-66, 1970.

48 Gunnlaugsson, G. H., Wychulis, A. R., Roland, C., and Ellis, F. H., Jr.: Analysis of the records of 1,657 patients with carcinoma of the esophagus and cardia of the stomach, Surg. Gynecol. Obstet. **130**:997-1005, 1970.

49 Marcial, V. A., Tomé, J. M., Ubiñas, J., Bosch, A., and Correa, J. N.: The role of radiation therapy in esophageal cancer, Radiology **87**:231-239, 1966.

50 Minielly, J. A., Harrison, E. G., Jr., Fontana, R. S., and Payne, W. S.: Verrucous squamous cell carcinoma of the esophagus, Cancer **20**:2078-2087, 1967.

51 Pearson, J. G.: The value of radiotherapy in the management of squamous oesophageal cancer, Br. J. Surg. **58**:794-798, 1971.

52 Rywlin, A. M., and Ortega, R.: Glycogenic acanthosis of the esophagus, Arch. Pathol. **90**:439-443, 1970.

53 Smithers, D. W.: The treatment of carcinoma of the oesophagus, Ann. R. Coll. Surg. Engl. **20**: 36-49, 1957.

54 Ushigome, S., Spjut, H. J., and Noon, G. P.: Extensive dysplasia and carcinoma in situ of esophageal epithelium, Cancer **20**:1023-1029, 1967.

Other tumors

55 Boyd, D. P., Meissner, W. A., Verlkoff, C. L., and Gladding, T. C.: Primary melanocarcinoma of the esophagus; report of a case, Cancer **7**:266-270, 1954.

56 Brenner, S., Heimlich, H., and Widman, M.: Carcinoid of esophagus, N. Y. State J. Med. **69**:1337-1339, 1969.

57 Flege, J. B., Jr., and Edmonds, T. T.: Granular cell myoblastoma of the esophagus, J. Thorac. Cardiovasc. Surg. **8**:217-220, 1969.

58 Fraser, G. M., and Kinley, C. E.: Pseudosarcoma with carcinoma of the esophagus, Arch. Pathol. **85**:325-330, 1968.

59 Heitzman, E. J., Heitzman, G. C., and Elliott, C. F.: Primary esophageal amyloidosis, Arch. Intern. Med. **109**:595-600, 1962.

60 Jang, G. C., Clouse, M. E., and Fleischner, F. G.: Fibrovascular polyp—a benign intraluminal tumor of the esophagus, Radiology **92**:1196-1200, 1969.

61 Piccone, V. A., Klopstock, R., LeVeen, H. H., and Sika, J.: Primary malignant melanoma of the esophagus associated with melanosis of the entire esophagus; first case report, J. Thorac. Cardiovasc. Surg. **59**:865-870, 1970.

62 Rojas, R. A. M., and Vallecillo, L. A.: Primary adenoid cystic carcinoma of the esophagus, Arch. Otolaryng. **70**:197-201, 1959.

63 Stout, A. P., Humphreys, G., and Rottenburg, L.: A case of carcinosarcoma of the esophagus, Amer. J. Roentgenol. Radium Ther. Nucl. Med. **61**:461-469, 1949.

64 Thoreson, W. E.: Secondary carcinoma of the esophagus as a cause of dysphagia, Arch. Pathol. **38**:82-84, 1944.

65 Yates, D. R., and Ross, L. G.: Paget's disease of the esophageal epithelium, Arch. Pathol. **86**:447-452, 1968.

Stomach

Methods of examination
Examination of surgical specimens

Partial or complete resections of the stomach received in the surgical pathology laboratory should be quickly placed in fixative because autolysis takes place rapidly. It is useful to pin the specimens on cork board in a 10% formalin solution. After fixation is complete, the sections can be taken carefully and all lesions can be diagrammatically recorded. If it is necessary to make sections of the entire mucosal surface, strips of gastric mucosa can be rolled up, pinned, placed again in 10% formalin, and embedded in paraffin. In this fashion, an entire lengthwise section of the mucosal surface of the stomach can be studied[1] (Fig. 385).

Tissue sections of all areas of the stomach should be obtained in order to demonstrate occult abnormalities that may exist. With tumors, it is important to take sections through the area of transition between normal and neoplastic mucosa. If a carcinoma is located close to the pylorus, it is imperative that a section be taken through the pylorus and adjacent duodenum. Both ends of the resected specimen should be sectioned and examined for tumor. Lymph nodes should be carefully dissected and placed in separate bottles for identification of specific lymph node groups. In cases of chronic peptic ulcer, multiple sections should be taken from the edges, as well as one or two from the base. A microscopic focus of carcinoma may be present in only one of them.

Cytology

Roentgenographic examination of the stomach is the most useful method for the detection of lesions of the stomach. However, it may not be possible for the radiologist to determine if the lesion is benign or malignant.[4] In such cases, gastric cytology has proved of most value.[5] The obtaining of a proper gastric specimen for cytology should be done only by properly trained personnel. The haphazard intubation of an improperly prepared patient by the house officer sometime during the day is a waste of time, effort, and money. Patients need to be properly prepared with overnight fasting, proper hydration, and overnight suction if there is any gastric obstruction to ensure a completely empty stomach at the time of the test. Vigorous lavage by saline or Ringer's solution gives as satisfactory or superior result as the use of mucolytic agents or abrasive methods.[4, 6, 12, 13]

The rather involved procedure for gastric cytology precludes its use as a general screening method for unselected patients. However, even in high-risk patients such as those with pernicious anemia or low hydrochloric acid, gastric cytology has been disappointing. MacDonald et al.[9] screened 500 patients with these conditions and found only three cases of carcinoma, only one of which was potentially curable. Similar results have been reported by Boon et al.[3] The method can be extraordinarily accurate, for several laboratories have reported positive results of 93% to 98%, with false positives usually less than 1%.[2, 6, 8, 11, 12] Lymphomas of the stomach are less readily detected by cytology, with rates of 40% to 64% being reported.[10, 13] There is no question that cytology is more accurate in determining the presence or absence of gastric cancer than is roentgenographic interpretation.[7, 11, 13] When both methods are combined, an accuracy of over 95% is possible in determining the presence of cancer.[8]

Gastroscopic biopsy

Gastroscopic biopsy has been used by Benedict[14] in the differential diagnosis of chronic gastritis, diffuse carcinoma, and lymphoma. He correlated the biopsy findings with the x-ray films and the surgical specimens. A positive biopsy is of great value, for it influences definitive therapy. A negative biopsy is of limited value. Areas of the stomach previously inaccessible to gastroscopic biopsy can now be easily reached with fiberoptic gastroscopes. The light microscopy, histochemistry, and electron microscopy of the normal stomach have been thoroughly investigated.[16, 17] The morphologic features of chronic gastritis have been well defined, quantitated, and successfully correlated with physiologic tests. Gastric biopsy can contribute to the diagnosis of hemochromatosis, amyloidosis, Crohn's disease, giant hypertrophic gastritis, malignant lymphoma, and eosinophilic gastritis.[18] The procedure is simple and the incidence of complications—particularly bleeding—extremely low. In the series of 1,226 biopsies reported by Joske et al.,[15] hemorrhage was seen in only ten cases (0.8%); in only two patients (0.16%) it was of sufficient severity to require transfusion.

Frozen section

Frozen sections of lesions in the stomach and the immediate areas may be helpful in determining the operative procedure. Microscopic examination of lymph nodes or of peritoneal implants far from the primary abdominal cancer may reveal metastatic carcinoma. Frozen section of a perforated gastric ulcer, particularly in an older person, may show carcinoma. In other instances, the radiologist may describe a lesion that the surgeon is not able to identify. Frozen section of generous biopsies of the questionable area shown by roentgenogram may be diagnostic. The diagnosis of diffuse carcinoma (so-called linitis plastica) is probably the most difficult problem that the surgical pathologist will encounter in frozen section material. The small size of the tumor cells, lack or inconspicuousness of glandular formations, and the marked inflammatory and fibroplastic reaction that accompanies this neoplasm are the responsible factors. We have had some success by staining the ethanol-fixed frozen sections in 1% alcian blue at pH 2.5 for one minute and using nuclear-fast red as counterstain. The tumor cells, which often show a distinct cytoplasmic staining, should be differentiated from mast cells, which also stain with this technique.

When an ulcerated lesion of the stomach is found by the surgeon, he must weigh the value of frozen section against the possibility of implantation of cancer by multiple biopsies of the ulcer. If the debatable ulcer is situated in the midportion or the distal half of the stomach and no evidence of neoplastic spread beyond the stomach exists, resection can be performed without need of gastrotomy and biopsy. If an ulcer is in the juxtaesophageal area, it has a greater likelihood of containing cancer. In this area, surgical therapy varies radically according to the nature of the ulcer. In this area specifically, biopsy and frozen section are necessary, and the risk of spread of cancer by gastrotomy and biopsy must be taken. Fortunately, the latter situation is encountered rarely.

Nonneoplastic lesions
Heterotopic pancreas

In 215 cases of heterotopic pancreas in the stomach reviewed by Palmer,[20] 120 presented clinically as a gastric mass, whereas seventy-four were found at autopsy or incidentally during laparotomy. Grossly, these lesions may form a hemispheric mass, a symmetrical cone, or a short cylindrical nipplelike projection. About three-fourths of them occur in the submucosal layer and about one-seventh in the muscular layer. The great majority have been found in the antrum (61%) and pylorus (24%).

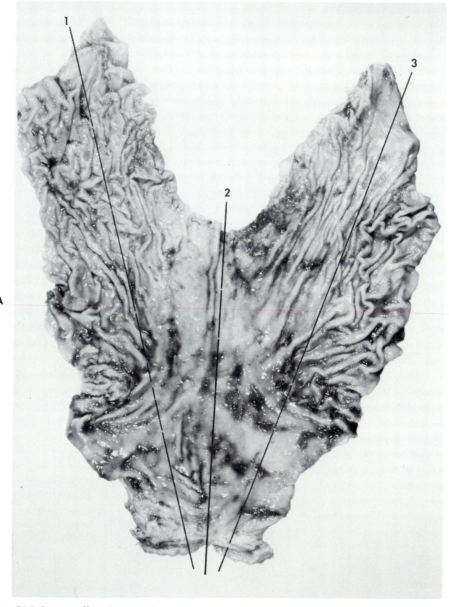

Fig. 385 Swiss-roll technique for examination of gastric mucosa. **A,** Three strips of mucosa are sectioned from anterior wall, lesser curvature, and posterior wall. **B,** Mucosa is rolled, pinned, and processed in routine manner. **C,** Microscopic appearance of specimen. (**A,** WU neg. 71-10615; **B,** WU neg. 71-10616; **C,** WU neg. 71-10694.)

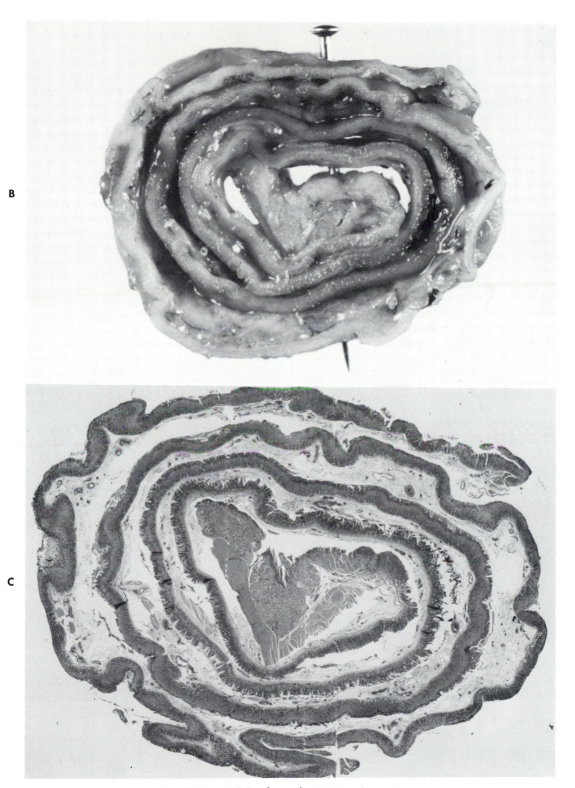

Fig. 385 cont'd For legend, see opposite page.

On section, they grossly resemble normal pancreas. When a nipplelike projection exists, single or multiple ducts may empty on the surface. This can be detected radiographically, and it is an important diagnostic sign.

The heterotopic tissue usually consists of pancreatic acini and ducts without islets. Brunner's glands may be present. We have seen carcinoma arising from heterotopic pancreas.[19] A closely related lesion has been described by Stewart and Taylor[21] as *adenomyoma*. It is composed of large ducts, Brunner's glands, and smooth muscle proliferation.

Hypertrophy of pylorus

Hypertrophy of the pylorus occurs predominantly in children. Usually no sections are submitted because cure is effected by a longitudinal division of the muscles (Ramstedt procedure).

In the adult, hypertrophy of the pylorus may occur as an idiopathic finding (80% in men). We agree with Lumsden and Truelove[25] that this is an extremely rare condition unless it is associated with some other abnormality. When the condition occurs primarily in the adult, it is associated with hypertrophy of the pyloric circular muscle fibers.[23, 26] Radiographically and clinically, a tumor may be suspected. In rare instances, the stomach is resected because of an erroneous diagnosis of neoplasm. Grossly and microscopically, all that is found is hypertrophy of pyloric muscle that ends abruptly at the duodenum, sometimes accompanied by a mild degree of fibrosis.[22] Chronic gastritis is usually present.[24] Although it is possible that some of the cases represent a persistence of the infantile form into adult life, we believe that in most instances the process is secondary to antral gastritis or peptic ulcer of the pyloric channel, which may have healed by the time of surgery.

Gastritis

The concept of chronic gastritis has been greatly clarified by the systematic use of endoscopic gastric biopsy.[30] The two main features of this disease are infiltration of the lamina propria by inflammatory cells and atrophy of the glandular epithelium. Plasma cells and lymphocytes (with occasional formation of follicles) predominate among the inflammatory cells, although eosinophils and neutrophils also may be present. If the inflammatory infiltrate is the only abnormality present, the condition is designated as *chronic superficial gastritis* or, better, as *chronic gastritis with no atrophy*. When glandular atrophy is present in the fundic mucosa, it can be quantitated as mild, moderate, or severe by roughly estimating the thickness of the glandular portion in relation to the thickness of the whole mucosa[38] (Fig. 386). Naturally, a properly oriented biopsy containing muscularis mucosae is needed to make this estimation. Increasing degrees of atrophy are commonly associated with cystic dilatation of glands, atypia of the crypt epithelium, and intestinal metaplasia. The latter is characterized by the appearance of goblet cells, brush border, Paneth cells, and a marked increase in the number of enterochromaffin cells.[36] If atrophy is seen in the absence of inflammatory changes, the condition may be designated as gastric atrophy, although in most cases this probably represents the end stage of a chronic atrophic gastritis. Grossly, atrophic gastritis produces a thin, smooth mucosa with undue prominence of submucosal vessels. We have found an excellent correlation between the degree of gastric atrophy as estimated by endoscopic biopsy and the results of the acid secretory tests. Conversely, the correlation of histology with symptomatology, radiology, and gastroscopy has been disappointing. We have found severe atrophic gastritis in asymptomatic individuals and a normal gastric mucosa in patients with persistent dyspepsia.

In most of the cases, the changes of chronic gastritis are diffuse. Joske et al.[30] examined two pieces of mucosa taken at the same time from different portions of

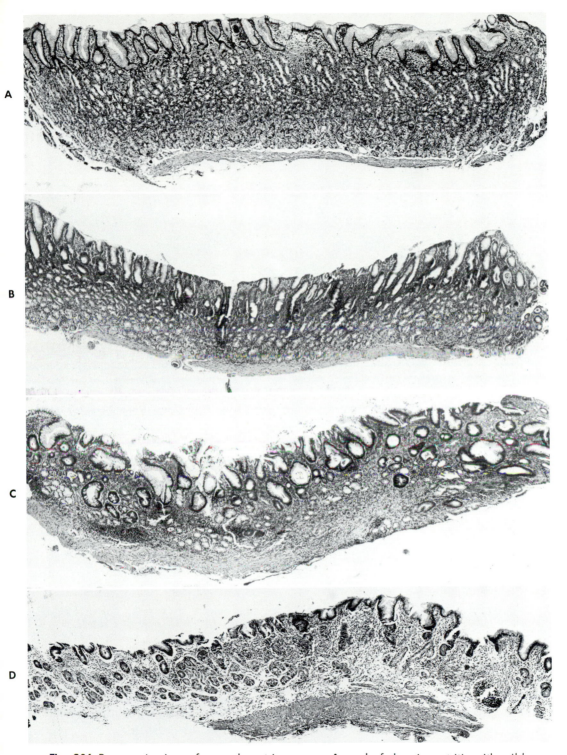

Fig. 386 Panoramic view of normal gastric mucosa, **A,** and of chronic gastritis with mild, **B,** moderate, **C,** and severe, **D,** degrees of atrophy. All of these biopsies were taken from fundic region. (**A** to **D,** ×40; **A,** WU neg. 72-6067; **B,** WU neg. 72-6069; **C,** WU neg. 72-6070; **D,** WU neg. 72-6071.)

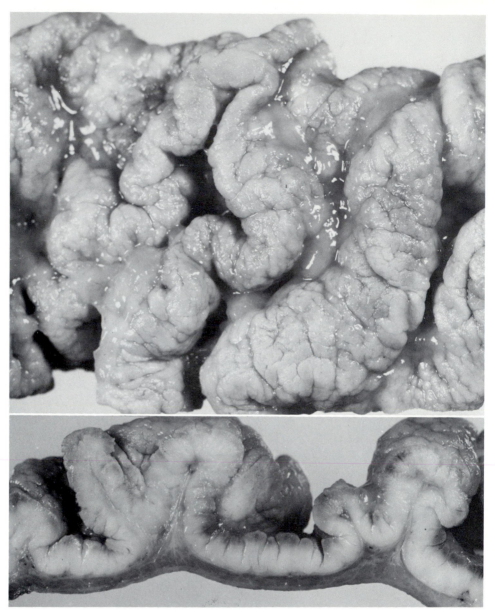

Fig. 387 Giant hypertrophic gastritis in 65-year-old woman. This gross pattern could easily be confused with malignant lymphoma. (WU negs. 59-5144 and 59-5143.)

the body of the stomach and found that in 536 (73.8%) the appearances of the two pieces were very similar. In other instances, the gastritis is patchy or "zonal," especially when secondary to a localized process such as carcinoma. Chronic atrophic gastritis is the rule in cases of gastric cancer, and in general its severity is proportional to the extent of the tumor.[29] Most cases of gastric peptic ulcer are associated with antral and fundal gastritis, whereas in duodenal ulcer the gastritis, if present at all, is often restricted to the antrum. Morson[34] studied the incidence and extent of intestinal metaplasia and found it greatest in stomachs removed for carcinoma, least in those with duodenal ulcer, and intermediate in cases of gastric ulcer.

In pernicious anemia, gastric biopsy may show chronic gastritis with severe atrophy or gastric atrophy without inflammation.[28] The changes are said to be restricted to the fundus and body of the stomach, whereas the antrum remains uninvolved. Carcinoma occurs with increased frequency in patients with pernicious anemia. Schell et al.[37] found all stages of transition from benign to malignant epithelium. When cancer appears, it is often multicentric, polypoid, and located in the fundus.

Hemorrhagic gastritis is an acute life-threatening condition usually engrafted on a background of chronic gastritis.[39] Alcoholism, anti-inflammatory drugs, and stress have been implicated as the precipitating factors. The appearance of the stomach at surgery is characteristic, with multiple, minute areas of hemorrhage throughout the entire mucosa. The microscopic appearance is not so dramatic as the surgical findings would anticipate. In some cases, multiple superficial erosions are found, but in many others the only abnormality seen in the biopsy is a chronic atrophic gastritis, with perhaps some extravasation of blood in the lamina propria. In Lulu and Dragstedt's series,[32] the overall mortality was 55%. They advocated vagotomy and high subtotal gastrectomy as the treatment of choice.

Menétrier[33] described, in a frequently quoted (and misquoted) paper published in 1888, two different gastric diseases under the common term *polyadenomes*.[35] The first, *polyadenomes polypeux*, is discussed later under gastric polyps (p. 378). The second, *polyadenomes en nappes*, is also known as giant hypertrophy of the gastric rugae and giant hypertrophic gastritis[27] (Fig. 387). It is to this variety that the term Menétrier's disease is usually attached. A localized and a diffuse form have been described. Hypochlorhydria or achlorhydria is the rule. Radiographically and grossly, the condition can be confused with malignant lymphoma and carcinoma. The disease often involves the greater curvature of the stomach and is characterized grossly by markedly hypertrophic rugae resembling cerebral convolutions. The transition between normal and diseased mucosa is always abrupt. Microscopically, the glands are markedly elongated and tortuous. Of twenty cases cases reported by Kenney et al.,[31] three had associated multiple endocrine adenomatosis. This finding suggests that the rugal hypertrophy may be the result of an as yet unidentified hyperfunctioning endocrine cell. It should be mentioned here that most of the cases diagnosed by radiologists and gastroscopists as "hypertrophic gastritis" will show normal stomach or atrophic gastritis on biopsy.

Peptic ulcer

Peptic ulceration occurs in the stomach and duodenum, as a marginal or jejunal ulcer after gastrojejunostomy, in association with Meckel's diverticulum, and in the lower third of the esophagus. Such ulceration occurs in the presence of hydrochloric acid. The physiologic mechanisms in the pathogenesis of peptic ulceration have been extensively studied by Dragstedt et al.[40] This information is presented well by Harkins.[43]

Acute ulceration of the stomach is a common finding at autopsy and is usually a terminal event. This acute ulceration may occur in any debilitating illness, in sepsis, or following surgery or trauma (stress ulcer), in patients with central nervous system injury or disease (Cushing's ulcer), as a complication of long-term steroid therapy (steroid ulcer), in patients with extensive burns (Curling's ulcer), and following the introduction of tubes into the stomach.[42, 46] If the ulcer involves only the mucosa, it can heal completely, but if part of the muscle is destroyed, it is replaced by fibrotic tissue, leaving a depressed pit. *Chronic ulcerations* of the stomach occur principally in the area of stomach normally lined by pyloric type of mucosa—i.e., the distal half,

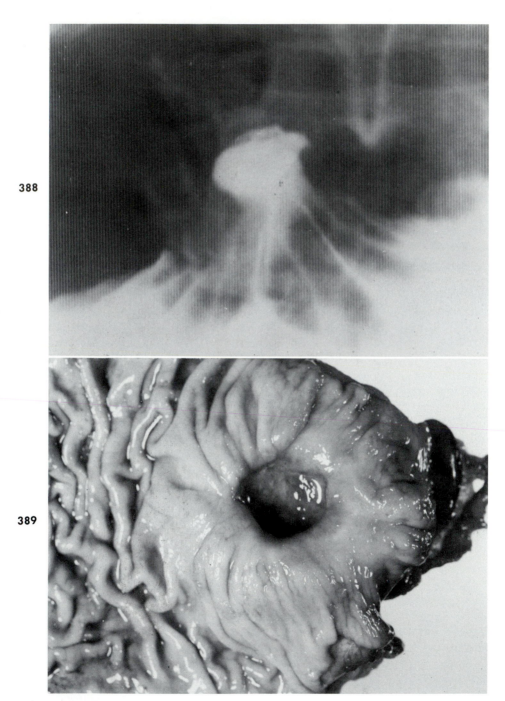

Fig. 388 Converging mucosal folds, so well seen in chronic ulcer shown in Fig. 389, can also be seen radiographically. (WU neg. 52-826.)
Fig. 389 Sharply delimited chronic gastric ulcer with converging folds of stomach mucosa extending right to margin of ulcer. Ulcer occurred in 53-year-old man. (WU neg. 58-495.)

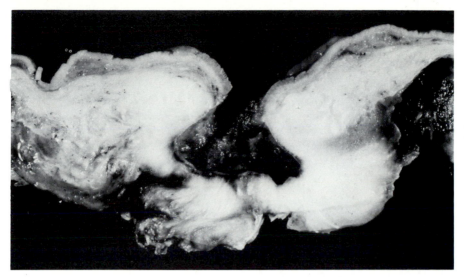

Fig. 390 Typical gross appearance of chronic peptic ulcer. Entire thickness of muscular layer has been destroyed.

especially along the lesser curvature (so-called Magenstrasse). However, they can occur anywhere in the stomach. It is interesting to note that even when located high in the fundus, they are usually surrounded by pyloric type of mucosa, probably as the result of a metaplastic process.

In the past, it was considered that a high percentage of all ulcers over 2.5 cm in diameter were cancer and that about 100% of the ulcers of the greater curvature and about 70% of those in the prepyloric area were cancer. In our experience, these statements have not been true. In forty-nine ulcers larger than 2.5 cm, only eighteen were malignant (37%). In twelve ulcers on the greater curvature, six were benign and six were malignant. In the prepyloric zone, there were thirty-seven ulcers, only eight of which were malignant (22%).[41] These statistics have great interest but in an individual patient are of little value.

Grossly, the benign ulcer of the stomach is sharply delineated. The converging folds of the stomach mucosa extend to the margin of the ulcer (Figs. 388 and 389). Grossly, it may be *impossible* to identify carcinoma in an ulcer that appears benign. From 10% to 15% of gastric carcinomas appear grossly to be benign ulcers. On sec-

tion of a benign ulcer, there is an undermining of the edges with complete fibrous replacement of the wall of the stomach by grayish white scar (Fig. 390). Proximally, the ulcer has overhanging edges. The distal edge has sloping borders. There is subserosal fibrosis on the surface of the stomach directly overlying the ulcer. In the vicinity of the ulceration, the lymph nodes may be enlarged. Any unusual marginal nodularity about the ulcer should suggest the presence of carcinoma. The transition of a benign ulcer to carcinoma occurs only rarely, and we have had difficulty in finding cases that would withstand critical clinical and pathologic analysis. These criteria will be discussed later.

Microscopically, the surface of a benign chronic ulcer shows purulent exudate and fibrinoid necrosis. Subserosal fibrosis, thick-walled vessels, and proliferated nerve bundles are present in the wall of the stomach near the ulcer. The deeper layers reveal organization of the exudate and fibrous connective tissue replacement of the muscle. The vascular changes are characterized by subendothelial fibrous proliferation and are secondary to the ulcer (Fig. 391). In the healing of a chronic gastric ulcer, deep epithelial heterotopia with

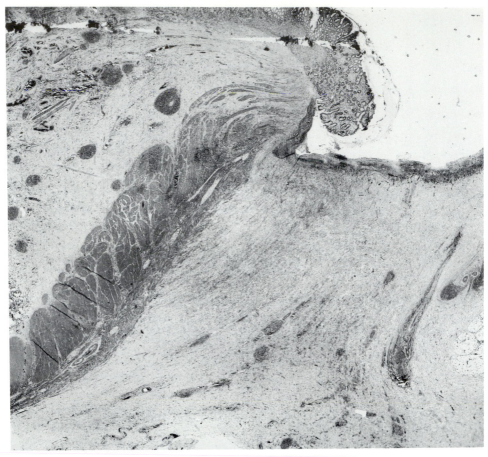

Fig. 391 Chronic ulcer of stomach. Base is completely replaced by fibrous tissue, proximal area has overhanging mucosal borders, and muscle has been displaced because of fibrosis. (WU neg. 58-838.)

penetration but without transgression of the muscle wall can occur. Such changes can be incorrectly diagnosed as carcinoma.[47]

The ratio of duodenal to gastric ulcer is 4:1. The mean acid output in patients with gastric ulcer is lower than that in normal individuals. However, the failure to obtain an acid response in an augmented histamine test practically rules out the diagnosis of benign peptic ulcer.[44] The most important clinical criterion for benign peptic ulcer is *complete* healing of the ulcer. Partial healing also can be seen in gastric carcinomas. The usual criterion for adequate healing is a reduction in crater size of at least 50% over a six-week to eight-week

period of intensive medical management. Unfortunately, when patients medically treated for peptic ulcer have been followed for a long enough period, recurrences have been found in 80% to 90%.[45]

Syphilis

Syphilis of the stomach is an extremely rare entity that radiographically and grossly simulates closely the linitis plastica type of carcinoma of the stomach. In the early stages the stomach feels soft, but later on it becomes firm. Ulceration first occurs almost invariably in the pyloric portion. The liver may show evidence of syphilis with hepar lobatum or stellate scars. In advanced syphilis, the stomach

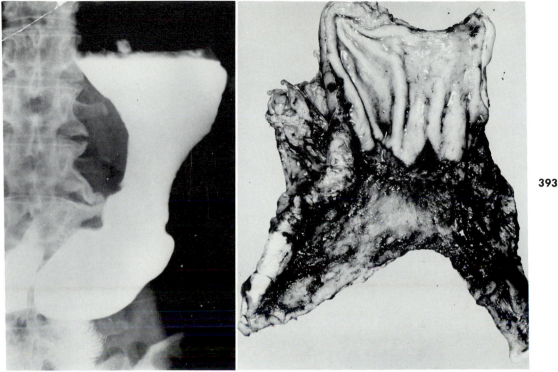

392

393

Fig. 392 Prominent deformity of stomach due to syphilis. (WU neg. 50-4531.)
Fig. 393 Resected stomach shown in Fig. 392. Note prominent deformities and areas of ulceration. Microscopic changes were compatible with, but not diagnostic of, syphilis. (WU neg. 50-4181.)

is shrunken, small in size, and has a so-called leather bottle appearance. There is great thickening of the wall.[48] The serology is positive.

The foregoing findings warrant exploration and frozen section. If several adequate frozen sections show only diffuse lymphoid infiltration and desmoplasia of the mucosal and submucosal tissue without evidence of tumor, the surgeon should withdraw unless the deformity is great enough to warrant resection (Figs. 392 and 393). In our four cases, the gross and microscopic findings were compatible with, but not diagnostic of, syphilis.

Although frozen section may differentiate syphilis from carcinoma of the linitis plastica type, resection is not indicated when such a differentiation is impossible. Patients with carcinoma of the linitis plastica type are not successfully treated by resection.[49] On the other hand, if the patient has syphilis, antisyphilitic therapy may be of great symptomatic value. Williams and Kimmelstiel[50] reported gumma and gummatoid lesions with proliferative endarteritis and phlebitis in some of their patients.

Other lesions

Inflammatory fibroid polyp of the stomach is the best name for lesions previously described under the name eosinophilic granuloma, neurofibroma, and hemangiopericytoma. These lesions are frequently associated with hypochlorhydria or achlorhydria. In nine of the ten patients reported by Helwig and Ranier,[57] the lesion was in the pyloric antrum. These lesions are probably not true neoplasms. Gross appearance is somewhat similar to a pyogenic granuloma (Fig. 394). Microscopically, this le-

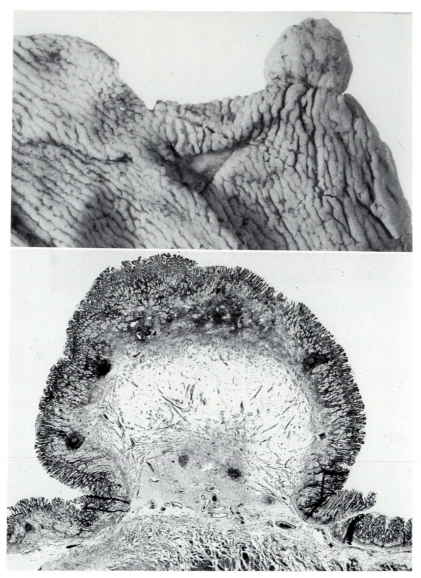

Fig. 394 Inflammatory fibroid polyp of stomach that was sharply delimited both grossly and microscopically. (AFIP 332975; from Helwig, E. B., and Ranier, A.: Inflammatory fibroid polyps of the stomach, Surg. Gynecol. Obstet. **96:**355-367, 1953; by permission of Surgery, Gynecology & Obstetrics.)

sion is located in the submucosa and is characterized by vascular and fibroblastic proliferation (often in a whorl-like arrangement) and a polymorphic inflammatory response, usually dominated by eosinophils.

Another condition associated with a large number of eosinophils is *diffuse eosinophilic gastroenteritis.* As the name implies, it is a diffuse process rather than

a well-circumscribed polypoid mass. There is no good evidence that these two conditions are related.[56] The latter involves the distal portion of the stomach and proximal portion of the duodenum and can cause pyloric obstruction. It may be associated with allergic phenomena and extreme eosinophilia.[60] Microscopically, edema and diffuse infiltration by eosino-

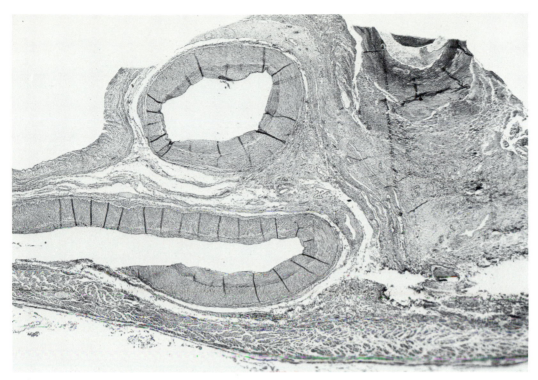

Fig. 395 Cirsoid aneurysm of vessel in wall of stomach which caused death from hemorrhage. (Low power; WU neg. 52-1831; Case 14655.)

phils is prominent. Necrotizing angiitis has been observed in some cases.[58] The lesion probably represents a local reaction to ingested allergen. Ashby et al.[51] concluded that many of their cases were secondary to infestation by *Eustoma rotundatum*, a parasite of the North Sea herring.

When making the diagnosis of diffuse eosinophilic gastroenteritis, it should be remembered that a mild to moderate number of eosinophils can sometimes be seen in other conditions, such as polyarteritis nodosa and Hodgkin's disease and even in peptic ulcers and carcinomas.

Tuberculosis has been reported.[52] Sirak[61] reported a noncaseating granulomatous lesion of the stomach microscopically suggesting *sarcoidosis.* Grossly, the stomach resembled the linitis plastica type of cancer.

Rarely, *hemorrhage* can occur from perforation of arteriosclerotic aneurysm of gastric vessels within the wall of the stomach (Fig. 395). Millard[59] collected seventeen instances of ruptured gastric aneu-

rysm. The etiology was arteriosclerotic, and there was a high fatality rate. However, three patients were saved by prompt surgical resection. On several occasions we have seen severe gastric hemorrhage occur because of rupture of small submucosal arteries (3 mm to 5 mm). These arteries were often located high on the lesser curvature. *Duplication* of the stomach can occur.[55] The large majority of **gastric diverticula** occur in a juxtacardiac position and are probably the result of anatomically weak areas. The remaining can occur anywhere else in the stomach and are commonly associated with another disease, such as peptic ulcer.[54]

Bezoars are occasionally seen as surgical specimens. The great majority fall into two categories: *trichobezoar*, which is composed of hair, and *phytobezoar*, composed of vegetable products. More than 85% of the latter are caused by ingestion of unripened persimmons.[53]

Radiation therapy to the upper portion

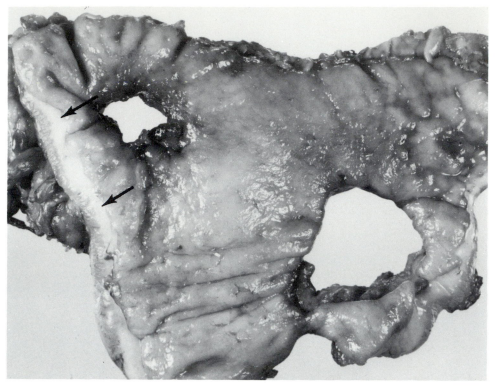

Fig. 396 Subtotal resection of stomach showing two large well-delimited ulcers. Arrows indicate prominent submucosal fibrosis. Patient had received intensive irradiation for Hodgkin's disease. (WU neg. 72-9770.)

of the abdomen can result in gastric ulcerations with little fibrous reaction which therefore makes them prone to perforation (Fig. 396).

Tumors
Smooth muscle tumors

Leiomyomas are common as an incidental autopsy finding. Meissner[64] found forty-four leiomyomas in twenty-three of fifty consecutive autopsies. They are often multiple and form small, well-defined homogeneous nodules. Smooth muscle tumors occur much less frequently clinically than carcinomas but are the most common benign neoplasm of the stomach. About 600 cases have been reported. They may arise from the muscularis propria, muscularis mucosae, or the muscle present in the blood vessel wall. They appear most commonly in the region of the pars media (40%) and antrum (25%).[65] They usually

are submucosal (about 60%) and grow toward the lumen of the stomach, where they make a smooth projection into the lumen (Fig. 397). In time, however, a central ulceration occurs that may penetrate deeply into the tumor. This may result in hematemesis.

Leiomyomas also may grow out from the serosal surface (30%). These smooth muscle tumors may become quite large. Although 20% occur near the pylorus, obstruction is rare. On section, they are well circumscribed and have a smooth, lobulated or whorled-silk appearance. An hourglass defect may occur at the cardia or pylorus if the tumor encircles the stomach. Areas of hemorrhage, necrosis, and calcification may be present.

Microscopically, most smooth muscle tumors show well-differentiated smooth muscle cells with a variable degree of hyalinized connective tissue. However, a rela-

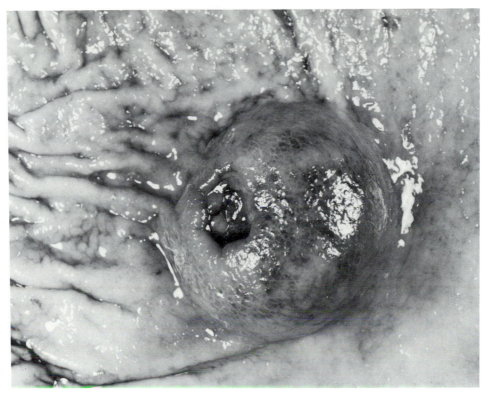

Fig. 397 Leiomyoma of stomach with central ulceration so characteristic of this benign neoplasm. (WU neg. 58-494.)

tively large number show a wide variation from the classical pattern. Peculiar features sometimes seen in gastric leiomyomas include extreme cellularity, presence of occasional large cells with bizarre hyperchromatic nuclei, marked diffuse vascularity, tumor cells of round rather than spindle shape, and regimentation of nuclei. Electron microscopic studies have shown that myofibrils are very sparse or even absent in most of the cases, in contrast to normal smooth muscle cells and uterine leiomyomas.[70] As a result, special stains at a light microscopic level, such as Masson's trichrome or Mallory's P.T.A.H., are usually of no help. This often results in a smooth muscle tumor being misdiagnosed as neurilemoma, fibroma, carcinoid tumor, glomus tumor, or sarcoma. A reasonably distinct variety of smooth muscle tumor is the so-called bizarre leiomyoblastoma[68, 69] (Fig. 398). It is characterized by round cells

with central nucleus and abundant clear cytoplasm. The latter is probably an artifact of fixation.[66] Areas of transition with more typical spindle cells are often present. The large majority of leiomyoblastomas follow a benign clinical course.[68, 69]

There is now fairly general agreement that the simple most important criterion for differentiating a leiomyoma from a leiomyosarcoma is the number of mitotic figures present.[63] Cellularity, hemorrhage, bizarre nuclei, necrosis, and large size are common accompanying features of malignant tumors, but they are not diagnostic per se. How many mitoses are needed per high-power field in order to call a smooth muscle tumor malignant is obviously arbitrary. Fortunately, most of these tumors are very cooperative: they have either few or no mitoses or a large number of them. However, smooth muscle tumors of the gastrointestinal tract have been known to appear

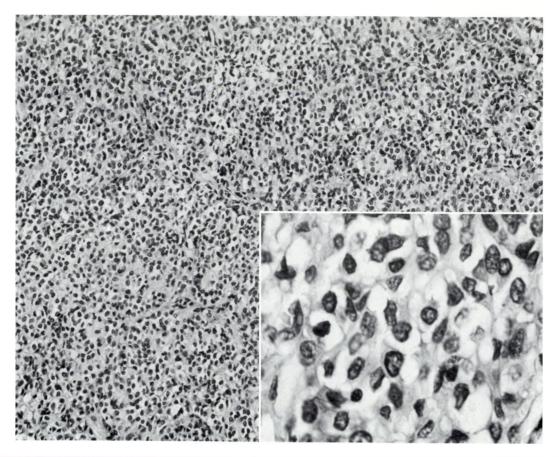

Fig. 398 Gastric leiomyoma of clear cell type, also known as bizarre leiomyoblastoma. Tumor has indistinct lobular configuration. **Inset** shows clear cytoplasm and well-defined cell margins. (×150; WU neg. 71-7565; **inset,** ×600; WU neg. 71-7566.)

perfectly benign under the microscope and behave as malignant neoplasms clinically. We have seen two such cases. It is therefore possible to underestimate as well as to overestimate the malignant potentialities. They do not usually metastasize to regional lymph nodes but spread distantly to the liver and lungs.[67] Giberson et al.[62] reported forty instances of leiomyosarcoma of the stomach. Twelve had metastases. The lymph nodes were involved in three, but only by direct extension.

These tumors may be diagnosed roentgenographically because of the smooth outline and central niche in the tumor. At the time of operation, the pathologist can easily make a gross diagnosis of smooth muscle tumor, but it is often impossible to tell with certainty whether the tumor is benign or malignant.

Certainly, enucleation of the tumor is not adequate. Conservative local resection of the neoplasm and stomach wall is the least that should be undertaken. Since this tumor tends to spread distantly without involvement of lymph nodes, wide resection of any lymph node area does not appear indicated.

Polyps

The nomenclature of gastric polyps is confusing, mainly because they have been usually regarded analogous to colonic polyps in microscopic appearance and natural history.[71, 73] This is unfortunate because the most common of the two main varieties

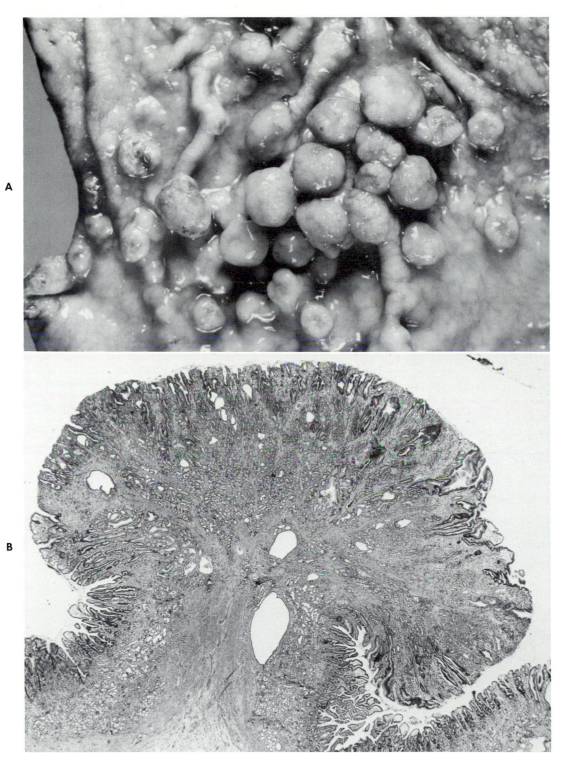

Fig. 399 Gastric polyps of "hyperplastic" type occurring in 65-year-old woman. **A,** Large sessile polyps of firm consistency occupy large portion of gastric mucosa. **B,** Panoramic microscopic view of one of polyps. Note cystic dilatation of glands and bundles of smooth muscle between glands. (**A,** WU neg. 73-364; **B,** ×5; WU neg. 73-459.)

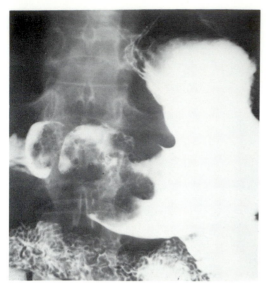

Fig. 400 Large polypoid lesion with filling defect in region of pylorus. (WU neg. 55-4778.)

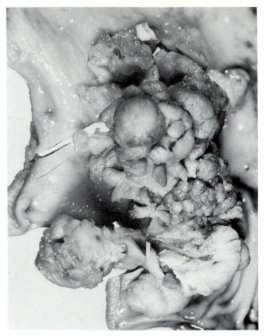

Fig. 401 Same lesion shown in Fig. 400. Subtotal gastric resection demonstrated polypoid lesion with focal carcinoma. There was no tumor in stalk and no lymph node metastases. Patient has remained well over five years. (WU neg. 55-4575.)

of gastric polyps has no exact counterpart in the large bowel. We are referring to the type variously called regenerative, inflammatory, hyperplastic, and hamartomatous, which corresponds to Menétrier's *polyadenomes polypeux*. This variety comprises 75% of all gastric polyps. They are randomly distributed in the stomach, are small and often multiple, and have a smooth or slightly lobulated contour. Microscopically, they are composed of hyperplastic glands of pyloric shape (often dilated or even cystic), fibrous stroma, inflammatory cells, and scattered smooth muscle bundles from the muscularis mucosae (Fig. 399). *Atypia is not present.* Coexisting carcinoma (not originating in the polyps) was seen in 8% of thirty-nine patients reported by Ming and Goldman[72] and in 28% of seventy-four cases studied by Tomasulo.[75]

The second type is the adenomatous polyp (Figs. 400 and 401). Usually antral in location, single, large, and with some papillary foci, it is composed of *atypical* glands with pseudostratified cells having nuclear abnormalities and numerous mitoses.[74] The microscopic appearance is practically the same as that of the colonic adenomatous polyp. Coexisting carcinoma

is seen in a large proportion of cases (59% in the series reported by Tomasulo).[75]

Carcinoma

The classification of carcinoma of the stomach is, of necessity, artifactual because practically all of these carcinomas arise from the mucus-secreting cells. In rare instances, carcinoma may arise from heterotopic pancreas. The classification of the carcinoma is of value only if it helps in diagnosis or prognosis.

Borrman[76] has a system of some merit that shows the gradual gradation between tumors that are fungating and growing mainly within the lumen (Fig. 402) and those that are deeply invasive and growing through the wall of the stomach. Tumors that evert and grow within the lumen have a much lower incidence of metastasis.

Lauren[77] divided his 1,344 cases of gastric carcinoma into two main histologic types: intestinal (53%) and diffuse (33%).

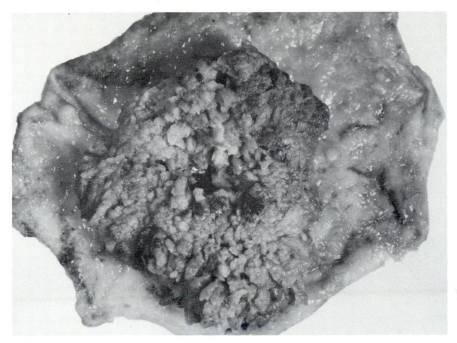

Fig. 402 Polypoid adenocarcinoma of stomach. Villous areas alternate with solid foci. Superficial stromal invasion was present. (WU neg. 70-6564.)

The remaining were heterogeneous in composition. The intestinal type is thought to arise from metaplastic epithelium, an assumption corroborated by electron microscopic studies.[78] As expected, the prognosis was worse in the diffuse variety.

The better defined clinicopathologic varieties of gastric carcinoma are as follows:

1 Adenocarcinoma—no specific type (60% to 80%)
2 Adenocarcinoma associated with peptic ulcer ("ulcer-cancer") (5% or less)
3 Adenocarcinoma — superficial spreading type (less than 5%)
4 Adenocarcinoma—linitis plastica type (less than 5%)
5 Carcinoma—adenosquamous ("adenoacanthoma") and epidermoid (less than 1%)

Adenocarcinoma—no specific type

There is wide variation in the gross appearance of carcinomas of the stomach. Unfortunately, most of the tumors grow extensively within the stomach, infiltrating a large portion of the wall. In many instances, the tumor spreads to the serosa and involves various node groups. They secrete variable amounts of mucin. Highly mucinous tumors have a gelatinous appearance. The secretion of the tumor cells is usually an acid mucosubstance, easily detected with alcian blue or colloidal iron stains, whereas in normal stomach neutral mucosubstances predominate.[79]

Adenocarcinoma associated with peptic ulcer ("ulcer-cancer")

The possible occurrence of carcinoma arising on the basis of a preexisting chronic peptic ulcer has been argued for years. Stout,[91] Gömöri,[82] Newcomb,[89] and others have accepted it, whereas equally prominent authorities, such as Mallory,[87] Palmer,[90] and Hebbel,[83] have denied it. It seems to us that the problem should be analyzed from two different aspects.

The first aspect is pathogenetic and can be proposed in the following way: Are there any pathologic criteria by which a gastric cancer can be assumed to have arisen from a peptic ulcer, and, if so, what are they? Malignant tumors with central ulceration without steep overhanging mar-

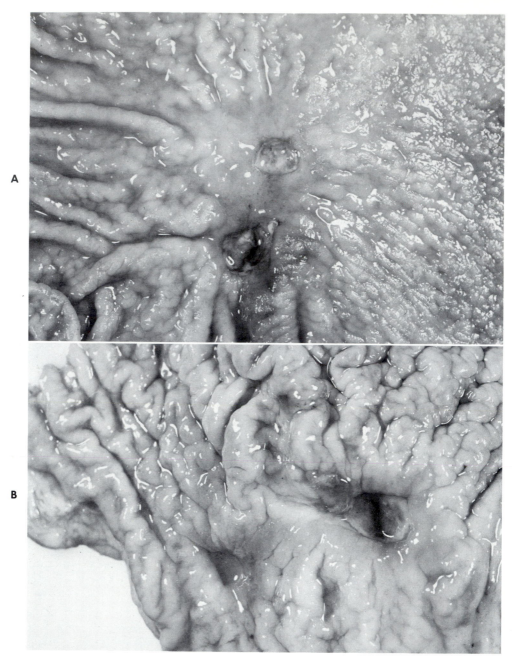

Fig. 403 Gross appearance of ulcers demonstrating difficulty in determining whether given ulcer is benign or malignant. **A,** Two sharply demarcated benign ulcers with converging mucosal folds. **B,** Two ulcers that do not look too dissimilar but in reality represent primary ulcerating carcinoma. (**A,** WU neg. 54-181; **B,** WU neg. 54-5518.)

gins, with neoplastic cells at the base, and with preservation of the muscle should obviously be considered primary ulcerating carcinomas (Fig. 403). Presence of carcinoma on both margins of an ulcer is also suggestive that the ulceration is secondary to the neoplasm. The main problem of interpretation resides with lesions having all the typical features of chronic peptic ulcer (such as convergence of rugal folds, sharp

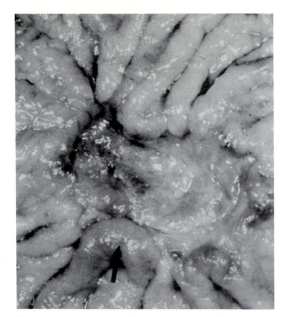

Fig. 404 Apparently benign chronic ulcer. Carcinoma, however, was found on one margin. Prominent fold seen at inferior margin of ulcer contained carcinoma (arrow). (EFSCH.)

demarcation, upward bending of the muscularis propria and fusion with the muscularis mucosae and a fibrous base with total replacement of the muscle, vascular obliterative changes, and absence of tumor) in which carcinoma is found *in only one margin* after subserially sectioning the lesion (Fig. 404). We encountered four such lesions in a consecutive series of sixty-one peptic ulcers. In these cases, did the carcinoma arise from the mucosa at one edge of the ulcer, or did the ulcer arise because of the carcinoma in an area of diminished resistance? There is simply no way to answer this question with the data presently available. We can only say that, if malignant change of a gastric ulcer happens at all, it must be an extremely rare occurrence.

The second aspect of this possible relationship is a practical one and regards the management of patients with symptoms and radiologic signs suggestive of peptic ulcer. Fortunately, there is now enough information to answer satisfactorily the three basic questions in this regard.[84]

1 How reliable are our diagnostic methods in differentiating a benign peptic ulcer from a carcinoma? The differential diagnosis between peptic ulcer and ulcerated carcinoma by radiographic examination is subject to error.[88] In published series of patients with lesions diagnosed radiographically as benign who were subsequently operated upon, carcinoma was found in 6.2% to 15.2%.[84] In our institution, five out of 101 ulcers diagnosed as benign proved histologically to be malignant, an error of 5%. Conversely, of ninety ulcerated lesions diagnosed as malignant or probably malignant, twenty-five were benign, an error of 28%. Blendis et al.[80] have shown that by using a combined approach with radiology, cytology, and gastrophotography, a high diagnostic accuracy can be achieved.

2 Of patients with a clinical and radiographic diagnosis of peptic ulcer who have been treated medically, how many will later be found to have gastric cancer? Of 473 cases followed for a minimum of ten years by Ihre et al.,[84] gastric cancer developed in only five (1.1%). In Jordan's series[85] of 111 patients who were followed for a minimum of five years, only two developed carcinoma.

3 Is the risk of developing gastric cancer greater among patients who have had surgical treatment for benign peptic ulcer than among the general population? This can be answered by saying that no statistically significant increase in mortality from gastric cancer has been detected in most series.[84, 86] Côté et al.[81] reported seventeen cases of gastric cancers developing many years after partial gastrectomy; twelve of the patients had had gastric ulcer and five duodenal ulcer.

Adenocarcinoma—superficial spreading type

The superficial spreading type of carcinoma forms a serpiginous-like ulcer that may reach a considerable size (to 54 sq cm)[93] (Fig. 405).

The definition of a superficial gastric cancer varies according to the authors. We

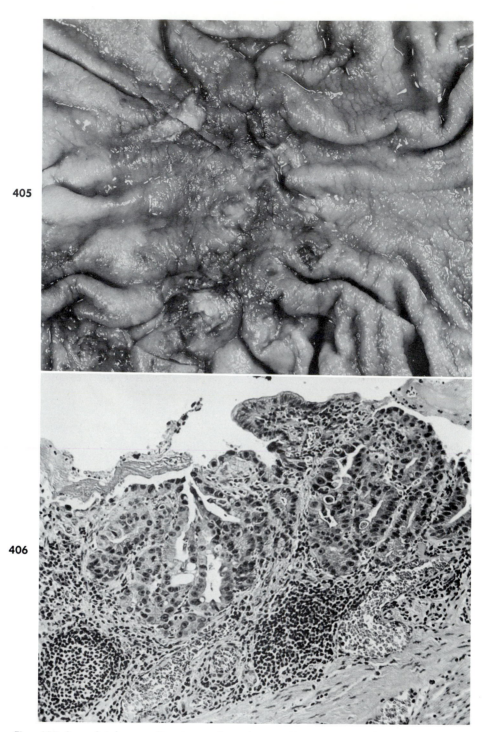

405

406

Fig. 405 Superficial spreading type of carcinoma. Margins are indistinct, and there was no penetration of muscular coats of stomach. (WU neg. 50-383.)

Fig. 406 Superficial spreading carcinoma. Note complete disorganization of lining glands. There was no penetration of muscular coat of stomach. Patient was alive and well thirteen years following gastrectomy. (×210; WU neg. 50-6002.)

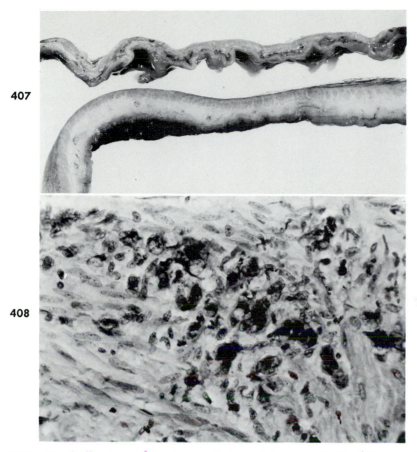

Fig. 407 Linitis plastica type of carcinoma of stomach compared with thickness of normal stomach. There is tremendous thickening of wall with tumor growing in dense fibrous tissue, which is well demonstrated in Fig. 408. (WU neg. 49-7107.)

Fig. 408 Linitis plastica type of carcinoma of stomach. These tumor cells represent small nests of carcinoma cells growing in dense connective tissue. (×400; WU neg. 50-689.)

agree that the term should be restricted to tumors that do not extend beyond the muscularis mucosae, which represents the anatomic boundary of the mucosa. Multiple foci of origin are common (Fig. 406). Lymph node metastases were found in five of 27 cases reviewed by Bragg et al.[92] Of eighteen patients available for five-year follow-up, only two had died as a consequence of gastric tumor.

Adenocarcinoma—linitis plastica type

The rare linitis plastica type of carcinoma of the stomach presents profound desmoplasia.[95] Gross alterations begin in the prepyloric area with perhaps some slight superficial ulceration. There is evi-

dence of pyloric obstruction as the wall of the stomach becomes thickened (Figs. 407 and 408). Sections of the wall of this thickened stomach show hypertrophy of the muscle with a great increase of grayish white submucosal tissue. There are thin, fine, grayish white areas of tissue infiltrating the muscle, often extending on the serosal surface. Lymph node involvement is usually present.

In the microscopic examination of carcinoma of the stomach, it is important to examine sections from the limits of the resection to determine whether or not tumor is present. If the tumor is close to the pylorus, a segment of duodenum should be submitted, for in these tumors the duodenum is invaded in about 50% of cases.[96] In the duodenum, tumor may be seen within the lymphatics, and it can be present in almost any layer except the mucosa. Carcinoma close to the esophagus commonly invades it.

Bilateral ovarian metastases are common and constitute the majority of the cases referred to as Krukenberg's tumor. In rare instances, extension of tumor cells through the muscle wall, probably by way of lymphatic vessels, may extend throughout the entire gastrointestinal tract.[94]

If carcinoma of the stomach is exceedingly undifferentiated, or if it is of the linitis plastica type, stains for epithelial mucin may be helpful. If this stain is positive, it proves carcinoma rather than a sarcoma. Of course, highly undifferentiated carcinoma may secrete no mucin.

Carcinoma—adenosquamous ("adenoacanthoma") and epidermoid

The adenosquamous and epidermoid varieties of carcinoma comprise a very small proportion of gastric cancer (between 0.4% and 0.7%). Straus et al.[97] found forty-one adenoacanthomas and forty-five pure epidermoid carcinomas of the stomach reported in the literature. Only cases surrounded by gastric mucosa in all sides can be accepted. Those extending to the lower end of the esophagus cannot be included, since an esophageal origin cannot be ruled out.

Clinicopathologic correlation

It is unfortunate that carcinoma of the stomach is so often incurable. If the tumor does not grow in the cardioesophageal or pyloric areas, there will be no obstruction, and the early symptoms may be vague and nonspecific: weight loss, anemia, and minimal gastrointestinal symptoms. In a few instances, the first sign of a carcinoma is the presence of pulmonary, hepatic, or lymph node metastases. The so-called Virchow's node (left supraclavicular) in carcinoma of the stomach is relatively infrequent.

Roentgenographic examination of the stomach will demonstrate the lesion in almost 100% of the cases, but in about 10% it will be impossible to determine whether the lesion is benign or malignant. Unfortunately, tumor spreads rather quickly in the stomach, through the wall, and to the abundant lymph nodes in both immediate and distant zones beyond the possibility of resection (para-aortic lymph nodes and those in the region of the celiac axis). Unsuspected extensive metastases to the liver are found frequently at operation.

The pathologic examination of the specimen should be thorough, for the findings are of great value in the estimation of prognosis.[99, 103] When carcinoma is found at the limit of the excision, the situation is hopeless. The microscopic pattern of the tumor is of little value in estimating prognosis. However, the depth of penetration of the carcinoma is of great importance, for the deeper the penetration, the greater the chance of metastasis. Furthermore, in groups of patients, the smaller the gastric cancer, the better the prognosis.[98] In a few instances in which superficial carcinomas are localized to the mucosa and submucosa, the results are excellent. With penetration of the muscular wall, the incidence of metastasis increases. If no lymph nodes are involved on thorough pathologic examination, over 50% of the patients may be expected to survive for five years. With involvement of lymph nodes, the prognosis is poor. Fewer than 10% of the patients survive five years.

The presence of a pushing border accompanied by degenerative changes and cellular infiltrate at the interface between the normal tissue and the cancer is a favorable prognostic sign. Unfortunately, this finding occurs rather infrequently.[102] There are also exceptions in which the pathologic findings show advanced disease but the patient persists in surviving despite them. The reasons for such survival are unknown.

Total gastrectomy used to be recommended for all patients with carcinoma of

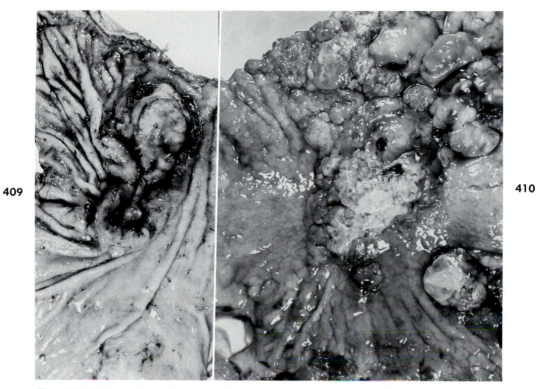

409

410

Fig. 409 Malignant lymphoma which presented as ulcer. (WU neg. 50-6055.)
Fig. 410 Diffuse involvement of stomach by malignant lymphoma. (WU neg. 50-390.)

the stomach. However, as Walters et al.[104] pointed out, an equally adequate resection of the nodes is possible by subtotal gastric resection. It is true that the operative mortality following total gastrectomy is now low in experienced hands and approaches that of subtotal gastrectomy, but the morbidity that develops in total gasrectomy is still high. Therefore, we believe that total gastrectomy in all patients is not justified. With tumor growing in the region of the cardioesophageal area or high on the lesser curvature, indications for total gastrectomy seem better advised.

Concepts of what constitutes a radical subtotal gastrectomy differ. Certainly in the past, the competent surgeon was more conservative than he would be today. Therefore, the meticulous study by McNeer et al.[101] of autopsied patients in whom subtotal gastrectomy had been done and local recurrence had developed is of limited value today in discussing the merits of radical subtotal gastrectomy versus total gastrectomy. It is unfortunate that the overall survival in all cases of gastric cancer in most series is in the neighborhood of 7%.[100] The most interesting change in this disease has been the marked decrease in incidence in some countries such as the United States.

Malignant lymphoma

Malignant lymphoma of the stomach may be a primary or a secondary manifestation. If primary, the tumors make up only a small percentage of all malignant tumors of the stomach. The majority are located in the distal half of the stomach.[109]

Grossly, this lesion has many patterns (Figs. 409 and 410). It has its inception in the submucosal lymphoid tissue or within the lamina propria and thus is submucosal in nature. There may be giant convolutions resembling cerebral convolutions and mimicking, to some extent, a

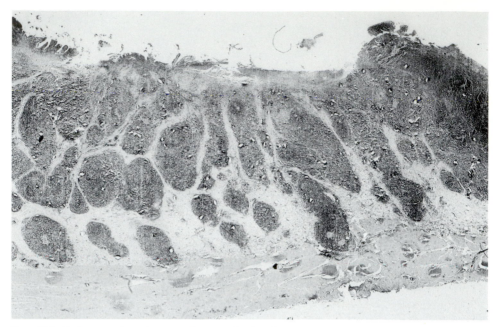

Fig. 411 Malignant lymphoma of stomach that has spread through wall and ulcerated surface. (Low power; WU neg. 50-5217.)

hypertrophic gastritis. There may be a tremendous lobulated mass with areas of superficial or deep ulceration. In twelve of thirty-four cases at Barnes Hospital, the lesion was polypoid.[108] This tumor does not usually involve the pylorus. It cannot be distinguished from carcinoma with certainty either grossly or radiographically.

Primary malignant lymphoma may remain restricted to the stomach, but it frequently involves regional nodes to form a voluminous mass. Microscopically, it can be any variation of malignant lymphoma (Fig. 411).

It is sometimes difficult to distinguish microscopically a histiocytic lymphoma from an undifferentiated small cell carcinoma. However, if there is no transition from normal to abnormal epithelium, if the muscularis mucosae is intact, if the cells contain no mucin, and if there is no suggestion of acinar pattern, the tumor is probably malignant lymphoma. Response to irradiation may be helpful in differentiating these two neoplasms.

Patients with malignant lymphoma may have a large palpable mass and still be in excellent physical condition. The diagnosis of malignant lymphoma is not usually made clinically or radiographically. The history often suggests peptic ulcer. At times, perforation can occur.

Malignant lymphoma of the stomach is more curable than carcinoma of the stomach, for cure can be effected by either surgery or appropriate irradiation or a combination of both.[106] Resection is usually done in operable patients, often with a clinical diagnosis of carcinoma. A biopsy is sometimes done in inoperable patients, and if malignant lymphoma is found and given radiotherapy, cure or long-term survival may result. There are about as many cases of malignant lymphoma cured by surgery as are cured by irradiation, but it is not known which method of treatment is best.

It is worth stressing that reactive lymphoid hyperplasia of the stomach may closely simulate lymphoma. We have had difficulty with this lesion, particularly when it has been present fairly deep in the muscle, but the presence of lymph follicle formation and distinct intermingling of other cells, such as plasma cells, commonly seen in chronic inflammation has been helpful. Naturally, the regional lymph nodes would show only hyperplasia. It is certain that this lesion accounts for some of the reported cures of malignant lymphoma of the stomach.[105] Often it is associated with a gastric or duodenal peptic ulceration.[107]

Other tumors

Gastric *carcinoid tumors* are microscopically and biologically similar to those seen in the lung, another foregut derivative.[121] They are usually argyrophil, but only rarely argentaffin. They can be multiple and associated with diffuse hyperplasia of argyrophil cells.[112] In some instances, the tumor has been found to secrete 5-hydroxytryptophan rather than serotonin.[118] Long-term survival is the rule, even in the presence of distant metastases.[115] It is now known that there are at least four different types of endocrine cells in the normal stomach.[116] A combined morphologic and biochemical study will be necessary to determine which of these cells is the common progenitor of carcinoid tumor. When making a diagnosis of gastric carcinoid tumor, it should be remembered that scattered argentaffin cells may be found in otherwise typical gastric carcinomas.[114]

Glomus tumors can occur in the stomach.[113] All of the reported cases have followed a benign clinical course.[111] Vascular leiomyoma, a much more common neoplasm, should always be considered in the differential diagnosis.

Plasma cell tumors,[117] *plasma cell granulomas,*[119] and *lipomas*[120] have been reported. We have seen an apparently benign gastric *fibrous histiocytoma* associated with severe anemia.[110] We also have seen a typical *"collision tumor,"* the two components being a well-differentiated adenocarcinoma and a malignant lymphoma of histiocytic type. *Metastatic carcinoma* may occur in the stomach from any widely disseminated neoplasm.

REFERENCES
Methods of examination
Examination of surgical specimens

1 Hebbel, R.: Chronic gastritis; its relation to gastric and duodenal ulcer and to gastric carcinoma, Am. J. Pathol. **19**:43-71, 1943.

Cytology

2 Ackerman, N. B.: An evaluation of gastric cytology; results of a nation-wide survey, J. Chronic Dis. **20**:621-626, 1967.

3 Boon, T. H., Schade, R. O. K., Middleton, G. D., and Reece, M.: An attempt at presymptomatic diagnosis of gastric carcinoma in pernicious anaemia, Gut **5**:269-270, 1964.

4 Brandborg, L. L.: Gastric exfoliative cytology; past, present, and future, Gastroenterology **55**:632-635, 1968.

5 Crozier, R. E., Middleton, M., and Ross, J. R.: Clinical application of gastric cytology, N. Engl. J. Med. **255**:1128-1131, 1956.

6 Foushee, J. H. S., Kalnins, Z. A., Dixon, F. R., Girsh, S., Morehead, R. P., O'Brien, T. F., Pribor, H., and Tattory, C.: Gastric cytology; evaluation of methods and results in 1,670 cases, Acta Cytol. (Baltimore) **13**:399-406, 1969.

7 Henning, N., Witte, S., and Bressel, D.: The cytologic diagnosis of tumors of the upper gastrointestinal tract (esophagus, stomach, duodenum), Acta Cytol. (Baltimore) **8**:121-130, 1964.

8 MacDonald, W. C., Brandborg, L. L., Taniguchi, L., and Rubin, C. E.: Gastric exfoliative cytology; an accurate and practical diagnostic procedure, Lancet **2**:83-86, 1963.

9 MacDonald, W. C., Brandborg, L. L., Taniguchi, L., Beh, J. E., and Rubin, C. E.: Exfoliative cytologic screening for gastric cancer, Cancer **17**:163-169, 1964.

10 Prolla, J. C., Kobayashi, S., and Krisner, J. B.: Cytology of malignant lymphomas of the stomach, Acta Cytol. (Baltimore) **14**:291-296, 1970.

11 Raskin, H. F., Kirsner, J. B., and Palmer, W. L.: Role of exfoliative cytology in the diagnosis of cancer of the digestive tract, J.A.M.A. **169**:789-791, 1959.

12 Schade, R. O. K.: Gastric cytology; principles, methods and results, London, 1960, Edward Arnold, Ltd., pp. 38-40.

13 Taebel, D. W., Prolla, J. C., and Kirsner, J. B.: Exfoliative cytology in the diagnosis of stomach cancer, Ann. Intern. Med. **63**:1018-1026, 1965.

Gastroscopic biopsy

14 Benedict, E. B.: Gastroscopic biopsy in the differential diagnosis of gastritis and carcinoma, N. Engl. J. Med. **245**:203-206, 1951.

15 Joske, R. A., Finckh, E. S., and Wood, I. J.: Gastric biopsy; a study of 1,000 consecutive successful gastric biopsies, Q. J. Med. **95**:269-294, 1955.

16 MacDonald, W. C., and Rubin, C. E.: Gastric biopsy; a critical evaluation, Gastroenterology **53**:143-170, 1967.

17 Rubin, W., Ross, L. L., Sleisenger, M. J., and

Jeffries, G. H.: The normal human gastric epithelia; a fine structural study, Lab. Invest. 19:598-626, 1968.

18 Whitehead, R.: Interpretation of mucosal biopsies from the gastrointestinal tract. In Dyke, S. C., editor: Recent advances in clinical pathology, ser. 5, London, 1968, J. & A. Churchill, Ltd., pp. 375-400.

Nonneoplastic lesions
Heterotopic pancreas

19 Goldfarb, W. B., Bennett, D., and Monafo, W.: Carcinoma in heterotopic gastric pancreas, Ann. Surg. 158:56-58, 1963.

20 Palmer, E. D.: Benign intramural tumors of the stomach; a review with special reference to gross pathology, Medicine (Baltimore) 30: 81-181, 1951 (extensive bibliography).

21 Stewart, M. J., and Taylor, A. L.: Adenomyoma of the stomach, J. Pathol. Bacteriol. 28:195-202, 1925.

Hypertrophy of pylorus

22 Bateson, E. M., Talerman, A., and Walrond, E. R.: Radiological and pathological observations in a series of seventeen cases of hypertrophic pyloric stenosis of adults, Br. J. Radiol. 42:1-8, 1969.

23 Du Plessis, D. J.: Primary hypertrophic pyloric stenosis in the adult, Br. J. Surg. 53: 485-492, 1966.

24 Hobson, A.: Hypertrophic pyloric stenosis in the adult, Br. Med. J. 1:99-100, 1948.

25 Lumsden, K., and Truelove, S. C.: Primary hypertrophic pyloric stenosis in the adult, Br. J. Radiol. 31:261-266, 1955.

26 Wellmann, K. F., Kagan, A., and Fang, H.: Hypertrophic pyloric stenosis in adults, Gastroenterology 46:601-608, 1964.

Gastritis

27 Bartlett, J. P., and Adams, W. E.: Generalized giant hypertrophic gastritis simulating neoplasm, Arch. Surg. 60:543-588, 1950.

28 Cox, A. J.: The stomach in pernicious anemia, Am. J. Pathol. 19:491-501, 1943.

29 Hebbel, R.: Chronic gastritis, its relation to gastric and duodenal ulcer and to gastric carcinoma, Am. J. Pathol. 19:43-71, 1943 (extensive bibliography).

30 Joske, R. A., Finckh, E. S., and Wood, I. J.: Gastric biopsy; a study of 1,000 consecutive successful gastric biopsies, Q. J. Med. 95: 269-294, 1955.

31 Kenney, F. D., Dockerty, M. B., and Waugh, J. M.: Giant hypertrophy of gastric mucosa, Cancer 7:671-681, 1954.

32 Lulu, D. J., and Dragstedt, L. R., II: Massive bleeding due to acute hemorrhagic gastritis, Arch. Surg. 101:550-554, 1970.

33 Menétrier, P.: Des polyadenomes gastriques et de leures rapports avec le cancer de l'estomac, Arch. Physiol. Norm. Pathol. 1:32-55, 236-262, Pl. III, 1888.

34 Morson, B. C.: Intestinal metaplasia of the gastric mucosa, Br. J. Cancer 9:365-376, 1955.

35 Palmer, E. D.: What Menétrier really said, Gastrointest. Endosc. 15:83-90 passim, 1968.

36 Rubin, W.: Proliferation of endocrine-like (enterochromaffin) cells in atrophic gastric mucosa, Gastroenterology 57:641-648, 1969.

37 Schell, R. F., Dockerty, M. B., and Comfort, M. W.: Carcinoma of the stomach associated with pernicious anemia, Surg. Gynecol. Obstet. 98:710-720, 1954.

38 Whitehead, R., Truelove, S. C., and Gear, M. W. L.: The histological diagnosis of chronic gastritis in fibreoptic gastroscope biopsy specimens, J. Clin. Pathol. 25:1-11, 1972.

39 Winawer, S. J., Bejar, J., McCray, R. S., and Zamcheck, N.: Hemorrhagic gastritis; importance of associated chronic gastritis, Arch. Intern. Med. 127:129-131, 1971.

Peptic ulcer

40 Dragstedt, L. R., Woodward, E. R., Linares, C. A., and Rosa, C. de la: The pathogenesis of gastric ulcer, Ann. Surg. 160:497-511, 1964.

41 Elliott, G. V., Wald, S. M., and Benz, R. I.: A roentgenologic study of ulcerating lesions of the stomach, Am. J. Roentgenol. Radium Ther. Nucl. Med. 77:612-622, 1957.

42 Fitts, C. D., Cathcart, R. S., III, Artz, C. P., and Spicer, S. S.: Acute gastrointestinal tract ulceration; Cushing's ulcer, steroid ulcer, Curling's ulcer and stress ulcer, Am. Surg. 37:218-223, 1971.

43 Harkins, H. N.: Stomach and duodenum. In Moyer, C. A., Rhoads, J. E., Allen, J. G., and Harkins, H. N.: Surgery, principles and practice, ed. 3, Philadelphia, 1965, J. B. Lippincott Co., chap. 29.

44 Kay, A. W.: An evaluation of gastric acid secretion tests, Gastroenterology 53:834-844, 1967.

45 Kukral, J. C.: Gastric ulcer; an appraisal, Surgery 63:1024-1036, 1968.

46 Pruitt, B. A., Jr., Foley, F. D., and Moncrief, J. A.: Curling's ulcer; a clinical-pathology study of 323 cases, Am. Surg. 172:523-539, 1970.

47 Stewart, M. J.: Cancer of the stomach: some pathological considerations, Br. J. Radiol. 20: 505-507, 1947.

Syphilis

48 Palmer, W. L., Schindler, R., Templeton, F. E., and Humphreys, E. M.: Syphilis of the stomach; case report, Ann. Intern. Med. 18: 393-406, 1943.

49 Saphir, O., and Parker, M. L.: Linitis plastica type of carcinoma, Surg. Gynecol. Obstet. **76:** 206-213, 1943.

50 Williams, C., and Kimmelstiel, P.: Syphilis of the stomach, J.A.M.A. **115:**578-582, 1940 (extensive bibliography).

Other lesions

51 Ashby, B. S., Appleton, P. J., and Dawson, I.: Eosinophilic granuloma of gastro-intestinal tract caused by herring parasite Eustoma rotundatum, Br. Med. J. **1:**1141-1145, 1964.

52 Clagett, O. T., and Walters, W.: Tuberculosis of the stomach, Arch. Surg. **37:**505-520, 1938.

53 Delia, C. W.: Phytobezoars (diospyrobezoars); a clinicopathologic correlation and review of six cases, Arch. Surg. **82:**579-583, 1961.

54 Eells, R. W., and Simril, W. A.: Gastric diverticula; report of thirty-one cases, Am. J. Roentgenol. Radium Ther. Nucl. Med. **68:** 8-14, 1952.

55 Goon, C. D.: Duplication of the stomach with extension into the chest, Am. Surg. **19:**721-727, 1953.

56 Heddle, S. B., Parrott, K. B., Paloschi, G. P. G., Prentice, R. S. A., Persyko, L., and Beck, I. T.: Diffuse eosinophilic gastroenteritis, Can. Med. Assoc. J. **100:**554-559, 1969.

57 Helwig, E. B., and Ranier, A.: Inflammatory fibroid polyps of the stomach, Surg. Gynecol. Obstet. **96:**355-367, 1953.

58 McCune, W. S., Gusack, M., and Newman, W.: Eosinophilic gastroduodenitis with pyloric obstruction, Ann. Surg. **142:**510-518, 1955.

59 Millard, M.: Fatal rupture of gastric aneurysm, Arch. Pathol. **59:**363-371, 1955.

60 Salmon, P. R., and Paulley, J. W.: Eosinophilic granuloma of the gastro-intestinal tract, Gut **8:**8-14, 1967.

61 Sirak, H. D.: Boeck's sarcoid of the stomach simulating linitis plastica, Arch. Surg. **69:**769-776, 1954.

Tumors
Smooth muscle tumors

62 Giberson, R. G., Dockerty, M. B., and Gray, H. K.: Leiomyosarcoma of the stomach; clinicopathologic study of 40 cases, Surg. Gynecol. Obstet. **98:**186-196, 1954.

63 Golden, T., and Stout, A. P.: Smooth muscle tumors of the gastrointestinal tract and retroperitoneal tissues, Surg. Gynecol. Obstet. **73:** 784-810, 1941.

64 Meissner, W. A.: Leiomyoma of the stomach, Arch. Pathol. **38:**207-209, 1944.

65 Palmer, E. D.: Benign intramural tumors of the stomach: a review with special reference to gross pathology, Medicine (Baltimore) **30:** 81-181, 1951 (extensive bibliography).

66 Salazar, H., and Totten, R. S.: Leiomyoblas-

toma of the stomach; an ultrastructural study, Cancer **25:**176-185, 1970.

67 Salmela, H.: Smooth muscle tumours of the stomach; a clinical study of 112 cases, Acta Chir. Scand. **134:**384-391, 1968.

68 Stout, A. P.: Bizarre smooth muscle tumors of the stomach, Cancer **15:**400-409, 1962.

69 Tallquist, G., Salmela, H., and Lindstrom, B. L.: Leiomyoblastoma of the stomach; a clinico-pathological study of 10 cases, Acta Pathol. Microbiol. Scand. **71:**194-202, 1967.

70 Welsh, R. A., and Meyer, A. T.: Ultrastructure of gastric leiomyoma, Arch. Pathol. **87:** 71-81, 1969.

Polyps

71 Marshak, R. H., and Feldman, F.: Gastric polyps, Am. J. Dig. Dis. **10:**909-935, 1965.

72 Ming, S.-C., and Goldman, H.: Gastric polyps; histogenetic classification and its relation to carcinoma, Cancer **18:**721-726, 1965.

73 Monaco, A. P., Roth, S. I., Castleman, B., and Welch, C. E.: Adenomatous polyps of the stomach; a clinical and pathological study of one hundred and fifty-three cases, Cancer **15:**456-467, 1962.

74 Rigler, L. G., and Kaplan, H. S.: Pernicious anemia and tumors of the stomach, J. Natl. Cancer Inst. **7:**327-332, 1947.

75 Tomasulo, J.: Gastric polyps; histologic types and their relationship to gastric carcinoma, Cancer **27:**1346-1355, 1971.

Carcinoma

76 Borrman, R.: Geschwülste des Magens und Duodenums. In Henke, F., and Lubarsch, O., editors: Handbuch der Speziellen Pathologischen Anatomie und Histologie, Berlin, 1926, Julius Springer, pp. **IV-L,**864-871.

77 Lauren, P.: The two histological main types of gastric carcinoma; diffuse and so-called intestinal type carcinoma, Acta Pathol. Microbiol. Scand. **64:**31-49, 1965.

78 Ming, S.-C., Goldman, H., and Freiman, D. G.: Intestinal metaplasia and histogenesis of carcinoma in human stomach; light and electron microscopic study, Cancer **20:**1418-1429, 1967.

Adenocarcinoma—no specific type

79 Lev, R.: The mucin histochemistry of normal and neoplastic gastric mucosa, Lab. Invest. **14:**2080-2100, 1965.

Adenocarcinoma associated with peptic ulcer ("ulcer-cancer")

80 Blendis, L. M., Beilby, J. O. W., Wilson, J. P., Cole, M. J., and Hadley, G. D.: Carcinoma of stomach; evaluation of individual and combined diagnostic accuracy of radi-

ology, cytology and gastrophotography, Br. Med. J. **1**:656-659, 1967.

81 Côté, R., Dockerty, M. B., and Cain, J. C.: Cancer of the stomach after gastric resection for peptic ulcer, Surg. Gynecol. Obstet. **107**: 200-204, 1958.

82 Gömöri, G.: Carcinoma arising from chronic gastric ulcer, Surg. Gynecol. Obstet. **57**:439-450, 1933.

83 Hebbel, R.: Superficial carcinoma of the stomach, Bull. Univ. Minnesota Hosp. **22**: 59-67, 1950.

84 Ihre, B. J. E., Barr, H., and Havermark, G.: Ulcer-cancer of the stomach; a follow-up study of 473 cases of gastric ulcer, Gastro-enterologia (Basel) **102**:78-91, 1964.

85 Jordan, S.: The relationship of gastric ulcer to gastric carcinoma, Cancer **3**:515-552, 1950 (panel discussion with George R. Pack as moderator).

86 Krag, E.: Long-term prognosis in medically treated peptic ulcer; a clinical, radiographical and statistical follow-up study, Acta Med. Scand. **180**:657-670, 1966.

87 Mallory, T. B.: Carcinoma in situ of the stomach and its bearing on the histogenesis of malignant ulcers, Arch. Pathol. **30**:348-362, 1940.

88 Nelson, S. W.: The discovery of gastric ulcers and the differentiated diagnosis between benignancy and malignancy, Radiol. Clin. North Am. **7**:5-25, 1969.

89 Newcomb, W. D.: The relationship between peptic ulceration and gastric carcinoma, Br. J. Surg. **20**:279-308, 1932.

90 Palmer, W. L.: Benign and malignant gastric ulcers: their relation and clinical differentiation, Ann. Intern. Med. **13**:317-338, 1939.

91 Stout, A. P.: The relationship of gastric ulcer to gastric carcinoma, Cancer **3**:515-552, 1950 (panel discussion with George R. Pack as moderator).

Adenocarcinoma—superficial spreading type

92 Bragg, D. G., Seaman, W. B., and Lattes, R.: Roentgenologic and pathologic aspects of superficial spreading carcinoma of the stomach, Am. J. Roentgenol. Radium Ther. Nucl. Med. **101**:437-446, 1967.

93 Golden, R., and Stout, A. P.: Superficial spreading carcinoma of the stomach, Am. J. Roentgenol. Radium Ther. Nucl. Med. **59**: 157-167, 1948.

Adenocarcinoma—linitis plastica type

94 Fernet, P., Azar, H. A., and Stout, A. P.: Intramural (tubal) spread of linitis plastica along the alimentary tract, Gastroenterology **48**:419-424, 1965.

95 Saphir, O.: Linitis plastica type of carcinoma, Surg. Gynecol. Obstet. **76**:206-213, 1943.

96 Zinninger, M. M.: Extension of gastric cancer in the intramural lymphatics and its relation to gastrectomy, Am. Surg. **20**:920-927, 1954.

Carcinoma—adenosquamous ("adenoacanthoma") and epidermoid

97 Straus, R., Heschel, S., and Fortmann, D. J.: Primary adenosquamous carcinoma of the stomach; a case report and review, Cancer **24**:985-995, 1969.

Clinicopathologic correlation

98 Comfort, M. W., Gray, H. K., Dockerty, M. B., Gage, R. P., Dornberger, G. R., Solis, J., Epperson, D. P., and McHaughton, R. A.: Small gastric cancer, Arch. Intern. Med. **94**:513-524, 1954.

99 Hawley, P. R., Westerholm, P., and Morson, B. C.: Pathology and prognosis of carcinoma of the stomach, Br. J. Surg. **57**:877-883, 1970.

100 Lumpkin, W. M., Crow, R. L., Jr., Hernandez, C. M., and Cohn, I., Jr.: Carcinoma of stomach; review of 1,035 cases, Ann. Surg. **159**: 919-931, 1964.

101 McNeer, G., VandenBerg, H., Donn, F. Y., and Bowden, L.: A critical evaluation of subtotal gastrectomy for the cure of cancer of the stomach, Ann. Surg. **134**:2-7, 1951.

102 Monafo, W. W., Jr., Krause, G. L., Jr., and Guerra Medina, J.: Carcinoma of the stomach; morphological characteristics affecting survival, Arch. Surg. **85**:754-762, 1962.

103 Steiner, P. E., Maimon, S. N., Palmer, W. L., and Kirsner, J. B.: Gastric cancer; morphologic factors in five-year survival after gastrectomy, Am. J. Pathol. **24**:947-969, 1948.

104 Walters, W., Gray, H. K., Priestly, J. T., and Waugh, J. M.: Report on surgery of stomach and duodenum for 1947, Mayo Clin. Proc. **23**: 554-562, 1948.

Malignant lymphoma

105 Faris, T. D., and Saltzstein, S. L.: Gastric lymphoid hyperplasia; a lesion confused with lymphosarcoma, Cancer **17**:207-212, 1964.

106 Joseph, J. I., and Lattes, R.: Gastric lymphosarcoma; clinicopathologic analysis of 71 cases and its relation to disseminated lymphosarcoma, Am. J. Clin. Pathol. **45**:653-669, 1966.

107 Perez, C. A., and Dorfman, R. F.: Benign lymphoid hyperplasia of the stomach and duodenum, Radiology **87**:505-510, 1966.

108 Snoddy, W.: Primary lymphosarcoma of the stomach, Gastroenterology **20**:537-553, 1952 (extensive bibliography).

109 Stobbe, J. A., Dockerty, M. B., and Bernatz, P. E.: Primary gastric lymphoma and its

grades of malignancy, Am. J. Surg. **112**:10-19, 1966.

Other tumors

110 Alerte, F.: Xanthofibroma of the stomach; report of a case with severe secondary hypochronic anemia, Arch. Pathol. **75**:99-104, 1963.

111 Appleman, H. D., and Helwig, E. B.: Glomus tumors of the stomach, Cancer **23**:203-213, 1969.

112 Black, W. C., and Haffner, H. E.: Diffuse hyperplasia of gastric argyrophil cells and multiple carcinoid tumors; a histochemical and ultrastructural study, Cancer **21**:1080-1099, 1968.

113 Kay, S., Callahan, W. P., Jr., Murray, M. R., Randall, H. T., and Stout, A. P.: Glomus tumors of the stomach, Cancer **4**:726-736, 1951.

114 Kubo, T., and Watanabe, H.: Neoplastic argentaffin cells in gastric and intestinal carcinomas, Cancer **27**:447-454, 1971.

115 Lattes, R., and Grossi, C.: Carcinoid tumors of the stomach, Cancer **9**:698-711, 1956.

116 Pearse, A. G. E., Coulling, I., Weavers, B., and Friesen, S.: The endocrine polypeptide cells of the human stomach, duodenum, and jejunum, Gut **11**:649-658, 1970.

117 Remigio, P. A., and Klaum, A.: Extramedullary plasmacytoma of stomach, Cancer **27**:562-568, 1971.

118 Sandler, M.: An atypical carcinoid tumour secreting 5-hydroxytryptophan, Lancet **1**:137-139, 1958.

119 Soga, J., Saito, K., Suski, N., and Sakai, T.: Plasma cell granuloma of the stomach, Cancer **25**:618-625, 1970.

120 Turkington, R. W.: Gastric lipoma. Report of a case and review of the literature, Am. J. Dig. Dis. **10**:719-726, 1965.

121 Williams, E. D.: The classification of carcinoid tumours, Lancet **1**:238-239, 1963.

Small bowel

DUODENUM
Diverticula

Diverticula of the duodenum occur in from 1% to 2% of all individuals. They are usually solitary, located in the second portion, and can attain a large size. They can produce obstructive jaundice, pancreatitis, duodenal obstruction, fistulas, hemorrhage, and perforation.[1]

Peptic ulcer

Peptic ulceration of the duodenum is one of the frequent lesions encountered in surgical pathology. Partial gastric resection may not encompass the ulcer, and only in a few instances is complete excision of the ulcer performed. Peptic ulceration probably occurs as a sequel to disturbed gastric function associated with significant psychologic stresses of life.[4, 5]

Grossly, this chronic single lesion is usually within 2 cm of the pylorus (Fig. 412), although it may occur in the second por-

tion of the duodenum.[3] When the ulcer is in the latter position, it may be the source of upper abdominal pain and bleeding yet not be discernible radiographically.

Peptic ulcer has well-defined margins sharply set off from the surrounding mucosa. At times, a large vessel with an open lumen may be seen at the base of the ulcer. Fibrosis of a healed ulcer may produce secondary diverticula and considerable shortening of the duodenum. Peptic ulcer of the duodenum does not become malignant.

Polypoid hamartoma of Brunner's glands

A rare lesion, polypoid hamartoma of Brunner's glands is characterized by a nodular proliferation of histologically normal Brunner's glands, accompanied by ducts and scattered stromal elements. It is probably not a true neoplasm. The most common location is the posterior wall at the junction between the first and second portions. It can be the cause of melena or duodenal obstruction.[2]

Adenocarcinoma

Most cases of duodenal carcinomas arise from the mucosa in the region of the ampulla. This entity is described under tumors of the periampullary region (Chapter 14). Carcinoma arising elsewhere in the duodenum is extremely rare. We have seen one carcinoma in the second portion of the duodenum arising from heterotopic pancreas.

JEJUNUM
Acute jejunitis

A rare entity, acute jejunitis occurs with equal frequency in men and women past 55 years of age. The pathogenesis is obscure, but Brynjulfsen[8] suggested that a virulent organism penetrates the intestinal wall through a mucosal flaw.

Grossly, the involved loop of bowel is sharply demarcated, and the inflammation present is mainly in the mucosa. There may be pus on the serosal surface (Fig.

413). The bowel itself is somewhat edematous and frequently slightly distended. It may involve the jejunum or the duodenum. The lymph nodes are often enlarged. Microscopically, there is frequently a widespread lymphangitis and lymphadenitis. The mesentery has a somewhat glassy appearance. Abscesses between folds of the mesentery have been observed.

Ulcer

Marginal ulcer, although it may be actually stomal in position, is usually situated on the wall of the jejunum away from the gastroenterostomy opening. This type of peptic ulcer is a complication of gastroenterostomy and of gastric resection (Billroth II) for duodenal ulcer. It is rarely seen after gastric resections for benign gastric ulcer or cancer of the stomach. It eventually occurs in a high proportion of patients who have gastroenterostomy alone for duodenal ulcer. Jejunal ulceration is more likely to occur after gastric resection for duodenal ulcer if the extent of the resection has been inadequate, if the entire antrum is not removed,[10] and if the afferent jejunal loop is of excessive length.

Ulceration of the small intestine not related to gastroduodenal pathology is an uncommon lesion. Most cases are due to the ingestion of enteric-coated tablets of potassium chloride. Grossly, a transverse area

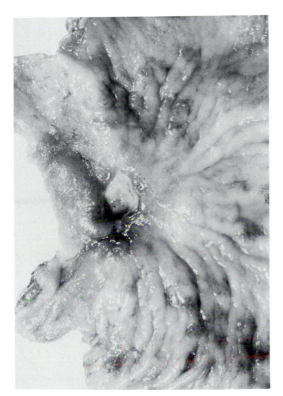

Fig. 412 Chronic penetrating ulcer of first portion of duodenum. (WU neg. 49-2144.)

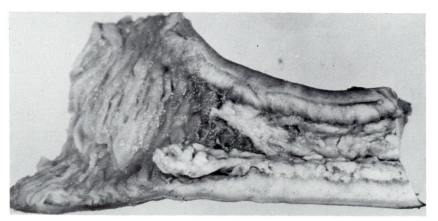

Fig. 413 Phlegmonous jejunitis. Note fibrin on mucosal surface of bowel. (WU neg. 50-5538.)

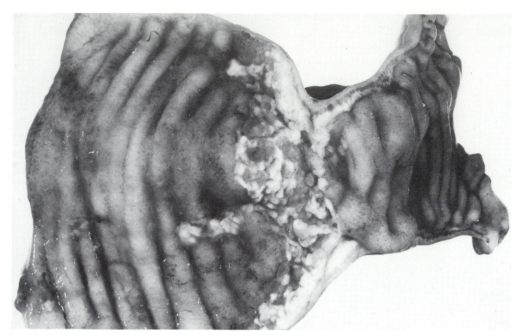

Fig. 414 Stenosing lesion of small bowel in patient who had taken enteric-coated tablets of potassium chloride. (From Allen, A. C., Boley, S. J., Schultz, L., and Schwartz, S.: Potassium-induced lesions of the small bowel, J.A.M.A. **193**:85-90, 1965; copyright 1965, American Medical Association.)

of ulceration is seen surrounded by congestion, hemorrhage, or edema[6] (Fig. 414). Obstruction, perforation, and hemorrhage are the commonest presenting signs. Microscopically, the changes are nonspecific and indistinguishable from those seen in the "idiopathic" form.[9] The latter designation is given to those ulcers in which no demonstrable etiology can be found. Diseases to be considered in the differential diagnosis include congenital abnormalities, mechanical disorders, vascular occlusions,[11] neoplasms, specific inflammations, radiation effect, islet cell tumor, celiac disease, and endometriosis.[9] As it is sometimes the case with peptic ulcers, idiopathic ulcers of the small bowel can be accompanied by a prominent lymphocytic and histiocytic reaction, which can be confused with malignant lymphoma.[7]

SMALL BOWEL
Malabsorption

The development of flexible peroral biopsy tubes has made it possible to biopsy the mucosa of the small intestine with a minimum of discomfort or risk. When the tube has reached the desired level, a tuft of mucous membrane is drawn into it by negative pressure. A small full-thickness mucosal biopsy can then be taken. There are many different biopsy tubes available for this purpose, such as the Carey capsule, the Rubin tube, and the Crosby capsule. In our institution, we use the latter. The incidence of serious complications, such as bleeding or perforation, has been negligible.[13]

Two basic requirements should be met in order to obtain the maximum possible information from a small bowel biopsy.

Fig. 415 Basic patterns of small bowel biopsies under dissecting microscope and their light microscopic counterparts. Light microscopic appearances are usually designated as **A**, normal; **B**, partial villous atrophy; **C** and **D**, subtotal villous atrophy. (Courtesy Dr. R. Whitehead, Oxford, England.)

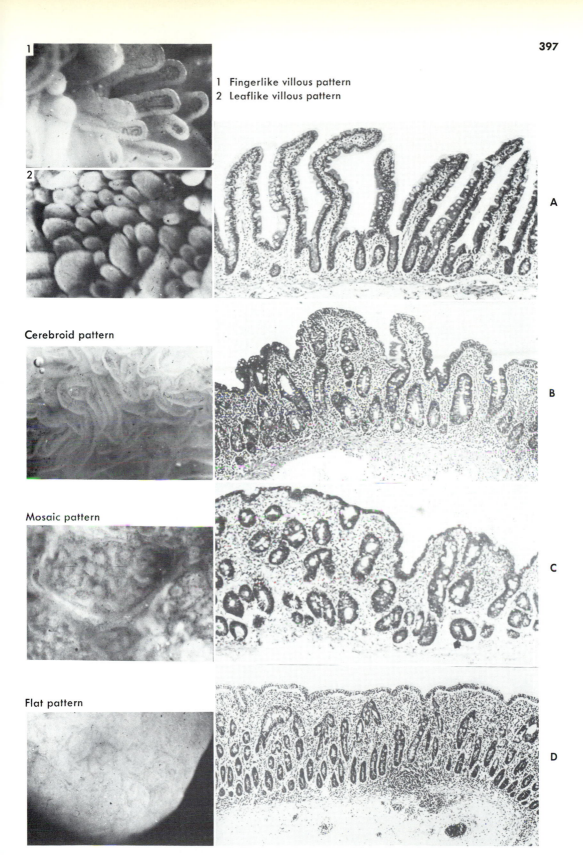

1 Fingerlike villous pattern
2 Leaflike villous pattern

A

Cerebroid pattern

B

Mosaic pattern

C

Flat pattern

D

Fig. 415 For legend, see opposite page.

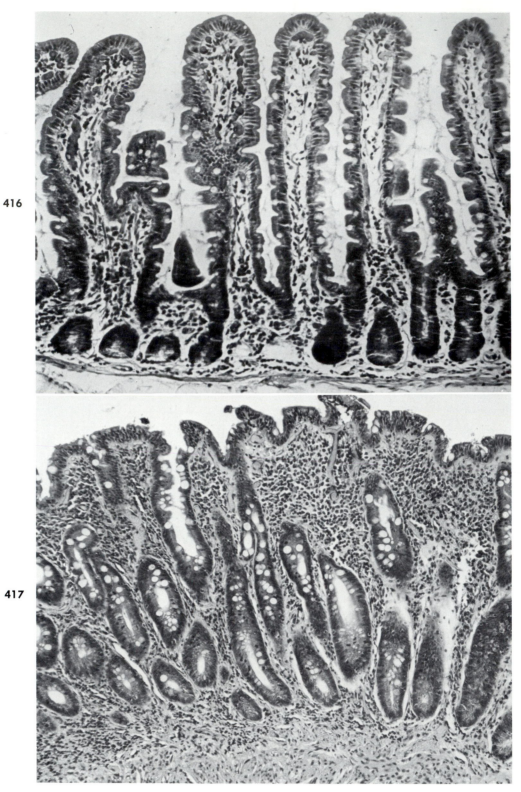

416

417

Fig. 416 and Fig. 417 For legends, see opposite page.

Since the morphology of the mucosa shows normal regional variations, it is important that biopsies are taken from approximately the same area in all patients. This is achieved by fluoroscopic control. The standard site of biopsy is a point slightly distal to the ligament of Treitz. Once the biopsy is obtained, it should be placed quickly on a flat surface, mucosal side up, with the aid of a dissecting microscope. Filter paper and Gelfoam are commonly used for this purpose. The mucosal appearance under the dissecting microscope should be recorded as part of the gross description. The five basic patterns are (1) villous, finger-like, (2) villous, leaflike or tonguelike, (3) convoluted, (4) mosaic, and (5) flat (Fig. 415). The information obtained is useful and gives a preliminary assessment of the mucosal state, but it should never replace an accurate light microscopic examination. More important, the handling of the mucosa during this procedure should be extremely gentle. Wiping away of adherent mucus should not be attempted.[35]

The tissue is fixed in formalin with the filter paper or Gelfoam attached to it to prevent curling. The filter paper should be removed during any one of the subsequent steps, whereas Gelfoam can be embedded in the paraffin block attached to the tissue. It is imperative that sections be cut at right angles to the mucosal surface.

The malabsorption syndrome can be the result of a large variety of organic and functional disorders.[19, 32] Small bowel biopsy is particularly useful in the evaluation of *celiac disease* (celiac sprue; nontropical sprue), a condition characterized by a totally flat mucosa and a dramatic clinical and morphologic response to removal of gluten from the diet.[26] Microscopically, the villi are atrophic or absent but the overall thickness of the mucosa is essentially normal (Figs. 416 and 417). It has become apparent in recent years that not all cases with total villous atrophy represent celiac disease. According to Rubin et al.,[26] the same morphologic appearance can be seen in dermatitis herpetiformis, kwashiorkor, and severe cases of tropical sprue. Weinstein et al.[31] have further segregated from classical celiac disease a type characterized by increased deposition of eosinophilic hyaline material within the lamina propria, which they have designated as *collagenous sprue.* Whether this is a specific entity or merely a morphologic variant of celiac disease is not clear at the present time. The pathogenesis of celiac disease is not known. Recent studies favor the theory that the villous atrophy results from a shortened life-span of jejunal epithelial cells.[25, 28]

A well-documented albeit rare complication of celiac disease is the development of intestinal malignant lymphoma. Whitehead[34] has shown that the process is gradual, beginning as a mixed cell infiltrate in the lamina propria, increasing number of atypical histiocytes, and ending as a full-blown malignant lymphoma. This course of events must be suspected in patients with a long history of celiac disease who develop reversal of the response to gluten withdrawal, fever, weight loss, abdominal pain, finger clubbing, bowel ulcerations, or sustained rise in serum IgA levels.

Tropical sprue is an altogether different condition.[20, 24] It has a definite geographic distribution, is relatively unaffected by gluten ingestion, and responds to folic acid, vitamin B_{12}, and tetracycline.[16] The morphologic changes are *nonspecific.* The large majority of cases show partial villous atrophy, although examples of both normal mucosa and total villous atrophy have been reported.

Whipple's disease (intestinal lipodystrophy) has a pathognomonic appearance

Fig. 416 Normal jejunal mucosa. Villi are delicate and tall. (×220; contributed by Dr. F. E. Pittman, New Orleans, La.)
Fig. 417 Celiac sprue with markedly atrophic villi. (×140; WU neg. 66-12074.)

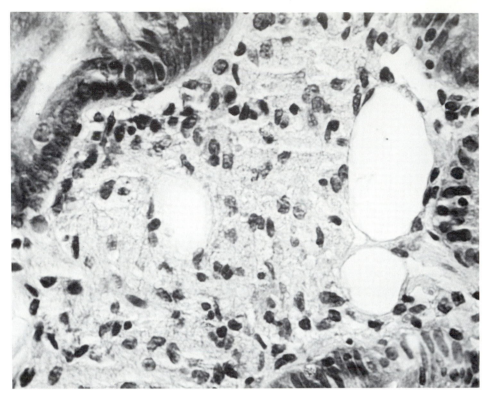

Fig. 418 Whipple's disease showing large foamy histiocytes in lamina propria of mucosa of small intestine. (×600; WU neg. 66-12077.)

in a jejunal biopsy. Large macrophages are seen crowding the lamina propria, distorting the villi and alternating with empty spaces (Fig. 418). Their cytoplasm contains large amounts of a diastase-resistant, PAS-positive material. This is due to the presence of bacilliform bodies, which also occur in the lumen, between the epithelial cells and in macrophages. They have been well demonstrated by electron microscopy[30] (Fig. 419), although attempts of culture have not given consistent results.

The disease is not restricted to the bowel. Macrophages of identical appearance have been identified in the rest of the alimentary tract, regional and peripheral lymph nodes,

heart, liver, spleen, adrenal glands, and nervous system.[15] The round empty spaces, which may be surrounded by giant cells and are also present in mesenteric lymph nodes, are seen to contain neutral fat by special stains. Their significance is obscure. It should be remembered that a similar change, although not accompanied by PAS-positive macrophages, is often seen in intra-abdominal lymph nodes of normal individuals, probably secondary to the ingestion of mineral oil.[12] Small bowel biopsy remains the best way to diagnose Whipple's disease. Biopsy of peripheral lymph nodes can be suggestive of the disease if the typical macrophages are present but is not pathog-

Fig. 419 Electron micrograph of macrophage in submucosa of small intestine in Whipple's disease. Nucleus, **N,** and nucleous, **nu,** are at top. Cytoplasm contains membrane-limited sacs, **S,** that are filled with dense spherical and rod-shaped bodies, **b,** intermixed with fine membranous profiles. These rods have been shown to have fine structural morphology of bacteria and may be responsible for disease. Material in these sacs is periodic acid–Schiff positive. (×15,000.)

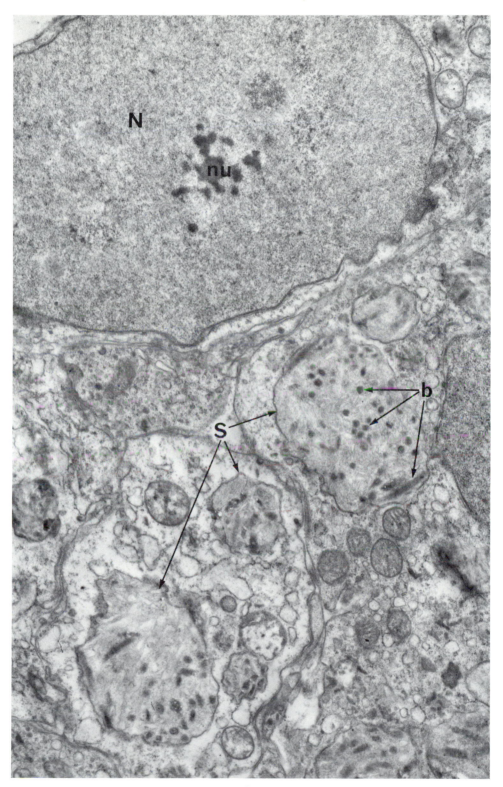

Fig. 419 For legend, see opposite page.

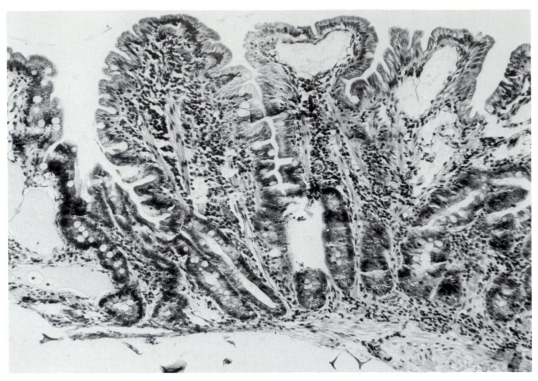

Fig. 420 Intestinal lymphangiectasia responsible for protein-losing enteropathy. (×140; WU neg. 66-12078.)

nomonic.[23] The interpretation of rectal biopsies is hampered by the fact that mucincontaining macrophages ("muciphages"), present in the lamina propria of 10% of all individuals, have a strong resemblance to the histiocytes of Whipple's disease, at least at a light microscopic level.[14]

Other diseases associated with malabsorption in which small bowel biopsy may be of value include **abeta-lipoproteinemia** (acanthocytosis), in which the apical villous cytoplasm shows striking vacuolation as a result of inability to synthesize betalipoprotein,[18] **agammaglobulinemic sprue,** characterized by total absence of plasma cells in the lamina propria,[21] **intestinal lymphangiectasia,** in which a protein-losing enteropathy develops probably as a result of the entrance of protein-rich fluid into the extracellular space of the lamina propria from the dilated lymphatic channels and subsequent drainage into the gut lumen[29] (Fig. 420), **amyloidosis, scleroderma,**[22] and **parasitic infestation,** such as

giardiasis,[36] hookworm disease,[27] strongyloidiasis,[35] and capillariasis.[33]

Peña and Whitehead[24a] studied the small bowel morphology in different types of disaccharide deficiencies. They found no detectable abnormality in isolated lactase deficiency. Whenever morphologic changes were present, *all* the disaccharidases measured—i.e., lactase, maltase, and sucrase were found to be depressed.

In **nodular lymphoid hyperplasia,** the entire small bowel is studded with well-circumscribed nodules of lymphoid tissue (Fig. 421). *Giardia lamblia* is usually present. Patients with this condition have low or absent IgA and IgM, decreased IgG, susceptibility to infections, and diarrhea with or without steatorrhea.[17]

Crohn's disease (regional ileitis)

Crohn's disease occurs with equal frequency in men and women in their twenties or thirties.[38] An increasing number of pediatric cases have been reported in re-

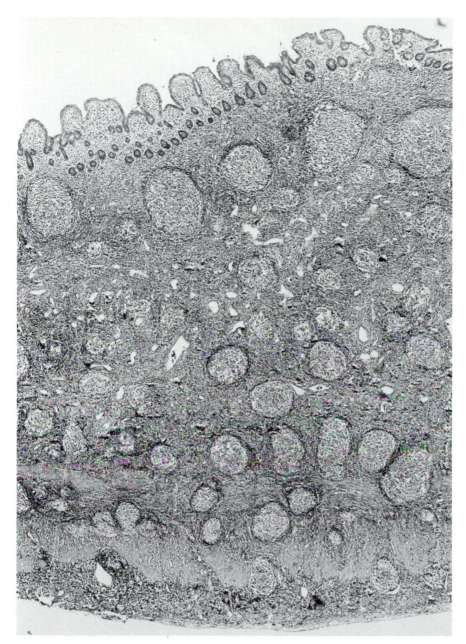

Fig. 421 Striking lymphoid hyperplasia of small bowel in patient with dysgammaglobulinemia. Involvement is mainly submucosal. (×34; WU neg. 72-223.)

cent years.[48] Often there is a background
of psychologic disturbances.

Grossly, the ileum is the usual site of
the disease, although all portions of the
small bowel can be involved. In the forty-
four patients reported by Dixon,[40] the ileum
was involved in forty-three. The duodenum
is rarely involved. We have seen eleven
cases, all but one associated with involvement of the distal portion of the small
bowel.[49] Even rarer is involvement of the
stomach.[41] We have recently diagnosed
a case in an endoscopic biopsy. Crohn's
disease also can involve the large bowel,

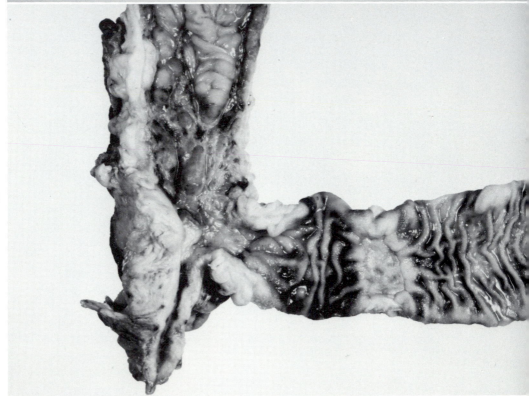

Fig. 422 Typical gross appearance of Crohn's disease involving terminal ileum. There are extensive ulceration, marked narrowing of lumen, and thickening of wall. Subserosal fat is prominent. Fistula is beginning to form (arrow). Disease stops abruptly at ileocecal valve. (WU neg. 71-7092.)

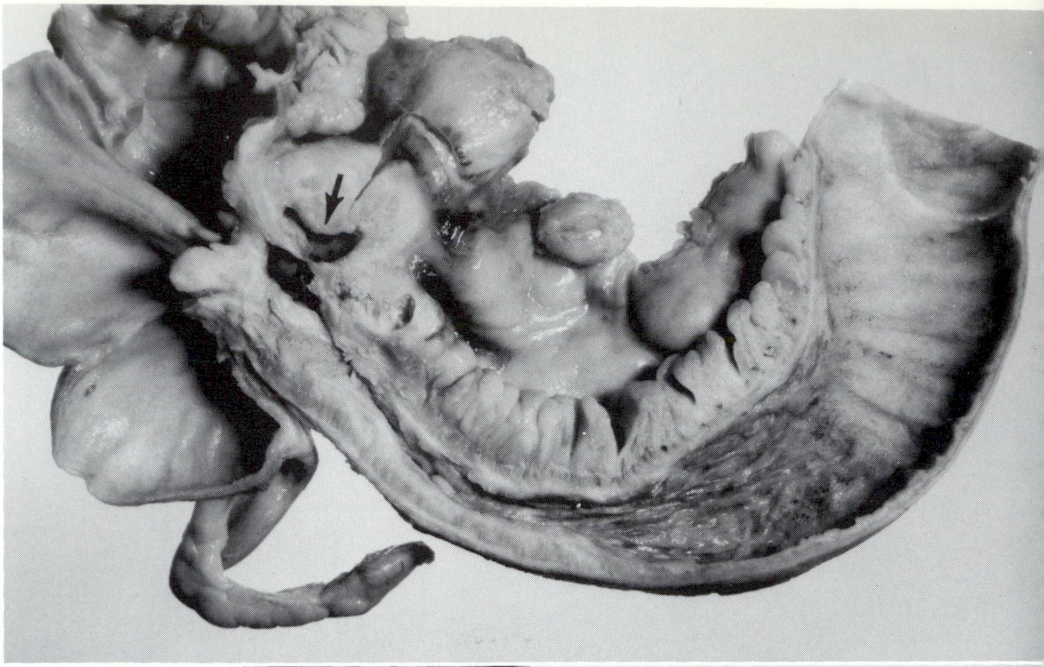

Fig. 423 Crohn's disease involving small bowel, cecum, appendix, and ascending colon. Longitudinal ulcerations and "skip areas" are two common features of this disease. (WU neg. 69-1571.)

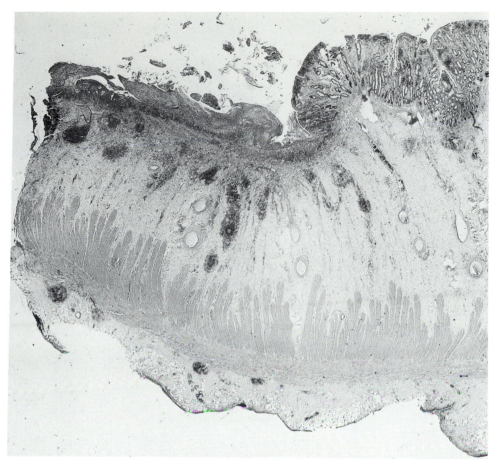

Fig. 424 Crohn's disease. There are ulceration, submucosal fibrosis, lymphadenoid nodules, dilatation of lymphatics, and subserosal fibrosis. (Low power; WU neg. 50-5222.)

as well as multiple sites in the small intestine. In a series of 297 cases mentioned by Morson,[46] 66% of the cases were restricted to the small bowel, 17% to the large bowel, and 17% had involvement of both segments. Each area may be poorly or sharply delimited.

Early in the disease, the involved small bowel has a soggy feeling and a reddish purple surface. When involvement of the bowel is chronic and severe, the impression on palpation has been compared to "an eel in rigor mortis."[39] Ulceration may be very prominent, and the lumen may

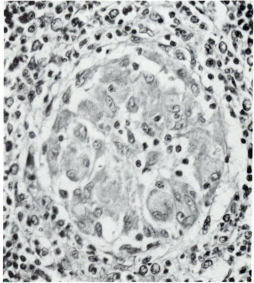

Fig. 425 Reticulum cell hyperplasia in lymph node as described by Blackburn et al.[37] (×400; WU neg. 51-6011.)

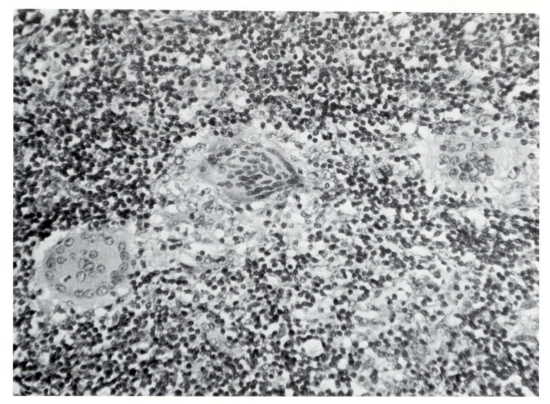

Fig. 426 Multinucleated giant cells in mesenteric lymph nodes of patient with Crohn's disease. (WU neg. 68-7089.)

be narrowed to 0.5 cm (Figs. 422 and 423). The bowel proximal to the obstruction may be dilated and hypertrophied.

In advanced stages of the process, there may be fistulas between loops of small bowel, between small and large bowel, between bowel and abdominal wall, and between bowel and bladder. Fibrosed mesentery produces irregularities in the contour of the bowel which may be somewhat corrugated. Later on, there may be subserosal fibrosis, shortening of the mesentery, and enlargement of the regional lymph nodes. Free perforation within the peritoneal cavity may occur.[45]

Microscopically, the earliest changes are those of submucosal edema. With prominent lymphadenoid hyperplasia, superficial ulceration may occur[37] (Fig. 424). The submucosal infiltrate is made up mainly of plasma cells, lymphocytes, and eosinophils. The submucosal and myenteric nerve plexuses are often prominent, probably due to edema of the bowel rather than to any intrinsic changes in the nerve plexuses.

Blackburn et al.[37] emphasized the changes in the lymphoid nodules and indicated that with the passage of time large pale cells develop in the germinal centers and are gradually replaced by sarcoidlike collections of giant cells that he calls "giant cell systems" (Fig. 425). These areas never become necrotic or caseous. The same changes may occur in the prominently enlarged regional lymph nodes (Fig. 426). The early submucosal thickening is due to lymphedema. Often the muscularis mucosae is hypertrophied.[47] Giant cells of foreign body type may be present (Fig. 427). With still further passage of time, intramural abscesses appear. Inflammatory changes result in fibrosis of the muscle and subserosa. The three pathologic changes of greater significance in the diagnosis of Crohn's disease, re-

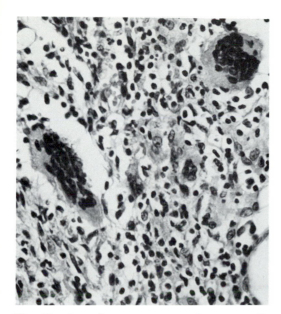

Fig. 427 Granulomatous area with giant cells in small intestinal lesions of Crohn's disease. (×400; WU neg. 51-6010.)

gardless of location, are transmural involvement, sarcoidlike granulomas (present in approximately 60% of the cases), and fissures. The latter are defined as slitlike ulcerations of sharp edges and narrow lumen, arranged perpendicularly to the mucosa and extending deeply into the submucosa and even the muscularis externa. The degree and extent of the pathologic features bear little relationship to prognosis.[43] The disease has an undulating yet progressive course. Complete spontaneous regression occurs rarely.

Crohn's disease can occur as a segmental involvement of the large bowel without involvement of the small bowel (Fig. 428). Unlike ulcerative colitis, it may be associated with skip areas. Frequently, it may involve the anus and be associated with fistulas.[44, 46] These anal lesions may be the first clinical manifestation of the disease.[42]

The treatment of choice of patients with

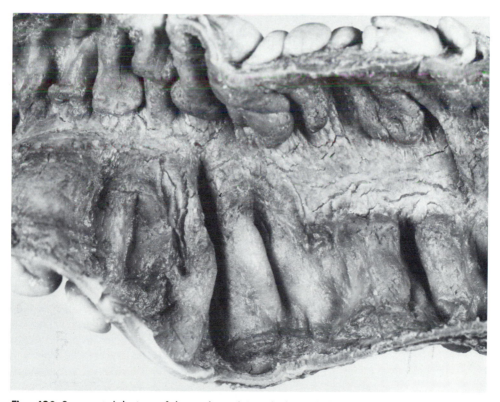

Fig. 428 Segmental lesion of large bowel in which pathologic findings were pathognomonic of Crohn's disease with transmural involvement and prominent giant cell systems in both bowel and regional lymph nodes. (WU neg. 67-3926.)

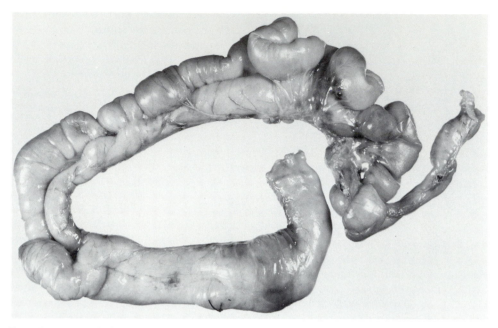

Fig. 429 Resected duplication of ileum in 5-month-old female infant. This duplication had common muscular wall except for one small point of communication where there was ulcer. Mucosal surface contained gastric mucosa with parietal cells. (WU neg. 58-568.)

regional ileitis is psychiatric and dietary in the absence of complications of disease. Surgical therapy is indicated with the development of partial or complete intestinal obstruction, internal or external fistulas, perforation with abscess, hemorrhage, and intractability despite medical management.

Specific operative procedures to be utilized in these patients should be individualized. However, resection of the involved small bowel seems preferable to sidetracking procedures when the condition of the patient is not critical. Resection should not be done in the early acute stage of regional ileitis that is commonly encountered at laparotomy for appendicitis. In these instances, appendectomy may be performed without fear of subsequent fistula formation if the cecum is not involved by an inflammatory process.

Congenital defects
Heterotopic pancreas

Heterotopic pancreas may undergo any pathologic changes seen in the normal pancreas. It consists mainly of ducts and lobular tissue usually without islet tissue. Blockage of the duct can occur where it empties into the intestinal tract, and this block can cause infection and fat necrosis. The duodenum is the most common location of this lesion particularly in the region of the ampulla of Vater.

Rare cases of islet cell tumors within heterotopic pancreas have been reported,[50] and we have seen carcinoma arising within it.

Duplication and atresia

Duplication and atresia of the gastrointestinal tract occur most often in the ileum (Fig. 429). Those of the colon and stomach also are not rare.

The *duplication* may be accompanied by inflammatory changes, and those of the small intestine may or may not extend to, and communicate with, the lumen of the large bowel.[53] Nearly all of them are incomplete. There is a common muscular wall between the gastrointestinal tract and the duplication. This prevents the surgeon from separating the duplication from the

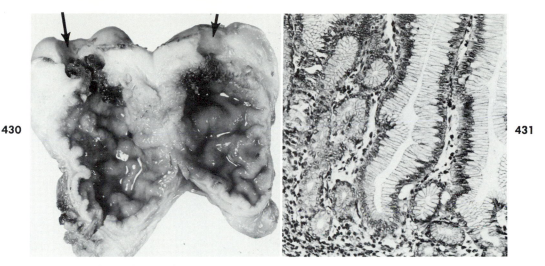

Fig. 430 Perforated Meckel's diverticulum. Arrows point to area of perforation. (WU neg. 48-4286.)

Fig. 431 Section from perforated Meckel's diverticulum illustrated in Fig. 430 to show normal gastric glands that contain parietal cells. (×85; WU neg. 48-4308.)

intact gastrointestinal tract. In other words, duplication must be treated either by resection of the area of gut including its duplication or by removal of its walls, which are not a part of the wall of the intact gut.

Intestinal atresia may arise in some cases on the basis of embryologic defects.[54] In others, mechanical injury to the vascular system of the bowel is probably the pathogenetic agent. This may result from intrauterine intussusception, isolated volvulus, or incarceration.[51]

Hirschsprung's disease, when involving the whole colon, may extend to the small intestine. The disease is associated with a high mortality, the most common complication being enterocolitis.[56]

Meckel's diverticulum

Meckel's diverticulum is found in 2% of all persons. It is more frequent in men (63%). Early in fetal life, the intestine communicates with the yolk sac for nourishment. By the fourth week, the opening has gradually narrowed to form a tubular structure known as the vitelline duct. At the 7 mm stage, the vitelline duct normally is obliterated by atrophy and forms a

fibrous cord. This fibrous cord between the umbilicus and the bowel is subsequently absorbed.

Failure of all or part of the vitelline duct to become obliterated accounts for the various types of vitelline duct abnormalities. A persistent fibrous cord may extend from a diverticulum to the umbilicus, to adjacent bowel, or to mesentery. The vitelline duct may remain patent throughout, causing an enteroumbilical fistula. Persistence of the proximal portion of the duct only constitutes Meckel's diverticulum. Because of the risk of complications, Meckel's diverticulum should be removed even when it is detected accidentally.[55]

Aberrant pancreatic tissue may be present in the wall of Meckel's diverticulum. Gastric, duodenal, or colonic mucosa occasionally forms part or all of the mucosal lining of the diverticulum (Figs. 430 and 431). The usual location is approximately 80 cm proximal to the ileocecal valve on the antimesenteric border.

The lengths of the diverticula vary from 1 cm to 8 cm. About 30% of patients have other congenital abnormalities. The diverticula may perforate, ulcerate, or in-

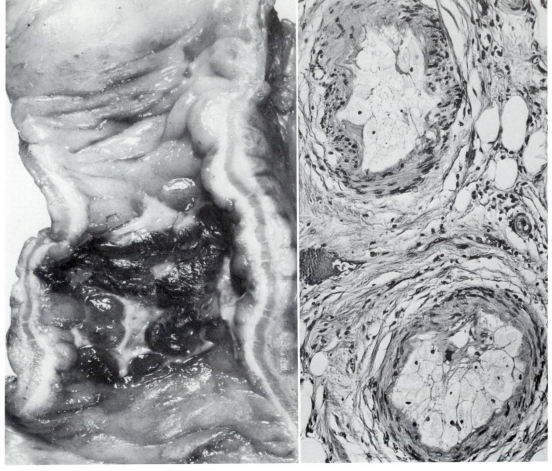

Fig. 432 Stenosing lesion of bowel with ulceration. Submucosal fibrosis is present, and muscular layer is well defined. (From Perkins, D. E., and Spjut, H. J.: Intestinal stenosis following radiation therapy, Am. J. Roentgenol. Radium Ther. Nucl. Med. **88:**953-966, 1962.)

Fig. 433 Irradiation effect in two small mesenteric arteries. Subintimal foam cells are present, changes that are almost specific for irradiation effect. (From Perkins, D. E., and Spjut, H. J.: Intestinal stenosis following radiation therapy, Am. J. Roentgenol. Radium Ther. Nucl. Med. **88:**953-966, 1962.)

tussuscept. Intestinal obstruction can occur from unabsorbed bands. Peptic ulceration of the ileum adjacent to Meckel's diverticulum is a common cause of massive hemorrhage in children.

A large variety of benign and malignant tumors have been reported arising from Meckel's diverticulum. The most common is carcinoid tumor.[57] Other tumors include villous adenoma, adenocarcinoma, leiomyoma, and leiomyosarcoma.[52]

Irradiation effect

Roentgentherapy of malignant tumors within the peritoneal cavity may cause damage to the intestinal tract, the amount of which depends on many factors. Damage occurs most frequently in patients treated for carcinoma of the cervix.

Grossly, the small bowel often appears fibrotic. The wall may be partially replaced by fibrous tissue, and the submucosa may be greatly thickened. In patients

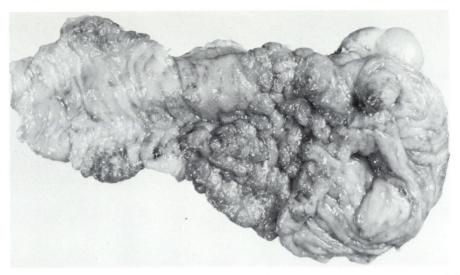

Fig. 434 Extreme lymphoid hyperplasia of ileum with intussusception in 4-year-old child. (WU neg. 55-7041.)

with advanced lesions, mucosal ulceration is often observed at the time of surgical resection.

Microscopically, early irradiation effect may be demonstrated by an increased production of mucus[60] and by nuclear changes in the lining epithelium. Later, submucosal edema that may be completely reversible occurs. If the damage is severe, fibrosis of the muscular wall and ulceration occur (Fig. 432). Infection often complicates the picture. The vascular changes are specific (Fig. 433) and can be recognized by the subendothelial deposition of lipid.[58] There may be necrosis, calcification, and thrombosis. These changes occur principally in the intima.

Frozen section is a reliable method in determining the degree of irradiation damage. This technique is of value to the surgeon in assessing whether or not the ends of the intestine after resection and anastomosis can be expected to heal.[59]

Intussusception

For the most part, intussusception occurs in the first two years of life. In over one-half the patients, it occurs in the first year. It is rare after the age of 5 years and is two or three times more common in the male child. During the first year of life,

the amount of lymphoid tissue in the ileo-cecal valve and the degree of projection of the valve into the cecum are at their maximum. Both decrease during the second year of life. There is a good correlation between the amount of lymphoid tissue in the last few inches of ileum and the incidence of ileocolic intussusceptions.

Lymphoid hyperplasia as a cause of intussusception may be overlooked because intussusceptions are frequently reduced, and advanced inflammatory changes obscure this condition in resection specimens. Bell and Steyn[61] found viruses in the lymph nodes of children with mesenteric adenitis and intussusception. This entire hypothesis has been supported by Perrin and Lindsay[62] and by Sarason et al.[64] We have seen an instance in which such focal lymphoid hyperplasia was erroneously considered to be a neoplasm and was resected (Fig. 434). Such lymphoid hyperplasia does not involve the muscularis.

Intussusception in the older age group is frequently accompanied by a pedunculated intraluminal tumor such as a lipoma. A length of intestine (the intussuscipiens) literally swallows part of the bowel just proximal to it. This swallowed portion (the intussusceptum) is drawn down within the intussuscipiens until it can go no

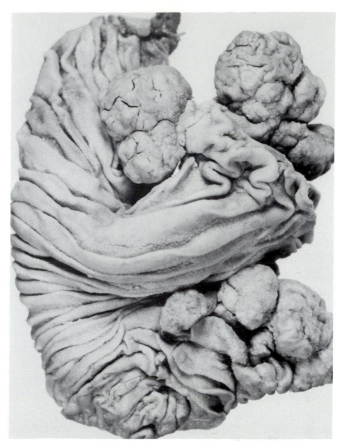

Fig. 435 Resected small bowel demonstrating multiple benign adenomatous polyps in 14-year-old boy with Peutz-Jeghers syndrome. He was well thirteen years later. (WU neg. 49-6157.)

farther because of traction of the mesentery. Traction and compression shut off circulation to the intussusceptum so that it becomes necrotic and sloughs. The upper ends of the intussuscipiens and the intussusceptum may become firmly united, and end-to-end anastomosis takes place. However, such an occurrence is extremely rare. The intussusceptive mass of intestine has a curved sausagelike form with concavity toward the mesenteric attachment at the spinal column.

If operation is performed early, manual reduction of the intussusception is possi-

ble. Resection is necessary when reduction is not feasible. Mortality is directly related to the time that elapses between onset and operation. In children, there is a rapid rise in mortality after the second day. In early uncomplicated cases, a barium enema may be used to reduce the intussusception.[63]

Tumors
Benign epithelial tumors

Benign tumors of epithelial origin of the small bowel are infrequent. We have seen rare polypoid tumors having the appear-

Fig. 436 Hamartomatous polyp of small bowel in 12-year-old girl. Tumor, which had caused intussusception, was not associated with other features of Peutz-Jeghers syndrome. **A,** Gross appearance of tumor, showing distinct lobulation, short stalk, and multiple small cysts. **B,** Panoramic view of microscopic section. Ramifying central stalk containing numerous muscle bundles supports florid epithelial proliferation. Many of glands show cystic dilatation. (**A,** WU neg. 73-2503; **B,** WU neg. 73-2935.)

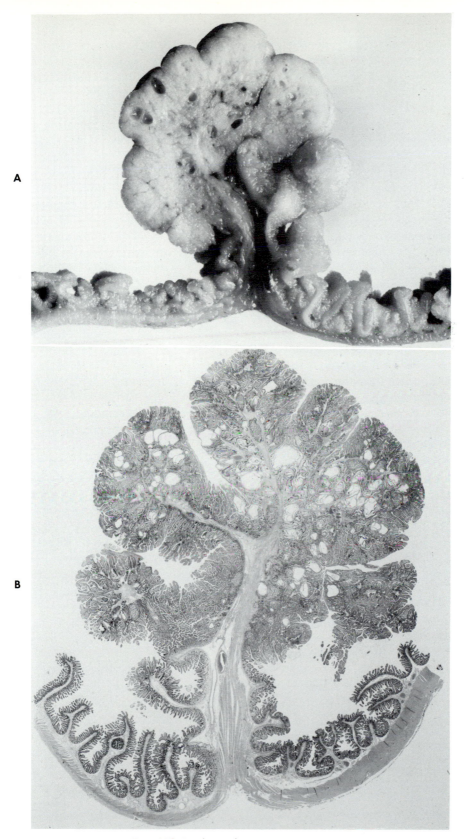

Fig. 436 For legend, see opposite page.

ance of villous adenoma or of adenomatous polyps of the large bowel. These polyps may be single or multiple, pedunculated or sessile (Fig. 435). The duodenum and jejunum are more often involved than the ileum.

Epithelial polyps of the small intestine are commonly present among patients having familial melanin pigmentation of the lips and oral mucosa (Peutz-Jeghers syndrome).[66, 74]

Grossly, these polyps do not differ from the usual adenomatous polyp, but microscopically they are much different. The epithelial elements in this type of polyp are supported by broad bands of smooth muscle fibers, thick in the center of the lesion but thinner on the periphery. Paneth and argentaffin cells are at the base of the tubules next to the muscular framework. We have seen identical lesions in the absence of the other components of the Peutz-Jeghers syndrome (Fig. 436). We believe, with Morson,[73] that this lesion is hamartomatous and perhaps represents a malformation of the muscularis mucosae. In these polyps all varieties of epithelial cells, columnar, goblet, Paneth, and argentaffin, are present. This microscopic pattern is similar wherever these polyps occur. The disordered epithelial pattern of these polyps which blends between the muscle bundles has, in the past, caused an erroneous diagnosis of cancer.

We have now seen three patients with both the Peutz-Jeghers syndrome and adenocarcinoma of the small intestine. Dozois et al.[69] collected eleven such cases from the world literature. Four of the tumors were located in the stomach, three in the duodenum, three in the large bowel, and one in the ileum. Seven of the patients had already died at the time of the reports.

Adenocarcinoma

Adenocarcinomas of the small bowel are similar to those of the large bowel. Grossly, they usually have a fairly typical napkin ring appearance and produce partial intestinal obstruction (Fig. 437). The bowel proximal to the tumor is frequently widely dilated. Microscopically, these tumors are usually moderately well-differentiated adenocarcinomas that have extended through all layers of the bowel to involve the regional lymph nodes. The prognosis is consequently extremely poor.

Smooth muscle tumors

Smooth muscle tumors of the small bowel may occur in any segment and may grow in any of the muscular layers, including the muscularis mucosae, either intraluminally or extraluminally. They produce signs and symptoms depending upon their gross pattern. Grossly, they are fairly well delineated. Smooth muscle tumors presenting intraluminally may be the source of occult or massive bleeding. They may have a central niche similar to those within the stomach. If they grow toward the mesentery, they may form a fairly large, bulky mass. They may be suspected of being malignant if they are cellular and soft. There are seldom any regional metastases, for these tumors tend to invade the bloodstream and metastasize distantly.

The microscopic differentiation between the benign and malignant smooth muscle tumor may be extremely difficult. The guidelines detailed in the discussion of smooth muscle tumors of stomach also can be applied to the small bowel lesion. Mitotic activity is the single most important microscopic feature, although by no means infallible (Figs. 438 to 440).

Lipoma

Lipomas of the small bowel characteristically grow in the submucosa and for that reason may cause signs and symptoms of intussusception. Grossly, they resemble lipomas seen in other locations, bulge upward into the mucosal surface, and in time may ulcerate. They do not undergo malignant change.

Malignant lymphoma

Malignant lymphomas may involve the bowel primarily or as part of a widely

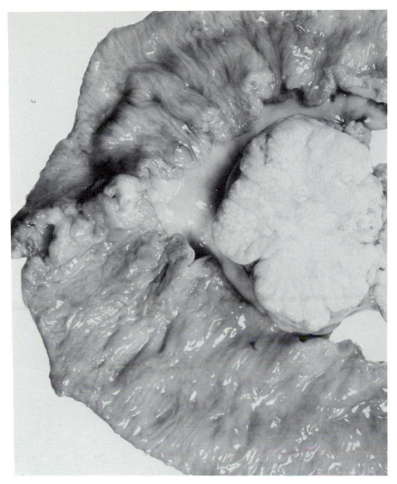

Fig. 437 Classical constricting adenocarcinoma of small bowel with large metastasis. This case, although hopeless, was found at time of exploratory laparotomy for gallbladder disease. (WU neg. 50-3798.)

disseminated process. They often occur in male children and have a poor prognosis. The terminal ileum and ileocecal valve region are the most common sites of involvement.

Grossly, these tumors have a rather characteristic garden hose appearance that is rather sharply delineated, forms a bulky tumor mass, and frequently involves the regional lymph nodes. Cross section of the tumor reveals the wall of the bowel to be completely replaced by homogeneous fish-flesh cellular tissue. The mucosal surface has often been completely destroyed. The extent of involvement, together with the gross appearance, should make the diagno-

sis (Fig. 441). Microscopically, all types of malignant lymphoma are seen, from the well-differentiated lymphocytic type to the histiocytic type, often designated as reticulum cell sarcoma.

Patients with malignant lymphoma of the small bowel, particularly children, do poorly, and only rare cases are ever cured either by surgery or by irradiation. Rarely, Hodgkin's disease and plasmacytoma can also involve the small bowel[68] (Fig. 442).

Carcinoid tumors

Carcinoid tumors occur mainly in the ileum but rarely may arise in other portions of the small bowel, even the duode-

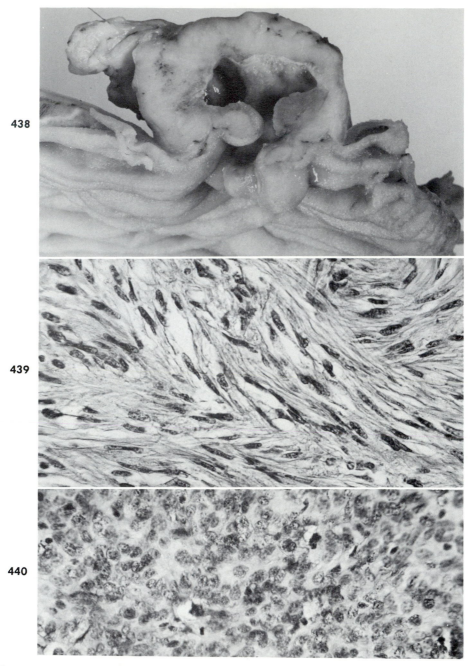

Fig. 438 Smooth muscle tumor of jejunum of long clinical duration that was grossly and microscopically thought to be benign. Note classical central excavation. (WU neg. 49-6469.)

Fig. 439 Same tumor illustrated in Fig. 438 showing well-differentiated smooth muscle cells. Mitotic figures were rare. (×510; WU neg. 52-2875.)

Fig. 440 Two years later, tumor shown in Figs. 438 and 439 locally recurred and metastasized to liver. Tumor was highly undifferentiated in liver, but other areas showed smooth muscle origin. (×500; WU neg. 52-2876.)

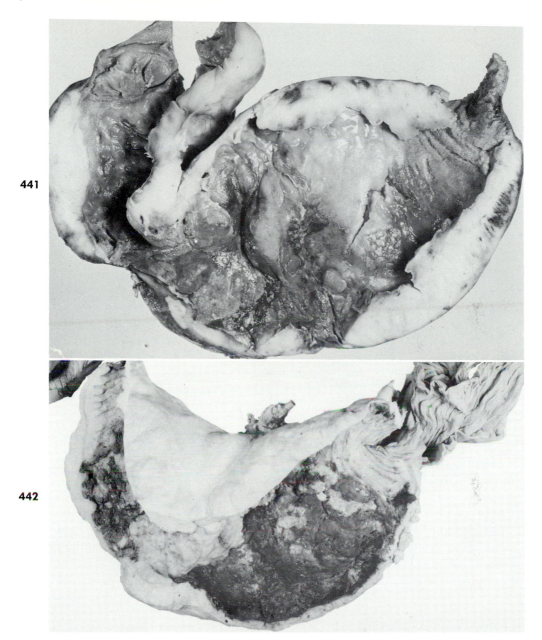

441

442

Fig. 441 Large malignant lymphoma of small bowel that replaced all layers. (WU neg. 49-2033.)
Fig. 442 Hodgkin's disease of small bowel. This process has destroyed entire wall of bowel and produced multiple areas of ulceration.

num. They are frequently multiple (16% to 34%), often associated with malignant gastrointestinal tumors of other microscopic types.[71] The mucosa is often intact over them. At times, they grow large enough to involve the entire wall of the bowel and with the accompanying fibrosis may "buckle" the bowel wall (Fig. 443). On section, they usually have a bright yellow color because of their increased fat content. Regional nodal and hepatic metastases may exist.

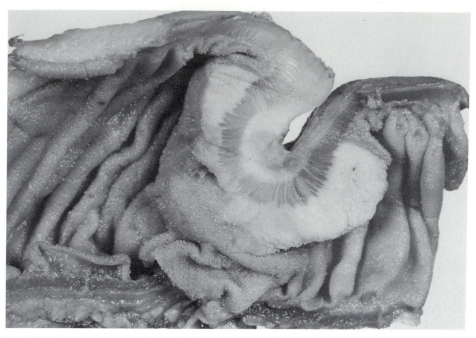

Fig. 443 Carcinoid tumor of small bowel. Note "buckling" of bowel wall with hypertrophy of muscle. Bulk of tumor lies above muscle. (WU neg. 49-4120; specimen contributed by Dr. W. Hall, Chambersburg, Pa.)

Microscopically, carcinoid tumors of the small bowel differ according to their site, which, in turn, is an expression of their embryologic development.[81] Those of distal duodenum and jejunoileum constitute the "classic" type. The pattern is that of solid masses of monotonous-appearing cells with small nuclei, inconspicuous cytoplasm, and fine nucleoli (Fig. 444). Mitotic figures are rare. Argentaffin and diazo reaction are usually positive, whereas the presence of acini and mucin secretion is quite rare. Carcinoid tumors of the proximal portion of the duodenum share with those of gastric and pulmonary origin a microscopic appearance characterized by trabecular arrangement and negative argentaffin and diazo reaction. The microscopic distinction with ectopic islet cell tumor may be impossible even after histochemical and electron microscopic examination.[80]

These tumors are malignant neoplasms that have a slow growth rate but eventually metastasize and cause the death of the patient. It is worthwhile to resect these tumors, even in the presence of metastases in the liver, because life may be prolonged several years by resection.[72]

The carcinoid syndrome is associated with carcinoid tumors that have metastasized to the liver.[75, 78, 79] The syndrome is characterized by cyanosis of the face and anterior part of the chest, intermittent hypertension, palpitation, and frequent watery stools. The main secretion of the tumor is serotonin (5-hydroxytryptamine).

Fig. 444 Characteristic pattern of carcinoid tumor growing just beneath thinned overlying epithelium. (Low power; WU neg. 49-1622.)

Fig. 445 Marked elastotic degeneration of branch of mesenteric artery associated with carcinoid tumor, which can be seen surrounding vessel. Both elastic laminae are affected. Patient was operated upon because of gangrene of small bowel. (Verhoeff–van Gieson; ×33; WU neg. 73-4270.)

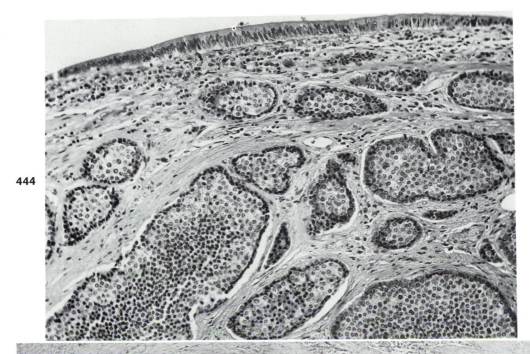

444

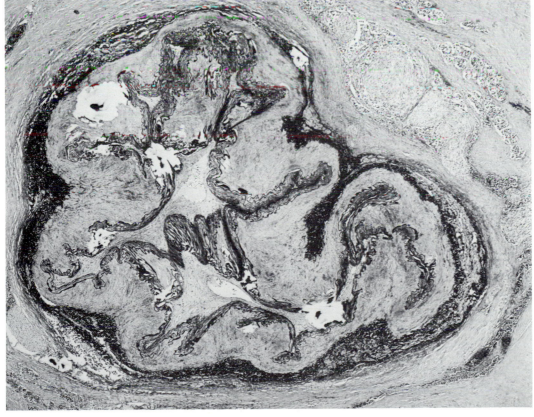

445

Fig. 444 and Fig. 445 For legends, see opposite page.

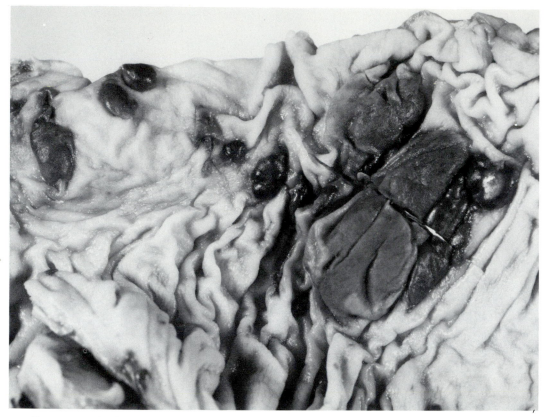

Fig. 446 Multiple hemangiomas of small bowel. Microscopically, they were of cavernous variety. (Courtesy Dr. W. C. Black, Albuquerque, N. M.)

This substance may be identified in the blood. In the urine it appears as 5-hydroxy-indolacetic acid.[77] These tumors have shown also to secrete kinins, prostaglandins, and histamine.[76] It is not yet clear which of these substances is the main one responsible for the symptoms and signs of the carcinoid syndrome.[67]

Rare complications of carcinoid tumor are gangrene of the small bowel secondary to obliterative elastic sclerosis of the mesenteric blood vessels (Fig. 445) and scleroderma-like lesions of the skin.[65, 70]

Other lesions

Benign *vascular tumors* of the small bowel may be single or multiple and may be associated with hemangiomas in other organs.[82, 85] They may bleed or perforate. Grossly, the lesion is not well delimited and on compression is soft and blanches.

The midjejunum is the most common location. Microscopically, a cavernous hemangioma is the most common variety (Fig. 446).

In *hereditary telangiectasia,* there are lesions of the mucous membrane and skin. These lesions are multiple, and severe gastrointestinal hemorrhage can occur from them. Smith et al.[86] reported 159 patients, twenty-one of whom had significant hemorrhage. Demonstration of these lesions at surgery is difficult, and surgical resection is usually not successful.

Nine examples of a peculiar benign tumor occurring almost exclusively in the second portion of the duodenum, especially in the proximity of the ampulla of Vater, have been described by Taylor and Helwig.[87] Most lesions are small, pedunculated and submucosal, with frequent ulceration of the overlying mucosa. The microscopic

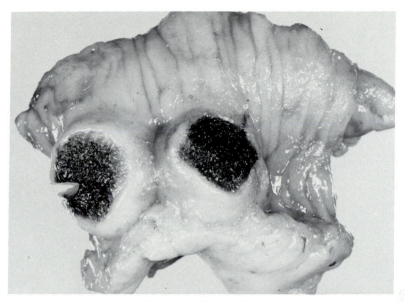

Fig. 447 Metastatic carcinoma involving small bowel. Tumor metastasis appeared first in submucosa and finally ulcerated surface. Note how normal mucosa extends to edge of ulceration. This finding helps to differentiate it from primary carcinoma. (WU neg. 50-5539.)

appearance is distinctive, with no exact counterpart elsewhere in the body. Epithelioid cells with radial arrangement and occasional ribbon formation alternate with compact nests of cells, spindle elements, and large cells with the appearance of ganglion cells. Argyrophil granules can usually be demonstrated. The microscopic appearance seems a combination of carcinoid tumor, chemodectoma, and ganglioneuroma. Kepes and Zacherias[83] have coined the name *gangliocytic paraganglioma* for this neoplasm. All cases so far published had followed a benign clinical course.

Rarely, *metastatic carcinoma* involves the small bowel and may cause symptoms of obstruction necessitating palliative resection (Fig. 447). Willbanks and Fogelman[88] performed palliative surgery on eighteen patients with *malignant melanoma* metastatic to the small and/or large bowel. All fourteen patients with multiple tumors died within one year, whereas among the four with apparently solitary metastasis, there was a five-year survivor. Small bowel obstruction can be caused also by *endometriosis*.[84]

REFERENCES
DUODENUM

1 Juler, J. L., List, J. W., Stemmer, E. A., and Connolly, J. E.: Duodenal diverticulitis, Arch. Surg. **99:**572-578, 1969.
2 ReMine, W. H., Brown, P. W., Jr., Gomes, M. M. R., and Harrison, E. G., Jr.: Polypoid hamartomas of Brunner's glands; report of six surgical cases, Arch. Surg. **100:**313-316, 1970.
3 Warmoes, F., and Rennewaert, M.: Frequency of ulcers of second portion of duodenum, Acta Gastroenterol. Belg. **12:**652-657, 1949.
4 Wolf, S.: Summary of evidence relating life situation and emotional response to peptic ulcer, Ann. Intern. Med. **31:**637-649, 1949.
5 Wolf, S., and Wolf, H. G.: Human gastric function, an experimental study of man and his stomach, London, 1943, Oxford University Press.

JEJUNUM

6 Allen, A. C., Boley, S. J., Schultz, L., and Schwartz, S.: Potassium-induced lesions of the small bowel, J.A.M.A. **193:**85-90, 1965.
7 Artinian, B., Lough, J. O., and Palmer, J. D.: Idiopathic ulcer of small bowel with pseudolymphomatous reaction; a clinicopathological study of six cases, Arch. Pathol. **91:**327-333, 1971.
8 Brynjulfsen, B. C.: Jejunitis acuta—ileitis regionalis acuta, Acta Chir. Scand. **96:**361-388, 1948.
9 Davies, D. R., and Brightmore, T.: Idiopathic

and drug-induced ulceration of the small intestine, Br. J. Surg. **57**:134-139, 1970.

10 Dean, A. C. B., and Mason, M. K.: The distribution of pyloric mucosa in partial gastrectomy specimens, Gut **5**:64-67, 1964.

11 Raf, L. E.: Ischaemic stenosis of the small intestine, Acta Clin. Scand. **135**:253-259, 1969.

SMALL BOWEL
Malabsorption

12 Boitnott, J. K., and Margolis, S.: Mineral oil in human tissues. II. Oil droplets in lymph nodes of the porta hepatis, Bull. Hopkins Hosp. **118**:414-422, 1966.

13 Bolt, R. J.: Methods of small-bowel biopsy, J.A.M.A. **188**:40-41, 1964.

14 Ekuan, J. H., and Hill, R. B., Jr.: Colonic histiocytosis; clinical and pathological evaluation, Gastroenterology **55**:619-625, 1968.

15 Enzinger, F. M., and Helwig, E. B.: Whipple's disease; a review of the literature and report of fifteen patients, Virchows Arch. Pathol. Anat. **336**:238-269, 1963.

16 Guerra, R., Wheby, M. S., and Bayless, T. M.: Long-term antibiotic therapy in tropical sprue, Ann. Intern. Med. **63**:619-634, 1965.

17 Hermans, P. E., Huizenga, K. A., Hoffman, H. N., Brown, A. L., and Markowitz, H.: Dysgammaglobulinemia associated with nodular lymphoid hyperplasia of the small intestine, Am. J. Med. **40**:78-89, 1966.

18 Isselbacher, K. J., Scheig, R., Plotkin, G. R., and Caulfield, J. B.: Congenital β lipoprotein deficiency: an hereditary disorder involving a defect in the absorption and transport of lipids, Medicine (Baltimore) **43**:347-361, 1964.

19 Jeffries, G. H., Weser, E., and Steisenger, M. H.: Malabsorption, Gastroenterology **56**:777-797, 1969.

20 Klipstein, F. A., and Baker, S. J.: Regarding the definition of tropical sprue, Gastroenterology **58**:717-721, 1970.

21 Kopp, W. L., Trier, J. S., Stiehm, E. R., and Foroozan, P.: "Acquired" agammaglobulinemia with defective delayed hypersensitivity, Ann. Intern. Med. **69**:309-317, 1968.

22 Levinson, J. D., and Kirsner, J. B.: Infiltrative diseases of the small bowel and malabsorption, Am. J. Dig. Dis. **15**:741-766, 1970.

23 Maizell, H., Ruffin, J. M., and Dobbins, W. O., III: Whipple's disease; a review of 19 patients from one hospital and a review of the literature since 1950, Medicine (Baltimore) **49**:175-205, 1970.

24 Menendez-Corrada, R.: Current views on tropical sprue and a comparison to nontropical sprue, Med. Clin. North Am. **52**:1367-1385, 1968.

24a Peña, A. S., and Whitehead, R.: Quoted by Whitehead.[35]

25 Rubin, W., Ross, L. L., Sleisenger, M. H., and Weser, E.: An electron microscopic study of adult celiac disease, Lab. Invest. **15**:1720-1747, 1966.

26 Rubin, C. E., Eidelman, S., and Weinstein, W. M.: Sprue by any other name, Gastroenterology **58**:409-413, 1970.

27 Sheehy, T. W., Meroney, W. H., Cox, R. S., and Soler, J. E.: Hookworm disease and malabsorption, Gastroenterology **42**:148-156, 1962.

28 Trier, J. S., and Browning, T. H.: Epithelial-cell renewal in cultured duodenal biopsies in celiac sprue, N. Engl. J. Med. **283**:1245-1250, 1970.

29 Waldmann, T. A.: Protein-losing enteropathy, Gastroenterology **50**:422-443, 1966.

30 Watson, J. H. L., and Haubrich, W. S.: Bacilli bodies in the lumen and epithelium of the jejunum in Whipple's disease, Lab. Invest. **21**:347-357, 1969.

31 Weinstein, W. M., Saunders, D. R., Tytgat, G. N., and Rubin, C. E.: Collagenous sprue; an unrecognized type of malabsorption, N. Engl. J. Med. **283**:1297-1301, 1970.

32 Weser, E., Jeffries, G. H., and Sleisenger, M. H.: Malabsorption, Gastroenterology **50**:811-828, 1966.

33 Whalen, G. E., Rosenberg, E. B., Strickland, G. T., Gutman, R. A., Cross, J. H., Watten, R. H., Uylangeo, C., and Dizou, J. J.: Intestinal capillariasis; a new disease in man, Lancet **1**:13-16, 1969.

34 Whitehead, R.: Primary lymphadenopathy complicating idiopathic steatorrhoea, Gut **9**:569-575, 1968.

35 Whitehead, R.: The interpretation and significance of morphological abnormalities in jejunal biopsies, J. Clin. Pathol. **24**(suppl. 5, Roy. Coll. Pathol.):108-124, 1971 (excellent review).

36 Yardley, J. H., Takano, J., and Hendrix, T. R.: Epithelial and other mucosal lesions of the jejunum in giardiasis; jejunal biopsy studies, Bull. Hopkins Hosp. **115**:389-406, 1964.

Crohn's disease (regional ileitis)

37 Blackburn, G., Hadfield, G., and Hunt, A. H.: Regional ileitis, St. Barth. Hosp. Rep. **72**:181-224, 1939.

38 Crohn, B. R., Ginzburg, L., and Oppenheimer, G. D.: Regional ileitis, J.A.M.A. **99**:1323-1329, 1932.

39 Dalziel, T. K.: Chronic interstitial enteritis, Br. Med. J. **2**:1068-1070, 1913.

40 Dixon, C. F.: Regional enteritis, Ann. Surg. **108**:857-866, 1938.

41 Fielding, J. F., Toye, D. K. M., Benton, D. C., and Cooke, W. T.: Crohn's disease of the stomach and duodenum, Gut **11**:1001-1006, 1970.

42 Gray, B. K., Lockhart-Mummery, H. E., and Morson, B. C.: Crohn's disease of the anal region, Gut **6**:515-524, 1965.

43 Gump, F. E., Sakellariadis, P., Wolff, M., and Broell, J. R.: Clinical-pathological investigation of regional enteritis as a guide to prognosis, Ann. Surg. **176**:233-242, 1972.

44 Lockhart-Mummery, H. E., and Morson, B. C.: Crohn's disease of the large intestine, Gut **5**:493-509, 1964.

45 Mogadam, M., and Priest, R. J.: Necrotizing enteritis in Crohn's disease of the small bowel, Gastroenterology **56**:337-341, 1969.

46 Morson, B.: Crohn's disease; lecture 2, Trans. Med. Soc. Lond. **86**:177-192, 1970 (excellent review).

47 Rappaport, H., Bourgoyne, F. H., and Smetana, H. F.: The pathology of regional enteritis, Milit. Surg. **109**:463-502, 1951.

48 Rubin, S., Lambie, R. W., and Chapman, J.: Regional ileitis in childhood, Am. J. Dis. Child. **114**:106-110, 1967.

49 Wise, L., Kyriakos, M., McCown, A., and Ballinger, W. F.: Crohn's disease of the duodenum, Am. J. Surg. **121**:184-194, 1971.

Congenital defects

50 de Castro Barbosa, J. J., Dockerty, M. B., and Waugh, J. M.: Pancreatic heterotopia, Surg. Gynecol. Obstet. **82**:527-542, 1946.

51 Halles, J. A., Jr.: Atresia of the small intestine; current concepts in diagnosis and treatment, Clin. Pediatr. (Phila.) **3**:257-262, 1964.

52 Haugen, O. A., Pegg, C. S., and Kyle, J.: Leiomyosarcoma of Meckel's diverticulum, Cancer **26**:929-934, 1970.

53 Ladd, W. E., and Gross, R. E.: Abdominal surgery of infancy and childhood, Philadelphia, 1941, W. B. Saunders Co.

54 Lynn, H. B., and Espinas, E. E.: Intestinal atresia; an attempt to relate location to embryologic processes, Arch. Surg. **79**:357-361, 1959.

55 Söderlund, S.: Meckel's diverticulum; a clinical and histologic study, Acta Chir. Scand. [Suppl.] **248**:1-233, 1959.

56 Walker, A. W., Kempson, R. L., and Ternberg, J. L.: Aganglionosis of the small intestine, Surgery **60**:449-457, 1966.

57 Weitzner, S.: Carcinoid of Meckel's diverticulum; report of a case and review of the literature, Cancer **23**:1436-1440, 1969.

Irradiation effect

58 Perkins, D. E., and Spjut, H. J.: Intestinal stenosis following radiation therapy, Am. J. Roentgenol. Radium Ther. Nucl. Med. **88**:953-966, 1962.

59 Sugg, W. L., Lawler, W. H., Ackerman, L. V., and Butcher, H. R., Jr.: Operative therapy for severe irradiational injury in the enteral and urinary tracts, Ann. Surg. **157**:62-70, 1963.

60 Warren, S., and Friedman, N. B.: Pathology and pathologic diagnosis of radiation lesions in the gastro-intestinal tract, Am. J. Pathol. **18**:499-513, 1942.

Intussusception

61 Bell, T. M., and Steyn, J. H.: Viruses in lymph nodes of children with mesenteric adenitis and intussusception, Br. Med. J. **1**:700-702, 1962.

62 Perrin, W. S., and Lindsay, E. C.: Intussusception; monograph based on 400 cases, Br. J. Surg. **9**:46-71, 1921.

63 Ravitch, M. M., and McCune, R. M., Jr.: Reduction of intussusception by barium enema; clinical and experimental study, Ann. Surg. **128**:904-917, 1948.

64 Sarason, E. L., Prior, J. T., and Prowda, R. L.: Recurrent intussusception associated with hypertrophy of Peyer's patches, N. Engl. J. Med. **253**:905-908, 1955.

Tumors

65 Anthony, P. P.: Gangrene of the small intestine—a complication of argentaffin carcinoma, Br. J. Surg. **57**:118-122, 1970.

66 Bartholomew, L. G., Moore, C. E., Dahlin, D. C., and Waugh, J. M.: Intestinal polyposis associated with mucocutaneous pigmentation, Surg. Gynecol. Obstet. **115**:1-11, 1962.

67 Dollinger, M. R., and Gardner, B.: Newer aspects of the carcinoid spectrum, Surg. Gynecol. Obstet. **122**:1335-1349, 1966.

68 Douglass, H. O., Jr., Sika, J. V., and LeVeen, H. H.: Plasmacytoma; a not so rare tumor of the small intestine, Cancer **28**:456-460, 1971.

69 Dozois, R. R., Judd, E. S., Dahlin, D. C., and Bartholomew, L. G.: The Peutz-Jeghers syndrome. Is there a predisposition to the development of intestinal malignancy? Arch. Surg. **98**:509-517, 1969.

70 Fries, J. F., Lindgren, J. A., and Bull, J. M.: Scleroderma-like lesions and the carcinoid syndrome, Arch. Intern. Med. **131**:550-553, 1973.

71 Kuiper, D. H., Gracie, W. A., Jr., and Pollard, H. M.: Twenty years of gastrointestinal carcinoids, Cancer **25**:1424-1430, 1970.

72 Moertel, C. G., Sauer, W. G., Dockerty, M. B., and Baggenstoss, A. H.: Life history of the carcinoid tumor of the small intestine, Cancer **14**:901-912, 1961.

73 Morson, B. C.: Some peculiarities in the histology of intestinal polyps, Dis. Colon Rectum **5**:337-344, 1962.

74 River, L., Silverstein, J., and Tope, J. W.: Benign neoplasms of the small intestine, Surg. Gynecol. Obstet. **102**:1-38, 1956. (Extensive bibliography.)

75 Sanders, R. J., and Axtell, H. K.: Carcinoids of the gastrointestinal tract, Surg. Gynecol. Obstet. **119**:369-380, 1964. (Extensive bibliography.)

76 Sandler, M., Williams, E. D., and Karim, S. M. M.: The occurrence of prostaglandins in amine-peptide-secreting tumours. In Mantegazza, P., and Horton, E. W., editors: Prostaglandins, peptides and amines, London and New York, Academic Press, Inc., pp. 3-7.

77 Sjoerdsma, A., Weissbach, H., and Udenfriend, S.: Simple test for diagnosis of metastatic carcinoid (argentaffinoma), J.A.M.A. **159**:397, 1955.

78 Thorson, A. H.: Studies on carcinoid disease, Acta Med. Scand. **161**(suppl. 334):1-132, 1958.

79 Thorson, A. H., Biorck, G., Bjorkman, G., and Waldenstrom, J.: Malignant carcinoid of the small intestine with metastases to the liver, valvular disease of the right side of the heart (pulmonary stenosis, and tricuspid regurgitation without septal defects), peripheral vasomotor symptoms, bronchoconstriction, and an unusual type of cyanosis, Am. Heart J. **47**:795-817, 1954.

80 Weichert, R., Reed, R., and Creech, O., Jr.: Carcinoid-islet cell tumors of the duodenum, Ann. Surg. **165**:660-669, 1967.

81 Williams, E. D., and Sandler, M.: The classification of carcinoid tumours, Lancet **1**:238-239, 1963.

Other lesions

82 Hansen, P. S.: Hemangioma of the small intestine, Am. J. Clin. Pathol. **18**:14-42, 1948.

83 Kepes, J. J., and Zacharias, D. L.: Gangliocytic paragangliomas of the duodenum; report of two cases with light and electron microscopic examination, Cancer **27**:61-70, 1971.

84 Kinder, C. H.: Acute small-bowel obstruction due to endometriosis, Br. J. Surg. **41**:550-552, 1953.

85 Shepherd, J. A.: Angiomatous conditions of the gastrointestinal tract, Br. J. Surg. **40**:409-421, 1953.

86 Smith, C. R., Jr., Bartholomew, L. G., and Cain, J. C.: Hereditary hemorrhagic telangiectasia and gastrointestinal hemorrhage, Gastroenterology **44**:1-6, 1963.

87 Taylor, H. B., and Helwig, E. B.: Benign nonchromaffin paragangliomas of the duodenum, Virchows Arch. Pathol. Anat. **335**:356-366, 1962.

88 Willbanks, O. L., and Fogelman, M. J.: Gastrointestinal melanosarcoma, Am. J. Surg. **120**:602-606, 1970.

Appendix

Appendicitis

The appendix is a vestigial organ serving no useful purpose in man. It frequently is the site of inflammation requiring its removal. Appendicitis is a disease occurring most frequently in young men but can occur in either sex at any age. It is a disease of the Western world and is common in Great Britain and America. In Asia and Africa, it is reported infrequently. This difference may be based on a dietary variance. Appendicitis occurs where the diet is reduced in bulk with diminished cellulose and high protein intake.[8]

The mucosa of the normal appendix has a light yellow tint, and its surface is smooth and glistening. Mucosal hemorrhages and hyperemia of surface vessels are usually related to operative trauma, whereas a fibrinous or purulent coating indicates invasive infection. In children from the age of 10 years to young adults, *diffuse lymphoid hyperplasia* may produce enough obstruction in the lumen to cause appendicitis and even intussusception[13, 15, 17] (Figs. 448 and 449).

In this country, about 3% of appendices removed show infestation with *Oxyuris vermicularis*.[4] These parasites are most often found in the appendices of children between the ages of 7 and 11 years. The infestation is not a causal agent of appendicitis but occurs with about the same frequency in normal appendices. The parasite wanders widely and frequently invades the lower female genital tract. From there, it may reach the peritoneal cavity by ascending along the uterus and fallopian tubes. Granulomas caused by this organism have been observed in the endometrium, fallopian tubes, ovaries, mesentery, and mesoappendix[3] (Fig. 450).

Wilkie[25] demonstrated in the rabbit that if fecal material is milked into the lumen of the appendix and then the appendix is ligated, the rabbit dies within twenty-four hours from a perforated gangrenous appendix. If the rabbit's appendix is free from infection and is ligated, mucocele alone results.

Wangensteen[23, 24] demonstrated in human beings that there is active secretion of fluid by the appendiceal mucosa. The highest secretory pressure was 126 cm of water after fourteen hours of obstruction. He found that under certain circumstances the balance between secretion and absorption was narrow. With fibrosis, there was diminished secretory capacity. This finding may be responsible, at least in part, for the diminished incidence of appendicitis in older people. A normal appendix is, therefore, more vulnerable to distention by partial obstruction than a fibrosed appendix.

Acute inflammation, particularly in the normal appendix, occurs when there is *secretion under pressure behind an obstruction* sufficient to impair the resistance of the normal wall to infection. This obstruction is usually a *fecalith*, but it may be a foreign body, a true calculus,[9] a gallstone, a carcinoma of the cecum, or a primary tumor of the appendix. With infection and dilatation beyond the area of the block, an inflammatory process may produce complete necrosis of the appendix with perforation and peritonitis. The obstructive type is more likely to lead to perforation.

425

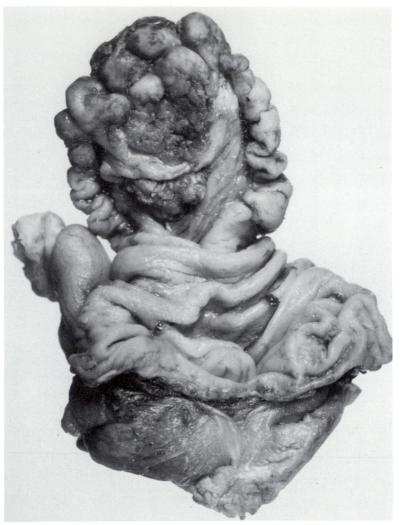

Fig. 448 Appendix from 4-year-old child in whom intussusception occurred. There is extreme lymphoid hyperplasia, and cuff of cecum is present. (WU neg. 70-7236.)

Nonobstructive appendicitis can be related to a generalized infection, particularly in the respiratory tract. It is possible that nonobstructive appendicitis in aged persons is due to diminished lymphatic tissue, a thin fibrous appendix, and vascular occlusion.[7, 22, 26] We have not seen primary vascular occlusive disease produce appendicitis.

Acute appendicitis

There is close correlation between the gross and microscopic findings in acute appendicitis. Therkelsen[21] reported 154 acute appendices: 125 demonstrated gross evidence of inflammation, twenty-five showed doubtful evidence of it, and four appeared normal. In apparently normal appendices, focal inflammation localized to a small area of mucosa may occur.

In acute appendicitis, the external surface shows fibrin and variable amounts of pus, and the mucosa often is necrotic and ulcerated. Frequently, a fecalith is impacted in the lumen. The process may become localized and form an appendiceal abscess. In the presence of an acute inflammatory process, secondarily infected thrombi may spread along the ileocolic and upper mesenteric veins.[6]

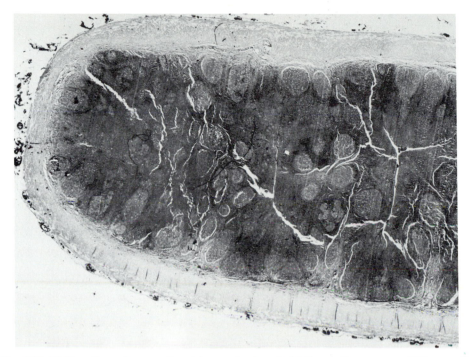

Fig. 449 Obliteration of appendiceal lumen by lymphoid tissue. (Low power; WU neg. 49-3706.)

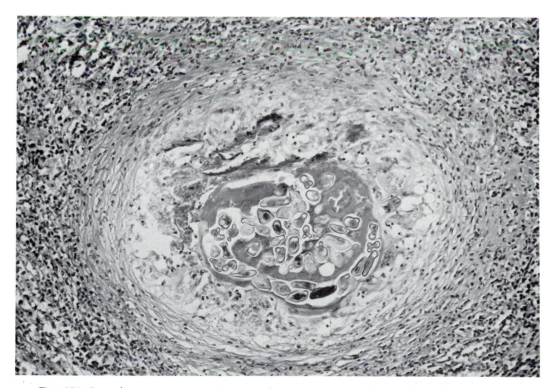

Fig. 450 Granulomatous reaction in appendiceal serosa secondary to *Oxyuris vermicularis* infestation in 6-year-old girl. Clinical diagnosis was acute appendicitis. (×150; WU neg. 72-229.)

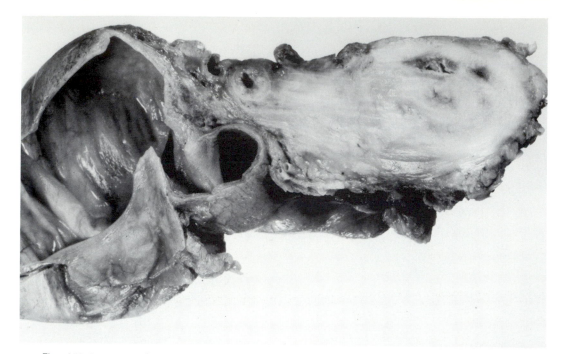

Fig. 451 Periappendicular abscess secondary to episode of acute appendicitis that occurred one month previously. Abscess was palpable clinically. (WU neg. 64-5085.)

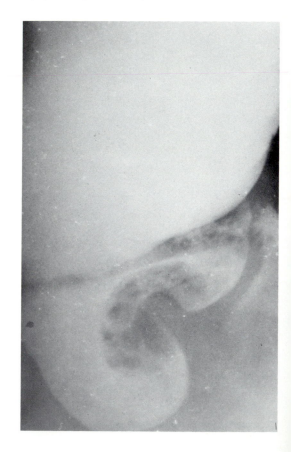

Microscopically, the diagnosis of appendicitis is relatively simple. In the *acute inflammatory processes,* minimal inflammation to necrosis and complete destruction of the wall of the appendix may exist. In the early lesion, neutrophils appear at the base of the crypt adjacent to a small defect in the epithelium. After this inflammatory process reaches the submucosa, it spreads quickly to the remaining appendix. Lymphangitis is usually widespread. In advanced stages, the mucosa may be destroyed, the wall necrotic, and the vessels thrombosed. Thrombosed vessels secondary to the acute process occurred in twenty-six of 100 cases reviewed by Remington and McDonald.[19] Pylephlebitis may originate in a thrombosed vessel of the diseased appendix and spread to the portal veins. The appendices of these persons will show pathologic alterations depend-

Fig. 452 Detailed view of defect in ileocecal area. Lesion was misinterpreted as carcinoma and was radically removed. (WU neg. 57-1352.)

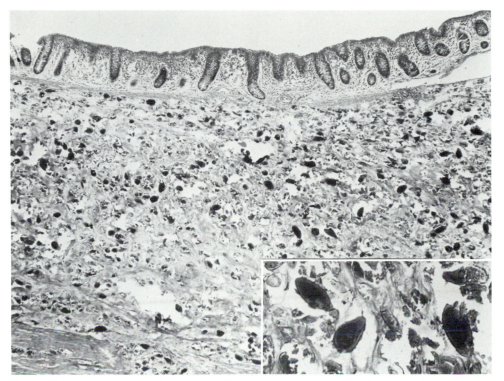

Fig. 453 Schistosomiasis of appendiceal submucosa covered by intact epithelium. **Inset** shows detail of parasite eggs. This involvement can cause appendicitis. (×30; **inset,** ×150.)

ing on the time interval between the acute attack and the operation.

Appendiceal abscess is usually in the right iliac fossa lateral to the cecum (Figs. 451 and 452). Variations in location are related to the site of the appendix. Large abscesses may perforate into the cecum or rectum or even extend to the skin surface.

Appendiceal granulomas composed of epithelioid cells, fibroblasts, and a large number of eosinophils, having a necrotic center, and surrounded by diffuse eosinophilic infiltration have been correlated by Stemmerman[20] with the presence of *Strongyloides stercoralis* in stool examinations.

Schistosomiasis and other parasitic infestations of the appendix are described by Collins[10] in his comprehensive review of diseases of this organ (Fig. 453).

We have seen a single instance of acute necrotizing arteritis in the vessels of the appendix (Fig. 454), probably on an allergic basis.

In the rare lesion of the appendix that occurs in the prodromal stage of measles, the patient develops appendicitis, and the microscopic examination shows proliferation of the endothelial cells with the presence of many multinucleated giant cells (Fig. 455). Similar changes have been reported in the tonsil. If the pathologist is astute enough to recognize these changes, he can tell the patient's physician that the child is about to break out into the characteristic rash of measles.[5, 12]

Clinicopathologic correlation

Acute appendicitis continues to be a frequent acute surgical illness treated in general hospitals. In 1886 Fitz,[11] through his thorough studies, demonstrated that the appendix was the origin of mysterious inflammation of the right iliac fossa. Three years later, McBurney[16] emphasized the principles of accurate early diagnosis and prompt surgical intervention. By 1900, the mortality rate had fallen to 35%. During

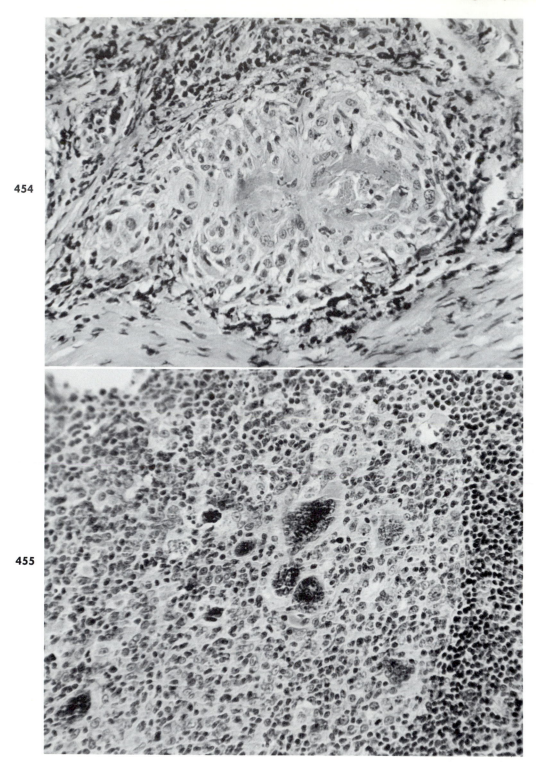

Fig. 454 Necrotizing arteritis of appendix in child with possible rheumatic fever. (×325; WU neg. 57-3371A.)
Fig. 455 Typical giant cells appearing in appendix of child in prodromal stage of measles. (×350; WU neg. 57-4625; courtesy Dr. J. L. Bonenfant, Quebec, Canada.)

the next three decades, it was further reduced to 5% as a result of dissemination of knowledge to the public and the physician concerning the symptoms and signs of acute appendicitis, the need for early surgical intervention, and the dangers of catharsis and morphine for undiagnosed abdominal pain.

In the following twenty-five years, a combination of improved surgical technique, better preoperative and postoperative care, advances in anesthesiology, and the development of effective antibacterial agents led to further declines in mortality to a fraction of 1%. The later reduction in risk was accomplished mainly in three classes of patients: those with perforation and peritonitis, the very young, and the very old.

Almond[2] reviewed all the appendices removed in adults in 1954 and all the appendices removed in children in 1954 and 1955 at Barnes Hospital and the St. Louis Children's Hospital, respectively. He found that the accuracy of diagnosis was 67% in adults and 90% in children. In spite of the fact that perforation had occurred in 31% of the adults and in 36% of the children, there were no deaths (Table 14). The mortality from perforated appendices is, in many instances, attributable to poor surgical therapy. It is granted that obstruction is the usual cause of appendicitis, and in this series of cases reviewed we could find objective evidence of such an obstruction in 34% of the patients (Table 15), a figure much lower than that quoted in the literature. We have looked carefully for local evidence of vascular etiology in aged patients but have yet to see a single instance that we could prove pathologically.

Obstructive appendicitis causes acute periumbilical colicky pain and reflex vomiting incident to increased intraluminal pressure (Figs. 456 to 458). Fever and leukocytosis develop with the onset of peritoneal inflammatory signs in the right lower quadrant of the abdomen. With inflammatory invasion of the muscle, perforation may finally occur, rarely with temporary relief of pain, soon followed by signs of peritonitis.

Acute appendicitis in children[18] and in aged persons[22, 26] may be mishandled because of failure to consider the diagnosis and because the findings are often atypical. Appendicitis can rarely be simulated by infarction of the greater omentum.[1]

"Chronic appendicitis"

There is no doubt that the appendix should be removed if the clinical signs and symptoms suggest the probability of appendicitis. Chronic appendicitis as a primary entity has been greatly disputed. There is no doubt that patients may develop classical signs of acute appendicitis which subside.

Table 14 Appendectomy for acute appendicitis

	Adults	Children	Total
All cases	121	99	220
Acute appendicitis	80 (66.6%)	89 (90.0%)	169
Perforated appendix	25 (31.2%)	32 (35.9%)	57 (33.7%)
Peritonitis	14 (17.5%)	21 (23.6%)	35 (20.7%)
Abscess	11 (13.7%)	11 (12.3%)	22 (13.0%)

Table 15 Mechanisms of obstruction in acute appendicitis

Type	Children	Adults	Total
Fecalith	23	23	46
Lymphoid hyperplasia	6	3	9
Dilatation (cause unknown)	8	11	19
			74

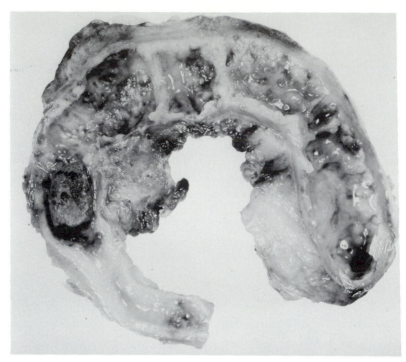

Fig. 456 Acute appendicitis distal to obstructing fecalith. (WU neg. 49-5325.)

Permanent changes may be found in appendices that have been infected. If gangrene has occurred, only a stump of the appendix may remain. In other instances in which an inflammatory process has destroyed the muscle, fibrous replacement is present. Of course, if the process was superficial and confined to the mucosa and submucosa, no changes will be found.

The symptoms and signs of chronic appendicitis are as vague and shadowy as the pathology. Primary chronic appendicitis as a pathologic or clinical entity is unlikely. This does not preclude the existence of appendiceal colic without acute inflammation. In the natural development of the appendix, fibrosis beginning at the tip takes place with aging. Such fibrosis does not cause symptoms.

Unfortunately, in some laboratories the pathologist is a willing accomplice to the surgeon who is liberal in his clinical diagnosis of chronic appendicitis. These pathologists never call an appendix normal. Rough handling and clamping of the ap-

pendix may produce hemorrhage, and with age there is an increase of fibrous tissue with diminished lymphoid tissue. Normally, there may be a collection of lymphocytes in the muscular wall of the appendix, and a rare plasma cell or eosinophil may be seen in the mucosa. Just because vague preoperative symptoms disappear is not necessarily evidence that the symptoms were in any way related to the appendix. As Hertzler[14] stated, "The anatomic structure of appendices commonly removed under the diagnosis of chronic appendicitis shows no variation from the appendices of individuals suffering from no abdominal complaint whatsoever."*

Tumors
So-called mucocele

In the condition designated mucocele, the appendix shows localized or diffuse globular enlargement. The lumen is di-

*From Hertzler, A. E.: An inquiry into the nature of chronic appendicitis, Am. J. Obstet. Gynecol. 11:155-170, 1926.

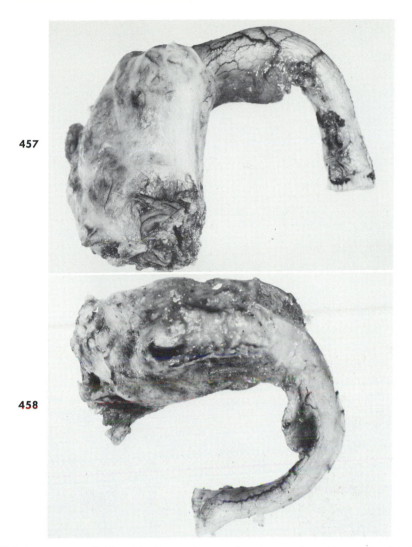

Fig. 457 Acute appendicitis with obstruction, perforation, and periappendiceal inflammation. (WU neg. 49-4993.)
Fig. 458 Large inflammatory mass that shows destruction of wall and fecalith in place. (WU neg. 49-4993.)

lated and contains large amounts of glairy mucus (Fig. 459). It is usually assumed that the changes are secondary to proximal obstruction of the lumen. Cheng's experimental model[27] is often quoted in this regard. He showed that if the lumen of the rabbit "appendix" is surgically occluded, dilatation of the distal portion with flattening of the epithelium and accumulation of mucus results. If the mucus is transplanted to the rabbit peritoneum, it acts as foreign material and in time is absorbed.

In our opinion, the term *mucocele* embraces a group of conditions having different morphology and pathogenesis.[33] In a few instances, the disease seems indeed to be the result of occlusion of the lumen, being analogous to that sometimes seen in the gallbladder. The epithelium is flat, atrophic, and devoid of any atypical features. In other cases, a localized focus of mucosal hyperplasia is seen, the appearance being indistinguishable from that of a hyperplastic colonic polyp. We feel that

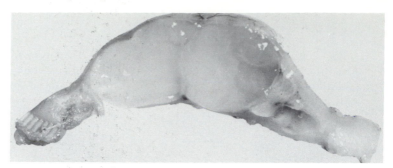

Fig. 459 Classic example of so-called mucocele of appendix still confined within lumen but showing extreme distention and thinning of wall. This was incidental finding in woman undergoing cholecystectomy. Microscopically, features were those of mucinous cystadenoma. (WU neg. 53-2882.)

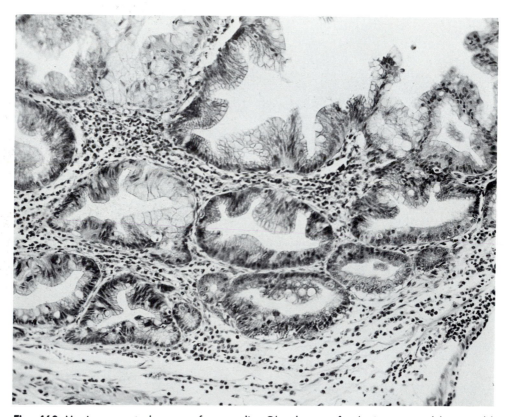

Fig. 460 Mucinous cystadenoma of appendix. Glands are of colonic type and have mild degree of atypia and tendency to papillary configuration. Most lesions designated as mucoceles belong to this category. (×150; WU neg. 55-6012.)

the remaining cases, which represent most of the lesions diagnosed as "mucoceles," are actually mucinous neoplasms of the appendix.[26a, 33]

The large majority of these mucinous neoplasms are benign—i.e., mucinous cystadenomas. They are lined by *atypical* mucinous epithelium with at least some areas of papillary configuration (Fig. 460). Secondary changes include thinning of the wall, extensive ulceration, and calcification. The latter may be evident radiographical-

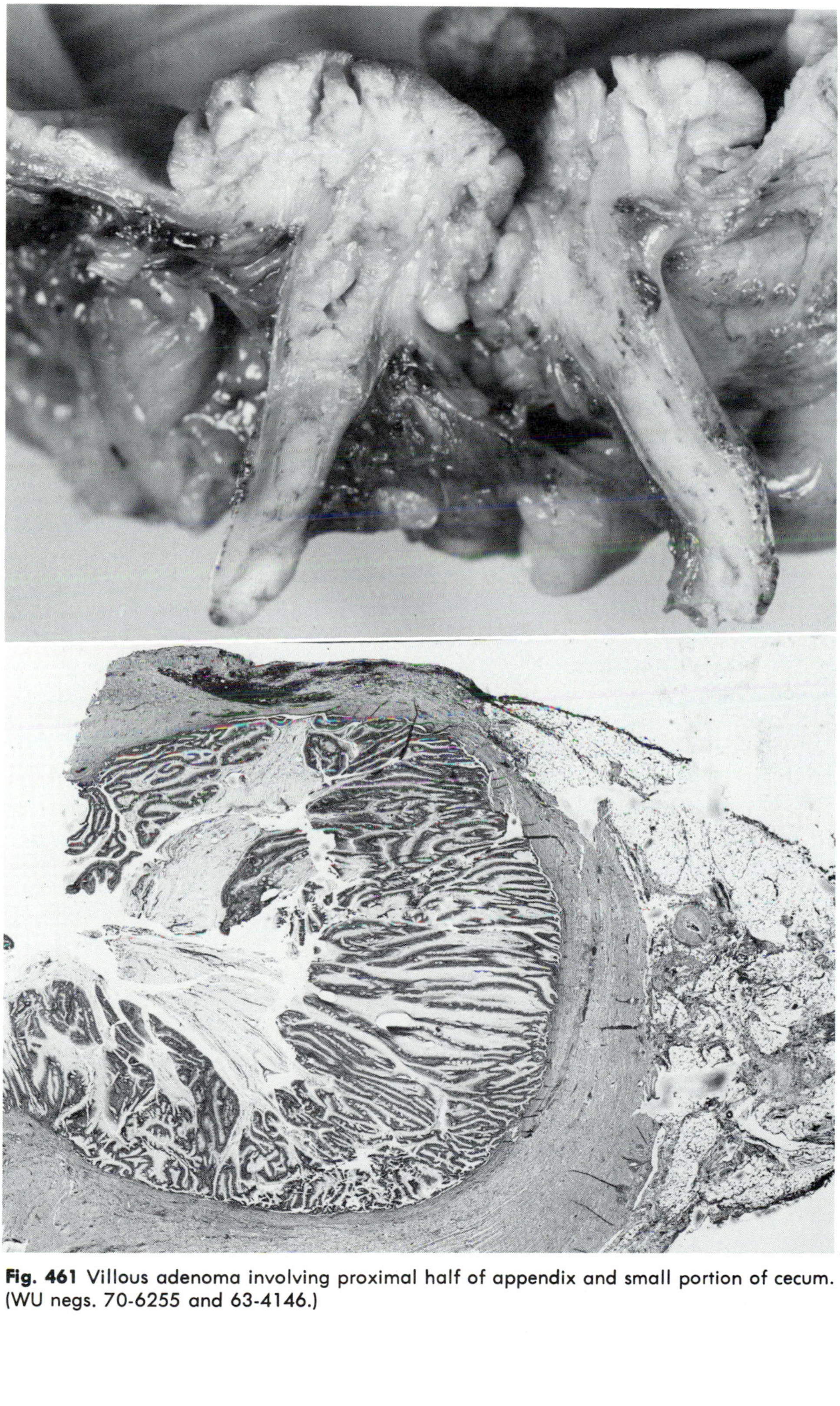

Fig. 461 Villous adenoma involving proximal half of appendix and small portion of cecum. (WU negs. 70-6255 and 63-4146.)

ly. As a result of increased intraluminal pressure, mucus may penetrate into the wall, reach the serosa, and appear as a periappendicular or retroperitoneal mass at operation. Removal of the appendix is curative, even in the presence of the latter complication. A certain proportion of these cases are associated with ovarian mucinous cystadenoma of strikingly similar microscopic appearance.[43] The malignant counterpart—i.e., mucinous cystadenocarcinoma—has the same gross appearance and many microscopic features in common with the benign form.[34, 46] The diagnosis of malignancy can be made if there is invasion of the appendiceal wall by atypical glands or, in the presence of peritoneal mucinous deposits, if these deposits contain clearly identifiable epithelial cells (whether atypical or not) admixed with the mucinous material. The latter condition, when generalized, is known as *pseudomyxoma peritonei*.[38] This process forms gelatinous nodules and in time may cause the death of the patient through infection or intestinal obstruction by invasion of the surrounding structures such as the bladder, the abdominal wall, and the intestine. We have not seen involvement above the diaphragm or metastases to lymph nodes. In three instances perforated malignant material spread into a hernial sac and was diagnosed by microscopic examination. Mucinous cystadenocarcinomas of the appendix may be associated with similar independent lesions of the ovary.[43] Radiotherapy may temporarily slow the growth of the metastatic tumor. Removal of as much of the tumor as possible may be helpful in prolonging life even for several years. However, peritonitis is frequent after such palliative operations. *Pseudomyxoma peritonei* indistinguishable from the one previously described can be the result of ovarian mucinous cystadenocarcinoma.

Adenocarcinoma

Few cases of primary adenocarcinoma of the appendix have been reported.[29, 37, 41] Adenocarcinomas of the cecum that have secondarily invaded the appendix have been erroneously reported as primary carcinoma. Carcinoma may be located in any part of the appendix. It may be an incidental finding grossly or even microscopically. The symptoms resemble acute appendicitis. Right hemicolectomy is the treatment of choice except for very superficial tumors of well-differentiated nature that can be cured by simple appendectomy.[45]

Classic villous adenoma can occur primarily in the appendix[30, 31] (Fig. 461).

Carcinoid tumor

Carcinoid tumors are found in about one out of every 300 routine appendectomies[42] and represent the most common tumor of the appendix. The peak incidence occurs in the third and fourth decades of life. In most of the cases, they are incidental findings, but they may be found associated with acute appendicitis as a result of obstruction of the lumen. In the 144 cases, reported by Moertel et al.,[42] 71% were located in the tip of the appendix, 22% in the body, and 7% in the base; 70% of the lesions were less than 1 cm in diameter, and only two measured 2 cm or more. Grossly, the tumors are firm, yellow, and fairly well circumscribed (Fig. 462).

Microscopically, the majority of the cases show solid nests of monotonous cells alternating with acinar and "ribbon" formation[40] (Fig. 463, A). Argentaffin and diazo reaction are almost always positive. Invasion of muscle and lymphatic vessels is the rule, and spread to the peritoneal surface is quite common. A second type of carcinoid tumor, which is often misdiagnosed as primary or metastatic carcinoma, is characterized by glandular formation without solid nests (Fig. 463, B). Mucin stains are positive, whereas argentaffin and diazo reactions are negative.[28] The lack of mitoses and atypia, orderly arrangement, and origin at the base of the glands should suggest this diagnosis. Electron microscopic examination will be diagnostic even with formalin-fixed material because of the presence of neurosecretory granules.[44]

We have also seen an appendiceal neoplasm composed of nests of well-differentiated mucin-positive signet ring cells infiltrating the entire thickness of the wall (Fig. 463, *C*). Argentaffin and argyrophil stains were positive in some of the tumor cells. Whether this tumor type should be designated as carcinoid is debatable, but it is important to remember that it follows the same indolent clinical course and is associated with the same good prognosis as the ordinary carcinoid tumor.[36, 45a]

Five (4.2%) of the patients in the series

ston,[35] the tumor produced ACTH in excess, resulting in a clinical picture of Cushing's syndrome.

Other lesions

Primary malignant lymphomas of the appendix have been reported.[49] We have observed ***metastases*** to the appendix ***from breast carcinoma.***[47]

Diverticula of the appendix are usually multiple. They are of the "false" type, arising in a weak area as a result of increased

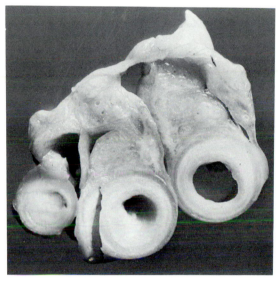

Fig. 462 Carcinoid tumor of appendix which blocked lumen and caused acute appendicitis. (WU neg. 52-4366.)

reported by Moertel et al.[42] had an associated carcinoid of the ileum, and nineteen (13%) had a second primary cancer. Metastatic spread of the appendiceal carcinoid is quite unusual and often limited to the regional lymph nodes. As a general rule, it is restricted to tumors greater than 2 cm in diameter. It is now well established that simple appendectomy is adequate therapy for this neoplasm even in the presence of serosal invasion, except for the very rare cases measuring 2 cm or more in diameter.[42] Only five cases of carcinoid syndrome secondary to appendiceal carcinoid tumor have been reported.[39] Liver metastases were present or suspected in every instance. In a case reported by John-

intraluminal pressure. Diverticulitis may occur, resulting in a clinical picture indistinguishable from acute appendicitis.[51]

Endometriosis and ***ectopic decidual reaction*** are sometimes seen as incidental findings beneath the serosa.

Granular cells, isolated or in clusters, are found in the musculature of the appendix in approximately 5% of the cases.[50] Their light and electron microscopic appearances are quite similar to those of the cells of so-called granular cell tumor. Sobel et al[52] have given convincing evidence that these cells represent altered smooth muscle cells.

Heterotopic gastric and ***esophageal*** tissue has been described by Droga et al.[48]

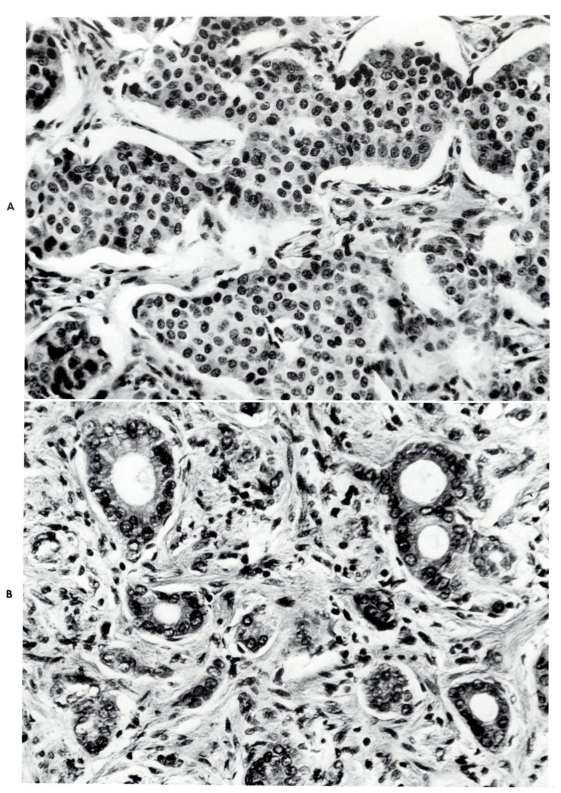

A

B

Fig. 463 For legend, see opposite page.

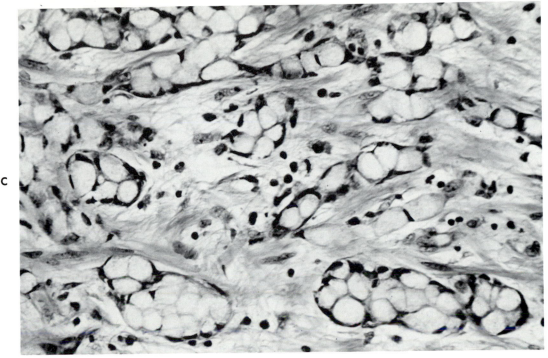

Fig. 463 A, Appendiceal carcinoid tumor of ordinary type. This variety usually contains argentaffin as well as argyrophil cells. **B,** Appendiceal carcinoid tumor forming well-defined glandular structures. In this variety, cells are often argyrophil but only rarely argentaffin. **C,** Tumor of appendix formed by nests of mucin-positive signet ring cells infiltrating entire wall. There is little stromal reaction to tumor, no cellular atypia, and no individual cell infiltration. Argentaffin and/or argyrophil cells can often be demonstrated. **(A** to **C,** ×350; **A,** WU neg. 73-4620; **B,** WU neg. 73-4619; **C,** WU neg. 73-4621.)

REFERENCES
Appendicitis

1 Alecce, A. A., Sullivan, S. G., and Ashworth, W.: Spontaneous idiopathic segmental infarction of the omentum, Ann. Surg. 142:316-320, 1955.

2 Almond, C.: Unpublished data, Division of Surgical Pathology, Washington University School of Medicine, St. Louis, Mo., 1956.

3 Arean, V.: Personal communication, 1969.

4 Ashburn, L. L.: Appendiceal oxyuriasis, Am. J. Pathol. 17:841-856, 1941.

5 Bonenfant, J. L.: Lésions appendiculaires au cours de la rougeole, Arch. Fr. Pediatr. 9:1-10, 1952.

6 Boyce, F. F.: Acute appendicitis and its complications, New York, 1949, Oxford University Press, Inc.

7 Boyce, F. F.: Special problems of acute appendicitis in middle and late life, Arch. Surg. 68:296-304, 1957.

8 Burkitt, D. P.: The aetiology of appendicitis, Br. J. Surg. 58:695-699, 1971.

9 Clark, L. P.: Calculi in the appendix, Br. J. Surg. 40:272-273, 1946.

10 Collins, D. C.: 71,000 human appendix specimens; a final report, summarizing forty years' study, Am. J. Proctol. 14:265-281, 1963.

11 Fitz, R. H.: Perforating inflammation of the vermiform appendix with special reference to its early diagnosis, Am. J. Med. Sci. 92:321, 1886.

12 Galloway, W. H.: Appendicitis in the course of measles, Br. Med. J. 2:1412-1414, 1957.

13 Gray, S. H., and Heifetz, C. J.: Lymphoid hyperplasia of appendix, Arch. Surg. 35:887-900, 1937.

14 Hertzler, A. E.: An inquiry into the nature of chronic appendicitis, Am. J. Obstet. Gynecol. 11:155-170, 1926.

15 Hwang, J. M. S., and Krumbhaar, E. B.: Amount of lymphoid tissue of human appendix and its weight at different age periods, Am. J. Med. Sci. 199:75-83, 1940.

16 McBurney, C.: Experience with early operative interference in cases of disease of vermiform appendix, N. Y. State J. Med. 50:676, 1889.

17 Nathans, A. A., Merenstein, H., and Brown, S. S.: Lymphoid hyperplasia of the appendix, Pediatrics 12:516-524, 1955.

18 Packard, G. B., and McLauthlin, C. H.: Acute appendicitis in children, J. Pediatr. **39**:708-714, 1951.

19 Remington, J. H., and McDonald, J. R.: Vascular thrombosis in acute appendicitis, Surgery **24**:787-792, 1948.

20 Stemmerman, G. N.: Eosinophilic granuloma of the appendix; a study of its relation to strongyloides infestation, Am. J. Clin. Pathol. **36**:524-531, 1961.

21 Therkelsen, F.: On histologic diagnosis of appendicitis, Acta Chir. Scand. **94**(suppl. 108):1-48, 1948.

22 Thorbjarnarson, B., and Loehr, W. J.: Acute appendicitis in patients over the age of sixty, Surg. Gynecol. Obstet. **125**:1277-1280, 1967.

23 Wangensteen, O. H.: The genesis of appendicitis in the light of the functional behavior of the vermiform appendix, Lancet **2**:491-506, 1939.

24 Wangensteen, O. H., and Dennis. C.: Experimental proof of the obstructive origin of appendicitis in man, Ann. Surg. **110**:629-647, 1939.

25 Wilkie, D. P. D.: The etiology of acute appendicular disease, Can. Med. Assoc. J. **22**:314-316, 1930.

26 Williams, J. S., and Hale, H. W., Jr.: Acute appendicitis in the elderly: review of 83 cases, Ann. Surg. **162**:208-212, 1965.

Tumors

26a Aho, A. J., Heinonen, R., and Laurén, P.: Benign and malignant mucocele of the appendix, Acta Chir. Scand. **139**:392-400, 1973.

27 Cheng, K. K.: An experimental study of mucocele of the appendix and pseudomyxoma peritonei, J. Pathol. Bacteriol. **61**:217-225, 1940.

28 Dische, F. E.: Argentaffin and non-argentaffin carcinoid tumours of the appendix, J. Clin. Pathol. **21**:60-66, 1968.

29 Edmonson, H. T., Jr., and Hobbs, M. L.: Primary adenocarcinoma of the appendix, Am. Surg. **33**:717-732, 1967.

30 Goldfarb, W. B., and Kempson, R. L.: Villous adenomas of the appendix, Surgery **55**:769-772, 1964.

31 Hameed, K.: Villous adenoma of the vermiform appendix with Cushing's syndrome; ultrastructural study of a case, Cancer **27**:681-686, 1971.

32 Hesketh, K. T.: The management of primary adenocarcinoma of the vermiform appendix, Gut **4**:158-168, 1963.

33 Higa, E., Rosai, J., Pizzimbono, C. A., and Wise, L.: Mucosal hyperplasia, mucinous cystadenoma and mucinous cystadenocarcinoma of the appendix; a reevaluation of appendiceal "mucocele," Cancer (in press, 1973).

34 Hilsabeck, J. R., Judd, E. S., Jr., and Woolner, L. B.: Carcinoma of the vermiform appendix, Surg. Clin. North Am. **31**:995-1011, 1951.

35 Johnston, W. H., and Waisman, J.: Carcinoid tumor of the vermiform appendix with Cushing's syndrome, Cancer **27**:681-686, 1971.

36 Klein, H. Z.: Mucinous carcinoid tumor of the vermiform appendix, Cancer (in press).

37 Lesnick, G., and Miller, D.: Adenocarcinoma of the appendix, Cancer **2**:18-24, 1949.

38 Little, J. M., Halliday, J. P., and Glenn, D. C.: Pseudomyxoma peritonei, Lancet **2**:659-663, 1969.

39 Markgraf, W. H., and Dunn, T. M.: Appendiceal carcinoid with carcinoid syndrome, Am. J. Surg. **107**:730-732, 1964.

40 Masson, P.: Carcinoids (argentaffin-cell tumors) and nerve hyperplasia of the appendicular mucosa, Am. J. Pathol. **4**:181-212, 1928.

41 Mauritzen, K.: Primary adenocarcinoma of the appendix; report of sixteen cases, Acta. Chir. Scand. **115**:447-456, 1958.

42 Moertel, C. G., Dockerty, M. B., and Judd, E. S.: Carcinoid tumors of the vermiform appendix, Cancer **21**:270-278, 1968.

43 Ries, E.: Pseudomyxoma peritonei, Surg. Gynecol. Obstet. **39**:569-579, 1924.

44 Rosai, J., and Rodriguez, H. A.: Application of electron microscopy to the differential diagnosis of tumors, Am. J. Clin. Pathol. **50**:555-562, 1968.

45 Steinberg, M., and Cohn, I., Jr.: Primary adenocarcinoma of the appendix, Surgery **61**:644-660, 1967.

45a Subbuswamy, S. G., Gibbs, N. M., Ross, C. F., and Morson, B. C.: Goblet cell carcinoid of the appendix, Cancer (in press, 1974).

46 Woodruff, R., and McDonald, J. R.: Benign and malignant cystic tumors of appendix, Surg. Gynecol. Obstet. **71**:750-755, 1940.

Other lesions

47 Bolker, H., and Shapiro, A. L.: Appendiceal metastasis in carcinoma of the breast, N. Y. State J. Med. **40**:219-220, 1940.

48 Droga, B. W., Levine, S., and Baker, J. J.: Heterotopic gastric and esophageal tissue in the vermiform appendix, Am. J. Clin. Pathol. **40**:190-193, 1963.

49 Galloway, W. H., and Owens, E. J.: Primary lymphosarcoma of appendix occurring in childhood, Br. Med. J. **2**:1387-1388, 1949.

50 Hausman, R.: Granular cells in musculature of appendix, Arch. Pathol. **75**:360-372, 1963.

51 Rabinovitch, J.: Diverticulosis and diverticulitis of the vermiform appendix, Ann. Surg. **155**:434-440, 1962.

52 Sobel, H. J., Marquet, E., and Schwarz, R.: Granular degeneration of appendiceal smooth muscle, Arch. Pathol. **92**:427-432, 1971.

Large bowel

Diverticulosis and diverticulitis

Diverticulosis and diverticulitis are rare in patients under 40 years old. About one in eight patients over 45 years of age has clinically detectable diverticulosis, but surgical complications occur in only 10% or less.[4] In autopsy studies, the incidence of diverticulosis is naturally higher. Hughes[3] found diverticula in ninety of 200 colons examined in Brisbane, Australia. When the cecal diverticula were excluded, the total incidence was 43%. The sigmoid colon was affected in 99% of the specimens. This was the only area of involvement in 41% of the cases; in 30%, the disease spread to the descending colon, in 4% to the transverse colon, and in 16% to the entire colon. Diverticulosis is extremely rare in underdeveloped countries. A high-residue diet seems to be the main protective factor. It probably acts by diminishing the efficiency of colonic segmentation, which is the mechanism responsible for mucosal herniation.[8] We agree with Morson[5] that a muscle abnormality is responsible, in part at least, for diverticular disease of the colon.

The muscle abnormality is the most consistent and striking abnormality in diverticular disease. The taeniae coli appear thick, assuming an almost cartilaginous consistency. The circular muscle is thick and has a corrugated or concertina-like appearance. In between these muscular corrugations the mouths of the diverticula are found as they penetrate the bowel wall to lie in the pericolic fat. These corrugations are interdigitating processes of circular muscle. They are not continuous around the circumference of the bowel wall, being only semicircular arcs of muscle confined to the two zones between the mesenteric and antimesenteric taeniae. Each arc consists of a double layer of circular muscle and the thin investing layer of longitudinal muscle. This appearance is always found in specimens without inflammatory changes and in those with a relatively slight amount of inflammation. But when there is extensive pericolic inflammation the accompanying extramural fibrosis seems to have a restricting effect on the normal freedom of movement of the sigmoid colon, leading to the most bizarre and irregular shapes and in particular to the formation of a fibromuscular tumor.*

Ulceration into a nutrient vessel may cause severe hemorrhage[7, 9] (Figs. 464 and 465). Diverticula may perforate and form pericolic abscesses. The diverticulum has a flasklike shape, fills with feces, and cannot empty because there is no muscle in the sac. In time, the hernia forces its way through the muscular layer and extends into the appendices epiploicae. In an obese person, it may be difficult to recognize diverticula at the time of operation. Secondary inflammatory changes may occur. Usually the tissues in the immediate area become adherent to the zone of threatened perforation. Acute free perforation is rare. An inflammatory mass usually forms that may be confused with carcinoma (Fig. 466). The spontaneous drainage into bladder or adjacent bowel of an abscess secondary

*From Morson, B. C.: The muscle abnormality in diverticular disease of the colon, Proc. R. Soc. Med. 56:798-800, 1963.

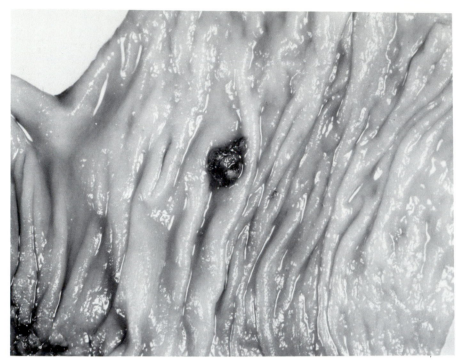

Fig. 464 Clot overlying orifice of uninflamed cecal diverticulum. Massively bleeding artery was open at neck of diverticulum. (WU neg. 64-8413.)

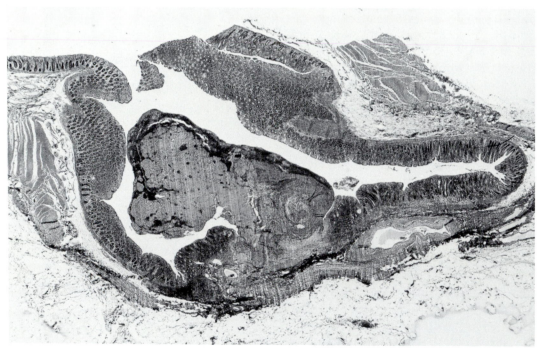

Fig. 465 Photomicrograph of diverticulum of large bowel from which massive hemorrhage occurred. There is thrombus overlying vessels. There is no inflammation present. (×14; WU neg. 72-5407.)

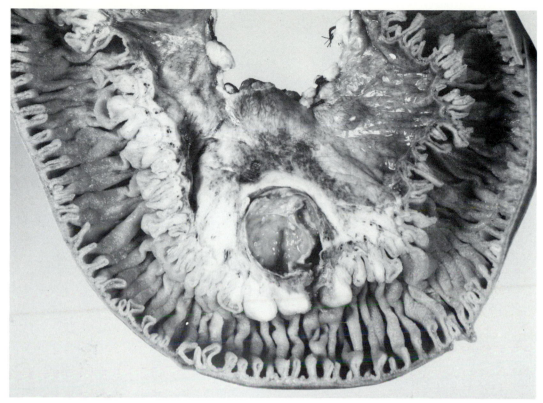

Fig. 466 In this colon with extensive diverticulosis, one of diverticula perforated and formed large inflammatory mass in mesentery. (WU neg. 67-4009.)

to diverticular perforation results in fistulas. Cecal diverticula should be separated from the ordinary case of diverticulosis. They are often solitary, not necessarily associated with sigmoid involvement, and frequently lack the muscular abnormalities always seen in the other locations.[3] Despite statements to the contrary in the literature, the large majority of cecal diverticula resemble microscopically colonic diverticula by the lack of smooth muscle in their walls. They may cause a firm, indurated mass in the region of the ileocecal valve and may be confused with cancer clinically and radiographically.[1, 6]

Diverticulitis usually involves a much longer segment of the bowel than does carcinoma (Figs. 467 and 468). The barium-filled colon has sawtooth serrations and a narrowed lumen. However, careful radiographic examination usually shows the mucosa to be intact. Pain, a common symptom of diverticular disease, may be of muscular origin or the result of inflammation.

Surgical resection is being performed more frequently in patients with the complications of diverticulitis such as perforation, obstruction, and hemorrhage. However, morbidity and mortality rates are

Table 16 Relationship of colic inflammation to the severity of regional complications of colonic resection*

Pathologic diagnosis	Number of patients	Number of postoperative complications	
		Fatal	Nonfatal
Diverticulosis	89	0	15
Diverticulitis	35	1	11
Perforation with abscess	28	2	13
Total	152	3	39

*From Giffin, J. M., Butcher, H. R., Jr., and Ackerman, L. V.: The surgical management of colonic diverticulitis, Arch. Surg. 94:619-626, 1967; copyright 1967, American Medical Association.

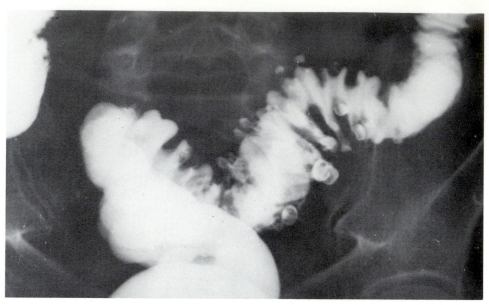

Fig. 467 Classic picture of diverticulosis. (WU neg. 57-990.)

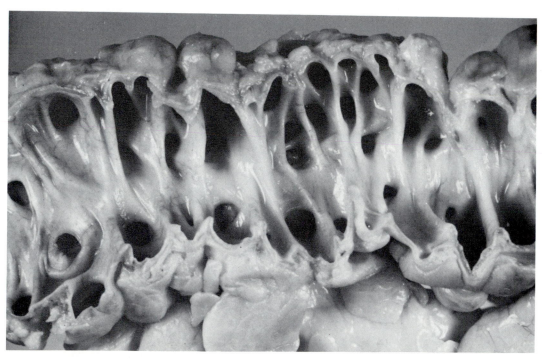

Fig. 468 Extensive diverticulosis of sigmoid colon with segmentation and shortening of bowel. Openings of diverticula can be seen clearly. Circular muscle is thick and corrugated. (WU neg. 71-10089.)

higher in these instances than when resections are performed for uncomplicated acute diverticulitis[2] (Table 16). Other indications are repeated attacks of diverticulitis while on a good medical regimen and the development of urinary symptoms.

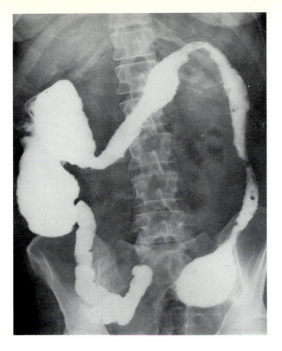

Urinary symptoms may imply impending sigmoid vesical fistula. Welch et al.[10] reported an operative mortality of 2.6% among 114 patients treated by resection.

Ulcerative colitis

For many years, the presence of a chronic inflammatory disease of the large bowel not attributed to a specific organism was equivalent to the diagnosis of ulcerative colitis. It is now apparent that many of these cases actually represented examples of Crohn's disease involving the colon, a condition also known as granulomatous

Fig. 469 Extensive narrowing of bowel wall with loss of haustrations from chronic ulcerative colitis. (WU neg. 48-5548.)

Table 17 Differences between ulcerative colitis and Crohn's disease (granulomatous colitis)

	Ulcerative colitis	Crohn's disease
Clinical		
Rectal bleeding	Common	Inconspicuous
Abdominal mass	Practically never	10% to 15%
Abdominal pain	Usually left-sided	Usually right-sided
Sigmoidoscopy	Abnormal in 95%	Abnormal in less than 50%
Free perforation	12%	4%
Colon carcinoma	5% to 10%	Very rare
Anal complications	Rare; minor	75%; fissures, fistulas, ulceration
Response to steroid therapy	75%	25%
Results of surgery	Very good	Fair
Ileostomy dysfunction	Rare	Common
Radiographic		
Sparing of rectum	Exceptional	90%
Involvement of ileum	Rare; dilated ("backwash ileitis")	Common; constricted
Strictures	Absent	Often present
Skip areas	Absent	Common
Internal fistulas	Absent	May be present
Longitudinal and transverse ulcers	Exceptional	Common
Fissuring	Absent	Common
Thumbprinting	Absent	Common
Morphologic		
Distribution of involvement	Diffuse; predominantly left-sided; mucosal and submucosal	Focal; predominantly right-sided; transmural
Mucosal atrophy and regeneration	Marked	Minimal
Cytoplasmic mucin	Diminished	Preserved
Lymphoid aggregates	Rare	Common
Edema	Minimal	Marked
Hyperemia	May be extreme	Minimal
Granulomas	Absent	Present in 60%
Fissuring	Absent	Present
Crypt abscesses	Common	Rare
Rectal involvement	Practically always	50%
Ileal involvement	Minimal; dilated not more than 10 cm	50%; constricted; transmural inflammation
Lymph nodes	Reactive hyperplasia	May contain granulomas

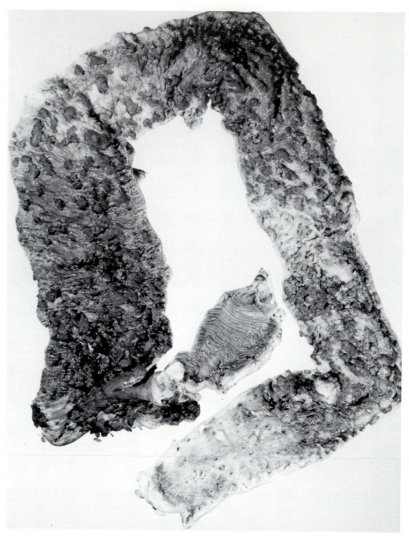

Fig. 470 Typical case of ulcerative colitis. Irregular ulcerations of geographic configuration surround small islands of residual mucosa which are hyperemic and covered by inflammatory exudate. (WU neg. 59-4551.)

colitis. The clinical, radiographic, and morphologic differences between these two diseases have now been clearly delineated (Fig. 469; Table 17). It has also become apparent that in a certain proportion of cases (approximately 10% in our experience), features of both conditions are present and the differential diagnosis becomes impossible. The occurrence of such cases, the occasional coexistence of typical Crohn's disease of the small bowel and ulcerative colitis of the large bowel in the same patient,[36] and the occurrence of both diseases in the same family[24] indicate that perhaps the distinction between these two entities has been drawn too rigidly.[20, 33] Be that as it may, there are enough clinical and pathologic differences in the majority of the cases to justify a separation which has prognostic and therapeutic implications.[30, 31, 37]

Ulcerative colitis occurs with equal frequence in both sexes. It appears most often in patients between 20 and 40 years of

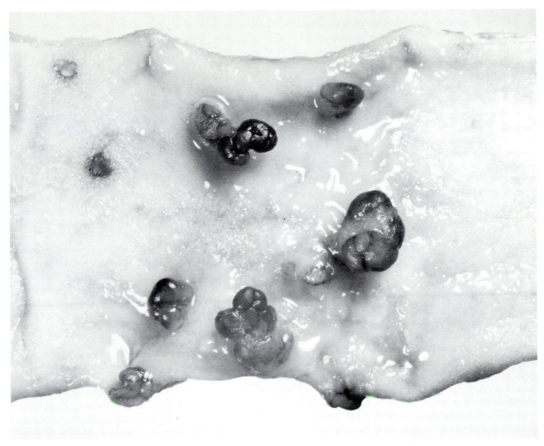

Fig. 471 Pseudopolyps associated with long-standing ulcerative colitis. These pseudopolyps do not become cancer, but they are reflection of advanced disease. (WU neg. 65-5036.)

age but may occur at any age. The etiology is unknown, but psychogenic disturbances seem to be important in many patients.[12] The gross appearance of the lesions varies with the stage of the disease.

The process is thought to begin most frequently in the rectosigmoid area, but it is possible that other areas also are affected early, since only the rectal zone is easily inspected through the sigmoidoscope. In some patients, the rectum remains the only portion of large bowel involved.[18] These patients are only rarely afflicted by the complications of the diffuse form, such as arthritis, uveitis, pyoderma gangrenosum, and cancer. In the diffuse form, any portion of the bowel can be affected. The process attacks the ileum in about one-third of the patients. This involvement is superficial, of little clinical importance, always in continuity with the colonic disease, and rarely spreads more than 10 cm from the ileocecal valve. The ileum is dilated, in striking contrast with the typical stenosis of Crohn's disease. The appendix is diseased in 20% to 60% of the cases. Anal lesions are seen in 10%. They are secondary to the diarrhea and may consist of midline dorsal fissures, skin excoriations, acute perianal and ischiorectal abscesses, and rectovaginal fistulas.[30]

Grossly, in the acute stage, the mucosal surface of the bowel is wet and glairy from blood and mucus, and petechial hemorrhages are often seen. Small and large ulcers often appear. They have an irregular

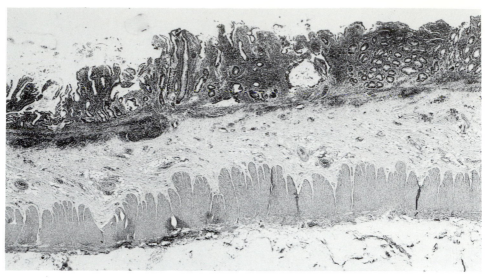

Fig. 472 Relatively quiescent area in chronic ulcerative colitis. Note that changes are restricted to mucosa and submucosa. (Low power; WU neg. 50-5411.)

outline, sometimes with a geographic configuration. Long longitudinal ulcers, especially if connected by transverse ulcers, are *not* a feature of ulcerative colitis.

Foci of residual inflamed mucosa and areas of granulation tissue, appearing as elevated nodules in an otherwise flat surface, are known as pseudopolyps (Figs. 470 and 471). They are typically small and multiple. Rarely, they can attain a large size and raise the clinical and radiographic suspicion of carinoma.[22]

In the end stages of the process, the entire bowel becomes fibrotic and is narrowed and shortened. Infrequently, cicatricial stenosis associated with an inflammatory mass may result in an erroneous clinical and radiographic diagnosis of carcinoma. We have seen extensive ulcerative colitis in a terminal and quiescent stage in which ulceration was absent, the mucosa was atrophic, and extensive submucosal fat deposition existed.

The essential lesion of ulcerative colitis is an excessive destruction of undifferentiated cells at the bases of the crypts of Lieberkühn.[27] As a result, the glands are irregular, atrophic ones alternating with others showing signs of regeneration. There is often a marked decrease in the amount

of cytoplasmic mucus present.[21] Inflammatory cells penetrate and destroy the villi and form small abscesses at their bases. With progression, these abscesses extend along the submucosa. Secondary intestinal changes occurring in ulcerative colitis start at the lumen and progress outward: mucosal regeneration, hypertrophy of the muscularis mucosae, submucosal fibrosis, fatty infiltration, muscular hypertrophy, and subserosal fibrosis.

When pus escapes in the submucosa, ulceration may develop, and mucosal bridges with underlying purulent exudate may form. Beneath the ulcers is granulation tissue containing abundant cells typical of chronic inflammation. The inflammatory process may either remain above the muscularis mucosae or involve the entire submucosa (Fig. 472).

McAuley and Sommers[28] reported an increase of mast cells in ulcerative colitis. Paneth cells are usually absent beyond the cecum. Watson and Roy,[35] however, reported their presence in the ascending transverse and descending colon of patients with ulcerative colitis. In a few patients, vascular changes involve the medium-sized submucosal arteries. Thrombosis may occur with changes identical to polyarteritis or thromboangiitis obliterans. These vascular alterations occur in about 10% of instances.

The duration of the disease may be prolonged, with many remissions and exacerbations. However, there is a high mortality in the first two years of the disease.[25] Nutritional deficiencies and anemia often accompany the disease.

Biopsy of the rectosigmoid and rectum in ulcerative colitis may yield useful information.[26] In known instances of ulcerative colitis, the biopsy may demonstrate an active process prior to clinical relapse.[34] These pathologic changes include crypt abscesses (Fig. 473) that are preceded by collections of polymorphonuclear leukocytes at the base of the crypts. Before the colectomy, a colon may be defunctionalized with an ileostomy or a colostomy. Such colons may show extreme narrowing of the lumen, atrophy of the components of the wall, and a great increase in the pericolic fat.[27] If the rectal biopsy of a patient with colitis is *microscopically* normal, the diagnosis of ulcerative colitis is extremely unlikely.[30] Some patients with ulcerative colitis have associated liver disease. This may consist of fatty infiltration, abscess, cirrhosis, cholangitis with pericholangitis, and, rarely, carcinoma of the biliary tract.[13, 29]

Frequent complications of ulcerative colitis are perforation with peritonitis and abscess, toxic megacolon, venous thrombosis (most often in the iliac vein), and cancer. After ten or more years of ulcerative colitis, carcinoma tends to develop at multiple sites in the colon (Fig. 474). Carcinoma occurred in ten of 226 patients reported by Kiefer et al.[23] Counsell and Dukes[11] emphasized the atypical gross appearance of the cancer and its rapid spread. The site of origin is almost always a flat rather than a polypoid mucosa. Morson[30] described the earliest gross change as a rather thick mucosa with a finely nodular or velvety surface configuration. (Fig. 475). Goldgraber et al.[19] emphasized the more even distribution of cancer, the mul-

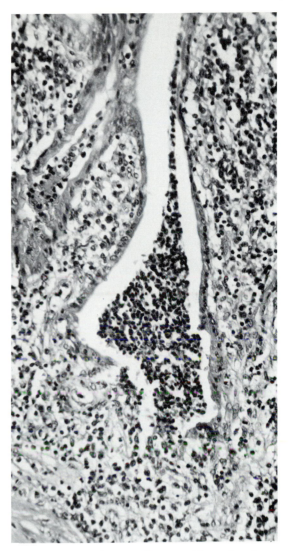

Fig. 473 Typical crypt abscess with perforation. This occurs in ulcerative colitis but is not a pathognomonic finding. (×265; WU neg. 62-8853.)

tiple foci of origin, the atypical gross appearance, and the fact that cancer occurring with ulcerative colitis tends to occur in younger persons. In sixty-three surgically treated patients with chronic ulcerative colitis, the incidence of carcinoma was 11.1%. In eleven patients who had chronic ulcerative colitis for more than ten years, five developed carcinoma. In 153 colectomy specimens reported by Dukes and Lockhart-Mummery,[15] eight demonstrated cancer.

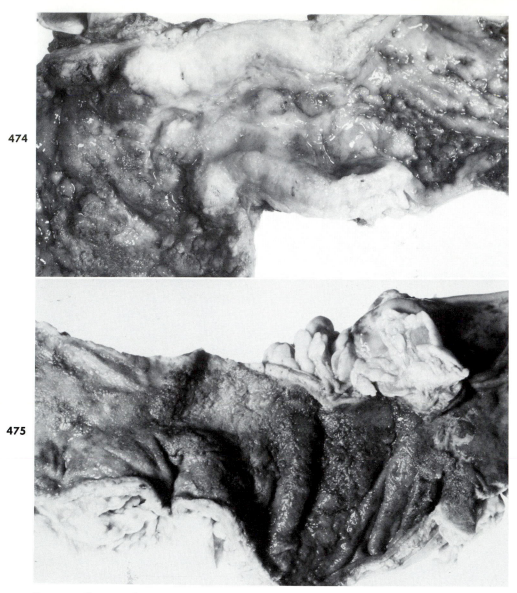

Fig. 474 Chronic ulcerative colitis with superimposed carcinoma in region of constriction. (WU neg. 66-1472.)
Fig. 475 Chronic ulcerative colitis with superimposed carcinoma. Area containing tumor is in center and appears as ill-defined thickened area of velvety appearance. Lesion was not detected radiographically. (WU neg. 64-10208.)

The risk of development of cancer in children with chronic ulcerative colitis appears to be a serious one. In the series of 396 children reported by Devroede at al.,[14] cancer developed in 3% by ten years, in 23% by twenty years, and in 43% by thirty-five years after the onset of ulcerative colitis. The risk of cancer developing in association with ulcerative colitis is higher when the first attack of colitis is severe, when the entire colon is involved, when the illness is continuous and unremitting, and when the disease begins in childhood.[16, 17]

Morson and Pang[32] described the presence of precancerous changes in the rec-

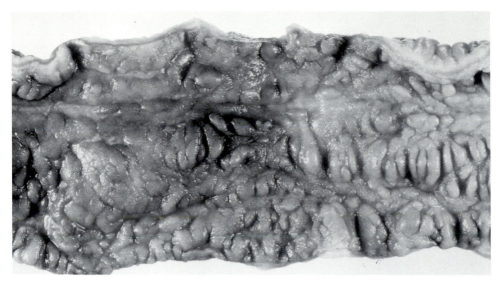

Fig. 476 Crohn's disease of large bowel. Extensive longitudinal ulcers joined by transverse ulcers separate edematous mucosa in patches, resulting in typical "cobblestone" appearance. (WU neg. 70-3574.)

tal mucosa of patients with ulcerative colitis harboring an invasive carcinoma elsewhere in the colon. Although this finding is of interest and can be of great help in an individual case, it is our opinion that a careful evaluation of the clinical features described previously remains the safest method for the assessment of cancer risk in this population.

Crohn's disease (granulomatous colitis)

Approximately 34% of all cases of Crohn's disease occur in the large bowel. In one-half of these, the ileum also is involved. Grossly, the segmental distribution of the lesions (with "skip" areas which can be demonstrated radiographically) and the preference for the right side of the colon are two important diagnostic features.[41] Other gross findings of significance include stricture formation, fissuring, cobblestone appearance, and transmural involvement (Fig. 476). Anal lesions are seen in 75% of the cases and may present as chronic fissures, fistulas, and ulceration. They can be the first clinical manifestation of Crohn's disease and are recognized microscopically by the presence of granulomas.[39] The microscopy of Crohn's

disease in the large bowel is not significantly different from that seen in the small bowel. Fissures, noncaseating granulomas (present in 60% of the cases), and transmural involvement are typical. The mucosa has a relatively normal appearance and retains a significant amount of mucus, even in areas immediately adjacent to ulcerations. Fistulas arising on the basis of fissuring are common. Although perianal fistulas can be seen in both Crohn's disease and ulcerative colitis, internal fistulas are virtually pathognomonic of the former. Complications of Crohn's disease include skin ulceration (of perianal skin, around colostomies and ileostomies, and elsewhere) and toxic megacolon. Jones[40] found eleven reported cases of colonic cancer associated with Crohn's disease and added four of his own. In contrast to ulcerative colitis, the risk of cancer in Crohn's disease is so small that it should not influence the management of this condition.[38]

Ischemic colitis

A rare disease, ischemic colitis has been confused in the past with Crohn's disease and ulcerative colitis. It is usually seen in

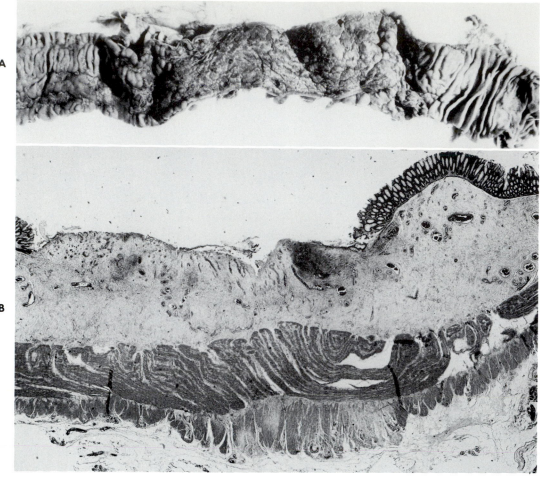

Fig. 477 Ischemic colitis involving portion of left colon in 70-year-old woman. **A,** Gross appearance of lesion. Note segmental nature and sharply circumscribed margins. **B,** Panoramic view of lesion, showing ulceration and marked vascularity of submucosa. (**B,** ×10; WU neg. 72-9821; **A** and **B,** courtesy Dr. B. Morson, London, England.)

patients past 50 years of age and is characterized by sudden onset of bleeding and abdominal pain. It is a segmental disease, the splenic flexure being the classical site of involvement, due to its relative paucity of blood supply. The rectum is almost never involved. Morson[43] has described three morphologic variants: infarct, transient ischemia, and ischemic stricture. The latter is more likely to be seen as a surgical specimen (Fig. 477). Microscopically, there is ulceration covered by granulation tissue, which extends into the submucosa and surrounds individual smooth muscle fibers of the muscularis mucosae.

Hemosiderin is abundant. Hyaline thrombi can be seen in the lumen of small vessels. Fissures, lymphoid follicles, and granulomas are absent.

Ischemic colitis occurs in patients with arteriosclerosis, diabetes, after vascular surgery, in association with collagen diseases (i.e., scleroderma and rheumatoid arthritis), and as a complication of birth control pills.[42]

Hirschsprung's disease (idiopathic megacolon)

The symptoms and signs of Hirschsprung's disease usually begin shortly after

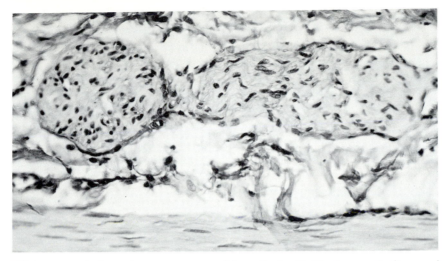

Fig. 478 Intramural plexus in narrow segment in patient with Hirschsprung's disease showing absence of ganglion cells. (×360; WU neg. 51-188.)

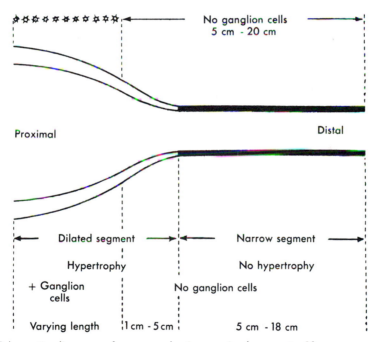

No ganglion cells
5 cm - 20 cm

Proximal

Distal

Dilated segment

Narrow segment

Hypertrophy

No hypertrophy

+ Ganglion
cells

No ganglion cells

Varying length   1 cm - 5 cm   5 cm - 18 cm

Fig. 479 Schematic diagram of gross and microscopic changes in fifteen cases of Hirschsprung's disease. (WU neg. 51-361; from Bodian, M., Stephens, F. D., and Ward, B. C. H.: Hirschsprung's disease and idiopathic megacolon, Lancet **1:**6-11, 1949.)

birth with gaseous distention and even acute intestinal obstruction. In the chronic form, the large bowel is hypertrophied and dilated proximal to an apparently normal colonic segment usually in the sigmoid.

The pathogenesis of this disorder is related to the lack of parasympathetic ganglion cells in the intramural and submucosal plexuses of the distal segment of the colon[48] (Fig. 478). Hypertrophied, disorganized nonmyelinated nerve fibers are seen instead in this location. The ganglion cells also are absent from a segment of the adjoining dilated colon[45] (Fig. 479). The distance in the proximal dilated segment in which ganglion cells are absent is variable. Complete absence from the entire proximal segment of the colon has been reported.[52] In such instances, the infant or young child may present with the clinical picture of partial or complete intestinal obstruction. When no mechanical obstruction is found at operation and there is no apparent cause for paralytic ileus, the cecum should be biopsied and examined by frozen section. If ganglion cells are absent, temporary ileostomy may be lifesaving if the small intestine is not also aganglionic.[46] Walker et al.[49] reported four cases of aganglionosis of the entire colon and portions of the small bowel. The infants presented with symptoms of intestinal obstruction without evidence of megacolon.

Frozen section is a practical method of determining the absence of ganglion cells and should be used to determine the level of transection of the bowel at operation. This procedure is facilitated if the surgeon gives the pathologist a rectangular piece of the entire muscular wall, so that the tissue can be properly oriented. In order that frozen section be reliable, the piece examined should be at least 4 cm long, and multiple serial sections should be taken.

We have checked the terminal rectum in patients without megacolon, and ganglion cells have always been observed. Since ganglion cells are normally scanty near the internal anal sphincter, biopsies should be taken at a point 2 cm above the anal valves in infants and 3 cm in older children.[44, 50] There may be instances in which biopsy of the rectum should be done in order to establish the diagnosis.[47] If so, it should be deep and adequate. In most instances, however, the clinical signs and the radiographic findings should be sufficient to make a presumptive diagnosis of megacolon.

The myenteric plexus is absent in the most distal part of the colon in all patients with congenital megacolon.[51] Bodian et al.[45] stated that there is lack of parasympathetic function and coordinated propulsive movement of the distal segment. Operative treatment for intractable megacolon is resection of the segment of the colon in which ganglion cells are absent with preservation of the sphincter and establishment of the upper colonic–anal anastomosis.

Plexiform neurofibromatosis may be associated with megacolon.

Tuberculosis

Most patients with secondary ulcerating tuberculosis of the colon do not require surgical therapy. Infrequently, stenosing lesions, particularly in the region of the cecum, accompany minimal pulmonary tuberculosis.[53] Grossly, the process involves the ileocecal area. There is ulceration with diffuse fibrosis extending through the wall, causing contraction and obstruction[55] (Fig. 480). A mass can be felt in approximately 50% of the cases.[54] Microscopically, the changes show typical tubercles and extensive desmoplasia. Demonstration of acid-fast bacilli, either by stain of the sections or culture, is needed in order to establish the diagnosis of tuberculosis. It should be remembered that the large majority of cases of granulomatous disease of the ileocecal area seen in the United States and in Engand represent examples of Crohn's disease.[56] Surgical resection is usually curative, although flare-up of the pulmonary lesion may take place.

Cytology

Raskin and Pleticka[57] have perfected the technique of colonic cytology. In eighty-seven patients with carcinoma, the disease was correctly identified in seventy (80.5%). In 438 patients with no tumor, there were apparently two false positives (0.45%). However, the technique employed to obtain the specimen, which involves extensive cleansing of the colon followed by a diagnostic enema with manipulation of the patient, has led to an unenthusiastic response from clinicians.

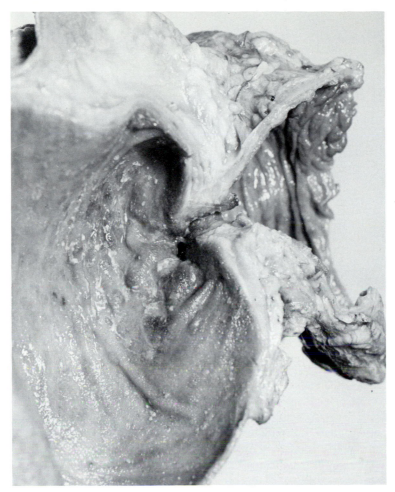

Fig. 480 Constricting tuberculous lesion at ileocecal valve occurring in young man. There was almost complete intestinal obstruction. Note extreme dilatation of small bowel on left with areas of tuberculous ulceration. After resection, patient completely recovered. (WU neg. 52-3256.)

Generally speaking, exfoliative cytology is of little practical value in the diagnosis of cancer of the large bowel.

Biopsy

A positive biopsy should be obtained before radical surgery for carcinoma of the rectum and rectosigmoid area is undertaken. It is imperative that sufficient representative material be taken. Small wisps of tissue are not adequate.

Although the gross pattern of a carcinoma is usually characteristic, inflammatory lesions can simulate cancer, and, conversely, innocent-appearing small le-

sions may prove to be undifferentiated carcinomas. Poorly differentiated malignant tumors usually are diagnosed easily, although only a few small islands of tumor cells may be present in the signet ring type of carcinoma.

It may be difficult to make a definite diagnosis of carcinoma in a well-differentiated tumor without evidence of invasion. Similarly, *endometriosis* may be called carcinoma erroneously unless the characteristic stroma is recognized (Fig. 511). Tissue from the edge of an ulcerative carcinoma may contain only hyperplastic colonic epithelium. Lymphoid polyp and

481

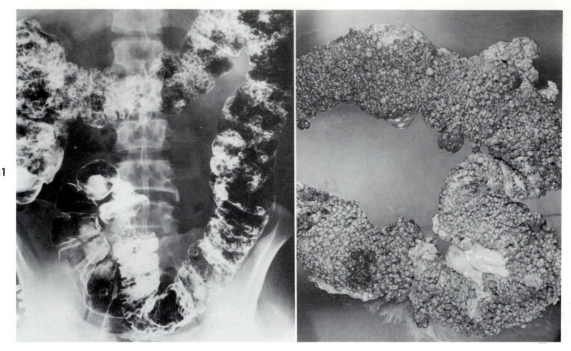

Fig. 481 Familial polyposis of entire bowel. (WU neg. 49-1718.)
Fig. 482 Extensive polyposis. There were four separate carcinomas present, but fortunately all 265 regional lymph nodes were negative. (WU neg. 49-6546.)

malignant lymphoma may be difficult to differentiate. Gafni and Sohar[60] demonstrated that rectal biopsy in amyloidosis is frequently positive. A definitive diagnosis was possible in twenty-six of thirty patients. These results are comparable to those obtained by renal biopsy and better than those from liver biopsy. It is important for the biopsy to include the submucosa, for this can be the only place of amyloid deposition.[62] An increased use of rectal biopsy for the diagnosis of storage diseases of the nervous system has been made in recent years in view of the fact that lesions similar to those in the brain may be seen in the ganglion cells of the myenteric plexus.[58, 61]

The cooperation of a surgeon skilled in taking tissue and the cooperation of an experienced pathologist make the biopsy diagnosis of lesions of the colon almost 100% accurate.[59] Lesions below the peritoneal reflection should be removed in toto where possible to facilitate their orienta-tion for section by the pathologist. Large villous adenomas should be biopsied from indurated areas because cancer may exist within them.

Tumors
Epithelial polyps

The colonic and rectal polyps included in this discussion are those of epithelial origin, which represent the large majority. They can be divided in five rather distinct categories, acknowledging the existence of occasional transitional forms.[65]

Adenomatous polyps are distributed throughout the large bowel, with 40% found in the right colon, 40% in the left colon, and 20% in the rectum.[63, 69] They may be sessile or pedunculated, may have a short or a long stalk, attached by a rather narrow base, and may be multiple or single. Knoblike projections are frequently seen on the surface. Microscopically, there is an increase in the number of glands and cells per unit area as compared to the normal

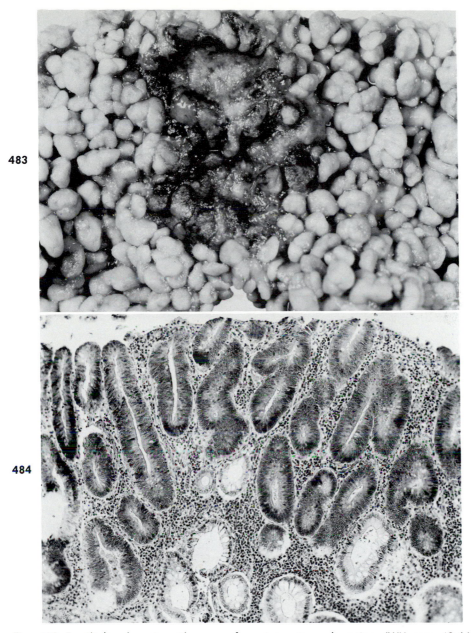

Fig. 483 Familial polyposis with area of carcinomatous ulceration. (WU neg. 49-6638.)
Fig. 484 Minimal alterations in surface glands of polyp in patient with familial polyposis. (×135; WU neg. 52-2481.)

mucosa. The cells are crowded, contain enlarged hyperchromatic nuclei, and have an increased number of mitoses.[75] Mucin production is usually scanty. The basement membrane is not thickened. The changes first affect the superficial portion of the

glands,[84] a fact substantiated by in vivo incorporation of tritiated thymidine.[67]

Focal areas of villous configuration are not infrequent in adenomatous polyps. Fung and Goldman[70] found them in 35% of 67 polyps by careful examination of multi-

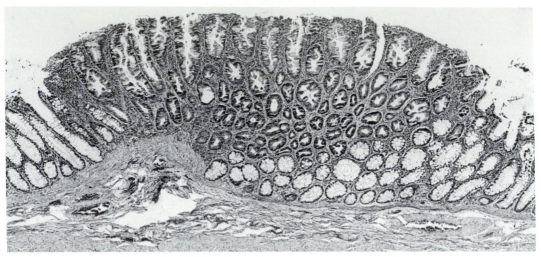

Fig. 485 Hyperplastic polyp of large bowel. Note maturation toward surface and serrated configuration of glands. (×33; WU neg. 72-1306.)

ple sections under a dissecting microscope. The incidence appeared to be related to the size of the polyp, reaching 75% in lesions larger than 1 cm. in diameter. The significance of this change has not been established, but it is our impression that the natural history of polyps with a mixed pattern approaches that of pure adenomatous polyps.

Familial polyposis of the large bowel is one entity that must be segregated from other polyps, despite the fact that the microscopic appearance of the individual lesions is indistinguishable from that of solitary adenomatous polyps. This inherited defect is an autosomal mendelian dominant characteristic with a high degree of penetrance.[83] The tumors in familial polyposis become manifest much earlier than the usual adenomatous polyp, usually in the second decade of life. Carcinomatous change in this lesion occurs some twenty years earlier than other cases of cancer, usually in the early thirties. Whether the cancer arises on the basis of a preexisting polyp or from the intervening normal mucosa is still a debated issue.

Grossly, the bowel is studded with polyps ranging anywhere from very slight elevations of the normal mucosa to large polypoid tumors. Malignant change is sug-

gested by fixation or ulceration of the surface (Figs. 481 to 484).

In rare instances, familial polyposis can involve the entire gastrointestinal tract.[86] Before considering this diagnosis in a given case, it should be remembered that most polypoid lesions of the ileum seen in patients with familial colonic polyposis represent foci of lymphoid hyperplasia.[76, 83] *Gardner's syndrome* is a familial condition in which adenomatous polyps of the large bowel are seen associated with multiple osteomas of the skull and mandible, multiple keratinous cysts of the skin, and soft tissue neoplasms, especially fibromatosis.[71] Carcinoma of the periampullary region has been described in twelve cases of this syndrome.[79]

Hyperplastic (metaplastic) polyps have only recently gained widespread acceptance as a specific type.[78] In the past, they have been misdiagnosed as either normal mucosa or adenomatous polyps. They are characteristically of very small size, rarely exceeding 5 mm in diameter. If a careful gross examination of the colonic mucosa is made, hyperplastic polyps will be found in 30% to 50% of the cases.[66] Their microscopic appearance is distinctive (Fig. 485). Elongated glands with papillary infoldings are seen, resulting in a sawtooth

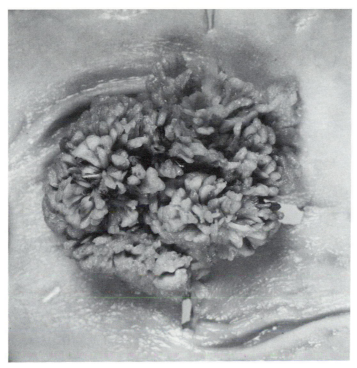

Fig. 486 Large villous adenoma of sigmoid colon. Note broad base of attachment and innumerable thin papillary projections. (WU neg. 65-874.)

configuration of the lumen. The mitotic activity is increased only at the base. Elsewhere, the epithelial cells have an inconspicuous basal nucleus and abundant cytoplasm filled with mucin. The basement membrane beneath the surface epithelium is thickened, a change that can be easily appreciated on hematoxylin-eosin–stained sections. These polyps do not become malignant.

Villous (papillary) adenoma is a distinctive, relatively infrequent type of polyp that usually is single and occurs in the rectum or rectosigmoid of older patients.[68] It eventually forms a large superficial neoplasm that may encircle the bowel. The consistency is so soft that the tumor can be missed completely on digital examination.[80] It has papillary villous projections and is usually attached by a wide base (Fig. 486). Villous adenomas are very rarely pedunculated. Therefore, if a biopsy of a polypoid lesion having a definite stalk shows villous areas, the most likely diagno-

sis is that of adenomatous polyp with focal villous change. Microscopically, these villous projections ramify through a long, papillary, crownlike growth (Fig. 487). In time, a high percentage of these lesions become malignant (Fig. 488). The recorded incidence has ranged from 35% to 70%.[64, 87]

Retention polyp is the most frequent colonic polyp seen in children, but it also may occur in adults. In the 158 patients reported by Roth and Helwig,[81] fifty-nine were over the age of 17 years. The polyp is usually single and located in the sigmoid colon or rectum.[73, 74]

Grossly, the retention polyp may be superficially ulcerated and on cross section has a cystic, latticelike appearance (Fig. 489). Microscopically, it shows inflammatory changes on the surface and mucus-containing cysts (Fig. 490). This type of polyp does not become malignant. These polyps may be sloughed and pass from the colon. It is unlikely that these lesions

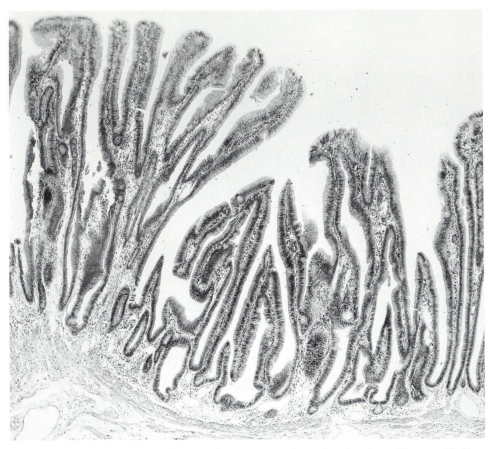

Fig. 487 Pattern of villous adenoma demonstrating long fronds of papillary epithelium springing directly from mucosal surface. (WU neg. 52-2858.)

are true neoplasms.[77] Rarely, multiple retention polyps are seen throughout the bowel. This condition can be life-threatening.[72, 85] It is closely related to the *Cronkhite-Canada syndrome* (multiple polyposis associated with ectodermal changes, such as alopecia, nail atrophy, and hyperpigmentation). Ruymann[82] has pointed out that the morphologic appearance of the lesions found in the latter condition is that of retention polyps. This was the case in the single patient with this condition that we have examined.

Peutz-Jeghers polyps have similar microscopic features to those seen in the small bowel. Lack of atypia, disorganization of glands, occurrence of several cell types (including Paneth cells), and the presence of smooth muscle fibers from the muscu-

laris mucosae are the most important features.

Treatment

There is no difficulty in the treatment of the retention polyps in children. Simple removal is sufficient. On the other hand, all untreated patients with familial polyposis eventually develop carcinoma of the colon. Therefore, even though the patient is young, total colectomy is indicated.[90]

The treatment of solitary polypoid lesions is influenced by their size and location (Figs. 491 to 494). Polyps below the peritoneal reflection can be removed through the proctoscope. If the stalk is free from cancer, the patient is cured. If a polypoid cancer or a polyp with a focal area of cancer within it does not show invasion

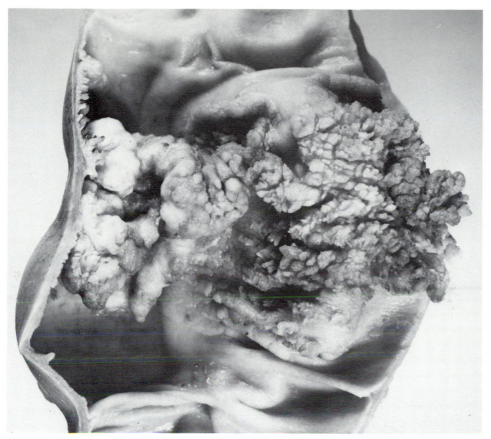

Fig. 488 Villous adenoma with large area of invasive carcinoma. Note difference between thin, delicate, papillary appearance of villous tumor (right) and solid, nodular configuration of malignant component (left). Regional lymph node metastases were present. (WU neg. 66-10290.)

of its stalk and lies above the muscularis mucosae, then metastases to regional lymph nodes practically never take place. Under extremely rare circumstances (two cases in our experience), such an event has occurred. In one instance, a polypoid cancer on a stalk beyond the peritoneal reflection was resected with a segment of bowel, and a portion of one lymph node was involved[88] (Fig. 495). Because this finding is rare, the general approach to therapy of polypoid lesions of the colon should not be altered.

If the polypoid lesion is located above the peritoneal reflection, the best treatment is resection of the segment of bowel (Fig. 496). The larger such lesions, the greater the likelihood that they are cancer.

Lesions greater than 3 cm in diameter are nearly always cancer.[89] The introduction of the flexible fiberoptic colonoscope may radically change the approach to the management of polypoid lesions of the large bowel. With this instrument, an experienced operator can remove in one piece, with minimum morbidity, polyps situated as proximally as the cecum.[91, 92] This technique avoids the periodic radiographic examinations needed if the polyp is left in situ and the laparotomy formerly required to excise it.

Villous adenomas should be removed in toto, preferably in one piece. This allows a proper orientation of the specimen, so that in the presence of focal carcinoma, the extent of the tumor can be assessed.

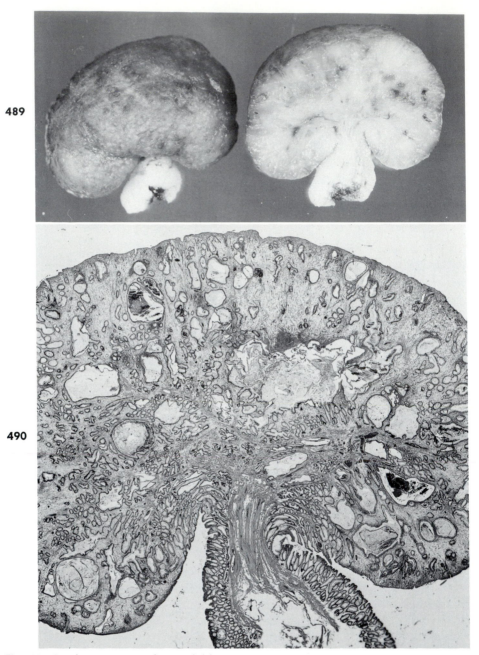

Fig. 489 Single retention polyp in child. Note cystic spaces. (WU neg. 50-6790.)
Fig. 490 Same polyp shown in Fig. 489 with overproduction of mucus and surface ulceration. This type of polyp does not become malignant. (Low power; WU neg. 51-144.)

This determination is of great importance in the decision as to whether further surgery is indicated.

Carcinoma

Data proving that carcinomas of the colon arise in preexisting adenomatous polyps do not as yet exist.[94] There is an abrupt change between the cancer and the adjacent colonic epithelium without evidence of transition. We subserially sectioned twenty-two colonic carcinomas 2 cm or less in diameter and found no evidence of preexisting adenomatous polyp.[111]

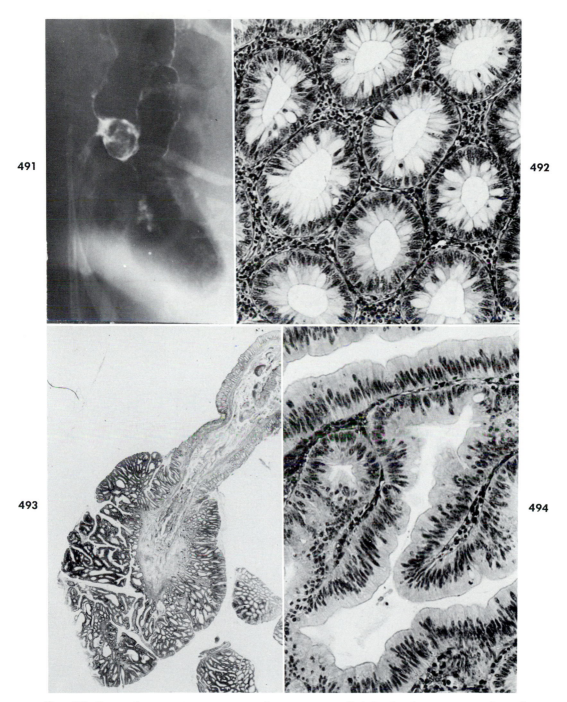

491

492

493

494

Fig. 491 Evacuation roentgenogram to demonstrate well-defined adenomatous polyp of splenic flexure. (WU neg. 48-6677.)

Fig. 492 Cross section of normal glands in polyp shown in Fig. 491 with some mitotic activity. (×150; WU neg. 48-6700.)

Fig. 493 Adenomatous polyp shown in Fig. 491 demonstrating well-defined pedicle. There is no evidence of infiltration of pedicle by carcinoma. (Low power; WU neg. 48-6703.)

Fig. 494 This section demonstrates deviation from normal glands shown in Fig. 492 with stratification of nuclei and beginning loss of nuclear polarity. (×150; WU neg. 48-6701.)

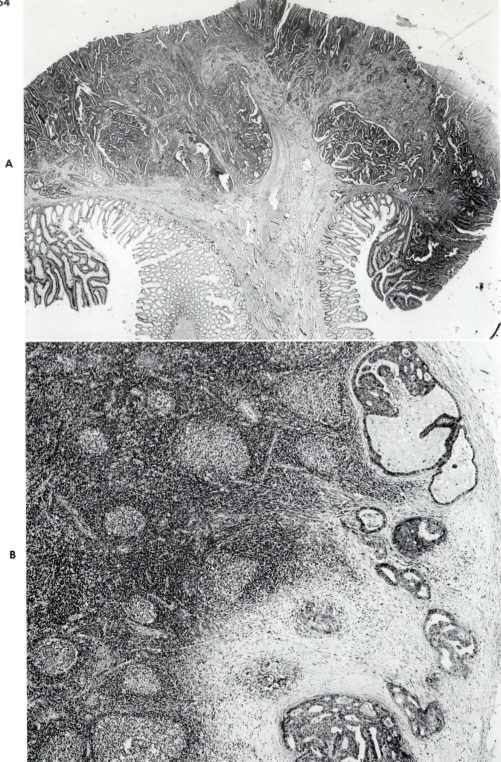

Fig. 495 Polypoid well-delimited cancer on stalk. There is no tumor in stalk, yet regional lymph node in immediate vicinity of stalk showed partial replacement by tumor. This is exceptionally rare occurrence. (**A,** WU neg. 64-335; **B,** WU neg. 64-338; **A** and **B,** courtesy Dr. F. T. Kraus, St. Louis, Mo.)

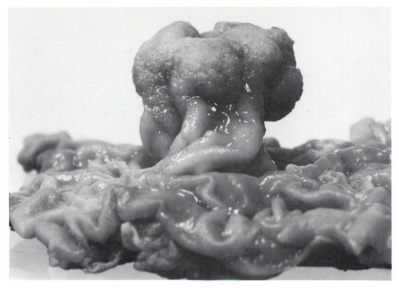

Fig. 496 Segmental resection of colon showing adenomatous polyp 2 cm in diameter. (WU neg. 60-2498.)

The distributions of polyps and carcinomas in the colon differ. Hultborn[107] found that only 20% of colonic polyps occur in the rectum, whereas 50% of colonic carcinomas are situated there. Furthermore, the incidence of carcinoma of the colon appears to be the same among patients with polyps as it is among those without polyps. We believe that a high percentage of all colonic carcinomas rise de novo in normal mucosa. They may be infiltrating or polypoid. If they are polypoid, then tissue sections will show obvious carcinoma at all levels (Fig. 497). If the cancer has not invaded the muscular wall of the colon, the incidence of lymph node metastases is low.

If a polypoid lesion has a focal area of cancer in its tip, removal of the polypoid mass is curative. Practically all benign adenomatous polyps show some degree of atypia, and in the past many pathologists used phrases such as "stratification of nuclei," "questionable carcinoma in situ," and "possible cancer." Many patients have had extensive operations because of such equivocation. The diagnosis of carcinoma of the colon is usually easy, and borderline epithelial alterations are unrelated to it.

The classification of carcinoma of the large bowel has little practical significance except for a few rare variants that have gross distinctions and a divergent clinical course and prognosis.

The usual *adenocarcinoma* of the large bowel is a bulky tumor with well-defined, rolled margins about an area of central ulceration. There is a sharp dividing line between the carcinoma and the normal bowel wall. In rare instances, intramural spread may be seen.[93] When these tumors are sectioned, grayish white tissue replaces the bowel wall. In some, this replacement is well demarcated. In others, fingers of tumor extend from the main mass. The pathologist should determine whether the tumor is confined to the wall or whether it has extended to the pericolic tissues. Large veins should be examined, for gross vein invasion may be seen rarely.[99] If the tumor secretes a large amount of mucin, it has a mucoid, glairy appearance, and lakes of mucin may separate the layers of bowel wall.

There is a rare type of carcinoma that is similar to the linitis plastica variant observed in the stomach.[108] This lesion exhibits poorly defined margins and a peb-

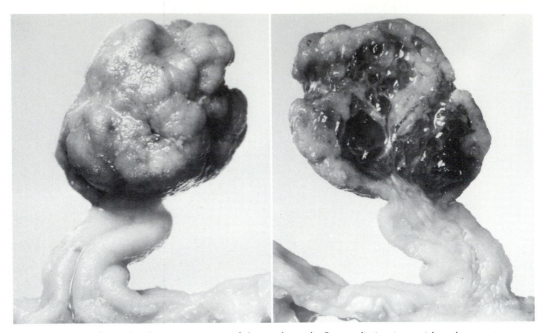

Fig. 497 Polypoid adenocarcinoma of large bowel. Gross distinction with adenomatous polyp is impossible. (WU negs. 69-6849 and 69-6850.)

bly mucosal surface that often is only superficially ulcerated (Figs. 498 to 500).

Dukes[97, 100] proposed a staging system for rectal carcinomas which can also be applied to cancers of the colon. It is widely used because of its direct relationship with prognosis. Stage A tumors involve the wall of the bowel only, Stage B tumors extend through the wall, and Stage C tumors have lymph node metastases. The five-year survival rates are 90%, 65%, and 20%, respectively. Among Stage A tumors, those limited to the mucosa and submucosa have a better prognosis than those that have penetrated the muscularis externa. Among Stage C neoplasms, the prognosis is worse for the tumors that, in addition to having nodal metastases, have extended beyond the wall.

Examination of specimen

The method of examination of large bowel specimens as proposed by Dukes[99] is probably the best. He fixes the specimen, makes a diagram to scale, and plots the distribution of the lymph nodes, putting them in separate bottles. Clearing the specimen is also accurate, producing an average of at least fifty lymph nodes,[96, 106] but we have found that such a time-consuming procedure is not practical.

Our modified method consists of opening the specimen, pinning it on corkboard, and placing it in formalin. After fixation, at least three or four sections are cut from the primary tumor. These sections extend through the entire thickness of the wall. The large veins are carefully examined. If there is any suggestion of tumor within them, sections are made. The nodes are dissected from the mesentery and divided into groups, each group being placed in a separate bottle. The nodes below the tumor are also isolated. These are obviously important nodes, for if tumor is found within them the prognosis is probably hopeless inasmuch as retrograde involvement means blockage of lymphatics at and above the level of the tumor. Likewise, the lymph nodes at the high point of the dissection where the vessels are ligated are also examined separately, for if tumor is found, it means the disease has spread beyond the resection. Lymph nodes are

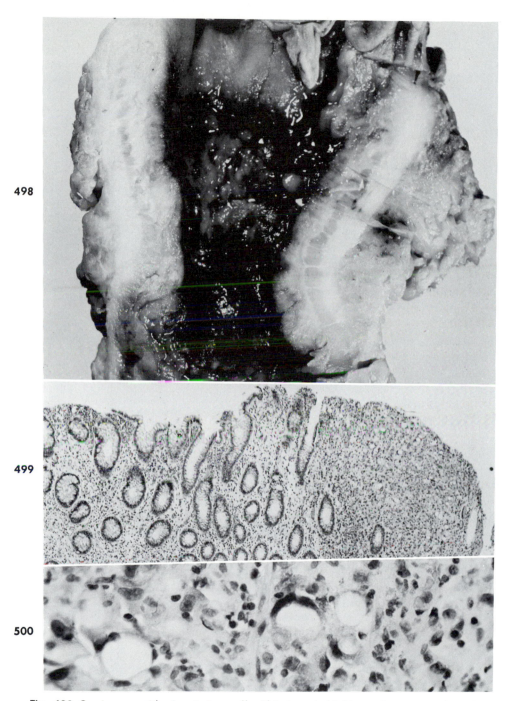

498

499

500

Fig. 498 Carcinoma with signet ring cells. This type is highly malignant, narrows lumen, and has pebbly mucosal surface and thickened muscular wall. (WU neg. 51-4682.)
Fig. 499 Biopsy of carcinoma illustrated in Fig. 498 showing small area effacing glands. (Low power; WU neg. 51-5362.)
Fig. 500 Area of biopsy illustrated in Fig. 499 showing signet ring tumor cells. There were many lymph nodes involved in surgical specimen.

also removed from the region of the tumor and from the area between the tumor and the high point of the dissection. Sections are taken from other polyps or lesions noted in the bowel. At times, each end of the specimen can be ligated after distending the bowel to about its normal lumen with 10% formalin. This serves to preserve the gross changes in the bowel in the same pattern as shown by roentgenogram. This method is often helpful in demonstrating lesions other than carcinoma.

Microscopic description

The usual carcinoma of the large bowel is a well-differentiated adenocarcinoma secreting variable amounts of mucin. In a few instances, there may be extremely large lakes of mucin with scattered collections of tumor cells. The rare variant of the so-called linitis plastica type of carcinoma shows retention of the mucin for the most part within and compressing the tumor cells, giving the nuclei a signet ring effect. In a few instances, areas of squamous change may be present. We have seen such alterations both in the cecum and in the lower rectum.

It is important that stains be used for the main sections of the tumor which will demonstrate the presence or absence of vein invasion. We use the Verhoeff–van Gieson, which stains smooth muscle yellow and brings out clearly the black elastic tissue. If vein invasion is demonstrated, the prognosis is extremely unfavorable. Also of prognostic importance is the presence or absence of perineurial invasion by the tumor and whether microscopic examination shows the tumor confined to the bowel wall or extending into the pericolic fat. If there is tumor present in the lymph nodes, it is wise to examine the tissue in the immediate vicinity of nodes, for tumor frequently extends beyond the lymph node capsule to invade surrounding veins. Rarely, bone formation occurs in slowly growing carcinomas of the rectum.[98]

We have seen several instances of local recurrence of colonic carcinoma at the suture line. Tumor has been apparently implanted on the raw surface at the time of operation. This was well shown in one case because tumor was present at the suture line, there was suture material intimately associated with the cancer, and no involved lymph nodes were present. Methods of avoiding this complication have been described by Goligher et al.[105] and Cole et al.[95]

Prognosis as related to pathologic findings

The prognosis in carcinoma of the large bowel is closely related to the pathologic findings (Table 18). About 75% of all

Table 18 Prognosis in carcinoma of large bowel based on pathologic findings

Excellent	Carcinoma in a polyp without invasion of stalk Carcinoma in villous adenoma limited to mucosa and submucosa Carcinoma limited to mucosa and submucosa (Only under exceptional circumstances do metastases develop in any of foregoing groups)
Good	Carcinoma limited to wall of bowel without lymph node metastases
Fair	Carcinoma with lymph node metastases limited to immediate area of tumor
Poor to hopeless	Signet ring mucin-secreting carcinoma Extensive lymph node metastases Gross or microscopic evidence of vein invasion Microscopic evidence of perineurial invasion Retrograde lymph node metastases (hopeless)

Poor differentiation parallels invasiveness (see Table 19) and thereby metastases
Exceedingly large carcinomas may have favorable outlook
Carcinomas located in rectosigmoid area have worse outlook than carcinomas located in right colon
Conservative surgical procedures prejudice cure
Cure by radical surgery is still possible in presence of fixation to other organs
Vein invasion usually does not occur until tumor has invaded wall of bowel

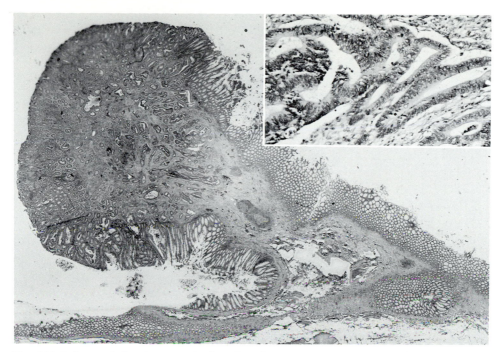

Fig. 501 Polyp with focal cancer. Stalk is free from involvement and therefore prognosis is excellent. **Inset** shows area of carcinoma. (WU neg. 58-233.)

carcinomas occur within or distal to the sigmoid colon. However, under the best circumstances, the cure rate is still relatively low. For instance, in 1,026 patients reported by Glenn and McSherry,[103] 92% were considered operable but in only 65% was a curative operation attempted. The five-year survival rate for this group of patients was 40.5%, which, in reality, was only 26% of the total group, or about one in four.

These dismal figures cannot improve further unless cancer is found at an earlier stage of its development. We believe that the only way to do this is to do appropriately timed proctoscopic examinations of both men and women over 40 years of age. Routine barium enemas are too expensive and not entirely without risk. Barium enemas (preferably air contrast) are well indicated in any patient with symptoms. Proctoscopic examinations should detect 75% of the cases. The discovery by Gold et al.[104] of a circulating antigen in patients with colonic carcinoma is a promising new approach to the diagnosis and management

of these tumors. The antigen, known as carcinoembryonic antigen or CEA, has been detected in 72% to 97% of patients with colonic cancer.[113, 114] It disappears after resection of the tumor and reappears in the event of recurrence or metastases. Its presence also has been described in carcinomas of stomach, pancreas, breast, and prostate gland. It is practically never found in normal individuals, although patients with chronic liver or renal disease may have it in small amounts.[114]

In the United States, at present, carcinoma of the large bowel is by far the commonest and most curable tumor of the gastrointestinal tract. The prognosis is excellent if focal microscopic cancer is discovered incidentally in a polyp (Fig. 501). The prognosis also correlates very well with Dukes' classification.[97] In his Stage A, with the tumor confined to the mucosa and submucosa, the prognosis is excellent. With invasion of the wall the prognosis becomes less favorable, and with involvement of the lymph nodes the five-year survival rate drops sharp-

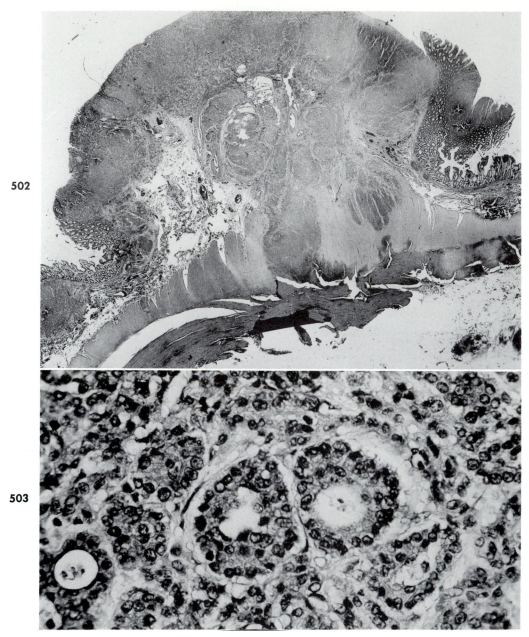

Fig. 502 Small carcinoma of rectum found on routine rectal examination. There were metastases to many nodes, with blood vessel and nerve sheath invasion. (Low power; WU neg. 51-145.)

Fig. 503 Same lesion shown in Fig. 502 demonstrating poorly differentiated adenocarcinoma. (×435; WU neg. 51-151.)

ly. We have seen *small*, highly undifferentiated carcinomas metastasize widely (Figs. 502 and 503). Conversely, we have seen circumferential carcinomas that were superficial, well differentiated, and without metastases. With vein invasion, the five-year survival is no more than 15%. Perineurial invasion is also a sign of advanced disease and usually is accompanied by other ominous pathologic findings.

Table 19 Relationship of histologic grades to incidence of lymphatic metastases (1,807 cases)*

Grade of tumor	Total cases	Cases with metastases	% with metastases
Low	109	35	18.4
Average	1,162	515	44.3
High	455	356	78.2

*From Dukes, C. E.: The surgical pathology of rectal cancer, J. Clin. Pathol. 2:95-98, 1949.

Table 20 Influence of lymphatic spread on five-year survival rate after excision of rectum*†

	Operation survivals	Alive at five years	% of five-year survivals
Without lymphatic metastases (A and B)	357	243	68.1
With lymphatic metastases (C)	359	94	26.2

*From Dukes, C. E.: The surgical pathology of rectal cancer, J. Clin. Pathol. 2:95-98, 1949.
†Based on all cases operated on at St. Mark's Hospital, 1928 to 1941, inclusive.

In groups of cases, the higher the grade, the worse the prognosis[101, 102] (Table 19).

The location and extent of lymph node involvement are also significant. Cures are possible when only those nodes in the immediate vicinity of the tumor are involved. The greater the number of lymph nodes involved, the worse the prognosis (Table 20).

In Spratt and Spjut's study,[112] if more than six lymph nodes contained metastatic cancer, less than 10% of the patients survived more than five years. If more than sixteen mesenteric lymph nodes contained cancer, all patients died within the five-year period. The former extent of involvement was not observed in cancers less than 2 cm in greatest diameter, and the latter extent of involvement was not observed in cancers less than 3 cm in diameter. Within these parameters, there was correlation between degree of lymph node involvement and size of the tumor.

If there is involvement of the lymph nodes in a retrograde fashion or if the tumor extends to the high point of the dissection, cure is practically never attained. Retrograde intramural spread of rectal cancer is fortunately rare. Quer et al.[109] studied eighty-nine specimens and found retrograde spread in only three.

The microscopic pattern of the tumor may show infiltrating or pushing margins. With pushing margins, there may be an inflammatory infiltrate at the interface between the tumor and the neighboring tissue. This infiltrate is often made up of plasma cells and lymphocytes and is associated with degenerative changes within the tumor. This change may be associated with huge tumors without metastases and indicates a good prognosis[112] (Fig. 504).

There is also some correlation between the location of the tumor within the bowel and prognosis. Carcinomas of the cecum tend to be less invasive and have a lower percentage of lymph node metastases. The carcinomas of the rectum and rectosigmoid area more quickly infiltrate the wall and metastasize more frequently. The type of operation also influences the outcome. An extensive resection of the tumor may cure certain persons who would die of cancer after less radical operations.

Adequate surgery for cancer of the large bowel varies with its location. If cancer is located below the peritoneal reflection, abdominoperineal resection is preferable to resections preserving the anus. For carcinoma in the cecal area, ileocolectomy is the operation of choice. When carcinomas are located in other portions of the bowel, the operations must be of sufficient scope to obtain the potentially involved regional lymph nodes.

Clinicopathologic correlation

Benign tumors may cause changes in bowel habits and, occasionally, gross or microscopic bleeding. Pedunculated and submucosal tumors may intussuscept. Villous adenomas may cause fluid and electrolyte depletion.[110]

Carcinoma of the large bowel often provokes diarrhea alternating with constipation. Complete large bowel obstruction

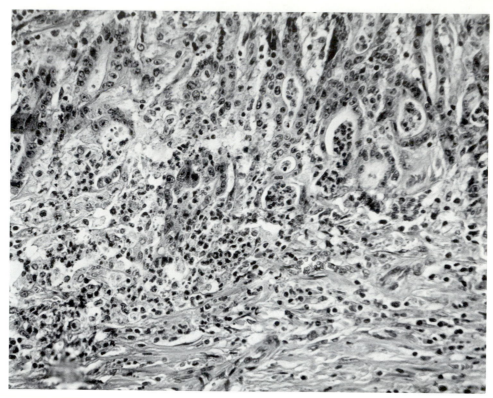

Fig. 504 Well-differentiated adenocarcinoma of large bowel with evidence of inflammatory response at interphase between tumor and surrounding tissue. This indicates good prognosis. (WU neg. 61-5207.)

develops most frequently when the carcinoma is situated in the sigmoid or left colon. Perforation of the colonic wall may appear at the site of the cancer. It is more frequent in the cecum in the presence of an obstructing carcinoma of the left colon. The patient with carcinoma of the cecum or ascending colon typically has no obstructive symptoms but suffers from anemia due to chronic blood loss. One out of four such patients develop signs of appendicitis (Fig. 505).

Malignant lymphoma

Malignant lymphomas are less frequently found in the large bowel than in the small bowel or stomach, but we have seen them in every portion of the large bowel. This tumor may produce prominent mucosal folds, distinct nodules, prominent ulceration, or a large mass. On section, extremely cellular gray tumor may be seen re-

placing muscle. On rare occasion, it presents as multiple small polyps distributed throughout the gastrointestinal tract. Frequently, there are large involved regional lymph nodes having the same characteristics as the primary tumor. The microscopic pattern varies to include all types of malignant lymphoma. It is rarely curable. We have not seen Hodgkin's disease involve the large bowel, although it has been reported by others.

Lymphoid polyp ("benign lymphoma")

Lymphoid polyps may be found infrequently in the rectal area. They are soft, superficial polyps usually covered by an intact, gray, smooth mucosa. In Helwig and Hanson's series,[116] forty were single and twenty-five were multiple. These submucosal lesions are made up of lymphoid tissue with follicle formation, a lobular

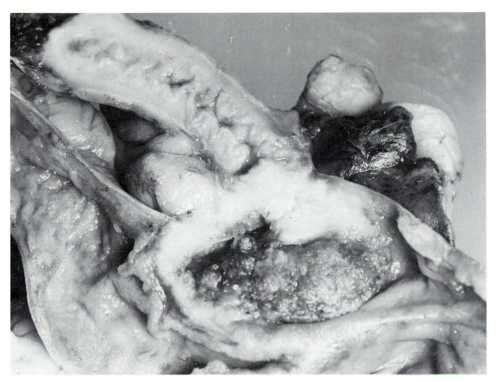

Fig. 505 Carcinoma blocking lumen of appendix which caused obstructive appendicitis. Patient entered hospital with signs and symptoms of acute appendicitis. At operation, large tumor mass was felt in region of cecum and ileocolectomy was done. (WU neg. 54-1796.)

pattern, and reaction centers. The tumor may distort the muscularis mucosae and even involve the muscularis propria.[115] A superficial or small biopsy could be incorrectly diagnosed as malignant lymphoma. The patient may complain of a mass, bleeding, or prolapse. Local excision is curative.

Carcinoid tumor

Carcinoid tumors of the large bowel are rare malignant neoplasms arising from cells of the enterochromaffin system.[120, 121] They occur in any portion of the large bowel. Those located in the colon tend to be large, extend deeply through the wall of the bowel, and involve the regional lymph nodes. They often have a light yellow color. In the rectum, they are often located in the anterior or lateral wall. The shape is spherical, and ulceration is usually lacking. Of the 147 cases of rectal carcinoid

examined by Caldarola et al.,[118] 105 measured less than 0.5 cm in diameter. Only three were associated with lymph node metastases, and all of these were larger than 2 cm in diameter. Multicentricity, a common finding in small bowel carcinoid tumors, is not a feature of rectal tumors. We know of only one case associated with the carcinoid syndrome. Microscopically, invasion of the stroma by small cells growing in a ribbon or festoon fashion is seen[123] (Fig. 506). Argentaffin and argyrophil reactions are usually negative,[117] although exceptions occur. Tumors smaller than 2 cm in diameter are best treated by local excision, whereas larger neoplasms (which are extremely rare) need a radical operation in view of their propensity for lymph node involvement.[118, 122] Rare combinations of carcinoid tumor and mucus-secreting adenocarcinoma have been described.[119]

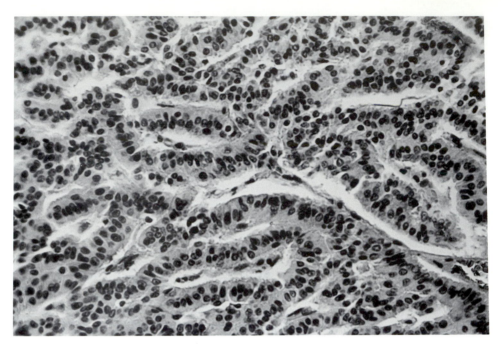

Fig. 506 Carcinoid tumor of rectum. Note typical pattern of festoons and ribbons. (×235; WU neg. 51-1222.)

Other lesions

Heterotopic gastric epithelium is rarely found in the rectum.[137]

Barium granulomas of the rectum and perirectal tissues can occur following barium enema. Barium escapes through a break in the mucosa produced by infection, tumor, foreign body, or trauma. The barium provokes a granulomatous reaction. The crystals may be seen under polarized light.[125]

Neonatal necrotizing enterocolitis is a condition of unknown etiology primarily affecting infants who are either premature or who have had exchange transfusions. It also may be seen as a complication of Hirschsprung's disease. Most cases begin in the first week of life and are manifest by abdominal distention, disappearance of bowel sounds, and passage of small amounts of blood-stained stool.[133a] The area of maximal involvement is the terminal ileum and ascending colon. The mucosa becomes necrotic and may partially slough off. Small submucosal gas-filled cysts are often present (Fig. 507); these can be detected

radiographically, an important diagnostic sign.[130a] Bowel perforation may occur. In these cases, resection of the perforated and necrotic bowel is indicated.[136]

Pneumatosis cystoides intestinalis may occur rarely in the large bowel, produce signs of intestinal obstruction, and lead to an incorrect radiographic diagnosis of cancer. Grossly, this lesion shows polypoid grapelike masses formed by submucosal gas-filled cysts (Fig. 508). Biopsy of the case shown in Fig. 508 demonstrated a submucosal cyst lined by giant cells and granulomatous changes in the stroma. These changes are diagnostic.[131] Two distinct age groups are affected. In infants, the disease is usually the result of an acute necrotizing enterocolitis and often has a fatal outcome.[136] In adults (mean age, **56** years), it follows a chronic, relatively benign clinical course.[132]

Colitis cystica profunda is a nonneoplastic condition associated with intramural mucus-containing cysts of the colon and rectum. This condition may present as a single polypoid mass or involve extensive

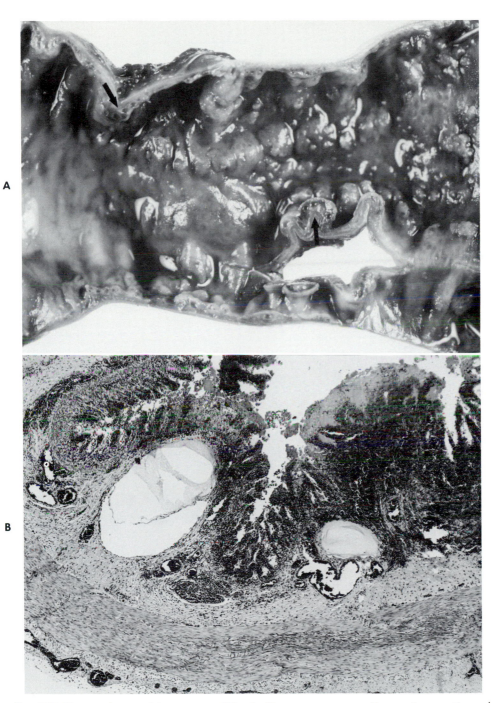

Fig. 507 Neonatal necrotizing enterocolitis. **A,** Gross appearance. Mucosa is necrotic and hemorrhagic. Numerous small gas-filled cysts are present (arrows). **B,** Microscopic appearance. There is extensive hemorrhagic infiltration of mucosa and loss of glandular epithelium. Two submucosal cysts can be seen. (**A,** WU neg. 73-7364; **B,** ×40; WU neg. 73-7490.)

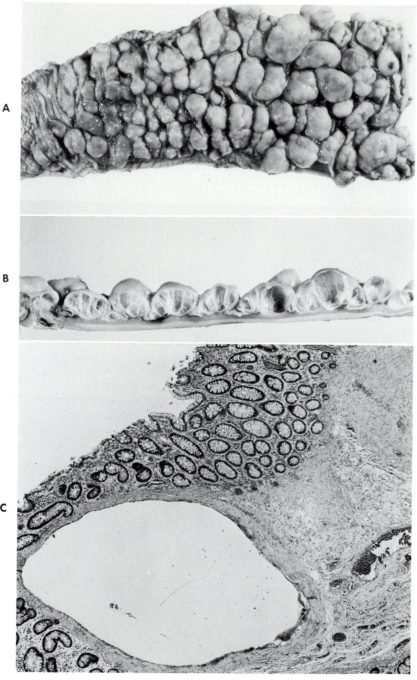

Fig. 508 **A** and **B,** Polypoid grapelike masses formed by submucosal gas-filled cysts. **C,**
Biopsy showing one of these small cysts surrounded by granulomatous changes in stroma.
(**A,** WU neg. 54-6278; **B,** WU neg. 54-6279; **C,** low power; WU neg. 55-587; **A** to **C,** from
Ramos, A. J., and Powers, W. E.: Pneumatosis cystoides intestinalis: report of a case, Am.
J. Roentgenol. Radium Ther. Nucl. Med. **77:**678-683, 1957.)

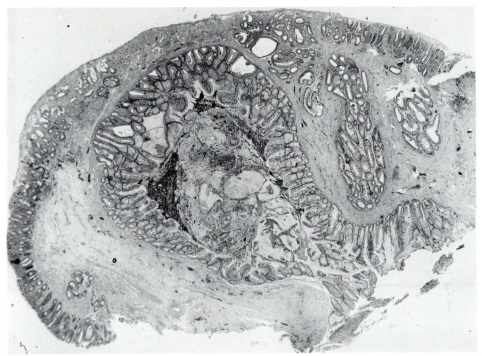

Fig. 509 Typical single polypoid mass in which clusters of normal glands are present beneath mucosa. Because of their location in large bowel and production of mucin, this architectural pattern may be mistaken for cancer. (WU neg. 67-2182.)

areas of the bowel[124, 127] (Fig. 509). The localized form, also known as hamartomatous inverted polyp,[124] is typically located in the rectum, 5 cm to 12 cm from the anal margin. It presents as a localized plaque, nodule, or polyp and is associated with chronic proctitis.[135] We agree with Wayte and Helwig[135] that in most cases it is the result of inflammation and ulceration of the bowel; this provides the means by which mucosa can extend along granulation tracts and thus form lakes of mucus in the submucosa. We have seen several of these cases which have been mistaken for a mucinous-producing carcinoma of the rectum or rectosigmoid. However, this mucin production is not accompanied by any epithelial abnormalities. We have seen the same displacement of normal mucous glands in severe irradiation change and in ulcerative colitis.

Rarely, *endometriosis* of the large bowel produces almost complete obstruction.[130] The presence of endometrial tissue within the wall of the bowel causes secondary smooth muscle hypertrophy[133] (Fig. 510). Endometriosis of the colon may be diagnosed at operation by frozen section. Endometrial glands present within the muscle are usually associated with endometrial stroma. This finding makes the pathologic diagnosis a simple one (Fig. 511).

Malakoplakia of the colon has been reported[134] (Fig. 512).

Lipomas of the large bowel are rare, invariably are submucosal, and therefore may intussuscept[129] (Figs. 513 and 514). *Lipomatosis* of the ileocecal valve may be mistaken for a tumor.[126] Occasional *leiomyomas* and *leiomyosarcomas* have been reported.[128] *Metastatic malignant tumors* occur as a part of a disseminated process. These tumors form disklike areas in which there is a central area of ulceration, but the normal mucosa extends to the ulcer, indirect evidence that it was first a metastasis in the submucosa. We have seen this occur particularly in malignant

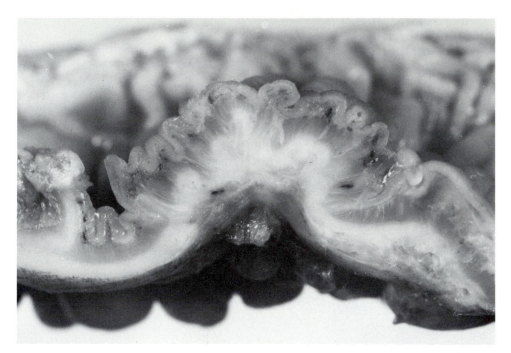

Fig. 510 Localized endometriosis of sigmoid producing partial obstruction. (WU neg. 66-2606.)

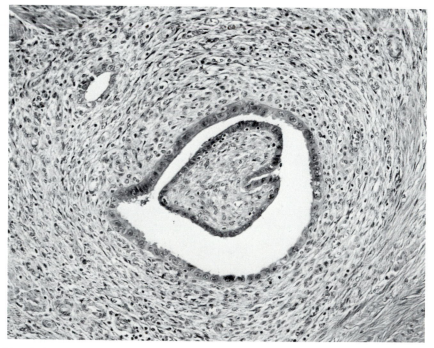

Fig. 511 Endometriosis of large bowel. Note endometrial glands surrounded by typical stroma. (×150; WU neg. 62-4211.)

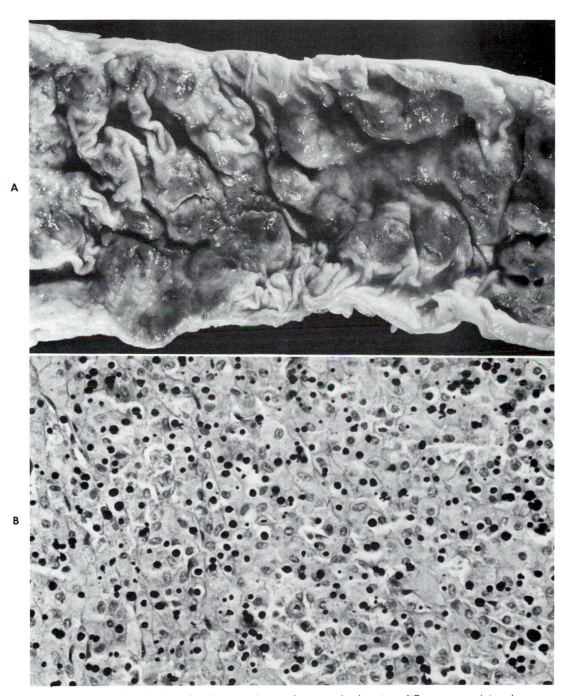

Fig. 512 Malacoplakia of colon. **A,** Gross photograph showing diffuse mucosal involvement and submucosal thickening. **B,** von Kossa's stain demonstrating innumerable Michaelis-Gutmann bodies among massive histiocytic infiltrate. (Courtesy Dr. J. Albores-Saavedra, Mexico City, Mexico.)

melanoma, malignant lymphoma, and primary carcinoma of the lung. Our most exotic case was the metastasis of a renal cell carcinoma to an intestinal carcinoid tumor. Grossly, it simulated an adenomatous polyp (Fig. 515).

REFERENCES
Diverticulosis and diverticulitis

1 Butler, D. B., and Miller, G. V.: Solitary diverticulitis of the cecum; report of case, Arch. Surg. 68:355-358, 1954.
2 Giffin, J. M., Butcher, H. R., Jr., and Ackerman, L. V.: The surgical management of colonic diverticulitis, Arch. Surg. 94:619-626, 1967.
3 Hughes, L. E.: Postmortem survey of diverticular disease of the colon. Part I. Diverticulosis and diverticulitis. Part. II. The muscular abnormality in the sigmoid colon, Gut 10:336-351, 1969.
4 Mailer, R.: Diverticula of the colon; a pathological and clinical study, Lancet 2:51-58, 1928.
5 Morson, B. C.: The muscle abnormality in diverticular disease of the colon, Proc. R. Soc. Med. 56:798-800, 1963.

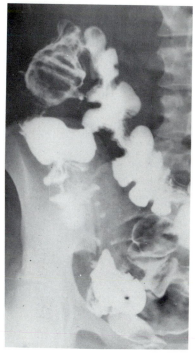

Fig. 513 Filling defect caused by lipoma. Lipomatosis of ileocecal valve may mimic carcinoma. (WU neg. 48-3832.)

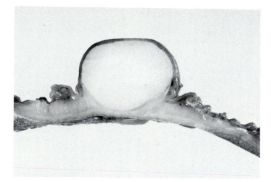

Fig. 514 Submucosal lipoma of sigmoid colon. Tumor is soft, yellow, and sharply circumscribed. (WU neg. 65-915.)

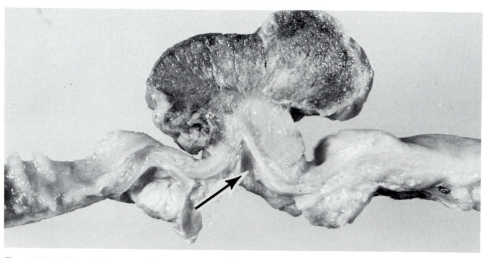

Fig. 515 Polypoid lesion of ileocecal area. Surface of lesion represents metastatic renal cell carcinoma, and base (arrow) represents primary carcinoid tumor. (WU neg. 61-6327.)

6 Nicholas, E. R., Frymark, W. B., and Raffensperger, J. R.: Acute cecal diverticulitis; report of 25 cases, J.A.M.A. **182**:157-160, 1962.

7 Noer, R. J.: Hemorrhage as a complication of diverticulitis, Ann. Surg. **141**:674-685, 1955.

8 Painter, N. S., and Burkitt, D. P.: Diverticular disease of the colon; a deficiency disease of western civilization, Br. Med. J. **2**:450-454, 1971.

9 Sorger, K., and Wacks, M. R.: Exsanguinating arterial bleeding associated with diverticulating disease of the colon, Arch. Surg. **102**: 9-14, 1971.

10 Welch, C. E., Allen, A. W., and Donaldson, G. A.: An appraisal of resection of the colon for diverticulitis of the sigmoid, Ann. Surg. **138**:332-343, 1953.

Ulcerative colitis

11 Counsell, P. B., and Dukes, C. E.: The association of chronic ulcerative colitis and carcinoma of the rectum and colon, Br. J. Surg. **39**:485-495, 1952.

12 Daniels, G. E.: Psychiatric aspects of ulcerative colitis, N. Engl. J. Med. **226**:178-184, 1942.

13 DeDombal, F. T., Goldie, W., Watts, J. McK., and Goligher, J. C.: Hepatic histologic changes in ulcerative colitis, Scand. J. Gastroenterol. **1**:220-227, 1966.

14 Devroede, G. J., Taylor, W. F., Sauer, W. G., Jackman, R. J., and Stickler, G. B.: Cancer risk and life expectancy of children with ulcerative colitis, N. Engl. J. Med. **285**:17-52, 1971.

15 Dukes, C. E., and Lockhart-Mummery, H. E.: Practical points in the pathology and surgical treatment of ulcerative colitis; a critical review, Br. J. Surg. **45**:25-36, 1957.

16 Edwards, F. C., and Truelove, S. C.: The course and prognosis of ulcerative colitis, Gut **4**:299-315, 1963 (excellent review).

17 Edwards, F. C., and Truelove, S. C.: The course and prognosis of ulcerative colitis. III. Complications, Gut **5**:1-22, 1964 (excellent review).

18 Folley, J. H.: Ulcerative proctitis, N. Engl. J. Med. **282**:1362-1364, 1970.

19 Goldgraber, M. B., Humphreys, E. M., Kirsner, J. B., and Palmer, W. L.: Carcinoma and ulcerative colitis, Gastroenterology **34**:809-839, 1958.

20 Goldman, J., Hinrichs, R., Glotzer, D. J., Gardner, R. C., and Zeitzel, L.: Ulcerative *versus* granulomatous colitis, Lab. Invest. **22**: 497-498, 1970.

21 Hellstrom, H. R., and Fisher, E. R.: Estimation of mucosal mucin as an aid in the differentiation of Crohn's disease of the colon and chronic ulcerative colitis, Am. J. Clin. Pathol. **48**:259-268, 1967.

22 Hinrichs, H. R., and Goldman, J.: Localized giant pseudopolyps of the colon, J.A.M.A. **205**:248-249, 1968.

23 Kiefer, E. D., Eytinge, D. J., and Johnson, A. C.: Malignant degeneration in chronic ulcerative colitis, Gastroenterology **19**:51-57, 1951.

24 Kirsner, J. B.: Ulcerative colitis; mysterious, multiplex, and menacing, J. Chronic Dis. **23**: 681-684, 1971.

25 Kirsner, J. B., Palmer, W. L., Maimon, S. N., and Ricketts, W. E.: Clinical course of chronic nonspecific ulcerative colitis, J.A.M.A. **137**: 922-928, 1948.

26 Lumb, G. D., and Protheroe, R. H. B.: Biopsy of the rectum in ulcerative colitis, Lancet **2**:1208-1210, 1955.

27 Lumb, G. D., and Protheroe, R. H. B.: Ulcerative colitis; a pathologic study of 152 surgical specimens, Gastroenterology **34**:381-407, 1958.

28 McAuley, R. L., and Sommers, S. C.: Mast cells in nonspecific ulcerative colitis, Am. J. Dig. Dis. **6**:233-236, 1961.

29 Morowitz, D. A., Glagov, S., Dordal, E., and Kirsner, J. B.: Carcinoma of the biliary tract complicating chronic ulcerative colitis, Cancer **27**:356-361, 1971.

30 Morson, B.: Current concepts of colitis; lecture 1, Trans. Med. Soc. Lond. **86**:159-176, 1970.

31 Morson, B.: Crohn's disease; lecture 2, Trans. Med. Soc. Lond. **86**:177-192, 1970.

32 Morson, B. C., and Pang, L. S. C.: Rectal biopsy as an aid to cancer control in ulcerative colitis, Gut **8**:423-434, 1967.

33 Schachter, H., Goldstein, M. J., Rappaport, H., Fennessy, J. J., and Kirsner, J. B.: Ulcerative and "granulomatous" colitis—validity of differential diagnostic criteria; a study of 100 patients treated by total colectomy, Ann. Intern. Med. **72**:841-851, 1970.

34 Truelove, S. C., and Richards, W. C. D.: Biopsy studies in ulcerative colitis, Br. Med. J. **1**:1315-1318, 1956.

35 Watson, A. J., and Roy, A. D.: Paneth cells in the large intestine in ulcerative colitis, J. Pathol. Bacteriol. **80**:309-316, 1960.

36 Whitehead, R.: Personal communication, 1971.

37 Wright, R.: Ulcerative colitis, Gastroenterology **58**:875-897, 1970 (extensive bibliography).

Crohn's disease (granulomatous colitis)

38 Farmer, R. G., Hawk, W. A., and Turnbull, R. B., Jr.: Carcinoma associated with mucosal ulcerative colitis, and with transmural colitis and enteritis (Crohn's disease), Cancer **28**:289-292, 1971.

39 Gray, B. K., Lockhart-Mummery, H. E., and Morson, B. C.: Crohn's disease of the anal region, Gut 6:515-524, 1965.

40 Jones, J. H.: Colonic cancer and Crohn's disease, Gut 10:651-654, 1969.

41 Lockhart-Mummery, H. E., and Morson, B. C.: Crohn's disease of the large intestine, Gut 5:493-509, 1964.

Ischemic colitis

42 Kilpatrick, Z. M., Silverman, J. F., Betancourt, E., Farman, J., and Lawson, J. P.: Vascular occlusion of the colon and oral contraceptives; possible relation, N. Engl. J. Med. 278:438-440, 1968.

43 Morson, B. C.: Ischaemic colitis, Postgrad. Med. J. 44:665-666, 1968.

Hirschsprung's disease (idiopathic megacolon)

44 Aldridge, R. T., and Campbell, P. E.: Ganglion cell distribution in the normal rectum and anal canal; a basis for the diagnosis of Hirschsprung's disease by anorectal biopsy, J. Pediatr. Surg. 3:475-490, 1968.

45 Bodian, M., Stephens, F. D., and Ward, B. C. H.: Hirschsprung's disease and idiopathic megacolon, Lancet 1:6-10, 1949.

46 Madsen, C. M.: Hirschsprung's disease, Springfield, Ill., 1964, Charles C Thomas, Publisher.

47 Swenson, O., Fisher, J. H., and MacMahon, H. E.: Rectal biopsy as an aid in the diagnosis of Hirschsprung's disease, N. Engl. J. Med. 253:632-635, 1955.

48 Swenson, O., Rheinlander, H. F., and Diamond, I.: Hirschsprung's disease; a new concept of the etiology, N. Engl. J. Med. 241:551-556, 1949.

49 Walker, A. W., Kempson, R. L., and Ternberg, J. L.: Aganglionosis of the small intestine, Surgery 60:449-457, 1966.

50 Weinberg, A. G.: The anorectal myenteric plexus; its relation to hypoganglionosis of the colon, Am. J. Clin. Pathol. 54:637-642, 1970.

51 Whitehouse, F. R., and Kernohan, J. W.: Myenteric plexus in congenital megacolon; study of eleven cases, Arch. Intern. Med. 82:75-111, 1948.

52 Zuelzer, W. W., and Wilson, J. L.: Functional intestinal obstruction on a congenital neurogenic basis in infancy, Am. J. Dis. Child. 75:40-64, 1948.

Tuberculosis

53 Fuchs, F.: Beitrage zur Chirurgischen Klinik der Darmtuberkulose, Beitr. Klin. Chir. 136:514-527, 1926.

54 Howell, J. S., and Knapton, P. J.: Ileo-caecal tuberculosis, Gut 5:524-529, 1964.

55 Inberg, K. R.: Cicatrizing intestinal tuberculosis and allied conditions, Acta Chir. Scand. 95:307-326, 1947.

56 Lee, F. D., and Roy, A. D.: Ileo-caecal granulomata, Gut 5:517-523, 1964.

Cytology

57 Raskin, H. F., and Pleticka, S. The cytologic diagnosis of cancer of the colon, Acta Cytol. (Baltimore) 8:131-140, 1964.

Biopsy

58 Brett, E. M., and Berry, C. L.: Value of rectal biopsy in pediatric neurology; report of 165 biopsies, Br. Med. J. 3:400-403, 1967.

59 Gabriel, W. B., Dukes, C. E., and Bussey, H. J. R.: Biopsy of the rectum, Br. J. Surg. 38:400-411, 1951.

60 Gafni, J., and Sohar, E.: Rectal biopsy for the diagnosis of amyloidosis, Am. J. Med. Sci. 240: 332-336, 1960.

61 Kamoshita, S., and Landing, B. H.: Distribution of lesions in myenteric plexus and gastrointestinal mucosa in lipidoses and other neurologic disorders of children, Am. J. Clin. Pathol. 49:312-318, 1968.

62 Kyle, R. A., Spencer, R. J., and Dahlin, D. C.: Value of rectal biopsy in the diagnosis of primary systemic amyloidosis, Am. J. Med. Sci. 251:501-506, 1966.

Tumors

Epithelial polyps

63 Arminski, T. C., and McLean, D. W.: Incidence and distribution of adenomatous polyps of the colon and rectum based on 1,000 autopsy examinations, Dis. Colon Rectum 7:249-261, 1964.

64 Bacon, H. E., and Eisenberg, S. W.: Papillary adenoma or villous tumor of the rectum and colon, Ann. Surg. 174:1002-1008, 1971.

65 Bussey, H. J. R.: Gastrointestinal polyposis, Gut 11:970-978, 1970.

66 Chapman, I.: Adenomatous polypi of large intestine; incidence and distribution, Ann. Surg. 157:223-226, 1963.

67 Cole, J. W., and McKalen, A.: Studies on the morphogenesis of adenomatous polyps in the human colon, Cancer 16:998-1002, 1963.

68 Ewing, M. R.: Villous tumors of the rectum, Ann. R. Coll. Surg. Engl. 6:413-441, 1950.

69 Feyrter, F.: Zur Geschwulstlehre (nach Untersuchungen am menschlichen Darm). I. Polypen und Krebs, Beitr. Pathol. Anat. 86:663-670, 1931.

70 Fung, C. H., and Goldman, H.: The incidence and significance of villous change in adenomatous polyps, Am. J. Clin. Pathol. 53:21-25, 1970.

71 Gardner, E. J.: Follow-up study of a family group exhibiting dominant inheritance for a

syndrome including intestinal polyps, osteomas, fibromas, and epidermal cysts, Am. J. Hum. Genet. 14:375-389, 1962.

72 Haggitt, R. C., and Pitcock, J. A.: Familial juvenile polyposis of the colon, Cancer 26:1232-1238, 1970.

73 Helwig, E. B.: Benign tumors of the large intestine—incidence and distribution, Surg. Gynecol. Obstet. 76:419-426, 1943.

74 Helwig, E. B.: Adenomas of the large intestine in children, Am. J. Dis. Child. 72:289-295, 1946.

75 Helwig, E. B.: The evolution of adenomas of the large intestine and their relation to carcinoma, Surg. Gynecol. Obstet. 84:36-49, 1947.

76 Helwig, E. B., and Hanson, J.: Lymphoid polyps (benign lymphoma) and malignant lymphoma of the rectum and anus, Surg. Gynecol. Obstet. 92:233-243, 1951.

77 Horrilleno, E. G., Eckert, C., and Ackerman, L. V.: Polyps of the rectum and colon in children, Cancer 10:1210-1220, 1957.

78 Lane, N., Kaplan, H., and Pascal, R. R.: Minute adenomatous and hyperplastic polyps of the colon: divergent patterns of epithelial growth with specific associated mesenchymal changes; contrasting roles in the pathogenesis of carcinoma, Gastroenterology, 60:537-551, 1971.

79 MacDonald, J. M., Davis, W. C., Crago, H. R., and Berk, A. D.: Gardner's syndrome and periampullary malignancy, Am. J. Surg. 113:425-430, 1967.

80 Ramirez, R. F., Culp, C. E., Jackman, R. J., and Dockerty, M. B.: Villous tumors of the lower part of the large bowel, J.A.M.A. 194:121-125, 1965.

81 Roth, S. I., and Helwig, E. B.: Juvenile polyps of the colon and rectum, Cancer 16:468-479, 1963.

82 Ruymann, F. B.: Juvenile polyps with cachexia; report of an infant and comparison with Cronkhite-Canada syndrome in adults, Gastroenterology 57:431-438, 1969.

83 Sachatello, C. R.: Familial polyposis of the colon; a four-decade follow-up, Cancer 28:581-587, 1971.

84 Valdes-Dapena, A., and Beckfield, W. J.: Adenomatous polyps of the large intestine, Gastroenterology 32:452-461, 1957.

85 Veale, A. M. O., McColl, I., Bussey, H. J. R., and Morson, B. C.: Juvenile polyposis coli, J. Med. Genet. 3:1-76, 1969.

86 Yonemoto, R. H., Slayback, J. B., Byron, R. L., Jr., and Rosen, R. B.: Familial polyposis of the entire gastrointestinal tract, Arch. Surg. 99:427-434, 1969.

87 Wheat, M. W., Jr., and Ackerman, L. V.: Villous adenomas of the large intestine; clinicopathologic evaluation of 50 cases of villous adenomas with emphasis on treatment, Ann. Surg. 147:476-487, 1958.

Treatment

88 Kraus, F. T.: Pedunculated adenomatous polyp with carcinoma in the tip and metastasis to lymph nodes, Dis. Colon Rectum 8:283-286, 1965.

89 Spratt, J., Moyer, C., and Ackerman, L. V.: Relationship of polyps of the colon to colonic cancer, Ann. Surg. 148:682-698, 1958.

90 Spratt, J. S., Jr., and Watson, F. R.: The rationale of practice for polypoid lesions of the colon, Cancer 28:153-159, 1971.

91 Williams, C., Muto, T., and Rutter, K. R. P.: Removal of polyps with fibreoptic colonoscope; a new approach to colonic polypectomy, Br. Med. J. 1:451-452, 1973.

92 Wolff, W. I., and Shina, H.: Polypectomy via the fiberoptic colonoscope; removal of neoplasms beyond reach of the sigmoidscope, N. Engl. J. Med. 288:329-332, 1973.

Carcinoma

93 Black, W. A., and Waugh, J. M.: The intramural extension of carcinoma of the descending colon, sigmoid, and recto-sigmoid, Surg. Gynecol. Obstet. 87:457-464, 1948.

94 Castleman, B., and Krickstein, H. I.: Do adenomatous polyps of the colon become malignant? N. Engl. J. Med. 267:469-474, 1962.

95 Cole, W. H., McDonald, G. O., Roberts, S. S., and Southwick, H. W.: Dissemination of cancer; prevention and therapy, New York, 1961, Appleton-Century-Croft, Inc.

96 Coller, F. A., Kay, E. B., and MacIntyre, R. S.: Regional lymphatic metastases of carcinoma of the colon, Ann. Surg. 114:56-76, 1941.

97 Dukes, C. E.: Histologic grading of rectal carcinoma, Proc. R. Soc. Med. 30:371-376, 1937.

98 Dukes, C. E.: Ossification in rectal cancer, Proc. R. Soc. Med. 32:1489-1494, 1939.

99 Dukes, C. E.: Cancer of the rectum; an analysis of 1,000 cases, J. Pathol. Bacteriol. 50:527-539, 1940.

100 Dukes, C. E.: Peculiarities in the pathology of cancer of the anorectal region, Proc. R. Soc. Med. 39:763-765, 1946.

101 Dukes, C. E.: The surgical pathology of rectal cancer, J. Clin. Pathol. 2:95-98, 1949.

102 Dukes, C. E.: The significance of the unusual in the pathology of intestinal tumors, Ann. R. Coll. Surg. Engl. 4:90-103, 1949.

103 Glenn, F., and McSherry, C. K.: Carcinoma of the distal large bowel; 32-year review of 1026 cases, Ann. Surg. 163:838-849, 1966.

104 Gold, P., and Freedman, S. O.: Specific carcino-embryonic antigens of the human digestive system, J. Exp. Med. 122:467-481, 1965.

105 Goligher, J. C., Dukes, C. E., and Bussey, H. J. R.: Local recurrences after sphincter-saving excisions for carcinoma of the rectum and rectosigmoid, Br. J. Surg. 39:199-211, 1951.

106 Grinnell, R. S.: The lymphatic and venous spread of carcinoma of the rectum, Ann. Surg. 116:200-216, 1942.

107 Hultborn, K. A.: The causal relationship between benign epithelial tumors and adenocarcinoma of the colon and rectum, Acta Radiol. 113:1-71, 1954.

108 Laufman, H., and Saphir, O.: Primary linitis plastica type of carcinoma of the colon, Arch. Surg. 62:79-91, 1951.

109 Quer, R. E., Dahlin, D. C., and Mayo, C. W.: Retrograde intramural spread of carcinoma of the rectum and rectosigmoid; a microscopic study, Surg. Gynecol. Obstet. 96:24-30, 1953.

110 Solomon, S. S., Moran, J. M., and Nabseth, D. C.: Villous adenoma of rectosigmoid accompanied by electrolyte depletion, J.A.M.A. 194:117-122, 1965.

111 Spratt, J. S., Jr., and Ackerman, L. V.: Small primary adenocarcinomas of the colon and rectum, J.A.M.A. 179:337-346, 1962.

112 Spratt, J. S., Jr., and Spjut, H. J.: Prevalence and prognosis of individual clinical and pathologic variables associated with colorectal carcinoma, Cancer 20:1976-1985, 1967.

113 Thompson, D. M. P., Krupey, J., Freedman, S. O., and Gold, P.: The radioimmunoassay of circulating carcinoembryonic antigen of the human digestive system, Proc. Natl. Acad. Sci. U.S.A. 64:161-167, 1969.

114 Zamcheck, N., Moore, T. L., Dhar, P., and Kupchik, H.: Immunologic diagnosis and prognosis of human digestive-tract cancer; carcinoembryonic antigens, N. Engl. J. Med. 286:83-86, 1972.

Lymphoid polyp ("benign lymphoma")

115 Cornes, J. S., Wallace, M. H., and Morson, B. C.: Benign lymphomas of the rectum and anal canal; a study of 100 cases, J. Pathol. Bacteriol. 82:371-382, 1961.

116 Helwig, E. B., and Hanson, J.: Lymphoid polyp (benign lymphoma) and malignant lymphoma of the rectum and anus, Surg. Gynecol. Obstet. 92:233-243, 1951 (extensive bibliography).

Carcinoid tumor

117 Black, W. C.: Enterochromaffin cell types and corresponding carcinoid tumors, Lab. Invest. 19:473-486, 1968.

118 Caldarola, V. T., Jackman, R. J., Moertel, C. G., and Dockerty, M. B.: Carcinoid tumors of the rectum, Am. J. Surg. 107:844-849, 1964.

119 Hernandez, F. J., and Reid, J. D.: Mixed carcinoid and mucus-secreting intestinal tumors, Arch. Pathol. 88:489-496, 1969.

120 Horn, R. C., Jr.: Carcinoid tumors of the colon and rectum, Cancer 2:819-837, 1949.

121 Pearson, C. M., and Fitzgerald, P. J.: Carcinoid tumors, a re-emphasis of their malignant nature, Cancer 2:1005-1025, 1949 (extensive bibliography).

122 Peskin, G., and Orloff, M.: A clinical study of 25 patients with carcinoid tumors of the rectum, Surg. Gynecol. Obstet. 109:673-682, 1959.

123 Stout, A. P.: Carcinoid tumors of the rectum derived from Erspamer's pre-enterochrome cells, Am. J. Pathol. 18:993-1009, 1942.

Other lesions

124 Allen, M. S., Jr.: Hamartomatous inverted polyps of the rectum, Cancer 19:257-265, 1966.

125 Beddoe, H., Kaye, S., and Kaye, S.: Barium granuloma of the rectum; report of case, J.A.M.A. 154:747-748, 1954.

126 Cabaud, P. G., and Harris, L. T.: Lipomatosis of the ileocecal valve, Ann. Surg. 150:1092-1098, 1959.

127 Epstein, S. E., Ascari, W. Q., Albow, R. C., Seaman, W. B., and Lattes, R.: Colitis cystica profunda, Am. J. Clin. Pathol. 45:186-201, 1966.

128 Golden, T., and Stout, A. P.: Smooth muscle tumors of the gastrointestinal tract and retroperitoneal tissues, Surg. Gynecol. Obstet. 73:784-810, 1941.

129 Haller, J. D., and Roberts, T. W.: Lipomas of the colon; clinicopathologic study of 20 cases, Surgery 55:773-781, 1964.

130 Kratzer, G. L., and Salvati, E. P.: Collective review of endometriosis of the colon, Am. J. Surg. 90:866-869, 1955.

130a Pochaczevsky, R., and Kassner, E. G.: Necrotizing enterocolitis of infancy, Am. J. Roentgenol. Radium Ther. Nucl. Med. 113:283-296, 1971.

131 Ramos, A. J., and Powers, W. E.: Pneumatosis cystoides intestinalis; report of a case, Am. J. Roentgenol. Radium Ther. Nucl. Med. 77:678-683, 1957.

132 Smith, B. H., and Welter, L. H.: Pneumatosis intestinalis, Am. J. Clin. Pathol. 48:455-465, 1967.

133 Spjut, H. J., and Perkins, D. E.: Endometriosis of the sigmoid colon and rectum, Am. J. Roentgenol. Radium Ther. Nucl. Med. 82:1070-1075, 1959.

133a Stevenson, J. K., Graham, C. B., Oliver, T.

K., Jr., and Goldenberg, V. E.: Neonatal necrotizing enterocolitis; a report of twenty-one
cases with fourteen survivors, Am. J. Surg.
118:260-272, 1969.

134 Terner, J. Y., and Lattes, R.: Malakoplakia of
colon and retroperitoneum, Am. J. Clin. Pathol. **44**:20-31, 1965.

135 Wayte, D. M., and Helwig, E. B.: Colitis
cystica profunda, Am. J. Clin. Pathol. **48**:
159-169, 1967.

136 Wilson, S. E., and Woolley, M. M.: Primary
necrotizing enterocolitis in infants, Arch.
Surg. **99**:563-566, 1969.

137 Wolff, M.: Heterotopic gastric epithelium in
the rectum; a report of three new cases with
a review of 87 cases of gastric heterotopia in
the alimentary canal, Am. J. Clin. Pathol.
55:604-616, 1971.

Anus

Anatomy

The anal canal is a tubular structure 3 cm to 4 cm in length extending from the perineal skin to the lower end of the rectum (Fig. 516). The junction between the anal canal and the perineal skin is known as the *anal verge*. The *dentate or pectinate line* marks the junction between the anal canal and the rectum. The segment of anal canal located immediately below this line exhibits a number of longitudinal folds known as *anal columns (of Morgagni).* Homologous structures in the lower rectum are designated *rectal columns (of Morgagni)* and the depressions between them as *rectal sinuses (of Morgagni).* The anal columns are connected at the dentate line by the *anal or semilunar valves* (transverse plicae). The latter form the inner boundary of minute pockets designated as *anal crypts (of Morgagni).*

The anal canal is lined by keratinized or nonkeratinized squamous epithelium, except for a circular zone, 0.3 cm to 1.1 cm in width, lined by transitional epithelium and thought to represent a remnant of the embryonal cloaca. This zone corresponds to the area of the anal columns and crypts. It is limited superiorly by the dentate line and inferiorly by the lower end of the anal valves. It has a glistening, wrinkled, membranous appearance which is often made discontinuous by the presence of the *anal papillae.* These are toothlike, raised projections located on top of the anal columns, extending upward onto the rectum and representing ridges of squamous mucosa directly joining the rectal mucosa. Both anal crypts and papillae show marked individual variations and are occasionally absent. The *anal ducts (glands)* discharge into the anal crypts and can extend upward or, more commonly, downward. They penetrate the sphincters and sometimes extend into the perianal fat[1, 2] (Fig. 517).

Embryologic defects

Anorectal anomalies occur in approximately 1 of every 1,800 births.[3] They are divided into three major types depending on the relationship of the lower bowel to the puborectalis component of the levator ani muscle.[4] *High or supralevator anomalies* (40%) have a serious prognosis because of severe obstruction, common association with other congenital anomalies (in vertebrae and urinary tract), and defective innervation of the pelvic muscles. A fistulous tract to the bladder, urethra, or vagina is often present. A complicated sacroabdominoperineal approach is needed for reconstruction. In *low or translevator anomalies* (40%), obstruction is rarely severe. The pelvic innervation is normal, and associated anomalies are rare. Fistulas may or may not be present. A simple perineal operation will cure most of these patients. *Intermediate anomalies* are rare (15%). An abdominoperineal approach is usually needed for reconstruction. The remaining varieties, quite rare, include *perineal groove* and *persistent anal membrane.*

Familiarity with the anatomic variants of anorectal anomalies and a thorough radiologic investigation (plain x-ray films, cystograms, and fistulograms) are essential for an accurate diagnosis and, therefore, a proper treatment. Unsuccessful operations lead to stricture and colonic obstruction (Fig. 518), which may eventually necessitate a permanent colostomy.

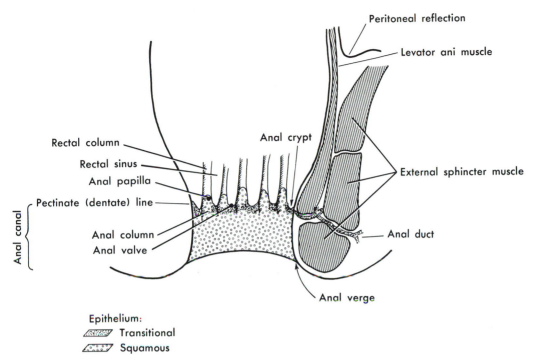

Fig. 516 Diagrammatic representation of normal anal structures. Cloacogenic carcinoma arises from small area of transitional epithelium.

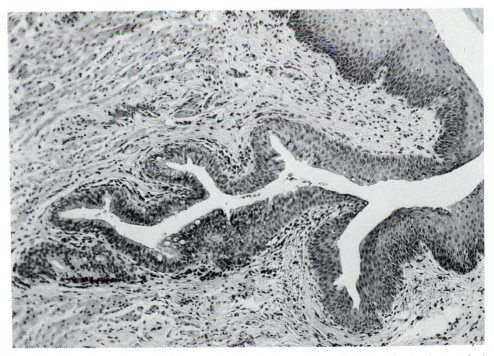

Fig. 517 Normal anal gland. It is penetrating into muscle and is lined by both stratified squamous and mucus-secreting cells. (×110; WU neg. 51-5610.)

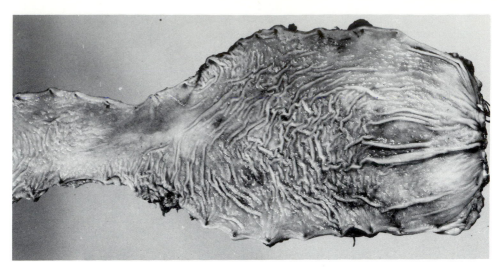

Fig. 518 A 10-year-old child with imperforate anus and absence of anal sphincter finally underwent abdominal perineal resection after multiple attempts to establish fecal continence through perineum. Marked dilatation of rectum was result of cicatricial obstruction. (WU neg. 62-1950.)

Fissure, ulcer, and fistula

An anal *fissure* is a single linear separation of the tissues of the anal canal extending through the mucous membrane. About 90% of anal fissures are found at the posterior commissure overlying the bifurcation of the sphincter as it divides to circle the rectum.

An anal *ulcer* is a chronic process, usually oval in shape, that extends into the muscular layer. Above it is a hypertrophied papilla, and behind this papilla is an infected crypt. External to the ulcer is a skin tag, the result of chronic edema and fibrosis surrounding the ulcer.

An anal *fistula* is an abnormal track having an internal opening within the anal canal, usually at the dentate line. The fistulous track may lead to the skin, or it may end blindly in the perianal soft tissues. The lining is made of granulation tissue, although epithelium may eventually grow at either end of the track. Most cases of fistula-in-ano are caused by an intersphincteric abscess originating in an anal duct[8, 10] and have a nonspecific microscopic appearance. On the other hand, anal fistulas may be a manifestation of tuberculosis,[9] Crohn's disease,[6] ulcerative colitis,[7] and actinomy-

cosis.[5] It is important therefore that tissue obtained from an anal fistula be examined microscopically in every case. The incidence of tuberculosis as a cause of anal fistulas has dropped from 16% to less than 1% at St. Mark's Hospital (London) in a fifty-year period.[9] The patients almost invariably show radiologic evidence of pulmonary tuberculosis. Fistulas due to Crohn's disease are often complex and painless, with irregular edges and with little induration. The diagnosis may be suggested by the presence of noncaseating granulomas, being careful not to confuse them with the foci of foreign-body reaction sometimes seen in nonspecific fistulas.

Hemorrhoids

Stasis of blood in the veins of the hemorrhoidal plexus is usually due simply to dependency. However, pathologic processes in the drainage path of those veins may cause secondary engorgement. Therefore, the presence of hemorrhoids may be an indication of some other process such as cirrhosis of the liver with portal hypertension, carcinoma of the rectum, leiomyoma of the uterus, or pregnancy.

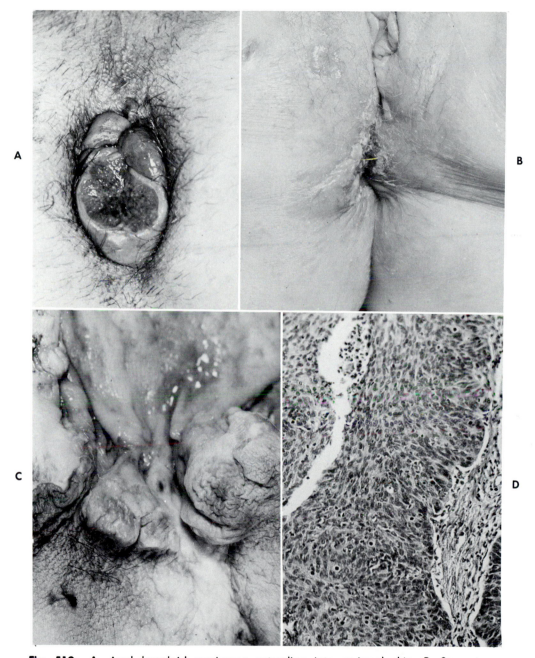

Fig. 519 A, Anal basaloid carcinoma extending into perianal skin. **B,** Same tumor showing excellent temporary results following irradiation. **C,** Tumor recurred locally, and abdominoperineal resection was done. Note irradiation effect in skin and narrowed anal canal. **D,** Microscopic appearance of persistent tumor. Note plexiform pattern and palisading of cells around border. Regional lymph nodes were negative. Patient died of disseminated disease four years following microscopic diagnosis. (**A,** WU neg. 49-5917; **B,** WU neg. 48-1714; **C,** WU neg. 50-1350; **D,** ×200; WU neg. 50-695.)

Hemorrhoids can be present either within or outside the anus. Thrombosis of these dilated veins is frequent. If the cause of venous obstruction is removed, the hemorrhoids may disappear, although in many instances resection is necessary. Inflammatory changes are secondary to surface ulceration rather than thrombosis.[11]

Microscopic examination of hemorrhoids rarely may show nonspecific granulomas, tuberculosis, malignant lymphoma, epidermoid carcinoma, or even malignant melanoma.

Tumors
Carcinoma

Anal carcinoma is an infrequent lesion. Grossly it appears near the mucocutaneous junction and grows either upward into the rectum and surrounding tissues or outward to the perianal tissues (Fig. 519, A to D). At times, the growth almost exactly simulates an adenocarcinoma of the rectum, and the correct diagnosis is made only with biopsy. Involvement of the perianal skin may be superficial with only surface ulceration and slightly elevated margins. Such lesions have been mistaken for an unusual inflammatory process. In other instances, a typical deeply ulcerated neoplasm with rolled edges is seen (Fig. 520). Local extension upward of the growth may burrow beneath the overlying epithelium only to ulcerate at a higher level. Because of the dual lymphatic supply of the pectinate line, regional lymph nodes along the rectum or in the inguinal areas may contain metastases.

Microscopically, carcinoma of the anus has been classically equated with squamous cell tumors of differing degrees of differentiation. The work of Grinvalsky et al.,[14] corroborated by many other authors,[15, 17, 19] indicates instead that two major tumor types exist.

The first is a bona fide *epidermoid carcinoma.* It comprises approximately 70% of all anal cancers and 90% of the cancers of those located in the anal skin.[18] It is similar in every respect to tumors of the same type occurring in other organs, such as the lung and esophagus.

The second type, called *basaloid* or *cloacogenic,* comprises 18% of all anal cancers. It is almost always located within the anal canal and presumably arises from the area of transitional epithelium of cloacogenic origin previously described. An important diagnostic microscopic feature is the presence of palisading at the periphery of the clumps of tumor cells, somewhat resembling the pattern seen in basal cell carcinomas of skin (Fig. 519, D). Foci of mucin secretion and squamous differentiation are often present.[17] Pang et al.[19] have found an excellent correlation between the degree of differentiation and prognosis: the five-year survival rate was 90%, 60%, and 0% for well-differentiated, moderately differentiated, and poorly differentiated tumors, respectively.

Of seventy-nine patients with epidermoid and basaloid carcinoma of the anus treated at Barnes Hospital and the Ellis Fischel State Cancer Hospital, thirty-one (39%) survived five years. No inguinal nodes were palpated in forty-one patients treated by abdominal perineal resection. Inguinal metastases became evident subsequently in only three patients. Therapeutic inguinal dissection was followed by five-year survival in all of these.[13] Usually, however, if the inguinal lymph nodes are involved, prognosis is poor.[16]

Klotz et al.[17] reviewed 373 cloacogenic carcinomas of the anal canal. This tumor was twice as frequent in women. Metastases occurred in 19% of the patients, and wide abdominal perineal resection produced a cure rate of 50%.

True basal cell carcinomas can occur at the anal margin and can be cured either by local excision or by irradiation.[21] We have seen granuloma inguinale confused clinically with epidermoid carcinoma (Fig. 521). Biopsy in such cases will exclude carcinoma. A definite diagnosis of granuloma inguinale can be made if Donovan bodies are found (Fig. 522).

Patients with long-standing lymphopath-

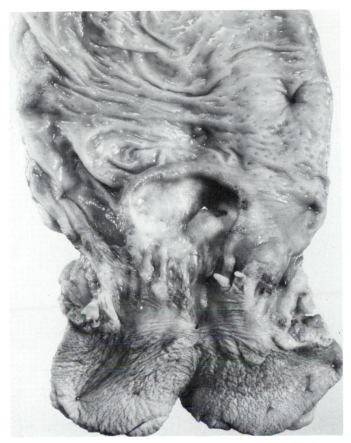

Fig. 520 Large excavated carcinoma involving dentate line and extending into rectal mucosa. Microscopically, it was of basaloid type. All twenty-six lymph nodes were free of tumor. Patient, 56-year-old white woman, is alive seven years after surgery without evidence of tumor recurrence. (WU neg. 65-3325.)

ia venereum with associated rectal stricture are prone to develop squamous metaplasia of the rectum and epidermoid carcinoma[20] (Fig. 523). Female patients with anal carcinoma have an increased incidence of carcinomas of the lower genital tract, particularly of the uterine cervix.[12]

Malignant melanoma

Approximately one anal melanoma is seen for every eight anal epidermoid carcinomas and one for every 250 rectal adenocarcinomas.[23] The tumor often begins at the pectinate line and grows into the rectal ampulla. It may extend a long way along the submucosa and emerge through the mucosa at a high point, thus simulating a primary rectal tumor.[22] Mul-

tiple polypoid masses may form and grow beneath the intact mucosa (Fig. 524). Because they are polypoid and smooth, they look benign and can be easily confused with thrombosed hemorrhoids. Rectal bleeding is the most common complaint. Microscopically, they are similar to those described under skin. The prognosis is invariably hopeless.

Other lesions

Paget's disease of the anus presents as an erythematous, ulcerated lesion of eczematoid appearance. It is a malignant neoplasm of the intraepidermal portion of apocrine glands, with or without associated dermal involvement. The latter was found in thirteen of thirty-eight cases studied by

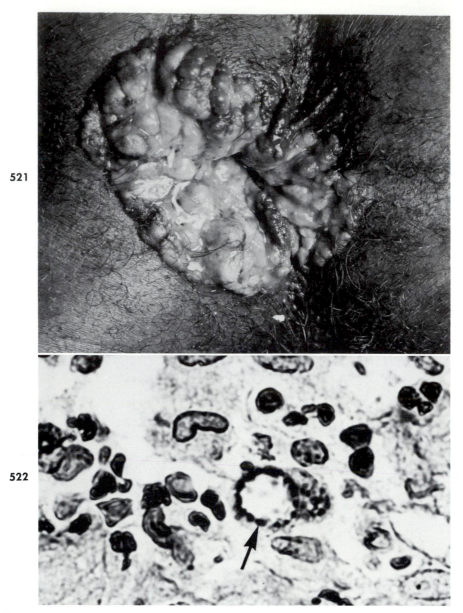

Fig. 521 Granuloma inguinale simulating carcinoma. (WU neg. 48-4599.)
Fig. 522 Donovan bodies (arrow) within cyst in cytoplasm of macrophage in patient with granuloma inguinale. (Warthin-Starry; high power; WU neg. 66-9158.)

Helwig et al.[25] Eleven patients had lymph node metastases, and all of them died of their disease. The cells of anogenital Paget's disease invariably contain acid mucosubstances, an important feature in the differential diagnosis with melanoma and Bowen's disease.

Metastases to the anal region often arise in rectal carcinomas. We have seen a patient with rectal carcinoma who developed metastases at the site of a recently performed hemorrhoidectomy.

Hidradenomas may arise from apocrine sweat glands in the anal area.[28] *Epidermoid cysts* also occur in the anus.[24] *Pseudotumors* may be produced by sclerosing

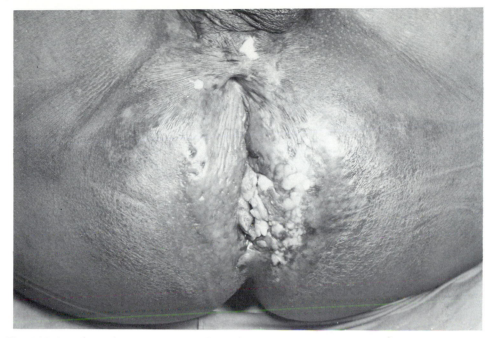

Fig. 523 Lymphopathia venereum with epidermoid carcinoma. Frei test was positive. (WU neg. 52-3301.)

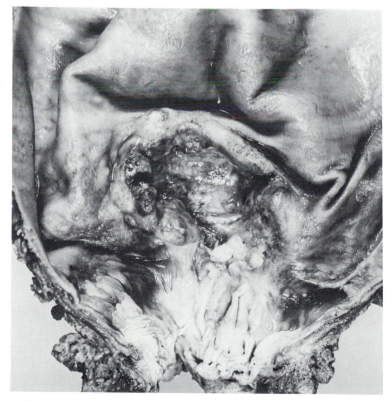

Fig. 524 Malignant melanoma growing into rectum to form polypoid mass. There were innumerable metastases. (WU neg. 50-4182.)

agents used to obliterate hemorrhoids. We have seen two cases of *eosinophilic granuloma* involving the perianal skin.[26] A case of *botryoid rhabdomyosarcoma* of the anus in a 2-month-old infant was reported by Sharp and Helwig.[27]

REFERENCES

Anatomy

1 Grinvalsky, H. T., and Helwig, E. B.: Carcinoma of the anorectal junction. I. Histological considerations, Cancer 9:480-488, 1956.
2 Klotz, R. G., Pamukooglu, T., and Souillard, D. H.: Transitional cloacogenic carcinoma of the anal canal, Cancer 20:1727-1745, 1967 (extensive bibliography).

Embryologic defects

3 Louw, J. H., Cywes, S., and Cremin, B. J.: Anorectal malformations — classification and clinical features, S. Afr. J. Surg. 9:11-20, 1971.
4 Santulli, T. V., Kiesewetter, W. B., and Bill, A. H. Jr.: Anorectal anomalies; a suggested international classification, J. Pediatr. Surg. 5:281-287, 1970.

Fissure, ulcer, and fistula

5 Fry, G. A., Martin, W. J., Dearing, W. H., and Culp, C. E.: Primary actinomycosis of the rectum with multiple perianal and perineal fistulae, Mayo Clin. Proc. 40:296-299, 1965.
6 Gray, B. K., Lockhart-Mummery, H. E., and Morson, B. C.: Crohn's disease of the anal region, Gut 6:515-525, 1965.
7 Lennard-Jones, J. E., Lockhart-Mummery, H. E., Chir, M., and Morson, B. C.: Clinical and pathological differentiation of Crohn's disease and proctocolitis, Gastroenterology 54:1162-1170, 1968.
8 Lilius, H. G.: Fistula-in-ano; an investigation of human foetal anal ducts and intramuscular glands and a clinical study of 150 patients, Acta Chir. Scand. [Suppl.] 383:1-88, 1968.
9 Logan, V. S.: Anorectal tuberculosis, Proc. R. Soc. Med. 62:1227-1230, 1969.
10 Parks, A. G., and Morson, B. C.: The pathogenesis of fistula-in-ano, Proc. R. Soc. Med. 55:751-754, 1962.

Hemorrhoids

11 Laurence, A. E., and Murray, A. J.: Histopathology of prolapsed and thrombosed hemorrhoids, Dis. Colon Rectum 5:56-61, 1962.

Tumors
Carcinoma

12 Cabrera, A., Tsukada, Y., Pickren, J. W., Moore, R., and Bross, I. D. J.: Development of lower genital carcinomas in patients with anal carcinomas; a more than casual relationship, Cancer 19:470-480, 1966.
13 Dillard, B. M., Spratt, J. S., Jr., Ackerman, L. V., and Butcher, H. R., Jr.: Epidermoid cancer of anal margin and canal; review of 79 cases, Arch. Surg. 16:772-776, 1963.
14 Grinvalsky, H. T., and Helwig, E. B.: Carcinoma of the anorectal junction. I. Histological consideration, Cancer 8:480-488, 1956.
15 Grodsky, L.: Current concepts on cloacogenic transitional cell anorectal cancers, J.A.M.A. 207:2057-2061, 1969.
16 Judd, E. S., Jr., and Burleigh, E. DeT., Jr.: Squamous-cell carcinoma of the anus; results of treatment, Surgery 37:220-228, 1955.
17 Klotz, R. G., Pamukooglu, T., and Souillard, D. H.: Transitional cloacogenic carcinoma of the anal canal, Cancer 20:1727-1745, 1967 (extensive bibliography).
18 Morson, B. C., and Pang, L. S. C.: Pathology of anal cancer, Proc. R. Soc. Med. 61:623-626, 1968.
19 Pang, L. S. C., and Morson, B. C.: Basaloid carcinoma of the anal canal, J. Clin. Pathol. 20:128-135, 1967.
20 Rainey, R.: The association of lymphogranuloma inguinale and cancer, Surgery 35:221-235, 1954.
21 Wittoesch, J. H., Woolner, L. B., and Jackman, R. J.: Basal cell epithelioma and basaloid lesions of the anus, Surg. Gynecol. Obstet. 104:75-80, 1957.

Malignant melanoma

22 Mason, J. K., and Helwig, E. B.: Ano-rectal melanoma, Cancer 19:39-50, 1966.
23 Morson, B. C., and Volkstädt, H.: Malignant melanoma of the anal canal, J. Clin. Pathol. 16:126-132, 1963.

Other lesions

24 Bonser, G. M., Raper, F. P., and Shuchsmith, H. S.: Epidermoid cysts in the region of the rectum and anus; a report of four cases, Br. J. Surg. 37:303-306, 1950.
25 Helwig, E. B., and Graham, J. H.: Anogenital (extramammary) Paget's disease; a clinicopathological study, Cancer 16:387-403, 1963.
26 Morales, A. R., Fine, G., Horn, R. C., Jr., and Watson, J. H. L.: Langerhans cells in a localized lesion of the eosinophilic granuloma type, Lab. Invest. 20:412-423, 1969.
27 Sharp, W. C., Jr., and Helwig, E. B.: Sarcoma botryoides (embryonal rhabdomyosarcoma) of the anus, J. Dis. Child. 97:845-848, 1959.
28 Teloh, H. A.: Apocrine adenoma of the anus, Cancer 7:367-372, 1954.

11 Major and minor salivary glands

Distribution of salivary gland tissue

Salivary gland tissue is distributed wide-ly. The major salivary glands are the parotid, submaxillary, and sublingual glands. The parotid gland is the largest, the submaxillary gland is about one-fourth its size, and the sublingual gland is about one-third the size of the submaxillary gland. The main duct of the parotid gland (Stensen's duct) empties into the oral cavity on the buccal mucosal surface. The ducts of both the submaxillary and sub-lingual glands open in the floor of the mouth.

Salivary gland tissue is present in many other locations, where it may give rise to inflammatory conditions, to benign tumors, and to malignant tumors. Its location in-fluences, to some extent, clinical signs and symptoms, pathology, and treatment. It can be found in the lips, more often in the upper than the lower lip, and is pres-ent throughout the oral cavity. Mucous glands are found in the buccal mucosa, gingiva, floor of the mouth, hard and soft palates, tonsillar areas, and tongue. The mucous-secreting glands of the trachea, bronchus, and the sinuses may be the site of tumors similar to those of the major salivary glands. Youngs and Scofield[3] have described eleven such cases, the most common location being along the medial border of the right sternocleidomas-toid muscle near the sternoclavicular joint. The majority of the cases were associated with cysts or sinus tracts, suggesting an embryologic relationship with the branchial apparatus.

Heterotopic salivary gland tissue can be found in lymph nodes within or near the parotid gland in both newborn infants and adults.[1] We have seen ectopic salivary gland tissue in the supraclavicular area on two occasions.[2]

Sialolithiasis

Calculi may form in the major ducts of the submaxillary, sublingual, and parotid glands. Those laminated calculi without a foreign body or bacterial nidus are com-posed of a crystalline compound apatite identified as carbonate apatite[4] (Fig. 525).

The stones are more frequently found in the ducts of the submaxillary gland than in those of the parotid gland be-cause the saliva is more supersaturated in

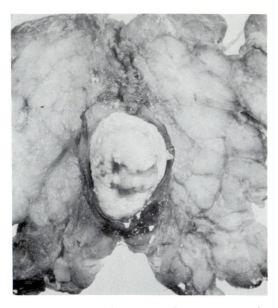

Fig. 525 Large radiopaque calculus within submaxillary gland. (WU neg. 48-4631.)

calcium salts.[5] The formation of calculi blocks secretion and produces swelling of the salivary gland tissue. If ductal obstruction persists, the gland becomes inflamed and indurated as acinar tissue is destroyed. With obstructed ducts of the submaxillary and lingual glands, tremendous induration can occur in the floor of the mouth that may be mistaken for neoplasm by palpation. The duct orifices become erythematous and swollen. Radiologic examination, including sialography, may demonstrate radiopaque obstructive masses. Microscopic examination of glands that have been affected by stones shows dilatation of ducts, at times squamous metaplasia of the epithelium, moderate to prominent chronic inflammation, and a variable destruction of acinar tissue (Fig. 526).

We have seen one instance in which

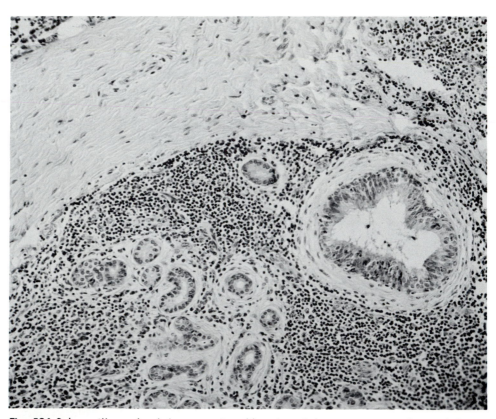

Fig. 526 Submaxillary gland demonstrating dilatation of ducts, acinar atrophy, and chronic inflammation. There were small stones in one of ducts leading to this area. (×150; WU neg. 57-3460A.)

there were numerous almost microscopic stones within small ducts with subsequent atrophy of the lobules. This process occurred in both parotid glands.

Irradiation effect

The submaxillary glands which are often included in the field of irradiation for tumors of the oral cavity, swell and become firm as a result of the radiation (Fig. 527). Microscopic examination shows decrease of acinar elements and the presence of chronic inflammatory cells in the interstitial tissue (Fig. 528). The lining of the duct epithelium may become squamous. Such changes are often mistaken clinically for metastatic carcinoma, leading to unnecessary radical therapy such as bilateral upper neck dissection.[6]

Mikulicz's disease

Mikulicz's disease (benign lymphoepithelial lesion) is characterized by an asymptomatic swelling of all or a combination of parotid, submaxillary, sublingual, and lacrimal glands.[13] This swelling slowly increases and can become quite striking. If the patient develops an infection, the process subsides only to recur. Mikulicz's

disease is one manifestation of a generalized symptom complex known as Sjögren's syndrome. Keratoconjunctivitis, xerostomia, rheumatoid arthritis, and hypergammaglobulinemia are common components of this syndrome.[9] Microscopically, the changes are similar in the salivary and lacrimal glands. There is preservation of the lobular architecture, abundant lymphoid tissue with germinal centers, and scattered "myoepithelial islands"[14] (Fig. 529). The latter appear as solid epithelial nests surrounded and occasionally infiltrated by lymphoid cells. They represent foci of myoepithelial proliferation within salivary ducts and are an important diagnostic feature.[11]

A rare complication of Mikulicz's disease is the development of malignant lymphoma within the involved salivary glands, later spreading to other structures.[7, 12, 15] Even rarer is the occurrence of what has been called the malignant variant of Mikulicz's disease.[10] We have seen several examples of this lesion, which

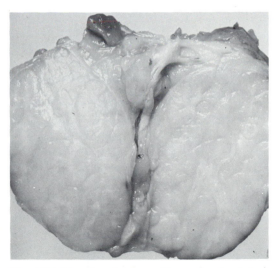

Fig. 527 Fibrosis of submaxillary gland related to irradiation. Note obliteration of normal pattern of salivary gland. (WU neg. 51-5879.)

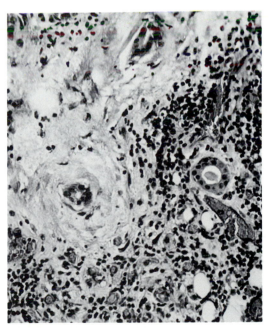

Fig. 528 Effect of irradiation on submaxillary gland. Note persistence of ducts, absence of acinar tissue, and presence of chronic inflammatory cells. (×230; WU neg. 50-686.)

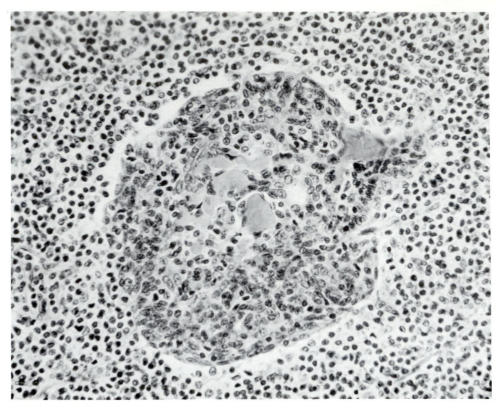

Fig. 529 Prominent myoepithelial proliferation of duct epithelium in patient with Mikulicz's disease. (×370; WU neg. 57-3679A; slide contributed by Dr. B. Castleman, Boston, Mass.)

is characterized by repeated local recurrences and eventually lymph node metastases. The low-power microscopic view is quite similar to that of Mikulicz's disease. High-power examination, however, reveals cytologic malignant features in the *epithelial component*, which are especially manifest in the specimens obtained from the recurrences. The patients present with a *unilateral* mass and lack the extrasalivary components of Sjögren's syndrome, two points to remember in the differential diagnosis. We prefer to think of this tumor as an undifferentiated carcinoma with lymphoid infiltration, unrelated to Mikulicz's disease.[8]

The generic term of Mikulicz's syndrome has been applied to the diffuse enlargement of salivary and lacrimal glands regardless of etiology. Mikulicz's disease, as just described, is the most common cause.

Malignant lymphoma, tuberculosis, sarcoidosis, and even syphilis occasionally are responsible.

Tumors
Benign tumors
Hemangioma

Capillary hemangioma is the most common salivary gland tumor in infants and children. It is often congenital and usually involves the parotid gland. It forms a diffuse, soft mass without fixation to the overlying skin. Microscopically, it is made up of anastomosing thin-walled capillaries growing between salivary ducts and acini. The solid proliferation of endothelial cells and the presence of mitotic figures may lead to a mistaken diagnosis of malignant tumor (Fig. 530). These lesions do not become malignant and can spontaneously regress.[16, 17]

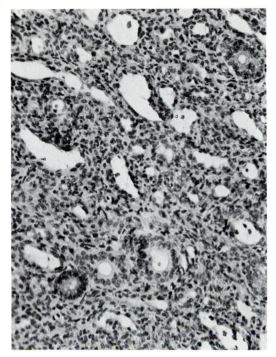

Fig. 530 Capillary hemangioma involving parotid salivary gland in child. Cellular hemangioma replaces salivary gland, but ducts can still be seen. (×210; WU neg. 50-688.)

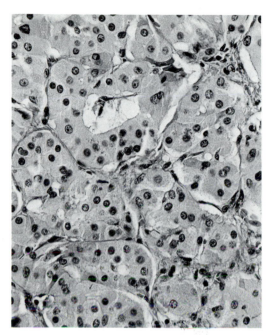

Fig. 531 Oxyphilic adenoma of parotid gland with large cells, granular cytoplasm, and uniform nuclei. This benign tumor arises from duct epithelium. (×400; WU neg. 52-2572.)

Lipoma and neurilemoma

Lipoma rarely involves the region of the parotid salivary gland. *Lipomatosis* is a diffuse nontumoral deposition of adipose tissue throughout the gland accompanied by enlargement of the organ. It has been seen with diabetes, cirrhosis, chronic alcoholism, malnutrition, and hormonal disturbances.[18] In some cases, this has been found to be preceded by hypertrophy of the serous acinar cells, interstitial edema, and ductular atrophy, a process known as *sialosis.*

Neurilemoma is a tumor of nerve sheath origin which, at times, can arise from one of the fine radicals of the facial nerve and be present in the region of the parotid salivary gland (see Chapter 23 for detailed description). It is a perfectly benign encapsulated neoplasm that often is incorrectly diagnosed as sarcoma when it occurs in the region of the parotid gland.[19] Failure to recognize this tumor as a benign neoplasm may result in needless sacrifice of the facial nerve.[20] We have now seen two instances in which this occurred.

Oxyphilic adenoma (oncocytoma) and papillary cystadenoma lymphomatosum (Warthin's tumor)

The oxyphilic adenoma and the papillary cystadenoma, benign neoplasms, should be discussed together because of their common histogenesis. Both arise from duct epithelium.

The *oxyphilic adenoma,* also called oncocytoma,[21, 23] grows slowly and does not become large. On microscopic examination, it is composed of large cells with eccentric nuclei and granular acidophilic cytoplasm (Fig. 531). The cytoplasm is granular because it is packed with mitochondria (Fig. 532). Some of these mitochondria contain large amounts of glycogen, whereas others are partitioned, suggesting division. This latter feature is apparently not seen in the

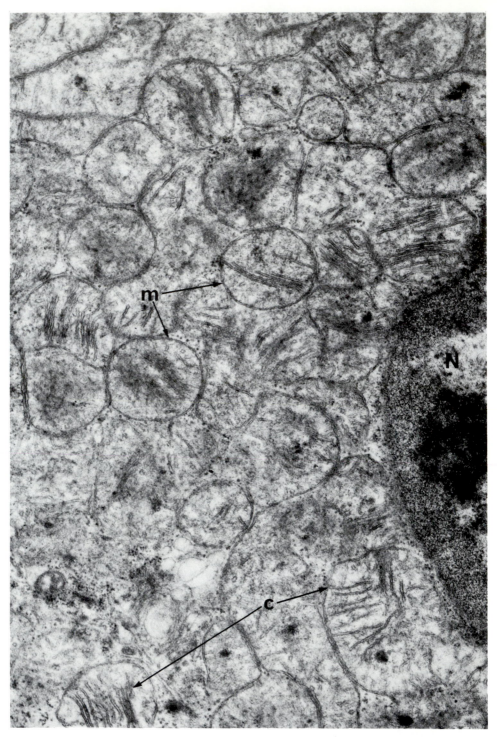

Fig. 532 Electron micrograph of mitochondria in oxyphilic adenoma. These cytoplasmic organelles are bounded by double membrane, **m.** From inner membrane, shelflike invaginations called cristae, **c,** extend into amorphous mitochondrial matrix. Enzymes of oxidative phosphorylation are concentrated in mitochondria. Portion of nucleus, **N,** is at right. (×31,000.)

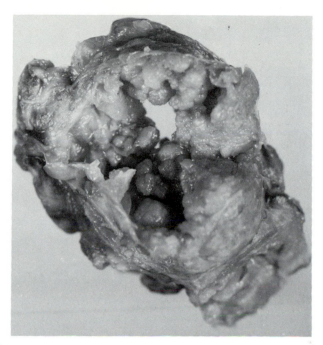

Fig. 533 Papillary cystadenoma lymphomatosum of parotid gland. Tumor has brownish gray color due to presence of lymphoid tissue. There are large cystic spaces present. (WU neg. 52-2950.)

mitochondria of the cells of Warthin's tumor.[27] Mitotic figures are absent, and cellular transition from normal lining cells of the ducts is seen. Focal collections of oncocytes may be seen in the normal gland adjacent to this tumor. Rarely, the entire gland is occupied by these nodules, a nonneoplastic process designated as oncocytosis.[30]

Simple excision is all that is necessary. These tumors do not become malignant and only rarely recur if incompletely removed. The differentiation between hyperplasia and tumor may be difficult. Oxyphilic cells increase in number with age. Although these tumors are predominantly within the parotid salivary gland, we have also seen such neoplasms within the submaxillary gland. A malignant variant of this tumor called oxyphilic carcinoma or malignant oncocytoma occurs.[22]

Papillary cystadenoma lymphomatosum differs from all other salivary gland tumors in two respects: it affects males in 80% to 90% of the cases and is bilateral in 10% to 15%. It comprises 70% of all bilateral salivary gland neoplasms.[29] Grossly, this

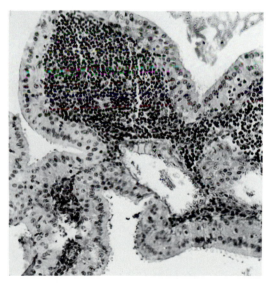

Fig. 534 Typical papillary cystadenoma lymphomatosum. Lymphoid tissue with germinal centers occurs beneath lining of large oxyphil cells. (Low power; WU neg. 48-6470.)

tumor rarely attains a large size. It does, however, become cystic and occasionally is fixed to the overlying skin and mistaken for a malignant neoplasm. On cross sec-

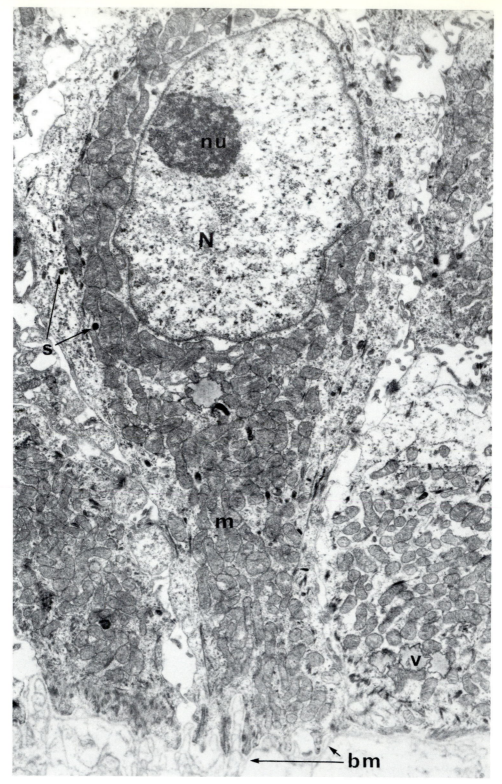

Fig. 535 Electron micrograph of oxyphil cells in epithelium of Warthin's tumor. Cell is set upon fine basement membrane, **bm.** Cytoplasm is packed with mitochondria, **m,** almost to exclusion of other organelles. Few vacuoles, **v,** containing lipid are present. Unidentified dense rods and spheres, **s,** are scattered through cytoplasm. Nucleolus, **nu,** is prominent. (×9,000.)

tion, it forms a cystic mass (Fig. 533). Between the fluid-filled cystic spaces, grayish lymphoid tissue can be seen.

Microscopically, lymphoid tissue is prominent, often with germinal centers. Covering the surface of this lymphoid tissue are large cells with granular cytoplasm similiar to the cells seen in oxyphilic adenoma (Fig. 534). Mucin-secreting cells and groups of sebaceous cells may be present. Occasionally, the lymphoid component is scanty or absent. By electron microscopy, the cytoplasm is packed with mitochondria[24] (Figs. 535 and 536).

There have been cases reported in the submaxillary gland, but it is probable that

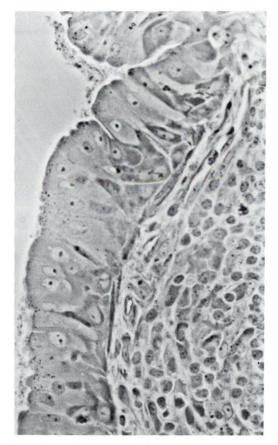

Fig. 536 Phase photomicrograph of Warthin's tumor of parotid gland. Fine lipid droplets in apical cytoplasm of pseudostratified columnar cells appear as black dots. Numerous mitochondria (Fig. 535) are barely discernible at this magnification. (×700.)

at least some of these represent tumors arising from the mandibular extension of the parotid salivary gland. Simple excision of these neoplasms is all that is necessary.[25, 28]

We have seen two instances of Warthin's tumor in which the whole neoplasm was necrotic, the appearance being that of a recent hemorrhagic infarct.[26]

Basal cell adenoma

Basal cell adenoma is a type of benign salivary gland tumor that has been recognized only recently. Grossly, it is encapsulated and often cystic. Solid, ductal, and trabecular structures are formed by epithelial cells. Typical features are the peripheral palisading of cells and the presence of abundant basal lamina material encircling the neoplastic nests, giving a pattern strongly reminiscent of dermal eccrine cylindroma and basal cell carcinoma[31] (Fig. 537). This tumor behaves in a benign fashion and must not be confused with adenoid cystic carcinoma.

Pleomorphic adenoma (mixed tumor)

Pleomorphic adenoma (mixed tumor) is the most frequent neoplasm of the salivary glands (Table 21). The incidence in the different glands is directly proportional to the volume of the gland. It is most frequent in women around 40 years of age but is also seen in children[33, 36] and in elderly persons of either sex.

Grossly, the tumor forms a rubbery, resilient mass that has a bosselated surface and may be large (Figs. 538 to 540). The consistency depends on the presence of cartilage and the degree of cellularity. Extensions of tumor invade the normal salivary gland tissue. On section, it has a somewhat glistening, mucoid appearance and, at times, zones of apparent cartilage. Bone is extremely rare.

Microscopically, there is no neoplasm that is so frequently diagnosed incorrectly as carcinoma by the neophyte in pathology. The bewildering pattern, the extreme cell-

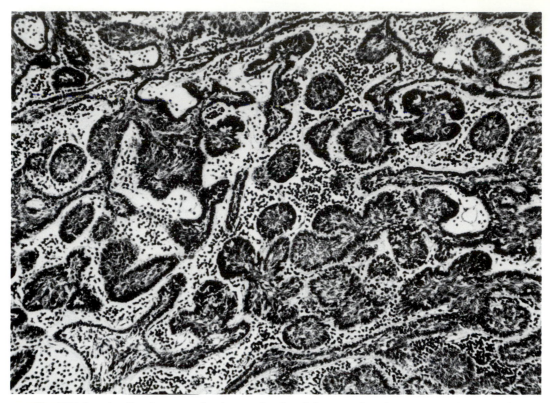

Fig. 537 Basal cell adenoma of salivary gland. Solid nests of uniform epithelial cells with prominent peripheral palisading can be seen. (×150; WU neg. 73-7482.)

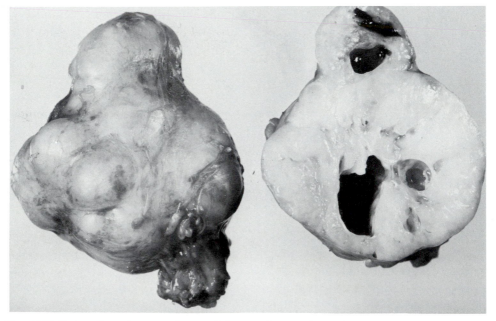

Fig. 538 External and cut surfaces of large pleomorphic adenoma of parotid salivary gland. Cut surface shows areas of cystic change, and external surface has typical bosselated appearance. (WU neg. 55-4349.)

ularity, the invasion of the capsule by the neoplasm all make it most confusing. The typical tumor is made up of glands that mimic the normal tubules of the gland. These glandular structures often have a double layer (Fig. 541). In the extremely well-differentiated tumor, keratinized epithelial plugs may be present within the lumen. There is a characteristic mucoid myxomatous stroma that may develop into cartilage.[39] This true cartilage developing from the connective tissue stroma is thought by Yates and Paget[40] to be related to an organizer produced by the epithelial elements. Two types of mucin may be formed: epithelial mucin from the glandlike areas and mesodermal mucus from the stroma.[32, 38] In the past the designation "semimalignant" was sometimes given to pleomorphic adenomas having areas of extreme cellularity (Fig. 542). However, follow-up studies have indicated that these tumors differ in no way from the ordinary variety. The adjective "semimalignant" therefore should be dropped. The rarity of mitotic figures and absence of necrosis are of help in the differential diagnosis with true malignant neoplasms. Something similar can be said of pleomorphic adeno-

mas having foci superficially resembling the adenoid cystic pattern. The presence of these foci does not influence the prognosis and therefore should be disregarded.

The *recurrence rate* of the pleomorphic adenoma depends on many factors, the most important of which is the operative treatment. In most series, it approaches 10%.[37] A high percentage of the recurrences appear during the first year following operation. Operation for recurrent tumor often fails. Further, recurrence is high (25%).[34] Surrounding the mass, other inconspicuous nodules may be attached to the main mass by threadlike filaments of neoplastic tissue. They may have the shape and the appearance of lymph nodes and be mistaken for nodal metastases by both the surgeon and the pathologist. Therefore, if the surgeon enucleates the tumor, small remnants will be left behind and, perhaps after many years, will recur. If the surgeon cuts through the tumor, he may implant it in the wound. We have seen such recurrences on numerous occasions. The microscopic pattern of the tumor is of no aid in estimating whether

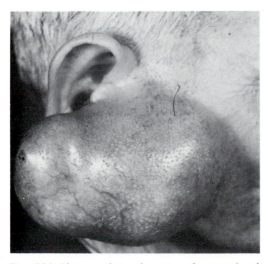

Fig. 539 Pleomorphic adenoma of parotid salivary gland of long duration. There was no ulceration or facial nerve paralysis. (WU neg. 50-3146.)

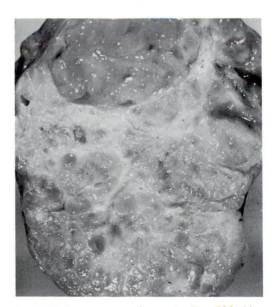

Fig. 540 Same tumor shown in Fig. 539. Note variegated appearance with areas of mucoid change and cartilage-like material. (WU neg. 50-3147.)

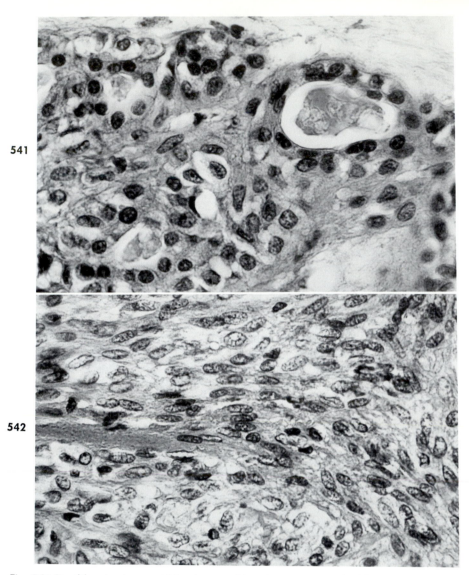

Fig. 541 Ductlike structures within pleomorphic adenoma. Note double cellular layer. (×380; WU neg. 51-801.)

Fig. 542 Area of prominent cellularity in pleomorphic adenoma. Such changes may be mistaken for malignancy. (×360; WU neg. 51-802.)

a given pleomorphic adenoma will or will not recur. The surgical removal must encompass the tumor so that there will be a margin of normal salivary gland tissue around its extracapsular removal. With this method of attack, the incidence of recurrence will be sharply reduced. Under exceptionally rare circumstances, a pleomorphic adenoma of ordinary benign microscopic appearance will metastasize to the lungs or other organs.[35]

Malignant tumors

Malignant tumors of the parotid salivary gland are much fewer in number than pleomorphic adenomas. The high-grade malignant varieties can be differentiated in most cases from the benign tumors on the basis of their clinical and gross characteristics (Fig. 543; Table 21). Unfortunately, this does not hold for the well-differentiated types, such as acinic cell carcinoma and low-grade mucoepider-

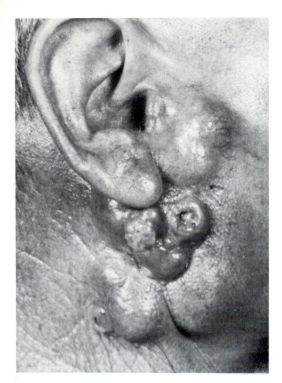

Fig. 543 Highly malignant salivary gland tumor. Note infiltration of skin with secondary ulceration. (EFSCH 48-10058.)

moid carcinoma. In these, the clinical presentation, as a rule, is indistinguishable from that of benign neoplasms.

Carcinoma in pleomorphic adenoma (malignant mixed tumor)

The incidence of malignant change in a pleomorphic adenoma is, to a great extent, influenced by the liberality of the pathologist. Recurrent pleomorphic adenomas are not usually malignant. They represent only persistence of a previously inadequately excised neoplasm. We believe that this is the usual cause rather than multiple foci of origin.

Usually the microscopic pattern of the recurrent or persistent tumor exactly mimics the previous excision (Figs. 544 and 545). Such recurrences may take up to fifty years to develop, but more often they recur repeatedly over a period of several decades. The highest percentage of local recrudescences appears in the first eighteen months following the primary operation.

There is no doubt that malignant transformation infrequently may take place in a pleomorphic adenoma (4.5% in the series reported by Moberger and Eneroth).[44] It is true that the proof of malignant change may be difficult. If a patient has a clinical history of a long-persisting tumor that suddenly begins to grow and microscopic examination shows an obvious malignant tumor and if there is no preexisting evidence of a benign tumor, it cannot be said that it arose in a pleomorphic adenoma purely on the basis of the clinical story. It is necessary to have microscopic evidence of a previously existing pleomorphic adenoma or to have malignant tumor and pleomorphic adenoma in the

Table 21 Differentiation between benign and malignant high-grade salivary gland tumors*

	Benign	Malignant
Clinical history		
Rate of growth	Slow (years)	Rapid (months)
Sex	More frequent in females	No essential difference
Age	Peak before 40 years of age	Peak about 50 years of age
Pain	Usually absent	Invariably present
Physical examination		
Fixation	Freely movable	Often fixed to skin, deep structures, bone
Facial nerve paralysis (parotid tumors)	Practically never	Common (about 33%)
Consistency	Firm, cystic, nodular	May be stony hard
Gross pathology	Well-circumscribed capsule; often shows cartilage	No capsule; invasion of bone and contiguous tissue
Metastases	Never	Rather frequent (lymph nodes, lungs, bone)

*From Ackerman, L. V., and del Regato, J. A.: Cancer, St. Louis, 1970, The C. V. Mosby Co.

same neoplasm. Such cases, in our experience, are few.[41]

Clinical evidences of malignant change in a pleomorphic adenoma are increase in growth, pain, facial paralysis, and other signs that accompany a primary malignant tumor of salivary gland origin. Microscopic evidence of malignant change includes prominence of the nuclei and nucleoli, many mitotic figures, some of them abnormal, and areas of infiltrative destructive growth.[43] Perineurial invasion and local and distant metastases indicate obvious cancer. Moberger and Eneroth[44] have pointed out that when a pleomorphic adenoma undergoes malignant transformation it can assume the appearance of any of the recognized variants of salivary gland carcinoma such as mucoepidermoid cancer and epidermoid cancer. The treatment is more dependent therefore on the type of carcinoma present

rather than on the fact that it arose from a pleomorphic adenoma.

In our experience, any pleomorphic adenoma that becomes malignant is usually one of extremely long duration that has been poorly treated by surgery and/or irradiation.[42]

Adenoid cystic carcinoma

The microscopic pattern of adenoid cystic carcinoma has certain well-defined characteristics. Nests and columns of cells are seen, often arranged concentrically around a glandlike space filled with PAS-positive material (Fig. 546). These are not true glandular spaces. They represent instead cavities containing replicated basal lamina material manufactured by the tumor cells.[49] The microscopic pattern is treacherous, for these tumors appear rather

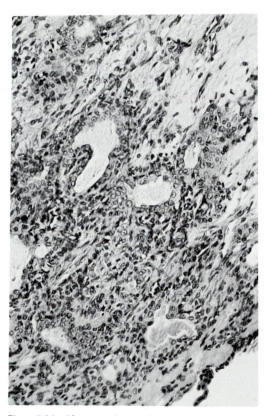

Fig. 544 Pleomorphic adenoma with typical microscopic pattern. (×200; WU neg. 52-2575.)

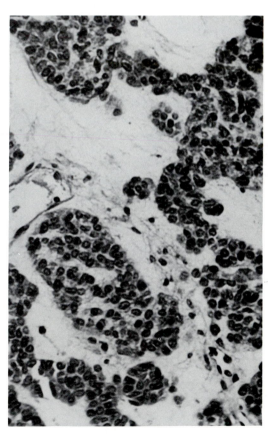

Fig. 545 Same tumor shown in Fig. 544 recurrent after nine-year interval. (×200; WU neg. 49-4000.)

benign. In our experience these neoplasms, if inadequately treated, inevitably cause death[18] (Fig. 547). Extreme microscopic variations may occur in which pseudoglandular spaces do not occur and only small nests of highly infiltrative tumor cells are seen. These cells may, on muci-

carmine stains, show small amounts of epithelial mucin. Such tumors stubbornly recur and show high proclivity for involvement of perineurial spaces[46, 47] (Fig. 548).

Adenoid cystic carcinomas frequently metastasize to the lungs without clinical evidence until seen on roentgenographic examination. If one of these tumors is diagnosed, a radical surgical approach should be used no matter how benign it appears under the microscope. Inoperable recurrences show excellent temporary regression to irradiation therapy.[45] This tumor often is incorrectly diagnosed as a carcinoma in pleomorphic adenoma.

Mucoepidermoid carcinoma

The mucoepidermoid tumor of the salivary glands has been well described by Foote and Becker.[50] Four cell types can be identified: mucin-producing, squamous, intermediate, and clear.[53] A low-grade type

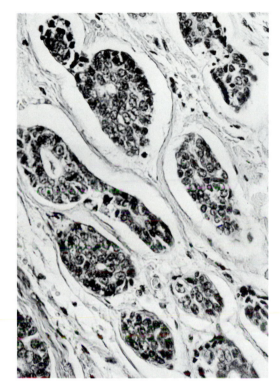

Fig. 546 Photomicrograph of adenoid cystic carcinoma of salivary gland. Note well-differentiated pattern. This tumor metastasized to lung. (×360; WU neg. 51-1954.)

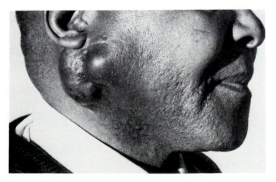

Fig. 547 Recurrent adenoid cystic carcinoma following conservative surgical therapy. Short time after reexcision, patient died as result of metastatic involvement to brain.

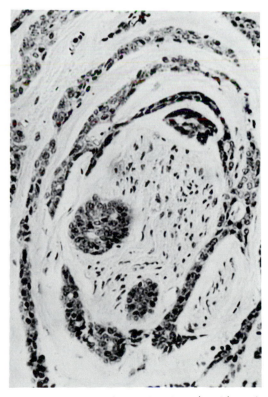

Fig. 548 Perineurial invasion in adenoid cystic carcinoma of salivary gland. (×320; EFSCH 43-1351.)

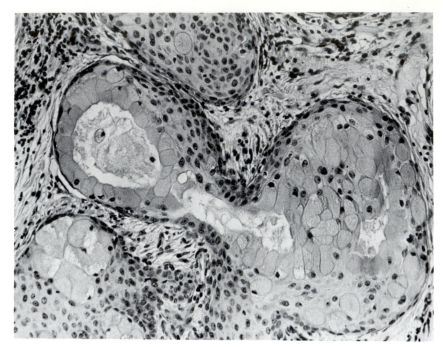

Fig. 549 Low-grade mucoepidermoid carcinoma. Well-differentiated squamous cells, together with mucin-producing cells, are present. (High power.)

and a high-grade type are described, with striking differences in prognosis.[51] The former presents grossly as a well-circumscribed mass having cystic areas with mucinous material. Microscopically, mucin-producing cells predominate (Fig. 549). The high-grade variety is grossly infiltrative and has less tendency to cyst formation. Atypical squamous cells predominate over the mucin-producing elements. When the keratin escapes into the interstitial tissue, it causes an inflammatory reaction.

In the series reported by Jakobsson et al.,[52] the determinate five-year survival rate was 98% for the low-grade variety and 56% for the high-grade type. Most of the latter showed their malignant behavior within the first five years following surgery, in contrast with the continuous fall in survival rate over a twenty-year period seen with adenoid cystic carcinoma and acinic cell adenocarcinoma.

Papillary adenocarcinoma

The papillary adenocarcinoma is a rare neoplasm. In the series reported by Blanck et al.,[54] it comprised 2.8% of all parotid tumors. In our experience, it grows large, has well-defined papillary structures, and may form mucin. Hemorrhage and necrosis are common in the large tumors (Fig. 550). This tumor can be confused with mucoepidermoid carcinoma, acinic cell carcinoma, and metastatic thyroid carcinoma. Blanck et al.[54] divided their cases into a high-grade and a low-grade variety on the basis of presence or absence of stromal invasion. The former had a poor prognosis, comparable to that of adenoid cystic carcinoma, whereas the latter did not differ prognostically from low-grade mucoepidermoid tumors.

Epidermoid carcinoma

Some epidermoid carcinomas probably arise from squamous metaplasia of the lining epithelium of the ducts. Overgrowth by the squamous component of mucoepidermoid carcinoma may be the origin of other tumors. At times, mucin stains may substantiate this supposition. These epidermoid carcinomas eventually infiltrate

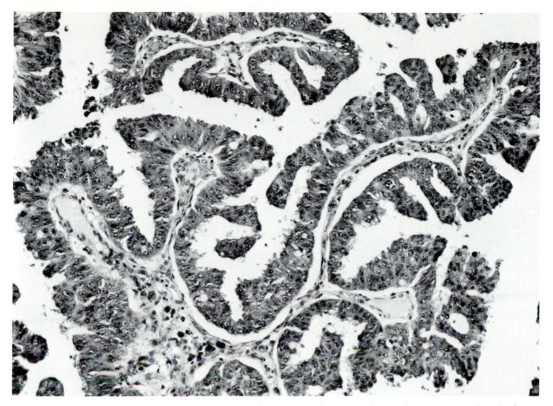

Fig. 550 Papillary adenocarcinoma of salivary gland. It was located in parotid gland of 65-year-old man. Note layering of cells and atypicality. (×150; WU neg. 73-4471.)

surrounding structures and grow rather rapidly.

Irradiation therapy may prove helpful. Many supposedly primary epidermoid carcinomas in reality represent metastases to nodes within the parotid salivary gland. These metastases arise frequently from an epidermoid carcinoma of the skin.

Acinic cell adenocarcinoma

Acinic cell adenocarcinoma is a rare, slowly growing carcinoma that at times closely resembles a renal cell carcinoma. The large majority of the cases are located in the parotid gland. Grossly, the tumors present as an encapsulated round mass with a solid, friable, grayish white cut surface. The tumor cells have a rather foamy cytoplasm (Figs. 551 and 552) but do not contain fat or epithelial mucin. Basophilic granularity of the cytoplasm, resembling that of the serous cells of salivary glands, is its most characteristic feature.[56] Glycogen is present in small amounts. Lymphoid tissue may be prominent. The ultrastructural patterns of this tumor have been studied by Echevarria.[55] It often is incorrectly diagnosed as metastatic carcinoma from the kidney and has even been described as an adenoma. In a series of thirty-seven cases examined by Eneroth and Jakobsson,[56] there was local recurrence in eleven and metastases in seven, four of them in regional lymph nodes. The determinate survival rate at five years was 89%, but it fell to 56% after twenty years. Radical surgical therapy is indicated. Neck dissection does not appear warranted.[57]

Carcinoma—unclassified

There remain a few highly undifferentiated carcinomas in which growth and infiltration are rapid. Usually their malignant nature is evident clinically. In a few

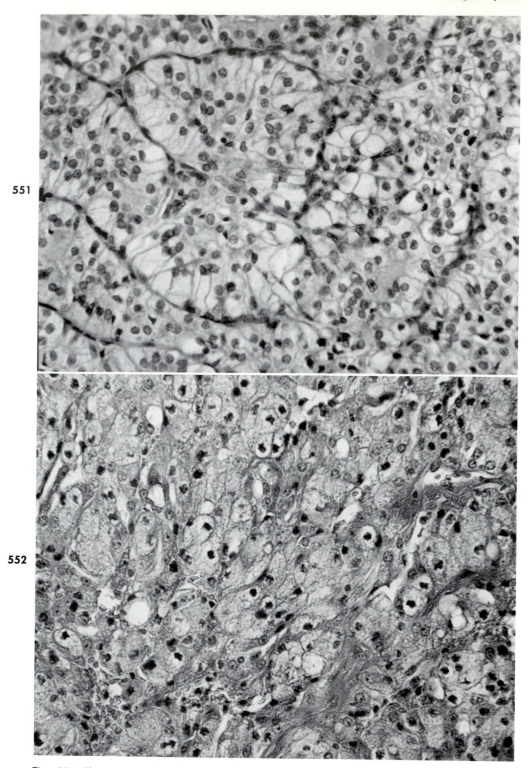

Fig. 551 Classic example of acinic cell adenocarcinoma occurring in 60-year-old woman. (×400; WU neg. 57-3160; slide contributed by Dr. W. Drake, St. Louis, Mo.)
Fig. 552 Acinic cell adenocarcinoma of parotid gland. Tumor cells are uniform and have small central nucleus and abundant basophilic cytoplasm which, in some places, appears granular and in others vacuolated. Mucin stain was negative. (×300; WU neg. 73-62.)

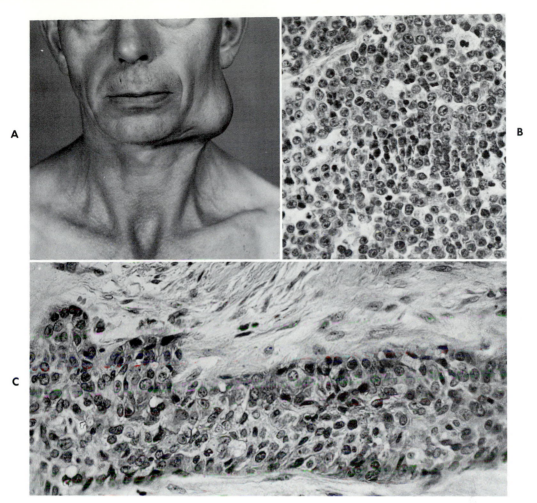

Fig. 553 A, Tumor of parotid salivary gland. There is no evidence of facial nerve paralysis. Tumor had been growing rather rapidly, and it was not known whether it was benign or malignant. **B,** Aspiration biopsy lesion illustrated in **A** showing highly undifferentiated malignant neoplasm. **C,** Same tumor shown in **A,** removed by radical resection, demonstrating ductal origin of neoplasm. **(A,** Courtesy Dr. F. Leidler, Houston, Texas; **B,** ×200; WU neg. 50-1421; **C,** ×200; WU neg. 50-1420.)

instances, however, we have seen highly undifferentiated carcinomas of the salivary gland that have grown rather slowly and produced a clinical picture suggesting a mixed tumor. This is the type of tumor which, in the past, was diagnosed as a sarcoma microscopically. Multiple sections often can prove the origin of this tumor from the epithelium of the ducts of the salivary glands (Fig. 553).

Malignant lymphoma

Malignant lymphomas occur primarily in the parotid salivary gland or the submax-illary gland but can arise in any of the salivary glands. Clinically, they present, more often than not, as unilateral masses instead of the diffuse enlargement seen in Mikulicz's disease. These lesions appear to grow slowly. The microscopic differentiation of lymphoid hyperplasia from true lymphoma may be extremely difficult. In this respect, these lesions resemble some of the lymphomas around the eye and its adnexa. Lymphomas may involve the salivary gland as a part of a disseminated process. Most of the cases are of the well-differentiated lymphocytic type, either nodular or diffuse.[58] Myoepithelial islands are not present. We have not seen Hodgkin's disease primary in the salivary glands.

Metastatic carcinoma

Metastatic cancer in the region of the parotid salivary gland can occur. It is particularly confusing there because of lymphoid tissue within the substance of the parotid gland. With growth of the tumor, a primary malignant neoplasm of the salivary gland can be mimicked exactly. The two tumors that most commonly metastasize to the parotid gland are epidermoid carcinoma of the skin and malignant melanoma.

Special considerations because of location

Tumors of the *parotid salivary gland* are of the highest significance and of great concern because of the intimate relation of the parotid gland to the facial nerve. The facial nerve may vary in its distribution.[65] The parotid is a bilobed structure with a broad superficial lobe and a smaller deep lobe, with the facial nerve running between the two lobes. Variations of this anatomy occur. A tumor involving the superior portion of the gland can be dissected free and the facial nerve saved. Complete removal of the parotid salivary gland with preservation of the facial nerve is possible.[59] Fortunately, most parotid tumors arise within the superficial lobe from either the tail (50%) or the anterior portion (25%) and can be safely removed by a superficial parotidectomy. The few cases that arise from the deep lobe often present as a pharyngeal mass without external evidence of tumor.[63]

In the treatment of malignant tumors of the salivary glands, plastic repair of the eyelid will be required subsequently. However, there should be no hesitation in sacrificing the facial nerve.

The most common tumor in the *submaxillary gland* area is a metastatic carcinoma in the submaxillary lymph nodes. The primary tumor usually arises within the oral cavity. If, however, there is a definite primary neoplasm of the submaxillary gland, it may be excised widely without fear of damage to nerves or other vital structures. The recurrence rate of submaxillary gland tumors is relatively high because of the gland's close relation to the mandible, which is the critical point in adequate removal of these neoplasms.

It must be remembered that a relatively high percentage of the tumors of the submaxillary gland are malignant as compared to the tumors of the parotid gland. In our series, one out of three parotid gland tumors was malignant, as compared to about an equal incidence of benign and malignant tumors in the submaxillary gland (Table 22).

In the series of 2,632 salivary gland tumors reported by Eneroth,[60] the incidence of malignancy was 17% for the parotid gland, 38% for the submaxillary gland, and 44% for the palate. He pointed out that a salivary gland tumor is twelve times more frequent in the parotid than in the submaxillary gland, a difference that cannot be explained on the basis of gland size alone. The most common malignant tumor of the parotid gland is mucoepidermoid carcinoma, followed by undifferentiated carcinoma and acinic cell carcinoma. On the other hand, adenoid cystic carcinoma comprises most submaxillary and palatal malignant salivary gland neoplasms. The prognosis of adenoid cystic carcinoma is directly dependent on its location, best when situated in the palate, intermediate when in the parotid gland, and worse in the submaxillary gland. The poor prognosis seen in the submaxillary location is shared by other tumor types.[61]

In the *lip*, salivary gland tumors usually occur in the upper lip because the mucous glands are most prominent there. They usually present as well-defined, rubbery, small tumors without ulceration. The diagnosis can often be made clinically. Careful excision is all that is necessary, since most of such neoplasms are benign.

Within the *oral cavity*, mixed tumors

can occur in any location, including gingiva, buccal mucosa, hard palate, soft palate, tonsillar area, and even tongue.[62] They

Table 22 Incidence of benign and malignant tumors of major salivary glands*

Parotid gland		
Pleomorphic adenoma		322
Primary benign	254	
Recurrent benign (persistent)	49	
Malignant	19	
Carcinoma		82
Epidermoid	30	
Acinic cell adenocarcinoma	2	
Undifferentiated	25	
Mucoepidermoid	25	
Adenocarcinoma		35
Simple	12	
Papillary	3	
Adenoid cystic	20	
Papillary cystadenoma lymphomatosum (Warthin's tumor)		34
Unilateral	30	
Bilateral	4	
Oxyphilic adenoma		4
Lipoma		1
Total in parotid gland		**478**
Submandibular gland		
Pleomorphic adenoma		31
Primary benign	25	
Recurrent benign (persistent)	5	
Malignant	1	
Carcinoma		12
Epidermoid	4	
Undifferentiated	6	
Mucoepidermoid	2	
Adenocarcinoma		12
Simple	1	
Adenoid cystic	11	
Papillary cystadenoma lymphomatosum (Warthin's tumor)		1
Total in submandibular gland		**56**
Other locations		
Pleomorphic adenoma		19
Primary benign	17	
Malignant	2	
Carcinoma		7
Undifferentiated	2	
Acinic cell adenocarcinoma	1	
Mucoepidermoid	4	
Adenocarcinoma		13
Simple	1	
Adenoid cystic	12	
Total in other locations		**39**
Grand total		**573**

*Surgical Pathology Laboratory, Washington University School of Medicine, St. Louis, Mo.

are distributed in frequency almost proportional to the amount of mucous glandular tissue. They are, therefore, most common in the hard palate.[64] For the most part, these tumors form rather firm, rubbery, nonulcerated masses. The diagnosis may not be suspected, and at times the incisional biopsy may be too superficial to reveal the tumor. Incisional biopsy, however, can make the diagnosis. Once the diagnosis is assured, the tumor should be excised, if possible, with a normal margin of tissue. All types of salivary gland tumors can occur in the oral cavity.[64]

Biopsy

We have already commented on the necessity of biopsy for tumors of salivary gland origin within the oral cavity, indicating the need for a small, deep incisional biopsy. There is usually little necessity for biopsy of submaxillary gland tumors. The greatest difficulty is in the region of the parotid salivary gland, where it would be helpful to know the exact pathology before embarking upon surgery. It is understandable that biopsy would not be required for the obviously malignant or obviously benign tumors. It is only in the borderline group that it is of such great importance.

Needle biopsy of salivary gland tumors for accurate diagnosis prior to contemplated surgery has been used. The microscopic diagnosis of squamous carcinoma, undifferentiated tumors, and pleomorphic adenomas is not difficult. However, on several occasions we have not been able to make the differential diagnosis between an adenoid cystic carcinoma and a benign neoplasm. Furthermore, we have demonstrated implantation along the needle tract. Therefore, we have found the use of this diagnostic procedure limited.

In several instances, careful incisional biopsy has been done. If the tumor proved to be malignant, then this area of biopsy could be encompassed by the subsequent surgical procedure.

We have also not hesitated to do frozen

section in some of these debatable salivary gland tumors. In some instances, we have been able to make a definitive diagnosis of a malignant or a benign salivary gland tumor. In the malignant group, particularly of the high-grade varieties, it is practically mandatory to combine the surgical procedure with a radical neck dissection. In one instance, fixation to the skin was present, and frozen section revealed a benign papillary cystadenoma rather than carcinoma. The interpretation of frozen section of salivary gland tumors is difficult and requires considerable experience and judgment.

Fig. 554 Distribution of recurrent tumor nodules (shown as black dots), as demonstrated by careful histologic study of reexcision of pleomorphic adenoma which, at time of first operation, had apparently been enucleated. Surgical scar measured 3.5 cm. (Courtesy Dr. F. Leidler, Houston, Texas.)

Clinicopathologic correlation

Recurrence in pleomorphic adenomas is almost entirely dependent on the adequacy of the primary operation. Inadequate procedures such as enucleation of the tumor and contamination of the operative field will be followed by a high recurrence rate

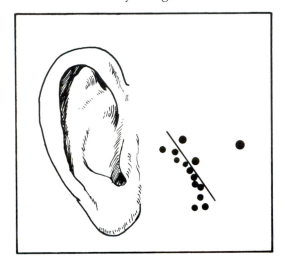

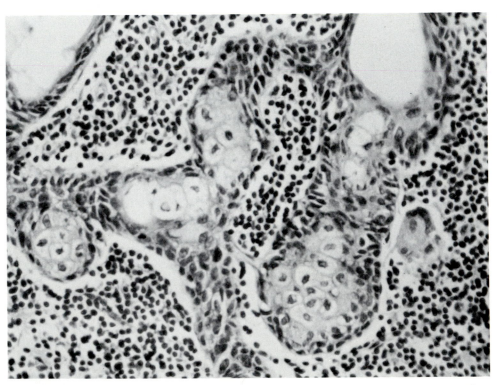

Fig. 555 Sebaceous gland hyperplasia associated with lymphocytic infiltration within parotid gland. (×440; WU neg. 57-98A.)

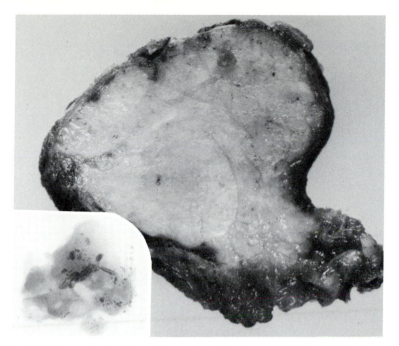

Fig. 556 Amyloid "tumor" of submaxillary gland. Lesion was bilateral. Note homogeneous, waxy appearance. **Inset,** X-ray appearance of surgical specimen, showing focal coarse foci of calcification. (WU neg. 72-678.)

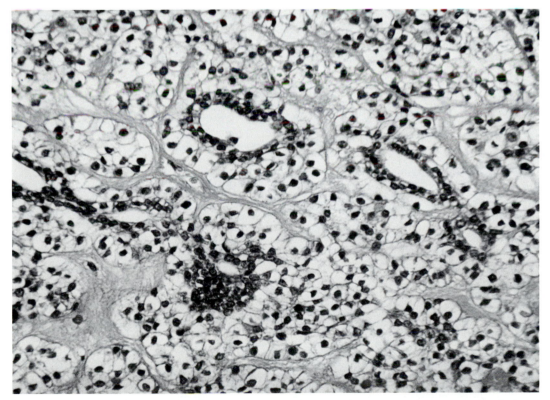

Fig. 557 Clear cell adenoma of parotid gland. Glandular formations are seen surrounded by large collections of clear cells. (×350; WU neg. 70-9779.)

(Fig. 554). This recurrence rate is more dependent on the quality of the surgery than on the microscopic pattern of the tumor. Recurrences may occur over an exceedingly long time period. All patients with pleomorphic adenomas must be followed for life. Few patients with pleomorphic adenomas ever die of this disease. In 296 traced patients followed at the Mayo Clinic, only four died of tumor.[66]

Primary irradiation therapy should be considered for an obviously inoperable tumor rather than inadequate resection followed by postoperative irradiation.

Other lesions

We have seen several other lesions that have been mistaken clinically for a neoplasm. These include a single instance of *cat-scratch disease* involving a lymph node within the parotid gland, two instances of *epidermal inclusion cysts* in the region of the parotid gland which were thought to be carcinoma, a *pilomatrixoma* clinically mistaken for pleomorphic adenoma, and finally an area of deep induration caused by a *healed abscess* that had been drained twenty years previously. *Sebaceous glands* are rarely included in the parotid gland (Fig. 555). They can be present in a variety of salivary gland tumors.[69] We have seen two instances of benign tumor which we designated as *sebaceous lymphadenoma*. The malignant counterpart of this condition (i.e., *sebaceous carcinoma*) has been described by Silver and Goldstein.[70] *Amyloidosis* can occur as part of a generalized process or as a localized pseudoneoplastic mass (so-called amyloid tumor) (Fig. 556). We have seen a case of *plasmacytoma* of the submaxillary gland, later developing typical bone x-ray changes of multiple myeloma.[68] Two congenital epithelial parotid tumors were designated as *embryoma* by Vawter and Tefft.[71] We have recently encountered three examples of a salivary gland tumor composed of small tubules surrounded by prominent clear cells in the position normally occupied by the myoepithelial cells (Fig. 557). The

behavior of this *clear cell adenoma* has been that of a benign neoplasm.

REFERENCES

Distribution of salivary gland tissue

1 Brown, R. B., Gaillard, R. A., and Turner, J. A.: Significance of aberrant or heterotopic parotid gland tissue in lymph nodes, Ann. Surg. 138:850-856, 1953.
2 Jernstrom, P., and Prietto, C. A.: Accessory parotid gland tissue at base of neck, Arch. Pathol. 73:473-480, 1962.
3 Youngs, L. A., and Scofield, H. H.: Heterotopic salivary gland tissue in the lower neck, Arch. Pathol. 83:550-556, 1967.

Sialolithiasis

4 Blatt, I. M., Denning, R. M., Zumberge, J. H., and Maxwell, J. H.: Studies in sialolithiasis, Ann. Otol. Rhinol. Laryngol. 67:595-617, 1958.
5 Husted, E.: Sialolithiasis, Acta Chir. Scand. 105:161-171, 1953.

Irradiation effect

6 Evans, J. C., and Ackerman, L. V.: Irradiated and obstructed submaxillary salivary glands simulating cervical lymph node metastasis, Radiology 62:550-555, 1954.

Mikulicz's disease

7 Anderson, L. G., and Talal, N.: The spectrum of benign to malignant lymphoproliferation in Sjögren's syndrome, Clin. Exp. Immunol. 9:199-221, 1971.
8 Arthaud, J. B.: Anaplastic parotid carcinoma ("malignant lymphoepithelial lesion") in seven Alaskan natives, Am. J. Clin. Pathol. 57:275-289, 1972.
9 Bloch, K. J., Buchanan, W. W., Wohl, M. J., and Bunim, J. J.: Sjögren's syndrome: a clinical, pathological and serological study of sixty-two cases, Medicine (Baltimore) 44:187-231, 1965 (extensive bibliography).
10 Gravanis, M. B., and Giansanti, J. S.: Malignant histopathologic counterpart of the benign lymphoepithelial lesion, Cancer 26:1332-1342, 1970.
11 Hamperl, H.: The myothelia (myoepithelial cells): normal state; regressive changes; hyperplasia; tumors, Curr. Top. Pathol. 53:161-220, 1970.
12 Miller, D. G.: The association of immune disease and malignant lymphoma, Ann. Intern. Med. 66:507-521, 1967.
13 von Mikulicz, J.: Concerning a peculiar symmetrical disease of the lacrimal and salivary glands, Med. Classics 2:165-186, 1937.
14 Morgan, W. S., and Castleman, B.: A clinico-

pathologic study of "Mikulicz's disease," Am. J. Pathol. **29**:471-503, 1953.

15 Talal, N., Sokoloff, L., and Barth, W. F.: Extrasalivary lymphoid abnormalities in Sjögren's syndrome (reticulum cell sarcoma, "pseudolymphoma," macroglobulinemia), Am. J. Med. **43**:50-64, 1967.

Tumors
Benign tumors
Hemangioma

16 Caldwell, R. A.: A case of congenital capillary hemangioma of the parotid gland, Br. J. Surg. **39**:261-263, 1951.

17 McFarland, J. A.: A congenital capillary angioma of the parotid gland, Arch. Pathol. **9**: 820-827, 1930 (extensive bibliography).

Lipoma and neurilemoma

18 Davidson, D., Leibel, B. S., and Berris, B.: Asymptomatic parotid gland enlargement in diabetes mellitus, Ann. Intern. Med. **70**:31-38, 1969.

19 Katz, A. D., Passy, V., and Kaplan, L.: Neurogenous neoplasms of major nerves of face and neck, Arch. Surg. **103**:51-56, 1971.

20 Roos, D. B., Byars, L. T., and Ackerman, L. V.: Neurilemomas of the facial nerve presenting as parotid gland tumors, Ann. Surg. **144**:258-262, 1956.

Oxyphilic adenoma (oncocytoma) and papillary cystadenoma lymphomatosum (Warthin's tumor)

21 Ackerman, L. V.: Oncocytoma of the parotid gland, Arch. Pathol. **36**:508-511, 1943.

22 Bazaz-Malik, G., and Gupta, D. N.: Metastasizing (malignant) oncocytoma of the parotid gland, Z. Krebsforsch. **70**:193-197, 1968.

23 Hamperl, H.: Benign and malignant oncocytoma, Cancer **15**:1019-1027, 1962.

24 McGavran, M. H.: The ultrastructure of papillary cystadenoma lymphomatosum of the parotid gland, Virchows Arch. Pathol. Anat. **338**: 195-202, 1965.

25 Meza-Chavez, L.: Oxyphilic granular cell adenoma of the parotid gland (oncocytoma); report of five cases and study of oxyphilic granular cells (oncocytes) in normal parotid glands, Am. J. Pathol. **25**:523-547, 1949.

26 Patey, D. H., and Thackray, A. C.: Infected adenolymphoma: a new parotid syndrome, Br. J. Surg. **57**:569-572, 1970.

27 Tandler, B., Hutter, R. V. P., and Erlandson, R. A.: Ultrastructure of oncocytoma of the parotid gland, Lab. Invest. **23**:567-580, 1970.

28 Thompson, A. S., and Bryant, H. C., Jr.: Histogenesis of papillary cystadenoma lymphomatosum (Warthin's tumor) of the parotid salivary gland, Am. J. Pathol. **26**:807-849, 1950.

29 Turnbull, A. D., and Frazell, E. L.: Multiple tumors of the major salivary glands, Am. J. Surg. **118**:787-789, 1969.

30 Schwartz, I. S., and Feldman, M.: Diffuse multinodular oncocytoma ("oncocytosis") of the parotid gland, Cancer **23**:636-640, 1969.

Basal cell adenoma

31 Batsakis, J. B.: Basal cell adenoma of the parotid gland, Cancer **29**:226-230, 1972.

Pleomorphic adenoma (mixed tumor)

32 Azzopardi, J. G., and Smith, O. D.: Salivary gland tumours and their mucins, J. Pathol. Bacteriol. **77**:131-140, 1959.

33 Byars, L. T., Ackerman, L. V., and Peacock, E.: Tumors of salivary gland origin in children; a clinical pathologic appraisal of 24 cases, Ann. Surg. **146**:40-52, 1957.

34 Frazell, E. L.: Clinical aspects of tumors of the major salivary glands, Cancer **7**:637-659, 1954.

35 Gerughty, R. M., Scofield, H. H., Brown, F. M., and Hennigar, G. R.: Malignant mixed tumors of salivary gland origin, Cancer **24**:471-486, 1969.

36 Krolls, S. O., Trodahl, J. N., and Boyers, R. C.: Salivary gland lesions in children; a survey of 430 cases, Cancer **30**:145-155, 1972.

37 Malett, K. J., and Harrison, M. S.: The recurrence of salivary gland tumours, J. Laryngol. Otol. **85**:439-448, 1971.

38 Quintarelli, G., and Robinson, L.: The glycosaminoglycans of salivary gland tumors, Am. J. Pathol. **51**:19-37, 1967.

39 Welsh, R. A., and Meyer, A. T.: Mixed tumors of human salivary gland; histogenesis, Arch. Pathol. **85**:433-447, 1968.

40 Yates, P. O., and Paget, G. E.: A mixed tumor of salivary gland showing bone formation with a histochemical study of the tumor mucoids, J. Pathol. Bacteriol. **64**:881-888, 1952.

Malignant tumors
Carcinoma in pleomorphic adenoma (malignant mixed tumor)

41 Beahrs, O. H., Woolner, L. B., Kirklin, J. W., and Devine, K. D.: Carcinomatous transformation of mixed tumors of the parotid gland, Arch. Surg. **75**:605-614, 1957.

42 Buxton, R. W., Maxwell, J. H., and Cooper, D. R.: Tumors of the parotid gland, Laryngoscope **59**:565-594, 1949.

43 Eneroth, C. M.: Histological and clinical aspects of parotid tumours, Acta Otolaryng. (Stockholm) **191**(suppl.):1-99, 1964 (extensive bibliography).

44 Moberger, J. G., and Eneroth, C.-M.: Malignant mixed tumors of the major salivary glands; special reference to the histologic

structure in metastases, Cancer **21**:1198-1211, 1968.

Adenoid cystic carcinoma

45 Baclesse, F.: Radiosensitivity and metastases observed in course of cylindromas and mixed tumors, Bull. Cancer (Paris) **29**:260-274, 1940-1941.
46 McDonald, J. R., and Havens, F. Z.: A study of malignant tumors of glandular nature found in the nose, throat and mouth, Surg. Clin. North Am. **28**:1087-1106, 1948.
47 Quattlebaum, F. W., Dockerty, M. B., and Mayo, C. W.: Adenocarcinoma, cylindroma type, of the parotid gland, Surg. Gynecol. Obstet. **82**:342-347, 1946.
48 Smith, L. C., Lane, N., and Rankow, R. M.: Cylindroma (adenoid cystic carcinoma), Am. J. Surg. **110**:519-526, 1965.
49 Tandler, B.: Ultrastructure of adenoid cystic carcinoma of salivary gland origin, Lab. Invest. **24**:504-512, 1971.

Mucoepidermoid carcinoma

50 Foote, F. W., and Becker, W. F.: Mucoepidermoid tumors of the salivary glands, Ann. Surg. **122**:820-844, 1945.
51 Healey, W. V., Perzin, K. H., and Smith, L.: Mucoepidermoid carcinoma of salivary gland origin; classification, clinical-pathologic correlation, and results of treatment, Cancer **26**:368-388, 1970.
52 Jakobsson, P. Å., Blanck, C., and Eneroth, C.-M.: Mucoepidermoid carcinoma of the parotid gland, Cancer **22**:111-124, 1968.
53 Woolner, L. B., Pettet, J. R., and Kirklin, J. W.: Mucoepidermoid tumors of major salivary glands, Am. J. Clin. Pathol. **24**:1350-1362, 1954.

Papillary adenocarcinoma

54 Blanck, C., Eneroth, C.-M., and Jakobsson, P. Å.: Mucus-producing adenopapillary (non-epidermoid) carcinoma of the parotid gland, Cancer **28**:676-685, 1971.

Acinic cell adenocarcinoma

55 Echevarria, R. A.: Ultrastructure of the acinic cell carcinoma and clear cell carcinoma of the parotid gland, Cancer **20**:563-571, 1967.
56 Eneroth, C.-M., and Jakobsson, P. A.: Acinic cell carcinoma of the parotid gland, Cancer **19**:1761-1772, 1966.
57 Godwin, J. T., Foote, F. W., Jr., and Frazell, E. L.: Acinic cell adenocarcinoma of the parotid gland; report of 27 cases, Am. J. Pathol. **30**:465-477, 1954.

Malignant lymphoma

58 Freedman, I.: Electron microscopy in head and neck oncology, Acta Otolaryngol. (Stockholm) **71**:115-122, 1971.

Special considerations because of location

59 Bailey, H.: The surgical anatomy of the parotid gland, Br. Med. J. **2**:245-248, 1948.
60 Eneroth, C.-M.: Incidence and prognosis of salivary-gland tumours at different sites; a study of parotid, submandibular and palatal tumours in 2632 patients, Acta Otolaryngol. (Stockholm) **263**:174-178, 1970.
61 Eneroth, C.-M., Hjertman, L., and Moberger, G.: Malignant tumours of submandibular gland, Acta Otolaryngol. (Stockholm) **64**:514-536, 1967.
62 Fine, G., Marshall, R. B., and Horn, R. C., Jr.: Tumors of the minor salivary glands, Cancer **13**:653-669, 1960.
63 Frazell, E. L.: Clinical aspects of tumors of the major salivary glands, Cancer **7**:637-659, 1954.
64 Hobaek, A.: Intraoral mucous- and salivary gland mixed tumors, Acta Radiol. **32**:229-247, 1949.
65 McCormack, L. J., Cauldwell, E. W., and Anson, B. J.: The surgical anatomy of the facial nerve; with special reference to the parotid gland, Surg. Gynecol. Obstet. **80**:620-630, 1945.

Clinicopathologic correlation

66 Kirklin, J. W., McDonald, J. R., Harrington, S. W., and New, G. B.: Parotid tumors; histopathology, clinical behavior, and end results, Surg. Gynecol. Obstet. **92**:721-733, 1951.

Other lesions

67 McGavran, M. H., Bauer, W. C., and Ackerman, L. V.: Sebaceous lymphadenoma of the parotid salivary gland, Cancer **13**:1185-1187, 1960.
68 Pascoe, H. R., and Dorfman, R. F.: Extramedullary plasmacytoma of the submaxillary gland, Am. J. Clin. Pathol. **51**:501-507, 1969.
69 Rawson, A. J., and Horn, R. C., Jr.: Sebaceous glands and sebaceous gland-containing tumors of parotid salivary gland, with consideration of histogenesis of papillary cystadenoma lymphomatosum, Surgery **27**:93-101, 1950.
70 Silver, H., and Goldstein, M. A.: Sebaceous cell carcinoma of the parotid region; a review of the literature and a case report, Cancer **19**:1773-1779, 1966.
71 Vawter, G. F., and Tefft, M.: Congenital tumors of the parotid gland, Arch. Pathol. **82**:242-245, 1966.

12 Liver

Biopsy

Needle biopsy of the liver is a useful diagnostic procedure. Its use may obviate a major operation or resolve an obscure medical diagnostic problem. The Menghini type of needle is the safest instrument to use and produces adequate specimens with a minimum of distortion.[4, 5] Rapid fixation and multiple, well-stained, thin (3μ to 4μ) sections are necessary for accurate interpretation. At the time of biopsy, provisions should be made for cultures and cytochemical or electron microscopic studies if the clinical situation suggests that they might provide valuable information. Normal baselines are available on which to evaluate minor morphologic alterations of the human hepatocyte.[3]

Needle biopsy is contraindicated when trained operators are not available, in patients with uncorrected bleeding disorders, and in patients with long-standing extrahepatic biliary obstruction. When performed by experienced operators, complications are unusual and mortality very rare. Menghini[4] reported a personal experience of 2,000 needle biopsies without mortality. Thaler[9] encountered one fatal complication for every 5,845 biopsies in a total of 23,382 cases, and Lindner[2] estimated on fatal case for every 6,615 biopsies in a total of 79,381.

The surgeon who plans biopsy of the liver should perform the formal incisional biopsy immediately upon entering the peritoneal cavity. If he delays biopsy until the end of an operative procedure, inflammatory infiltration and distortion of the parenchyma beneath the liver capsule and even infarction caused by abdominal retractors may be present. Long surgical procedures produce focal areas of hepatic necrosis microscopically.[8] The subcapsular area is not representative of the entire organ. Marked fibrosis in this portion of the liver may coexist with minimal or no changes in the remaining parenchyma. Therefore the operator should perform not only incisional biopsy, but also a deeper parenchymal needle biopsy in all diagnostically difficult cases. If it is the surgeon's belief that only one type of biopsy is indicated, the deep needle biopsy is preferred.

The indications for liver biopsy can be divided into four major categories: (1) diagnosis of cases in which clinical and laboratory studies are equivocal, (2) evaluation of the degree of the morphologic

521

damage present, (3) monitoring of the evolution of a disease and its response to therapy, and (4) determination of hepatic involvement in systemic disorders—metabolic, granulomatous, or neoplastic. Generally speaking, in patients with acute jaundice, the clinical and laboratory findings often provide a definitive diagnosis. It is in patients with chronic jaundice or hepatomegaly that needle biopsy is most often required for the diagnosis.[1]

We have found needle biopsy highly useful in acute viral hepatitis, chronic active hepatitis, cirrhosis, alcoholic hepatitis, primary and metastatic neoplasms, granulomatous processes, hemochromatosis, and amyloidosis.

Difficulties arise in classifying types of cirrhosis, in separating intrahepatic from extrahepatic cholestasis, in evaluating neonatal jaundice, and in recognizing certain types of drug-induced hepatic damage. However, even in these disease processes, accurate diagnosis can often be made if clinical and laboratory data are carefully correlated with histologic changes.

The pathologist should not attempt diagnosis by needle biopsy without having all clinical and laboratory data available. Such information is required because the cellular findings in various liver diseases vary with the stage of the process and actually shade from one disease process to another.

There is good correlation between the clinical state of the patient and the liver function tests, but very little between either of these two parameters and the microscopic appearance of the liver.[7] It is not uncommon to encounter prominent structural derangement of the liver parenchyma in a patient with only minimal clinical evidence of liver disease. As Popper et al.[6] emphasized, the morphologic changes in the liver persist long after there has been pronounced clinical and laboratory improvement.

Viral hepatitis

Needle biopsy is not necessary for the diagnosis of acute viral hepatitis unless the clinical and laboratory findings are atypical. Histologically, the disease is panlobular. It manifests itself by a combination of degenerative, inflammatory, and regenerative changes.[12, 18] The former are mainly represented by isolated liver cell necrosis in the form of "acidophilic (Councilman-like) bodies." These are necrotic hepatocytes, often found free in tissue spaces or even in sinusoids.[20] Balloon degeneration of hepatocytes is also common. This is probably the result of extreme dilatation of the granular endoplasmic reticulum.[27] The inflammatory changes consist of periportal mononuclear (mainly lymphocytic) inflammation and diffuse hyperplasia of Kupffer cells (Fig. 558). Neutrophils and eosinophils are scanty or absent. Evidence of regeneration is seen even in early stages of the disease in the form of anisocytosis, mitotic activity, and increase in the number of binucleate hepatocytes. None of these changes are, by themselves, diagnostic of viral hepatitis. In approximately 50% of the cases, central cholestasis is present. If the other changes are minimal, the differentiation from extrahepatic biliary obstruction or drug-induced changes may be difficult. Inconstant changes of acute viral hepatitis include accumulation of ceroid and iron in macrophages and proliferation of bile ducts.[25] The electron microscopic appearance of acute viral hepatitis has been well described.[26, 27, 30]

Cooper et al.[15] showed that anicteric viral hepatitis is not only frequent but often becomes chronic and may progress to significant liver damage. In a small percentage of cases of viral hepatitis, the parenchymal necrosis affects a group of adjacent hepatocytes within a lobule and is therefore designated as confluent or submassive. It may be centrilobular or extend from centrilobular areas to portal tracts. The collapse of these foci leads to the condensation of the existing connective tissue fibers, a process designated as bridging. Over 50% of the patients with this finding either die or develop cirrhosis.[14, 16] For the still rarer instances in which the necrosis involves the whole lobule, the terms massive ne-

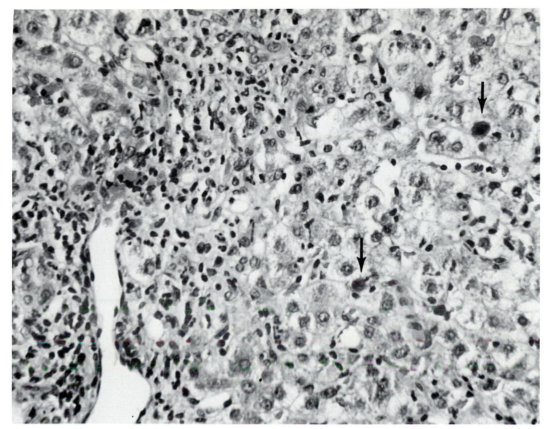

Fig. 558 Viral hepatitis six months following administration of blood transfusions in 36-year-old woman. Australia antigen was present. Liver shows marked inflammatory portal inflammation and panlobular disease, evidenced by hyperplasia of Kupffer cells, swollen hepatocytes, and scattered acidophilic bodies (arrows). (×350; WU neg. 73-366.)

crosis and *fulminant hepatitis* have been used.[11, 21] It should be emphasized that not all cases of massive liver necrosis are of viral origin. Diverse drugs, anesthetizing agents, and shock may result in similar changes.[10]

Approximately one-half of the patients with acute viral hepatitis have circulating Australia antigen (hepatitis-associated antigen or HB-Ag) which probably represents the protein coat or capsid material of a small virus.[28] Its discovery has rendered obsolete the classical division of viral hepatitis into an "infectious" form and a "serum" form. It now appears that there are at least two viruses that can cause the disease, both of which can be transmitted by two or more routes of infection. One of these viruses (called MS-2) can be detected by the presence of the Aus-

tralia antigen; the other(s) cannot.[24, 29] In about 95% of the cases, this antigen disappears four to five weeks after the onset of symptoms.[13] Persistence for more than thirteen weeks was encountered by Nielsen et al.[22] in 4.3% of their patients, all of whom developed complications.

Iwarson et al.[19] found that patients with Australia antigen in their serum had more pronounced parenchymal cell damage and more prominent Kupffer cell hyperplasia than Australia antigen–negative patients. Conversely, the latter group had a higher incidence of intrahepatic cholestasis. This antigen can be demonstrated by immunofluorescence in the liver and in extrahepatic locations.[23] In an electron microscopic study of six immunosuppressed renal transplant recipients who developed Australia antigen–associated hepatitis, Huang[17]

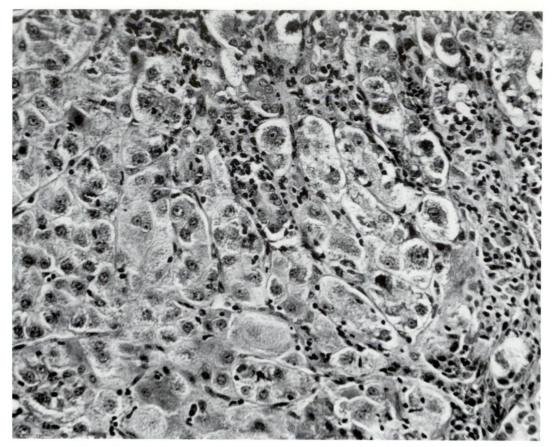

Fig. 559 Chronic active hepatitis in 28-year-old man. Portal inflammatory infiltrate disrupts limiting plate and surrounds individual hepatocytes, some of which exhibit degenerative changes. (×300; WU neg. 73-68.)

found viruslike particles of 230Å size in five. He believes this finding to be diagnostic for HAA hepatitis.

The possible outcomes of acute viral hepatitis are total resolution (over 80%), death in acute hepatic insufficiency in the patients with massive necrosis, chronic persistent hepatitis, chronic active hepatitis, postnecrotic scarring, and cirrhosis.

Chronic persistent and chronic active hepatitis

Chronic hepatitis has been defined as an inflammatory process of the liver lasting longer than one year and lacking the nodular regeneration and distorted architecture of cirrhosis. Two types have been described. The distinction between them, although not always possible, is de-

sirable in view of their different natural course.[31, 35] This is mainly based on microscopic criteria, since clinical and laboratory data may be very similar in the two conditions.

Chronic persistent hepatitis appears to be, in most cases, a sequel of acute viral hepatitis. In most series, the majority of the patients are Australia antigen–positive.[40] The disease follows a benign clinical course, without apparent progression to either chronic active hepatitis or cirrhosis.[32, 35] Microscopically, it shows in minor degree all of the features of acute viral hepatitis. Although portal inflammation is regularly present, this does not extend to the periportal areas. The lobular architecture is preserved and fibrosis is minimal or absent.

Chronic active hepatitis, also known as chronic aggressive hepatitis, appears to be a syndrome rather than a single disease.[34, 38, 39, 41] From 10% to 25% of the cases are positive for the Australia antigen. Most of the patients are males with an antecedent episode of acute viral hepatitis.[37, 42] In this instance, chronic active hepatitis probably represents a progression of the viral infection, particularly of the type with a confluent pattern of necrosis.[33] About 15% of the cases are negative for the Australia antigen but positive for the LE test. This group, mainly represented by young females, is probably the expression of a "collagen disease" with lupuslike features.[36] The larger group (60% to 75%) is comprised of patients who are negative for both the Australia antigen and the LE test. The majority probably represent sequelae of acute viral hepatitis.

The prognosis of chronic active hepatitis is poor. Cirrhosis develops in the majority of patients. Microscopically, intense inflammatory reaction, often rich in plasma cells, spreads from the portal tracts into the periportal areas. Together with the accompanying fibrosis, it destroys the limiting plate and results in the formation of periportal hepatocytic islets (Fig. 559). The architecture is altered, but there is no nodular regeneration. Periportal unicellular necrosis ("piecemeal necrosis") is a regular finding. Intralobular changes are of minimal degree—an important diagnostic feature.

Chronic nonpurulent destructive pericholangitis

A rare disease, chronic nonpurulent destructive pericholangitis has many clinical and pathologic similarities with chronic active hepatitis.[43, 45] It can be differentiated from the latter by the presence of xanthomatous changes, granulomas, and copper deposition and by the reduction or absence of bile ducts.[44] So-called primary biliary cirrhosis represents the end-stage of this condition.

Drug-induced and toxic hepatitis

The range of hepatic alterations that can occur as a result of iatrogenic or toxic injuries is extensive.[49, 49a] Hepatocellular degeneration, cholestasis, steatosis, pigmentary disturbances, vascular reactions, fibrosis, cirrhosis, and neoplasms can all occur, singly or in combination. A morphologic classification of the type of injury is desirable, because it may relate to the prognosis and give an indication to the type of agent involved, although considerable overlap exists.

A picture of *pure cholestasis,* unaccompanied by inflammatory features, is classically described in association with anabolic steroids (i.e., methyltestosterone), although many other agents also can produce it, such as psychotherapeutic agents (i.e., chlorpromazine), anticonvulsants (i.e., diphenylhydantoin), oral contraceptives, antibiotics (i.e., erythromycin estolate), and antineoplastic agents (i.e., methotrexate, 6-mercaptopurine).[47] The resulting picture, which can be confused clinically with extrahepatic biliary obstruction, is characterized microscopically by the presence of bile plugs in dilated canaliculi and bile pigment in hepatocytes of the centrilobular area. The rest of the lobule and portal tracts are unaffected.

Portal and periportal inflammation is the most common drug-induced lesion. A large variety of drugs can cause it, including most of those mentioned in connection with pure cholestasis, particularly the phenothiazines.[48] Microscopically, a mixed inflammatory infiltrate, sometimes rich in eosinophils, permeates the portal spaces and spreads into the peripheral portion of the lobules. Proliferated bile ductules are common. Fibrosis and "piecemeal necrosis" may result in a picture of chronic active hepatitis. Associated cholestasis, usually centrilobular, is seen in about 70% of the cases.[50] Intralobular hepatocytes may show some pleomorphism and rare acidophilic bodies but are for the most part unremarkable.

Panlobular inflammation, resulting in a

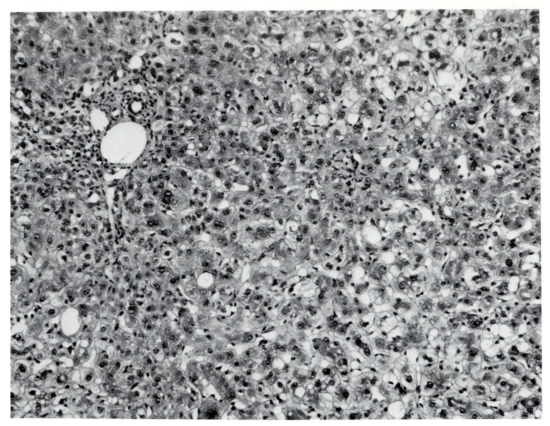

Fig. 560 Drug-induced hepatitis secondary to methotrexate administration in 14-year-old girl with acute lymphocytic leukemia. Liver function tests improved when drug was withdrawn but returned to previous abnormal values when it was readministered. There is portal and lobular inflammation, as well as prominent ballooning degeneration. These changes are difficult to distinguish from those of viral hepatitis. (×150; WU neg. 73-71.)

clinical and microscopic picture strikingly similar to viral hepatitis, has been seen secondarily to the administration of mono-amino-oxidase inhibitors, cincophene, the anesthetic halothane, iproniazid, amino-salicylic acid, PAS, phenylbutazone, zoxazolamide, and several other drugs[46, 50] (Fig. 560). As in the cases of acute viral hepatitis, the necrosis may be spotty, confluent, or massive. In 23% of 150 cases with massive hepatic necrosis reviewed by Trey et al.,[52] fulminant hepatic failure occurred within twenty-one days after exposure to halothane anesthesia. As Popper et al.[50] emphasized, in the individual patient it is often difficult to determine whether hepatic injury of this type is drug induced or the result of an intercurrent viral hepatitis.[46]

Nonspecific reactive hepatitis, to be discussed below, is probably the commonest form of liver reaction to drugs, although is rarely seen in biopsy specimens because of the absence or insignificance of its clinical and laboratory manifestations.

Steatosis not accompanied by necrosis or inflammation has been described following the administration of intravenous tetracycline and corticosteroids.[47, 51]

Zonal necrosis is usually an expression of toxic reaction. It involves practically every person exposed to the agent and is usually dose-dependent. The necrosis resulting from carbon tetrachloride, tannic acid, halothane, copper, and *Amanita phalloides* intoxication is usually centrilobular, whereas that due to intoxication with ferrous sulfate or "phosphorus" has a predominantly peripheral distribution.[53]

Alcohol-induced hepatic changes

It has been fairly well documented that the ingestion of moderate to large amounts of alcohol may lead directly or indirectly to a variety of hepatic abnormalities, of which acute alcoholic hepatitis, steatosis, and cirrhosis are the most important.[62, 69, 69a] Rubin and Lieber[70] demonstrated the direct hepatotoxic effect of alcohol isocaloric substitution for carbohydrate in young nonalcoholic volunteers. This rapidly led to steatosis, preceded ultrastructurally by focal cytoplasmic degradation and alterations in mitochondria and endoplasmic reticulum. Lane and Lieber[63] obtained similar results. Liver biopsies from chronic alcoholics are abnormal in 90% of the cases,[57] but in these circumstances it is usually impossible to separate the direct effects of alcohol from those resulting from dietary deficiency. The ultrastructural alterations seen in hepatocytes of alcoholics were well described and beautifully illustrated by Ma.[65]

The *steatosis* that follows alcohol ingestion is a reversible condition usually asymptomatic. However, it may result in jaundice and even death from hepatic insufficiency.[64] It is unlikely that liver fat accumulation per se is responsible for the development of cirrhosis.

Acute alcoholic hepatitis can be superimposed on a liver with previous fatty metamorphosis, in a liver with cirrhosis, or in a previously normal organ. It is invariably the result of a prolonged bout with John Barleycorn. The microscopic changes are characteristic. In addition to the cirrhosis, which may or may not be present, there is extensive cellular degeneration and necrosis and inflammatory reaction. Some degree of steatosis is always present. Cholestasis is common. Marked sclerosis of the centrilobular sinusoids and veins may be present and lead to partial obliteration of the venous outflow tract.[58] The most important feature is the presence of Mallory's bodies in the cytoplasm of hepatocytes, often surrounded by a cluster of neutrophil leukocytes (Fig. 561). These represent a peculiar form of hepatocellular degeneration and can be seen in hepatic diseases other than those induced by alcohol, such as infantile cirrhosis and hepatoma.[66, 67, 71] By light microscopy, they appear as round or elongated cytoplasmic acidophilic clumps, often serpentine and located in a perinuclear position. Luxol-fast blue stains them a deep blue color.[55, 68] Their ultrastructural appearance is that of a filamentous network not particularly related with any cellular organelle.[72] Former claims of their possible origin from mitochondria have not been substantiated.[54, 56, 73]

Clinically, acute alcoholic hepatitis can be confused with extrahepatic biliary obstruction.[60] Hardison and Lee[61] found a mortality rate of 33% in their series of eighty-seven patients. In our experience, this has been considerably lower. It is likely that repeated bouts of acute alcoholic hepatitis rather than the steatosis per se, is the primary event in the development of Laennec's cirrhosis.[59]

Nonspecific reactive hepatitis

As the name indicates, nonspecific reactive hepatitis is a nonspecific hepatic reaction to a variety of infectious and toxic agents. Microscopically, the main change is a mild intralobular and/or portal inflammation, sometimes accompanied by mild proliferation of bile ducts and Kupffer cells and very rare necrotic hepatocytes. A subsiding viral hepatitis may exhibit a microscopic appearance indistinguishable from that of nonspecific reactive hepatitis.

Extrahepatic biliary obstruction

Needle biopsy has been used in an effort to differentiate between intrahepatic and extrahepatic cholestasis. The distinction can usually be made in long-standing cases, but in the early stages the changes are often not diagnostic.[80-82] Significant intrahepatic cholestasis can occur in acute viral, drug-

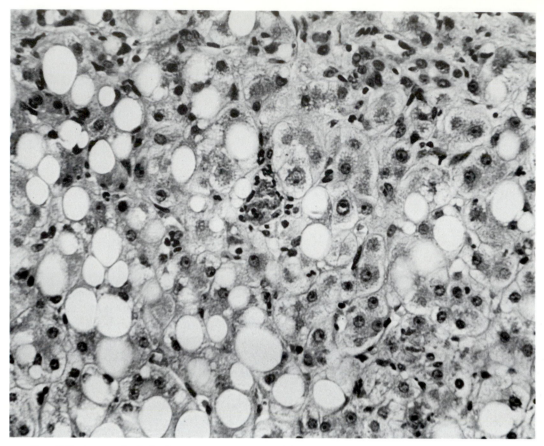

Fig. 561 Acute alcoholic hepatitis in 52-year-old woman. Large clump of Mallory's alcoholic hyalin can be seen in center, surrounded by cluster of neutrophils. There is also extensive fatty metamorphosis. (×350; WU neg. 73-66.)

induced, and acute alcoholic hepatitis and in the immediate postoperative period in patients with massive hemorrhage.[74, 77] Presence of cholestasis in interlobular ducts, bile lakes, and bile infarcts can be regarded as almost pathognomonic of extrahepatic obstruction but are only rarely seen in early cases (Fig. 562). Features favoring extrahepatic cholestasis include concentric fibrosis around interlobular bile ducts, neutrophilic infiltration of the portal spaces, acute or chronic cholangitis, a marked degree of cholangiolar proliferation, and focal lobular necrosis with neutrophil reaction.[75, 78] Conversely, the presence of more than an occasional acidophilic body in the areas of cholestasis, increased number of mitotic figures or binucleated forms among the hepatocytes,

and eosinophils within sinusoids favor an intrahepatic process.[79] Acidophilic bodies at the limiting plates or eosinophils in the portal areas are less significant, since they may be present in extrahepatic obstruction with ascending infection.[76] Acute cholangiolitis, pseudoxanthomatous changes, and the degree of cholestasis in the canaliculi, hepatocytes, and, to a certain extent, even in the cholangioles have little value in the differential diagnosis.

Jaundice in neonatal period

The three most important causes of neonatal jaundice persisting or appearing after the first or second week of life are biliary atresia, neonatal hepatitis, and galactosemia, in that order of frequency.[84]

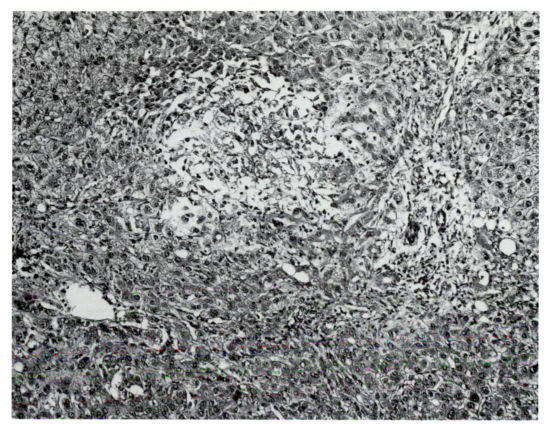

Fig. 562 Needle biopsy taken from 75-year-old woman with progressive jaundice shows large "bile infarct," a pathognomonic sign of extrahepatic biliary obstruction. At laparotomy, metastatic adenocarcinoma was found in region of porta hepatis. (×150; WU neg. 73-65.)

Less common etiologies include toxoplasmosis, congenital syphilis, cytomegalovirus disease, herpes simplex, and infectious mononucleosis.[87] The major problem facing the pediatrician and the pathologist is the urgent identification of the patients with extrahepatic biliary destruction who might benefit from early surgical therapy, even if correction of the atresia can be made in only 5% of the cases. A clinical distinction can be made in the majority of the patients, but in approximately 10% this is not possible. For the latter, needle or open biopsy of the liver may be extremely helpful.[85]

In cases of congenital biliary atresia, there is considerable ductal and ductular proliferation and distortion, mild degenerative changes in the hepatocytes, and medial hypertrophy of hepatic artery branches. Portal fibrosis occurs in approximately one-half of the patients, portal and/or lobular inflammation in 25%, and partial giant cell transformation in 25%.[83, 85, 86] In cases of hepatitis, signs of hepatocellular damage and inflammation are constant. The bile ducts and ductules are normal or only minimally proliferated and show no distortion. Portal fibrosis is absent or minimal, and changes in the branches of the hepatic artery are rare. Giant cell transformation varies from marked to negligible.

We believe that the degree of changes in the bile ducts and ductules is the most important differential feature. Conversely, we feel that the diagnostic value of giant cell transformation has been overemphasized and is responsible for most of the diagnostic errors made in the past.

Functional defects of bilirubin metabolism

Bilirubin originates from the conversion of the heme moiety of hemoglobin and other hemoproteins through a complex enzymatic mechanism. The circulating bilirubin, which is mainly albumin-bound, is then carried to the sinusoidal surface of the hepatocytes. The unbound fraction is transported through the cell membrane, probably by a specific carrier mechanism, bound within the cytoplasm of the hepatocytes to cytoplasmic acceptor proteins and converted to a water-soluble conjugate by the action of several microsomal enzymes, particularly glucuronyl transferase. *This conjugation step is essential for the biliary excretion of bilirubin.* The last step is the secretion of the conjugated bilirubin, which proceeds against a large concentration gradient and is little understood at the present time.[95]

The process is complicated but nevertheless highly efficient. Exceptionally, one or another of these enzymatic steps is defective and the result is a jaundice with little or no hepatic morphologic alterations, save for some accumulation of bile pigment. Most of these conditions are congenital and familial.[94a] The better defined varieties are the following:

1 *With accumulation of unconjugated bilirubin*
   a *Gilbert's syndrome,* possibly the result of a defect in the transport across the liver cell membrane from the plasma to the liver cell or a reduction in the concentration or binding forces of intrahepatic acceptor proteins. Glucuronyl transferase activity is normal. The jaundice is chronic and intermittent, and the disease follows a benign clinical course.[93]
   b *Crigler-Najjar syndrome,* secondary to defective conjugation of bilirubin as a result of a congenital absence or gross reduction of glucuronyl transferase. The jaundice is lifelong. In severe cases, it is associated with bilirubin encephalopathy and frequently results in death at an early age.[90]
   c *Lucey-Driscoll syndrome,* believed to be the consequence of inhibition of glucuronyl transferase by a substance derived from the mother's milk, possibly a steroid hormone.
2 *With accumulation of conjugated bilirubin*
   a *Dubin-Johnson syndrome,* the result of an undetermined defect in the secretion of conjugated bilirubin.[89] A pigment with the histochemical and ultrastructural appearance of lipofuscin is present in the hepatocytes in large amounts.[92]
   b *Rotor's syndrome,* a probably related disorder in which pigment deposition is lacking.[91]

Many patients with familial hyperbilirubinemia do not fit neatly into one of these categories. In some instances, the serum bilirubin is alternatively conjugated and unconjugated.[94] Pigment indistinguishable from that seen in the Dubin-Johnson syndrome has been described in association with Gilbert's syndrome.[88]

In general, the contribution of the surgical pathologist to the diagnosis and management of this group of diseases is small and mainly limited to the exclusion of intrahepatic anatomic causes for the jaundice. There is no anatomic lesion in any, save for accumulation of pigment. No cholestasis exists.

Cirrhosis

The three basic anatomic features of cirrhosis are (1) degeneration or necrosis of hepatocytes, (2) fibrosis, and (3) nodular hepatic regeneration. Many classifications of cirrhosis have been proposed, none of which is entirely satisfactory.[99, 101, 107] We avoid terms such as nutritional and posthepatitic cirrhosis, because their etiologic connotations are rarely justified. Anatomically, three major categories of cirrhosis can be recognized: monolobular, multilobular, and mixed (monolobular and multilobular).[100]

In *monolobular cirrhosis,* the fibrous septa enclose a lobule or a portion of a lobule. In the most common variety of this form, no substructure can be recognized in the nodules. The fibrous septa are thin, and there is a greater or lesser degree of fatty metamorphosis of the hepatocytes. This variety of monolobular cirrhosis, often

designated as *Laennec's* or *portal,* can be
seen in chronic alcoholism, hemochromatosis, and galactosemia. Indian infantile cirrhosis also belongs to this category.[105] It is
also possible that viral hepatitis may lead
to this morphologic variety or cirrhosis.
Cardiac cirrhosis is a rare variety of monolobular cirrhosis in which the fibrous septa
join central veins, leaving a portal tract
in the center of the nodule. It can be seen
secondary to constrictive pericarditis, tricuspid incompetence, or hepatic vein occlusion. In *biliary cirrhosis,* another variant
of monolobular cirrhosis, the fibrous strands
join portal tracts, and central veins remain
in the center of the nodules. The secondary
type is the result of extrahepatic biliary
obstruction, almost always associated with
some degree of ascending infection. So-
called primary biliary cirrhosis has been
mentioned in the discussion of chronic
nonpurulent destructive pericholangitis.

The nodules of **multilobular cirrhosis**
contain several hepatic lobules enclosed
by thick fibrous septa. Therefore, several
portal tracts and central veins can be
identified in them.[96] It is usually assumed
that the areas of fibrosis occur in places
formerly the site of confluent hepatic
necrosis—hence the term postnecrotic cirrhosis. The cirrhosis developing as a complication of acute viral hepatitis, active
chronic hepatitis, toxic necrosis, hepa-
tolenticular degeneration (Wilson's disease), thorium dioxide (Thorotrast) deposition, and alpha-1-antitrypsin deficiency
are of this type.[97] In the latter condition,
PAS-positive globular material may be
found in the cytoplasm of the hepatocytes.[104] Many cases of cirrhosis occurring
in chronic alcoholics are also of this variety.
It is certainly possible that they represent
the complication of an intercurrent subclinical viral or toxic hepatitis but seems
most likely that in most cases they develop
from monolobular cirrhosis by a process
of continuing regeneration.[103] In general,
the longer the established history of
alcoholism, the greater the possibility that
a multilobular cirrhosis will be found.[102]

The microscopic diagnosis of cirrhosis by
needle biopsy is more accurate in the
monolobular than in the multilobular form.
In the latter, the specimen may contain
material from the inside of one of the
large nodules and therefore exhibit little
or no fibrosis.[98, 106] If the diagnosis of cirrhosis can be made, it is still often difficult
to accurately classify it as to the type.[96]

Granulomatous hepatitis

The differential diagnosis of granulomas
found in liver biopsies involves a large
number of conditions.[108] In our experience,
sarcoidosis, histoplasmosis, and tuberculosis are the most common. Other infectious
diseases include brucellosis, tularemia, Q
fever, secondary syphilis, leprosy, toxoplasmosis, and kala-azar. We have also
seen hepatic noncaseating granulomas in
patients with Hodgkin's disease. In some
instances, the liver was also involved by
the malignant process, but in others it was
not (Chapter 20). These should be differentiated from the foreign body granulomas secondary to bile, cholesterol, mineral
oil, or other materials and with the portal
granulomas often seen in association with
primary biliary cirrhosis. Unfortunately,
in a large percentage of the cases (over
95% in our experience), the etiology of
liver granulomas remains undetermined
despite the most careful investigations.

Abscess

Metastatic foci may occur in the liver
during systemic inflammatory processes.
The most important inflammatory complication from the surgical standpoint is *pyle-*
phlebitic abscess secondary to acute appendicitis with periappendiceal spread.
Infected thrombi in the radicals of the
portal system travel to the liver, resulting
in multiple abscesses in the liver parenchyma. The etiology of this condition often
is not recognized because it is overshadowed by the other clinical symptoms. The
patients are extremely ill with spiking
fever. Pylephlebitic abscesses are very rare
today.

Amebic abscesses are relatively uncommon in this country. They are secondary to lesions of the gastrointestinal tract and are recognized only after tissue study. Clinically, amebic abscess is often missed, since 25% to 50% of the patients lack a history of dysentery, and amebae are detected in the stool in only 12% of the cases. Amebae may be found in fresh material from the abscess wall, even by needle biopsy.[109]

Echinococcus cyst

Echinococcus disease of the liver is rare in the United States but frequent in Iceland, Australia, Turkey, South America, and New Zealand.[111-113] Hydatid disease is caused by the larval or cystic stage of the dog tapeworm. Four species of the parasite have been identified: *Echinococcus granulosis* (by far the commonest), *Echinococcus oligarthrus*, *Echinococcus patagonicus,* and *Echinococcus multilocularis.*[113] Its definitive hosts are dogs, wolves, cats, and other carnivora. The intermediate or cystic stage is present in sheep, hogs, and cows, but man or other mammals can become infected.

The most common sites of echinococcus cysts are the liver (60% to 70% of patients) and the lung, but they can occur in many other locations. We have seen them in the spleen, soft tissue (Fig. 1147), bone, breast, brain, and spinal extradural space. When the cyst is viable, the skin and complement fixation tests are often positive, and eosinophilia is frequent, even if of mild degree. Death of the parasite is accompanied by collapse of the wall and calcification. At this stage, the skin test is of little value, and eosinophilia may be absent or not over 5%.[110] Rupture of a hepatic or splenic cyst into the peritoneal cavity may result in a fatal anaphylactic reaction or in the formation of innumerable small granulomas closely resembling peritoneal tuberculosis. The diagnosis is made by identifying fragments of germinal membrane or scolices in their center. Hepatic echinococcus cysts also can rupture inside the gallbladder or through the diaphragm into the pleural space and lung.

Grossly, hydatidosis of the liver is usually of the unilocular type. The cysts average 1 cm to 7 cm in diameter. About 75% are in the right lobe, the majority on the inferior surface extending downward into the peritoneal cavity. Histologic examination of a section from the cyst wall is diagnostic. It is formed by an outer *chitinous* layer and an inner *germinal* layer and is surrounded by granulation tissue or a fibrous capsule. The neighboring liver parenchyma often shows pressure atrophy and a moderately intense portal infiltrate in which eosinophils may be prominent. The viable cyst is filled with colorless fluid, which contains daughter cysts and brood capsules with scolices. The latter can be easily identified after macerating a portion of the germinal layer in saline solution.

Nonparasitic cysts

Nonparasitic cysts of the liver may be solitary or multiple. The former most commonly affect women between 40 and 60 years of age and are usually found in the anteroinferior surface of the right lobe.[119] There is no familial incidence or cystic disease of other organs. The cysts may attain a diameter of 10 cm or more. Although usually intrahepatic, they may be pedunculated. Grossly, solitary cysts have a well-developed fibrous wall varying in thickness from 0.5 mm to 2 cm. The cavity may be unilocular or multilocular and may contain clear fluid or bile. The lining of the cyst is flattened bile duct epithelium. Pressure atrophy of the surrounding hepatic parenchyma is common. Complications include necrosis, calcification, torsion, and hemorrhage.[114, 117] The pathogenesis is not known. It is possible that at least in some instances the cysts develop as a result of local obstruction of biliary ducts. Surgical excision is the treatment of choice.[115, 116]

Polycystic liver disease is accompanied by cysts of the kidneys in 60% of the cases.[118, 119] In approximately 5% of the patients, cysts of pancreas, spleen, or lung are present as well. A definite familial incidence has been demonstrated.

Congenital hepatic fibrosis

The presenting sign of congenital hepatic fibrosis is usually hematemesis or hepatomegaly in a child or adolescent, accompanied by minimal or no signs of liver dysfunction.[121, 123] A familial history can be elicited in about one-half of the cases. At operation, the liver appears markedly enlarged and extremely firm. Grossly visible cysts are rare or absent. Microscopically, wide bands of fibrous tissue containing large numbers of bile ducts are seen traversing a normal parenchyma. Marked regional variations in the intensity of the changes are often seen. The proliferated bile ducts may be collapsed, normal sized, or markedly dilated. Only a few contain bile. No abnormalities of the lobular architecture or of the hepatocytes can be detected.

Portal hypertension develops in 50% to 70% of the patients. This constitutes one of the more clear-cut indications for portosystemic shunt. A renal disease characterized by cystic dilatation of the collecting tubules coexists in 33% of the sporadic cases and in 70% of the familial cases.[120, 122] Among the seventy-seven patients with congenital hepatic fibrosis reviewed by Sommerschild et al.,[124] the mortality rate was 50%, with death mainly from chronic renal insufficiency and massive variceal hematemesis.

Tumors and tumorlike conditions
Bile duct hamartoma and adenoma

Bile duct hamartomas present grossly as multiple, small, whitish nodules scattered throughout the liver. They may be mistaken for metastatic carcinoma by the operating surgeon. Microscopically, they appear as a focal disorderly collection of bile ducts and ductules surrounded by abundant fibrous stroma.[133] True bile duct adenomas are usually solitary. They appear as solid tumors or as cystadenomas. Warvi[175] reviewed sixty-two cases of solid bile duct adenomas, thirty-eight of which were surgically excised. Grossly, they appear as well-circumscribed wedgelike white masses, sometimes with a central depression, closely resembling metastatic carcinoma.[156] More than a hundred cases of bile duct cystadenomas have been collected.[128, 157]

Mesenchymal hamartoma

A rare benign lesion, mesenchymal hamartoma is restricted to infants, in whom it appears as a solitary, spherical, reddish nodule. Microscopically, the main component is a well-vascularized mature connective tissue intermixed with elongated branching bile ducts. The low-power appearance is quite reminiscent of fibroadenoma of the breast.[174]

Focal nodular hyperplasia

We have seen several examples of focal nodular hyperplasia, which usually presents as a large, solitary, gray-white, solid mass beneath the capsule, sometimes pedunculated.[120, 177] On cut section, a white depressed area of fibrosis is seen in the center, with broad strands radiating from it to the periphery in a stellate configuration (Fig. 563). Microscopically, *all the components of the normal liver lobule are present.* The cellular morphology and relationship between hepatocytes and bile ducts are essentially those of normal liver, both by light and electron microscopic criteria.[139, 148] Fibrosis bridging portal tracts resembles the pattern of cirrhosis.[131] This lesion often presents in childhood and is invariably asymptomatic.[165] The differential diagnosis should be made with liver cell adenoma,[161] well-differentiated hepatocarcinoma, and partial nodular transformation of the liver, a rare entity associated with portal hypertension.[169]

We also have seen a diffuse form of this lesion in which almost every lobule is affected, but there is no fibrosis.[173]

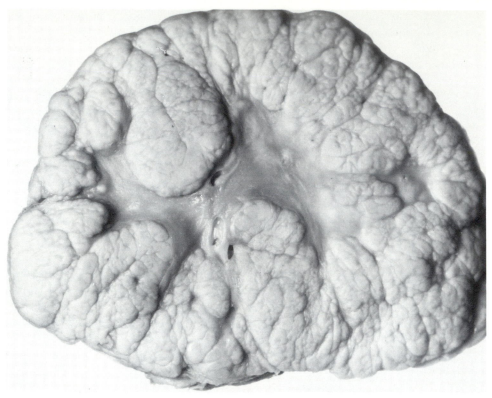

Fig. 563 Focus of nodular hyperplasia removed from liver of 20-year-old woman. Mass measured 5 cm × 5 cm × 8.5 cm. Note typical central scar wtih stellate configuration. (WU neg. 66-12024.)

Liver cell adenoma

In our experience, true adenomas of the liver are exceptional. Grossly, they have a well-defined capsule and a different color than the surrounding liver. The typical central scar of nodular hyperplasia is absent (Fig. 564). Microscopically, the tumor is composed of well-differentiated hepatocytes with abundant eosinophilic granular cytoplasm. *There are no portal triads or central veins,* and there is no connection with the biliary system. Multiple sections should be carefully evaluated to rule out a well-differentiated liver cell carcinoma. Search for blood vessel invasion is particularly important. Not infrequently, the morphologic differential diagnosis is impossible, and only the clinical course establishes the true nature of the lesion.

Liver cell carcinoma (hepatoma)

Liver cell carcinoma has a high incidence in all African countries south of the Sahara and in Southeast Asia.[144] This may be due, at least partially, to the ingestion of *aflatoxins,* metabolic products of the growth of the ubiquitous fungus *Aspergillus flavus.*[126] Infection with hepatotrophic viruses also has been implicated. Although rare in this country, hepatoma is seen sufficiently often to have clinical importance. Men are more often affected than women. The rare cases occurring in children should be differentiated from the more common hepatoblastoma. About 50% of the cases are associated with cirrhosis and undoubtedly are causally related with it. The cirrhosis is usually of the multilobular or postnecrotic type (including hemochromatosis) in the United

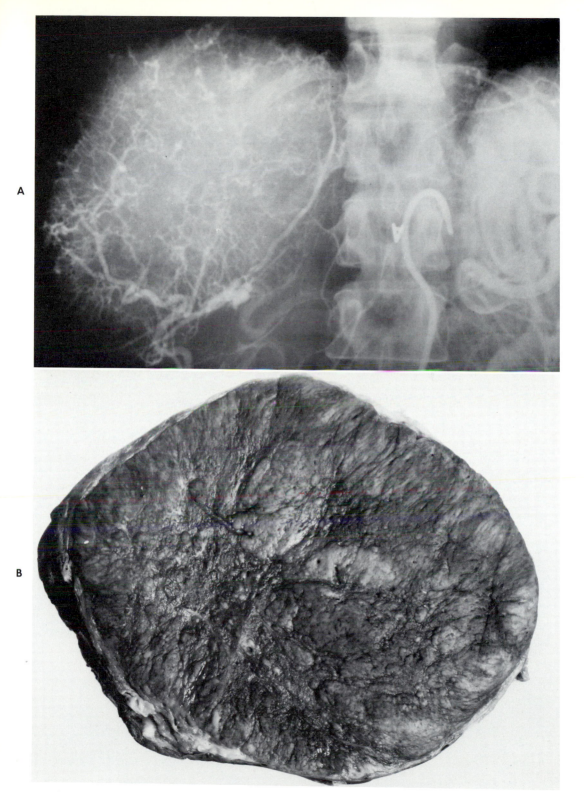

Fig. 564 A, Arteriogram showing large well-vascularized mass in right lobe of liver in 43-year-old white woman. **B,** Gross appearance of lesion. Tumor is well encapsulated and irregularly lobulated. Microscopicaly, it was composed throughout by well-differentiated hepatocytes. Diagnosis was liver cell adenoma. Patient is alive and well three years following partial hepatectomy. (**A,** WU neg. 68-11196; **B,** WU neg. 68-11128.)

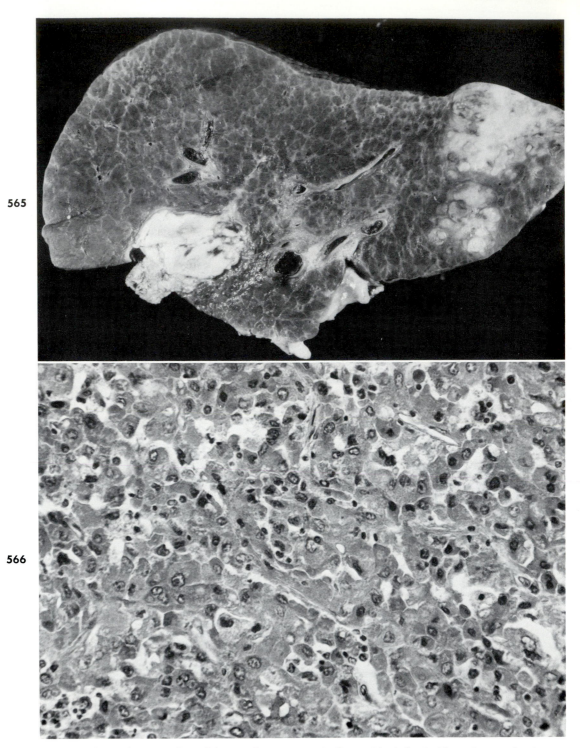

565

566

Fig. 565 Multicentric foci of liver cell carcinoma in liver with cirrhosis. There is portal vein thrombosis by tumor. As is usually the case, cirrhosis is of multilobular (postnecrotic) type. (Courtesy Dr. J. Murray, Johannesburg, South Africa.)
Fig. 566 Liver cell carcinoma. Tumor cells resemble hepatocytes but have obvious features of malignancy. (×350; WU neg. 73-178.)

States as well as in Africa and Latin America.[138, 143, 149] A case of liver cell carcinoma associated with biliary cirrhosis secondary to congenital bile duct atresia was reported by Deoras and Dicus.[136] Several cases have been seen following the administration of thorium dioxide suspension (Thorotrast), the average latent period being twenty years.[171] It is important to separate the tumors associated with cirrhosis from the others because in the former there is usually widespread involvement, making resection impossible.

Grossly, liver cell carcinoma may present as a single large mass, as multiple nodules, or as diffuse liver involvement. Portal vein thrombosis is found in a high proportion of cases[125] (Fig. 565). Microscopically, the poorly differentiated tumors show great pleomorphism, bizarre mitotic figures, and tumor giant cells.[137, 160] The nuclei and nucleoli are prominent, and the cytoplasm is scanty and basophilic (Fig. 566). Tumor cells often line vascular sinuses, and they may contain bile pigment. These are two important diagnostic features. The pattern of growth may be trabecular, tubular, or solid.[141] Blood vessel invasion is frequent. In the well-differentiated neoplasms, an occasional focus of enlarged hyperchromatic nuclei, an atypical mitotic figure, or a blood vessel with a tumor thrombus may be the only clue to the malignant nature of the lesion. The ultrastructure of this neoplasm has been well described by Ruebner et al.[166]

Hepatomas are sometimes associated with systemic manifestations such as hypoglycemia, erythrocytosis, hypercalcemia, the carcinoid syndrome, and several others.[153, 162]

Hepatomas quickly permeate the liver through the portal venous system, spread to the lung, and grow into the pulmonary arterial tree. Local invasion of the diaphragm often occurs. Metastases to regional lymph nodes also are common. Rarely, wide dissemination through the bloodstream takes place, with the development of extensive bone metastases.

Alpha-fetoprotein can be detected by immunodiffusion in a large percentage of patients with liver cell carcinoma.[159, 163] The incidence of positivity is higher in places in which hepatoma is endemic (more than 75%) than in Europe or the United States (40% to 60%). The tests also may be positive with malignant gonadal tumors and, rarely, with metastatic carcinomas to the liver, hepatitis, and posttraumatic liver regeneration. According to Ruoslahti et al.,[167] who developed a highly sensitive radioimmunoassay for the detection of alpha-fetoprotein, increases over one hundred times normal levels are diagnostic of liver carcinoma if a malignant gonadal tumor can be excluded.

Needle biopsy into a hepatoma may result in fatal intra-abdominal hemorrhage. The only effective treatment of liver cell carcinoma is complete resection, but this is possible only for single well-localized tumors.[145] In the presence of cirrhosis and in patients with metastases to the hilum, there is no chance of cure.

Cholangiocarcinoma

Malignant tumors of bile ducts are less common than those of liver cells and are not so frequently associated with cirrhosis. They may arise within developmental cysts.[176] Microscopically, they have a bile duct pattern but do not contain bile (Fig. 567). The ductlike structures are lined by cuboidal or columnar cells and are accompanied by abundant connective tissue stroma. The delicate vascular stroma of hepatoma is absent. Some primary malignant hepatic tumors consist of both hepatocytes and bile duct cells, the former usually predominating.

Hepatoblastoma

Hepatoblastoma, a highly malignant tumor, occurs almost exclusively in infants, although isolated cases in older children and adults have been reported.[132] It has no relationship with cirrhosis. An association with a variety of congenital abnormalities has been reported.[145] Willis' conten-

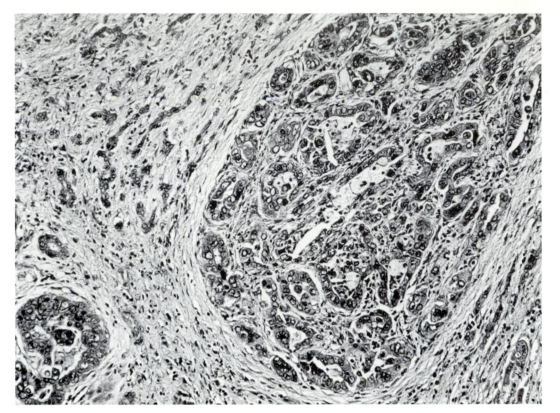

Fig. 567 Cholangiocarcinoma. Tumor was entirely intrahepatic. Glandular structures grow in cellular nests, separated by fibrous stroma containing strands of less differentiated tumor cells. Bile pigment is absent. (×175; WU neg. 73-689.)

tion that hepatoblastoma is a tumor distinct from hepatoma has received ample confirmation by the work of Ishak and Glunz.[145] Grossly, hepatoblastoma is solid, well circumscribed, and more often solitary than multiple. Microscopically, the main elements are epithelial.[127] Some closely resembling hepatocytes are arranged in irregular laminae which are two cells thick, as in the fetal liver (Fig. 568). Others have an embryonal appearance, contain numerous mitoses, and are sometimes arranged in ribbons, rosettes, or papillary formations. By electron microscopy, even the better differentiated cells are more immature than those of liver cell carcinoma.[146, 155] Foci of extramedullary hematopoiesis are often identified within the tumor. Some hepatoblastomas contain in addition a stromal component that may be undifferentiated or develop into bone or cartilage

(Fig. 569). This results in an appearance quite reminiscent of Wilms' tumor. There is no difference in clinical behavior between the "epithelial" and "mixed" varieties. The microscopic difference between hepatoblastoma and hepatoma are outlined in Table 23. Hepatoblastoma metastasizes early to regional nodes, lung, and brain.[145] In some cases, it has resulted in virilization as a result of ectopic sex hormone production.[130, 150]

Vascular tumors

Hemangioma is the most common benign tumor of the liver. In most cases, it is found incidentally at laparotomy or autopsy. Occasionally, it grows large enough to form a clinically apparent mass. Shumacker[170] reviewed fifty-six cases of large hepatic hemangiomas. Complications of these tumors include spontaneous bleed-

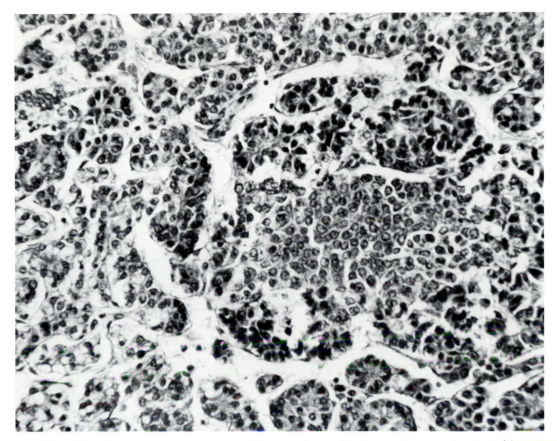

Fig. 568 Microscopic appearance of "pure" hepatoblastoma. Tumor cells resemble embryonal hepatocytes in different stages of development. (×350; WU neg. 73-182.)

ing with rupture and sequestration of platelets resulting in thrombocytopenic purpura.[142] It usually projects only slightly above the cut surface, but it may be pedunculated. On section, the spongy appearance and dark red color are characteristic. Microscopically, most liver hemangiomas are of the cavernous type, constituted by widely dilated nonanastomotic vascular spaces lined by flat endothelial cells and supported by fibrous tissue. Thrombi in different stages of organization are often encountered.

In children, most hemangiomas are quite cellular and often are designated as *hemangioendotheliomas* (Fig. 570). In the series reported by Dehner and Ishak,[135] 87% of the cases were diagnosed prior to 6 months of age. The tumors can be solitary or multiple. The latter are not infrequently associated with hemangiomas in other sites, particularly skin.[152] They are associated with a high mortality rate, largely as a result of hepatic failure or congestive heart failure.[135] Microscopically, the blood vessels of hemangioendotheliomas are lined by one or more layers of plump endothelial cells. The lumen is small or collapsed in most vessels, although focal cavernous foci can sometimes be identified.

We regard hepatic vascular tumors having freely anastomosing channels lined by hyperchromatic and pleomorphic endothelial cells as malignant and designate them as *angiosarcomas.* Most cases occur in adults, but well-documented cases in infants are also on record.[127, 147] Many of the adult cases have appeared following the use of thorium dioxide suspension

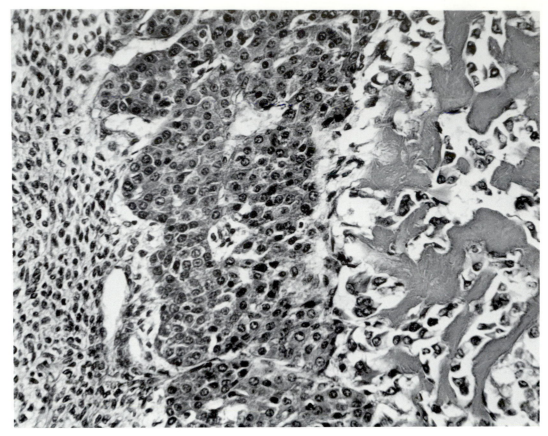

Fig. 569 Hepatoblastoma of mixed type. Tumor is composed of spindle cells of embryonal appearance (left), solid cords of hepatocytes (center), and malignant osteoid (right). (×300; W.U. neg. 73-180.)

(Thorotrast), the average latent period being approximately twenty years.[164] We also have seen a case following prolonged arsenic administration. These angiosarcomas, also known as Kupffer cell sarcomas, are invariably fatal.[134]

Metastatic tumors

Primary malignant tumors of the gallbladder, extrahepatic bile ducts, pancreas, and stomach frequently involve the liver by direct extension. Distant metastases from carcinomas of the large bowel, kidney, pancreas, stomach, lung, and breast appear with appalling frequency. Sarcomas, too, may metastasize to the liver. Unfortunately, practically all malignant neoplasms grow well in liver parenchyma.

Grossly, metastatic carcinoma in the liver forms discrete masses that may locally elevate the capsule and appear as poorly defined yellow or gray masses. Central necrosis with umbilication occurs in the larger nodules. *The absence of visible nodules on the external surface of the liver does not rule out the possibility of metastatic involvement.* We have seen several cases in which large metastases were completely hidden within the parenchyma.[140]

Many benign lesions may have a gross appearance indistinguishable from metastatic carcinoma. This is true of fibrous scars, healed tubercles from ancient hematogenous dissemination, granulomas of tuberculous, syphilitic, or other etiology, bile duct hamartoma, and nodular hyperplasia. Therefore, *it is imperative that a microscopic confirmation be obtained in*

Table 23 Morphologic comparison between epithelial type of hepatoblastoma and liver cell carcinoma (hepatoma)*

Histologic findings	Hepato-blastoma	Liver cell carcinoma (hepatoma)
Tumor mass	Single	Single or multiple
Pseudocapsule	Present	Usually absent
Trabeculae	Usually two cells thick	Usually many cells thick
Canaliculi	Present	Present
"Light and dark" pattern	Present	Usually absent
Size of cells compared to uninvolved hepatocytes	Smaller	Larger
Pleomorphism	Absent to minimal	Present
Tumor giant cells	Absent	Present
Multinucleated tumor cells	Absent	Present
Bile formation	Present	Present
Glycogen	Present	Present or absent
Fat	Present	Present or absent
Cytoplasmic globular and other inclusions	Absent	Present or absent
Extramedullary hematopoiesis	Present	Absent
Associated cirrhosis	Absent	Present or absent

*From Ishak, K. G., and Glunz, P. R.: Hepatoblastoma and hepatocarcinoma in infancy and childhood, Cancer **20:**396-422, 1967.

every patient in whom liver metastases are detected at laparotomy, regardless of how typical they might seem grossly to the surgeon or the pathologist.

Naturally, the finding of multiple hepatic metastases at exploration for carcinoma of the stomach, pancreas, or large bowel makes all surgical attempts of only palliative value. In carefully selected patients with a single blood-borne metastatic lesion or with direct extension into the liver by a neighboring malignant tumor, partial hepatectomy may result in long-term palliation and, exceptionally in cure.[151] Resection of hepatic metastases is particularly worthwhile in patients with metastatic carcinoid because of the dramatic amelioration of the symptoms of the carcinoid syndrome often achieved.[158]

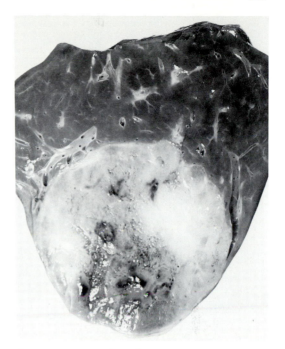

Fig. 570 Hemangioendothelioma of liver occurring in child. It was removed successfully. (WU neg. 54-5739.)

Other tumors

True liver *teratomas* are exceptional.[154] The majority are benign. We have seen three cases of *malignant mesenchymoma* in children, mainly composed of a mixture of highly atypical stromal elements.[172] Both of these entities need to be differentiated from the more common hepatoblastoma with an osseous or cartilaginous stromal component.

Malignant lymphoma in the liver is practically always the expression of a generalized disease. *Fibrosarcomas* have been reported.[168]

REFERENCES
Biopsy

1 Edmonson, H. A., and Peters, R. L.: Diagnostic problems in liver biopsies, Pathol. Annu. **2:**213-242, 1967.
2 Lindner, H.: Grenzen und Gefahren der perkutanen Leberbiopsie mit der Menghini-Nadel: Erfahrungen bei 80,000 Leberbiopsien, Deutsch Med. Wschr. **92:**1751-1757, 1967.
3 Ma, M. H., and Biempica, L.: The normal human liver cell; cytochemical and ultrastructural studies, Am. J. Pathol. **62:**353-375, 1971.

4 Menghini, G.: One-second needle biopsy of the liver, Gastroenterology 35:190-199, 1958.

5 Menghini, G.: One-second biopsy of the liver; problems of its clinical application, N. Engl. J. Med. 283:582-585, 1970.

6 Popper, H., Steigman, F., Meyer, K. A., Kozoll, D. D., and Franklin, M.: Correlation of liver function and liver structure, Am. J. Med. 6:278-291, 1949.

7 Post, J., and Rose, J. V.: Clinical, functional, and histologic studies in Laennec's cirrhosis of the liver, Am. J. Med. 8:300-313, 1950.

8 Sunzel, H., and Zettergren, L.: Histological liver lesions developing during abdominal operations, Gastroenterologia (Basel) 105:45-55, 1966.

9 Thaler, H.: Uber Vorteil und Risiko der Leberbiopsiemethode nach Menghini, Wien Klin. Waschenschr. 76:533-538, 1964.

Viral hepatitis

10 Babior, B. M., and Davidson, C. S.: Postoperative massive liver necrosis; a clinical and pathological study, N. Engl. J. Med. 276:645-652, 1967.

11 Baggenstoss, A. H.: Pathological anatomy of hepatitis, J.A.M.A. 165:1099-1107, 1957.

12 Bianchi, L.: Morphologic features in biopsy diagnosis of acute viral hepatitis, Prog. Liver Dis. 3:236-251, 1970.

13 Blumberg, B. S., Sutnick, A. I., London, W. T., and Millman, I.: Australia antigen and hepatitis, N. Engl. J. Med. 283:349-354, 1970.

14 Boyer, J. L., and Klatskin, G.: Pattern of necrosis in acute viral hepatitis; prognostic value of bridging (subacute hepatic necrosis), N. Engl. J. Med. 283:1063-1071, 1970.

15 Cooper, W. C., Gershon, R. K., Sun, S-C., and Fresh, J. W.: Anicteric viral hepatitis; a clinicopathological follow-up study in Taiwan, N. Engl. J. Med. 274:585-595, 1966.

16 Desmet, V. J., de Groote, J., and van Damme, B.: Acute hepatocellular failure; a study of 17 patients treated with exchange transfusion, Hum. Pathol. 3:167-182, 1972.

17 Huang, S.: Hepatitis-associated antigen hepatitis; an electron microscopic study of viruslike particles in liver cells, Am. J. Pathol. 64:483-492, 1971.

18 Ishak, K. G.: Viral hepatitis: the morphologic spectrum. In Gall, E. A., and Mostofi, F. K., editors: The Liver (International Academy of Pathology Monograph No. 13), Baltimore, 1973, The Williams & Wilkins Co.

19 Iwarson, S., Lundin, P., and Hermodsson, S.: Liver morphology in acute viral hepatitis related to the hepatitis B antigen, J. Clin. Path. 25:850-855, 1972.

20 Klion, F. M., and Schaffner, F.: The ultra-structure of acidophilic "Councilman-like" bodies in the liver, Am. J. Pathol. 48:755-767, 1966.

21 Lucke, B.: I. The pathology of fatal epidemic hepatitis. II. The structure of the liver after recovery from epidemic hepatitis, Am. J. Pathol. 20:471-619, 1944.

22 Nielsen, J. O., Dietrichson, O., Elling, P., and Christoffersen, P.: Incidence and meaning of persistence of Australia antigen in patients with acute viral hepatitis: development of chronic hepatitis, N. Engl. J. Med. 285:1157-1160, 1971.

23 Nowoslawski, A., Krawczynski, K., Brzosko, W., and Madalinski, K.: Tissue localization of Australia antigen immune complexes in acute and chronic hepatitis and liver cirrhosis, Am. J. Pathol. 68:31-50, 1972.

24 Prince, A. M., Hargrove, R. L., Szmuness, W., Cherubin, C. E., Fontana, V. J., and Jeffries, G. H.: Immunologic distinction between infectious and serum hepatitis, N. Engl. J. Med. 282:987-991, 1970.

25 Review by an International Group: Morphological criteria in viral hepatitis, Lancet 1:333-337, 1971.

26 Ruebner, B. H., and Slusser, R. J.: Hepatocytes and sinusoidal lining cells in viral hepatitis; an electron microscopic study, Arch. Pathol. 86:1-11, 1968.

27 Schaffner, F.: The structural basis of altered hepatic function in viral hepatitis, Am. J. Med. 49:658-668, 1970.

28 Shulman, N. R.: Hepatitis-associated antigen, Am. J. Med. 49:669-692, 1970.

29 Sutnick, A. I., London, W. T., Millman, I., Coyne, V. E., and Blumberg, B. S.: Viral hepatitis; revised concepts as a result of the study of Australia antigen, Med. Clin. North Am. 54:805-817, 1970.

30 Wills, E. J.: Acute infective hepatitis; fine structural and cytochemical alterations in human liver, Arch. Pathol. 86:184-207, 1968.

Chronic persistent and chronic active hepatitis

31 Alpert, L. I., and Vetancourt, R.: Chronic hepatitis; a clinicopathologic study of 75 cases, Arch. Pathol. 88:593-601, 1969.

32 Becker, M. D., Baptista, A., Scheuer, P. J., and Sherlock, S.: Prognosis of chronic persistent hepatitis, Lancet 1:53-56, 1970.

33 Boyer, J. L., and Klatskin, G.: Pattern of necrosis in acute viral hepatitis; prognostic value of bridging (subacute hepatic necrosis), N. Engl. J. Med. 283:1063-1071, 1970.

34 Bulkey, B. H., Heizer, W. D., Goldfinger, S. E., and Isselbacher, K. J.: Distinctions in chronic active hepatitis based on circulating hepatitis-associated antigen, Lancet 2:1323-1326, 1970.

35 de Groote, J., Desmet, V. J., Gedigk, P., Korb, G., Popper, H., Poulsen, H., Scheuer, P. J., Schmid, M., Thaler, H., Uehlinger, E., and Wepler, W.: A classification of chronic hepatitis, Lancet **2**:626-628, 1968.

36 Doniach, D., Walker, J. G., Roitt, I. M., and Berg, P. A.: "Autoallergic" hepatitis, N. Engl. J. Med. **282**:86-88, 1970.

37 Gitnick, G. L., Gleich, G. J., Schoenfield, L. J., Baggenstoss, A. H., Sutnick, A. I., Blumberg, B. S., London, W. T., and Summerskill, W. H. J.: Australia antigen in chronic liver disease with cirrhosis, Lancet **2**:285-288, 1969.

38 Mistilis, S. P.: Natural history of active chronic hepatitis. II. Pathology, pathogenesis and clinicopathological correlation, Aust. Ann. Med. **17**:277-288, 1968.

39 Mistilis, S. P., Skyring, A. P., and Blackburn, C. R. B.: Natural history of active chronic hepatitis. I. Clinical features, course, diagnostic criteria, morbidity, mortality and survival, Aust. Ann. Med. **17**:214-223, 1968.

40 Shulman, N. R.: Hepatitis-associated antigen, Am. J. Med. **49**:669-691, 1970.

41 Sherlock, S.: Waldenstrom's chronic active hepatitis, Acta Med. Scand. **445**(suppl.):426-433, 1966.

42 Wright, R., McCollum, R. W., and Klatskin, G.: Australia antigen in acute and chronic liver disease, Lancet **2**:117-121, 1969.

Chronic nonpurulent destructive pericholangitis

43 Hoffbauer, F. W.: Primary biliary cirrhosis: observations on the natural course of the disease in 25 women, Am. J. Dig. Dis. **5**:348-383, 1960.

44 Ishak, K. G.: Hepatic pathology; short course in pathology, Meeting of the International Academy of Pathology, Washington, D. C., March, 1973.

45 Rubin, E., Schaffner, F., and Popper, H.: Primary biliary cirrhosis: chronic nonsuppurative destructive cholangitis, Am. J. Pathol. **46**:387-407, 1965.

Drug-induced and toxic hepatitis

46 Babior, B. M., and Davidson, C. S.: Hepatitis: drug or viral? Am. J. Med. **41**:491-496, 1966.

47 Ishak, K. G.: Hepatic pathology; short course in pathology, Meeting of the International Academy of Pathology, Washington, D. C., March, 1973.

48 Ishak, K. G., and Irey, N. S.: Hepatic injury associated with the phenothiazines; clinicopathologic and follow-up study of 36 patients, Arch. Pathol. **93**:283-304, 1972.

49 Klatskin, G.: Toxic and drug-induced hepatitis. In Schiff, L., editor: Diseases of the liver, Philadelphia, 1969, J. B. Lippincott Co., p. 498.

49a Popper, H.: Drug-induced liver injury. In Gall, E. A., and Mostofi, F. K., editors: The liver (International Academy of Pathology Monograph No. 13), Baltimore, 1973, The Williams & Wilkins Co.

50 Popper, H., Rubin, E., Gardiol, D., Schaffner, F., and Paronetto, F.: Drug-induced liver disease, Arch. Intern. Med. **115**:128-136, 1965.

51 Schultz, J. C., Adamson, J. S., Jr., Workman, W. W., and Norman, T. D.: Fatal liver disease after intravenous administration of tetracycline in high dosage, N. Engl. J. Med. **269**:999-1004, 1963.

52 Trey, C., Lipworth, L., Chalmers, T. C., Davidson, C. S., Gottlieb, L. S., Popper, H., and Saunders, S. J.: Fulminant hepatic failure; presumable contribution of halothane, N. Engl. J. Med. **279**:798-801, 1968.

53 Wepler, W., and Opitz, K.: Histologic changes in the liver biopsy in *Amanita phalloides* intoxication, Hum. Pathol. **3**:249-254, 1972.

Alcohol-induced hepatic changes

54 Albukerk, J., and Duffy, J. L.: Origin of alcoholic hyaline; an electron microscopic study, Arch. Pathol. **93**:510-517, 1972.

55 Becker, B. J. P.: The nature of alcoholic hyalin; a histochemical study, Lab. Invest. **10**:527-534, 1963.

56 Biava, C.: Mallory alcoholic hyalin: a heretofore unique lesion of hepatocellular ergastoplasm, Lab. Invest. **13**:301-320, 1964.

57 Christoffersen, P., and Nielsen, K.: Histological changes in human liver biopsies from chronic alcoholics, Acta Pathol. Microbiol. Scand.(A)**80**:557-565, 1972.

58 Edmonson, H. A., Peters, R. L., Reynolds, T. B., and Kuzma, O. T.: Sclerosing hyaline necrosis of the liver in the chronic alcoholic; a recognizable clinical syndrome, Ann. Intern. Med. **59**:646-673, 1963.

59 Gerber, M. A., and Popper, H.: Relation between central canals and portal tracts in alcoholic hepatitis; a contribution to the pathogenesis of cirrhosis in alcoholics, Hum. Pathol. **3**:199-207, 1972.

60 Green, J., Mistilis, S., and Schiff, L.: Acute alcoholic hepatitis; a clinical study of fifty cases, Arch. Int. Med. **112**:67-78, 1963.

61 Hardison, W. G., and Lee, F. I.: Prognosis in acute liver disease of the alcoholic patient, N. Engl. J. Med. **275**:61-66, 1966.

62 Isselbacher, K. J., and Greenberger, N. J.: Metabolic effects of alcohol on liver, N. Engl. J. Med. **270**:351-356, 402-410, 1964.

63 Lane, B. P., and Lieber, C. S.: Ultrastructural alterations in human hepatocytes following

ingestion of ethanol with adequate diets, Am. J. Pathol. **49**:593-603, 1966.

64 Lieber, C. S., and Rubin, E.: Alcoholic fatty liver, N. Engl. J. Med. **280**:705-708, 1969.

65 Ma, M. H.: Ultrastructural pathologic findings of the human hepatocyte. I. Alcoholic liver disease, Arch. Pathol. **94**:554-571, 1972.

66 Nayak, N. C., Sagreiya, K., and Ramalingaswami, V.: Indian childhood cirrhosis; the nature and significance of cytoplasmic hyaline of hepatocytes, Arch. Pathol. **88**:631-637, 1969.

67 Norkin, S. A., and Campagna-Pinto, D.: Cytoplasmic hyaline inclusions in hepatoma, Arch. Pathol. **86**:25-32, 1968.

68 Norkin, S. A., Weitzel, R., Campagna-Pinto, D., MacDonald, R. A., and Mallory, G. K.: "Alcoholic" hyalin in human cirrhosis; histochemical studies, Am. J. Pathol. **37**:49-61, 1960.

69 Popper, H., and Schaffner, F.: Structural studies in alcohol and drug induced liver injury. In Engel, A., and Larsson, T., editors: Alcoholic cirrhosis and other toxic hepatopathias, Stockholm, 1970, Nordiska Bokhandelns Förlag.

69a Rubin, E.: The spectrum of alcoholic liver injury. In Gall, E. A., and Mostofi, F. K., editors: The liver (International Academy of Pathology Monograph No. 13), Baltimore, 1973, The Williams & Wilkins Co.

70 Rubin, E., and Lieber, C. S.: Alcohol-induced hepatic injury in nonalcoholic volunteers, N. Engl. J. Med. **278**:869-876, 1968.

71 Smetana, H. F., Hadley, G. G., and Sirat, S. M.: Infantile cirrhosis: an analytical review of the literature and a report of 50 cases, Pediatrics **28**:107-127, 1961.

72 Smuckler, E. A.: The ultrastructure of human alcoholic hyalin, Am. J. Clin. Pathol. **49**:790-797, 1968.

73 Yokoo, H., Minick, O. T., Batti, F., and Kent, G.: Morphologic variants of alcoholic hyalin, Am. J. Pathol. **69**:25-40, 1972.

Extrahepatic biliary obstruction

74 Ballard, H., Bernstein, M., and Farrar, J. T.: Fatty liver presenting as obstructive jaundice, Am. J. Med. **30**:196-201, 1961.

75 Gall, E. A., and Dobrogorski, O.: Hepatic alterations in obstructive jaundice, Am. J. Clin. Pathol. **41**:120-139, 1964.

76 Ishak, K. G.: Hepatic pathology; short course in pathology, Meeting of the International Academy of Pathology, Washington, D. C., March, 1973.

77 Kantrowitz, P. A., Jones, W. A., Greenberger, N. J., and Isselbacher, K. J.: Severe postoperative hyperbilirubinemia simulating obstructive jaundice, N. Engl. J. Med. **276**:591-598, 1967.

78 Rubin, E.: Interpretation of the liver biopsy, Gastroenterology **45**:400-412, 1963.

79 Shorter, R. G.: Liver biopsy; an atlas of histologic appearances, New York, 1961, Pergamon Press.

80 Shorter, R. G., and Baggenstoss, A. H.: Extrahepatic cholestasis. I. Histologic changes in hepatic interlobular bile ducts and ductules in extrahepatic cholestasis, Am. J. Clin. Pathol. **32**:1-4, 1959.

81 Shorter, R. G., and Baggenstoss, A. H.: Extrahepatic cholestasis. II. Histologic features of diagnostic importance, Am. J. Clin. Pathol. **32**:5-9, 1959.

82 Shorter, R. G., and Baggenstoss, A. H.: Extrahepatic cholestasis. III. Chronology of histologic changes in the liver, Am. J. Clin. Pathol. **32**:10-17, 1959.

Jaundice in the neonatal period

83 Bennett, D. E.: Problems in neonatal obstructive jaundice, Pediatrics **33**:735-748, 1964.

84 Brent, R. L. (with contributions by Arey, J. B., Blanc, W. A., Craig, J. M., Gellis, S. S., Harris, R. C., Kaye, R., Landing, B. H., Newton, W. A., Jr., Sass-Kortasak, A., Stowens, D., Yakovac, W. C., and Zuelzer, W. W.): Persistent jaundice in infancy, J. Pediatr. **61**:111-144, 1962.

85 Brough, A. J., and Bernstein, J.: Liver biopsy in the diagnosis of infantile obstructive jaundice, Pediatrics **43**:519-526, 1969.

86 Kasai, M., Yakovac, W. C., and Koop, C. E.: Liver in congenital biliary atresia and neonatal hepatitis; a histopathologic study, Arch. Pathol. **74**:152-162, 1962.

87 Zuelzer, W. W., and Brown, A. K.: Neonatal jaundice; a review, Am. J. Dis. Child. **10**:87-127, 1961.

Functional defects of bilirubin metabolism

88 Barth, R. F., Grimley, P. M., Berk, P. D., Bloomer, J. R., and Howe, R. B.: Excess lipofuscin accumulation in constitutional hepatic dysfunction (Gilbert's syndrome); light and electron microscopic observations, Arch. Pathol. **91**:41-47, 1971.

89 Butt, H. R., Anderson, V. E., Foulk, W. T., Baggenstoss, A. H., Schoenfield, L. J., and Dickson, E. R.: Studies of chronic idiopathic jaundice (Dubin-Johnson syndrome): evaluation of large family with trait, Gastroenterology **51**:619-630, 1966.

90 Crigler, J. F., and Najjar, V. A.: Congenital familial nonhemolytic jaundice with kernicterus, Pediatrics **10**:169-179, 1952.

91 Dollinger, M. R., Brandborg, L. L., Sartor, V. E., and Bernstein, J. M.: Chronic familial hyperbilirubinaemia, Gastroenterology **52**:875-881, 1967.

92 Dubin, I. N., and Johnson, F. B.: Chronic idiopathic jaundice with unidentified pigment in liver cells; a new clinicopathologic entity with report of 12 cases, Medicine (Baltimore) **33**:155-197, 1954.

93 Foulk, W. T., Butt, H. R., Owen, C. A., Whitcomb, F. F., and Mason, H. L.: Constitutional hepatic dysfunction (Gilbert's disease): its natural history and related syndromes, Medicine (Baltimore) **38**:25-42, 1959.

94 Salter, J.: Another variant of constitutional familial hepatic dysfunction with permanent jaundice and with alternating serum bilirubin relations, Acta Hepatosplenol. **13**:38-47, 1966.

94a Johnson, F. B.: Genetic disorders of bilirubin metabolism. In Gall, E. A., and Mostofi, F. K., editors: The liver (International Academy of Pathology Monograph No. 13), Baltimore, 1973, The Williams & Wilkins Co.

95 Schmid, R.: Bilirubin metabolism in man, N. Engl. J. Med. **287**:703-709, 1972.

Cirrhosis

96 Baggenstoss, A. H.: Postnecrotic cirrhosis: morphology, etiology and pathogenesis, Prog. Liver Dis. **1**:14-38, 1961.

97 Baggenstoss, A. H., Soloway, R. D., Summerskill, W. H. J., Elveback, L. R., and Schoenfield, L. J.: Chronic active liver disease; the range of histologic lesions, their response to treatment, and evolution, Hum. Pathol. **3**:183-207, 1972.

98 Braunstein, H.: Needle biopsy of the liver in cirrhosis: diagnostic efficiency as determined by postmortem sampling, Arch. Pathol. **62**:87-95, 1956.

99 Gall, E. A.: Posthepatitic, postnecrotic and nutritional cirrhosis; a pathological analysis, Am. J. Pathol. **36**:241-271, 1960.

100 Ishak, K. G.: Hepatic pathology; short course in pathology, Meeting of the International Academy of Pathology, Washington, D. C., March, 1973.

101 Popper, H.: What are the major types of hepatic cirrhosis? In Ingelfinger, F. J., et al., editors: Controversy in internal medicine, Philadelphia, 1966, W. B. Saunders Co., pp. 233-243.

102 Rubin, E., and Popper, H.: The evolution of human cirrhosis deduced from observations in experimental animals, Medicine (Baltimore) **46**:163-183, 1967.

103 Rubin, E., Krus, S., and Popper, H.: Pathogenesis of postnecrotic cirrhosis in alcoholics, Arch. Pathol. **73**:288-299, 1962.

104 Sharp, H. L., Bridges, R. A., Krivit, W., and Frier, E. F.: Cirrhosis associated with alpha-antitrypsin deficiency; a previously unrecognized inherited disorder, J. Lab. Clin. Med. **73**:934-939, 1969.

105 Singh, A., Jolly, S. S., and Kumar, L. R.: Indian childhood cirrhosis, Lancet **1**:587-591, 1961.

106 Soloway, R. D., Baggenstoss, A. H., Schoenfield, L. J., and Summerskill, W. H. J.: Observer error and sampling variability tested in evaluation of hepatitis and cirrhosis by liver biopsy, Am. J. Dig. Dis. **16**:1082-1086, 1971.

107 Steiner, P. E.: Precision in the classification of cirrhosis of the liver, Am. J. Pathol. **37**:21-47, 1960.

Granulomatous hepatitis

108 Guckian, J. C., and Perry, J. E.: Granulomatous hepatitis; analysis of 63 cases and review of the literature, Ann. Intern. Med. **65**:1081-1100, 1966.

Abscess

109 Keeley, K. J., Schamaman, A., and Scott, A.: Definitive diagnosis of amoebic liver abscess; value of liver biopsy, Br. Med. J. **10**:375-376, 1962.

Echinococcus cyst

110 Hudson, P. L.: Echinococcus disease; report of three cases of calcified cysts of the liver, South. Med. J. **38**:584-589, 1945.

111 Kahn, J. B., Spruance, S., Harbottle, J., Connor, P., and Schultz, M. G.: Echinococcosis in Utah, Am. J. Trop. Med. Hyg. **21**:185-188, 1972.

112 Katz, A. M., and Pan, C-T.: Echinococcus disease in the United States, Am. J. Med. **25**:759-770, 1958.

113 Williams, J. F., Lopez, A. H., and Trejos, A.: Current prevalence and distribution of hydatidosis with special reference to the Americas, Am. J. Trop. Med. Hyg. **20**:224-236, 1971.

Nonparasitic cysts

114 Ackman, F. D., and Rhea, L. J.: Non-parasitic cysts of the liver: their clinical and pathological aspects, Br. J. Surg. **18**:648-654, 1931.

115 Claggett, O. T., and Hawkins, W. J.: Cystic disease of the liver, Ann. Surg. **123**:111-118, 1946.

116 Maingot, R.: Solitary non-parasitic cyst of the liver, Br. Med. J. **2**:867-868, 1940.

117 Montgomery, A. H.: Solitary nonparasitic cysts of the liver in children, Arch. Surg. **41**:422-435, 1940.

118 Moschcowitz, E.: Nonparasitic cysts (congenital) of the liver with a study of aberrant bile ducts, Am. J. Med. Sci. **131**:674-699, 1906.

119 Peltokallio, V.: Non-parasitic cysts of the liver; a clinical study of 117 cases, Ann. Chir. Gynaecol. Fenn. **174**(suppl.):7-63, 1970.

Congenital hepatic fibrosis

120 Boichis, H., Passwell, J., David, R., and Miller, H.: Congenital hepatic fibrosis and nephronophthisis, Q. J. Med. **42**:221-233, 1973.

121 Boley, S. J., Arlen, M., and Mogilner, L. J.: Congenital hepatic fibrosis causing portal hypertension in children, Surgery **54**:356-360, 1963.

122 Bradford, W. D., Bradford, J. W., Porter, F. S., and Sidbury, J. B.: Cystic disease of the liver and kidney with portal hypertension, Clin. Pediatr. **7**:299-306, 1968.

123 Kerr, D. N., Harrison, C. V., Sherlock, S., and Walker, R. M.: Congenital hepatic fibrosis, Q. J. Med. **30**:91-117, 1961.

124 Sommerschild, H. C., Langmark, F., and Maurseth, K.: Congenital hepatic fibrosis; report of two new cases and review of the literature, Surgery **73**:53-58, 1973.

Tumors and tumorlike conditions

125 Albacete, R. A., Matthews, M. J., and Saini, N.: Portal vein thromboses in malignant hepatoma, Ann. Intern. Med. **67**:337-348, 1967.

126 Alpert, M. E., and Davidson, C. S.: Mycotoxins; a possible cause of primary carcinoma of the liver, Am. J. Med. **46**:325-327, 1969.

127 Baggenstoss, A. H.: Pathology of tumors of liver in infancy and childhood. In Pack, G. T., and Islami, A. H., editors: Tumors of the liver, Vol. 26 of Recent results in cancer research, Heidelberg-Berlin, New York, 1970, Springer-Verlag.

128 Beattie, D. A., and Robertson, H. D.: A case of simple cyst of the liver with an analysis of 62 other cases, Lancet **2**:674-677, 1932.

129 Begg, C. F., and Berry, W. H.: Isolated nodules of regenerative hyperplasia of the liver; the problem of their differentiation from neoplasm, Am. J. Clin. Pathol. **23**:447-463, 1953.

130 Behrle, F. C., Mantz, F. A., Jr., Olson, R. L., and Trombold, J. C.: Virilization accompanying hepatoblastoma, Pediatrics **32**:265-271, 1963.

131 Benz, E. J., and Baggenstoss, A. H.: Focal cirrhosis of liver: its relation to so-called hamartoma (adenoma, benign hepatoma), Cancer **6**:743-755, 1953.

132 Carter, R.: Hepatoblastoma in the adult, Cancer **23**:191-197, 1969.

133 Chung, E. B.: Multiple bile-duct hamartomas, Cancer **26**:287-296, 1970.

134 DaSilva Horta, J.: Late lesions in man caused by colloidal thorium dioxide (Thorotrast); a new case of sarcoma of the liver 22 years after the injection, Arch. Pathol. **62**:403-418, 1956.

135 Dehner, L. P., and Ishak, K. G.: Vascular tumors of the liver in infants and children; a study of 30 cases and review of the literature, Arch. Pathol. **92**:101-111, 1971.

136 Deoras, M. P., and Dicus, W.: Hepatocarcinoma associated with biliary cirrhosis; a case due to congenital bile duct atresia, Arch. Pathol. **86**:338-341, 1968.

137 Edmonson, H. A., and Steiner, P. E.: Primary carcinoma of the liver; a study of 100 cases among 48,900 necropsies, Cancer **7**:462-503, 1954.

138 Gall, E. A.: Primary and metastatic carcinoma of the liver; relationship to hepatic cirrhosis, Arch. Pathol. **70**:226-232, 1960.

139 Garancis, J. C., Tang, T., Panares, R., and Jurevics, I.: Hepatic adenoma; biochemical and electron microscopic study, Cancer **24**:560-568, 1969.

140 Goligher, J. C.: Operability of carcinoma of rectum, Br. Med. J. **2**:393-397, 1941.

141 Hamperl, H.: The classification of liver tumors. In Pack, G. T., and Islami, A. H., editors: Tumors of the liver, Vol. 26 of Recent results in cancer research, Heidelberg-Berlin-New York, 1970, Springer-Verlag.

142 Hendrick, J. G.: Hemangioma of the liver causing death in a newborn infant, J. Pediatr. **32**:309-310, 1948.

143 Higginson, J.: Pathogenesis of liver cancer in the Johannesburg area (S. Africa) (symposium on cancer of the liver among African Negroes, August, 1956, in Kampala, Uganda), Acta Un. Int. Cancer **13**:590-598, 1957.

144 Higginson, J.: The epidemiology of primary carcinoma of the liver. In Pack, G. T., and Islami, A. H., editors: Tumors of the liver, Vol. 26 of Recent results in cancer research, Heidelberg-Berlin-New York, 1970, Springer-Verlag.

145 Ishak, K. G., and Glunz, P. R.: Hepatoblastoma and hepatocarcinoma in infancy and childhood, Cancer **20**:396-422, 1967.

146 Ito, J., and Johnson, W. W.: Hepatoblastoma and hepatoma in infancy and childhood, light and electron microscopic studies, Arch. Pathol. **87**:259-266, 1969.

147 Kauffman, S. L., and Stout, A. P.: Malignant hemangioendothelioma in infants and children, Cancer **14**:1186-1196, 1961.

148 Kay, S., and Talbert, P. C.: Adenoma of the liver, mixed type (hamartoma); report of 2 cases, Cancer **3**:307-315, 1950.

149 Lopez-Corella, E., Ridaura-Sanz, C., and Albores-Saavedra, J.: Primary carcinoma of the liver in Mexican adults, Cancer **22**:678-685, 1968.

150 McArthur, J. W., Toll, G. D., Russfield, A. B., Reiss, A. M., Quinby, W. C., and Baker, W. H.: Sexual precocity attributable to ectopic gonadotropin secretion by hepatoblastoma, Am. J. Med. **54**:390-403, 1973.

151 McKenzie, A. D., and Wilson, J. W.: Hepatic resection for blood borne metastases from large bowel carcinoma: case report and re-

view of literature, Can. J. Surg. **13**:159-162, 1970.

152 McLean, R. H., Moller, J. H., Warwick, W. J., Satran, L., and Lucas, R. V., Jr.: Multinodular hemangiomatosis of the liver in infancy, Pediatrics **49**:563-573, 1972.

153 Margolis, S., and Homcy, C.: Systemic manifestations of hepatoma, Medicine (Baltimore) **51**:381-391, 1972.

154 Misugi, K., and Reiner, C. B.: A malignant true teratoma of liver in childhood, Arch. Pathol. **80**:409-412, 1965.

155 Misugi, K., Okajima, H., Misugi, N., and Newton, W. A., Jr.: Classification of primary malignant tumors of liver in infancy and childhood, Cancer **20**:1760-1771, 1967.

156 Mixter, C. G., and Mixter, C. G., Jr.: Liver nodules encountered at laparotomy: significance and treatment, Ann. Surg. **138**:230-239, 1953.

157 Montgomery, A. H.: Solitary nonparasitic cysts of the liver in children, Arch. Surg. **41**:422-435, 1940.

158 Mosenthal, W. T.: Resection of massive liver metastases in the malignant carcinoid syndrome, Surg. Clin. North Am. **43**:1253-1262, 1963.

159 O'Conor, G. T., Tatarinov, Y. S., Abelev, G. I., and Uriel, J.: A collaborative study for the evaluation of a serologic test for primary liver cancer, Cancer **25**:1091-1098, 1970.

160 Patton, R. B., and Horn, R. C.: Primary liver carcinoma; autopsy study of 60 cases, Cancer **17**:757-768, 1964.

161 Phillips, M. J., Langer, B., Stone, R., Fisher, M. M., and Ritchie, S.: Benign liver cell tumors; classification and ultrastructural pathology, Cancer **32**:463-470, 1973.

162 Primack, A., Wilson, J., O'Conor, G. T., Engelman, K., and Canellos, G. P.: Hepatocellular carcinoma with the carcinoid syndrome, Cancer **27**:1182-1189, 1971.

163 Purves, L. R., Bersohn, I., and Geddes, E. W.: Serum alpha-fetoprotein and primary cancer of the liver in man, Cancer **25**:1261-1270, 1970.

164 Rakov, H. L., Smalldon, T. R., and Derman, H.: Hepatic hemangioendotheliosarcoma; report of a case due to thorium, Arch. Int. Med. **112**:173-178, 1963.

165 Ramchand, S., Suh, H. S., and Gonzalez-Crussi, F.: Focal nodular hyperplasia of the liver, Can. J. Surg. **13**:22-26, 1970.

166 Ruebner, B. H., Gonzalez-Licea, A., and Slusser, R. J.: Electron microscopy of some human hepatomas, Gastroenterology **53**:18-30, 1967.

167 Ruoslahti, E., Seppala, M., Vuopio, P., Saksela, E., and Peltokallio, P.: Radioimmunoassay of alpha-fetoprotein in primary and secondary cancer of the liver, J. Natl. Cancer Inst. **49**:623-630, 1972.

168 Shallow, T. A., and Wagner, F. B., Jr.: Primary fibrosarcoma of the liver, Ann. Surg. **125**:439-446, 1947.

169 Sherlock, S., Feldman, C. A., Moran, B., and Scheuer, P. J.: Partial nodular transformation of liver with portal hypertension, Am. J. Med. **40**:195-203, 1966.

170 Shumacker, H. B., Jr.: Hemangioma of the liver, Surgery **11**:209-222, 1942.

171 Smoron, G. L., and Battifora, H. A.: Thorotrast-induced hepatoma, Cancer **30**:1252-1259, 1972.

172 Stanley, R. J., Dehner, L. P., and Hesker, A. E.: Primary malignant mesenchymal tumors (mesenchymoma) of the liver in childhood; an angiographic-pathologic study of three cases, Cancer **32**:973-984, 1973.

173 Steiner, P. E.: Nodular regenerative hyperplasia of the liver, Am. J. Pathol. **35**:943-953, 1959.

174 Sutton, C. A., and Eller, J. L.: Mesenchymal hamartoma of the liver, Cancer **22**:29-34, 1968.

175 Warvi, W. N.: Primary tumors of the liver, Surg. Gynecol. Obstet. **80**:643-650, 1945.

176 Willis, R. A.: Carcinoma arising in congenital cysts of the liver, J. Pathol. Bacteriol. **55**:492-495, 1943.

177 Wilson, T. S., and Macgregor, J. W.: Focal nodular hyperplasia of the liver: the solitary cirrhotic liver nodule, Can. Med. Assoc. J. **100**:567-572, 1969.

13 Gallbladder

Congenital abnormalities
Cholelithiasis
Cholesterosis
Acute cholecystitis
Chronic cholecystitis
Tumors

Congenital abnormalities

Congenital abnormalities of the gallbladder are of many types. They include duplication, absence, anomalous positions, and the presence of heterotopic tissues.[2] There are many anomalous arrangements of the extrahepatic bile ducts and their adjoining arteries (Fig. 571). No pathologic significance can be ascribed to the "phrygian cap" deformity, which represents a redundant fundus that may become adherent to the body of the gallbladder.[6]

In *congenital atresia* of the bile ducts, the gallbladder and extrahepatic ducts may be completely absent or may be represented by a fibrous cord without a lumen. If there are no extrahepatic ducts, the liver will contain a few small bile ducts that may not even communicate with bile canaliculi. No large intrahepatic ducts will be present. Obviously, operative procedures are of no value under these circumstances. If the common duct is partially patent, it may be dilated and amenable to an operation that will improve biliary drainage.

Frozen section and gross inspection of the liver can determine the presence or absence of such ducts. Only a small percentage of infants with biliary duct atresia can be helped by anastomosis of a dilated intrahepatic or extrahepatic duct to an adjacent segment of proximal gastrointestinal tract. Rarely, dilated hepatic ducts traverse the lesser peritoneal cavity.[5]

Choledochal cyst is the most common cause of obstructive jaundice in children beyond infancy. It represents a focal dilatation of the common bile duct, which may secondarily obstruct the other biliary ducts or even the duodenum. Microscopically, it is lined by columnar epithelium. The pathogenesis is unknown.

Continued from opposite page.

8, Very dangerous anomaly of entire hepatic artery which follows cystic duct to gallbladder before turning into liver. Accidental ligation of entire hepatic artery was almost always fatal before advent of penicillin and chlortetracycline, and it is still hazardous.

9, Anomalous bile duct entering gallbladder through its bed in liver. Cholecystectomy in such instances is usually followed by profuse drainage of bile and is likely to result in fatal peritonitis unless external drainage is afforded.

10, Anomalous insertion of cystic duct into right hepatic duct. Section of right hepatic duct caudad to its junction with cystic duct can easily be mistaken for cystic duct and ligated, thus shutting off drainage of right lobe of liver into intestine.

11, Anomalous arrangement of right hepatic duct in which it enters gallbladder so that all of bile from right lobe of liver must drain through cystic duct.

(From Rhoads, J. E.: Liver, gallbladder and bile passages. In Rhoads, J. E., Allen, J. G., Harkins, H. N., and Moyer, C. A.: Surgery; principles and practice, ed. 4, Philadelphia, 1970, J. B. Lippincott Co.)

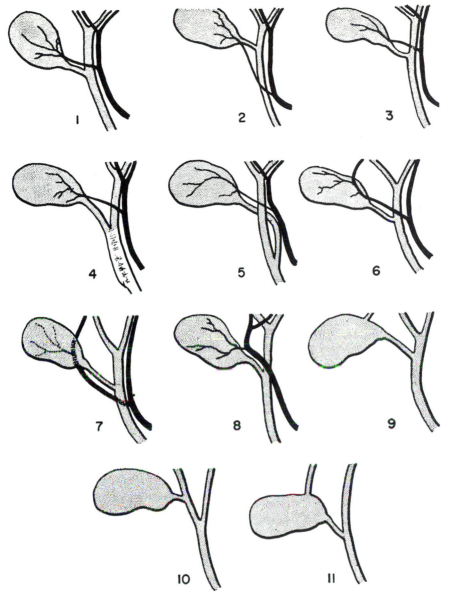

Fig. 571 Normal and anomalous arrangements of extrahepatic bile ducts and their adjoining arteries.

1, Normal arrangement.

2, Caudad origin of cystic artery (frequent variation).

3, Placement of cystic artery posterior to common hepatic duct.

4, Long cystic duct attached to common hepatic duct for some distance prior to confluence to form common bile duct.

5, Long cystic duct passing behind common hepatic duct and joining it medially at lower level.

6, Normal ductal system with anomalous right hepatic artery reaching gallbladder wall, where it gives off cystic artery and then turns into liver. In this anomaly, which is not rare, right hepatic artery is often ligated either with cystic duct or as separate structure erroneously identified as cystic artery.

7, Anomalous right hepatic artery in posterior position presenting same dangers as mentioned in 6.

Continued on opposite page.

Heterotopic tissues occurring in the gall-bladder include gastric mucosa, pancreas,[4] and even thyroid epithelium.[3] Most cases of heterotopic gastric mucosa present in the gallbladder neck or in the adjacent cystic duct as a small well-defined intra-mural nodule.[1]

Cholelithiasis

The pathogenesis of lithiasis is compli-cated by the interplay of innumerable factors. Stones in the gallbladder are more frequent in women than in men (ratios quoted being about 4:1). About 20% of them contain sufficient calcium to be radiopaque. About 50% of the nonopaque stones are manifest only by nonvisualiza-tion of the gallbladder by cholecystogra-phy. The others show as a negative shadow when the gallbladder concentrates the dye. The incidence of stones in the general population of the United States is 11%, as determined by the Framingham study.[7] Torvik and Höivik[13] report a frequency of 19.5% in autopsy material from Scandi-navia. The incidence increases with age until at 60 years about one out of every four women has stones.

Gallstones vary considerably in chemi-cal composition, the basic constituents being cholesterol, calcium bilirubinate, and calcium carbonate, either alone or in combination.[12] *Pure gallstones,* composed of only one of the substances mentioned, comprise 10% of the cases and include the following three types: cholesterol stones, calcium bilirubinate stones, and calcium carbonate stones.

Cholesterol stones are single, spheroidal, and coarsely nodular and have a trans-lucent bluish white color. On fracture, the stone shows large, flat crystals (Fig. 572). Most cholesterol stones are found in mul-tiparous women. This is probably related to the fact that cholesterol metabolism is altered during pregnancy and with the clinical observation that signs and symp-toms of cholelithiasis often develop short-ly after pregnancy.[8] However, no correla-tion exists between the presence of choles-

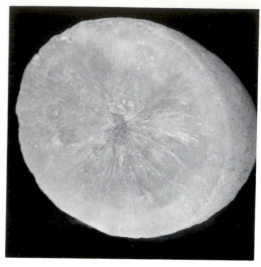

Fig. 572 Cross section of solitary, pure choles-terol stone showing typical crystalline structure. (WU neg. 52-4949.)

terol stones in the gallbladder and the level of cholesterol in the blood.

Calcium bilirubinate stones are multiple, small, brown to jet black, faceted stones, measuring 2 to 5 mm in diameter. Hemolyt-ic jaundice of the congenital type in which a long-continued increase of circulating bilirubin is present is associated with such stones in about one-half of the patients.[9] Stones of this type also form in sickle cell anemia. Greene and Snell[10] found ex-perimentally that an augmented rate of excretion of this pigment in the bile occurs by an increase in concentration rather than from an increase in volume of the bile. *Cal-cium carbonate stones* are amorphous and grayish white.

The gallbladder containing pure gall-stones shows little or no inflammatory re-action if the cystic duct is not obstructed. The finding of only pigment stones in the gallbladders of younger persons should arouse suspicion of hemolytic diseases.

Mixed gallstones (80% of all stones) con-sist of various combinations of cholesterol, calcium bilirubinate, and calcium carbon-ate. Their size and number vary. They are usually multiple, faceted, and laminated. Chronic cholecystitis is almost always present (Fig. 573). Several crops may be

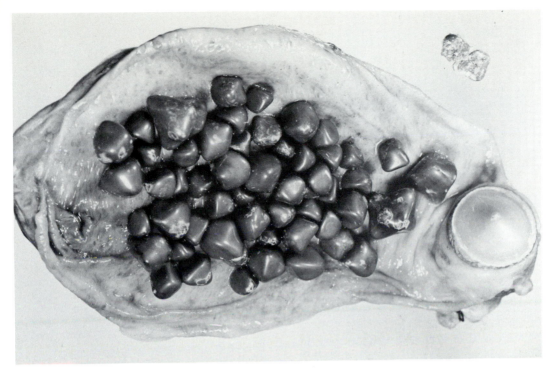

Fig. 573 Numerous stones of mixed type in chronically inflamed gallbladder. There is also large combined stone totally occluding cystic duct. (WU neg. 52-5034.)

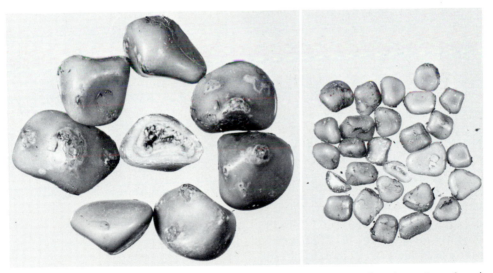

Fig. 574 Typical mixed stones with two different sizes suggesting that formation of each crop of stones occurred at different time. (WU neg. 52-4864.)

present, suggesting that the causes for their formation may operate at different times (Fig. 574).

Combined gallstones (10%) are characteristically large and single. They may have a pure nucleus with a mixed shell or the reverse. *Barrel stones,* a type of combined stones, are usually two in number, large, and faceted on one surface, and the thick-walled gallbladder is closely

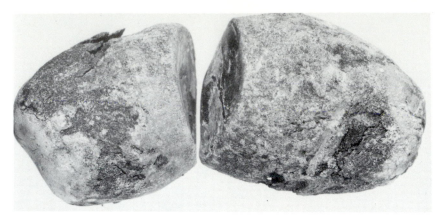

Fig. 575 Two typical barrel stones of combined type faceted on only one surface. These stones completely filled thick-walled gallbladder. (WU neg. 52-4431.)

wrapped around them (Fig. 575). Combined stones are always accompanied by chronic inflammation of the gallbladder and occasionally with biliary fistulas.

Gallstones are formed in the gallbladder and may escape from the gallbladder into the cystic and extrahepatic ducts. Their independent formation in the extrahepatic ducts is rare.[11] Choledocholithiasis and common duct obstruction by stone nearly always are secondary to cholecystolithiasis. The appearance of symptoms of common duct lithiasis some time after cholecystectomy for stone is nearly always caused by stones overlooked at the time of operation. However, the occasional finding of multiple small intrahepatic stones suggests that they may be formed in the hepatic duct system exclusive of the gallbladder.

Cholesterosis

Cholesterosis of the gallbladder has a characteristic pathologic pattern and occurs, for the most part, in multiparous women. Its pathogenesis is thought to be based on metabolic changes. Cholesterol is increased in the blood and bile during pregnancy, but at the time cholesterosis is discovered the blood cholesterol usually is normal. The bile salts keep cholesterol in solution. It is thought that if the bile salts fall below a certain level, precipitation of cholesterol occurs. However, Carter et al.[15] showed that about 80% of noncalculous gallbladders have a bile salt level

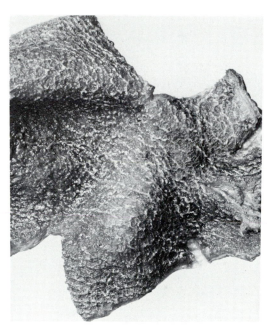

Fig. 576 Cholesterosis of gallbladder. Small yellow flecks are present along mucosal ridges. (WU neg. 52-4429.)

below that necessary to keep cholesterol in solution, yet no stones have been formed. Stasis is certainly a factor.

Gallbladders with cholesterosis are otherwise normal. We have not seen coexistence of cholesterosis and advanced inflammatory changes. This may indicate that the inflammatory process induces in some way the resorption of the cholesterol deposits. Grossly, the mucosa is prominently congested, and yellow flecks of lipid are con-

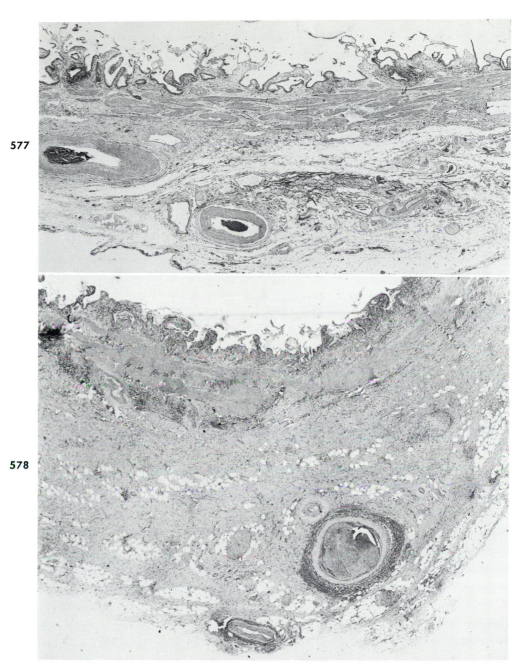

Fig. 577 Minimal chronic inflammatory changes in gallbladder with cholesterosis and small stone in cystic duct. Note that thickening is in subserosal area. (Low power; WU neg. 52-4491.)

Fig. 578 Advanced chronic cholecystitis. There is extreme subserosal fibrosis. and recent thrombus can be seen within a vessel. (Low power; WU neg. 52-4551.)

fined to the prominences of the ridges as longitudinal, linear streaks[16] (Fig. 576). This prominent congestion and the yellow flecks are the cause for the inelegant name

"strawberry" gallbladder. The bile is usually concentrated, clear, and dark. Chemical analysis demonstrates a high concentration of cholesterol.

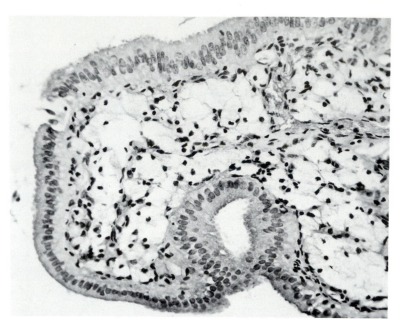

Fig. 579 Cholesterosis of gallbladder. Large foamy cells can be seen beneath normal epithelium of a villus. (×400; WU neg. 50-976.)

Microscopically, minimal to moderate chronic inflammation is seen in the subserosal tissue. Usually, such inflammatory changes are observed only when there are small stones in the cystic duct (Figs. 577 and 578). Lipid-filled foamy cells are present in the tips of the villi (Fig. 579). Boyd[14] demonstrated that this fat contains esters of cholesterol.

Acute cholecystitis

Before discussing acute cholecystitis, the role of bacterial infection in acute and chronic cholecystitis should be mentioned. Drennan[21] demonstrated bacteria in only nineteen of 100 inflamed gallbladders. Feinblatt[23] emphasized that bacterial peritonitis as a complication of acute cholecystitis is rare. If a gallbladder perforates, which is infrequent, the peritoneal reaction results from the bile salts rather than from bacterial infection. In an acutely distended gallbladder, bile may leak through the intact wall and cause the so-called bile peritonitis, a condition with an ominous prognosis.

Free perforation into the peritoneal cavity is a relatively rare occurrence in our institution but relatively common in others. The differences may be explained, in part, by the failure of some surgeons to operate upon patients promptly after onset of symptoms of gallbladder disease. If patients who recover from attacks of cholecystitis or biliary colic are not operated upon, the series will contain predominantly patients with major complications of this disease, including those with free perforations of the gallbladder. In a study reported by van der Linden and Sunzel,[30] one-half of 140 patients with acute cholecystitis had early operation (within twenty-four hours), whereas the remaining had delayed operation (two months later). The patients in the latter group had more protracted fever, hospital stay, and loss of time from work, and four of them came back before the two-month period with a new episode of acute cholecystitis.

Andrews[17] demonstrated that so-called empyema of the gallbladder usually consists of milky fluid which is an emulsion of calcium carbonate or an emulsion of amorphous or crystalline cholesterol. Womack and Bricker[31] demonstrated that the injection of concentrated bile into the gallbladder produces acute cholecystitis. If cholesterol or pigment stones lie free within the gallbladder, no inflammation is produced. Inflammatory changes in the gallbladder usually occur only when a single stone or stones are impacted in or around the cystic duct.[28] This was the case in eighty-nine of ninety-three patients with acute cholecystitis reported by Hallendorf et al.[25] Such impaction may interfere with the venous supply of the gallbladder by obstructing tortuous venous channels surrounding the cystic duct. This may cause congestion of the gallbladder wall and even hemorrhagic infarction. Under such circumstances, the primary insult to the gallbladder is aseptic and bacterial invasion occurs only secondarily. Proliferation of gas-forming organisms in the gallbladder wall results in the condition called *emphysematous* or *acute gaseous cholecystitis.*[18]

In children, gallbladder disease is rare. Of thirty-four cases reported by Hanson et al.,[26] fifteen had associated hemolytic disorders. Stones in the common duct are also unusual, and therefore jaundice in a child practically never indicates choledocholithiasis.[29] Furthermore, if acute cholecystitis occurs, it is often associated with some systemic infection such as hemolytic streptococcal septicemia or typhoid fever.[24]

Chronic follicular cholecystitis, a rare condition, is characterized by diffuse formation of lymph follicles in all layers of the gallbladder.[22]

In acute cholecystitis, the clinical symptoms and signs are those of an acute inflammation in the right upper quadrant of the abdomen.[27] Grossly, there is marked edema of the wall of the gallbladder. The mucosa has an angry grayish red color. *The pathogenesis is related to a stone impacted in the cystic duct.* Microscopic examination shows acute inflammation, subserosal edema, and often fresh thrombi within small veins. In keeping with the chemical rather than bacterial nature of the inflammation,

the tissue response is characterized in most cases by edema, hyperemia, extravasation of red blood cells, and widespread fibroblastic proliferation rather than by the customary polymorphonuclear infiltrate. The mucosa may be intact or show focal or extensive areas of ulceration.

Occasionally, a gallbladder removed because of acute inflammation will show fibrinoid necrosis of the muscular arteries, indistinguishable from that seen in polyarteritis nodosa.[19, 20] However, some of these patients remain asymptomatic thereafter, indicating that the vascular changes are not always part of a systemic disease.

Chronic cholecystitis

Chronic cholecystitis is rarely seen in the absence of lithiasis, although pure stones of the cholesterol and calcium birubinate types may be present without chronic cholecystitis. Thickening of the subserosal area is always present, sometimes to a striking degree. In most instances, stones are of the mixed or combined type (Figs. 573 and 580). Ulceration of the mucosa is infrequent.

Microscopically, the mucosa shows minimal to moderate chronic inflammation. It may be atrophic or normal or show diffuse hyperplastic changes.[36] The number of enterochromaffin cells is increased, sometimes to a striking degree.[33] Deposits of lipid in the intramural tissues are frequent, and stones may form in the wall.[51] The muscle may be hypertrophied, with mucosal diverticula (Rokitansky-Aschoff sinuses) penetrating its layers. Halpert[39] believes that Rokitansky-Aschoff sinuses do not occur in the normal human gallbladder, but with inflammation the continuity of the muscular wall is lost and the mucosa herniates into the perimuscular layer (Fig. 581). Luschka ducts have been described as ductlike structures lined by cuboidal epithelium found in the outermost layer of the gallbladder wall. They have a fibrous wall and do not communicate with the lumen of the gallbladder.

Robertson and Ferguson[45] believe that

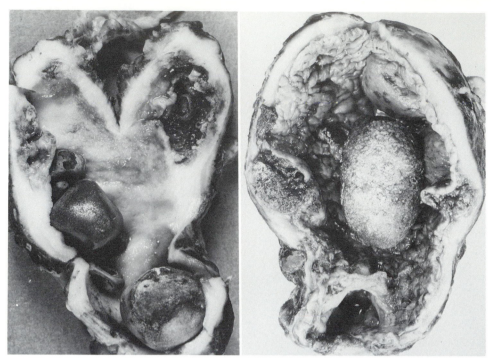

Fig. 580 Two gallbladders with advanced chronic cholecystitis. In both, subserosal portions are greatly thickened. In one, there is ulceration of mucosal surface. One gallbladder shows single large stone, and other shows multiple faceted stones. (WU negs. 50-2765 and 49-4576.)

the terms Luschka's crypts and Rokitansky-Aschoff sinuses should be abandoned and that diverticula of the gallbladder be substituted. They found such diverticula in about one-half of all gallbladders removed from patients over 30 years of age. Most of them communicated with the lumen of the gallbladder, but some were cut off from the gallbladder and became cysts with budlike branches (Fig. 582). These crypts can contain bile, bile pigment, cholesterol crystals, or true biliary calculi. Exaggerated examples of gallbladder diverticulosis associated with muscular hypertrophy have been dignified with the impressive but inaccurate names of *adenomyoma*, when focal, and *adenomyomatosis*, when diffuse.[41] The latter is identical to the cholecystitis glandularis proliferans described by King.[42] The localized form may involve any segment of the organ, but in most cases is located in the fundus, where it results in a sharply circumscribed

lesion[32] (Fig. 583). If stones have become impacted in the cystic duct, hemorrhagic infarction of the wall can occur ("gangrenous cholecystitis"). Bacterial invasion is secondary to such vascular alterations.

Small stones frequently travel through the cystic duct to become impacted in the ampulla of Vater or terminal third of the common duct, where they cause severe colic and intermittent obstructive jaundice.

It has often been argued that all gallbladders that contain stones should be removed surgically because of the risk of cancer, this being greater (5% to 10%) than the operative mortality (1% to 3%).[38] This argument lacks validity. At the Cleveland Clinic, Russell and Brown[46] reported twenty-nine cases of carcinoma of the gallbladder between 1932 and 1948. During this same time period, there were 1,488 cholecystectomics, which made the incidence of carcinoma only 1.9%.

The reasons for removing a gallbladder

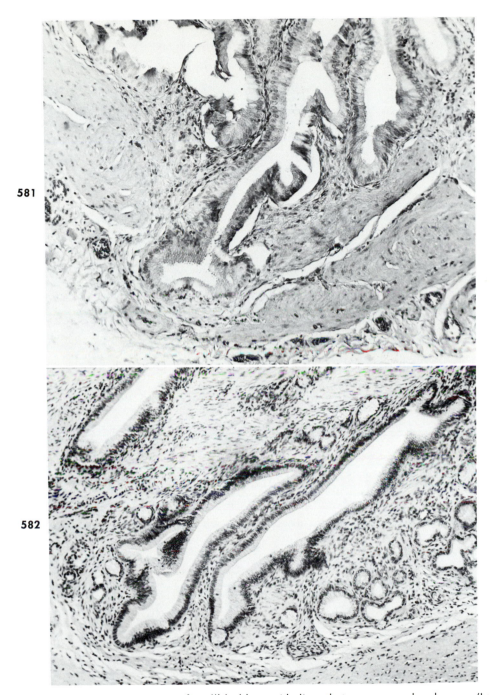

Fig. 581 Deep penetration of gallbladder epithelium between muscular layers. (Low power; WU neg. 49-5461.)
Fig. 582 Blindly ending ducts with budlike branches deep in gallbladder wall. (Low power; WU neg. 48-5173.)

containing stones are concerned with the serious inflammatory and obstructive complications that arise from them and not

with the possibility of associated cancer.[52] Truesdell[48] did exploratory laparotomies on 500 women for conditions other than

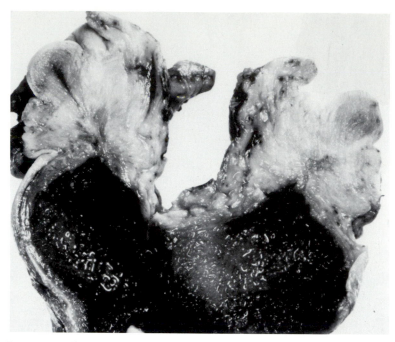

Fig. 583 Gallbladder with "adenomyoma" of fundus. (WU neg. 66-3278.)

gallbladder disease. Most of the patients had been pregnant sometime in the past. They were, therefore, a favorable group to have gallstones. He palpated the region of the gallbladder in this group and found fifty (or 10%) to have gallstones. Subsequent history and follow-up demonstrated that in only six were these truly silent stones. Lund[44] followed 526 nonoperative cases and demonstrated that one-third to one-half of the patients subsequently developed severe symptoms or complications from lithiasis. He concluded that prophylactic removal of the gallbladder containing stones is indicated in all patients who are good surgical risks.

Gallstones may lead to *internal biliary fistulas* that are usually located between the gallbladder and the duodenum, the gallbladder and the colon, or the common bile duct and the duodenum. Over 90% of the cases reported in the literature were in these locations.[49] These fistulas are created by the formation of inflammatory adhesions between the gallbladder and adjacent organs and the subsequent erosion of a stone through the gallbladder or the common duct into the gastrointestinal tract. Continuing choledochal obstruction contributes to the persistence of the fistula.[40] Fistulas are diagnosed by a roentgenogram of the abdomen when air can be seen in the extrahepatic biliary system. Moreover, a gastrointestinal series or a barium enema may reveal the unexpected outlining of the biliary tree. Fistulas may also become evident if the patient vomits or passes a large gallstone. With cholecystocolic fistulas, infection often is severe. Repair of these fistulas requires cholecystectomy and closure or resection of the involved portion of bowel.

Strictures of the common duct are usually caused by operative trauma in which the duct is excised or ligated inadvertently. Anatomic variations of the ducts and blood vessels may cause such an operative error.[35, 37] Strictures also occasionally are the result of infection following operation.[34] Their repair is a difficult surgical procedure. When the ends of the duct can be located, excision of the stricture and end-to-end anastomosis[43] or anastomosis of the duct to the duodenum[50] are recommended. At times, it may be necessary to anastomose the cut end of the

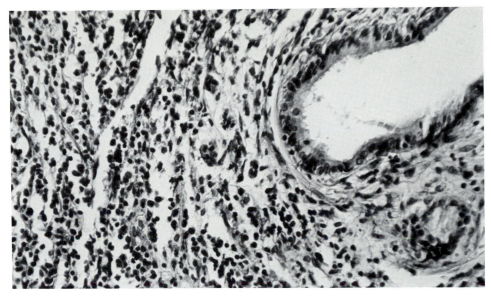

Fig. 584 Prominent chronic inflammatory change surrounding cystic bile duct. Note intact mucosa. This lesion occurred in 46-year-old black woman. Continuous T-tube drainage will often relieve process. (×285; WU neg. 62-233; slide contributed by Dr. W. B. Sorrell, Montgomery, Ala.)

hepatic duct to the jejunum.[43] Cole et al.[34] recommended the use of Roux-en-Y choledochojejunostomy for many strictures of the common duct.

Sclerosing cholangitis of the extrahepatic bile ducts is relatively rare, of unknown etiology, and accompanied by diffuse thickening of the wall. The mucosa remains intact. The common duct alone may be involved, but the hepatic ducts can also be inflamed[47] (Fig. 584) (Chapter 14).

Tumors

Christensen and Ishak[55] analyzed 180 benign tumors and pseudotumors of the gallbladder. The latter included three inflammatory polyps, all associated with chronic cholecystitis; twenty-one "cholesterol polyps," multilobular and yellow, composed of aggregates of foamy histiocytes covered by an intact mucosa; and eighteen examples of adenomatous or adenomyomatous hyperplasia. All of the fifty-one true benign neoplasms were adenomas, twenty-two of them having a papillary configuration (Fig. 585).

Cancer of the gallbladder and the extrahepatic ducts is an extremely serious disease. Carcinoma of the terminal third of the common bile duct is discussed in the chapter on pancreas and periampullary region. In a few instances, cancer may arise from the hepatic duct or at the confluence of the cystic and hepatic ducts.[64] Some of these tumors are extremely well differentiated with relatively slow growth, but most are discovered in an advanced stage (Figs. 586 and 587). They occur predominantly in women (ratio 5:1) usually past 50 years of age. An increased incidence of bile duct carcinoma has been reported in patients with ulcerative colitis.[57]

Russell and Brown[62] reported twenty-nine cases of carcinoma of the gallbladder among 1,488 cholecystectomies (an incidence of 1.9%). During this period (1932 to 1948), a diagnosis of cholelithiasis by roentgenologic examination was made in 4,459 persons. Thus, in the presence of cholelithiasis, the incidence of carcinoma was 0.66%.

Carcinoma may not be diagnosed clinically, but at the time of exploration of the gallbladder for stones, the diagnosis usually is evident. Even when it is possible to resect the gallbladder in the presence of carcinoma, practically no patients

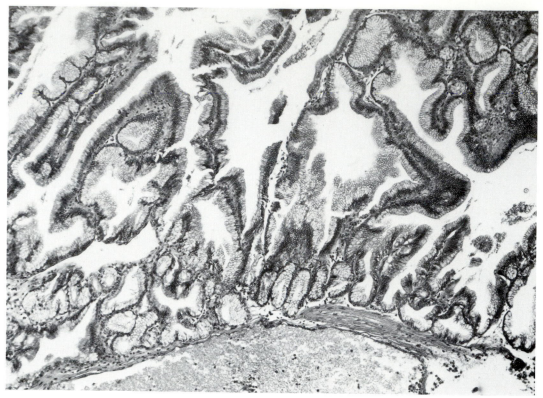

Fig. 585 Papillary adenoma of gallbladder. Tumor, which was seen in cholecystogram, measured 2 cm in diameter. (×90; WU neg. 71-5462.)

are cured.[61, 63] The only patients ever cured are those few in whom early cancer was found unexpectedly upon pathologic examination. Frank and Spjut[60] studied sixteen such "inapparent" carcinomas. Eleven of the patients died with clinical or pathologic evidence of metastatic carcinoma. No relation was found between the location or size of the tumor and the prognosis. All the long-term survivors had well-differentiated papillary adenocarcinomas, as was also the case in the series reported by Appleman et al.[54] (Figs. 588 and 589).

Microscopically, a gallbladder containing cancer shows extreme fibrosis of its wall. Gallstones are present in 80% to 90% of the cases (Fig. 590). The diagnosis is often missed grossly in the absence of an ulcerating, obviously cancerous mass. This indicates the need for microscopic examination of every excised gallbladder. We have seen several patients in whom an unexpected metastatic tumor was found

in the liver or bile ducts sometime following the removal of a gallbladder thought to have only cholelithiasis and cholecystitis on gross examination by the surgeon. The carcinomas are either adenocarcinoma (Fig. 587) or squamous carcinoma. Squamous carcinoma occurs from metaplasia of columnar epithelium of the gallbladder. The adenocarcinoma may secrete variable amounts of mucin. This is mainly sialomucin in character in contrast to the predominantly sulfomucin type secreted by the normal, inflamed, or obstructed gallbladder.[59] Rare undifferentiated forms, simulating sarcoma, also occur.[53]

Unfortunately, these carcinomas spread through the wall of the gallbladder and invade the liver, pericolic tissues, and lymph nodes and even infiltrate the duodenum. Because of such extensions, it is nearly always impossible to excise them completely.

Carcinoid tumors of the gallbladder have

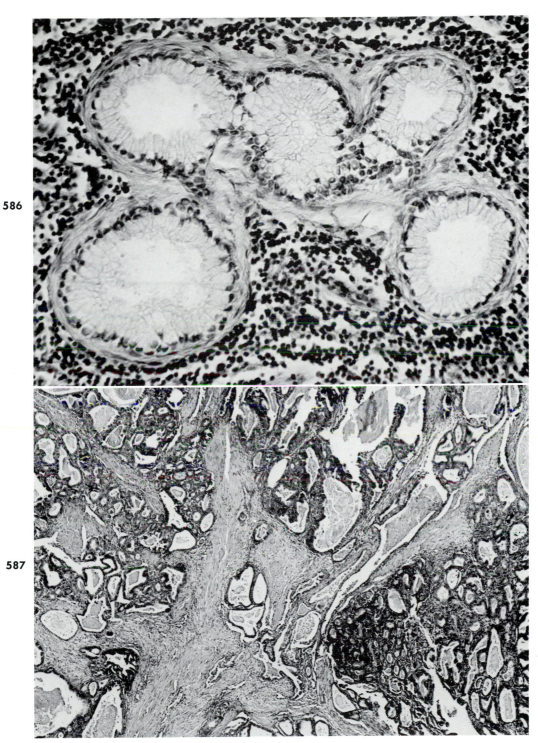

Fig. 586 Extremely well-differentiated adenocarcinoma metastatic to lymph node. Tumor arose from hepatic duct, but it was six years before patient died of this cancer. (×300; WU neg. 67-2377; slide contributed by Dr. R. E. Johnson, Columbia, Mo.)
Fig. 587 Adenocarcinoma of gallbladder showing extensive infiltration of muscular wall. (×38; WU neg. 69-3950.)

been reported.[56] There are five published cases of **granular cell tumor** of the extrahepatic bile ducts, three of them occurring in the common bile duct and two in the

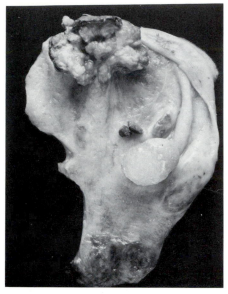

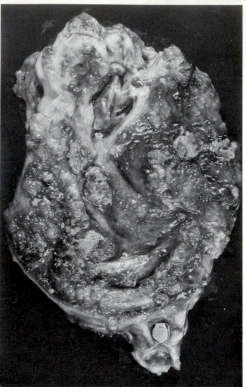

Fig. 588 Polypoid adenocarcinoma 2.5 cm in diameter in fundus. Stones are also present. Patient was well eight years after cholecystectomy. (From Appleman, R. M., Morlock, C. G., Dahlin, D. C., and Adson, M. A.: Long term survival in carcinoma of the gallbladder, Surg. Gynecol. Obstet. **117:**459-464, 1963; by permission of Surgery, Gynecology & Obstetrics.)

Fig. 589 Diffuse multicentric papillary carcinoma. Despite penetration of lesion through muscle in several areas, patient has survived five years after cholecystectomy. Note stone in cystic duct. (From Appleman, R. M., Morlock, C. G., Dahlin, D. C., and Adson, M. A.: Long term survival in carcinoma of the gallbladder, Surg. Gynecol. Obstet. **117:**459-464, 1963; by permission of Surgery, Gynecology & Obstetrics.)

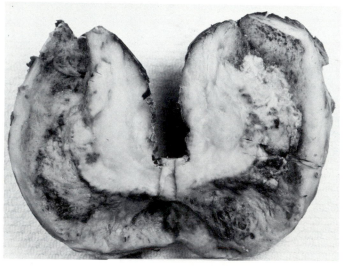

Fig. 590 Epidermoid carcinoma of gallbladder with almost complete replacement of wall and infiltration of surrounding structures. Stones were present.

cystic duct.[65] ***Embryonal rhabdomyosarcoma*** of the "sarcoma botryoides" type is
the most common malignant tumor of
extrahepatic bile ducts in children. Grossly,
it has a deceptively benign soft polypoid
appearance. Microscopically, undifferentiated spindle cells concentrate beneath an
intact epithelium. Cross striations may or
may not be present. The prognosis is extremely poor.[58]

REFERENCES

Congenital abnormalities

1 Christensen, A. H., and Ishak, K. G.: Benign
 tumors and pseudotumors of the gallbladder;
 report of 180 cases, Arch. Pathol. 90:423-432,
 1970.
2 Corcoran, D. B., and Wallace, K. K.: Congenital anomalies of the gall bladder, Am. Surg.
 20:709-725, 1954.
3 Curtis, L. E., and Sheahan, D. G.: Heterotopic tissues in the gallbladder, Arch. Pathol.
 88:677-683, 1969.
4 Järvi, O., and Meurman, L.: Heterotopic gastric mucosa and pancreas in the gallbladder
 with reference to the question of heterotopias
 in general, Ann. Acad. Sci. Fenn. 106:(suppl.
 22):1-42, 1964.
5 Moore, T. C.: Congenital atresia of the extrahepatic bile ducts; report of thirty-one proved
 cases, Surg. Gynecol. Obstet. 96:215-225, 1953.
6 Ober, W. B., and Wharton, R. N.: On the
 "Phrygian cap," N. Engl. J. Med. 255:571-572,
 1956.

Cholelithiasis

7 Friedman, G. D., Kannel, W. B., and Dawber,
 T. R.: The epidemiology of gallbladder disease; observations in the Framingham study,
 J. Chronic Dis. 19:273-292, 1966.
8 Gerwig, W. H., and Thistlethwaite, J. R.: Cholecystitis and cholelithiasis in young women following pregnancy, Surgery 28:983-996, 1950.
9 Giffin, H. Z.: Hemolytic jaundice: a review of
 seventeen cases, Surg. Gynecol. Obstet. 25:152-
 161, 1917.
10 Greene, C. H., and Snell, A. M.: Studies in the
 metabolism of the bile. II. The sequence of
 changes in the blood and bile following the
 intravenous injection of bile and its constituents, J. Biol. Chem. 78:691-713, 1928.
11 Madden, J. L., Vanderheyden, L., and Kanda-
 laft, S.: The nature and surgical significance
 of common duct stones, Surg. Gynecol. Obstet. 126:2-8, 1968.
12 Small, D. M.: Gallstones, N. Engl. J. Med.
 279:588-592, 1968.
13 Torvik, A., and Höivik, B.: Gallstones in an
 autopsy series, Acta Chir. Scand. 120:168-
 174, 1960.

Cholesterosis

14 Boyd, W.: Studies in gall-bladder pathology,
 Br. J. Surg. 10:337-356, 1923.
15 Carter, R. F., Greene, C. H., Twiss, J. R., and
 Hotz, R.: Etiology of gallstones, Arch. Surg.
 39:691-710, 1939.
16 Illingworth, C. F. W.: Cholesterosis of the gallbladder; a clinical and experimental study, Br.
 J. Surg. 17:203-229, 1929.

Acute cholecystitis

17 Andrews, E.: Pathologic changes of diseased
 gallbladders, Arch. Surg. 31:767-793, 1935.
18 Bigler, F. C.: Acute gaseous cholecystitis, Am.
 J. Med. 29:181-186, 1960.
19 Bohrat, M. G., and Bodon, G. R.: Isolated
 polyarteritis nodosa of the gallbladder, Am.
 Surg. 36:681-685, 1970.
20 Dillard, B. M., and Black, W. C.: Polyarteritis
 nodosa of the gallbladder and bile ducts, Am.
 Surg. 36:423-427, 1970.
21 Drennan, J. G.: A bacteriological study of the
 fluid contents of 100 gallbladders removed at
 operation, Ann. Surg. 76:482-487, 1922.
22 Estrada, R. L., Brown, N. M., and James, C.
 E.: Chronic follicular cholecystitis; radiological,
 pathological and surgical aspects, Br. J. Surg.
 48:205-209, 1958.
23 Feinblatt, H. M.: The infrequency of primary
 infection in gallbladder disease, N. Engl. J.
 Med. 199:1073-1078, 1928.
24 Glenn, F., and Hill, M. R., Jr.: Primary gall
 bladder disease in children, Ann. Surg. 139:
 302-311, 1954.
25 Hallendorf, L. C., Dockerty, M. B., and
 Waugh, J. M.: Gangrenous cholecystitis; a
 clinical and pathologic study of 100 cases,
 Surg. Clin. North Am. 28:979-998, 1948.
26 Hanson, B. A., Mahour, G. H., and Woolley,
 M. M.: Diseases of the gallbladder in infancy
 and childhood, J. Pediatr. Surg. 6:277-283,
 1971.
27 Lahey, F. H.: Acute cholecystitis, Surg. Clin.
 North Am. 32:837-845, 1952.
28 Mechling, R. S., and Watson, J. R.: The solitary gallstone, Surg. Gynecol. Obstet. 91:404-
 408, 1950.
29 Ulin, A. W., Nosal, J. L., and Martin, W. L.:
 Cholecystitis in childhood; report of a case
 with common duct stone, J.A.M.A. 147:1443-
 1444, 1951.
30 van der Linden, W., and Sunzel, H.: Early
 versus delayed operation for acute cholecystitis;
 a controlled clinical trial, Am. J. Surg. 120:7-
 13, 1970.
31 Womack, N. A., and Bricker, E. M.: Pathogenesis of cholecystitis, Arch. Surg. 44:658-
 676, 1942.

Chronic cholecystitis

32 Beilby, J. O.: Diverticulosis of the gall bladder; the fundal adenoma, Br. J. Exp. Pathol. **48:** 455-461, 1967.

33 Christie, A. C.: Three cases illustrating the presence of argentaffin (Kultschitzky) cells in human gall-bladder, J. Clin. Pathol. **7:**318-321, 1954.

34 Cole, W. H., Ireneus, C., and Raynolds, J. T.: Strictures of the common duct, Ann. Surg. **133:**684-695, 1951.

35 Eisendrath, D. N.: Anomalies of the bile ducts and blood vessels, J.A.M.A. **71:**864-866, 1918.

36 Elfving, G., Silvonen, E., and Tier, H.: Mucosal hyperplasia of the gallbladder in cases of cholecystolithiasis, Acta Chir. Scand. **135:** 519-522, 1969.

37 Flint, E. R.: Abnormalities of the right hepatic, cystic, and gastro-duodenal arteries, and of the bile ducts, Br. J. Surg. **10:**509-519, 1923.

38 Graham, E. A., Cole, W. H., Copher, G. H., and Moore, S.: Disease of the gall bladder and bile ducts, Philadelphia, 1928, Lea & Febiger.

39 Halpert, B.: Morphological studies on the gallbladder. II. The "true Luschka ducts" and "Rokitansky-Aschoff sinuses" of human gallbladder, Bull. Hopkins Hosp. **41:**77-103, 1927.

40 Hicken, N. F., and Coray, Q. B.: Spontaneous gastrointestinal biliary fistulas, Surg. Gynecol. Obstet. **82:**723-730, 1946.

41 Jutras, J. A., and Levesque, H. P.: Adenomyoma and adenomyomatosis of gallbladder; radiologic and pathologic correlations, Radiol. Clin. North Am. **4:**483-500, 1966.

42 King, E. S. J.: Cholecystitis glandularis and diverticula of the gall bladder, Br. J. Surg. **41:** 156-161, 1953.

43 Lahey, F. H., and Pyrtek, L. J.: Experience with the operative management of 280 strictures of the bile ducts, Surg. Gynecol. Obstet. **91:**25-56, 1950.

44 Lund, J.: Surgical indication in cholelithiasis; prophylactic cholecystectomy elucidated on the basis of long-term follow up on 526 nonoperated cases, Ann. Surg. **151:**153-162, 1960.

45 Robertson, H. E., and Ferguson, W. J.: The diverticula (Luschka's crypts) of the gall-bladder, Arch. Pathol. **40:**312-333, 1945.

46 Russell, P. W., and Brown, C. H.: Primary carcinoma of the gall bladder, Ann. Surg. **132:** 121-128, 1950.

47 Schwartz, S. I., and Dale, W. A.: Primary sclerosing cholangitis; review and report of six cases, Arch. Surg. **77:**439-451, 1958.

48 Truesdell, E.: Frequency and future of gall stones believed to be quiescent or symptomless, Ann. Surg. **119:**232-245, 1944.

49 Waggoner, C. M., and LeMone, D. V.: Clinical and roentgen aspects of internal biliary fistulas; report of twelve cases, Radiology **53:**31-41, 1949.

50 Walters, W.: Physiologic studies in cases of strictures of the common bile duct, Ann. Surg. **130:**448-454, 1949.

51 Weismann, R. E., and McDonald, J. R.: Cholecystitis, Arch. Pathol. **45:**639-657, 1948.

52 Wenchert, A., and Robertson, B.: The natural course of gallstone disease; eleven-year review of 781 nonoperated cases, Gastroenterology **50:**376-381, 1966.

Tumors

53 Appleman, H. D., and Coopersmith, N.: Pleomorphic spindle-cell carcinoma of the gallbladder; relation to sarcoma of the gallbladder, Cancer **25:**535-541, 1970.

54 Appleman, R. M., Morlock, C. G., Dahlin, D. C., and Adson, M. A.: Long term survival in carcinoma of the gallbladder, Surg. Gynecol. Obstet. **117:**459-464, 1963.

55 Christensen, A. H., and Ishak, K. G.: Benign tumors and pseudotumors of the gallbladder; report of 180 cases, Arch. Pathol. **90:**423-432, 1970.

56 Christie, A. C.: Three cases illustrating the presence of argentaffin cells in the human gall bladder, J. Clin. Pathol. **7:**318-321, 1954.

57 Converse, C. F., Reagan, J. W., and DeCosse, J. J.: Ulcerative colitis and carcinoma of the bile ducts, Am. J. Surg. **121:**39-45, 1971.

58 Davis, G. L., Kissane, J. M., and Ishak, K. G.: Embryonal rhabdomyosarcoma (sarcoma botryoides) of the biliary tree; report of five cases and review of the literature, Cancer **24:** 333-342, 1969.

59 Esterly, J. R., and Spicer, S. S.: Mucin histochemistry of human gallbladder; changes in adenocarcinoma, cystic fibrosis, and cholecystitis, J. Nat. Cancer Inst. **40:**1-10, 1968.

60 Frank, S. A., and Spjut, H. J.: Inapparent carcinoma of the gallbladder, Am. Surg. **33:** 367-372, 1967.

61 Jones, C. J.: Carcinoma of the gall bladder; a clinical and pathologic analysis of 50 cases, Ann. Surg. **132:**110-120, 1950.

62 Russell, P. W., and Brown, C. H.: Primary carcinoma of the gall bladder, Ann. Surg. **132:** 121-128, 1950.

63 Solan, M. J., and Jackson, B. T.: Carcinoma of the gall-bladder; a clinical appraisal and review of 57 cases, Br. J. Surg. **58:**593-597, 1971.

64 Whelton, M. J., Petrelli, M., George, P., Young, W. B., and Sherlock, S.: Carcinoma at the junction of the main hepatic ducts, Q. J. Med. **38:**211-230, 1969.

65 Whitmore, J. T., Whitley, J. P., LaVerde, P., and Cerda, J. J.: Granular cell myoblastoma of the common bile duct, Am. J. Dig. Dis. **14:**516-520, 1969.

14 Pancreas and periampullary region

Acute and chronic pancreatitis

Pancreatitis has been and still is a clinical enigma and the subject of much controversy. Its pathogenesis is unknown.[13] Experimental work has been hampered by the fact that most laboratory animals do not suffer naturally from this illness. In fact, it has not been produced in animals except by direct pancreatic trauma or by creating a closed duodenal loop.[19]

Between 1920 and 1930, the diagnosis of pancreatitis was infrequently considered except at operation or at postmortem examination, both of which permitted pathologic examination. In the early 1930's, the association of elevation of the serum amylase level with the pathologic findings of pancreatitis was repeatedly observed. The concept grew that an elevated serum amylase level alone would be adequate evidence of acute pancreatitis.[10] As operations decreased in number, the mortality associated with increase of serum amylase (and presumably, therefore, acute pancreatitis) also decreased.

Duodenal ulcer, volvulus, gangrenous cholecystitis, ruptured aortic aneurysm, and mesenteric thrombosis also may be accompanied by elevation of the serum amylase level, often at a higher value than that seen in pancreatic disease.[1] If these conditions are treated conservatively under the mistaken diagnosis of pancreatitis, the patients may die because they are not operated on. Even with early exploration of patients with an elevated serum amylase level, it is often difficult to detect any disease process in the pancreas at all. For instance, in sixty-seven patients explored within six weeks of an attack of presumed pancreatitis (fifty having a serum amylase level of 1,000 or more Somogyi units), forty-three had biliary lithiasis with a grossly normal pancreas, five had lithiasis and pancreatitis, and only one had pancreatitis alone.[3] Consequently, the concept that nonoperative treatment of pancreatitis is associated with a lower mortality than is operative therapy is fallacious when based on these figures. These studies also suggest that the nonoperative treatment has not in any way influenced the usual unfavorable course of patients with hemorrhagic or necrotizing pancreatitis.

Obviously, the mortality from pancreatitis will be less if patients with an elevated serum amylase level incident to biliary lithiasis are erroneously included among those with true fulminant hemorrhagic pancreatitis. From 80% to 90% of patients with elevated serum amylase levels have gallstones.

Since conservative treatment is of questionable benefit in severe pancreatitis and since serious lesions other than pancreatitis may cause an elevated serum amylase level, reevaluation of the operative treatment is indicated based on the following principles outlined by Bernard et al.[3] Immediate operation should be performed for signs of evident surgical catastrophe despite elevation of serum amylase levels. Operation should be considered in the patient who remains status quo or in whom the clinical condition worsens after a period of improvement, and elective exploration of the common bile duct should be performed at the optimal time in the clinical course of all patients who suffer from abdominal pain coupled with serum amylase elevation.

If careful examination of the pancreas at operation is correlated with clinical findings and coupled with pancreatic biopsy, our understanding of this complex problem might be clarified immeasurably.

The pancreas is occasionally involved by the mumps virus.[4] Longmire[12] cited two cases in which postmortem examination showed the same degree of pancreatitis in both the pancreas and heterotopic pancreas. The heterotopic pancreas was located in Meckel's diverticulum in one case and in the jejunum in the other.

Opie's famous case[16] (1901) demonstrated pancreatitis associated with a small stone lodged in the ampulla. The stone had converted the common bile duct and the main pancreatic duct (duct of Wirsung) into a common channel so that bile might have passed into the pancreatic duct and produced pancreatitis.

The theory that bile activates trypsinogen so that trypsin may digest the duct wall and allow pancreatic enzymes to digest the adjacent parenchyma is as yet unproved. Lipase splits fat and allows calcium soaps to form. Trypsin has the capacity to cause necrosis of the vessel walls, leading to hemorrhage.

Although Opie's observation[16] was valid, the formation of a common channel with a stone impacted in the ampulla occurs in only a small percentage of patients with pancreatitis (less than 5%). As Dragstedt et al.[8] pointed out, the union of the pancreatic duct and the bile duct to form an ampulla must occur at a sufficient distance from the duodenal opening to permit obstruction of the orifice without obstruction of either duct. The stone must be just the right size, for if it is too small, it will not block the ampullary opening, and if it is too large, it will block either or both the common bile duct and the main pancreatic duct. In 1919, Archibald[2] demonstrated experimentally that spasm of the sphincter of Oddi might produce a common channel.

Many studies have been made on autopsied cases to determine how often the anatomic setup would permit the common channel theory to operate. There are many anatomic variations in the ampullary area in which the formation of a common channel is not possible. These include separation of common and pancreatic ducts by a septum and independent emptying of the pancreatic duct into the duodenum. The consensus indicates that a common channel is possible in 50% to 60% of cases. Howard and Jones[11] studied 150 fresh specimens of pancreas, duodenum, and common duct. When the papilla of Vater was obstructed by a small calculus or clamped by a hemostat, fluid injected into the common bile duct regurgitated into the duct of Wirsung in eighty-one (54%) of the 150 specimens. Fresh rather than fixed specimens give the most accurate findings.

The pancreatic duct is visualized in about 25% of the patients having postoperative T-tube cholangiograms. If the common duct T tube is in place and pancreatic secretin is injected intravenously, almost pure pancreatic juice comes from the T tube.[5, 7] If spasm of the sphincter of Oddi is produced by morphine and if radiopaque material is injected through the T tube into the common duct, the whole pancreatic system may be visualized. Nitrites relax the sphincter. Hydrochloric acid causes spasm.

Chemical studies of bile coming from the common duct or gallbladder often show pancreatic ferments. Bile may be seen in the peripancreatic tissues of pa-

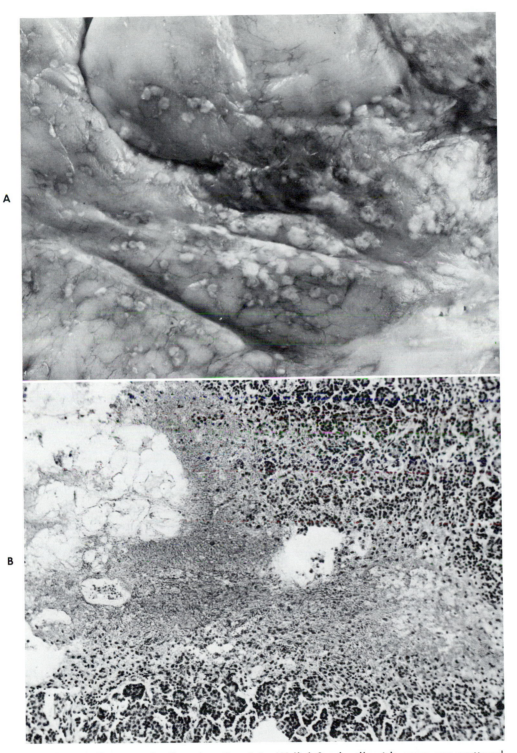

Fig. 591   A, Fat necrosis of pancreatic origin. Well-defined yellowish areas are scattered over mesentery. **B,** Fat necrosis in pancreas. (**A,** WU neg. 49-2145; **B,** ×140; WU neg. 49-5441.)

tients operated on for pancreatitis, possibly because of rupture of a pancreatic duct. These findings show that the common channel functions during life so that bile may enter the pancreatic duct system.

The secretory pressure of the gallbladder, bile ducts, and pancreatic ducts varies under different conditions. Pancreatitis often occurs after a heavy meal or in alcoholics. The anatomic arrangement of the duct of Santorini is important, for it has no sphincter, and if it communicates with the main duct of Wirsung, the biliary tract pressure would dominate. In Howard and Jones' anatomic study,[11] the duct of Santorini did not communicate with the duct of Wirsung in fifty-four (36%) of 150 specimens. This arrangement was present in forty-four of the eighty-one cases in which reflux could be demonstrated but in only ten of the seventy-nine cases in which no reflux occurred.

Rich and Duff[17] suggested that *increased secretion in the presence of partial block* of the ductal system may cause rupture of ductules and acini with liberation of pancreatic enzymes into the pancreas. They supported this attractive thesis by demonstrating partial squamous metaplasia of the ducts that might cause such a block. Such squamous metaplasia, however, occurs commonly in the apparently normal pancreas of older persons.

Pancreatitis may occur with tumors of the periampullary area or in the head of the pancreas. We have seen rare instances of pancreatitis accompanying primary vascular lesions of polyarteritis. Chronic pancreatitis is associated with alcoholism in approximately 75% of the cases.[20] The gross appearance is that of a nodular, hard, misshaped pancreas which may be either enlarged or atrophic. Microscopically, dilation of ducts, squamous metaplasia, interlobar fibrosis, and destruction of the acinar tissue are the predominant features. A rare hereditary form of pancreatitis manifesting during childhood and inherited as an autosomal mendelian dominant trait has been described by Comfort and Steinberg.[6] About 7% of hyperparathyroid patients develop chronic pancreatitis as a result of the hypercalcemia.[15] After an operation, particularly in the region of the pancreas, the patient may die suddenly and be found to have an extensive pancreatitis. Operative trauma may be the cause of such pancreatitis. Of seventy cases of postoperative pancreatitis reported by White et al.,[21] the original operation had included exploration of the common bile duct in twenty-eight and gastric resection in seventeen. In sixteen patients, the surgical procedure was such that the possibility of local trauma could be excluded. Unsuspected pancreatitis also may be found at autopsy (Fig. 591).

Chronic pancreatitis with lithiasis usually is diagnosed by roentgenologic examination or a postmortem examination rather than in a surgical pathology specimen. The two patients reported by MacKenzie[14] were alcoholics and had intractable pain, calcification of the pancreas, and pancreatic insufficiency. Stones form most often in the duct of Wirsung within 2 cm to 4 cm of the ampulla of Vater.[9] They represent a calcified mass of inspissated pancreatic secretion. Of the forty-five cases reviewed by Stobbe et al.,[18] the calculi were restricted to a small portion of the gland in twenty-two. Of these, none had symptoms of pancreatic origin, none had hyperparathyroidism, and only one patient had a history of alcoholism. The pathogenesis seemed to be related to narrowing or occlusion of the pancreatic ducts. Of the twenty-three patients with multiple diffuse calculi, six had hyperparathyroidism, three had associated pancreatic carcinoma, and 10 had a history of alcoholism. In all of the latter, a peculiar "mucoid" alteration of the ductal epithelium was described.

Annular pancreas

In annular pancreas, a rare embryologic abnormality (about ninety cases reported), the ventral anlage of the pancreas fails to rotate properly.[22, 25] Encirclement of the duodenum by pancreatic parenchyma may constrict it. Pancreatitis may develop in association with the anomaly.[23] The duct in the annular pancreas originates anteriorly, courses to the right over the duodenum and then posteriorly and to the left behind the duodenum, passing near the common duct.[24] These anatomic variations have to be kept in mind when operation is contemplated.

Heterotopic pancreas

Heterotopic pancreas is not rare.[27] Busard and Walters[26] found almost 550 cases in the literature. It is most common in the duodenum, stomach, and jejunum but also occurs in the ileum, Meckel's diverticulum, gastric and intestinal diverticula, gallbladder and bile ducts, omentum, and many other locations. We have seen a case in the ampulla of Vater that resulted in severe obstructive jaundice.

Grossly, heterotopic pancreas suggests normal pancreas. Microscopically, however, islet tissue is usually absent. Every pathologic change that occurs in the pancreas can occur in heterotopic pancreas.[28] Heterotopic pancreas in the stomach may cause hemorrhage, ulceration, or pyloric obstruction.

Pseudocysts

Congenital cysts of the pancreas are rare and usually are associated with cysts of other viscera such as liver or kidney. Pseudocysts are related to pancreatitis, trauma, and, rarely, to neoplastic duct obstruction. Blockage of ducts leads to an accumulation of secretion and cyst formation. These cysts often become large, spread beyond the substance of the pancreas into the lesser peritoneal cavity, and present through the gastrocolic or gastrohepatic ligament. They do not have an epithelial lining. The fluid within them has a high amylase content.

If the cyst cannot be excised, marsupialization of the cavity and sump drainage appear to be safe and effective. More re-cently, cystogastrostomy and cystojejunostomy have been recommended.[31] However, late complications such as hemorrhage and perforation have occurred.[30] The splenic artery is the most common source of intracystic hemorrhage which can be massive and result in sudden death.[29]

Tumors
Cytology

Duodenal drainage for cytologic examination is a somewhat complicated technical procedure. Tumors of the pancreatic duct, duodenum, and bile duct system can all shed tumor cells that can be aspirated. Intravenous secretin is used to enhance pancreatic secretion. The accuracy, unfortunately, is poor.[32, 33] Nieburgs et al.[34] found a positive cytology in twenty-three of seventy-three patients with pancreatic carcinoma, four of seven with a common duct cancer, and three of five with gallbladder cancer. However, there were twenty-four false positive diagnoses in 196 patients. Raskin et al.[35] reported positive results in thirty-seven of seventy-one patients with pancreatic cancer (52%). This technique is indicated in patients in whom there is a clinical suspicion of cancer. A positive result may force surgical exploration, but it should never be used as the only diagnosis if radical surgery such as a Whipple procedure is contemplated (Fig. 592). Frozen section must confirm the diagnosis. Raskin et al.[35] have obtained the highest level of diagnostic accuracy (Table 24).

Table 24 Location of ninety-five tumors with results of cytologic examination*

Site	Cytology negative	Cytology positive
Pancreas	34	37
Bile duct	5	5
Gallbladder	6	3
Duodenal—primary	0	2
Duodenal—metastatic	0	3
	45	50

*From Raskin, H. F., Moseley, R. D., Jr., Kirsner, J. B., and Palmer, W. L.: Carcinoma of the pancreas, biliary tract and liver, II, CA **11**:166-181, 1961.

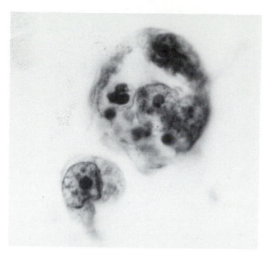

Fig. 592 Cluster of tumor cells obtained from duodenal lavage which led to diagnosis of adenocarcinoma. At operation, tumor was found to be primary in terminal third of common bile duct. (×1,250; WU neg. 67-567.)

Frozen section

Frozen sections for lesions of the periampullary area and pancreas are often difficult. A correct diagnosis requires the cooperative efforts of both the pathologist and the surgeon. Both of them should remember that the operative mortality for carcinoma of the head of the pancreas and periampullary area is still very high (10%) even in the hands of experienced surgeons.[37, 39] They must recognize that carcinoma in the head of the pancreas is practically never cured by surgery (no three-year survivals at Barnes Hospital), whereas favorable results may follow resection of tumors of the ampulla and the mucosal surface of the duodenum. The pathologist should not make a diagnosis of carcinoma from a frozen section unless he is absolutely certain.

There are many reasons for the difficulty in making a frozen section diagnosis. Sections can easily be taken from an area of the head of the pancreas containing no tumor. It may be difficult to distinguish well-differentiated adenocarcinoma from normal pancreatic ducts, but perineurial invasion, if present, is unequivocal evidence of carcinoma. Chronic pancreatitis simulates carcinoma because it makes the head of the pancreas hard. This hardness is due to inflammation and fibrous fixing of the lobules, but representative sections should be easy to interpret. Accessory pancreatic ducts forming acini may be present between muscle bundles and may be interpreted erroneously as carcinoma.[38] Pancreatitis with obstruction of the ducts may lead to almost complete disappearance of pancreatic lobules, leaving the dilated ducts, fibrous tissue, inflammation, and islet tissue. The fibrosis and inflammation cause so much distortion that the lesion may look malignant. With experience, however, frozen section is highly accurate.[40] With some degree of obstructive jaundice and no microscopic evidence of carcinoma in the head of the pancreas, it is mandatory that the duodenum be opened and explored. A carcinoma arising in the ampulla often forms a papillary mass, and sections taken from the surface may demonstrate well-differentiated papillary glandular lesions. The latter finding does not mean that the tumor is benign, for deep sections usually show more undifferentiated areas. If the carcinoma arises from the terminal third of the common bile duct, it may be difficult to obtain representative tissue.

During exploration of the jaundiced patient in whom obvious metastases are not present, securing histologic proof of carcinoma can be difficult. The head of the pancreas should be mobilized and carefully palpated, and the common duct should be exposed and its size determined. If a mass is felt in the head of the pancreas away from the ampullary region, direct incisional biopsy should be done. Experience is required to avoid the common duct, the gastroduodenal artery, and the portal vein.

If frozen section of the specimen shows only fibrosis and the common duct is dilated, the duct should be explored. If choledocholithiasis is not present to explain the findings, then duodenotomy should follow. *Dilatation of the common duct and of the gallbladder in the presence of jaun-*

dice, and in the absence of biliary tract stones, is almost always caused by carcinoma. Transduodenal biopsy or biopsy of the head of the pancreas should be performed, with care being taken to prevent duodenal spillage or excessive bleeding from the biopsy site so that possible seeding of the surrounding area by tumor cells can be avoided. In order to avoid hemorrhage and possible implantation and in order to secure tissue from the depths of the pancreas, we use needle biopsy and, like Coté et al.,[36] have found it accurate and free from complications.

Once the diagnosis of cancer is established, the type of operation, whether radical or palliative, should be determined. This depends on the degree of tumor spread as well as on its origin, whether ampullary or pancreatic. If a radical operation is contemplated, it is important to determine whether or not the portal vein is free of neoplastic invasion. Exposure of the portal vein above and below the pancreas is carried out, and the pancreas is dissected free of the anterior surface of the portal vein by careful blunt dissection. This is possible only in the absence of neoplastic involvement of the portal vein. If this maneuver shows the portal vein to be free of tumor, the head of the pancreas should then be resected. Even though the anterior surface of the portal vein is found to be free of tumor, cancer may occasionally invade the posterior wall of the portal vein from the region of the uncinate process. It is very difficult to determine whether or not the latter exists prior to the performance of a major portion of the resection. If the cancer is found inoperable because of invasion of the portal vein or local metastases, cholecystojejunostomy is all that is indicated.

Benign lesions of ampulla

The diagnosis of fibrosis of the papilla of Vater is sometimes made in patients with right upper abdominal pain in whom a "pinpoint ampullary opening" is found at operation.[41, 43] More often than not, the microscopic sections show no significant abnormalities. In our experience, clear-cut inflammatory or fibrotic changes in the papilla of Vater have always been associated with chronic gallbladder or pancreatic disease.

Benign tumors of the ampulla are extremely rare. A few instances of adenomas have been described.[42] We have seen an adenomyoma (Fig. 593) and a few inflammatory polyps (Fig. 594) causing partial biliary obstruction. Both of these lesions are nonneoplastic and can be treated by local resection.

Carcinoma of periampullary region exclusive of pancreas

Carcinomas are much less frequent in the periampullary region than in the pancreas. In spite of a low incidence, however, they are important because they are much more curable than carcinomas of the head of the pancreas. Tumors of this area can arise from the terminal third of the common bile duct, from the lining epithelium of the intestinal mucosa, from the true ampulla, and, under exceedingly rare circumstances, from Brunner's glands (Fig. 595).

Grossly, carcinoma of the terminal third of the common bile duct usually infiltrates the surrounding tissues and replaces the wall of the bile duct, extending upward beneath its mucosa and downward into the wall of the duodenum. The opened common bile duct is greatly thickened, and its mucosal surface has a granular appearance.

In carcinomas that arise from the ampulla or from the lining epithelium of the distal segment of the common bile duct, soft papillary masses usually develop in the duodenal lumen which, because of their softness, may not be felt through the unopened duodenum (Fig. 596). Grossly, they show a papillary, somewhat arborescent surface. Near their base, they are often quite firm. Duodenostomy with frozen sec-

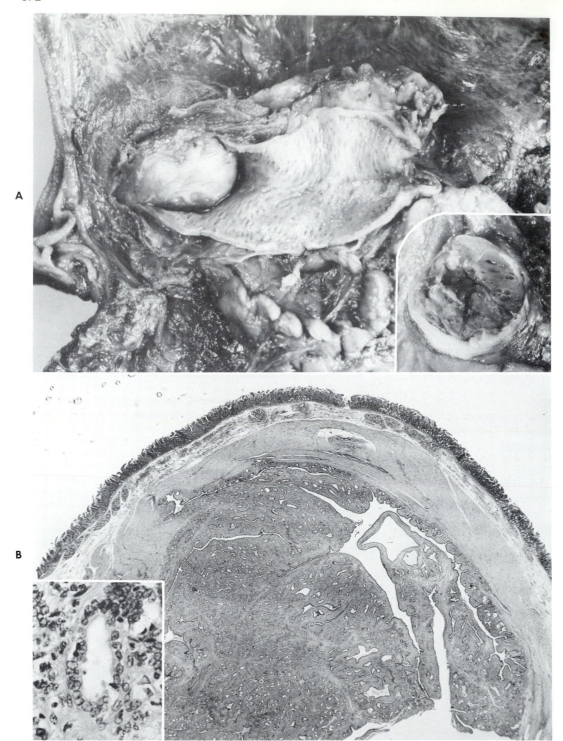

Fig. 593 A, Adenomyoma of ampulla of Vater resulting in obstructive jaundice. Common bile duct shows marked dilatation. **Inset,** Cross section of lesion demonstrating its well-encapsulated nature. It could have been easily enucleated. Instead, Whipple procedure was carried out under clinical impression of malignant neoplasm. **B,** Photomicrograph of same specimen. Glands and stroma intermingle in manner reminiscent of breast fibro-adenoma. **Inset** demonstrates benign appearance of glands. (**A,** WU neg. 71-8341; **inset,** WU neg. 71-8342; **B,** WU neg. 71-8656; **inset,** WU neg. 71-8657.)

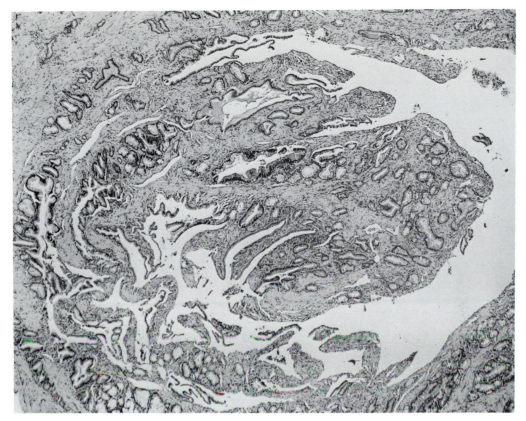

Fig. 594 Inflammatory polyp of ampulla producing almost complete obstructive jaundice. Removal resulted in complete relief of symptoms. (WU neg. 52-193.)

tion is needed to make the diagnosis. The biopsy should not be too superficial. Otherwise, the malignant nature of the tumor may be underestimated.

Microscopically, carcinoma of the terminal third of the common bile duct is usually a fairly well-differentiated adenocarcinoma, rarely an epidermoid carcinoma. The papillary tumors of the ampulla or intestine are made up of well-defined glands resembling the lining epithelium of the mucosa of the intestine (Figs. 597 and 598, A). The deeper portions of these tumors are often poorly differentiated (Fig. 598, B). Perineurial invasion may be present.

In the study of specimens from the periampullary region, the main pancreatic duct and the common bile duct must be dissected carefully to preserve their anatomic relationships. Sections should be carefully oriented so that the extent and origin of

tumor can be delineated. It is imperative also to search for lymph nodes in the specimen.

Miller et al.[44] reported thirty carcinomas arising from the ampullary area. Although these tumors appeared to be locally resectable, the seven patients surviving transduodenal resection were either dead or dying at the time of the report. By contrast, of the fourteen patients with carcinoma of the ampulla surviving radical resection, seven were living without disease. A recent review of the cases of ampullary carcinoma seen at our institution showed that about 80% were associated with regional lymph node metastases. The overall five-year survival rate was 33%. All patients with negative lymph nodes were cured.[45]

Islet cell tumors

Islet cell tumors make up a small fraction of all pancreatic neoplasms.[54]

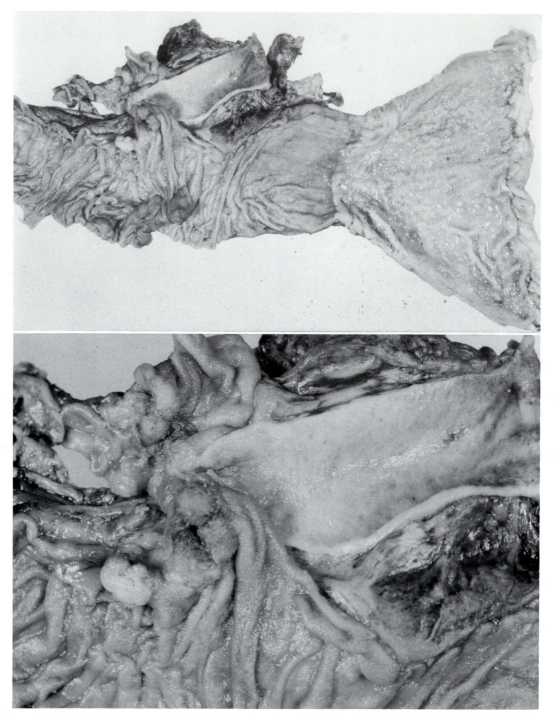

Fig. 595 Carcinoma of periampullary region. Patient, 63-year-old man, developed jaundice, chills, fever, and weight loss. Roentgenographic examination showed deformity in region of ampulla of Vater. One-stage pancreatoduodenectomy was done, and pathologic examination demonstrated polypoid tumor at ampulla of Vater. Tumor was fairly well differentiated, and there was no evidence of metastases. Patient died three years after operation of recurrent tumor in upper abdomen. (WU negs. 59-948 and 59-949.)

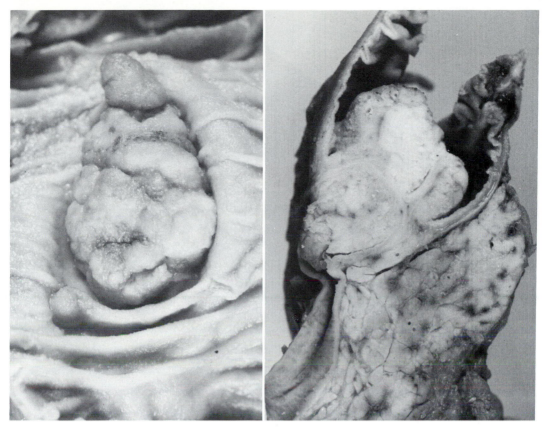

Fig. 596 Papillary adenocarcinoma of periampullary area in 67-year-old woman. Tumor resulted in obstructive jaundice and partial duodenal obstruction. (WU negs. 71-11073 and 71-11075.)

Most occur in adults, although a few in children and even in newborn infants have been described.[66] The most common location is the body and tail of the organ, correlating with a greater islet concentration in these locations. Grossly, the more cellular tumors have a pinkish cast and may resemble spleen or a congested lymph node (Fig. 599). They do not have a well-defined capsule. Other tumors, presumably longer standing, have a large amount of fibrous tissue and may even contain calcium and bone. Amyloid is rarely present.[58] Microscopically, most of the tumor cells resemble normal islet cells. They may be arranged in solid nests, ribbons, or festoons and are separated by a highly vascular stroma. Nuclear aberrations and mitoses are common. They should not be used as a criterion for malignancy. Actually, the only morphologic features that show a good correlation with metastatic spread and which should therefore be present for a diagnosis of islet cell carcinoma to be made are stromal invasion and tumor thrombi in the wall of veins. We have seen several islet cell carcinomas that have been confused with ductal adenocarcinoma because of the presence of glandular structures. They were discovered in a review of five-year survivors of Whipple's operation for pancreatic adenocarcinoma. Islet cell carcinomas are slow-growing tumors. For instance, in the first reported case of nonfunctioning islet cell tumor, vein invasion was the only evidence of malignancy. Liver metastases were first detected five years after the original operation, and the patient lived another five years following this discovery.[70, 71] Metastases are re-

Fig. 597 Papillary carcinoma of ampulla. (Low power; WU neg. 48-6338.)

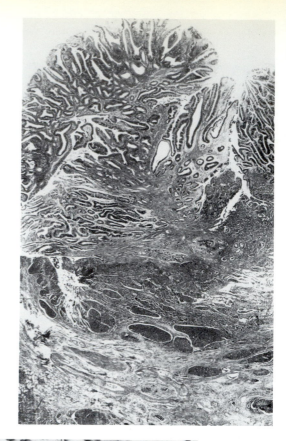

stricted to peripancreatic lymph nodes and liver in the majority of the cases (Fig. 600). Resection is justified even in incurable cases because of the long-term symptomatic relief that can be achieved. In some instances of islet cell hyperfunction, the pathologic examination will demonstrate diffuse hyperplasia of the islets of Langerhans, with preponderance of one or another of the different cell types, instead of a well-defined tumor mass.

Islet cell tumors may be nonfunctioning, at least at the level of clinical detection.

Fig. 598 **A,** Section taken from surface of tumor illustrated in Fig. 597 showing only questionable evidence of carcinoma with stratification of cells and loss of nuclear polarity. **B,** Sections from deepest portion of tumor shown in Fig. 597 illustrating highly undifferentiated carcinoma. (**A,** ×400; WU neg. 48-6332; **B,** ×400; WU neg. 48-6333.)

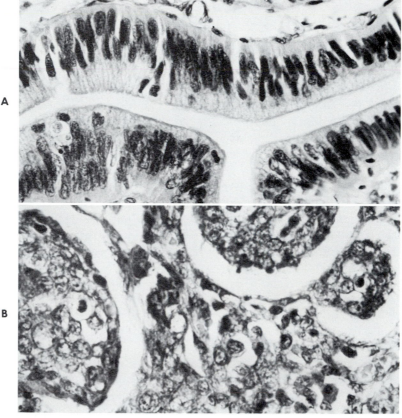

Most commonly, they present with an endocrine abnormality resulting from the secretion of insulin, gastrin, secretin-like hormone, glucagon, serotonin, ACTH, ADH, MSH, or a combination of these.[65] The majority of the islet cell tumors secreting more than one hormone are malignant. It is important to emphasize at this point that routine formalin-fixed, paraffin-embedded material is totally inadequate for the proper study of these neoplasms. Portions of the tumor tissue must be fixed in Bouin's or Zenker's solution and in glutaraldehyde, the first for the performance of special stains and the second for electron microscopic study (Fig. 601). Other portions should be frozen in order to have material available for immunofluorescent staining and biochemical assays.

Insulin-secreting **beta cell tumors** constitute the most common and better known variety of functioning islet cell tumors. The symptoms are the same as those resulting

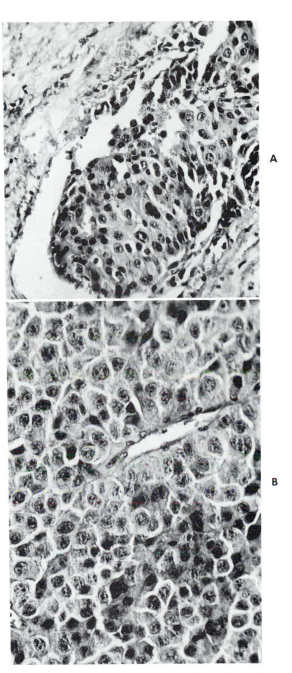

A

B

Fig. 600 A, Islet cell cancer, with blood vessel invasion, that measured 9 cm × 3.5 cm in diameter and weighed 500 gm. It contained bone and showed dense, incomplete fibrotic capsule. There were signs of hyperinsulinism. **B,** Eight years later, symptoms recurred. Patient was explored and tumor found to be present in liver. Patient died few months later. Well-differentiated tumor cells may be seen replacing liver parenchyma. (**A,** ×400; WU neg. 52-1833A; **B,** ×320; WU neg. 52-1834.)

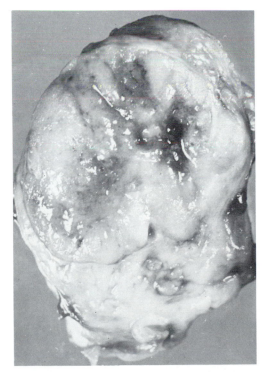

Fig. 599 Functioning, partially encapsulated, islet cell adenoma of pancreas. (WU neg. 51-1694.)

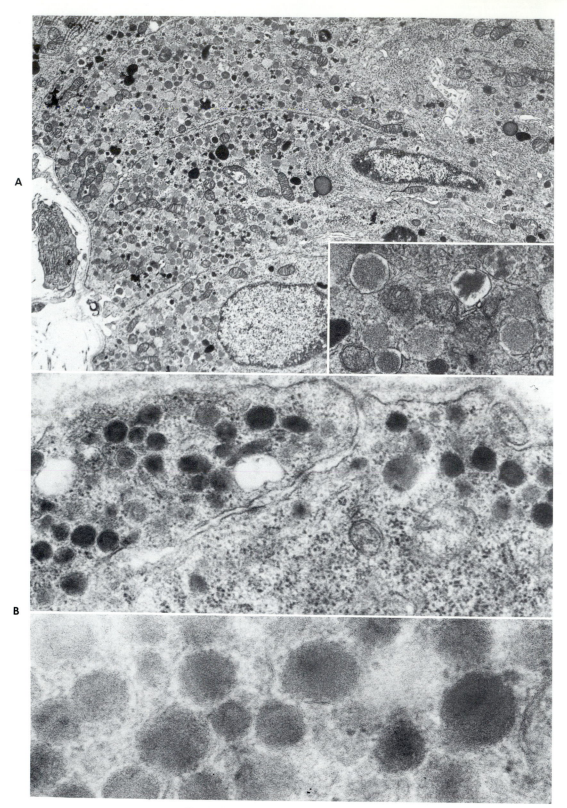

Fig. 601 For legend, see opposite page.

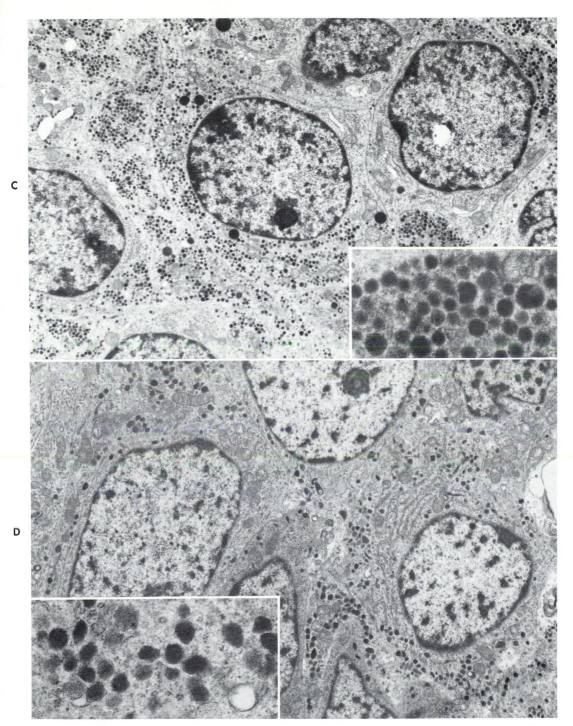

Fig. 601 Electron microscopic appearance of different types of islet cell tumors. **A,** Beta cell tumor. Many of granules have irregular or crystalline content. **B,** Alpha cell tumor. Granules are large and have dense peripheral nucleoid. **C,** Ulcerogenic tumor. Granules are similar to those of diarrheogenic tumor and of normal gastrin cells. Most tumors from patients with Zollinger-Ellison syndrome have this appearance. **D,** Ulcerogenic tumor having larger and more pleomorphic granules. This variety is uncommon in our experience. (Courtesy Dr. M. Greider, St. Louis, Mo., and Dr. M. H. McGavran, Hershey, Pa.)

from an overdose of insulin: mental confusion, weakness, fatigue, and convulsions. The Whipple triad should be fulfilled for a clinical diagnosis of islet cell tumor to be tenable. This triad consists of (1) symptoms and signs of hypoglycemia, usually induced by fasting or exercise, (2) fasting blood sugar levels below 50 mg%, and (3) relief of symptoms by the administration of glucose. Intravenous tolbutamide tests and determinations of circulating insulin levels are useful tests for the diagnosis of insulinomas.[63] Circulating proinsulin-like material has been detected by Gutman et al.[57] Celiac arteriography has proved extremely useful in the localization of these neoplasms, which may otherwise prove quite elusive at surgical exploration.[52] Only 10% of insulin-producing tumors are malignant if the criteria of infiltration and/or metastases are adhered to. The malignant variety is associated with a shorter history and a more pronounced hypoglycemia. In the series reported by Laroche et al.,[59] 94% were solitary and 6% multiple, all of the latter being benign. About 70% of the single adenomas had a diameter of 1.5 cm or less, the smallest measuring 4 mm. If the diagnosis of hyperinsulinism is reasonably certain and the surgical exploration fails to reveal a neoplasm, a subtotal pancreatectomy is justified. Of thirty-three patients reported by Laroche et al.[59] in whom this operation was performed, the tumor was found in the resected specimen in fifteen. In about 2% of the cases, insulin-producing islet cell tumors are found outside the pancreas, usually in the duodenal wall. In a small percentage of cases, tumors of other endocrine glands also are present.

Extrapancreatic neoplasms can rarely be associated with hypoglycemia that disappears on removal of the tumor. The secretion of an insulin-like hormone has been implicated. Approximately 50% of the lesions have been hepatomas or fibrosarcomas, and approximately 53% have been found in the liver or retroperitoneum. Most of them have been extremely large.[67]

Several examples of glucagon-secreting *alpha cell tumors,* first reported by McGavran et al.,[61] are now recorded[60] (Fig. 602). The tumor cells have the ultrastructural appearance of alpha cells. The relationship between the secretion of glucagon and the diabetes that most of these patients have is still problematic.

Ulcerogenic islet cell tumors result in the Zollinger-Ellison syndrome as a result of excessive production of gastrin. The syndrome is characterized by gastric hyperacidity with gastric, duodenal, or jejunal ulcers.[49, 53] Diarrhea is seen in one-third of the patients as a result of the excessive gastric secretion. Although the original reports emphasized the atypical location of the ulcers, this has not been substantiated in recent series. Radioimmunoassay of gastrin is the most useful test to confirm the diagnosis.[62] Other endocrine gland tumors are found in 20% to 40% of these patients.[46] Wermer[69] has made the interesting observation that if the Zollinger-Ellison syndrome is unaccompanied by other endocrine abnormalities, the pancreatic tumor will be solitary in practically every case. Conversely, patients with associated endocrine tumors (so-called multiple endocrine adenoma syndrome) often have multiple islet cell neoplasms.[46] The solitary neoplasms are malignant in approximately 60% of the patients, whereas the incidence and degree of malignancy is much lower in multiple tumors.[46]

There is still debate regarding the cell of origin of this neoplasm. It is not an alpha cell, as early reports had suggested. Some authors believe that the histochemical and fine structural features are those of delta cells.[47] Our findings indicate that the electron microscopic appearance is not that of either alpha, beta, or delta cells but rather that of the gastrin-producing cells of the gastric antrum.[55, 56] Whether cells with this morphologic appearance are normally present in the human pancreas has not been established with certainty. This histogenetic problem is further complicated by the fact that immofluorescent stain using anti-

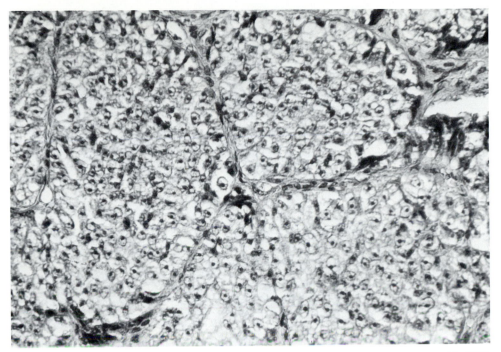

Fig. 602 Glucagon-secreting alpha-cell carcinoma of pancreas. (×300; WU neg. 66-437.)

human gastrin is positive for the normal gastrin-producing cells of the gastric antrum and for the pancreatic delta cells but generally not for the tumor cells associated with Zollinger-Ellison syndrome.[55] If the tumor cannot be removed entirely, total gastrectomy is the indicated therapy.

Twenty-seven cases of *diarrheogenic islet cell tumors* associated with a cholera-like syndrome in the absence of gastric hypersecretion have been described.[48, 68] A hormone with biologic properties similar to secretin has been detected in some instances.[50, 72] The morphologic, histochemical, and fine structural features of diarrheogenic tumors are indistinguishable from those of the ulcerogenic tumors.[56] In a review of fifty-six islet cell tumors, we found that the presence of a *gyriform* pattern of growth (reminiscent of giant distorted Langerhans' islets) was a feature of tumors of either alpha or beta origin. Conversely, all but one of the tumors containing glandular structures were of either ulcerogenic or diarrheogenic type. We found no consistent microscopic differences

between the tumors that gave rise to metastases and those that did not.[56]

Carcinoid syndrome with elevated serotonin levels has been described in patients with islet cell tumors, sometimes in association with hyperinsulinism.[51, 64]

Carcinoma

Carcinomas of the pancreas occur in either the head or close to the head in about two-thirds of the patients and in the body and tail in the other third.

Carcinomas of the body and tail grow insidiously, provoke widespread metastases, and often produce bizarre clinical signs and symptoms. Peripheral venous thrombi occur in about 25% of the patients.[77, 81] These tumors are only rarely operable and therefore are not often available as surgical specimens.

Carcinoma of the head of the pancreas, because of its strategic location in relation to the main extrahepatic ducts, usually causes progressive jaundice that is associated with pain in at least one-half the patients.

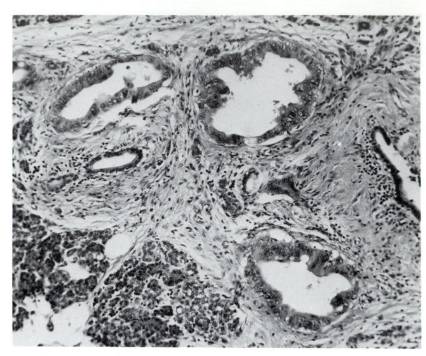

Fig. 603 Well-differentiated adenocarcinoma arising from pancreatic duct with resultant fibrosis of lobular tissue. (×70; WU neg. 48-6476.)

Grossly, these tumors are poorly delineated and quite firm and on cross section usually are yellowish gray. A high percentage of them arise from the epithelium of the ducts rather than from the acini, so that the involved ducts frequently become greatly dilated and plugged with necrotic tumor. This dilation may extend for a considerable distance beyond the main mass of the tumor. Because of ductal occlusion, the surrounding lobular tissue may be completely destroyed. The islet tissue is usually well preserved, resulting in an appearance designated as insular pancreas. However, atrophic or hypertrophic changes may occur. Most commonly, destruction of a variable amount of islet tissue mass results in a subclinical or overt diabetic picture. Rarely, hypertrophy of the islets occurs distal to a ductal adenocarcinoma and produces hypoglycemia.[78] In a few instances, the tumor arises from the acinar epithelium and completely obliterates the architecture of the pancreas without causing dilatation of the pancreatic ducts. Gambill[74] found significant pancreatitis in twenty-six (10%) of 255 patients with pancreatic or ampullary carcinoma. The presence of pancreatitis resulted in a considerable delay in the diagnosis of carcinoma.

Microscopically, the tumors that arise from the duct of the pancreas are often well-differentiated adenocarcinomas. It may be difficult to decide whether or not a malignant tumor is present (Fig. 603). Close attention must be given to the cytologic details. The neoplastic epithelium lining the ducts shows considerable stratification, loss of nuclear polarity, unusual nuclear changes, and mitotic aberrations. This neoplastic epithelium may extend to the point of transection of the pancreas. The carcinomas that arise from the acinar epithelium are made up of solid nests of cells that usually resemble the cells of normal acini. Highly pleomorphic carcinomas with areas of sarcomatoid appearance have been described by Sommers and Meissner.[80] Kay and Harrison[76] examined a case exhibiting osteoid formation, and we have seen two cases having an appear-

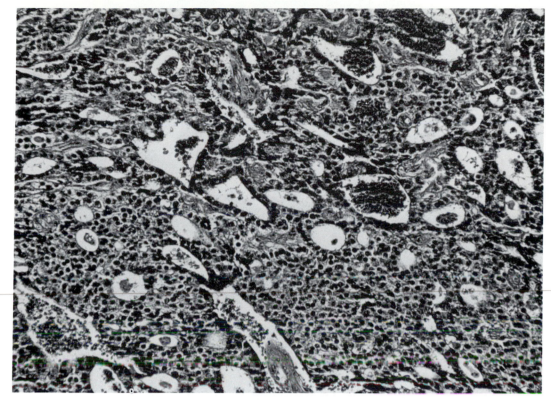

Fig. 604 Pancreatic carcinoma of infantile type. Tumor cells are uniform and form well-defined glands. (×175; WU neg. 73-7483.)

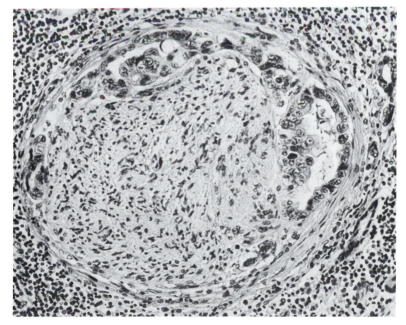

Fig. 605 Perineurial invasion in well-differentiated adenocarcinoma of pancreas. (High power; WU neg. 48-6337.)

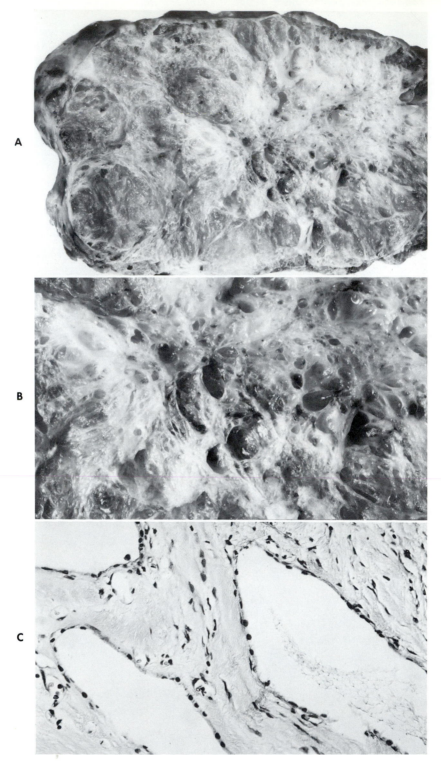

Fig. 606 **A,** Pancreatic cystadenoma in 65-year-old woman. Tumor measured 14 cm × 12 cm × 8 cm and was located within body of pancreas. **B,** Close-up view demonstrating multiple cysts separated by fibrous stroma. **C,** Same lesion shown in **A** and **B** demonstrating cysts, flattened epithelium, and fibrous stroma. (**A,** WU neg. 66-12770; **B,** WU neg. 66-12772; **C,** ×275; WU neg. 67-436.)

ance quite reminiscent of giant cell tumor of bone.[79] We also have seen two examples of a well-differentiated epithelial tumor, partially solid and partially papillary, occurring in children[73] (Fig. 604). Although on light microscopic appearance the possibility of islet cell origin was considered, electron microscopic studies have shown that this neoplasm is of ductal origin.[75] This tumor may attain a large size, extend outside the pancreas, and give rise to liver metastases.

Because carcinoma of the head of the pancreas extends along the ducts and invades the surrounding tissues and often the perineurial spaces and regional nodes, radical surgery is usually not feasible and practically never results in cure (Fig. 605). Palliative bypass operations result in similar survival times with much less operative mortality. On the other hand, ampullary carcinomas should be treated by Whipple's procedure whenever possible, since a significant number of cases can be cured by this operation.

Cystadenoma and cystadenocarcinoma

Cystadenomas of the pancreas are rare, slowly growing, true neoplasms that occur predominantly in women. They usually arise in the body or tail of the pancreas, where they may become extremely large. Diabetes may be associated with these lesions if the abundant islet cell tissue of the tail of the pancreas is destroyed by the tumor.

On section, the tumors are usually multiloculated (Fig. 606). The trabeculae between the locules may show calcification, which appears in a radiating pattern radiologically.[84] Fluid within the locules is often viscid or gelatinous.

Microscopically, these tumors are lined by cuboidal or tall columnar epithelium that resembles the lining epithelium seen in pseudomucinous cysts of the ovary. These tumors arise from duct epithelium.[83] They are usually benign but in rare instances are malignant.[85] A case of carcinoid tumor arising in the wall of a cyst-

adenoma was described by Persaud and Walrond.[86] Excision is the treatment of choice.[82]

REFERENCES
Acute and chronic pancreatitis

1 Adams, J. T., Libertino, J. A., and Schwartz, S. I.: Significance of an elevated serum amylase, Surgery 63:877-884, 1968.

2 Archibald, E.: Experimental production of pancreatitis in animals as result of resistance of common duct sphincter, Surg. Gynec. Obstet. 28:529-545, 1919.

3 Bernard, H. R., Criscione, J. R., and Moyer, C. A.: Pathologic significance of serum amylase concentration, Arch. Surg. 79:311-316, 1959.

4 Brown, M., and Smiley, R. K.: Chronic pancreatitis with steatorrhea following mumps with acute pancreatitis, Am. J. Dig. Dis. 17:280-282, 1950.

5 Colp, R., and Doubilet, H.: The operative incidence of pancreatic reflux in cholelithiasis, Surgery 4:837-846, 1938.

6 Comfort, M. W., and Steinberg, A. G.: Pedigree of a family with hereditary chronic relapsing pancreatitis, Gastroenterology 21:54-63, 1952.

7 Doubilet, H.: Pancreatic reflux deliberately produced, Surg. Gynecol. Obstet. 84:710-715, 1947.

8 Dragstedt, L. R., Haymond, H. E., and Ellis, J. C.: Pathogenesis of acute pancreatitis (acute pancreatic necrosis), Arch. Surg. 28:232-291, 1934.

9 Edmondson, H. A., Bullock, W. K., and Mehl, J. W.: Chronic pancreatitis and lithiasis, Am. J. Pathol. 26:37-55, 1950.

10 Elman, R.: Acute interstitial pancreatitis, Surg. Gynecol. Obstet. 57:291-309, 1933.

11 Howard, J. M., and Jones, R., Jr.: The anatomy of the pancreatic ducts; the etiology of acute pancreatitis, Am. J. Med. Sci. 214:617-622, 1947.

12 Longmire, W.: Personal communication, 1952.

13 McCutcheon, A. D.: A fresh approach to the pathogenesis of pancreatitis, Gut 9:296-310, 1968.

14 MacKenzie, W. C.: Pancreatitis, Ann. R. Coll. Surg. Engl. 15:220-235, 1954 (extensive bibliography).

15 Mixter, C. G., Jr., Keynes, M., and Cope, O.: Further experience with pancreatitis as a diagnostic clue to hyperparathyroidism, N. Engl. J. Med. 266:265-272, 1962.

16 Opie, E. L.: The etiology of acute hemorrhagic pancreatitis, Bull. Hopkins Hosp. 12:182-188, 1901.

17 Rich, A. R., and Duff, G. L.: Experimental and pathologic studies on the pathogenesis of acute

hemorrhagic pancreatitis, Bull. Hopkins Hosp. **58**:212-260, 1936.

18 Stobbe, K. C., ReMine, W. H., and Baggenstoss, A. H.: Pancreatic lithiasis, Surg. Gynecol. Obstet. **131**:1090-1099, 1970.

19 Strack, R., Dreizin, D. H., Ketyer, S., and Lazaro, E. J.: Duodenal reflux in the genesis of acute pancreatitis, Can. J. Surg. **10**:68-74, 1967.

20 Strum, W. B., and Spiro, H. M.: Chronic pancreatitis, Ann. Intern. Med. **74**:264-277, 1971.

21 White, T. T., Morgan, A., and Hopton, D.: Postoperative pancreatitis; a study of seventy cases, Am. J. Surg. **120**:132-137, 1970.

Annular pancreas

22 Baker, J. W., and Wilhelm, M. C.: Annular pancreas: report of surgical case with two-year follow up, Gastroenterology **15**:545-549, 1950.

23 Gross, R. E., and Chisholm, T. C.: Annular pancreas producing duodenal obstructions, Ann. Surg. **119**:759-769, 1944.

24 Lehman, E. P.: Annular pancreas as a clinical problem, Ann. Surg. **115**:574-585, 1942.

25 Tendler, M. J., and Ciuti, A.: The surgery of annular pancreas; a summary of sixty patients operated upon, Surgery **38**:298-310, 1955.

Heterotopic pancreas

26 Busard, J. M., and Walters, W.: Heterotopic pancreatic tissue, Arch. Surg. **60**:674-682, 1950.

27 de Castro Barbosa, J. J., Dockerty, M. B., and Waugh, J. M.: Pancreatic heterotopia, Surg. Gynecol. Obstet. **82**:527-542, 1946.

28 Chapman, B. M., Vogel, W. F., and Schomaker, T. P.: Massive gastric hemorrhage associated with aberrant pancreas in stomach, Gastroenterology **8**:367-374, 1947.

Pseudocysts

29 Greenstein, A., DeMaio, E., and Nabsetch, D. C.: Acute hemorrhage associated with pancreatic pseudocysts, Surgery **69**:56-62, 1971.

30 Rhoads, J. E.: In Rhoads, J. E., Allen, J. G., Harkins, H. N., and Moyer, C. A.: Surgery; principles and practice, ed. 4, Philadelphia, 1970, J. B. Lippincott Co., pp. 939-942.

31 Shumacker, H. B., Jr.: Internal drainage of pancreatic cysts by Roux-Y cystjejunostomy, Ann. Surg. **139**:63-66, 1954.

Tumors
Cytology

32 Henning, N., Witte, S., and Bressel, D.: The cytologic diagnosis of tumors of the upper gastrointestinal tract (esophagus, stomach, duodenum), Acta Cytol. (Baltimore) **8**:121-130, 1964.

33 Lemon, H. M., and Byrnes, W. W.: Cancer of the biliary tract and pancreas diagnosed from cytology of duodenal aspirations, J.A.M.A. **141**:254-257, 1949.

34 Nieburgs, H. E., Dreiling D. A., Rubio, C., and Reisman, H.: The morphology of cells in duodenal-drainage smears: histologic origin and pathologic significance, Am. J. Dig. Dis. **7**:489-505, 1962.

35 Raskin, H. F., Moseley, R. D., Jr., Kirsner, J. B., and Palmer, W. L.: Carcinoma of the pancreas, biliary tract and liver. Part II, CA **11**:166-181, 1961.

Frozen section

36 Coté, J., Dockerty, M. G., and Priestley, J. T.: An evaluation of pancreatic biopsy with the Vim-Silverman needle, Arch. Surg. **79**:588-596, 1959.

37 Longmire, W. P., Jr., and Marable, S. A.: Clinical experiences with major hepatic resections, Ann. Surg. **154**:460-464, 1961.

38 Loquvam, G. S., and Russell, W. O.: Accessory pancreatic ducts of the major duodenal papilla, Am. J. Clin. Pathol. **20**:305-313, 1950.

39 Newton, W. T.: Mortality and morbidity associated with resection of pancreaticoduodenal cancers, Am. Surg. **27**:74-79, 1961.

40 Spjut, H. J., and Ramos, A. J.: An evaluation of biopsy-frozen section of the ampullary region and pancreas: a report of 68 consecutive patients, Ann. Surg. **146**:923-930, 1957.

Benign tumors of ampulla

41 Acosta, J. M., Civantos, F., Nardi, G. L., and Castleman, B.: Fibrosis of the papilla of Vater, Surg. Gynecol. Obstet. **124**:787-794, 1967.

42 Cattell, R. B., and Prytek, L. J.: Premalignant lesions of the ampulla of Vater, Surg. Gynecol. Obstet. **90**:21-30, 1950.

43 Shingleton, W. W., and Gamburg, D.: Stenosis of the sphincter of Oddi, Am. J. Surg. **119**:35-37, 1970.

Carcinoma of periampullary region exclusive of pancreas

44 Miller, E. M., Dockerty, M. B., Wollaeger, E. E., and Waugh, J. M.: Carcinoma in the region of the papilla of Vater, Surg. Gynecol. Obstet. **92**:172-182, 1951.

45 Pizzimbono, C. A., Dehner, L. P., and Wise, L.: Ampullary carcinoma; clinicopathologic evaluation of 43 cases, Ann. Surg. (in press).

Islet cell tumors

46 Ballard, H. S., Frame, B., and Hartsock, R. J.: Familial multiple endocrine adenoma-peptic ulcer complex, Medicine (Baltimore) **43**:481-516, 1964.

47 Cavallero, C., Solcia, E., and Sampietro, R.: Cytology of islet tumours and hyperplasias associated with the Zollinger-Ellison syndrome, Gut 8:172-177, 1967.

48 Cerda, J. J., Raffensberger, E. C., and Rawnsley, H. M.: Cholera-like syndrome and pancreatic islet cell tumors, Med. Clin. North Am. 54:567-575, 1970.

49 Christlieb, A. R., and Schuster, M. M.: Zollinger-Ellison syndrome; a clinical appraisal based on a review of the literature, Arch. Intern. Med. 114:381-388, 1964.

50 Cleator, I. G., Thomson, C. G., Sircus, W., and Coombes, M.: Bio-assay evidence of abnormal secretin-like and gastrin-like activity in tumor and blood in cases of "choleraic diarrhea," Gut 11:206-211, 1970.

51 Dollinger, M. R., Ratner, L. H., Shamoian, C. A., and Blackbourne, B. D.: Carcinoid syndrome associated with pancreatic tumors, Arch. Intern. Med. 120:575-580, 1967.

52 Dunn, D. C.: Diabetes after removal of insulin tumours of pancreas: a long-term follow-up survey of 11 patients, Br. Med. J. 2:84-87, 1971.

53 Ellison, E. H., and Wilson, S. D.: The Zollinger-Ellison syndrome updated, Surg. Clin. North Am. 47:1115-1124, 1967.

54 Frantz, V. K.: Tumors of the pancreas. In Atlas of tumor pathology, Sect. VII, Fasc. 27 and Fasc. 28, Washington, D. C., 1959, Armed Forces Institute of Pathology.

55 Greider, M., and McGuigan, J. E.: Electron microscopic identification of the gastrin cell of the human antral mucosa by means of immunocytochemistry, Gastroenterology 63:572-583, 1972.

56 Greider, M. H., Rosai, J., and McGuigan, J. E.: The human pancreatic islet cells and their tumors. II. Ulcerogenic and diarrheogenic tumors, Cancer (in press).

57 Gutman, R. A., Lazarus, N. R., Penhos, J. C., Fajans, S., and Recant, L.: Circulating proinsulin-like material in patients with functioning insulinomas, N. Engl. J. Med. 284:1003-1008, 1971.

58 Heitz, P., Steiner, H., and Halter, F.: Multihormonal, amyloid-producing tumor of the islets of Langerhans in a twelve-year-old boy; clinical, morphological and biochemical data and review of the literature, Virchows Arch. [Pathol. Anat.] 353:312-324, 1971.

59 Laroche, G. P., Ferris, D. O., Priestley, J. T., Scholz, D. A., and Dockerty, M. B.: Hyperinsulinism: surgical results and management of occult functioning islet cell tumor; review of 154 cases, Arch. Surg. 96:763-771, 1968.

60 Lomsky, R., Langr, F., and Vortel, V.: Demonstration of glucagon in islet cell adenomas of the pancreas by immunofluorescent technic, Am. J. Clin. Pathol. 51:245-250, 1969.

61 McGavran, M. H., Unger, R. H., Recant, L., Polk, H. C., Kilo, C., and Levin, M. E.: A glucagon-secreting alpha-cell carcinoma of the pancreas, N. Engl. J. Med. 274:1408-1414, 1966.

62 McGuigan, J. E., and Trudeau, W. L.: Immunochemical measurement of elevated levels of gastrin in the serum of patients with pancreatic tumors of the Zollinger-Ellison variety. N. Engl. J. Med. 278:1308-1313, 1968.

63 Marks, V.: Progress report; diagnosis of insulinoma, Gut 12:835-843, 1971.

64 Patchefsky, A. S., Solit, R., Phillips, L. D., Craddock, M., Harrer, W. V., Cohn, H. E., and Kowlessar, O. D.: Hydroxyindole-producing tumors of the pancreas; carcinoid-islet cell tumor and oat cell carcinoma, Ann. Intern. Med. 77:53-61, 1972.

65 Rawlinson, D. G.: Electron microscopy of an ACTH-secreting islet cell carcinoma, Cancer 31:1015-1019, 1973.

66 Robinson, M. J., Clarke, A. M., Gold, H., and Connelly, J. F.: Islet cell adenoma in the newborn: report of two patients, Pediatrics 48:232-236, 1971.

67 Silverstein, M. N.: Tumor hypoglycemia, Cancer 23:142-144, 1969.

68 Stoker, D. J., and Wynn, V.: Pancreatic islet cell tumour with watery diarrhoea and hypokalaemia, Gut 11:911-920, 1970.

69 Wermer, P.: Duality of pancreatogenous peptic ulcer (correspondence), N. Engl. J. Med. 278:397-398, 1968.

70 Whipple, A. O.: Pancreatoduodenectomy for islet cell carcinoma, Ann. Surg. 121:847-852, 1945.

71 Whipple, A. O.: Personal communication, 1952.

72 Zollinger, R. M., Tompkins, R. K., Amerson, J. R., Endahl, G. L., Kraft, A. R., and Moore, F. T.: Identification of the diarrheogenic hormone associated with non-beta islet cell tumors of the pancreas, Ann. Surg. 168:502-521, 1968.

Carcinoma

73 Frable, W. J., Still, W. J. S., and Kay, S.: Carcinoma of the pancreas, infantile type; a light and electron microscopic study, Cancer 27:667-673, 1971.

74 Gambill, E. E.: Pancreatitis associated with pancreatic carcinoma: a study of 26 cases, Mayo Clin. Proc. 46:173-177, 1971.

75 Hamoudi, A. B., Misugi, K., Grosfield, J. L., and Reiner, C. B.: Papillary epithelial neoplasm of pancreas in a child; report of a case with electron microscopy, Cancer 26:1126-1134, 1970.

76 Kay, S., and Harrison, J. M.: Unusual pleo-

morphic carcinoma of the pancreas featuring production of osteoid, Cancer **23**:1158-1162, 1969.

77 Lafler, C. J., and Hinerman, D. L.: A morphologic study of pancreatic carcinoma with reference of multiple thrombi, Cancer **14**:944-952, 1961.

78 McBee, J. W., Lanza, F. L., and Erickson, E. E.: Hypoglycemia due to obstruction of pancreatic excretory ducts by carcinoma, Arch. Pathol. **81**:287-291, 1966.

79 Rosai, J.: Carcinoma of pancreas simulating giant cell tumor of bone; electron microscopic evidence of its acinar cell origin, Cancer **22**:333-344, 1968.

80 Sommers, S. C., and Meissner, W. A.: Unusual carcinomas of the pancreas, Arch. Pathol. **58**: 101-111, 1954.

81 Sproul, E. E.: Carcinoma and venous thrombosis: the frequency of association of the carcinoma in the body or tail of the pancreas with multiple venous thrombosis, Am. J. Cancer **34**:566-585, 1938.

Cystadenoma and cystadenocarcinoma

82 Benson, R. E., and Gordon, W.: Cystadenoma of the pancreas; with presentation of one case and review of twenty-eight cases collected from the medical literature, Surgery **21**:353-361, 1947.

83 Glenner, G. G., and Mallory, G. K.: The cystadenoma and related nonfunctional tumors of the pancreas; pathogenesis, classification and significance, Cancer **9**:980-996, 1956.

84 Haukohl, R. S., and Melamed, A.: Cystadenoma of pancreas, Am. J. Roentgenol. Radium Ther. Nucl. Med. **63**:234-245, 1950.

85 Jemerin, E. E., and Samuels, N. A.: Cystadenoma of pancreas, Ann. Surg. **127**:158-170, 1948.

86 Persaud, V., and Walrond, E. R.: Carcinoid tumor and cystadenoma of the pancreas, Arch. Pathol. **92**:28-30, 1971.

15 Adrenal gland and related paraganglia

Introduction

The cortex and the medulla of the adrenal gland have entirely different origins. The cortex arises from mesoderm, whereas the medulla arises from ectodermal chromaffin tissue. Except for cases of heterotopia, cortical tissue is seen only within the anatomic confines of the adrenal gland. On the other hand, islands of chromaffin tissue morphologically identical to that present in the adrenal medulla are normally found along the abdominal aorta. The most important of these is the Zuckerkandl's body, situated close to the angle formed by the anterior aortic wall and the origin of the inferior mesenteric artery. Excellent reviews of the anatomy and pathology of the adrenal gland are available.[1, 2]

Lesions of adrenal cortex

Heterotopia

Heterotopic adrenal cortical tissue has been reported in numerous locations. The most common site is the area adjacent to the adrenal gland. It occurs occasionally in the region of the celiac plexus,[4] within the kidney substance, along the course of the spermatic and ovarian veins, within the testes[3, 5] or the ovary, in the broad ligament near the ovary, or close to the tail of the epididymis. Stout[6] has seen heterotopic adrenal tissue in the canal of Nuck, in hernial and hydrocele sacs, in the mesentery of the appendix, and in the retroperitoneal area. Whether it ever occurs in the liver is doubtful.

Congenital hyperplasia

Congenital hyperplasia, an inborn error of metabolism, occurs with equal frequency in males and females and is transmitted by an autosomal recessive gene. It is responsible for the large majority of cases of adrenogenital syndrome developing within the first year of life. In approximately 95% of congenital hyperplasias, the basic defect is an absence of the enzyme 21-hydroxylase, which results in the accumulation of 17OH-progesterone and its catabolite pregnanetriol and in a deficiency of cortisol. The clinical picture is usually that of a pure virilizing syndrome, although in approximately 30% of the patients electrolyte disturbances occur.[9] The

589

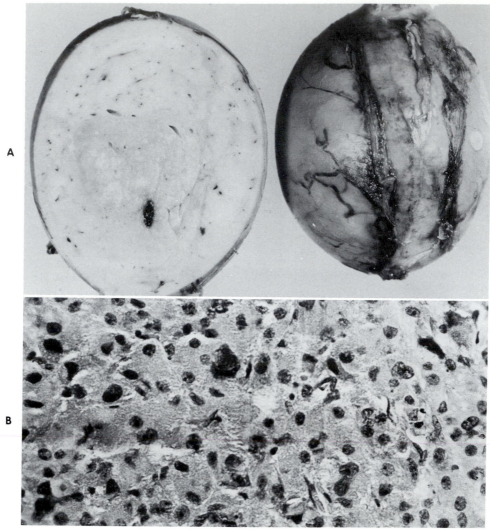

Fig. 607 **A,** Small cortical adenoma of adrenal gland that was causing virilizing signs. This tumor was identified by perirenal air insufflation. **B,** Same tumor illustrated in **A** showing large cells and atypical nuclei. Virilizing signs and symptoms rapidly regressed. Patient has remained well for over ten years. (**A,** WU neg. 49-6852; **B,** ×480; WU neg. 49-6714.)

second most frequent form is due to a deficiency of 11-hydroxylase and is characterized by virilization and hypertension. Three other variants, all exceptionally rare, have been described.[7] The pathologic change is the same in all types and is characterized by diffuse cortical hyperplasia, especially of the zona reticularis. The treatment consists of replacement with cortisol and surgical correction of the external sexual organs.[8]

Acquired hyperplasia

Acquired hyperplasia, which is always bilateral, may result in a diffuse or in a nodular ("adenomatous") enlargement of the adrenal gland. It is a frequent autopsy finding. Cortical nodules greater than 3 mm in size were encountered in 216 (2.86%) of 7,437 consecutive autopsies by Commons and Callaway.[10] These nodules do not have clinical significance. They increase in number with age but are not correlated with hypertension, diabetes, or cardiovascular disease. The symptomatic form of cortical hyperplasia can be ascribed in some cases to pituitary hyperfunction and in others to the presence of an ACTH-producing neoplasm. In the majority of the cases, however, the pathogenesis remains "idiopathic."

Adenoma

Adenomas are usually solitary and well encapsulated. On section, they often show a homogeneous yellow surface (Fig. 607, A). Foci of necrosis and hemorrhage are rare. Occasionally, adenomas have a dark brown or even black color because of the presence of large amounts of lipofuscin.[11] Adenomas are characteristically small neoplasms that rarely exceed 50 gm in weight, a point to remember in the differential diagnosis with carcinoma.[12] Microscopically, they may resemble the appearance of the zona fasciculata, the zona glomerulosa, or, more commonly, a combination of both. Occasional bizarre nuclear forms can be seen, as in most other endocrine neoplasms (Fig. 607, B). However, *mitoses are exceptionally rare or absent.*

Carcinoma

Adrenal cortical carcinoma is usually large and may weigh as much as 1,000 gm before discovery. A palpable adrenal cortical neoplasm is malignant in practically every instance. The cut surface shows a variegated pattern, many of the nodules being soft and friable. Areas of necrosis and hemorrhage are frequent (Fig. 608, A and B). They may result in fever and simulate an infectious disease.[15] A capsule may be present but is often infiltrated by tumor. Microscopically, it may be very difficult to decide whether a given tumor is benign or malignant. Many of the tumor cells closely resemble the adrenal cortical cells. Large cells with abundant acidophilic cytoplasm and bizarre hyperchromatic nuclei appear, as well as multinucleated forms[13] (Fig. 608, C). The two most reliable microscopic signs of malignancy are tumor invasion of blood vessels and the presence of numerous mitotic figures. Adrenal cortical cancer is generally a highly malignant neoplasm. One-half of the thirty-eight patients studied by Lipsett et al.[14] died within two years of the onset of symptoms. The most common sites of metastatic involvement are liver (60%), regional lymph nodes (40%), and lungs (40%).[13]

Clinicopathologic correlation

Acquired hyperplasia, adenoma, and carcinoma may be "nonfunctioning," at least at a clinical level, or, more commonly, be the cause of a variety of syndromes resulting from the secretion of excessive amounts of corticosteroid hormones. A fairly accurate prediction regarding the morphologic type of abnormality in the adrenal gland can be made by knowing the clinical syndrome plus the age and sex of the patient.

Nonfunctioning lesions

Whereas instances of cortical hyperplasia and adenomas are found commonly at postmortem examination of asymptomatic individuals,[16] most of the nonfunctioning adrenal cortical lesions seen as surgical specimens are carcinomas. The majority of these occur in the older age groups.[17] The finding of a cortical adenoma in a hypertensive patient does not, in itself, imply any causal relationship.

Aldosteronism

In primary aldosteronism, the excessive amount of secreted aldosterone results in urinary loss of potassium, retention of sodium, hypertension, and muscle weakness.[19] The adrenal lesion is an adenoma in the large majority of cases, cortical hyperplasia being responsible for the remaining. The adenoma is usually unilateral, solitary (91%), and small. In the series of eighteen cases reported by Neville and Symington,[21] 60% of the tumors weighed less than 6 gm. The cut surface has a homogenous golden yellow or yellow-brown color. Microscopically, one would expect these adenomas to

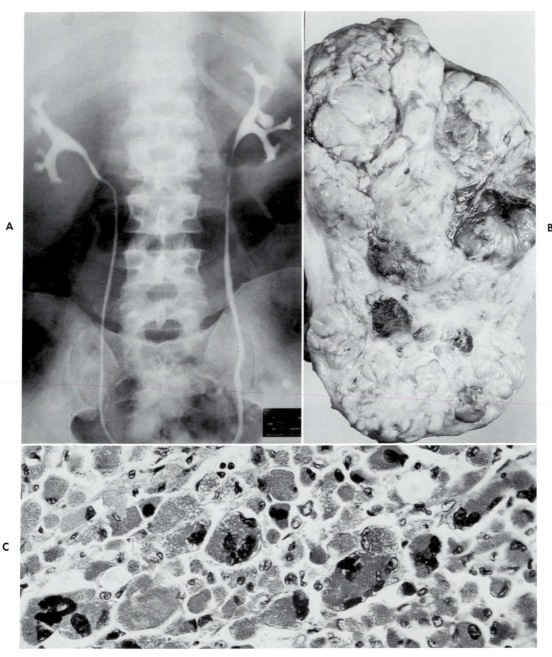

Fig. 608 **A,** Retrograde pyelogram of 47-year-old man with large asymptomatic tumor of right adrenal gland displacing right kidney. **B,** Same lesion illustrated in **A** showing large, bright yellow tumor (weight, 900 gm), encapsulated, with areas of necrosis. **C,** Same tumor shown in **A** and **B** demonstrating large cells with considerable variations in size and with many bizarre nuclei. There were tumor cells lying free within veins. This finding was significant, for two years after surgical removal patient developed pulmonary metastases. (**A,** WU neg. 50-2916; **B,** WU neg. 50-2656; **C,** ×450; WU neg. 50-2838.)

have an appearance similar to that of the zona glomerulosa, since this is the area in which aldosterone is produced in the normal adrenal gland. Although this is the case on occasion, most of the tumor cells resemble those of the zona fasciculata or have characteristics intermediate between zona glomerulosa and zona fasciculata cells (so-called "hybrid cells"). This combination of cell types also is evident on electron microscopic examination. Thus the cells of an aldosteronoma studied by Reidbord and Fisher[23] had mitochondria with lamellar cristae, characteristic of the zona glomerulosa, as well as mitochondria with cristae of the tubulovesicular types, as in the normal zona fasciculata. The zona glomerulosa of the nontumoral gland is often atrophic, although it may be normal or even hyperplastic.[22]

In the few reported cases where a cortical adrenal carcinoma has resulted in increased aldosterone production, secretion of other steroid hormones was also found, thus excluding them as cases of primary aldosteronism according to the rigid criteria proposed by Conn.[18]

Proper evaluation of a patient suspected of having primary aldosteronism includes pharmacologic exploration of the renin-angiotensin-aldosterone system[19, 20] and radiographic examination of the adrenal glands, especially arteriography, in order to differentiate it from cases of renovascular and essential hypertension.

Cushing's syndrome

Approximately 80% of patients with Cushing's syndrome are females, and the majority are adults. In 20%, the syndrome occurs before puberty (Figs. 609 and 610). The pathologic anatomy of the adrenal gland may be that of hyperplasia (Fig. 611), carcinoma, or adenoma, in that order (Table 25). The hyperplasia may, in turn, be the result of pituitary hyperfunction or ACTH-producing tumors or be present without a detectable cause. In cases of tumor, the remaining adrenal cortex often shows signs of atrophy (Fig. 612). Most cases of Cushing's syndrome in adults are due to hyperplasia, whereas carcinoma is the most common cause in children.[25, 26] The presence of a large adrenal mass in a patient with Cushing's syndrome is practically always indicative of carcinoma. Similarly, cases of Cushing's syndrome associated with obvious changes of virilization and markedly increased excretion of 17-ketosteroids are almost always due to cortical carcinoma. Schteingart et al.[30] consider the latter finding to be the most reliable biochemical sign of malignancy.

Most carcinomas are easily demonstrated by routine intravenous pyelography because of their large size. In contrast, the adenomas usually require arteriography for their localization. In eighty-one cases of Cushing's syndrome reviewed by Neville and Symington[27] the adrenal pathology was hyperplasia in sixty-nine cases, carci-

Table 25 Neoplasms in Cushing's syndrome*†

	Cases	Adrenal adenoma	Adrenal carcinoma	Cortical hyperplasia, pituitary tumor	Cortical hyperplasia, other tumor	Cortical hyperplasia, no tumor anywhere	Cortical hyperplasia, pituitary status not known, no other tumor
Barnes Hospital	74	9 (12.2%)	11 (14.9%)	11 (14.9%)	15 (20.3%)	3 (4.0%)	31 (41.8%)
Literature 1940-1962‡	178	18 (10.1%)	32 (18.0%)	29 (16.3%)	26 (14.6%)	6 (3.4%)	67 (37.6%)
Total	224	21 (9.4%)	41 (18.3%)	39 (17.4%)	33 (14.7%)	8 (3.6%)	82 (36.6%)

*From O'Neal, L. W.: Pathologic anatomy in Cushing's syndrome, Ann. Surg. **160:**860-869, 1964, and O'Neal, L. W.: Surgery of the adrenal glands, St. Louis, 1968, The C. V. Mosby Co.
†Percentages in parentheses.
‡J. Clin. Endocrinol. Metab., vols. 1-22, 1941-1962; Am. J. Med., vols. 1-33, 1946-1962; N. Engl. J. Med., vols. 222-267, 1940-1962; J. Pathol. Bacteriol., vols. 50-83, 1940-1962; Acta Endocrinol., vols. 1-41, 1948-1962.

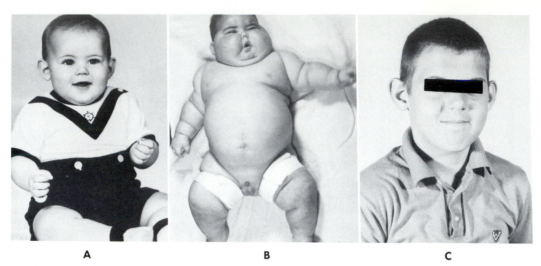

    A   **B**   **C**

Fig. 609 Child with Cushing's syndrome seven months before development of tumor, **A,** with tumor at 17 months of age, **B,** and ten years later, **C.** (**A,** WU neg. 56-599; **B,** WU neg. 56-358; **A** and **B,** from Heinbecker, P., O'Neal, L. W., and Ackerman, L. V.: Functioning and nonfunctioning adrenal cortical tumors, Surg. Gynecol. Obstet. **105:**21-33, 1957; by permission of Surgery, Gynecoolgy & Obstetrics; **C,** courtesy Dr. L. W. O'Neal, St. Louis, Mo.)

noma in seven, and adenoma in five. All of the carcinomas presented with the "mixed" type of Cushing's syndrome. Electron microscopic studies of cells from hyperplastic adrenal glands associated with Cushing's syndrome have shown mitochondria with tubulovesicular configuration of the cristae, consistent with elements of the zona fasciculata.[29]

In an increasingly large number of patients with Cushing's syndrome, the adrenal cortical hyperplasia is secondary to the presence of an ACTH-producing neoplasm. An excellent critical review of the pathology of these neoplasms has been made by Azzopardi and Williams.[24] In contrast to the prevailing opinion that almost any type of tumor may result in the production of Cushing's syndrome, nearly all acceptable cases fall into four main categories: (1) oat cell carcinoma of lung, (2) endocrine tumors of foregut origin, such as carcinoid tumor of the lung, medullary carcinoma of the thyroid gland, and carcinoid tumor of the thymus, (3) pheochromocytoma and related tumors, and (4) certain ovarian tumors. The first two account for more than 90% of the acceptable cases.

In this group of patients, hypokalemic alkalosis, skin pigmentation, edema, and severe diabetes mellitus occur more frequently than in the cases due to a primary adrenal lesion. Confirmation that the tumor is related to the Cushing's syndrome requires remission of the syndrome after tumor resection and demonstration of an ACTH-like substance by immunofluorescence or biochemical assay. Upton and Amatruda[31] have demonstrated that some of these tumors secrete not only ectopic ACTH but also a group of tumor peptides that stimulate the secretion of ACTH from the pituitary gland, thus contributing to the ectopic ACTH syndrome.

In a patient with Cushing's syndrome without identifiable tumor, adrenal exploration should be transabdominal. If one adrenal gland is found to be atropic, there is probably a tumor on the opposite side (Fig. 612). However, if one adrenal gland is normal or hyperplastic, the other gland may still contain a tumor. We have not found frozen sections helpful in determining whether a given adrenal gland is normal or atrophic. If adrenal hyperplasia is the cause of Cushing's syndrome, a total

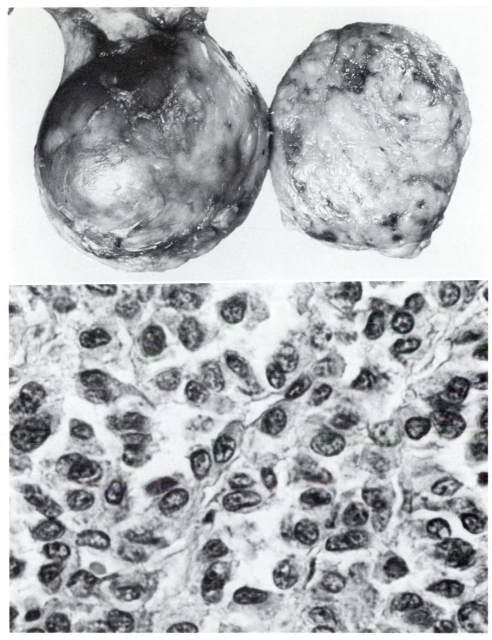

Fig. 610 Appearance of tumor causing Cushing's syndrome in patient shown in Fig. 609. This was cortical tumor, possibly malignant, with considerable pleomorphism. (×560; WU negs. 56-709 and 57-3686; from Heinbecker, P., O'Neal, L. W., and Ackerman, L. V.: Functioning and nonfunctioning adrenal cortical tumors, Surg. Gynecol. Obstet. **105**:21-33, 1957; by permission of Surgery, Gynecology & Obsterics.)

bilateral adrenalectomy should be performed.

Adrenogenital syndrome

Excess androgens secreted by an adrenal lesion bring about changes toward adult masculinity in male or female children and toward masculinity in female adults (Fig. 613). About 50% of the cases occur before puberty, and 80% of the patients are female.[34] Patterson[36] devised a simple chemical test that is helpful in differen-

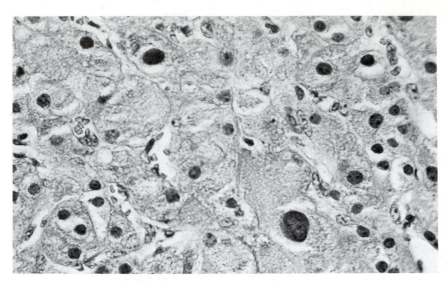

Fig. 611 Adrenal cortical hyperplasia in patient with Cushing's syndrome. Note large cells with bizarre nuclei. Mitoses are absent. (×400; WU neg. 52-2480.)

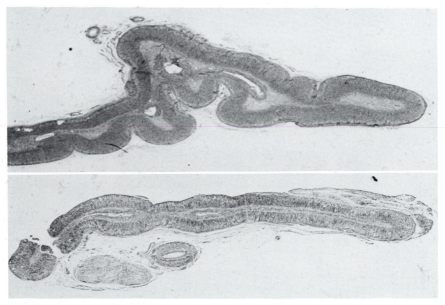

Fig. 612 Contrast between normal adrenal gland from 5-month-old girl and markedly atrophic adrenal gland that was contralateral to functioning carcinoma in 7-month-old girl. (Low power; WU negs. 56-5919 and 56-5920.)

tiating virilizing adrenal tumors from cases of adrenal hyperplasia, interstitial cell tumor of the testis, and Sertoli-Leydig cell tumor of the ovary. It is based on the finding of a specific 17-ketosteroid hormone designated as dehydroisoandrosterone. The rarest form of endocrine abnormality caused by an adrenal cortical tumor is feminization in a male adult accompanied by increase output of 17-ketosteroids. Practically all of these tumors are malignant.[33] Young patients succumb rapidly to the disease, whereas older individuals survive slightly longer. The most common cause of virilization in childhood is congenital adrenal hyperplasia. However, if

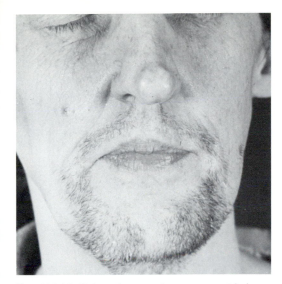

Fig. 613 Virilizing changes in woman with huge adrenal cortical tumor weighing over 1,000 gm. Microscopically, tumor appeared similar to one shown in Fig. 608, **C.** Patient remained free from recurrence for five years but in sixth year died of recurrent disease. (EFSCH 47-10379.)

an adrenal tumor is present, it will be a carcinoma in the majority of instances.[32, 35] On the other hand, virilization of adrenal origin in female adults is more often the result of a benign tumor than of a malignant one (Fig. 607). If the features of virilization are accompanied by those of Cushing's syndrome, there is a high probability that the lesion is a carcinoma.

Lesions of adrenal medulla
Neuroblastoma and related tumors

Neuroblastomas occur most often in the adrenal medulla of young children but are also seen in heterotopic areas such as the regions adjacent to the adrenal glands and, at times, in the posterosuperior portion of the mediastinum.

Grossly, these tumors are hemorrhagic and are small more often than large. They frequently contain foci of calcification (Fig. 614). Microscopically, there are

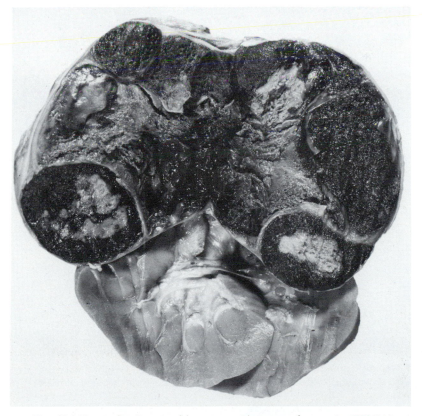

Fig. 614 Hemorrhagic neuroblastoma with zones of necrosis. (EFSCH.)

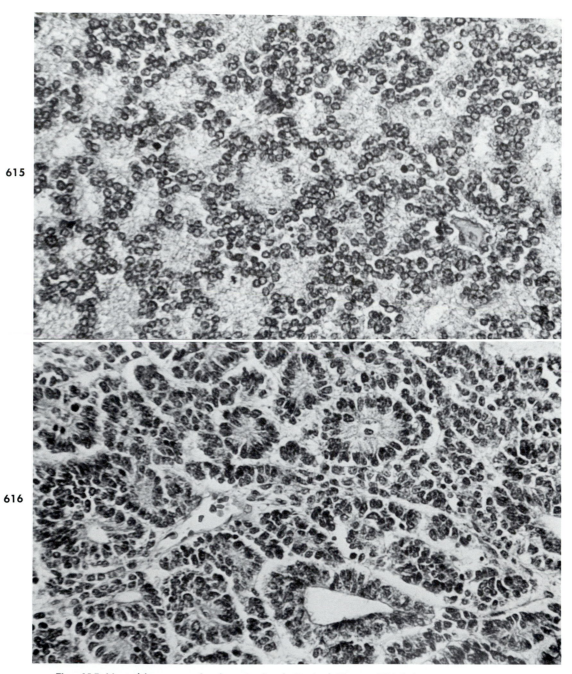

615

616

Fig. 615 Neuroblastoma of adrenal gland. Typical Homer Wright's rosettes are present throughout. Area encircled by nuclei contains fine network of neurofibrillary material. (×350; WU neg. 73-1354.)
Fig. 616 Wilms' tumor of kidneys shown for sake of comparison. Although some of smaller glands resemble neuroblastic rosettes, they can be differentiated by presence of central lumen with clear-cut cytoplasmic border. (×350; WU neg. 73-2954.)

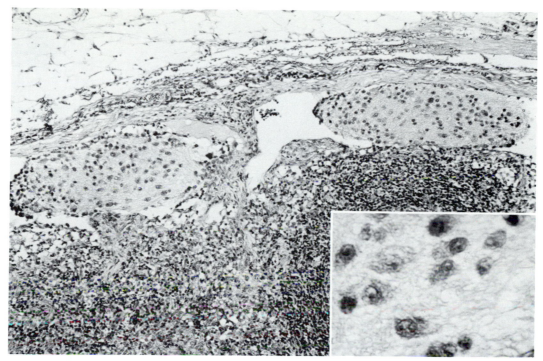

Fig. 617 Ganglioneuroblastoma metastatic in retroperitoneal lymph node. Two tumor nodules distend peripheral sinus. Primary tumor was located in adrenal gland. **Inset,** Higher magnification of tumor cells. Weblike material interposed between nuclei is important diagnostic feature. (×175; WU neg. 73-690; **inset,** ×600; WU neg. 73-691.)

collections of cells with uniform, deeply staining nuclei slightly larger than lymphocytes. There is little cytoplasm, and cytoplasmic outlines are poorly defined. Necrosis usually is present, leaving viable tumor cells grouped around blood vessels. True rosettes may or may not be present. These are characterized by a collection of tumor cells not related to blood vessels and arranged around a central lumen filled with a filamentous material (Figs. 615 and 616). The latter is composed of a tangled mass of neurites, as revealed by silver stains and electron microscopy. Better-differentiated zones in which the nuclei are larger and have fine chromatin are frequent. This correlates with an increased survival rate.[37, 39] In *ganglioneuroblastomas* there is a fine, fibrillar, cobwebby network between masses of cells (Fig. 617). This material is an important diagnostic feature of these neoplasms and is made of large numbers of neurites emanating from the tumor cells, with occasional formation of synaptic junc-

tions[40] (Fig. 618). Focal areas of calcification may be seen[41] (Fig. 619). Collections of ganglion cells which are often multinucleated can be seen in areas that are even better differentiated. Grossly, these tumors have a more homogeneous appearance and firmer consistency than neuroblastomas (Fig. 620).

Infrequently, well-differentiated *ganglioneuromas* occur similar to those described in the posterior portion of the mediastinum. Tumors of a similar nature may arise in any of the heterotopic locations mentioned.

Occasionally, small adrenal neuroblastomas are seen as incidental findings at autopsy.[38] The fact that in most reported cases the infants were less than 3 months of age suggests that many of the tumors may resolve spontaneously.

Pheochromocytoma

Pheochromocytomas may secrete norepinephrine, epinephrine, or both.[42] About 200 endocrinologically active cases have

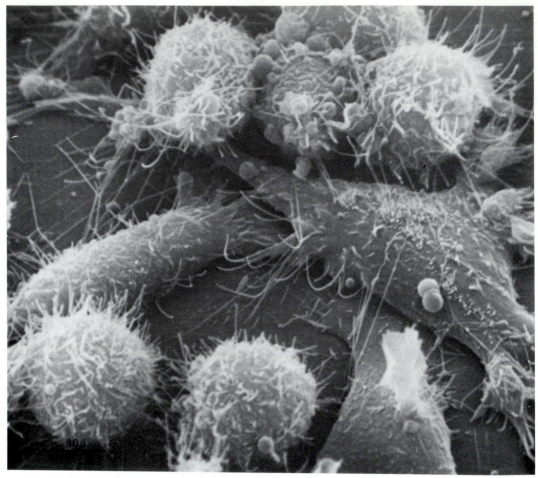

Fig. 618 Scanning electron micrograph of established line of mouse neuroblastoma that first appeared in sympathetic ganglion of A/J mouse. Spherical cells are probably in G_1 phase of cell cycle. Others are in late G_1 or S. Filiform cytoplasmic prolongations are extremely numerous. Some probably correspond to dendrites and axons. (×3,000; courtesy Dr. V. Fonte and Dr. K. Porter, Boulder, Colo.)

been reported. Pheochromocytoma has been called "the 10% tumor"—approximately 10% are malignant, 10% are bilateral (Fig. 621), and 10% are extra-adrenal. When extra-adrenal, they usually secrete only norepinephrine, since the adrenal cortex seems necessary for the methylation of this hormone to epinephrine. The most common locations of extra-adrenal pheochromocytoma are the retroperitoneal area (including the region of the Zuckerkandl's body), mediastinum, and urinary bladder.[48, 54] Norepinephrine-secreting endocrine tumors have been described in the region of the carotid body and glomus jugulare.[55] These are better designated as *paragangliomas.*

Occasionally, pheochromocytomas are associated with neurofibromatosis[51] or occur within the same family. Familial cases of pheochromocytoma associated with hyperparathyroidism, medullary carcinoma of the thyroid gland, and occasionally Cushing's disease are known as Sipple's syndrome or multiple endocrine adenomatosis Type II. This is inherited as a mendelian autosomal dominant.[56] Seven cases of pheochromocytoma associated with cerebellar hemangioblastoma were reviewed by Nibbelink et al.[53]

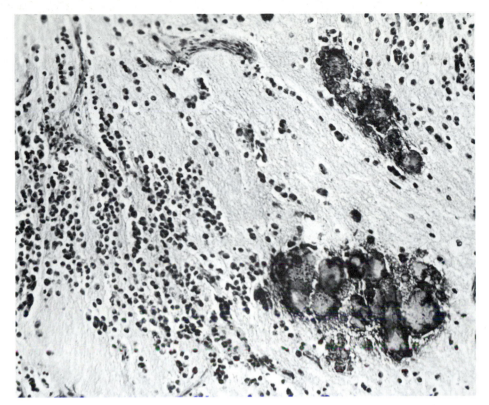

Fig. 619 Typical ganglioneuroblastoma demonstrating focal areas of calcification, cob-webby material, and collections of cells with deep-staining nuclei. (×200; WU neg. 54-1495.)

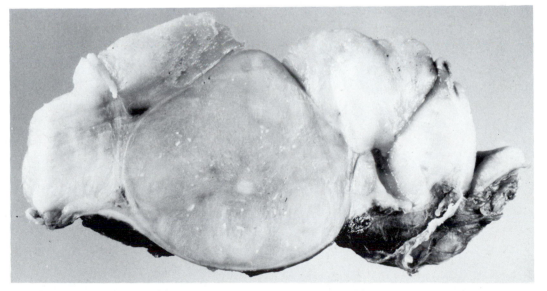

Fig. 620 Ganglioneuroblastoma excised from retroperitoneum of 5-year-old white boy. Dominant pattern was that of well-differentiated ganglion and Schwann cells, with only few clumps of neuroblasts being identified. (WU neg. 70-4615.)

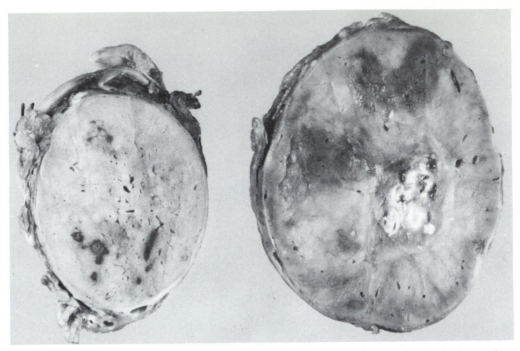

Fig. 621 Bilateral pheochromocytomas in 12-year-old girl. Patient also had signs of primary hyperparathyroidism. (WU neg. 61-11268.)

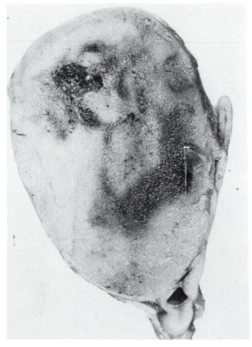

Fig. 622 Hemorrhagic yellowish white pheochromocytoma. Remnant of normal adrenal gland can be seen. Tumor appeared in patient with Recklinghausen's disease. (WU neg. 50-2610.)

Grossly, these tumors vary in size from a few grams to 2,000 gm. They are invariably encapsulated, usually soft, and, on section, yellowish white to reddish brown (Fig. 622). They are extremely well vascularized and can be well demonstrated by selective arteriography (Fig. 623). The larger tumors often have areas of necrosis, hemorrhage, and cyst formation. The adrenal gland usually is compressed or incorporated within the tumor. More than one tumor may be present. Ganem and Cahill[49] reported tumor in the adrenal gland and retroperitoneal space. Cragg[46] reported concurrent tumors of the left carotid body and both Zuckerkandl bodies.

Microscopically, tumor cells vary considerably in size and shape and have a finely granular and basophilic or eosinophilic cytoplasm. The nuclei are usually round or oval with prominent nucleoli (Fig. 624). Individual cells often are suggestive of ganglion cells. The tumor, if immersed in dichromate solution, takes on a characteristic dark brown appearance. This is the base of the chromaffin reaction.

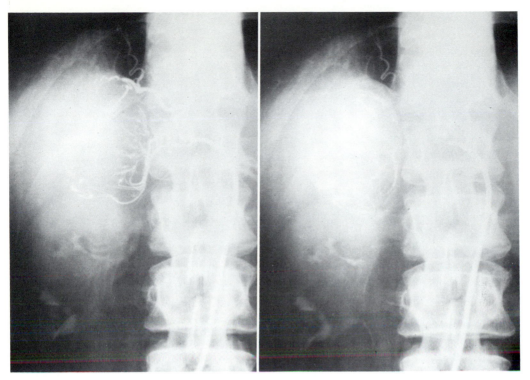

Fig. 623 Arteriographic demonstration of adrenal pheochromocytoma, early and late arterial phases. Latter shows typical "tumor stain." (From Meaney, T. F., and Bronocore, E.: Selective arteriography as a localizing and provocative test in the diagnosis of pheochromocytoma, Radiology **87**:309-314, 1966.)

It should be emphasized that in order to obtain consistent results, the tumor tissue should be fresh and the pH of the dichromate solution should be kept between 5 and 6.[50] By electron microscopic study, granules of norepinephrine and epinephrine type are present[57] (Fig. 625).

Elevated basal metabolic rate, as well as diabetic type of sugar tolerance curves, may indicate a pheochromocytoma. Duncan et al.[47] suggested that when diabetes mellitus, hypermetabolism, and hypertension are encountered together, pheochromocytoma should be considered.

The treatment of pheochromocytoma is excision. Colston[45] uses an upper abdominal transverse incision.

The clinical signs and symptoms of the hormonally active pheochromocytoma are the same as those produced by the injection of large amounts of epinephrine.[43] Of 176 pheochromocytomas reviewed by Calkins et al.,[44] only forty were shown to be hormonally active. Hypertensive attacks are usually intermittent but at times may be sustained, particularly in children.[52] They may be brought on by massaging the area of the tumor. Frequently at operation crises occur through handling. Histamine injection is probably contraindicated as a diagnostic procedure because of the severity of the hypertension likely to occur following its use.

Clinicopathologic correlation

Biochemical tests that measure urinary catecholamines are valuable in the diagnosis of tumors of neural crest origin, including both differentiated and undifferentiated tumors (ganglioneuroma, ganglioneuroblastoma, neuroblastoma, and pheochromocytoma). Tests for catecholamines, although invariably positive for these tumors, show considerable variation in the amount secreted.[59, 65, 68] Diarrhea is seen as a complication of ganglioneuroma more

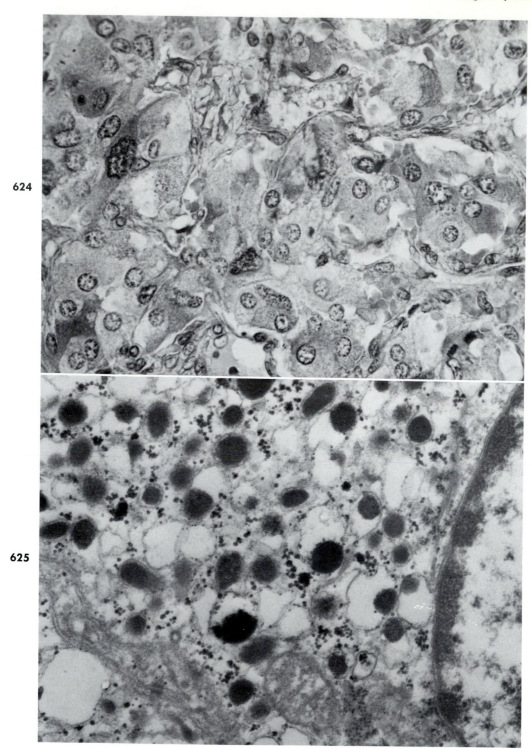

Fig. 624 Functioning pheochromocytoma. Note delicate vessels surrounding groups of cells and lack of mitotic activity. Intense granularity of cytoplasm is due to positive reaction to chromate. (×600; WU neg. 58-4083.)

Fig. 625 Electron micrograph of functioning adrenal pheochromocytoma. Numerous neurosecretory granules are present. (Uranyl acetate—lead citrate; ×33,700.)

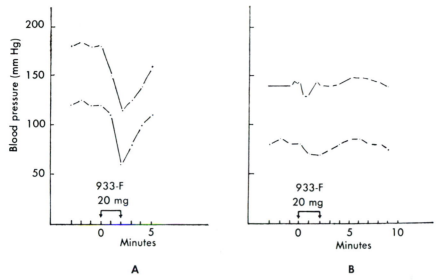

Fig. 626 Chart to demonstrate diagnostic value of drug 933-F in patient with pheo-chromocytoma (male; age, 37 years; weight, 55 kg). **A,** Effect before operation. **B,** Effect after operation. (WU neg. 50-1569; from Calkins, E., Dana, G. W., Seed, J. C., and Howard, J. E.: On piperidylmethyl-benzodioxane [933-F], hypertension, and pheochromocytoma, J. Clin. Endocrinol. Metab. **10:**1-11, 1950.)

commonly than of neuroblastoma. The pathogenesis is unclear.[61] Twenty-six cases of neuroblastoma have been reported in which a variety of developmental defects have been found.[66] These have involved different systems, without a consistent pattern emerging.

Tumors of the sympathetic nervous system occur primarily in children. Usually the more differentiated the tumor, the better the prognosis.[62] For instance, all ganglioneuromas are curable. For a given type of tumor, children under 2 years of age have the best prognosis. The main determinants of prognosis in neuroblastoma are differentiation and location of the tumor, age of the patient, findings at operation, and treatment received.[64] Of the patients reviewed by Gross et al.,[60] 88% of those whose tumor could be totally excised were cured of their disease.

Tumors originating in the mediastinum can often be effectively controlled (Fig. 627). Of thirty-six patients with tumors of the sympathetic nervous system whom we have followed for at least two years, twenty have survived without recurrence and seven-

teen have lived five years or longer. All nine patients whose tumors were mediastinal are living and well. In three of the thirty-six patients the tumors showed evidence of maturation to a more mature histologic type. This phenomenon has been demonstrated in tissue culture[58] (Fig. 628).

Patients may be cured even when liver metastases or bone marrow involvement exists[64, 67] (Fig. 629). Murray and Stout[63] have shown that tissue culture of neuroblastoma may make an absolute diagnosis within twenty-four hours because neurites become recognizable.

Other adrenal lesions

Cysts arising in the adrenal gland may be clinically confused with a retroperitoneal neoplasm due to their occasionally large size (up to 30 cm in diameter). They are sometimes bilateral. Microscopically, the wall is composed of partially calcified fibrous tissue without an epithelial lining. The content may be cloudy or blood-colored fluid. The mechanism of formation is often impossible to ascertain. Massive hemorrhage and cystic degeneration of a pri-

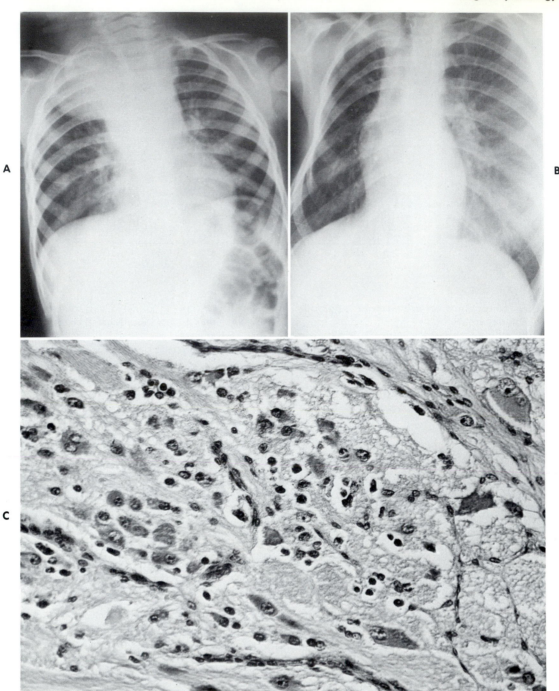

Fig. 627 **A,** Female infant, 17 months old, had tumor of right superior mediastinum. At exploratory thoracotomy, tumor was unresectable. Postoperatively, 2,800 R was given to neoplasm and adjacent mediastinum. **B,** Follow-up x-ray film of chest demonstrates decreased volume of right lung with shifting of mediastinum. Bony structures are not so well developed as on left side. **C,** Photomicrograph of ganglioneuroblastoma shows admixture of ganglion cells and neuroblasts. Patient remains well fifteen years later. (**A,** WU neg. 53-2782; **B,** WU neg. 65-6446; **C,** ×300; WU neg. 66-7571; **A** to **C,** from Perez, C. A., Vietti, T., Ackerman, L. V., Eagleton, M. D., and Powers, W. E.: Tumors of the sympathetic nervous system in children; an appraisal of treatment and results, Radiology **88:**750-760, 1967.)

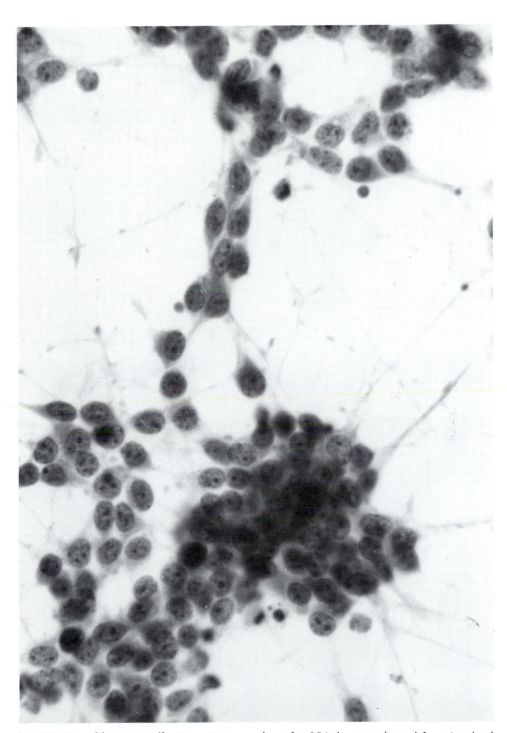

Fig. 628 Neuroblastoma cells, in continuous culture for 354 days, explanted from involved lymph node of 2-year-old girl from tissue obtained one hour postmortem. Note small nuclei, sparse cytoplasm, and many unipolar beaded axons extending from cell bodies. (×650; courtesy Dr. M. Goldstein, St. Louis, Mo.)

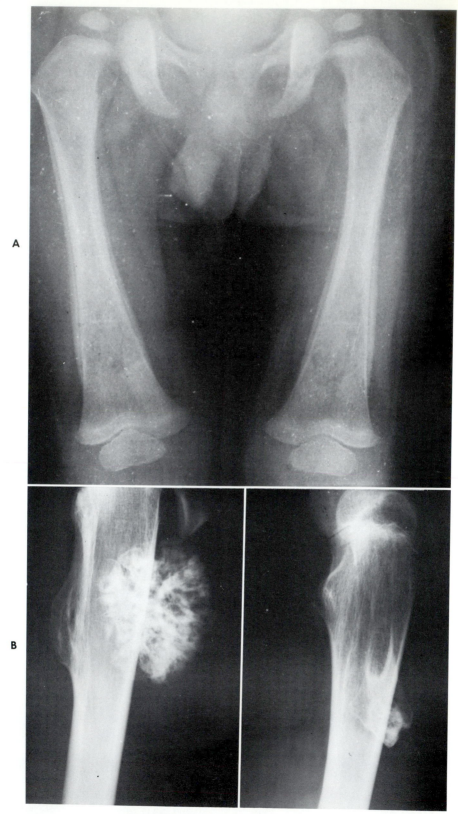

A

B

Fig. 629 For legend, see opposite page.

mary neoplasm are considered the two most likely explanations.[69]

Presence within the adrenal gland of adult fat containing active bone marrow elements is referred to as *myelolipoma.*[70] This is almost always a microscopic incidental finding at autopsy and only exceptionally will attain a size large enough to be detected clinically.[71] In contrast to other extramedullary foci of hematopoiesis in adults, which are usually an expression of a hematologic disease, adrenal myelolipoma is practically always accompanied by a normal bone marrow.

Tumors of related paraganglia

The paraganglion system is formed by numerous collections of neuroepithelial cells scattered throughout the body.[79, 82, 111, 114] The most conspicuous member of the group is the adrenal medulla, a neuroeffector system connected with the orthosympathetic system. Extra-adrenal paraganglia can be divided in two broad categories: those related to the parasympathetic system (ninth, tenth, and possibly third and fifth nerves) and those connected with the orthosympathetic system. The former are usually nonchromaffin, are concentrated in the head, neck, and mediastinum, and seem to have a chemoreceptor function. The latter are chromaffin, predominate along the thoracolumbar para-aortic region, and probably represent lesser homologues of the adrenal medulla.

Tumors arising from these structures are best called *paragangliomas.*[72, 77] The term chemodectoma is too restrictive, since it can be properly applied only to carotid and aortic body tumors. Paragangliomas which are obviously chromaffin and are associated with clinical evidence of norepinephrine and/or epinephrine secretion also can be designated as *extra-adrenal pheochromocytomas.* It is likely that most of the latter arise from orthosympathetic-related paraganglia, whereas most of the nonchromaffin, nonfunctioning tumors probably originate from parasympathetic-related organs. Unfortunately, it is often impossible on morphologic grounds to distinguish between these two types or to predict whether a tumor is functioning or not.[84, 95]

Paragangliomas have been found in practically every site in which normal paraganglia are known to occur, their description sometimes preceding that of the corresponding normal structure (Figs. 630 and 631; Table 26). A definite familial incidence has been detected.[115] Paragangliomas occurring bilaterally or affecting two or more paraganglia simultaneously have been reported.[90] Their microscopic appearance is practically the same regardless of location. Well-defined nests of cuboidal cells are separated by highly vascularized fibrous septa (Fig. 632, *B* and *C*). The individual cells have a moderately abundant granular cytoplasm. As with many other endocrine tumors, bizarre nuclei and vascular invasion are sometimes found. They should not be taken as evidence of malignancy. Mitoses are exceptional. A faint chromaffin reaction can sometimes be obtained in optimally fixed material, thus indicating that the designation of "nonchromaffin" is not always accurate. Argentaffin and

Fig. 629 In 1951, 13-month-old boy had neuroblastoma of right posterior mediastinum with numerous metastases to skull and long bones. X-ray films of both femurs showed periosteal bone proliferation with involvement of medullary canal. Patient received 2,000 R to mediastinum, 1,000 R to femurs, and 800 R to both tibias, left arm, and forearm. **B,** In 1964, twelve years after therapy, osteochondroma can be seen in distal portion of right femur and questionable low-grade chondrosarcoma in distal segment of left femur. Patient is alive and well eighteen years after therapy and five years following removal of cartilaginous tumors. (**A,** WU neg. 53-1459; **B,** WU negs. 66-667 and 66-668; **A** and **B,** from Perez, C. A., Vietti, T., Ackerman, L. V., Eagleton, M. D., and Powers, W. E.: Tumors of the sympathetic nervous system in children; an appraisal of treatment and results, Radiology **88:**750-760, 1967.)

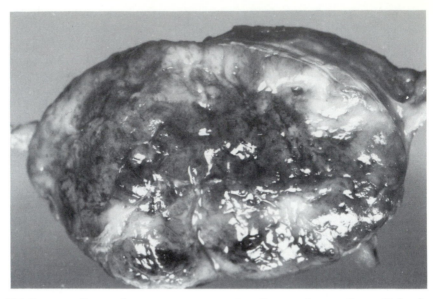

Fig. 630 Paraganglioma of vagus nerve measuring 5 cm × 4 cm × 2 cm. Stub of vagus nerve can be seen at inferior margin. (WU neg. 69-1739.)

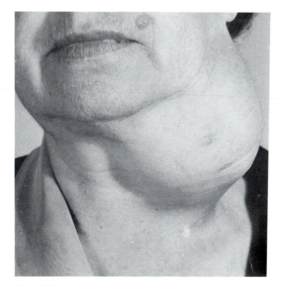

Fig. 631 Large, pulsating paraganglioma (carotid body tumor) in neck that had been present for many years. There were symptoms of obstruction. (Courtesy Dr. J. B. Brown, St. Louis, Mo.)

Table 26 Reported sites of occurrence of paraganglioma and their approximate frequency

Location	Approximate number of reported cases	References
Carotid body	600	78, 83, 100, 106
Glomus jugulare/ glomus tympanicum	300	94, 105, 107
Paraganglion intravagale	44	93, 99
Aortic body and other mediastinal paraganglia	35	102, 104, 113
Lung	25	88, 91
Retroperitoneum	21	101
Orbit	5	110
Tongue	<5	74
Urinary bladder	<5	85
Gallbladder	<5	97
Nasal cavity	<5	98
Larynx and trachea	<5	76, 116
Heart	<5	81
Pineal gland*	<5	108
Duodenum*	12	89, 109

*The place of these tumors in the paraganglioma category is still uncertain.

argyrophil cells can be regularly demonstrated by the del Rio Hortega techniques,[73] but only rarely with the Fontana-Masson or Masson-Hamperl methods as applied to paraffin-embedded material.

Treatment of freeze-dried preparations or tumor imprints with formaldehyde vapors induces a bright fluorescence indicative of catecholamines. This extremely sensitive and relatively easy technique should be

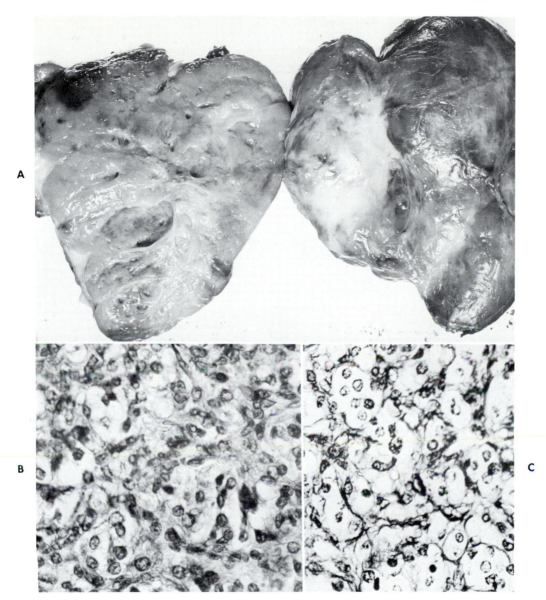

Fig. 632   A, Tumor shown in Fig. 631 was resected, and it was found necessary to remove segment of carotid artery. Gross specimen illustrated encapsulated neoplasm. It had vascular, grayish pink color and weighed 140 gm. **B,** Same tumor illustrated in **A** showing its cellularity, organoid pattern, and lack of mitotic activity. **C,** Same tumor illustrated in **A** stained with Wilder reticulin stain. Note that nests of tumor cells are encircled by reticulin fibers. (**A,** WU neg. 51-5003; **B,** ×460; WU neg. 51-5609; **C,** ×460; WU neg. 51-5609.)

routinely applied to this family of neoplasms.[80]

Ultrastructurally, the tumor cells contain large numbers of cytoplasmic neurosecretory granules of similar appearance to those seen in normal paraganglia.[75, 86] Biochemical assays have demonstrated the presence of norepinephrine and/or epinephrine.[103]

Most paragangliomas follow a benign clinical course. The incidence of malignancy is in the range of 10%—i.e., quite similar to that of adrenal pheochromocytomas.[87, 112] We know of no definite criteria by which to separate microscopically the benign from the malignant form.

The *neoplasms of the carotid body* arise at the bifurcation of the common carotid artery and become closely adherent to it (Figs. 631 and 632). This firm adherence is often misinterpreted by the surgeon as a sign of malignancy. Arteriography demonstrates them particularly well because of their rich vascularity. Grossly, this tumor usually is not large. Often the clinical diagnosis is not made until its characteristic location is determined at operation. Frozen section should make the diagnosis. The high operative risk and high morbidity formerly associated with the removal of a carotid body tumor have now markedly reduced as a result of improved operative techniques and the use of arterial substitutes.[92]

Alveolar soft part sarcoma, a rare malignant neoplasm of soft tissue designated in the past as malignant nonchromaffin paraganglioma, has probably no relation with this group of tumors.[96] It is discussed in Chapter 23.

REFERENCES

Introduction

1 O'Neal, L. W.: Surgery of the adrenal glands, St. Louis, 1968, The C. V. Mosby Co.
2 Symington, T.: Functional pathology of the human adrenal gland, Baltimore, 1969, The Williams & Wilkins Co.

Lesions of adrenal cortex
Heterotopia

3 Dahl, E. V., and Bahn, R. C.: Aberrant adrenal cortical tissue near the testis in human infants, Am. J. Pathol. **40:**587-598, 1962.
4 Graham, L. S.: Celiac accessory adrenal glands, Cancer **6:**149-152, 1953.
5 Nelson, A. A.: Accessory adrenal cortical tissue, Arch. Pathol. **27:**955-965, 1939.
6 Stout, A. P.: Personal communication.

Congenital hyperplasia

7 Hsia, D. Y.-Y.: Inborn errors of metabolism. Part 1: Clinical aspects, Chicago, 1966, Year Book Medical Publishers, pp. 245-255.
8 Jones, H. W., Jr., and Verkauf, B. S.: Surgical treatment in congenital adrenal hyperplasia; age at operation and other prognostic factors, Obstet. Gynecol. **36:**1-10, 1970.

9 New, M. I.: Congenital adrenal hyperplasia, Pediatr. Clin. North Am. **15:**395-407, 1968.

Acquired hyperplasia

10 Commons, R. R., and Callaway, C. P.: Adenomas of the adrenal cortex, Arch. Intern. Med. **81:**37-41, 1948.

Adenoma

11 Macadam, R. F.: Black adenoma of the human adrenal cortex, Cancer **27:**116-119, 1971.
12 Schtenigart, D. E., Oberman, H. A., Friedman, B. A., and Conn, J. W.: Adrenal cortical neoplasms producing Cushing's syndrome; a clinicopathologic study, Cancer **22:**1105-1013, 1968.

Carcinoma

13 Huvos, A. G., Hajdu, S. I., Brasfield, R. D., and Foote, F. W., Jr.: Adrenal cortical carcinoma; clinicopathologic study of 34 cases, Cancer **25:**354-361, 1970.
14 Lipsett, M. B., Hertz, R., and Ross, G. T.: Clinical and pathophysiologic aspects of adrenocortical carcinoma, Am. J. Med. **35:**374-383, 1963.
15 Wood, K. F., Lus, F., and Rosenthal, F. D.: Carcinoma of the adrenal cortex without endocrine effects, Br. J. Surg. **45:**41-50, 1957.

Clinicopathologic correlation
Nonfunctioning lesions

16 Hedeland, H., Östberg, G., and Hokfelt, B.: On the prevalence of adrenocortical adenomas in an autopsy material in relation to hypertension and diabetes, Acta Med. Scand. **184:**211-214, 1968.
17 Huvos, A. G., Hajdu, S. I., Brasfield, R. D., and Foote, F. W., Jr.: Adrenal cortical carcinoma; clinicopathologic study of 34 cases, Cancer **25:**354-361, 1970.

Aldosteronism

18 Alterman, S. L., Dominguez, C., Lopez-Gomez, A., and Lieber, A. L.: Primary adrenocortical carcinoma causing aldosteronism, Cancer **24:**602-609, 1969.
19 George, J. M., Wright, L., Bell, N. H., Bartter, F. C., and Brown, R.: The syndrome of primary aldosteronism, Am. J. Med. **48:**343-356, 1970.
20 Luetscher, J. A., Weinberger, M. H., Dowdy, A. J., and Nokes, T. W.: Effects of sodium loading, sodium depletion and posture on plasma aldosterone concentration and renin activity in hypertensive patients, J. Clin. Endocrinol. Metab. **29:**1310-1318, 1969.
21 Neville, A. M., and Symington, T.: Pathology of primary aldosteronism, Cancer **19:**1854-1868, 1966.

22 O'Neal, L. W., Kissane, J. M., and Hartroft, P. M.: The kidney in endocrine hypertension; Cushing's syndrome, pheochromocytoma and aldosteronism, Arch. Surg. **100:** 498-505, 1970.

23 Reidbord, H., and Fisher, E. R.: Aldosteronoma and nonfunctioning adrenal cortical adenoma; comparative ultrastructural study, Arch. Pathol. 88:155-161, 1969.

Cushing's syndrome

24 Azzopardi, J. G., and Williams, E. D.: Pathology of "nonendocrine" tumors associated with Cushing's syndrome, Cancer 22:274-286, 1968.

25 Gilbert, M. G., and Cleveland, W. W.: Cushing's syndrome in infancy, Pediatrics 46:217-229, 1970.

26 Loridan, L., and Senior, B.: Cushing's syndrome in infancy, J. Pediatr. 75:349-359, 1969.

27 Neville, A. M., and Symington, T.: The pathology of the adrenal gland in Cushing's syndrome, J. Pathol. Bacteriol. 93:19-35, 1967.

28 O'Neal, L. W.: Pathologic anatomy in Cushing's syndrome, Ann. Surg. 160:860-869, 1964.

29 Reidbord, H., and Fisher, E. R.: Electron microscopic study of adrenal cortical hyperplasia in Cushing's syndrome, Arch. Pathol. 86:419-426, 1968.

30 Schteingart, D. E., Oberman, H. A., Friedman, B. A., and Conn, J. W.: Adrenal cortical neoplasms producing Cushing's syndrome; a clinicopathologic study, Cancer 22:1005-1013, 1968.

31 Upton, G. V., and Amatruda, T. T., Jr.: Evidence for the presence of tumor peptides with corticotropin-releasing-factor-like activity in the ectopic ACTH syndrome, N. Engl. J. Med. 285:419-424, 1971.

Adrenogenital syndrome

32 Burrington, J. D., and Stephens, C. A.: Virilizing tumors of the adrenal gland in childhood: report of eight cases, J. Pediatr. Surg. 4:291-302, 1969.

33 Gabrilove, J. L., Sharma, D. C., Wotiz, H. H., and Dorfman, R. I.: Feminizing adrenocortical tumors in the male; a review of 52 cases including a case report, Medicine (Baltimore) 44:37-79, 1965.

34 Heinbecker, P., O'Neal, L. W., and Ackerman, L. V.: Functioning and nonfunctioning adrenal cortical tumors, Surg. Gynecol. Obstet. 105:21-33, 1957.

35 Kenny, F. M., Hashida, Y., Askari, H. A., Sieber, W. H., and Fetterman, G. H.: Virilizing tumors of the adrenal cortex, Am. J. Dis. Child. 115:445-458, 1968.

36 Patterson, J.: Diagnosis of adrenal tumours; a new chemical test, Lancet 2:580-581, 1947.

Lesions of adrenal medulla

Neuroblastoma and related tumors

37 Fortner, J., Nicastri, A., and Murphy, M. L.: Neuroblastoma: natural history and results of treating 133 cases, Ann. Surg. 167:132-142, 1968.

38 Guin, G. H., Gilbert, E. F., and Jones, B.: Incidental neuroblastoma in infants, Am. J. Clin. Pathol. 51:126-136, 1969.

39 Mäkinen, J.: Microscopic patterns as a guide to prognosis of neuroblastoma in childhood, Cancer 29:219-228, 1972.

40 Misugi, K., Misugi, N., and Newton, W. A., Jr.: Fine structural study of neuroblastoma, ganglioneuroblastoma and pheochromocytoma, Arch. Pathol. 86:160-170, 1968.

41 Wahl, H. R., and Craig, P. E.: Multiple tumors of sympathetic nervous system: report of a case showing a distinct ganglioneuroma, a neuroblastoma and a cystic calcifying ganglioneuroblastoma, Am. J. Pathol. 14:797-807, 1938.

Pheochromocytoma

42 Beer, E., King, F. H., and Prinzmetal, M.: Pheochromocytoma with demonstration of pressor (adrenalin) substance in the blood preoperatively during hypertensive crises, Ann. Surg. 106:85-91, 1937.

43 Calkins, E., and Howard, J. E.: Bilateral familial pheochromocytoma with paroxysmal hypertension: successful surgical removal of tumors in two cases with discussion of certain diagnostic procedures and physiologic considerations, J. Clin. Endocrinol. Metab. 7:475-492, 1947.

44 Calkins, E., Dana, G. W., Seed, J. C., and Howard, J. E.: On piperidylmethyl-benzodioxane (933-F), hypertension, and pheochromocytoma, J. Clin. Endocrinol. Metab. 10:1-11, 1950.

45 Colston, J. A. C.: Surgical aspects of bilateral familial pheochromocytoma, J. Urol. 59:1036-1060, 1948.

46 Cragg, R. W.: Concurrent tumors of the left carotid body and of both Zuckerkandl bodies, Arch. Pathol. 18:635-645, 1934.

47 Duncan, L. E., Jr., Semans, J. H., and Howard, J. E.: Adrenal medullary tumors (pheochromocytoma) and diabetes mellitus: disappearance of diabetes after removal of the tumor, Ann. Intern. Med. 20:815-821, 1944.

48 Fries, J. G., and Chamberlin, J. A.: Extra-adrenal pheochromocytomas; literature review and report of cervical pheochromocytoma, Surgery 63:268-279, 1968.

49 Ganem, E. J., and Cahill, G. F.: Pheochromocytomas coexisting in adrenal gland and retroperitoneal space, with sustained hypertension, N. Engl. J. Med. 238:692-697, 1948.

50 Kennedy, J. S., Symington, T., and Woodger, B. A.: Chemical and histochemical observations in benign and malignant phaeochromocytoma, J. Pathol. Bacteriol. 81:409-418, 1961.

51 Knudson, A. G., Jr., and Amromin, G. D.: Neuroblastoma and ganglioneuroma in a child with multiple neurofibromatosis; implications for the mutational origin of neuroblastoma, Cancer 19:1032-1037, 1966.

52 Moore, T. C., and Shumacker, H. B.: Adrenalin-producing tumors in childhood, Ann. Surg. 143:256-265, 1956.

53 Nibbelink, D. W., Peters, B. H., and McCormick, W. F.: On the association of pheochromocytoma and cerebellar hemangioblastoma, Neurology 19:455-460, 1969.

54 Overholt, R. H., Ramsay, B. H., and Meissner, W. A.: Intrathoracic pheochromocytoma, Dis. Chest 17:55-62, 1950.

55 Parkinson, D.: Intracranial pheochromocytomas (active glomus jugulare); case report, J. Neurosurg. 31:94-100, 1969.

56 Sarosi, G., and Doe, R. P.: Familial occurrence of parathyroid adenomas, pheochromocytoma, and medullary carcinoma of the thyroid with amyloid stroma (Sipple's syndrome), Ann. Intern. Med. 68:1305-1309, 1968.

57 Tannenbaum, M.: Ultrastructural pathology of adrenal medullary tumors, Pathol. Annu. 1970, pp. 145-172.

Clinicopathologic correlation

58 Goldstein, M. N., Burdman, J. A., and Journey, L. J.: Long-term tissue culture of neuroblastomas. II. Morphologic evidence for differentiation and maturation, J. Natl. Cancer Inst. 32:165-199, 1964.

59 Greer, M., Anton, A. H., Williams, C. M., and Echevarria, R. A.: Tumors of neural crest origin, Arch. Neurol. 13:139-148, 1965.

60 Gross, R. E., Farber, S., and Martin, L. W.: Neuroblastoma smypatheticum; a study and report of 217 cases, Pediatrics 23:1179-1191, 1959.

61 Hamilton, J. R., Radde, I. C., and Johnson, G.: Diarrhea associated with adrenal ganglioneuroma; new findings related to the pathogenesis of diarrhea, Am. J. Med. 44:453-463, 1968.

62 Mäkinen, J.: Microscopic patterns as a guide to prognosis of neuroblastoma in childhood, Cancer 29:219-228, 1972.

63 Murray, M. R., and Stout, A. P.: Distinctive characteristics of the sympathicoblastoma cultivated in vitro, Am. J. Path. 23:429-442, 1947.

64 Perez, C. A., Vietti, T. J., Ackerman, L. V., Kulapongs, P., and Powers, W. E.: Treatment of malignant sympathetic tumors in children:

clinicopathological correlation, Pediatrics 41:452-462, 1968.

65 Sunderman, F. W.: Measurements of vanilmandelic acid for the diagnosis of pheochromocytoma and neuroblastoma, Am. J. Clin. Pathol. 42:481-497, 1964.

66 Sy, W. M., and Edmonson, J. H.: The developmental defects associated with neuroblastoma; etiologic implications, Cancer 22:234-238, 1968.

67 Vogel, J. M., Coddon, D. R., Simon, N., and Gitlow, S. E.: Osseous metastases in neuroblastoma; a 17-year survival, Cancer 26:1354-1360, 1970.

68 Voorhess, M. L., and Gardner, L. I.: Studies of catecholamine excretion by children with neural tumors, J. Clin. Endocrinol. Metab. 22:126-133, 1962.

Other adrenal lesions

69 Hodges, F. V., and Ellis, F. R.: Cystic lesions of the adrenal glands, Arch. Pathol. 66:53-58, 1958.

70 McDonnell, W. V.: Myelolipoma of adrenal, Arch. Pathol. 61:416-419, 1956.

71 Newman, P. H., and Silen, W.: Myelolipoma of the adrenal gland; report of the third case of a symptomatic tumor and review of the literature, Arch. Surg. 97:637-639, 1968.

Tumors of related paraganglia

72 Abell, M. R., Hart, W. R., and Olson, J. R.: Tumors of the peripheral nervous system, Hum. Pathol. 1:503-551, 1970.

73 Barroso-Moguel, R., and Costero, I.: Argentaffin cells of the carotid body tumor, Am. J. Pathol. 41:389-402, 1962.

74 Bertogalli, D., Calearo, C., and Pignataro, O.: Les paragangliomes non-cromatophiles à siège rare; a propos de deux observations personelles (paragangliome du pneumogastrique cervical et paragangliome de la base de la langue), Ann. d'Otolaryngol. (Paris) 76:688-699, 1959.

75 Biscoe, T. J., and Stehbens, W. E.: Ultrastructure of the carotid body, J. Cell Biol. 30:563-578, 1966.

76 Blanchard, C. L., and Saunders, W. H.: Chemodectoma of the larynx, Arch. Otolaryngol. 61:472-474, 1955.

77 Brantigan, C. O., and Katase, R. Y.: Clinical and pathologic features of paragangliomas of the organ of Zuckerkandl, Surgery 65:898-905, 1969.

78 Conley, J. J.: Carotid body tumor; review of 29 cases, Arch. Otolaryngol. 81:187-193, 1965.

79 Coupland, R. E.: The chromaffin system. In Handbook of experimental pharmacology. Vol. 33: Catecholamines (Blaschko, H., and Mus-

chall, E., subeditors), New York, 1972, Springer-Verlag.

80 DeLellis, R. A., and Roth, J. A.: Norepinephrine in a glomus jugulare tumor; histochemical demonstration, Arch. Pathol. **92**:73-75, 1971.

81 Del Fante, F. M., and Watkins, E., Jr.: Chemodectoma of the heart in a patient with multiple chemodectomas and familial history; case report and survey of literature, Lahey Clin. Found. Bull. **16**:224-229, 1967.

82 Elliott, G. B.: Glomus-like bodies on the superior mesenteric artery, Can. Med. Assoc. J. **92**:1303-1305, 1965.

83 Farr, H. W.: Carotid body tumors; a 30 year experience at Memorial Hospital, Am. J. Surg. **114**:614-619, 1967.

84 Glenner, G. G., Crout, J. R., and Roberts, W. C.: A functional carotid-body-like tumor, Arch. Pathol. **73**:230-240, 1962.

85 Glucksman, M. A., and Persinger, C. P.: Malignant non-chromaffin paraganglioma of the bladder, J. Urol. **89**:822-825, 1963.

86 Grimley, P. M., and Glenner, G. G.: Histology and ultrastructure of carotid body paragangliomas; comparison with the normal gland, Cancer **20**:1473-1488, 1967.

87 Hamberger, C.-A., Hamberger, C. B., Wersäll, J., and Wågermark, J.: Malignant catecholamine-producing tumour of the carotid body, Acta Pathol. Microbiol. Scand. **69**:489-492, 1967.

88 Heppleston, A. G.: A carotid-body-like tumour in the lung, J. Pathol. Bacteriol. **75**:461-464, 1958.

89 Kepes, J. J., and Zacharias, D. L.: Gangliocytic paragangliomas of the duodenum; report of two cases with light and electron microscopy examination, Cancer **27**:61-70, 1971.

90 Kipkie, G. F.: Simultaneous chromaffin tumors of the carotid body and the glomus jugularis, Arch. Pathol. **44**:113-118, 1947.

91 Korn, D., Bensch, K., Liebow, A. A., and Castleman, B.: Multiple minute pulmonary tumors resembling chemodectomas, Am. J. Pathol. **37**:641-672, 1960.

92 Lahey, F. H., and Warren, S. W.: A long term appraisal of carotid body tumors with remarks on their removal, Surg. Gynecol. Obstet. **92**:481-491, 1951.

93 Lattes, R.: Nonchromaffin paraganglioma of ganglion nodosum, carotid body and aortic-arch bodies, Cancer **3**:667-694, 1950.

94 Lattes, R., and Waltner, J. G.: Nonchromaffin paraganglioma of the middle ear (carotid-body-like tumor; glomus-jugulare tumor), Cancer **2**:447-468, 1949.

95 Levit, S. A., Sheps, S. G., Espinosa, R. E., Remine, W. H., and Harrison, E. G.: Catecholamine-secreting paraganglioma of glomus-

jugulare region resembling pheochromocytoma, N. Engl. J. Med. **281**:805-812, 1969.

96 Marshall, R. B., and Horn, R. C., Jr.: Nonchromaffin paraganglioma; a comparative study, Cancer **14**:779-787, 1961.

97 Miller, T. A., Weber, T. R., and Appelman, H. D.: Paraganglioma of the gallbladder, Arch. Surg. **105**:637-639, 1972.

98 Moran, T. E.: Nonchromaffin paraganglioma of the nasal cavity, Laryngoscope **72**:201-206, 1962.

99 Murphy, T. E., Huvos, A. G., and Frazell, E. L.: Chemodectomas of the glomus intravagale: vagal body tumors, nonchromaffin paragangliomas of the nodose ganglion of the vagus nerve, Ann. Surg. **172**:246-255, 1970.

100 Oberman, H. A., Holtz, F., Sheffer, L. A., and Magielski, J. E.: Chemodectomas (nonchromaffin paragangliomas) of the head and neck; a clinicopathologic study, Cancer **21**:838-851, 1968.

101 Olson, J. R., and Abell, M. R.: Nonfunctional, nonchromaffin paragangliomas of the retroperitoneum, Cancer **23**:1358-1367, 1969.

102 Patcher, M. R.: Mediastinal nonchromaffin paraganglioma; a clinicopathological study based on 8 cases, J. Thorac. Cardiovasc. Surg. **45**:152-160, 1963.

103 Pryse-Davies, J., Dawson, I. M. P., and Westbury, G.: Some morphologic, histiochemical and chemical observations on chemodectomas and the normal carotid body, including a study of the chromaffin reaction and possible ganglion cell elements, Cancer **17**:185-202, 1964.

104 Rosai, J., and Mettler, E. A.: Quimiodectoma de mediastino, Rev. Asoc. Med. Arg. **79**:242-246, 1965.

105 Rosenwasser, H.: Glomus jugulare tumors, Arch. Otolaryngol. **88**:1-40, 1968.

106 Shamblin, W. R., ReMine, W. H., Sheps, S. G., and Harrison, E. G.: Carotid body tumor (chemodectoma); clinicopathologic analysis of 90 cases, Am. J. Surg. **122**:732-739, 1971.

107 Shermer, K. L., Pantius, E. E., Dziabis, M. D., and McQuistan, R. J.: Tumors of the glomus jugulare and glomus tympanicum, Cancer **19**:1273-1280, 1966.

108 Smith, W. T., Hughes, B., and Ermocilla, R.: Chemodectoma of the pineal region, with observations of the pineal body and chemoreceptor tissue, J. Pathol. Bacteriol. **92**:69-76, 1966.

109 Taylor, H. B., and Helwig, E. B.: Benign nonchromaffin paragangliomas of the duodenum, Virchows Arch. Pathol. Anat. **335**:356-366, 1962.

110 Thacker, W. C., and Duckworth, J. K.: Chemodectoma of the orbit, Cancer **23**:1233-1238, 1969.

111 Walters, G.: Catecholamine-secreting tumours. In Dyke, S. C., editor: Recent advances in clinical pathology, ser. 5, Boston, 1968, Little, Brown and Co.

112 Whimster, W. F., and Masson, A. F.: Malignant carotid body tumor with extradural metastases, Cancer **26**:239-244, 1970.

113 Wilkinson, R., and Forgan-Smith, R.: Chemodectoma in relation to the aortic arch (aortic body tumour), Thorax **24**:488-491, 1969.

114 Winkler, H., and Smith, A. D.: Phaeochromocytoma and other catecholamine-producing tumours. In Handbook of experimental pharmacology Vol. 33: Catecholamines (Blaschko, H., and Muschall, E., subeditors), New York, 1972, Springer-Verlag.

115 Zacks, S. I.: Chemodectomas occurring concurrently in the neck (carotid body), temporal bone (glomus jugulare) and retroperitoneum; report of a case with histochemical observations, Am. J. Pathol. **34**:293-309, 1958.

116 Zeman, M. S.: Carotid body tumor of the trachea, glomus jugularis tumor, tympanic body tumor, nonchromaffin paraganglioma, Ann. Otol. Rhinol. Laryngol. **65**:960-962, 1956.

16 Genitourinary tract

Kidney
Bladder

Kidney

Pathologic examination

Partial or complete nephrectomy is indicated for a variety of infectious, degenerative, and neoplastic conditions. Before the kidney is opened, careful search should be made for aberrant vessels and any ureteral constriction, particularly at the ureteropelvic junction. The gross examination of renal specimens containing neoplasms must determine by dissection of hilar vessels whether or not a tumor is growing within the venous lumina. Any narrowing or plaques within the renal artery should be recorded. The capsule of the kidney should be stripped, and the kidney should be transected to expose the entire renal pelvis. The character of stones should be determined chemically. Roentgenograms may be helpful.[1] In a group of patients with nephrolithiasis and hypercalcuria studied by Goldman et al.,[2] 7% had hyperparathyroidism. Sections for microscopic study should be large enough to include the cortex, medulla, and pelvis. Multiple 5 mm-thick sections of the entire specimen should be studied grossly so that small unsuspected lesions will not be overlooked.

Cytology

The material submitted for cytologic study usually consists of bladder washings. Catheterized urine is superior to voided specimens since the cells appear better preserved. Tumor cells from the kidney may originate in a renal cell or transitional cell carcinoma. If the transitional cells in the specimen are undifferentiated, carcinoma may be recognized. If normal-ap-

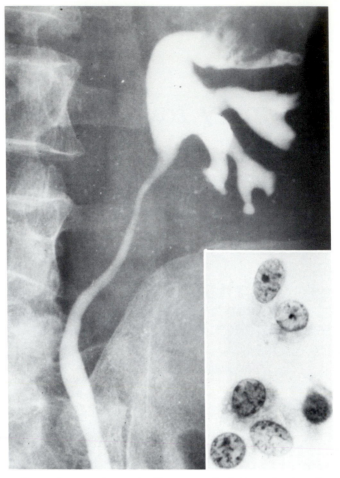

Fig. 633 Retrograde pyelogram demonstrating ragged, destroyed calyx. Tumor cells were obtained by catheterization and, as shown in inset, represent transitional cell carcinoma of intermediate grade. They can be recognized as tumor cells because of irregular distribution of chromatin in nuclei. (WU neg. 66-1983; **inset,** WU neg. 67-3096.)

pearing transitional cells are found, a well-differentiated transitional cell carcinoma may still exist.

In patients with keratinizing squamous carcinoma arising from the renal pelvis or ureter, carcinoma cells can usually be recognized with ease. These lesions, however, are rare. Because the cells of renal cell carcinoma usually contain large amounts of fat, Daut and McDonald[4] suggested the staining of cells found in the urine for fat in order to distinguish between this tumor and the transitional cell carcinoma. Focal hyperplasia of renal tubular epithelium may produce cells in

the urine that are mistaken for carcinoma. Tumor cells from renal cell carcinoma do not exfoliate until late in the evolution of the tumor. Wilms' tumor is practically never diagnosed by cytology because tumor cells are rare in the urinary stream.

We have concluded that cytology is unreliable for diagnosing renal cell carcinoma and well-differentiated tumors of the renal pelvis and ureter. It seems to be of practical value only in the few undifferentiated transitional and keratinizing squamous carcinomas of the renal pelvis and ureter (Figs. 633 and 634). Urinary cytology has been used to diagnose early rejection phe-

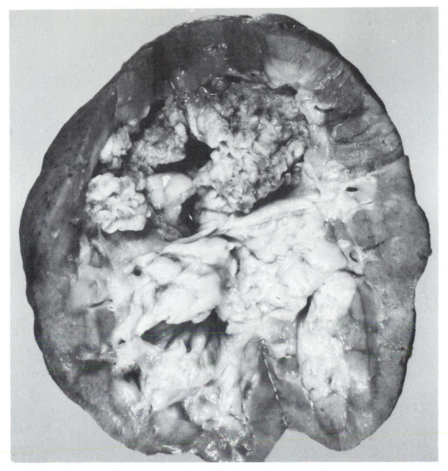

Fig. 634 Same tumor illustrated in Fig. 633. It is large papillary transitional cell carcinoma involving upper pelvis and calyces. (WU neg. 66-1897.)

nomena in kidney transplants since, in some cases, the cytologic evidence of rejection precedes other clinical and laboratory parameters.[3]

Biopsy

Incisional renal biopsy during the course of an operation is rarely indicated. If the lesion should be carcinoma, implantation is a distinct risk. On the other hand, percutaneous renal biopsy has become a routine procedure for the evaluation of medical renal diseases in most large medical centers. Its usefulness as a diagnostic and investigative tool has been amply demonstrated.[10, 12-14] In skilled hands, the procedure is at least as safe as percutaneous liver biopsy. Hematuria is a fairly common complication but is usually transient and rarely necessitates transfusion. Nephrectomy to control bleeding has not been necessary in our institution. Uncommon complications include hypertension due to perirenal hematoma, arteriovenous fistula, and sepsis. In some 4,000 biopsies, the mortality was 0.12%.[6]

There are relative and absolute contraindications to the procedure. Chief among the latter are lack of an experienced operator, presence of a solitary kidney, and hemorrhagic diathesis. Relative contraindications include inability of the patient to cooperate, azotemia, extreme hypertension, advanced calcific arteriosclerosis, renal neoplasm, and sepsis.

Portions of the specimen can be pro-

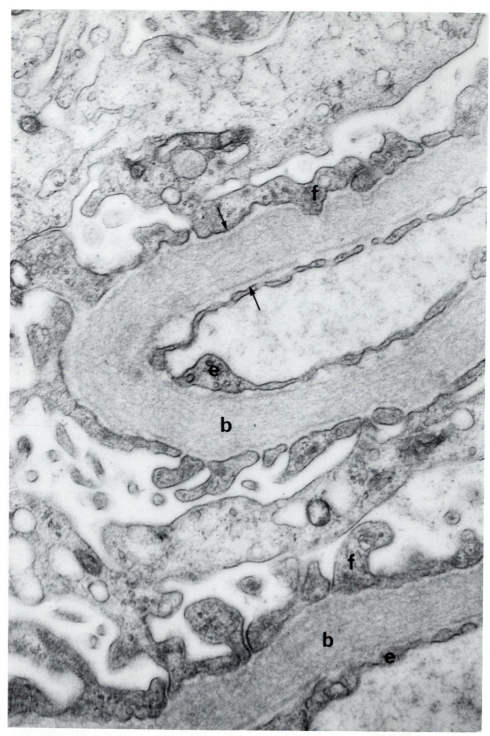

Fig. 635 Thickened basement membrane, **b,** in portions of two glomerular loops from kidney biopsy of patient with lupus erythematosus. Occasional foot processes of Bowman's epithelial cells, **f,** show fusion. No changes in endothelial cells, **e,** or fibrinoid deposits can be seen. (×31,600; courtesy Dr. S. Anderson and Dr. D. Johnston, St. Louis, Mo.)

cessed for electron microscopy (Fig. 635) and others quick frozen for histochemical and immunofluorescent studies.[5, 8] If the possibility of infection is contemplated, a small fragment of the biopsy should be placed in a sterile container and then ground in culture broth. Material for light microscopy should be fixed immediately. We find 10% buffered neutral formalin a satisfactory fixative as well as one that allows considerable flexibility in choice of stains. Sections should be cut as thin as possible (2μ to 4μ). Multiple serial sections should be made routinely—otherwise focal lesions may go undetected. In addition to the routine hematoxylin-eosin stain, it is useful to stain slides with Alcian blue–PAS, Gomori's silver methenamine, and Masson's trichrome. If a portion of the biopsy has been embedded in epoxy resins for electron microscopic study, the pathologist should make full use of this material by examining by light microscopy sections cut from these blocks.[7] The low thickness obtainable allows a sharpness of detail not possible with paraffin-embedded material. The block should not be improvidently cut through lest metachromatic stains or other preparations should prove necessary. An adequate specimen contains five to ten glomeruli and corresponding cortical tissue. The adequacy of a needle biopsy can be roughly estimated if the clinician who takes the biopsy examines the specimen with a hand lens to determine the amount of cortex present.

Kellow[11] found a correlation between random needle-aspirated and routine histologic sections in 84% of diffuse nephropathies and in 51% of focal disease. The choice between percutaneous puncture or, as done in some centers,[9] puncture of the kidney exposed by a small preliminary incision appears not to affect the success or adequacy of the biopsy as much as the operator's experience in the technique chosen. Pirani and Salinas-Madrigal[13] emphasized the importance of using a methodic approach in the microscopic examination of renal biopsies. Glomeruli,

tubules, vessels, and interstitium should be evaluated separately, and the changes present should be assessed as to type and degree.

There are several categories in which morphologic information obtained from renal biopsy may prove clinically useful:

1 Acute renal failure
2 Nephrotic syndrome
3 Systemic diseases in which renal involvement has important prognostic implications
4 Verification of the presence of absence of renal lesions in asymptomatic patients in whom a routine laboratory examination has disclosed unsuspected proteinuria or microscopic hematuria
5 Examination of asymptomatic relatives of patients with renal diseases associated with a high familial incidence
6 Evaluation of patients with renal transplants
7 Examination of prospective renal donors to be certain that the kidney has no occult diseases

Glomerulonephritis

Several forms of glomerulonephritis are recognized. The distinction is mainly based on the light microscopic appearance, although a correlation with the etiologic agent involved can sometimes be made. The available data indicate that immunologic mechanisms are the mediators of this disease, particularly the deposition of immune complexes and fixation of antiglomerular basement membrane antibody.[19, 34, 36]

Acute proliferative glomerulonephritis is, in most cases, secondary to group A streptococcal infection, although several other agents have been implicated.[16] It affects primarily children but can be seen in any age group.

In the classical clinical presentation, there are hypertension, hematuria, and oliguria after an upper respiratory infection. Microscopically, *all* of the glomeruli are affected. They are enlarged and show mesangial and endothelial proliferation, a

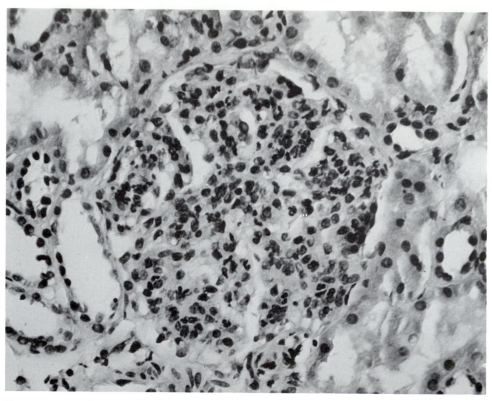

Fig. 636 Renal biopsy from 10-year-old girl with acute glomerulonephritis. Note diffuse hypercellularity of glomerular tuft. More than usual number of polymorphonuclear leukocytes are present. (×350; WU neg. 67-4639.)

variable degree of leukocytic (and sometimes eosinophilic) infiltration, ischemia, and accentuation of the lobular pattern[42] (Fig. 636). Red blood cells, leukocytes, and a granular proteinaceous material can be seen in the Bowman's space. There are no necrosis and no thickening of the peripheral capillary basement membrane. Immune complexes containing immunoglobulins, several components of the complement system, and fibrin can be regularly demonstrated by immunofluorescence.[30, 36, 39] Ultrastructurally, their counterparts are electron-dense deposits, often appearing as subepithelial dome-shaped "humps" over inflamed stalk areas.[20, 24] The severity of the glomerular changes shows good correlation with the glomerular filtration rate but not with the degree of hematuria or proteinuria.[27] As a rule, the glomerular changes subside after a period of

four to six weeks, although hypercellularity of the stalks, increased PAS-positive mesangial matrix, and lobular distortion may remain for several years.[29] Extraglomerular changes include edema and inflammation of the interstitium and hyaline droplets and granular casts in the tubules.

Total recovery is obtained in almost 100% of patients with epidemic poststreptococcal glomerulonephritis. In the sporadic cases, total recovery can be expected in 90% of the children and 70% of the adults.[21, 22, 37] This difference may be due to the fact that of the sporadic cases clinically diagnosed as acute glomerulonephritis, 10% to 15% actually represent acute exacerbations of a chronic disease.[23] There is an excellent correlation between the microscopic findings at the time of the initial attack and the ultimate outcome.[20, 32] Presence of more than occasional epithe-

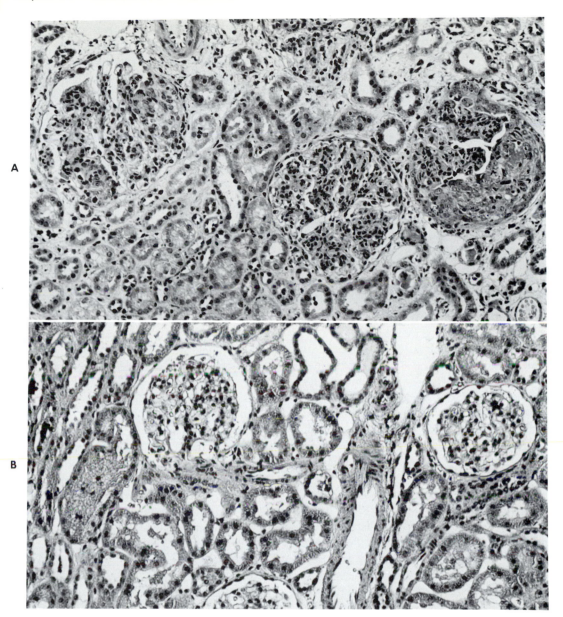

Fig. 637 **A,** Renal biopsy in 11-year-old boy with acute renal insufficiency. Diffuse acute glomerulonephritis is present. Many glomeruli (like one on right) show epithelial proliferation often associated with rapidly progressive clinical course. **B,** Two and one-half years later, following continuous course of anticoagulant therapy, patient is asymptomatic. Blood pressure, blood urea nitrogen, and creatinine are normal. Glomeruli seen in this biopsy are essentially normal, except for minor mesangial hypercellularity. (**A,** ×175; WU neg. 73-953; **B,** ×175; WU neg. 73-954.)

lial crescents should be regarded as an ominous prognostic sign. Cases with a marked degree of lobular stalk hyperplasia have a greater tendency to clinical chronicity.[29] Heptinstall[27] found capillary thrombosis, scarring, focal crescent formation, and greater interstitial reaction more commonly in cases with persistent proteinuria than in others.

In *rapidly progressive glomerulonephri-*

tis (also known as malignant glomerulonephritis and proliferative glomerulonephritis with extensive epithelial crescents), the clinical course is very rapid, usually resulting in death from renal failure in a few weeks or months.[15] The main microscopic change is the presence of extensive and numerous epithelial crescents in the glomeruli, which have arisen from proliferation of the visceral and/or parietal layers of Bowman's capsule. This is accompanied by fibrin deposition and occasionally by focal necrosis of portions of the glomerular tuft.[33] These changes develop in a matter of days and lead to collagen deposition and obliteration of the tufts. Exceptionally, the crescents disappear and normal renal function is reestablished[35] (Fig. 637). These morphologic changes can be seen in proliferative glomerulonephritides of diverse etiologies, such as poststreptococcal glomerulonephritis, acute lupus glomerulonephritis, Goodpasture's syndrome, polyarteritis nodosa, and the Schönlein-Henoch syndrome, but in most cases the condition is idiopathic.[42] According to Leonard et al.,[32] the prognosis is somewhat better in cases of poststreptococcal etiology than in others.

It is not clear yet whether **membranoproliferative glomerulonephritis** is a specific entity or a peculiar variant of poststreptococcal glomerulonephritis, although the former seems more likely.[31, 42] It usually presents in older children and young adults with asymptomatic hematuria or the nephrotic syndrome and slowly progresses to renal failure. It is often associated with depression of the serum complement and is unaffected by therapy.[18] Microscopically, it shows hypercellularity (produced by mesangial and endothelial proliferation) *and* diffuse thickening of the peripheral capillary wall.[17] This is probably due to circumferential extension of both mesangial cytoplasm and matrix into the peripheral portion of the capillary loops.[38] In later stages, the morphologic picture is that of a **lobular glomerulonephritis** as a result of the formation of sclerotic nodules in one

or more centrilobular areas of the tuft. Mandalenakis et al.[38] believe that membranoproliferative and lobular glomerulonephritis represent two microscopic variants of the same disease entity and suggest that they be designated as **mesangioproliferative glomerulonephritis.**

Chronic glomerulonephritis is not a specific entity but rather the end stage of several different forms of glomerulonephritis. The microscopic changes represent a combination of the nephritic process and those due to hypertension. All or almost all of the glomeruli are affected. Hyalinized tufts, adhesions between the tuft and Bowman's capsule, scattered cellular or fibrosed epithelial crescents, and concentric fibrosis of Bowman's capsule can all be encountered. Secondary changes in the tubules, interstitium, and vessels are invariable. The differential diagnosis with chronic pyelonephritis may be difficult. The main criteria to be used in this distinction are summarized in Table 27.

Focal glomerulonephritis is the most common cause of asymptomatic hematuria of renal origin.[26, 26a, 41] The disease is *focal* in the sense that it involves only some of the glomeruli (half or less of those present in biopsy) and *local* (or *segmental*) in that it affects only part (usually less than half) of the glomerulus.[27a] The involved portion of the glomerulus shows mesangial and endothelial proliferation, sometimes associated with thrombi, adhesions, and foci of epithelial proliferation. In later stages, these areas appear as foci of fibrosis, often adherent to Bowman's capsule. If the changes are minor and necrosis is absent, the prognosis is excellent[25] (Fig. 638). In the more severe cases, a typical nephrotic syndrome may develop.[43] In the presence of focal glomerulonephritis, every effort should be made to identify the etiologic agent, since similar changes can be seen in lupus erythematosus, polyarteritis nodosa, Wegener's granulomatosis, Schönleich-Henoch syndrome, Goodpasture's syndrome, and bacterial endocarditis (Fig. 639). The changes of focal glomerulone-

Table 27 Differential diagnosis between chronic glomerulonephritis and chronic pyelonephritis*

	Chronic glomerulonephritis	Chronic pyelonephritis
Gross	Kidneys both involved	May be unilateral, or one more affected than other
	Fine granularity	Coarse scarring or finer nodularity
	Pelvis and calyces not deformed	Deformity of pelvis and calyces
	Reduction in size of kidney usually moderate but may be considerable	Kidneys often considerably reduced
Microscopic	Diffuse involvement	Patchy involvement except in cases with gross reduction
	Glomeruli affected throughout kidney	Glomerular changes usually confined to scars except when severe hypertension is present
	Membranous thickening of tuft in certain forms	Membranous thickening of tuft rarely seen
	Proliferative tuft lesions common	Proliferative tuft lesions rare except with hypertension and renal failure
	Changes in Bowman's capsule not usually seen until late in disease (organized crescents excepted)	Relatively greater involvement of Bowman's capsule
	Tubular loss in relation to sclerosed glomeruli; no large tracts with complete loss	Tubular loss not confined to areas with glomerular sclerosis; large tracts with complete loss
	No thyroid-like areas except on minor scale	Thyroid-like areas which may be extensive
	Hypertrophy of remaining tubules	Hypertrophy not usually pronounced
	Polymorphs not usual (may occur terminally)	Polymorphs often seen
	Interstitial fibrosis fine and throughout kidney	Interstitial fibrosis coarse and mainly confined to scars
	Cellular infiltrates seldom great	Cellular infiltrate frequent and may be considerable
	Plasma cells infrequent	Plasma cells common
	Vascular changes usually moderate	Vascular changes may be extreme
	Pelvis seldom inflamed	Pelvis inflamed
	Necrotizing papillitis not seen	Necrotizing papillitis in diabetes and with obstruction

*From Heptinstall, R. H.: Pathology of the kidney, Boston, 1966, Little, Brown and Co.

phritis should be differentiated from foci of irregular resolution of inflammation in diffuse proliferative glomerulonephritis and the focal glomerular changes sometimes seen in association with severe hypertension and with the idiopathic nephrotic syndrome.

Nephrotic syndrome

There are several renal diseases that can lead to the nephrotic syndrome—i.e., the combination of proteinuria, hypoalbuminemia, and edema, often associated with hyperlipidemia and lipiduria.[61] In adults, the most common cause is *glomerulonephritis* (Fig. 640). All forms of the disease can be responsible, except perhaps the rapidly progressive type. Also common in this age group is a condition formerly designated as membranous glomerulonephritis and currently known as *membranous* (or *epimembranous*) *nephropathy*.[51] This term actually embraces a group of diseases having as a common denominator the presence of a marked uniform and diffuse thickening of the glomerular capillary walls, not accompanied by proliferative changes (Fig. 641). Ultrastructurally, irregular deposits, probably representing antigen-antibody complexes, are seen between the basement membrane and the epithelial cells. Fusion of the cell processes of the podocytes is also present. In thin sections stained with PAS or Gomori's

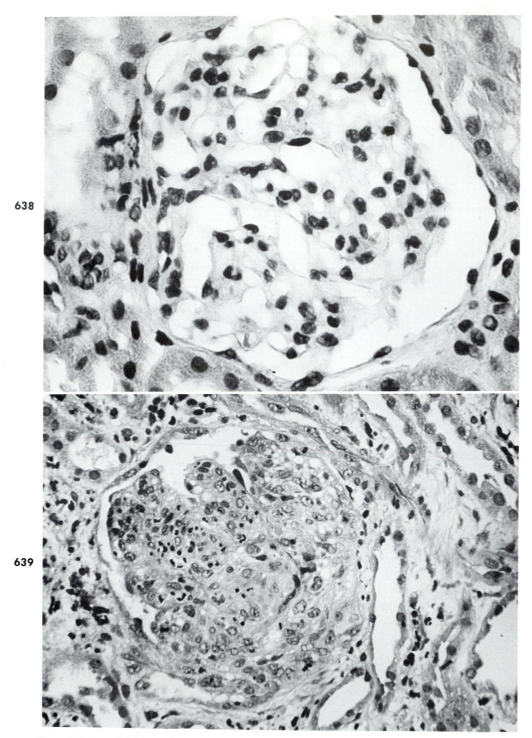

Fig. 638 Renal biopsy from 19-year-old woman with recurrent microscopic hematuria. Only lesion is minimal segmental hypercellularity of glomerular tuft. Patient remains well. (×600; WU neg. 67-4634.)

Fig. 639 Renal biopsy from 8-year-old boy with clinical features of the Schönlein-Henoch syndrome and renal insufficiency. This extensive but still focally accentuated glomerulonephritis bespeaks ominous prognosis. (×350; WU neg. 67-5637.)

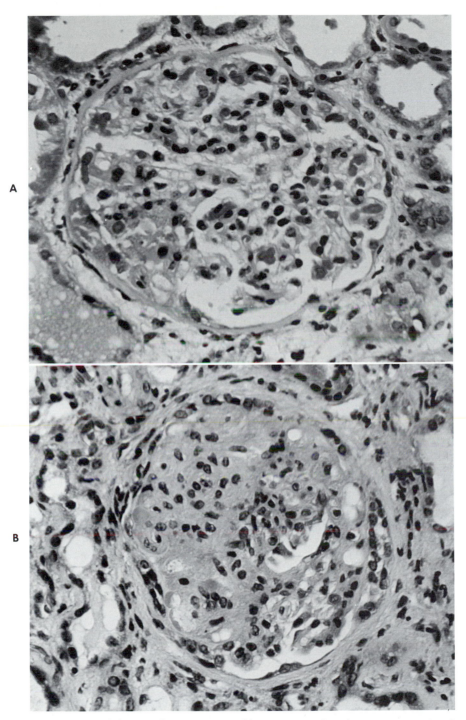

Fig. 640 A, Renal biopsy from 19-year-old woman with edema, proteinuria, hypo-albuminemia, hypercholesterolemia, and hematuria. Microscopic picture is that of acute proliferative glomerulonephritis. Presence of focal necrosis with nuclear debris and of epithelial proliferation are unfavorable signs. **B,** One year later, patient has full-blown nephrotic syndrome. Renal biopsy shows diffuse chronic glomerulonephritis with varying changes of glomerular obliteration. (**A,** WU neg. 71-8661; **B,** WU neg. 71-8662.)

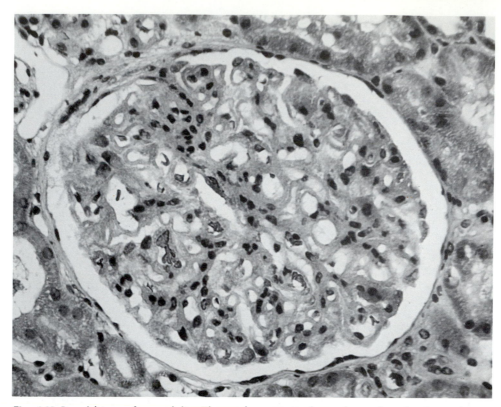

Fig. 641 Renal biopsy from adult with membranous nephropathy and nephrotic syndrome. Glomerulus is of normal cellularity, and basement membranes are uniformly thickened. (×350; WU neg. 67-5635.)

methenamine-silver, "spikes" can be seen extending from the basement membrane externally toward the epithelial cells. Most cases of membranous nephropathy are idiopathic, but others are secondary to lupus erythematosus, syphilis, hypersensitivity to drugs, or renal vein thrombosis.[45, 46, 72] The latter should be suspected if the membranous glomerular changes are associated with marked interstitial edema, neutrophilic margination in the glomerular capillaries, or peritubular venous thrombi.[60, 67, 72] In later stages, tubular atrophy out of proportion to the degree of the glomerular lesion may be the only finding suggestive of this condition. Electron microscopy can be helpful in the differential diagnosis between the idiopathic form and those secondary to lupus erythematosus or renal vein thrombosis.[66] It is also useful in distinguishing an early membranous nephropathy with only equiv-

ocal light microscopic changes from a lipoid nephrosis. This distinction is extremely important because of the markedly different natural history of these two diseases, which are totally unrelated.[68] Idiopathic membranous nephropathy slowly progresses to renal failure in the large majority of patients, unaffected by therapy.[70]

Lipoid nephrosis (also known as Earle's epithelial cell disease, minimal lesion, foot process disease, and true, pure, or nil nephrosis) is by far the commonest pathologic change in children with the nephrotic syndrome,[57] but it can also appear in adulthood.[59] By light microscopy, practically no abnormalities can be detected in the glomeruli in most instances (Fig. 642). However, electron microscopy of active cases regularly shows extensive foot process obliteration in the podocytes. In the absence of electron-dense deposits, the latter finding is diagnostic of this condi-

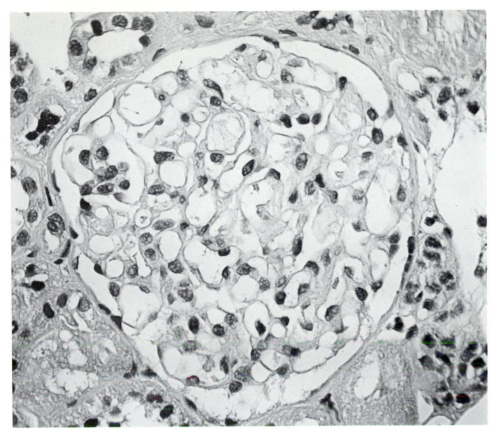

Fig. 642 Renal biopsy from child with idiopathic nephrotic syndrome. Basement membranes are not thickened and glomerulus is essentially normal by light microscopy. Dilatation of capillary loops is typical. (×550; WU neg. 67-2858.)

tion. Focal glomerulosclerosis is rarely detected in light microscopic sections but is a quite common ultrastructural finding.[74] If severe and extensive, it may exceptionally lead to renal insufficiency.[58] The tubules show features common to all of the diseases associated with the nephrotic syndrome—lipoid vacuolation and hyaline droplet degeneration.

Lipoid nephrosis responds well to steroids.[47, 64, 76] Development of resistance is often associated with focal areas of capillary collapse and sclerosis.[74]

Lupus nephropathy is another cause of nephrotic syndrome. Systemic lupus erythematosis involves the kidney in 50% to 70% of the cases.[52] Three major forms of the disease can be recognized.[44, 49, 69] In the first, already alluded to and comprising approximately one-sixth of the cases, the clinical and pathologic features are those of a membranous nephropathy, and the evolution is toward chronic renal insufficiency. In the second type, designated by Pollack et al.[69] as "minimal glomerular involvement," there are only minimal changes in the glomeruli by light microscopy and basement membrane irregularities (but no deposits) by electron microscopy (Fig. 635). The prognosis is excellent. The third type of lupus involvement of the kidney is manifested by a proliferative glomerulonephritis, which can be diffuse but is most often focal. Any one of the following changes can be seen, singly or in combination: mesangial and endothelial proliferation, epithelial crescents, neutrophilic infiltration, "wire loops," hyaline

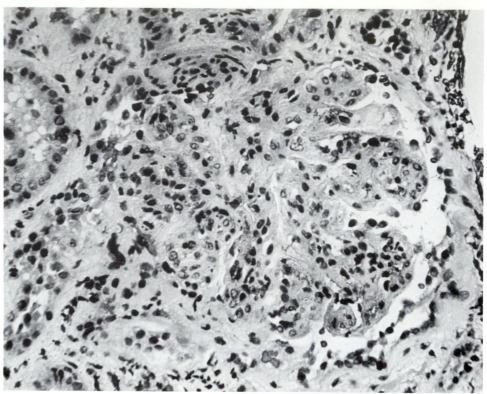

Fig. 643 Renal biopsy showing lupus glomerulonephritis. Lobular hypercellularity, focal hyaline thickening of basement membranes, and glomerular adhesions are present. (×340; WU neg. 67-5636.)

thrombi, and foci of lobular necrosis impregnated with nuclear dust (Fig. 643). None of these features are specific for the disease. Hematoxylin bodies are, but they can be identified only in a minority of cases. By immunoflourescence, deposits of immunoglobulins, fibrin, and complement components can be demonstrated in the active cases[63, 71] (Fig. 644). Ultrastructurally, electron-dense deposits are irregularly scattered beneath the endothelium and in the mesangium.[53] Some have a peculiar fingerprint pattern.[56] Clusters of cytoplasmic microtubules resembling myxoviruses are regularly present in the endothelial cells of glomerular and peritubular capillaries. None of these fine structural features can be regarded as specific for lupus nephropathy.[55, 75]

According to Seymour et al.[74] and Baldwin et al.,[44] the degree and extent of inflammatory changes correlate well with the ultimate outcome. In general, diffuse proliferative lesions follow a relentlessly progressive course, whereas those showing only focal involvement tend to respond favorably to therapy. This often coincides with a diminution and decreased density of the deposits seen with the electron microscope.

Other causes of nephrotic syndrome include amyloidosis and diabetes mellitus. In *amyloidosis,* the typical deposits accumulate in the mesangium and beneath the endothelium of the glomerulus, as well as in the wall of blood vessels and interstitium (Fig. 645). Dichroism after Congo red staining is regarded as the most specific test for amyloid.[50] Electron microscopy sometimes demonstrates amyloid deposits which are inapparent by light microscopy but are severe enough to produce proteinuria.[65]

Diabetic nephropathy involves the arterioles as well as the glomeruli.[54] The former show marked subendothelial hya-

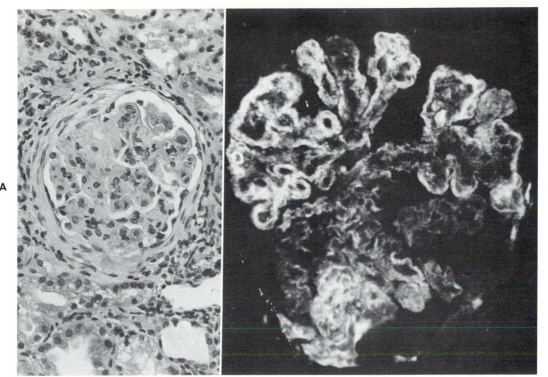

Fig. 644 Lupus nephrophathy in young woman with positive LE test and antinuclear antibody titer of 1:512. Patient died from renal insufficiency two months after this biopsy was taken. **A,** Routine section shows irregular thickening of basement membrane, "wire loops," and fibrosis of Bowman's capsule. **B,** Same specimen shown in **A** after "staining" for $B1_c$ globulin (C'3) in immunofluorescence preparation. Glomerular loops are unevenly infiltrated by immune complex deposits. Heavier infiltration is in "wire loops." Similar pattern was obtained after "staining" for IgG. (**A,** ×240; **B,** ×420; **A** and **B,** courtesy Dr. F. G. Germuth, Jr., St. Louis, Mo.)

line thickening. It is said that its presence in *both* afferent and efferent arterioles is specific for diabetes. The glomerular involvement is manifested by sclerosis, which can be diffuse or nodular (Fig. 646). This is the result of an increase of mesangial matrix *and* thickening of the peripheral capillary walls as a result of excess of basement membrane.[48, 62] Less significant changes include the so-called "exudative" lesions, characterized by the presence of eosinophilic masses in Bowman's space. They probably represent entrapped plasma proteins.[73]

Acute renal failure

Among the many renal diseases that may present with a clinical picture of acute renal failure, the most common are rapidly progressive glomerulonephritis, diffuse proliferative glomerulonephritis, accelerated (malignant) hypertension, acute tubular necrosis, symmetrical cortical necrosis, and toxic nephropathy. In all of these conditions, information provided by renal biopsy is extremely helpful in guiding the choice of therapeutic modalities and evaluating the ultimate prognosis. A good percentage of patients with predominantly interstitial lesions recover, whereas the prognosis is more variable in those with vascular or glomerular involvement. A very poor prognosis can be expected in the patients with accelerated hypertension and rapidly progressive glomerulonephritis.[79] Patients with diffuse proliferative glomerulonephritis of streptococcal etiology have a significantly better prognosis.[77]

The pathologic diagnosis of symmetrical

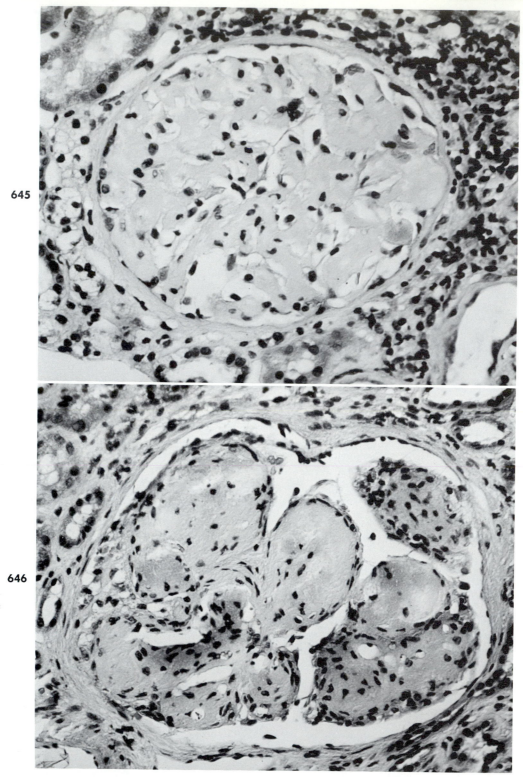

Fig. 645 Renal biopsy from patient with systemic amyloidosis. (×350; WU neg. 67-4638.)
Fig. 646 Renal biopsy showing nodular intercapillary glomerulosclerosis. Patient had latent but undiagnosed diabetes mellitus. (×300; WU neg. 67-4635.)

renal cortical necrosis, in contrast with acute tubular necrosis, is prognostically very ominous, although occasional survival with impaired renal function has been reported. The lesion predominantly affects parturient women, although cases have been reported following exanthemas of childhood, oligemic episodes in infancy (diarrhea), snake bite, in the course of the "hemolytic uremic syndrome," and complicating hypovolemic shock (other than obstetric) in adults. Hypoperfusion of the renal cortex followed by paralytic vasodilation have been incriminated in the pathogenesis of the lesion.

Tissues from the living patient are limited to percutaneous or open renal biopsies and require careful evaluation since the prognosis is so poor. Good specimens demonstrate ischemic necrosis of confluent areas of cortex. At the margins of these areas (subcapsular and at the corticomedullary junction), a mantle of hyperemic but viable renal parenchyma is demonstrable. In long-standing cases, resorption of devitalized tissue, usually with dystrophic calcification at the margins, is demonstrable.[78]

Renal transplant

The kidney is the organ most commonly transplanted in man. More than 5,000 renal transplants are on record.[88] Technically, the operation is relatively easy. The greatest difficulty resides in the prevention and control of the immunologic response of the recipient against the graft, which is mediated both by cellular and humoral mechanisms. The greater the differences in the histocompatibility (transplantation) antigens between the graft and the recipient, the stronger the immunologic attack.[87] In cases of rejection, renal biopsy may provide important information for the management of the patient.[81]

Three clinicopathologic forms of transplant rejection have been described: hyperacute, acute, and chronic.

In *hyperacute rejection,* humoral mechanisms are operative, represented by preexisting cytotoxic antibodies. The changes may occur within minutes of opening the anastomosis. Microscopically, massive cortical necrosis, widespread arteriolar and capillary thrombosis, and marked accumulation of neutrophils within glomerular and peritubular capillaries are the main features.[83, 89]

The *acute rejection,* which occurs within the first sixty days following the operation, is often well managed with immunosuppressive therapy. It is probably induced by a combination of cellular and humoral mechanisms. The microscopic interpretation of the changes present may be difficult, since the picture varies according to the severity and type of immunologic reaction, the modifications resulting from the therapy, and the degree of surgery-related injury. The main change is interstitial lymphocytic infiltration, often centered around blood vessels. The arteries may show fibrinoid necrosis, thrombosis, intimal fibrosis, or muscle cell hyperplasia. Dense deposits can be demonstrated ultrastructurally beneath the endothelium of the glomerular capillaries. They contain immunoglobulins (mainly IgM) and complement compounds.[85, 86] Proliferative glomerular changes also can be observed.[84] Necrotizing vascular changes and deposits of IgG are ominous prognostic signs.[80]

In *chronic rejection,* the obliterative vascular changes predominate, although focal fibrinoid necrosis may still be encountered. These alterations closely resemble those seen in accelerated (malignant) hypertension. Lymphocytic infiltration, fibrosis, tubular atrophy, and diffuse thickening of the glomerular basement membrane also are commonly observed.[84] A clinical picture of nephrotic syndrome may develop in these patients.[82]

Renal hypertension

Goldblatt[96] demonstrated in dogs that sustained hypertension could be produced by reduction of the arterial blood supply to one kidney. This was later found to be secondary to the increased secretion by the injured kidney of *renin*, a proteolytic enzyme that acts on a circulating plasma globulin (angiotensinogen) to produce an-

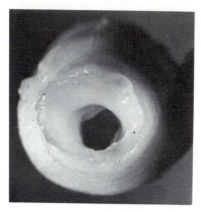

Fig. 647 Eccentric arteriosclerotic plaque in renal artery causing almost complete obstruction and hypertension. This was resected and arterial continuity reestablished. (WU neg. 61-6675.)

giotensin I, which is subsequently converted into an active pressor polypeptide (angiotensin II) by another enzyme. The site of elaboration and storage of renin is the juxtaglomerular apparatus. Hyperplasia and hypergranularity of these cells is regularly found in an ischemic kidney, whereas in the contralateral organ there is usually hypoplasia and hypogranularity. Crocker[95] found very little correlation between the juxtaglomerular cell count and the clinical response following surgery under these circumstances. However, if bilateral juxtaglomerular cell hypoplasia is found in the absence of parenchymal renal disease or bilateral renal artery stenosis, this can be taken as evidence of essential hypertension and a poor surgical response can be anticipated.

Many pathologic processes involving the human kidney can result in hypertension.

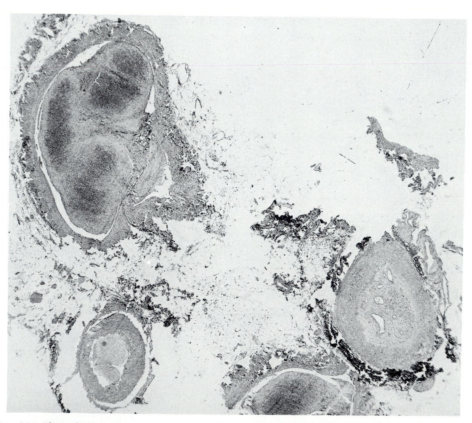

Fig. 648 Thrombosis of branches of renal artery and vein. These thrombi are of three months' duration. (Low power; WU neg. 58-806.)

They can be divided in three main categories: renovascular, renal parenchymal, and urinary tract obstruction. In the first, the hypertension is produced through the renin-angiotensin system, but this may not be the case for the other two categories.

Renovascular disease is the most common cause of renal hypertension. This includes arteriosclerotic narrowing and occlusion (Figs. 647 and 648), fibromuscular dysplasia[94, 98, 99, 102] (Fig. 649), poststenotic renal artery aneurysm,[90] traumatic thrombosis, embolism, aortic or renal coarctation, aberrant renal arteries, arteriovenous fistula,[100] and extrinsic compression.[93] The kidney in these cases shows varying degrees of nephrosclerotic atrophy, sometimes associated with segmental infarct or infarcts (Fig. 650). Total renal infarct does not result in hypertension.

Occlusion of the major renal artery rarely leads to total infarction of the kidney. Collateral vascular supply from capsular or adrenal vessels usually suffices for viability of irregularly defined areas of cortex. The presence of ischemic necrosis in more than one renal lobule not clearly confined to cortical elements bespeaks occlusion of a major renal artery.

The most common renal parenchymal diseases leading to hypertension are pyelonephritis and hydronephrosis (Fig. 651). Burns[92] reviewed his cases of hypertension and pyelonephritis and found that in those patients in whom hypertension had been relieved by nephrectomy, severe sclerosis of the renal artery was always present. If the kidney removed for pyelonephritis associated with hypertension shows prominent arteriolar disease, the chances are

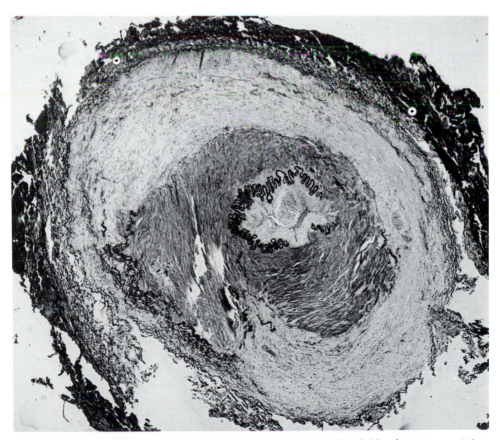

Fig. 649 Fibromuscular dysplasia of renal artery with only slitlike lumen remaining. Patient, 42-year-old woman, had hypertension. Segment of artery was removed and continuity reestablished. (×40; WU neg. 63-71.)

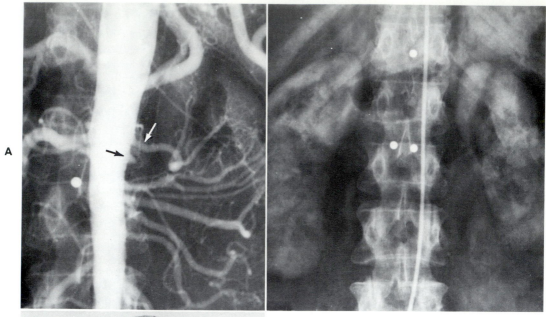

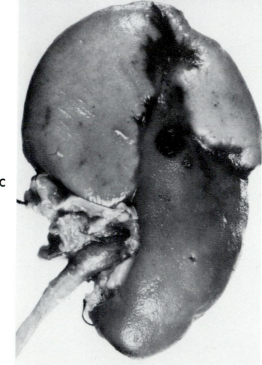

Fig. 650 Patient, 50-year-old woman, had sustained hypertension secondary to vascular lesion of left kidney. Increased levels of renin were demonstrated in blood from left renal vein. **A,** Arterial phase of arteriogram showing total occlusion of one renal artery (black arrow). An upper (polar) renal artery is patent (white arrow). **B,** Capillary phase of arteriogram demonstrating marked decrease in size of affected kidney. **C,** Surgically excised left kidney shows extensive infarct of area supplied by occluded artery. (**A,** WU neg. 72-2864; **B,** WU neg. 72-2784; **C,** WU neg. 72-2785.)

high that similar changes will be present in the opposite kidney and that hypertension will not be relieved permanently.

In the presence of a surgically correctable lesion of the renal artery, every effort should be made in preserving the corresponding kidney, which is potentially the least damaged one.[91] In the patients with parenchymal renal disease, the offending kidney needs to be removed. This often relieves the hypertension. It has been difficult, however, to select accurately those patients who will benefit from nephrectomy. Although the blood pressure frequently falls after removal of the kidney, it may soon return to the preoperative level. It has been stated that at least a year needs to lapse before results of the operation can be properly evaluated.

Recent large series of surgically treated patients have cooled the enthusiasm of for-

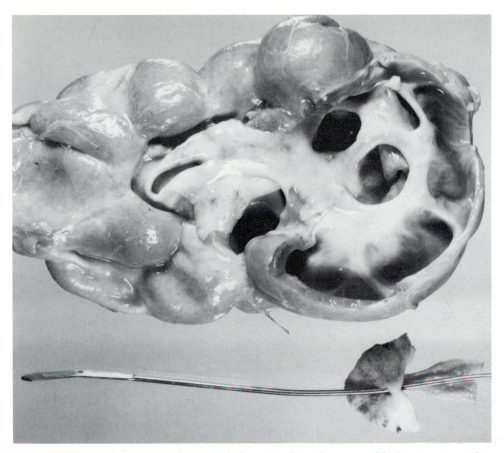

Fig. 651 Kidney of 15-year-old girl with hypertension. There was block at ureteropelvic junction resulting in hydronephrosis. (WU neg. 64-7373.)

mer days. In a study of 115 hypertensive patients with renal artery lesions reported by Shapiro et al.,[101] forty-three underwent surgery. Six years later, only eleven patients (28%) were normotensive or markedly improved. The authors concluded that the overall mortality from hypertensive disease had been scarcely modified by surgery.

Bartter's syndrome is characterized by elevated plasma renin, hyperplasia of the juxtaglomerular apparatus, hyperaldosteronism, and hyperkalemia but *no hypertension*. Goodman et al.[97] suggested that the primary defect in some patients is impairment of proximal sodium reabsorption.

Cystic lesions

Congenital cystic lesions of the kidney are important surgical problems.[103] In infants, they come to clinical attention by producing palpable masses. The vast majority of abnormal abdominal masses in newborn infants are renal, and most of these *in newborn infants* are benign.[104]

Renal dysplasia

Renal dysplasia is the commonest benign lesion involving the kidneys of newborn infants. It may also become apparent in older children or even adults, in whom it is usually fortuitously demonstrated. It is usually unilateral, although bilateral cases are occasionally encountered. The renal involvement may be total, segmental, or focal. Associated malformations are common, particularly absence or atresia of the ureter. Cardiovascular and gastrointestinal defects also are found in a significant proportion of cases. This condition has also

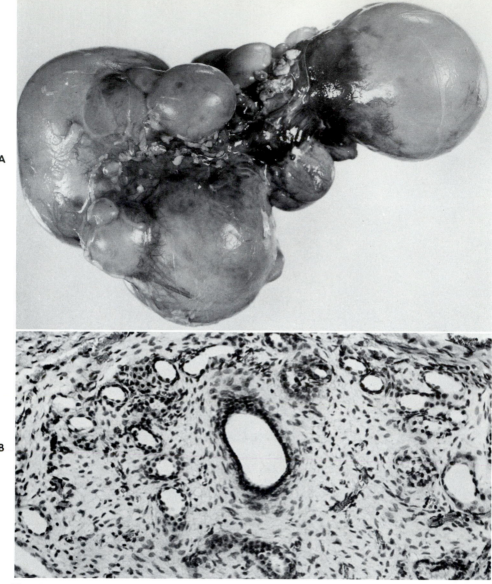

Fig. 652 **A,** Dysplastic kidney of 17-day-old infant. Opposite kidney appeared normal by pyelogram. **B,** Same kidney illustrated in **A** showing embryonic-like connective tissue and tubules. (**A,** WU neg. 49-5299; **B,** ×230; WU neg. 50-329.)

been designated as congenital unilateral multicystic disease of the kidney.[109]

A dysplastic kidney consists of an irregular aggregate of thin-walled cysts and loose fibrous stroma (Fig. 652, A). Microscopically, the lesion consists of cystic spaces lined by columnar or cuboidal epithelium, disorderly ductules, and immature mesenchymal stroma in which nodules of cartilage are often present[106] (Fig. 652, B).

Beyond infancy, dysplastic kidneys and other renal malformations present clinically with complications such as hydronephrosis, pyelonephritis, or calculus more commonly than as a cause of hypertension or chronic renal insufficiency.

Congenitally abnormal kidneys can also be the site of various types of specific infections such as tuberculosis and neoplasms.[107, 108] On occasion, kidneys with congenital abnormalities result in a mistaken clinical and radiographic diagnosis of Wilms' tumor.[105]

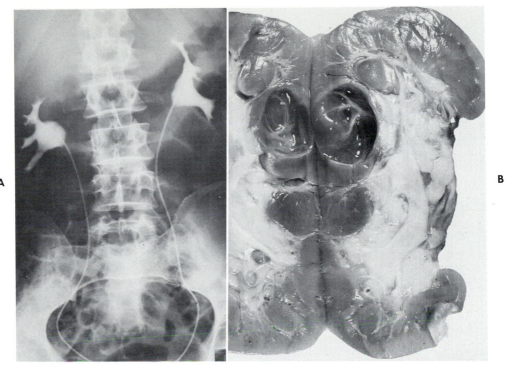

Fig. 653 A, Retrograde pyelogram. Note distortion of superior calyx of left kidney. Patient had hematuria, and differential diagnosis between cyst and tumor could not be made. **B,** Left kidney shown in **A** after removal demonstrating small cyst rather than neoplasm. (**A,** WU neg. 49-7135; **B,** WU neg. 49-7079.)

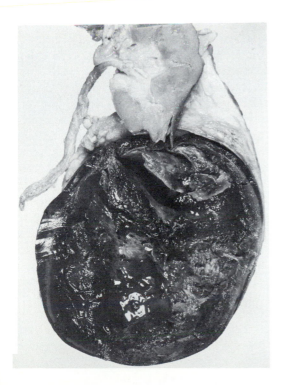

Simple cyst

A familiar renal lesion, the simple cyst is lined by a single layer of often discontinuous cuboidal epithelium. It contains clear yellow fluid and displaces renal parenchyma. The noncommittal designation of *simple cyst* circumvents exceptions to such terms as "solitary" cyst (simple cysts are, in fact, usually multiple), "cortical" cysts (simple cysts occur in the medulla as well as in cortex), and "serous" cysts (the content of uncomplicated simple cysts is protein-poor and not usually characterized as "serous").

Simple cysts are common findings at autopsy. One or more gross renal cysts are present in probably one-half of all individuals 50 years of age or older. The rarity of such lesions in infants and chil-

Fig. 654 Single large hemorrhagic cyst of lower pole of kidney. Carcinoma was present in it. Secondary calcification can occur in such lesions. (WU neg. 51-199.)

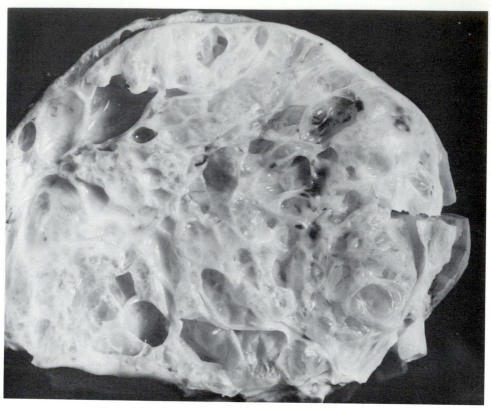

Fig. 655 Multilocular cyst from young girl. Patient had received course of irradiation therapy for presumed Wilms' tumor. When mass failed to regress, nephrectomy disclosed this lesion. (WU neg. 61-1804.)

dren[111, 112] supports an acquired rather than congenital mode of pathogenesis. In view of their frequency in older individuals, simple renal cysts are very rarely responsible for clinical symptoms. Presence of a mass, rupture, hemorrhage, or torsion occasionally calls attention to simple cysts. Most such lesions are detected by roentgenographic studies of the urinary system undertaken for unrelated conditions (Fig. 653). A few are calcified.[110] At least one-third of all renal cysts with hemorrhagic contents are actually cystic carcinomas[112] (Fig. 654).

Multilocular cyst

The multilocular cyst, an uncommon but distinctive lesion, may become clinically evident at any age (Fig. 655). Clinical manifestations result from the presence of a mass or, not uncommonly, from ureteral obstruction by one of the daughter locules.

Grossly, it is sharply delineated from the uninvolved renal parenchyma. On microscopic examination, the outer wall of the cyst contains fascicles of smooth muscle. Delicate septa divide the lesion into discrete daughter locules. The lining epithelium varies in appearance in the different cysts, ranging from tall cuboidal to an extremely flat type resembling endothelium.[114] In the past, the latter feature has often resulted in an erroneous diagnosis of lymphangioma. The stroma between the cysts may be cellular and simulate Wilms' tumor. Boggs and Kimmelstiel,[113] suggesting a developmental origin, designate such lesions "multilocular cystic nephroma."

Polycystic renal disease

Two distinct varieties of polycystic renal disease exist, both of which are hereditary

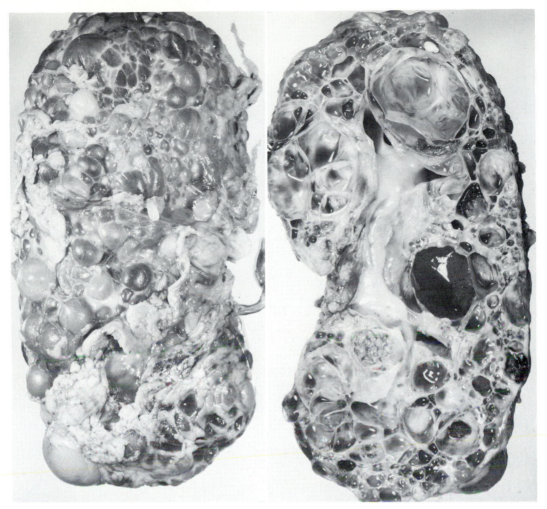

Fig. 656 External and cut surface of surgically excised kidney with adult polycystic disease. It weighed 3.850 gm. Patient, 32-year-old woman on chronic dialysis, developed left flank pain, dysuria, and fever. (WU negs. 72-941 and 72-942.)

and bilateral.[119] The *infantile variety*, which is the least common of the two, is seen exclusively in infants. It is only rarely a surgical problem and often leads to death in the first weeks or months of life.[120] The *adult variety* may be discovered shortly after birth but is more likely to be diagnosed after the patient is 30 years of age. In a large series reported by Bell,[115] only two cases were diagnosed in patients between the ages of 1 month and 25 years.

Because the polycystic condition usually is bilateral, it is not amenable to surgery. Renal complications are frequent and include pyelonephritis, lithiasis, tuberculosis,

and neoplasm. Rarely, this condition may be predominantly unilateral in either adult or child. Nine of 150 cases collected by Sieber[123] and eleven of sixty-four studied by Bell[115] were unilateral.

Grossly, the kidney retains its normal shape but may show all degrees of cystic degeneration ranging from a few isolated cysts to a kidney that is completely honeycombed (Fig. 656). In infancy, the kidneys are usually riddled with fairly uniform small cysts. In adults, these cysts are larger and vary greatly in size. In advanced disease, the cysts involve both the cortex and the medulla. The cysts frequently com-

Table 28 Differential features of various cystic lesions of the renal parenchyma*

Name	Incidence	Heredity	Age	Laterality
Renal dysplasia	Common	Usually none	Infancy	Usually unilateral; occasionally bilateral, segmental, or focal
Polycystic renal disease Adult	Fairly common	Dominant	Usually adults	Bilateral
Infantile	Rare	Recessive	Infancy and childhood	Bilateral
Congenital hepatic fibrosis	Rare	Recessive	Adolescents	Bilateral
Medullary cystic disease Sponge kidney	Fairly common	None	Adults	Usually bilateral
Uremic medullary cystic disease	Very rare	Suggestive	Adults	Bilateral
Simple cyst	Common	None	Adults	Usually unilateral
Multilocular cyst	Very rare	None	Any	Unilateral

*Adapted from Kissane, J. M.: Congenital malformations. In Heptinstall, R. H.: Pathology of the kidney, Boston, 1966, Little, Brown and Co.

municate with the calyces in adults but rarely in children. Studies on the chemical composition of the cyst's fluid suggest that the cysts are connected to patent nephrons and that they might contribute to renal function.[116, 117] The amount of normal parenchyma varies widely. The degree of cystic change is not always the same in both kidneys.

The microscopic appearance of the polycystic kidney varies. The glomeruli in the subcapsular areas frequently appear normal. In the young child, the connective tissue appears embryonic.

In the embryo, the ureter and the wolffian duct fuse with the metanephric blastema. The tubules that form the collecting tubules divide and subdivide repeatedly and finally connect with the convoluted tubules. Ribbert's theory (1900) is that

there is no union in polycystic disease. Kampmeier[118] feels that there is a persistence of fetal cysts formed from the first two generations of the detached convoluted tubules. Osathanondh and Potter[121] have conducted detailed nephron dissections that support neither of these hypotheses, and the pathogenesis remains unknown.

The prognosis following surgical removal of a polycystic kidney is obviously dependent on the function of the remaining kidney. If there is decrease of renal function demonstrated before operation, the prognosis is poor. Of thirty-one patients reported by Walters and Braasch,[124] eighteen were living from one to nineteen years after operation. The youngest patient, operated on at the age of 21 months, had been living over fourteen years at the time of the report.

Gross features	Microscopic features	Associated malformations	
		Genitourinary	Other
...en irregularly cystic, not ...iform	Immature tubules and ductules; mesenchymatous stroma; cartilage	Common; absent or atretic ureter	Common: cardiovascular; gastrointestinal
...ge bosselated kidneys; ...herical cysts in cortex ...d medulla	Various lining; some normal parenchyma	None	Cysts in liver, etc.; aneurysms, other cardiovascular; central nervous system; D, trisomy, etc.
...ge, smooth kidneys; ...iform or cylindrical cysts ...cortex and medulla	Nondescript lining; foci of normal nephrons	None	Cysts and aberrant ductules in liver; cysts in pancreas, spleen
...ttered spherical cysts	As adult type	None	Hepatic fibrosis with cysts or abnormal ductules; aneurysms (one pedigree)
...sts in tips of papillae	Various epithelial linings; calculi	None	None
...sts at corticomedullary ...ction; contracted cortex ...h cysts	Periglomerular and interstitial fibrosis	None	None
...gle or few cysts, usually ...tical	Nondescript lining	None	None
...cumscribed multilocular ...t; thick capsule	Smooth muscle in capsule; cellular mesenchyme in trabeculae	None	None

A third of the patients with the adult form of polycystic renal disease have cysts of the liver, which are usually small and devoid of clinical significance. Another well-documented association is between polycystic kidneys and cerebral artery aneurysms.[122] The differential diagnostic features of the various cystic diseases of the kidneys are summarized in Table 28.

Hydronephrosis

Hydronephosis or dilatation of the renal pelvis follows partial block of urinary outflow. Complete block (ligature) produces acute renal atrophy without significant ureteropelvic dilatation. Partial block can occur at any level in the urinary tract. The most common is nodular hyperplasia of the prostate. Various malignant lesions may partially block one or both ureters, the most frequent being carcinoma of the prostate, bladder, or cervix. Rarely, carcinoma of the ovary or rectum, and more rarely, leiomyoma of the uterus cause hydronephrosis.

Aberrant vessels at the juncture of the ureter and the pelvis may cause obstruction. These arteries may arise from the aorta or independently from the ovarian, spermatic, or iliac arteries. An aberrant vessel is often the cause of hydronephrosis in children (Fig. 651). White and Wyatt[126] reported thirty such cases. Ostling[125] believes that congenital ureteropelvic fixation may cause stricture. Poorly administered irradiation to the pelvic organs may produce sufficient ureteral injury to cause hydronephrosis.

Grossly, the hydronephrotic kidney may show any degree of dilatation (Figs. 657

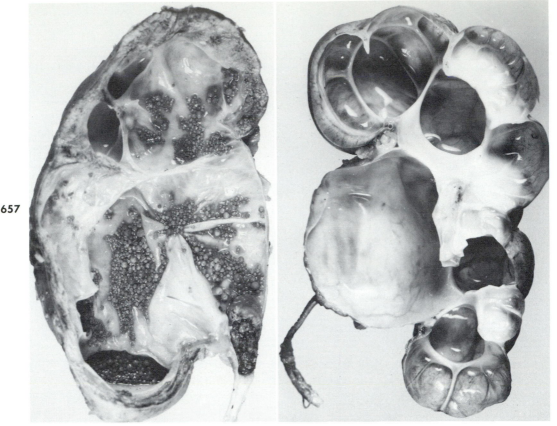

657

658

Fig. 657 Kidney with massive hydronephrosis and innumerable stones (largest blocking ureteropelvic junction) in 78-year-old woman who also had beta cell tumor of pancreas. (WU neg. 68-8799.)

Fig. 658 Massive hydronephrosis in 37-year-old man secondary to obstruction of ureteropelvic junction. In contrast to dyplastic kidney, wide communication between different cavities exists. (WU neg. 72-11069.)

and 658). On section, the dilated kidney may contain 300 ml to 500 ml of urine. The calyces are blunted, and the cortex is narrowed (Fig. 659). Even when the renal collecting system is sufficiently obstructed so that it is not visualized by pyelography, renal function (indicated by subsequent dye excretion) likely will return if the obstruction is removed or if the urinary stream is diverted before complete parenchymal destruction occurs.

Microscopically, in early hydronephrosis, the tubules are slightly dilated, a change which is replaced by atrophy in later stages of the disease. The glomeruli appear normal. They seem more numerous than

normal because of parenchymal compression and atrophy. The hydronephrosis in kidneys removed surgically is usually advanced. In it, the tubules become extremely atrophic, and the glomeruli become hyalinized and sometimes difficult to recognize. The renal cortex may be only a few millimeters thick. In this situation, hydronephrosis is often complicated by pyelonephritis.

Megaloureter

Progressive hydroureter and hydronephrosis complicate lumbosacral meningomyelocele because of impaired parasympathetic innervation. Grotesque dilatation

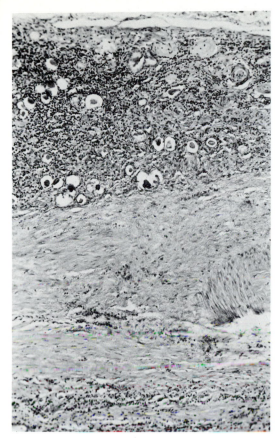

Fig. 659 Entire width of kidney. Note compression of cortex to small band made up of hyalinized glomeruli, fibrous tissue, and obliterated tubules. Pelvis shows focal hyperplasia of smooth muscle and slight chronic inflammation. (×100; WU neg. 49-6718.)

of ureters occurs as a component of the "triad syndrome" (congenital absence of abdominal muscles, obstructive uropathy, and cryptorchism). Hydroureter is an uncommon accompaniment of aganglionic megacolon. There is no functional or morphologic support for the suggestion that hydroureter in these instances results from absence of autonomic ganglia in the ureters or bladder. Ganglia are not normally present within the ureteral or vesical muscularis except along the intramural course of the ureters and in the vesical neck.

Progressive, often asymmetric, dilatation of the ureters associated with dilatation and hypertrophy of the bladder without morphologically demonstrable obstruction has been designated the megacystis-megaureter syndrome. Residual urine, vesicoureteral reflux, and recurrent infections of the urinary tract are clinical and roentgenographic features.[127] The syndrome has been attributed to fibroelastic contracture of the bladder neck (Marion's disease), but definitions of the syndrome are inexact and even such a basic epidemiologic aspect as sex incidence varies widely among reported series.

The pathogenesis of the disorder is not known, but symptoms are usually ameliorated by surgical procedures that improve vesical drainage (e.g., Y-V plasty). Snippets of tissue from such procedures are generally unrewarding to pathologic study.

Pyelonephritis

Pyelonephritis may be acute or chronic. There are three peaks of incidence: infancy and childhood, the childbearing age, and old age.[134] When the process is unilateral, it is a surgical problem. When it is acute, other complications such as perirenal infection may occur.

Chronic pyelonephritis is the most common disease of the kidney for which nephrectomy is done and one of the commonest causes of chronic renal insufficiency in the United States. It is also the most frequent renal disease found at autopsy.[129] It is frequently associated with congenital or acquired obstructive lesions of the lower urinary tract (Fig. 660), although it also may occur in the absence of any demonstrable obstruction. Chronic pyelonephritis is, by definition, an infectious disease. The organisms most commonly implicated are those of the coliform group, such as *Escherichia, Aerobacter,* and *Paracolon* bacilli.[130] It is likely that most of the so-called abacterial pyelonephritides are the result of prior asymptomatic bacterial infection. For instance, Aoki et al.[128] demonstrated by immunofluorescence the presence of a bacterial antigen shared by most strains of Enterobacteriaceae in the kidney from six

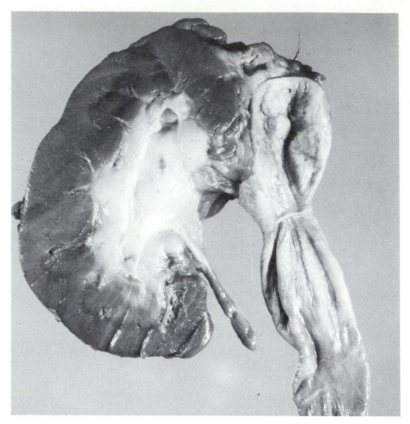

Fig. 660 Duplication of right pelvis and ureter. Anomalous ureter draining upper pole is markedly dilated and inflamed. Patient, 59-year-old man, presented with mass in the upper pole of right kidney. (WU neg. 71-4588.)

of seven patients with "abacterial" pyelonephritis. This causative factor has been well demonstrated experimentally. A ureter was partially blocked in a rabbit, and bacteria were introduced into the bloodstream. Infection then localized in the blocked kidney but not in the other kidney. When the block was removed, the infection cleared.[135]

In human beings the same sequence occurs. In children the block is often on a congenital basis. Pyelonephritis in young girls occurs because of the straight, shortened urethra. In women, cancer of the cervix is often a cause. In the older age groups, there are multiple causes of obstruction. In men, the main causes are cancer and nodular hyperplasia of the prostate gland. The anterior third of the male urethra always contains bacteria so that catheterization may result in infection.

Such infection may travel to the kidney by the lumen of the ureter.

In acute pyelonephritis, grossly the kidney is larger than normal and often has an adherent capsule. If the pyelonephritis is recent, there may be small yellow abscesses observed beneath the stripped capsule. On section, there are numerous small abscesses in the cortex and prominent linear bands in the medulla, indicating pus in the tubules (Fig. 661, *A*). The pelvis is infected. Microscopically, diffuse inflammation is present in the pelvis and between the tubules (Fig. 661, *B*). At times, confluent abscesses occur. Various renal areas may show varying stages of infection.

In chronic pyelonephritis, grossly the kidney is small, occasionally weighing only 60 gm to 80 gm. The capsule strips with great difficulty because of flat, irregular, wedged scars on the surface. Infrequently,

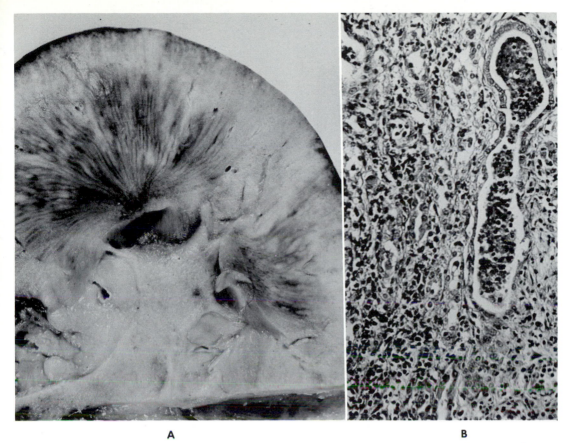

A   B

Fig. 661 **A**, Surgical specimen of kidney from patient with slight hydronephrosis and acute pyelonephritis. Note linear streaks in medulla due to pus within tubules. **B**, Same kidney illustrated in **A** showing masses of polymorphonuclear leukocytes within tubules. Note interstitial inflammation. (**A**, WU neg. 49-5678; **B**, ×230; WU neg. 50-378.)

the gross appearance will show no wedge-shaped scars, the small kidney having a finely granular external surface. This type of gross alteration also may be observed in experimental pyelonephritis. Usually there is some hydronephrosis. Stones may or may not be present. On cross section the cortex is irregular, and the calyces are blunted. According to Heptinstall,[133] a deformed calyx with an overlying parenchymal scar is the *only* gross feature specific for this condition and the most important for its differentiation from an ischemic kidney.

The most striking microscopic feature of chronic pyelonephritis is the patchy distribution of the lesions. In the affected areas, changes are present in the glomeruli, tubules, interstitium, and vessels. The glomeruli may show thickening of Bow-

man's capsule and even concentric fibrosis *outside* the capsule (periglomerular fibrosis). The glomerular tuft may be collapsed or hyalinized, a change of probably ischemic nature, often associated with concentric fibrosis *inside* Bowman's capsule. The tubules are destroyed or atrophic. Many are dilated and contain homogeneous eosinophilic casts. The interstitium is infiltrated by a variable number of lymphocytes, plasma cells, and other inflammatory cells. Fibrosis is always present. The arteries may be normal, but in most cases they show medial and intimal thickening. The pelvis, which is always inflamed, often contains lymphoid follicles. *Renal papillary necrosis* most frequently occurs in diabetics or in patients with obstructive uropathy. There are infarctlike

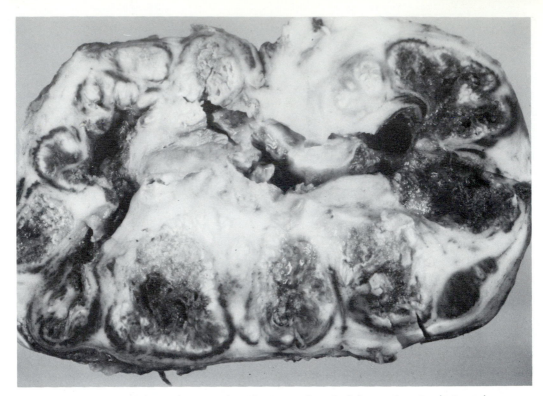

Fig. 662 Extreme hydronephrosis with wide areas of cortical destruction simulating tuberculosis. This is classic chronic pyelonephritis with xanthogranulomatous changes.

zones of necrosis of the papillae extending upward into the pyramids. These necrotic papillae may be passed and identified in the urinary sediment. On occasion, the diagnosis has been made by intrepid needle biopsy. Pyelograms show ragged calyces, ring shadows, and clubbing.[131]

Xanthogranulomatous pyelonephritis is a distinct type of renal infection characterized by massive enlargement, lithiasis, hydronephrosis, and the appearance of yellow lobulated masses replacing the architecture of the kidney and extending into the pelvis and the perirenal fat (Fig. 662). Microscopically, granulomas are prominent with multinucleated giant cells and foam cells. This condition occurred three times among 222 kidneys removed for various inflammatory conditions.[132] It may be confused clinically, grossly, and microscopically with renal cell carcinoma.[136] Pathologically, it also can be confused with malakoplakia, which may extend from the pelvis into the renal parenchyma.

Radiation nephritis

Irradiation damage to one or both kidneys results in *radiation nephritis*. This may cause hypertension, renal insufficiency, and death. With the use of megavoltage and with fuller knowledge of the danger, such changes may be avoided in the future.[137, 138]

The kidney damaged by irradiation is often reduced in size, with an adherent capsule. Microscopically, it usually shows intense intertubular damage, specific vascular alterations, and, at times, widespread sclerosis with isolation of glomeruli (Figs. 663 and 664). Fibrinoid necrotic lesions of the arterioles can also occur.

Pyelitis and ureteritis cystica

Hinman and Cordonnier[139] demonstrated that pyelitis and ureteritis cystica are the result of chronic inflammation of variable etiology. They believe that their development is due to chronic inflammation of

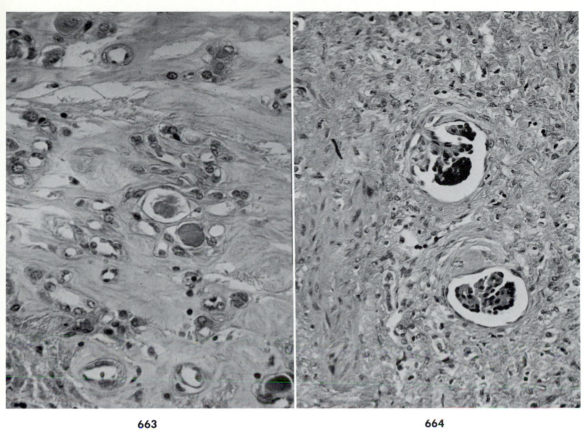

663   664

Fig. 663 Radiation nephritis with extensive sclerosis and remaining atrophic tubules. (WU neg. 59-3463.)

Fig. 664 Radiation nephritis with complete fibrosis of renal parenchyma with persistence of two glomeruli. (WU neg. 57-4651.)

the mucous membrane followed by downward proliferation of the surface epithelium. These buds of epithelium become pinched off possibly by the upgrowing connective tissue and form epithelial cell nests. Degeneration occurs centrally, and a cystic structure forms (Fig. 665). This lesion may be diagnosed by identifying peculiar mottled bubblelike defects in the ureterogram.

Pelvic lipomatosis

Pelvic lipomatosis must be differentiated from a true lipoma of the kidney. The former consists of fatty replacement of normal tissue and an increase of fat in the hilus of the kidney. This replacement occurs whenever there is atrophy of the kidney. It is present quite frequently in as-

sociation with chronic pyelonephritis and renal lithiasis.[140, 141]

Grossly, there is diffusely distributed fat in the region of the hilus, and the remaining kidney is atrophic (Fig. 666, A). Microscopically, mature fat is present. Clinically, extensive lipomatosis associated with lithiasis may stimulate renal neoplasm because of the filling defects usually seen pyelographically (Fig. 666, B).

Lithiasis

Primary renal stones are defined as those which occur in the absence of renal abnormality, persistent infection, or metabolic disease. Practically all renal stones develop within the renal pelvis, often in a major or minor calyx.

In Randall's study[144] of 1,154 pairs of

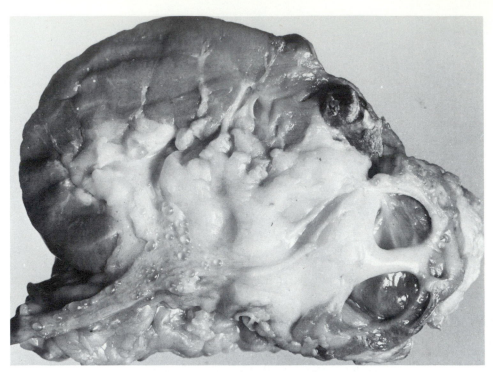

Fig. 665 Kidney with hydronephrosis and prominent ureteritis cystica. (WU neg. 53-1346.)

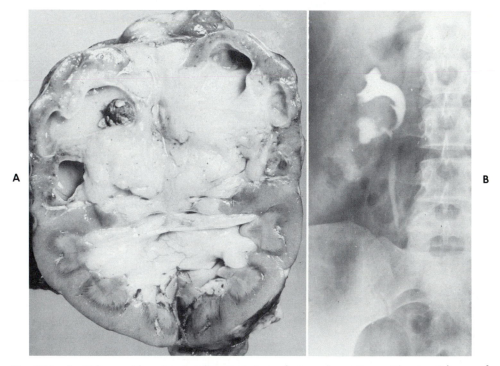

Fig. 666   A, Kidney with extensive lipomatosis and stone formation without evidence of neoplasm. **B,** Retrograde pyelogram from same case demonstrating pyelographic deformity. Malignant tumor was seriously considered. (**A,** WU neg. 48-3792; **B,** WU neg. 48-3845.)

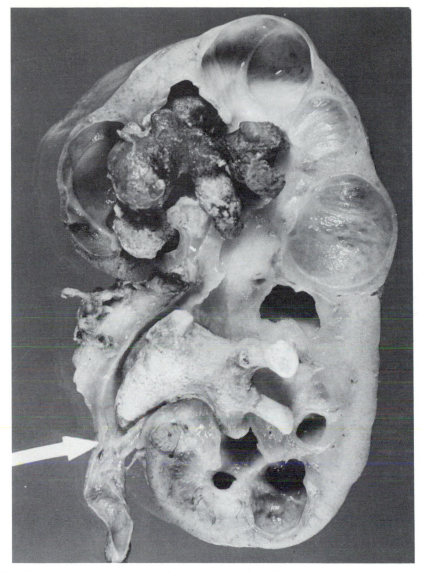

Fig. 667 Kidney with staghorn calculi, hydronephrosis, chronic pyelonephritis, and almost complete obstruction of ureter at ureteropelvic junction. (WU neg. 50-3971.)

kidneys, 227 (19.6%) showed calcium salt deposition in one or more renal papillae, and sixty-five showed a renal calculus attached to a renal papilla. These calculi were subepithelial and represented a plaque of calcium salt in the interstitial tissue. The first deposition of calcium salt was in the basement membrane of the walls of the collecting tubules. A primary renal calculus obtains its freedom by the plaque tearing away. It is interesting that the chemical composition of the calculus may consist of two entirely different substances. The one that is deposited secondarily depends upon the saturation of chemicals in the urinary stream.

Calculi arise from pathogenic conditions within the renal papillae, and damage to the collecting tubules and the supporting interstitial tissue follows. With attempted repair, calcium salt is deposited intratubularly or extratubularly. Interstitial deposition of calcium salt is much slower than its intratubular deposition. Intersti-

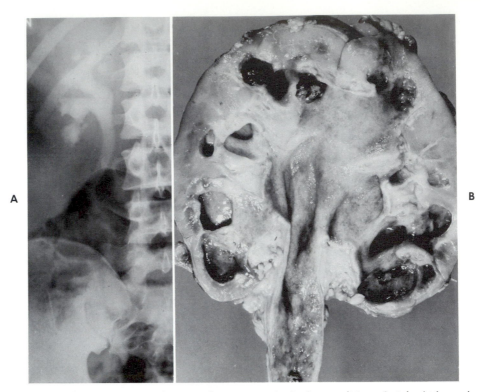

Fig. 668 **A,** Intravenous pyelogram showing marked abnormalities of right kidney due to tuberculosis. **B,** Same kidney shown in **A.** Note extensive destruction of kidney by tuberculosis with formation of cavities communicating with pelvis. Note involvement of ureter. Such kidney does not heal. (**A,** WU neg. 49-6236; **B,** WU neg. 47-3510.)

tially, calcium carbonate and calcium phosphate may be identified. Ulceration of the surface of the papilla acts as the nidus upon which urinary salts crystallize. Intratubular calcium phosphate calculi may be associated with secondary infarction of the papillae. Vitamin A deficiency may damage the renal tubular epithelium sufficiently to cause secondary calcium salt deposition. In hyperparathyroidism, intratubular type of damage occurs.

Randall's theory explains the origin of calculi that have arisen on papillae.[145] Carr[143] has a theory related to the lymphatics. He believes that the formation of stones is facilitated when the lymphatic drainage of the kidney is either overloaded or blocked. He thinks that the obstructing point is where the lymph duct leaves the kidney substance and enters the renal sinus at the calyceal fornices. If growth of stones occurs at this point, there will be necrosis

of the membrane separating the concretion from the lumen of the calyx, allowing seepage of urine into the area of calcification. This facilitates further growth of the stone by deposition of urinary salts. If there is reversal of lymphatic flow, microliths may flow backward and collect at the tip of the renal papillae, forming a Randall plaque. Carr[143] emphasized that these deposits first occur outside the tubules. A stone forming in a calyx indicates that the lymphatic duct from the lobule has been either obstructed or overloaded. Therefore partial nephrectomy for stone should include a whole segment of kidney, so that further stones will not form in the diseased segment. Carr's attractive theory was supported by the use of diffraction roentgen-ray analysis.

Renal stones may be recognized not only by their gross appearance (Fig. 667) but also by their radiologic changes. With alkaline urine, the stones contain calcium, ammonium, phosphorus, and magnesium. In hyperparathyroidism, the stones are made up of calcium and phosphorus, but if there is infection, they become coated with magnesium and ammonium phosphates.[142] With an acid urine, calcium oxalate forms stones with a crystalline structure radiating to a central point. Phosphorus stones grow in size by concentric layers.

Tuberculosis

Practically all renal tuberculosis is hematogenous in origin. The infection usually originates from foci in the lung, but in a few instances it may arise from bone lesions or secondary to a paravertebral abscess.

Tuberculous lesions appear initially in the cortex of the kidney, usually within the glomeruli. At this stage, the infection is bilateral.[150] The lesions either completely heal and become fibrous scars[151] or, more often, progress in one kidney but remain

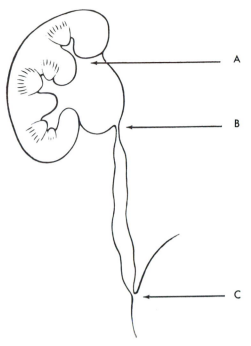

Fig. 669 Danger sites for fibrosis of "healing" are neck of calyx, **A**, ureteropelvic junction, **B**, and ureterovesical region, **C**. (From Hanley, H. G.: The indications for surgery in renal tuberculosis, Br. J. Surg. **45**:10-15, 1957.)

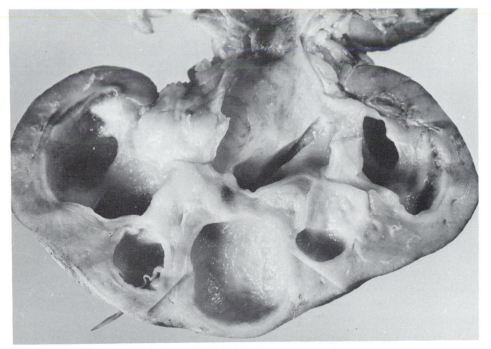

Fig. 670 Almost complete healing of tuberculosis of kidney. There is still extreme destruction with hydronephrosis, but there is no gross evidence of active disease. Fibrosis at ureteropelvic junction is present. (WU neg. 56-5140.)

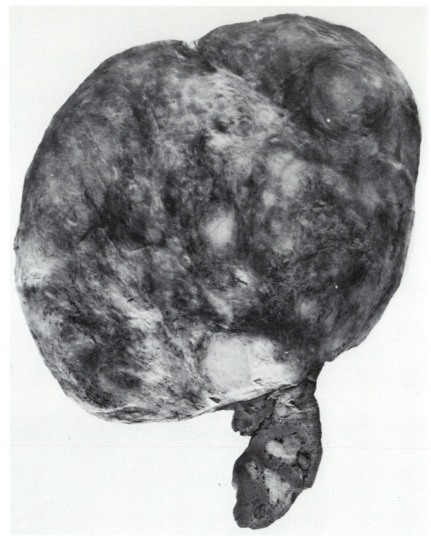

Fig. 671 Fetal hamartoma involving upper pole of kidney. This lesion is more solid, firm, and homogeneous than Wilms' tumor. (Courtesy Dr. H. Rodriguez, Mexico City, Mexico.)

stationary in the other. In fifty-six patients with renal tuberculosis reported by Auerbach,[146] forty-one showed unilateral involvement. With further spread, the apices of the pyramids and the walls of the calyces of the kidney are involved, possibly because infected tuberculous urine is retained in the smaller crevices.[152] When the urine contains tubercle bacilli, the kidney always has a tuberculous focus which, at times, is difficult to identify.

Tuberculosis in a kidney may vary from minute areas of ulceration near the tips of the papillae to wide zones of caseation that may coalesce to form huge cavitating masses, with only a shell of normal kidney (Fig. 668).

The change that has occurred in the pathology of tuberculosis due to the new antimicrobial agents has been reported by Hanley.[149] In the fibrosis of healing, block can occur at the neck of the calyx, the ureteropelvic junction, and the ureterovesical region (Fig. 669). With isoniazid therapy, the necrotic material is absorbed. Vascularization of the edges of the lesion occurs with less fibrosis. The vascularization may facilitate the effects of isoni-

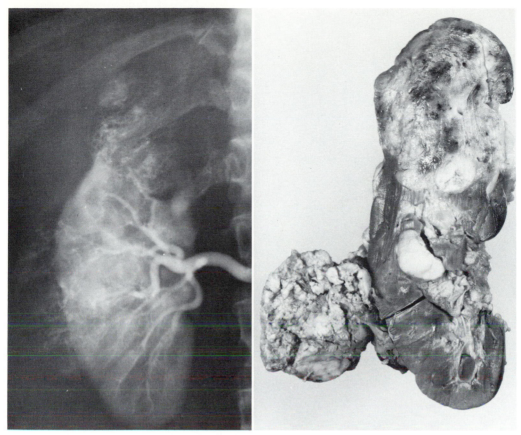

Fig. 672 Multiple angiomyolipoma. Contralateral kidney of patient, 51-year-old woman, also was affected. Lesion was confused clinically and radiographically with renal cell carcinoma. (WU negs. 70-2759 and 70-3391.)

azid.[147] With absorption of the caseous material, there is rapid clinical improvement. Grossly, the specimen may show healing evidenced by absence of caseation and a smooth pelvis. It may show also a fibrotic ureteropelvic block (Fig. 670). The incidence of tuberculosis with calculi is only 1%.[148]

Benign tumors

The benign tumors of the kidney make up less than 5% of all renal neoplasms. The *perirenal lipoma* may become huge.[163] Grossly and microscopically, it resembles lipomas elsewhere. Rarely, *leiomyomas* of the kidney capsule may produce masses that are confused with more common renal neoplasms.

Fetal hamartoma is a benign congenital renal tumor that is often confused with Wilms' tumor.[160] Grossly, it is solid, yellowish gray to tan, with a whorled configuration reminiscent of uterine leiomyoma (Fig. 671). Microscopically, an extremely cellular growth of spindle cells is the predominant feature. These probably represent primitive mesenchymal cells with the capacity to differentiate toward fibroblasts and smooth muscle cells.[153, 158] Mitoses are usually present and can be numerous. Entrapped glomeruli and other normal renal structures are often identified.[154] There is no capsule separating the tumor from the uninvolved parenchyma. The benign nature of this lesion has been amply demonstrated.[166]

Angiomyolipoma is a rare neoplasm composed of an intimate mixture of fat, blood

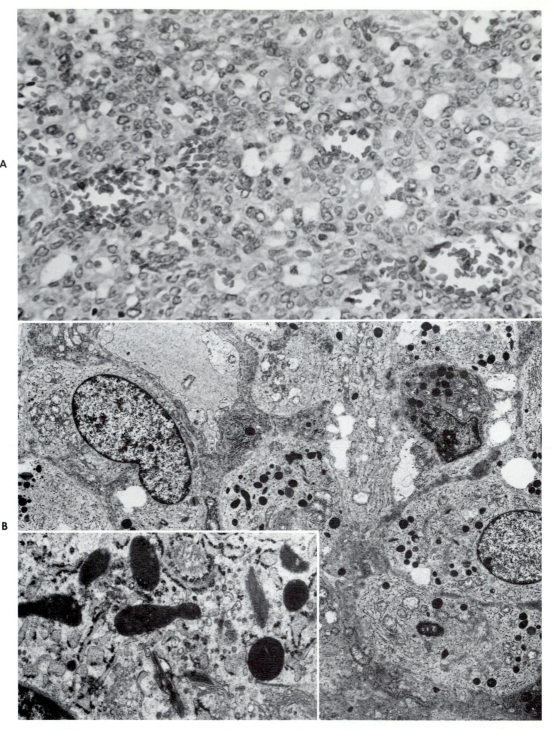

Fig. 673 **A,** Renin-producing juxtaglomerular cell tumor. Light microscopic appearance is strongly reminiscent of hemangiopericytoma. **B,** Fine structural appearance of same tumor shown in **A.** Tumor cells contain numerous secretory granules. **Inset,** Higher magnification of granules. Some are diamond shaped, identical to those seen in normal juxtaglomerular cells. This case has been reported by Conn et al.[155] (**A,** X350; WU neg. 73-3406; **B,** uranyl acetate–lead citrate; ×2,200; **inset,** uranyl acetate–lead citrate; ×19,000; **A, B,** and **inset,** courtesy Dr. M. R. Abell, Ann Arbor, Mich.)

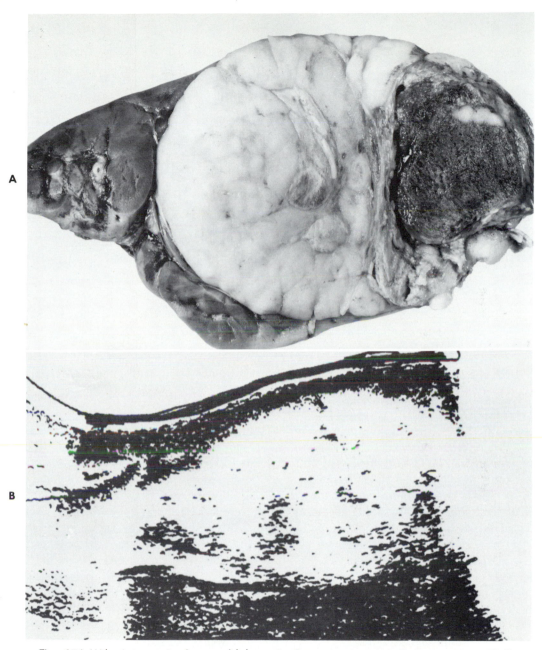

Fig. 674 Wilms' tumor in 3-year-old boy. **A,** Gross appearance of cross section. Well-circumscribed solid white mass replaces most of renal parenchyma. Several foci of hemorrhage and necrosis are present. **B,** Ultrasound scan of kidney shown in **A.** Lower pole appears normal. Tumor appears as large solid mass with scattered irregular echoes corresponding to areas of necrosis. (**A,** WU neg. 73-2364; **B,** courtesy Dr. E. Cubillo, St. Louis, Mo.)

vessels, and smooth muscle. Grossly, this tumor may show a striking resemblance to renal cell carcinoma because of its yellow color, intratumoral hemorrhages, and frequent extrarenal growth[159] (Fig. 672).

Multiple tumors were found in ten of the thirty-two patients reported by Farrow et al.[157] Five of them were bilateral. Microscopically, the cellularity, hyperchromatism, pleomorphism, and moderate mitotic

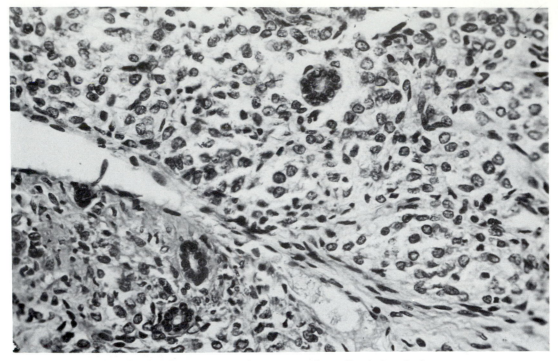

Fig. 675 Wilms' tumor showing typical stroma and small tubules. Such pattern suggests embryonic renal tissue. Patient died one year following nephrectomy as consequence of massive local recurrence. (×400; WU neg. 50-330.)

activity of the smooth muscle component may result in a mistaken diagnosis of leiomyosarcoma. The blood vessels are tortuous and thick walled and frequently lack an elastic tissue lamina.[165] Neurologic and/or cutaneous findings diagnostic or suggestive of tuberous sclerosis can be found in approximately one-third of patients with renal angiomyolipoma. The incidence is higher in cases of multiple or bilateral tumors. It has been estimated that about 80% of patients with the complete or severe form of tuberous sclerosis have renal tumors of this type.[156]

Three cases of renin-secreting *juxtaglomerular cell tumors* have been reported.[161, 164] The microscopic appearance is reminiscent of hemangiopericytoma. Intracytoplasmic granules are found with Bowie's stain and electron microscopy; and large amounts of renin can be demonstrated by bioassay of the tumor[155] (Fig. 673).

Small *adenomas* are often diagnosed in the arteriosclerotic or contracted kidney.

However, whether small yellowish areas of focal renal tubular hyperplasia should be called adenomas is questionable. When these lesions become larger, they may be dignified by this designation.

Adenomas of varying size also are frequently found incidentally at autopsy. Mintz and Gaul[162] examined sixty-one kidneys (fifty-eight otherwise abnormal) containing sixty-nine small circumscribed lesions, practically all less than 5 cm in diameter. There were forty-seven papillary cystadenomas, seven so-called fetal adenomas, and seven adrenal rests.

Malignant tumors
Wilms' tumor

Wilms' tumor of the kidney (embryoma or adenomyosarcoma) is seen primarily in infants. At least 50% of the cases occur before the age of 3 years and 90% before the age of 10 years. However, there are also well-documented cases in adults.[172, 178]

An association between Wilms' tumor

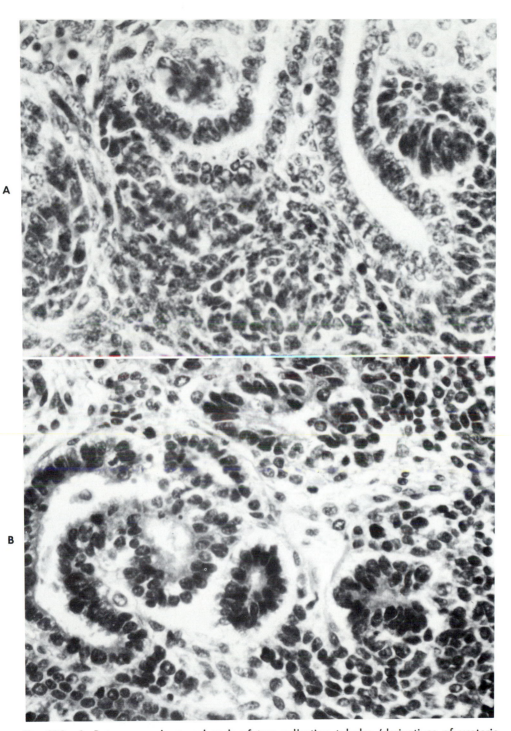

Fig. 676 A, Between and around ends of two collecting tubules (derivatives of ureteric bud) is nephrogenic blastema differentiating into glomerular capsule and renal tubules. **B,** Structures in Wilms' tumor that bear striking resemblance to developing metanephric tubules in embryonal renal blastema. (**A** and **B,** ×500; AFIP 218935-213 and 218935-214; from Lucké, B., and Schlumberger, H. G.: Atlas of tumor pathology, Sect. VIII, Fasc. 30, Washington, D. C., 1957, Armed Forces Institute of Pathology.)

and aniridia, hemihypertrophy, and other congenital anomalies has been documented.[173, 177] Geschickter and Widehorn[174] believe that Wilms' tumor probably arises from embryonic nephrogenic tissue and represents a loss of the factors controlling normal developmental processes in the growth zone of the renal cortex in either fetal life or in the first few months after birth.

These tumors are usually large (over 250 gm), well delineated, and firm and appear to have a definite capsule (Fig. 674). When rigid criteria are employed, the incidence of synchronous or subsequent contralateral involvement is probably less than 5%.[179, 180] In truly congenital cases, both kidneys may be entirely replaced by tumor tissue.

On section, they are often grayish white, are sharply circumscribed, and contain areas of hemorrhage. Only rarely do they invade the renal pelvis or ureter. Hematuria is infrequent. When advanced, Wilms' tumor invades veins, the renal capsule, the adrenal gland, and, later, the small bowel, large bowel, liver, and vertebrae. The most common sites of metastatic involvement are the lungs, liver, retroperitoneum, peritoneum, and mediastinum.

Microscopically, the tumor is variably but fundamentally characterized by the formation of abortive or embryonic glomerular and/or tubular structures surrounded by an immature spindle cell stroma.[169] The latter component often predominates. Smooth and striated muscle are frequently present. Lucké and Schlumberger[175] emphasized the close similarities of the tubules formed in Wilms' tumor with normal developing metanephric tubules (Figs. 675 and 676). The glomeruloid structures formed by this neoplasm are also strikingly similar to normal developing glomeruli by both light and electron microscopic criteria.[167] We have seen several cases of Wilms' tumor mainly composed of small undifferentiated cells which were confused with neuroblastoma. In children, the differential diagnosis should also include fetal hamartoma, whereas in adults the main sources of confusion are various sarcomas and sarcomatoid renal cell carcinomas.

It is now accepted that Wilms' tumor originates primarily from cells of the metanephric blastoma, although the occasional participation of neural elements remains a possibility.[176]

The prognosis of Wilms' tumor depends upon the presence of large vein involvement or penetration of the capsule. The microscopic pattern is unrelated to prognosis. The first clinical indication of this tumor usually is the presence of a large mass felt by the mother when handling the child. The current therapy for Wilms' tumor consists of excision of the involved kidney followed by radiation therapy to the tumor bed and chemotherapy. A cure rate of over 80% in unilateral Wilms' tumor has been achieved.[168, 170, 171] Even patients with bilateral tumors have been salvaged.[179]

Renal cell carcinoma

Renal cell carcinomas are usually not discovered until they are sufficiently advanced to cause either a mass or hematuria. The large majority occur in adults, but occasional examples in children have been recorded.[184, 189] Arteriography may be very helpful in delimiting a small carcinoma of the kidney (Fig. 677). These tumors often are well delineated, appear in the cortex, and, on section, are pseudoencapsulated and have a golden yellow color. On occasion, only a small portion is connected with the cortex, the bulk of the tumor appearing as an extrarenal mass. Because of their cellularity, hemorrhage, necrosis, and calcification are common (Fig. 678). It is not uncommon for renal cell carcinoma to undergo massive necrotic and degenerative changes, a mural nodule remaining as the only evidence of the real nature of the lesion (Fig. 679). Sometimes even this disappears, and the diagnosis is made only on microscopic examination. *Cortical cysts composed of a*

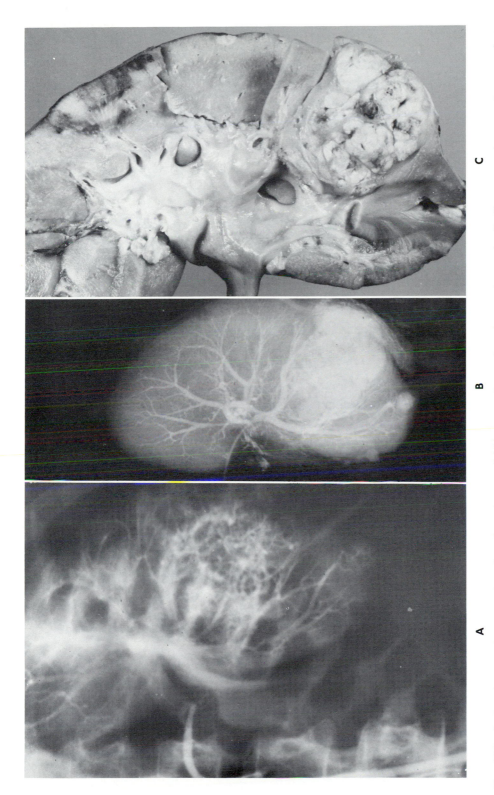

A

B

C

Fig. 677 A, Arteriogram demonstrating site of carcinoma of kidney as shown by abnormal vessels. **B,** These vessels are, of course, better seen in arteriogram after removal of kidney. **C,** Gross specimen demonstrating well-delimited renal cell carcinoma. (**A,** WU neg. 65-2228; **B,** WU neg. 65-2227; **C,** WU neg. 65-2326.)

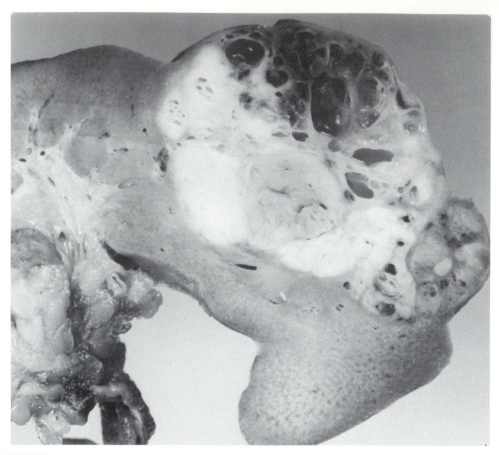

Fig. 678 Small circumscribed renal cell carcinoma extending through capsule. Lesion had bright yellow color, was hemorrhagic, and did not involve renal pelvis. There was no hematuria. (WU neg. 62-2104.)

fibrous (often partially calcified) capsule and containing a grumous, yellow, necrotic material represent, in most cases, necrotic renal cell carcinomas. These tumors often invade the renal pelvis. The presence or absence of vein invasion is the most important factor in prognosis. Capsular and pelvic invasion, poor differentiation, and pleomorphism are also unfavorable prognostic signs.[181, 193] On the other hand, size of the tumor at operation bears no relation to survival once the growth is 5 cm or greater in diameter.[191] In general, tumors measuring less than 5 cm in diameter do not metastasize.[182] However, exceptions to this rule do appear. Very small tumors may invade the renal vein and cause distant metastases. Conversely, large carcinomas

of the kidney have been seen without evidence of metastasis for long periods.

Microscopically, renal cell carcinomas show evidence of origin from renal tubules, best demonstrated in very small tumors in which transition from tubules to tumor can be seen. As in normal renal tubules, the tumor cells often show hyaline droplets and phagocytosis of broken-down blood pigment. Neutral fat and glycogen are practically always found in greater or lesser degree. On the other hand, mucin is absent. We have seen only one exception to this rule (Fig. 680). Various patterns appear. The cells may be granular or clear and may show papillary formation. As Gottesman et al.[188] emphasized, large sections or multiple sections usually

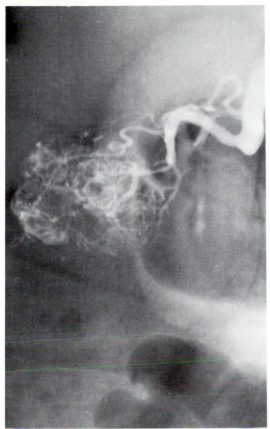

show diverse variations in the same tumor, a feature that renders subclassifications based on morphologic pattern of little significance. On occasion, a renal cell carcinoma may show typical areas alternating with others having a pleomorphic spindle cell and a giant cell appearance resembling sarcoma. Farrow et al.[186] examined thirty-seven of these "sarcomatoid" renal cell carcinomas, three of which also had areas resembling osteosarcoma. We have seen this type of renal cell carcinoma metastasizing diffusely to the bones and simulating microscopically a multicentric fibrosarcoma.

Renal cell carcinoma is sometimes associated with systemic manifestations such as fever, hepatosplenomegaly, and hepatic dysfunction.[192, 194, 197] It also can produce hypercalcemia as a result of the production

Fig. 679 Renal cell carcinoma illustrating phenomenon of massive necrosis not uncommonly seen with this neoplasm. Mural nodule of residual cancer was clearly demonstrated by arteriography. (WU negs. 72-10702, 72-10704, and 72-10829.)

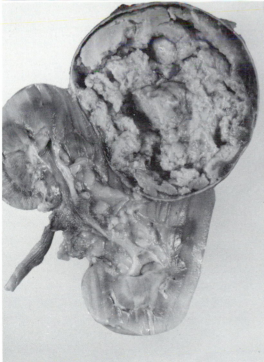

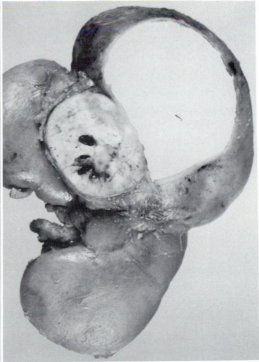

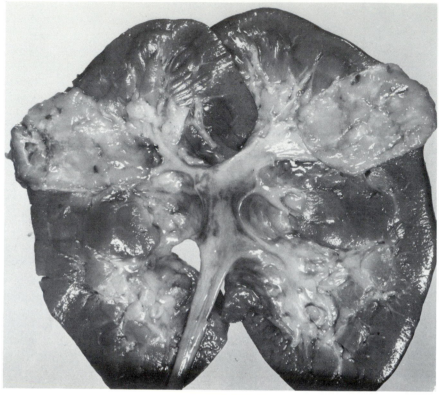

Fig. 680 Well-circumscribed mucin-producing renal cell carcinoma. (Courtesy Dr. F. Leidler, Houston, Texas.)

of a parathormone-like hormone[187] and polycythemia secondary to the secretion of an erythropoietic-stimulating substance.[190]

Renal cell carcinomas metastasize through the bloodstream, often to the lung. They frequently metastasize to bones, particularly the pelvis and the femur, where they may be mistaken for primary bone tumors. Aspiration of these metastatic masses, however, may show the characteristic pattern of renal cell carcinoma. The aspirated cells usually show well-defined cellular outlines, a central nucleus, and foamy cytoplasm that contains sudanophilic material and glycogen. Metastases may appear in unusual locations. We have seen them in the gingiva, larynx, and bronchus. They may masquerade as primary soft tissue sarcomas. We have several such cases in which the renal tumor was not detectable either clinically or radiographically at the time the metastasis was dis-

covered and became obvious only months or years later.

Renal cell carcinoma is the most common "recipient" of the curious phenomenon of metastasis of a cancer into another cancer. Lung carcinoma is the most common "donor," the resulting microscopic appearance leading to interesting problems of interpretation.[183]

Another of the many peculiarities of renal cell cancer is its occasional regression in the absence of all treatment, a phenomenon found also with gestational choriocarcinoma, malignant melanoma, and neuroblastoma and, in lesser proportion, with several other tumors.[185]

In most cases, renal cell carcinoma should be approached surgically in a radical manner. The kidney, its surrounding fat, and Gerota's fascia should be removed en bloc with the periaortic nodes adjacent to the renal hilum. Approximately 30%

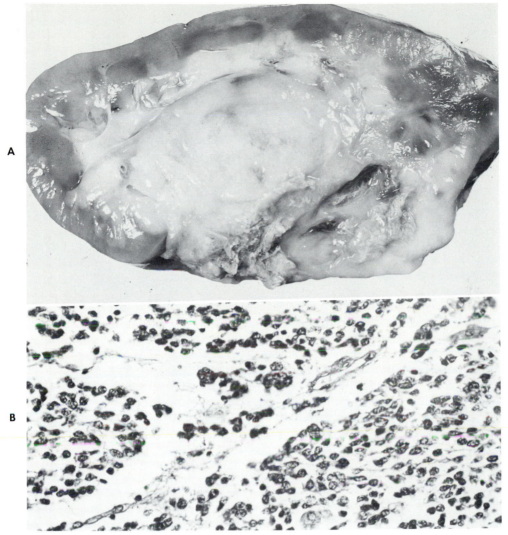

Fig. 681   A, Tumor extensively involving pelvis and, to slight extent, parenchyma. **B,** Same tumor shown in **A** demonstrating undifferentiated neoplasm with cells suggesting origin from sympathetic nervous system. (**A,** WU neg. 49-2147; **B,** ×400; WU neg. 50-331.)

of renal cell cancers involve perinephric fat and/or regional lymph nodes.[196] When such nodal involvement is operable and the nodes are removed, the survival rate appears to be remarkably good.[195]

Other malignant tumors

We have seen several malignant tumors involving the kidney of young adults that have a microscopic appearance suggestive of *neuroblastoma* (Fig. 681). Alternately, they could be interpreted as variants of

Wilms' tumor with massive overgrowth of the neural component.

Sarcomas of various types can arise within the kidney. In a review of twenty-six primary renal sarcomas, Farrow et al.[198] found fifteen leiomyosarcomas, five malignant hemangiopericytomas, five liposarcomas, and one rhabdomyosarcoma. It is possible, however, that some of these neoplasms (particularly liposarcomas) arose in the perirenal soft tissues and only secondarily invaded the kidneys.

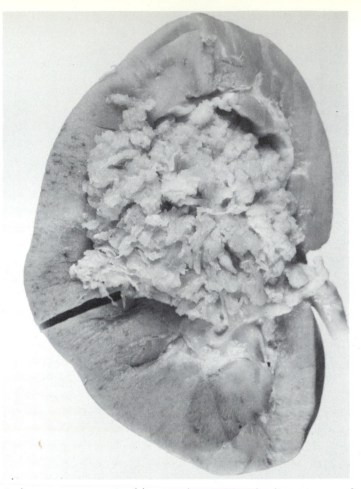

Fig. 682 Typical gross appearance of low-grade transitional cell carcinoma of renal pelvis in 49-year-old woman with gross painless hematuria. Only minimal stromal invasion was present. (WU neg. 70-9553.)

Renal involvement by *malignant lymphoma* is almost always the expression of a generalized process.[199] Tumors of the histiocytic type (reticulum cell sarcomas) predominate.[198] Exceptionally, *plasma cell myelomas* diffusely infiltrate the renal parenchyma.[198]

Metastatic carcinoma can involve the kidney as a part of a disseminated process, but we have seen few instances in which this involvement was of surgical significance.

Tumors of pelvis and ureter
Transitional cell carcinoma

Transitional cell carcinomas of the renal pelvis are relatively rare tumors.[207] They form soft grayish red masses with smooth

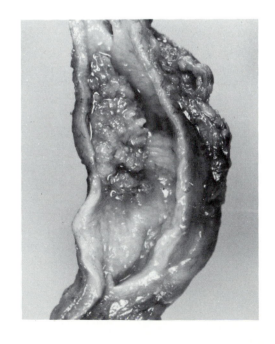

Fig. 683 Transitional cell carcinoma of right ureter in 68-year-old woman. Note typical papillary configuration. (WU neg. 68-11010.)

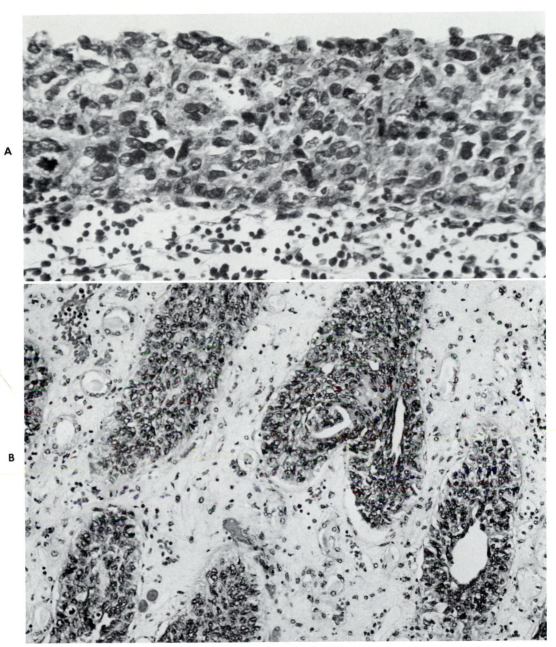

Fig. 684 **A,** Transitional cell carcinoma of renal pelvis. In this area, tumor is intraepithelial, but there were foci of stromal invasion elsewhere. **B,** Extension of tumor shown in **A** into collecting tubules, reminiscent of extension into endocervical glands by in situ carcinoma of uterine cervix. This finding is very unusual. (**A,** WU neg. 72-6554; **B,** WU neg. 72-6555.)

glistening surfaces and exactly resemble the transitional cell tumors of the bladder (Fig. 682). Necrosis is uncommon. They often diffusely involve the entire renal pelvis and form arborescent masses that may extend down the ureter. Similar tumors rarely are primary in the ureter[202, 208, 211] (Fig. 683).

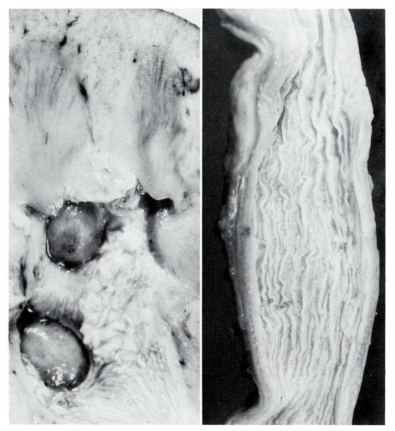

Fig. 685 **A,** Kidney with hydronephrosis, chronic pyelonephritis, leukoplakia, stone formation, and kerantinizing epidermoid carcinoma. **B,** Epidermoid carcinoma can be seen clearly but was not suspected prior to pathologic examination. (**A,** WU neg. 49-4321; **B,** WU neg. 49-4320.)

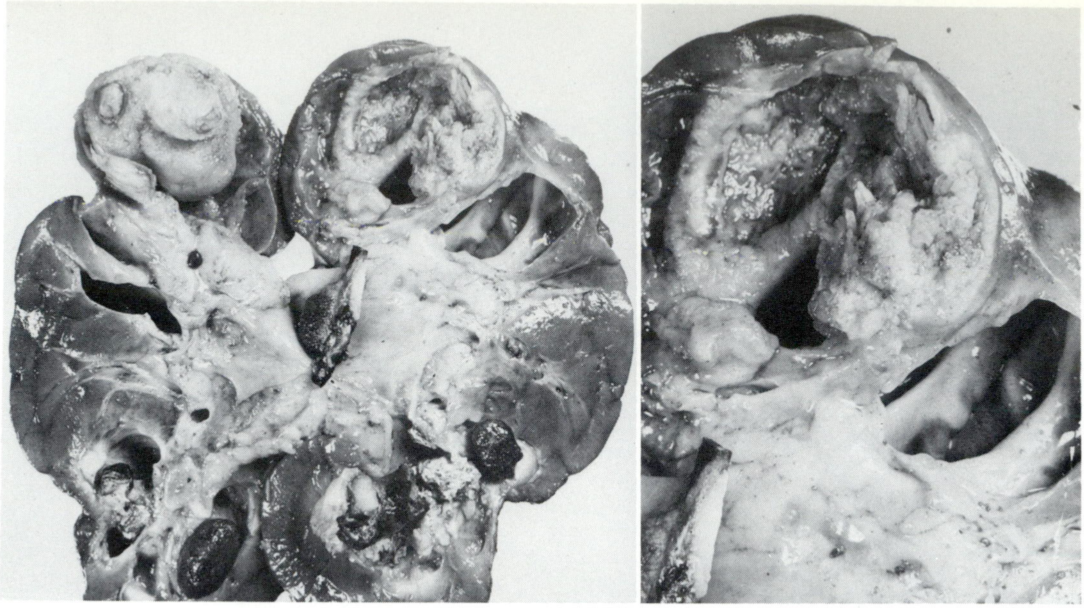

Fig. 686 Extensive leukoplakia of renal pelvis and ureter without stones. (WU negs. 50-6792 and 50-6791.)

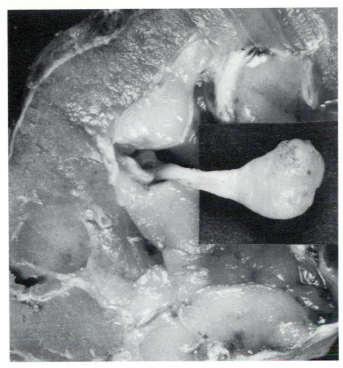

Fig. 687 Benign fibroepithelial polyp emerging from lower calyx of left kidney in 61-year-old woman. Tumor caused hematuria, and total nephrectomy was done. (WU neg. 72-11203.)

Microscopically, these carcinomas form branching masses of transitional cells supported by a delicate connective tissue stroma containing many blood vessels. The tumor may extend proximally along the collecting tubules (Fig. 684). The extreme cellularity and vascularity of these tumors cause the profuse hematuria. Usually these tumors are well differentiated rather than poorly differentiated, although both extremes occur.

Because these tumors implant along the ureter, it is imperative that this structure, including its intramural portion, be resected with the kidney. When the intramural portion is not resected, recurrence of the tumor within this bladder segment often occurs.[206]

Adenocarcinoma

As in the urinary bladder, it is not rare for transitional cell carcinomas of the pelvis or ureter to have small pools of mucin admixed with the tumor cells. These tumors should not be called adenocarcinomas. The term adenocarcinoma should be reserved for the rare neoplasms that not only secrete abundant mucin but also form unquestionable glandular structures.[201, 209]

Epidermoid carcinoma

The keratinized epidermoid carcinoma of the renal pelvis is a rare tumor associated usually with infection and renal calculi. Because of infection and calculi, a preoperative diagnosis is practically never made. Gahagan and Reed[204] found that the preoperative diagnosis in 106 patients was incorrect in all instances. The carcinoma is found to be advanced either at operation or when the specimen is examined.

Gross section of the specimen usually shows extensive pyelonephritis with multiple abscesses and renal stones. The necrotic and ulcerated neoplasm destroys and displaces renal parenchyma (Fig. 685).

Invariably, extension into surrounding tissue and involvement of distant nodes and other organs have occurred. Forty-eight of 100 cases reviewed by Gahagan and Reed[204] were associated with clinically evident stones. It is thought that there is some relation between the presence of leukoplakia and stones and the presence of epidermoid carcinoma. We have seen extensive leukoplakia without stones (Fig. 686). The prognosis for this group of patients is extremely poor.

Other tumors

Other tumors of the pelvis and ureter are exceptional. The benign lesions include a probably nonneoplastic condition designated as *fibroepithelial polyp* (Fig. 687), *angiomas, leiomyomas,* and *neurofibromas.*[200, 203, 205] The least rare nonepithelial malignant tumor of the ureter seems to be *leiomyosarcoma.*[210]

REFERENCES

Pathologic examination

1 Boyce, W. H., and King, J. S., Jr.: Crystal-matrix interrelations in calculi, J. Urol. **81:** 351-365, 1959.
2 Goldman, L., Gordon, G. S., and Chambers, E. L.: Changing diagnostic criteria for hyperparathyroidism, Ann. Surg. **146:**407-416, 1957.

Cytology

3 Bossen, E. H., Johnston, W. W., Amatulli, J. and Rowlands, D. T., Jr.: Exfoliative cytopathologic studies in organ transplantation. III. The cytologic profile of urine during acute renal allograft rejection, Acta Cytol. (Baltimore) **14:**176-181, 1970.
4 Daut, R. V., and McDonald, J. R.: Diagnosis of malignant lesions of the urinary tract by means of microscopic examination of centrifuged urinary sediment, Mayo Clin. Proc. **22:** 382-386, 1947.

Biopsy

5 Churg, J., and Grishman, E.: Ultrastructure of immune deposits in renal glomeruli, Ann. Intern. Med. **76:**479-486, 1972.
6 Dodge, W. F., Daeschner, C. W., Jr., Brennan, J. C., Rosenberg, H. S., Travis, L. B., and Hopps, H. C.: Percutaneous renal biopsy in children. I. General considerations, Pediatrics **30:**287-296, 1962.
7 Eastham, W. N., and Essex, W. B.: Use of tissues embedded in epoxy resin for routine histological examination of renal biopsies, J. Clin. Pathol. **22:**99-106, 1969.
8 Germuth, F. G., Jr., and Rodriguez, E.: Immunopathology of the renal glomerulus; immune complex deposit and antibasement membrane disease, Boston, 1973, Little, Brown and Co.
9 Hamburger, J., Crosnier, J., and Montera, H.: In "Entretiens de Bichat," Paris, 1960, L'expansion scientifique française, p. 455.
10 Heptinstall, R. H.: Pathology of the kidney, Boston, 1966, Little, Brown and Co.
11 Kellow, W. F.: Evaluation of the adequacy of needle biopsy specimens of the kidney; an autopsy study, Arch. Intern. Med. **104:**353-359, 1959.
12 Muehrcke, R. C., and Pirani, C. L.: Renal biopsy; an adjunct in the study of kidney disease. In Black, D. A. K., editor: Renal disease, ed. 3, Oxford, 1972, Blackwell Scientific Publications.
13 Pirani, C. L., and Salinas-Madrigal, L.: Evaluation of percutaneous renal biopsy. In Sommers, S. C., editor: Pathology annual, vol. 3, New York, 1968, Appleton-Century-Crofts, pp. 249-296.
14 Seymour, A. E., Spargo, B. H., and Penksa, R.: Contributions of renal biopsy studies to the understanding of disease, Am. J. Pathol. **65:**550-588, 1971.

Glomerulonephritis

15 Bacani, R. A., Velasquez, F., Kanter, A., Pirani, C. L., and Pollak, V. E.: Rapidly progressive (nonstreptococcal) glomerulonephritis, Ann. Intern. Med. **69:**463-485, 1968.
16 Burkholder, P. M., and Bradford, W. D.: Proliferative glomerulonephritis in children; a correlation of varied clinical and pathologic patterns utilizing light, immunofluorescence, and electron microscopy, Am. J. Pathol. **56:** 423-466, 1969.
17 Burkholder, P. M., Marchand, A., and Krueger, R. P.: Mixed membranous and proliferative glomerulonephritis; a correlative light, immunofluorescence, and electron microscopic study, Lab. Invest. **23:**459-479, 1970.
18 Cameron, J. S.: Glomerulonephritis, Br. Med. J. **21:**781-810, 1970.
19 Dixon, F. J.: The pathogenesis of glomerulonephritis, Am. J. Med. **44:**493-498, 1968.
20 Dodge, W. F., Spargo, B. H., Bass, J. A., and Travis, L. B.: The relationship between the clinical and pathologic features of poststrepto-

coccal glomerulonephritis; a study of the early natural history, Medicine (Baltimore) **47:**227-267, 1968.

21 Dodge, W. F., Spargo, B. H., Travis, L. B., Spivastava, R. N., Carvajal, H. F., DeBeaukelaer, M. M., Longley, M. P., and Menchaca, J. A.: Poststreptococcal glomerulonephritis; a prospective study in children, N. Engl. J. Med. **286:**273-278, 1972.

22 Earle, D. P.: Natural history of acute glomerulonephritis in adults. In Metcoff, J., editor: Acute glomerulonephritis, Boston, 1967, Little, Brown and Co., pp. 3-14.

23 Edelmann, C. M. Jr., Greifer, I., and Barnett, H. L.: The nature of kidney disease in children who fail to recover from apparent acute glomerulonephritis, J. Pediatr. **64:**879-887, 1964.

24 Faith, G. C., and Trump, B. F.: The glomerular capillary wall in human kidney disease: acute glomerulonephritis, systemic lupus erythematosus, and preeclampsia-eclampsia; comparative electron microscopic observations and a review, Lab. Invest. **15:**1682-1719, 1967.

25 Ferris, T. F., Gorden, P., Kashgarian, M., and Epstein, F. H.: Recurrent hematuria and focal nephritis, N. Engl. J. Med. **276:**770-775, 1967.

26 Glasgow, E. F., Moncrieff, M. W., White, R. H. R.: Symptomless haematuria in childhood, Br. Med. J. **2:**687-692, 1970.

26a Hendler, E. D., Kashgarian, M., and Hayslett, J. P.: Clinicopathological correlations of primary haematuria, Lancet **1:**458-463, 1972.

27 Heptinstall, R. H.: Pathology of the kidney, Boston, 1966, Little, Brown and Co.

27a Heptinstall, R. H., and Joekes, A. M.: Focal glomerulonephritis; a study based on renal biopsies, Q. J. Med. **28:**329-346, 1959.

28 Herdman, R. C., Pickering, R. J., Michael, A. F., Vernier, R. L., Gerwuz, H., and Good, R. A.: Chronic glomerulonephritis associated with low serum complement (chronic hypocomplementemic glomerulonephritis), Medicine (Baltimore) **49:**207-226, 1970.

29 Jennings, R. B., and Earle, D. P.: Post-streptococcal glomerulonephritis: histopathologic and clinical studies of the acute, subsiding acute, and early chronic latent phases, J. Clin. Invest. **40:**1525-1595, 1961.

30 Koffler, D., and Paronetto, F.: Immunofluorescent localization of immunoglobulins, complement, and fibrinogen in human disease. II. Acute, subacute, and chronic glomerulonephritis, J. Clin. Invest. **44:**1665-1671, 1965.

31 Lawrence, J. R., Pollak, V. E., Pirani, C. L., and Kark, R. M.: Histologic and clinical evidence of post-streptococcal glomerulonephritis

in patients with the nephrotic syndrome, Medicine (Baltimore) **42:**1-24, 1963.

32 Leonard, C. D., Nagle, R. B., Striker, G. E., Cutler, R. E., and Scribner, B. H.: Acute glomerulonephritis with prolonged oliguria; an analysis of 29 cases, Ann. Intern. Med. **73:**703-711, 1970.

33 Lewis, E. J., Cavallo, T., Harrington, J. T., and Cotran, R. S.: An immunopathologic study of rapidly progressive glomerulonephritis in the adult, Hum. Pathol. **2:**185-208, 1971.

34 McCluskey, R. T.: Evidence for immunologic mechanisms in several forms of human glomerular diseases, Bull. N. Y. Acad. Med. **46:**769-788, 1970.

35 McCluskey, R. T., and Baldwin, D. S.: Natural history of acute glomerulonephritis, Am. J. Med. **35:**213-230, 1963.

36 McCluskey, R. T., Vassalli, P., Gallo, G., and Baldwin, D. S.: An immunofluorescent study of pathogenic mechanisms in glomerular diseases, N. Engl. J. Med. **274:**695-701, 1966.

37 McCrory, W. W.: Natural history of acute glomerulonephritis in children. In Metcoff, J., editor: Acute glomerulonephritis, Boston, 1967, Little, Brown and Co., pp. 3-14.

38 Mandalenakis, N., Mendoza, N., Pirani, C. L., and Pollak, V. E.: Lobular glomerulonephritis and membranoproliferative glomerulonephritis; a clinical and pathologic study based on renal biopsies, Medicine (Baltimore) **50:**319-355, 1971.

39 Morel-Maroger, L., Leathem, A., and Richet, G.: Glomerular abnormalities in nonsystemic diseases; relationship between findings by light microscopy and immunofluorescence in 433 renal biopsy specimens, Am. J. Med. **53:**170-184, 1972.

40 Pirani, C. L., and Salinas-Madrigal, L.: Evaluation of percutaneous renal biopsy. In Sommers, S. C., editor: Pathology annual, vol. 3, New York, 1968, Appleton-Century-Crofts, pp. 249-296.

41 Rapoport, A., Davidson, D. A., Deveber, G. A., Ranking, G. N., and McLean, C. R.: Idiopathic focal proliferative nephritis associated with persistent hematuria and normal renal function, Ann. Intern. Med. **73:**921-928, 1970.

42 Seymour, A. E., Spargo, B. H., and Penksa, R.: Contributions of renal biopsy studies to the understanding of disease, Am. J. Pathol. **65:**550-588, 1971.

43 West, C. D., McAdams, A. J., and Northway, J. D.: Focal glomerulonephritis in children, J. Pediatr. **73:**184-194, 1968.

Nephrotic syndrome

44 Baldwin, D. S., Lowenstein, J., Rothfield, N. F., Gallo, G., and McCluskey, R. T.: The clinical course of the proliferative and mem-

branous forms of lupus nephritis, Ann. Intern. Med. 73:929-942, 1970.

45 Becker, C. G., Becker, E. L., Maher, J. F., and Schreiner, G. E.: Nephrotic syndrome after contact with mercury, Arch. Intern. Med. 110:178-186, 1962.

46 Braunstein, G. D., Lewis, E. J., Galvanek, E. G., Hamilton, A., and Bell, W. R.: The nephrotic syndrome associated with secondary syphilis; an immune deposit disease, Am. J. Med. 48:643-648, 1970.

47 Cameron, J. S.: Histology, protein clearances, and response to treatment in the nephrotic syndrome, Br. Med. J. 4:352-356, 1968.

48 Churg, J., and Dachs, S.: Diabetic renal disease. In Sommers, S. C., editor: Pathology annual, vol. 1, New York, 1966, Appleton-Century-Crofts, pp. 148-171.

49 Comerford, F. R., and Cohen, A. S.: The nephropathy of systemic lupus erythematosus; an assessment by clinical, light and electron microscopic criteria, Medicine (Baltimore) 46: 425-473, 1967.

50 Cooper, J. J.: The evaluation of current methods for the diagnostic histochemistry of amyloid, J. Clin. Pathol. 22:410-413, 1969.

51 Ehrenreich, T., and Churg, J.: Pathology of membranous nephropathy, In Sommers, S. C. editor: Pathology annual, vol. 3, New York, 1968, Appleton-Century-Crofts, pp. 145-186.

52 Estes, D., and Christian, C. L.: Renal histologic findings in systemic lupus erythematosus, Mayo Clin. Proc. 44:630-633, 1969.

53 Faith, G. C., and Trump, B. F.: The glomerular capillary wall in human kidney disease: acute glomerulonephritis, systemic lupus erythematosus, and preclampsia-eclampsia; comparative electron microscopic observations and a review, Lab. Invest. 15:1682-1719, 1966.

54 Gellman, D. D., Pirani, C. L., Soothill, J. F., Muehrcke, R. C., and Kark, R. M.: Diabetic nephropathy; clinical and pathologic study based on renal biopsies, Medicine (Baltimore) 38:321-367, 1959.

55 Grauscz, H., Earley, L. E., Stephens, B. G., Lee, J. C., and Hopper, J., Jr.: Diagnostic import of virus-like particles in the glomerular endothelium of patients with systemic lupus erythematosus, N. Engl. J. Med. 283:506-511, 1970.

56 Grishman, E., Porush, J. C., Rosen, S. M., and Churg, J.: Lupus nephritis with organized deposits in the kidneys, Lab. Invest. 16:717-725, 1967.

57 Habib, R., and Kleinknecht, C.: The primary nephrotic syndrome of childhood; classification and clinicopathologic study of 406 cases, Pathol. Annu. 6:414-474, 1971.

58 Hayslett, J. B., Krassier, L. S., Bensch, K. G., Kashgarian, M., and Epstein, F. H.: Progression of "lipoid nephrosis" to renal insufficiency, N. Engl. J. Med. 281:181-187, 1969.

59 Hopper, J., Jr., Ryan, P., Lee, J. C., and Rosenau, W.: Lipoid nephrosis in 31 adult patients; renal biopsy study by light, electron and fluorescence microscopy with experience in treatment, Medicine (Baltimore) 49:321-341, 1970.

60 Karafin, L., and Stearns, T. M.: Renal vein thrombosis in children, J. Urol. 92:91-97, 1964.

61 Kark, R. M., Pirani, C. L., Pollak, V. E., Muehrcke, R. C., and Blainey, J. D.: The nephrotic syndrome in adults; a common disorder with many causes, Ann. Intern. Med. 49:751-774, 1958.

62 Kawano, K., Arakawa, A., McCoy, J., Porch, J., and Kimmelstiel, P.: Quantitative study of glomeruli; focal glomerulonephritis and diabetic glomerulosclerosis, Lab. Invest. 21:269-275, 1969.

63 McCluskey, R. T., Vassalli, P., Gallo, G., and Baldwin, D. S.: An immunofluorescent study of pathogenic mechanisms in glomerular diseases, N. Engl. J. Med. 274:695-701, 1966.

64 Miller, R. B., Harrington, J. T., Ramos, C. P., Relamn, A. S., and Schwartz, W. B.: Long-term results of steroid therapy in adults with idiopathic nephrotic syndrome, Am. J. Med. 46:919-929, 1969.

65 Movat, H. Z.: The fine structure of the glomerulus in amyloidosis, Arch. Pathol. 69:323-332, 1960.

66 Muehrcke, R. C., Mandal, A. K., Gotoff, S. P., Isaacs, E. W., and Volini, F. I.: The clinical value of electron microscopy in renal disease, Arch. Intern. Med. 124:170-176, 1969.

67 Pirani, C. L., Pollak, V. E., Pritchard, J. C., and Burnett, R. G.: Renal vein thrombosis; light and electron microscopic observations. In Vostal, J., and Richet, G.: Proceedings of the Second International Congress of Nephrology, Amsterdam, 1964, Excerpta Medica Foundation, pp. 457-460.

68 Pollak, V. E., Rosen, S., Pirani, C. L., Muehrcke, R. C., and Kark, R. M.: Natural history of lipoid nephrosis and of membranous glomerulonephritis, Ann. Intern. Med. 69:1171-1196, 1968.

69 Pollak, V. E., and Pirani, C. L.: Renal histologic findings in systemic lupus erythematosus, Mayo Clin. Proc. 44:630-644, 1969.

70 Rosen, S.: Membranous glomerulonephritis: current status, Hum. Pathol. 2:209-231, 1971.

71 Rothfield, N., Ross, A., Minta, J. O., and Lepow, I. H.: Glomerular and dermal deposition of properdin in systemic lupus erythematosus, N. Engl. J. Med. 287:681-685, 1972.

72 Rosenmann, E., Pollak, V. E., and Pirani, C. L.: Renal vein thrombosis in the adult; a clinical and pathological study based on renal biopsies, Medicine (Baltimore) **47**:269-335, 1968.

73 Salinas-Madrigal, L., Pirani, C. L., and Pollak, V. E.: Glomerular and vascular "insudative" lesions of diabetic nephropathy; electron microscopic observations, Am. J. Pathol. **59**:369-397, 1970.

74 Seymour, A. E., Spargo, B. H., and Penksa, R.: Contributions of renal biopsy studies to the understanding of disease, Am. J. Pathol. **65**:550-588, 1971.

75 Tisher, C. C., Kelso, H. B., Robinson, R. R., Gunnells, J. C., and Burkholder, P. M.: Intraendothelial inclusions in kidneys of patients with systemic lupus erythematosus, Ann. Intern. Med. **75**:537-547, 1971.

76 White, R. H. R., Glasgow, E. F., and Mills, R. J.: Clinicopathological study of nephrotic syndrome in children, Lancet **1**:1353-1359, 1970.

Acute renal failure

77 Leonard, C. D., Nagle, R. B., Striker, G. E., Cutler, R. E., and Scribner, B. H.: Acute glomerulonephritis with prolonged oliguria, Ann. Intern. Med. **73**:703-711, 1970.

78 Rieselbach, R. E., Klahr, S., and Bucher, N. S.: Diffuse bilateral cortical necrosis; a longitudinal study of the functional characteristics of residual nephrosis, Am. J. Med. **42**:457-468, 1967.

79 Sevitt, L. H., Evans, D. J., and Wrong, O. M.: Acute oliguric renal failure due to accelerated (malignant) hypertension, Q. J. Med. **40**:127-144, 1971.

Renal transplant

80 Busch, G. J., Reynolds, E. S., Galvanek, E. G., Braun, W. E., and Dammin, G. J.: Human renal allografts; the role of vascular injury in early graft failure, Medicine (Baltimore) **50**:29-83, 1971.

81 Corson, J. M.: The pathologist and the kidney transplant, Pathol. Annu. **7**:251-292, 1972.

82 Harlan, W. R., Jr., Holden, K. R., Williams, G. M., and Hume, D. M.: Proteinuria and nephrotic syndrome associated with chronic rejection of kidney transplants, N. Engl. J. Med. **277**:769-776, 1967.

83 Kissmeyer-Nielsen, F., Olsen, S., Petersen, V. P., and Fjeldborg, O.: Hyperacute rejection of kidney allografts, associated with pre-existing humoral antibodies against donor cells, Lancet **2**:662-665, 1966.

84 Lindquist, R. R., Guttmann, R. D., Merrill, J. P., and Dammin, G. J.: Human renal allografts; interpretation of morphologic and im-

munohistochemical observations, Am. J. Pathol. **53**:851-881, 1968.

85 McPhaul, J. J. Jr., Dixon, F. J., Brettschneider, L., and Starzl, T. E.: Immunofluorescent examination of biopsies from long-term renal allografts, N. Engl. J. Med. **282**:412-417, 1970.

86 Porter, K. A., Andres, G. A., Calder, M. W., Dossetor, J. B., Hsu, K. C., Rendall, J. M., Seegal, B. C., and Starzl, T. E.: Human renal transplants. II. Immunofluorescent and immunoferritin studies, Lab. Invest. **18**:159-171, 1968.

87 Russell, P. S., and Winn, H. J.: Transplantation, N. Engl. J. Med. **282**:786-793, 848-854, 896-906, 1970.

88 Taylor, H. E.: Pathology of organ transplantation in man, Pathol. Annu. **7**:173-199, 1972.

89 Williams, G. M., Hume, D. M., Hudson, R. P. Jr., Morris, P. J., Kano, K., and Milgrom, F.: "Hyperacute" renal-homograft rejection in man, N. Engl. J. Med. **279**:611-618, 1968.

Renal hypertension

90 Abeshouse, B. S.: Aneurysm of the renal artery; report of two cases and review of the literature, Urol. Cutan. Rev. **55**:451-463, 1951.

91 Brown, J. J., Owen, K., Peart, W. S., Robertson, J. I. S., and Sutton, D.: The diagnosis and treatment of renal-artery stenosis, Br. Med. J. **2**:327-338, 1960.

92 Burns, E.: Unilateral renal disease and hypertension, Calif. Med. **79**:415-419, 1953.

93 Crocker, D. W.: Renal artery stenosis. In Sommers, S. C., editor: Pathology annual, vol. 3, New York, 1968, Appleton-Century-Crofts, pp. 187-211.

94 Crocker, D. W.: Fibromuscular dysplasias of renal artery, Arch. Pathol. **85**:602-613, 1968.

95 Crocker, D. W.: Bilateral juxtaglomerular cell counts in renal hypertension, Arch. Pathol. **93**:103-108, 1972.

96 Goldblatt, H.: The renal origin of hypertension, Springfield, Ill., 1948, Charles C Thomas, Publisher.

97 Goodman, A. D., Vagnucci, A. H., and Hartroft, P. M.: Pathogenesis of Bartter's syndrome, N. Engl. J. Med. **281**:1435-1439, 1969.

98 Harrison, E. G. Jr., Hunt, J. C., and Bernatz, P. E.: Morphology of fibromuscular dysplasia of the renal artery in renovascular hypertension, Am. J. Med. **43**:97-112, 1967.

99 McCormack, L. J.: Vascular changes in hypertension, Med. Clin. North Am. **42**:247-257, 1961.

100 Mangiardi, J. L., Santemma, E. E., and Sullivan, J. J., Jr.: Arteriovenous fistula of the kidney, Am. Heart J. **65**:549-554, 1963.

101 Shapiro, A. P., Perez-Stable, E., Scheib, E. T., Bron, K., Moutsos, S. E., Berg, G., and Mis-

age, J. R.: Renal artery stenosis and hypertension, Am. J. Med. 47:175-193, 1969.

102 Wylie, E. J., Perloff, D., and Wellington, J. S.: Fibromuscular hyperplasia of the renal arteries, Ann. Surg. 156:592-609, 1962.

Cystic lesions

103 Kissane, J. M.: Development of the kidney. In Heptinstall, R. H.: Pathology of the kidney, Boston, 1966, Little, Brown and Co., pp. 43-61.

104 Longino, L. A., and Martin, L. W.: Abdominal masses in the newborn infant, Pediatrics 21:596-604, 1958.

Renal dysplasia

105 Black, W. C., and Ragsdale, E. F.: Wilms' tumor, Am. J. Roentgenol. Radium Ther. Nucl. Med. 103:53-60, 1968.

106 Ericsson, N. O., and Ivemark, B. I.: I. Renal dysplasia and pyelonephritis in infants and children. II. Primitive ductules and abnormal glomeruli, Arch. Pathol. 66:255-263, 264-269, 1958.

107 Ladewig, P., and Eser, S.: Malignant tubular adenoma in a horseshoe kidney, J. Pathol. Bacteriol. 57:405-411, 1945.

108 McGinn, E. J., and Wickham, J. M.: Wilms' tumor in a horseshoe kidney, J. Urol. 56:520-524, 1946.

109 Vellios, F., and Garrett, R. A.: Congenital unilateral multicystic disease of the kidney; a clinical and anatomic study of 7 cases, Am. J. Clin. Pathol. 35:244-254, 1961.

Simple cyst

110 Daniel, W. W. Jr., Hartman, G. W., Witten, D. M., Farrow, G. M., and Kelalis, P. P.: Calcified renal masses; a review of 10 years experience at the Mayo Clinic, Radiology 103:503-508, 1972.

111 Harpster, C. M., Brown, T. H., and Delcher, A.: Solitary unilateral large serous cysts of the kidney with report of two cases and review of the literature, J. Urol. 11:157-175, 1924.

112 Heplar, A. B.: Solitary cysts of the kidney, Surg. Gynecol. Obstet. 50:668-687, 1930.

Multilocular cyst

113 Boggs, L. K., and Kimmelstiel, P.: Benign multilocular cystic nephroma; report of two cases of so-called multilocular cyst of the kidney, J. Urol. 76:530-541, 1956.

114 Powell, T., Schackman, R., and Johnson, M. D.: Multilocular cysts of the kidney, Br. J. Urol. 23:142-152, 1951.

Polycystic renal disease

115 Bell, E. T.: Renal disease, ed. 2., Philadelphia, 1950, Lea & Febiger, pp. 87-116.

116 Bricker, N. S., and Patton, J. F.: Cystic disease of the kidneys; a study of dynamics and chemical composition of cyst fluid, Am. J. Med. 18:207-219, 1955.

117 Gardner, K. D., Jr.: Composition of fluid in 12 cysts of a polycystic kidney, N. Engl. J. Med. 281:985-988, 1969.

118 Kampmeier, O. F.: Hitherto unrecognized mode of origin of congenital renal cysts, Surg. Gynecol. Obstet. 36:208-216, 1923.

119 Kissane, J. M.: Congenital malformations. In Heptinstall, R. H.: Pathology of the kidney, Boston, 1966, Little, Brown and Co.

120 Lieberman, E., Salinas-Madrigal, L., Gwinn, J. L., Brennan, L. P., Fine, R. N., and Landing, B. H.: Infantile polycystic disease of the kidneys and liver; clinical, pathological and radiological correlations and comparison with congenital hepatic fibrosis, Medicine (Baltimore) 50:277-318, 1971.

121 Osathanondh, V., and Potter, E. L.: Pathogenesis of polycystic kidneys, Arch. Pathol. 77:459-512, 1964.

122 Poutasse, E. F., Gardner, W. J., and McCormack, L. J.: Polycystic kidney disease and intracranial aneurysm, J.A.M.A. 154:741-744, 1954.

123 Sieber, F.: Ueber Cystennieren bei Erwachsenen, Deutsch. Z. Chir. 79:406-507, 1905.

124 Walters, W., and Braasch, W. F.: Surgical aspects of polycystic kidney; report of 85 surgical cases, Surg. Gynecol. Obstet. 58:647-650, 1934.

Hydronephrosis

125 Ostling, K.: The genesis of hydronephrosis, Acta Chir. Scand. 86(Suppl. 72):1-122, 1942.

126 White, R. R., and Wyatt, G. M.: Surgical importance of the aberrant vessel in infants and children, Am. J. Surg. 58:48-57, 1942.

Megaloureter

127 Malek, R. S., Kelalis, P. P., Burke, E. C., and Stickler, G. B.: Simple and ectopic ureterocele in infancy and childhood, Surg. Gynecol. Obstet. 134:611-616, 1972.

Pyelonephritis

128 Aoki, S., Imamura, S., Aoki, M., and McCabe, W. R.: "Abacterial" and bacterial pyelonephritis; immunofluorescent localization of bacterial antigen, N. Engl. J. Med. 281:1375-1382, 1969.

129 Beeson, P. B.: Factors in the pathogenesis of pyelonephritis, Yale J. Biol. Med. 28:81-104, 1955.

130 Coleman, P. N., and Taylor, S.: Coliform infection of the urinary tract, J. Clin. Pathol. 2:134-137, 1949.

131 Garrett, R. A., Norris, M. S., and Vellios, F.:

Renal papillary necrosis: a clinicopathologic study, J. Urol. **72**:609-617, 1954.

132 Ghosh, H.: Chronic pyelonephritis with xanthogranulomatous change, Am. J. Clin. Pathol. **25**:1043-1049, 1955.

133 Heptinstall, R. H.: Pathology of the kidney, Boston, 1966, Little, Brown and Co.

134 Keefer, C. S.: Pyelonephritis: its natural history and course, Bull. Hopkins Hosp. **100**:107-131, 1957.

135 Mallory, G. K., Crane, A. R., and Edwards, J. E.: Pathology of acute and of healed experimental pyelonephritis, Arch. Pathol. **30**:330-347, 1940.

136 Rios-Dalenz, J. L., and Peacock, R. C.: Xanthogranulomatous pyelonephritis, Cancer **19**:289-296, 1966.

Radiation nephritis

137 Luxton, R. W.: Radiation nephritis, Q. J. Med. **22**:215-242, 1953.

138 Luxton, R. W.: Radiation nephritis; a longterm study of 54 patients, Lancet **2**:1221-1224, 1961.

Pyelitis and ureteritis cystica

139 Hinman, F., and Cordonnier, J.: Cystitis follicularis, J. Urol. **34**:302-308, 1935.

Pelvic lipomatosis

140 Hamm, F. C., and DeVeer, J. A.: Fatty replacement following renal atrophy or destruction, J. Urol. **41**:850-866, 1939.

141 Young, H. H.: Lipomatosis or destructive fat replacement of renal cortex; report of 11 cases, J. Urol. **29**:631-644, 1933.

Lithiasis

142 Albright, F., and Reifenstein, E. C., Jr.: The parathyroid glands and metabolic bone disease; selected studies, Baltimore, 1948, The Williams & Wilkins Co.

143 Carr, R. J.: A new theory on the formation of renal calculi, Br. J. Urol. **26**:105-117, 1954.

144 Randall, A.: Origin and growth of renal calculi, Ann. Surg. **105**:1009-1027, 1937.

145 Randall, A.: The etiology of primary renal calculus, Int. Abstr. Surg. **71**:209-240, 1940; in Surg. Gynecol. Obstet., Sept., 1940.

Tuberculosis

146 Auerbach, O.: The pathology of urogenital tuberculosis, Int. Clin. **3**:21-61, 1940.

147 Dick, J. C.: Effect of isoniazid on tuberculous lesions of the kidneys, Lancet **1**:808-817, 1953.

148 Greenberger, A. J., and Greenberger, M. E.: Urogenital tuberculosis associated with pulmonary tuberculosis, Med. Clin. North Am. **20**:787-810, 1936.

149 Hanley, H. G.: The indications for surgery in renal tuberculosis, Br. J. Surg. **45**:10-15, 1957.

150 Medlar, E. M.: Causes of renal infection in pulmonary tuberculosis, Am. J. Pathol. **2**:401-414, 1926.

151 Reichle, H. S., and Work, J. L.: Incidence and significance of healed miliary tubercles in the liver, spleen and kidneys, Arch. Pathol. **28**:331-339, 1939.

152 Wegelin and Wildbolz: Anatomische Untersuchungen von Frühstadien der chronischen Nierentuberkulose, Z. Urolog. Chir. **2**:201-240, 1913-1914.

Benign tumors

153 Bogdan, R., Taylor, D. E. M., and Mostofi, F. K.: Leiomyomatous hamartoma of the kidney; a clinical and pathologic analysis of 20 cases from the Kidney Tumor Registry, Cancer **31**:462-467, 1973.

154 Bolande, R. P., Brough, A. J., and Izant, R. J., Jr.: Congenital mesoblastic nephroma of infancy; report of 8 cases and relationship to Wilms' tumor, Pediatrics **40**:272-278, 1967.

155 Conn, J. W., Cohen, E. L., Lucas, C. P., McDonald, W. J., Mayor, G. H., Blough, W. M., Jr., Eveland, W. C., Bookstin, J. J., and Lapides J.: Primary reninism; hypertension, hyperreninemia, and secondary aldosteronism due to renin-producing juxtaglomerular cell tumors, Arch. Intern. Med. **130**:682-696, 1972.

156 Critchley, M., and Earl, C. J. C.: Tuberose sclerosis and allied conditions, Brain **55**:311-346, 1932.

157 Farrow, G. M., Harrison, E. G., Jr., Utz, D. C., and Jones, D. R.: Renal angiomyolipoma; a clinicopathologic study of 32 cases, Cancer **22**:564-570, 1968.

158 Favara, B. E., Johnson, W., and Ito, J.: Renal tumors in the neonatal period, Cancer **22**:845-855, 1968.

159 Hajdu, S. I., and Foote, F. W., Jr.: Angiomyolipoma of the kidney; report of 27 cases and review of the literature, J. Urol. **102**:396-401, 1969.

160 Kay, S., Pratt, C. B., and Salzberg, A. M.: Hamartoma (leiomyomatous type) of the kidney, Cancer **19**:1825-1832, 1966.

161 Lee, M. R.: Renin-secreting kidney tumours; a rare but remediable cause of serious hypertension, Lancet **2**:254-255, 1971.

162 Mintz, E. R., and Gaul, E. A.: Kidney tumors; some causes of poor end results, N. Y. State J. Med. **39**:1405-1411, 1939.

163 Pfeiffer, G. E., and Gandin, M. M.: Massive perirenal lipoma with report of a case, J. Urol. **56**:12-27, 1946.

164 Robertson, P. W., Klidjian, A., Harding, L. K., and Walters, G.: Hypertension due to a renin-

secreting renal tumour, Am. J. Med. 43:963-976, 1967.

165 Tweeddale, D. N., Dawe, C. J., McDonald, J. R., and Culp, O. S.: Angiolipoleiomyoma of the kidney, Cancer 8:764-770, 1955.

166 Wigger, H. J.: Fetal hamartoma of kidney; a benign, symptomatic, congenital tumor, not a form of Wilms' tumor, Am. J. Clin. Pathol. 51:323-337, 1969.

Malignant tumors
Wilms' tumor

167 Balsaver, A. M., Gibley, C. W., Jr., and Tessmer, C. F.: Ultrastructural studies in Wilms' tumor, Cancer 22:417-427, 1968.

168 Bannayan, G. A., Huvos, A. G., and D'Angio, G. J.: Effect of irradiation on the maturation of Wilms' tumor, Cancer 27:812-818, 1971.

169 Bodian, M., and Rigby, C. C.: The pathology of nephroblastoma. In Riches, E., editor: Tumours of the kidney and ureter, Baltimore, 1964, The Williams & Wilkins Co., pp. 219-234.

170 D'Angio, G. J.: Management of children with Wilms' tumor, Cancer 30:1528-1533, 1972.

171 Farber, S.: Chemotherapy in the treatment of leukemia and Wilms' tumor, J.A.M.A. 198:826-836, 1966.

172 Farrow, G. M., Harrison, E. G., Jr., and Utz, D. C.: Sarcomas and sarcomatoid and mixed malignant tumors of the kidney in adults, Cancer 22:545-563, 1968.

173 Fraumeni, J. F., Jr., Geiser, C. F., and Manning, M. D.: Wilms' tumor and congenital hemihypertrophy; report of five new cases and review of literature, Pediatrics 40:886-898, 1967.

174 Geschickter, C. F., and Widehorn, H.: Nephrogenic tumors, Am. J. Cancer 22:620-658, 1934.

175 Lucké, B., and Schlumberger, H. G.: Tumors of the kidney, renal pelvis and ureter. In Atlas of tumor pathology, Sect. VIII, Fasc. 30, Washington, D. C., 1957, Armed Forces Institute of Pathology.

176 Masson, P.: The role of the neural crests in the embryonal adenosarcomas of the kidney, Am. J. Cancer 33:1-32, 1938.

177 Miller, R. W., Fraumeni, J. F., and Manning, M. D.: Association of Wilms' tumor with aniridia, hemihypertrophy and other congenital malformations, N. Engl. J. Med. 270:922-927, 1964.

178 Olsen, B. S., and Bischoff, A. J.: Wilms' tumor in an adult, Cancer 25:21-25, 1970.

179 Ragab, A. H., Vietti, T. J., Crist, W., Perez, C., and McAllister, W.: Bilateral Wilms' tumor; a review, Cancer 30:983-988, 1972.

180 Scott, L. S.: Bilateral Wilms' tumor, Br. J. Surg. 42:513-516, 1955.

Renal cell carcinoma

181 Arner, O., Blanck, C., and von Schreeb, T.: Renal adenocarcinoma: morphology, grading of malignancy, prognosis; study of 19 cases, Acta Chir. Scand. [Suppl.] 346:11-51, 1965.

182 Bell, E. T.: Renal disease, ed. 2, Philadelphia, 1950, Lea & Febiger, p. 436.

183 Campbell, L. V., Jr., Gilbert, E., Chamberlain, C. R., Jr., and Watne, A. L.: Metastases of cancer to cancer, Cancer 22:635-643, 1968.

184 Dehner, L. P., Leestma, J. E., and Price, E. B., Jr.: Renal cell carcinoma in children; a clinicopathologic study of 15 cases and review of the literature, J. Pediatr. 76:358-368, 1970.

185 Everson, T. C.: Spontaneous regression of cancer, Ann. N. Y. Acad. Sci. 114:721-735, 1964.

186 Farrow, G. M., Harrison, E. G., Jr., and Utz, D. C.: Sarcomas and sarcomatoid and mixed malignant tumors of the kidney in adults, Cancer 22:545-563, 1968.

187 Goldberg, M. F., Tashjian, A. H., Jr., Order, S. E., and Dammin, G. J.: Renal adenocarcinoma containing a parathyroid hormone-like substance and associated with marked hypercalcemia, Am. J. Med. 36:805-814, 1964.

188 Gottesman, J., Perla, D., and Elson, J.: Pathogenesis of hypernephroma, Arch. Surg. 24:722-751, 1932.

189 Grabstald, H.: Renal cell cancer. I. Incidence, etiology, natural history, and prognosis. II. Diagnostic findings. III. Types of treatment, N. Y. State J. Med. 64:2539-2545; 2658-2671; 2771-2782, 1964.

190 Hewlett, J. S., Hoffman, G. C., Senhauser, D. A., and Battle, J. D., Jr.: Carcinoma of the kidney producing multiple hormones, J. Urol. 106:820-822, 1971.

191 Kay, S.: Renal carcinoma; a 10-year study, Am. J. Clin. Pathol. 50:428-432, 1968.

192 Kiely, J. M.: Hypernephroma; the internist's tumor, Med. Clin. North Am. 50:1067-1983, 1966.

193 Rafla, S.: Renal cell carcinoma; natural history and results of treatment, Cancer 23:26-40, 1970.

194 Ramos, C. V., and Taylor, H. B.: Hepatic dysfunction associated with renal carcinoma, Cancer 29:1287-1292, 1972.

195 Robson, C. J., Churchill, B. M., and Anderson, W.: The results of radical nephrectomy for renal cell carcinoma, Trans. Am. Assoc. Genitourin. Surg. 60:122-126, 1968.

196 Skinner, D. G., Colvin, R. B., Vermillion, C. D., Pfister, R. C., and Leadbetter, W. F.: Diagnosis and management of renal cell carcinoma; a clinical and pathologic study of 309 cases, Cancer 28:1165-1177, 1971.

197 Walsh, P. N., and Kissane, J. M.: Nonmetastatic hypernephroma with reversible

hepatic dysfunction, Arch. Intern. Med. **122**:212-222, 1968.

Other malignant tumors

198 Farrow, G. M., Harrison, E. G., Jr., and Utz, D. C.: Sarcomas and sarcomatoid and mixed malignant tumors of the kidney in adults, Cancer **22**:545-563, 1968.

199 Richmond, J., Sherman, R. S., Diamond, H. D., and Craver, L. F.: Renal lesions associated with malignant lymphomas, Am. J. Med. **32**:184-207, 1962.

Tumors of pelvis and ureter

200 Abeshouse, B. S.: Primary benign and malignant tumors of the ureter; a review of the literature and report of one benign and twelve malignant tumors, Am. J. Surg. **91**:237-271, 1956.

201 Ackerman, L. V.: Mucinous adenocarcinoma of the pelvis of the kidney, J. Urol. **55**:36-45, 1946.

202 Bloom, N. A., Vidone, R. A., and Lytton, B.: Primary carcinoma of the ureter; a report of 102 new cases, J. Urol. **103**:590-598, 1970.

203 Compere, D. E., Begley, H. E., Issacks, H. F., Franzier, T. H., and Dryden, C. B.: Ureteral polyps, J. Urol. **79**:209-214, 1958.

204 Gahagan, H. Q., and Reed, W. K.: Squamous cell carcinoma of the renal pelvis; three case reports and review of literature, J. Urol. **62**:139-151, 1949.

205 Kao, V. C. Y., Graff, P. W., and Rappaport, H.: Leiomyoma of the ureter; a histologically problematic rare tumor confirmed by immunohistochemical studies, Cancer **24**:535-542, 1969.

206 Kimball, F. N., and Ferris, H. W.: Papillomatous tumor of the renal pelvis associated with similar tumors of the ureter and bladder; review of literature and report of two cases, J. Urol. **31**:257-304, 1934.

207 McDonald, J. R., and Priestley, J. T.: Carcinoma of renal pelvis; histopathologic study of seventy-five cases with special reference to prognosis, J. Urol. **51**:245-258, 1944.

208 McIntyre, D., Pyrah, L. N., and Raper, F. P.: Primary ureteric neoplasms; report of 40 cases, Br. J. Urol. **37**:160-191, 1965.

209 Suzuki, H., and Milam, D. F.: Primary mucus-producing adenomatous tumor—adenocarcinoma of renal pelvis; a case report and review of literature, Arch. Pathol. **84**:468-473, 1967.

210 Werner, J. R., Klingersmith, W., and Denko, J. V.: Leiomyosarcoma of the ureter; case report and review of literature, J. Urol. **82**:68-71, 1959.

211 Whitlock, G. F., McDonald, J. R., and Cook, E. N.: Primary carcinoma of the ureter; a pathologic and prognostic study, J. Urol. **73**:245-253, 1955.

Bladder

Biopsy

All bladder tumors should be biopsied. The urologist should not fulgurate a papillary tumor without biopsy because it appears benign. It is true that tumors wholly composed of delicate papillary fronds are often well differentiated, but exceptions occur. It is therefore better practice to biopsy the tumor before fulguration. Small biopsies should be sectioned at various levels. The biopsy often shows a lower grade of tumor than is found in the excised lesion. Even large biopsies may not be representative of the most undifferentiated part of the tumor. These undifferentiated areas are not necessarily at the base of the tumor. The pathologist should state whether or not the tumor invades the muscle in the bladder wall. This is of great prognostic value and influences operative therapy.

Cytology

Exfoliative cytology is of little practical value in the initial evaluation of bladder tumors because of their accessibility to formal biopsy. Exceptions are the cases associated with extensive chronic inflammation in which the biopsy may be negative because of sampling and in the exceptional case of a carcinoma hidden in a bladder diverticulum.[4] Melamed et al.[2a] found positive cytology in seventeen of twenty-five patients with carcinoma in situ of the bladder mucosa. This lesion may remain static for up to five years before progression takes place. Another drawback of cytology is the fact that well-differentiated (Grades I and II) lesions are often missed because of the close similarity of the cells with those of the normal bladder mucosa. However, Esposti et al.[1] recognized cytologically 86% of sixty-three cases of Grade II and Grade IV cancers from the first samples of urine and bladder washings. The greater significance of cytology of the urinary bladder is in the follow-up evaluation of patients who have received surgical or radiotherapeutic treatment for bladder carcinoma.[2] In some cases, the recurrence may not become clinically apparent until more than one year after the malignant cells have been detected in the urine.[3] Reichborn-Kjennerud and Hoeg[5] found malignant cells in the urine of seven patients from eleven to twenty-three months before recurrent tumor could be demonstrated at cytoscopy. Although radiation therapy may result in atypia of normal cells, a pathologist with the basic knowledge of the morphology of irradiation effect who is provided with accurate clinical information is unlikely to be confused. Esposti et al.[1] identified 88% of the eighty-six cases of bladder carcinoma recurring or persisting after supervoltage radiation therapy.

Examination of cystectomy specimens

We have found it very useful to examine specimens of total cystectomy by the inflation technique. After tying the ureters, a Foley or similar catheter is introduced through the urethra; the cavity is washed two or three times, distended with 10%

formalin, and immersed into a large jar containing formalin. Following fixation for twelve to sixteen hours, the specimen is bisected and sections are taken.

The tumor in cystectomy specimens must be sectioned carefully through the entire bladder wall. Other pertinent information frequently is obtained by sectioning areas of bladder epithelium uninvolved by the bladder tumor. Since the entire bladder epithelium may have been exposed to the same carcinogenic agent, examination of apparently normal mucosa may be rewarding. Special stains (Verhoeff–van Gieson) may demonstrate blood vessel invasion. Careful search for lymph nodes should be made in the loose tissue around the bladder.

Interstitial (Hunner's) cystitis

The classical clinical description of interstitial (Hunner's) cystitis is that of a female adult with an ulcerative process and marked submucosal edema resulting in prominent lower abdominal, suprapubic, or perineal pain and urinary frequency, all unresponsive to medical therapy.[6, 7] Smith and Dehner[8] microscopically examined twenty-eight cases considered representative of this nebulous condition. In contrast to previous reports, they found a similar sex incidence and a higher incidence of frequency and hematuria than of abdominal pain. Microscopically, ulceration of the mucosa covered by fibrin and necrotic material was always present. The underlying submucosa and muscularis showed edema and a nonspecific inflammatory infiltrate with numerous mast cells. The lesions occurred anywhere in the bladder, with no predilection for a particular site.

Tuberculosis

Tuberculosis is the most frequent of the rare granulomatous infections of the bladder. It invariably develops from secondary foci, most often in the kidney. Tuberculous lesions usually are found in the region of the trigone. They are superficial and small, with a floor of soft caseous material and a peripheral hyperemic zone. The most prominent involvement is often found at the ureteral orifice. With further progression, multiple ulcers coalesce to form larger ones that produce much fibrosis and involve the underlying musculature. Tuberculosis of the kidney was present in thirty-six of fifty patients with tuberculosis of the bladder reported by Auerbach.[9] Secondary involvement of the prostate gland also may occur.

Cystitis glandularis (cystica)

A common bladder condition, cystitis glandularis (cystica) results from metaplastic changes of the transitional epithelium as originally described by von Limbeck[12] (1887) and von Brunn[11] (1893). Focal proliferation of the basal epithelial layer produces solid nests that grow downward into the lamina propria. They are usually designated as von Brunn's islands.[15] Later, glandular metaplasia develops within them, and the progressive accumulation of mucin results in the formation of a central cystic area. Cells assume a concentric radiating pattern with basally situated nuclei and clear apical cytoplasm containing abundant mucin[17] (Fig. 688). Finally, cysts lined by flattened epithelium develop. These changes are always the expression of a chronic inflammatory process. They are particularly prominent in neurogenic bladder, in which the metaplastic glands may show an appearance strongly resembling colonic epithelium.[16] Grossly, cystitis glandularis presents an irregular mamilated appearance that may be confused cystoscopically with carcinoma.[13] The trigone is the area most commonly affected, although rare instances of involvement of the entire bladder mucosa have been reported.[10] Similar changes are practically always found in the renal pelvis and ureters. The lesion may regress completely if the underlying etiologic factor is removed.[14] We do not make a distinction between cystitis glandularis and cystitis cystica, since we consider them as expressions of the same pathologic change.[18]

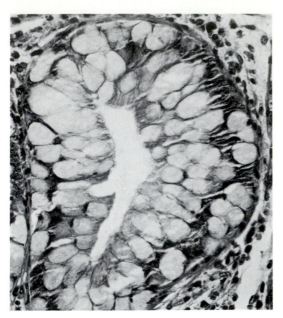

Fig. 688 Cystitis glandularis with formation of mucin-producing glands. (×225; WU neg. 49-6717.)

Endometriosis

Endometriosis is a rare condition of the bladder that has been reported approximately fifty times.[19] The localized form (endometrioma) occurs beneath an intact mucosa and has a bluish cast. This lesion undergoes cyclic change during the menstrual cycle. Forty-two of forty-six patients reported by Moore et al.[20] had had previous pelvic surgery or some disease of the female reproductive system. In twenty-one patients, the endometrioma could be palpated in the base of the bladder. Rarely, intraureteral endometriosis occurs.[21]

Diverticula

Diverticula of the bladder develop because of partial urinary obstruction in the urethra or bladder neck. Long-standing increased muscular contractions required to empty the bladder cause mucosal herniation in areas of congenital weakness. The most common locations are above the trigone on the posterior wall, the region of the urethral orifice, and the site of an obliterated urachus. Invariably, the diverticula are associated with a thick-

Table 29 Types of obstruction resulting in bladder diverticula*

	Cases	%
Nodular prostatic hyperplasia	153	66.52
Median bar	34	14.78
Contracted internal urethral orifice	18	7.82
Carcinoma of prostate	17	7.39
Stricture of urethra	5	2.19
Congenital valves in posterior urethra	3	1.30

*From Kretschmer, H. L.: Diverticula of the urinary bladder; a clinical study of 236 cases, Surg. Gynecol. Obstet. 71:491-503, 1940; by permission of Surgery, Gynecology & Obstetrics.

ened bladder wall. The types of obstruction that were responsible for the formation of diverticula in 236 patients (229 males and seven females)[23] are shown in Table 29. Free spontaneous perforation of bladder diverticula is extremely uncommon.[25]

The communication into the bladder is usually large but may be pinpoint in size.[27] The wall of the diverticulum usually consists of fibrous tissue with a little or no muscle. Squamous metaplasia of the lining epithelium often occurs if there is associated infection. The rather frequent occurrence of carcinoma within diverticula may relate to the obstruction, "leukoplakia," and chronic inflammation occurring in them. Diverticula may contain stones.[26]

Abeshouse and Goldstein[22] reviewed eighty-nine cases of malignant neoplasms occurring in diverticula. There were thirty-five unclassified carcinomas, nineteen papillary carcinomas, sixteen squamous carcinomas, and one adenocarcinoma. Kretschmer and Barber[42] had ten cases in which carcinoma was found within the diverticulum. These diverticula were locally resected, and in nine patients the tumor recurred locally.

Carcinoma
Transitional cell carcinoma

Aniline dye workers are known to develop carcinoma of the bladder rather more frequently than other persons.[31]

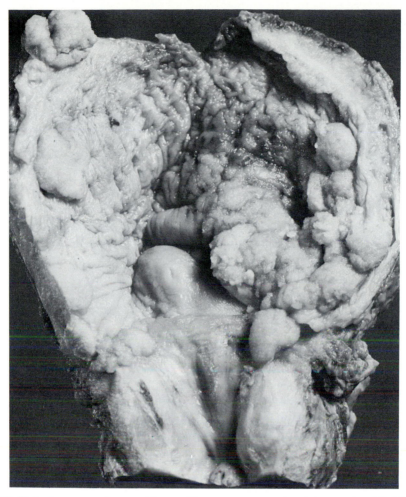

Fig. 689 Cystectomy specimen with papillomatous tumor involving entire bladder with area of invasion. (WU neg. 50-4918.)

Tumors of the bladder can be produced experimentally by aniline dyes.[35, 36] Barsotti and Vigliani[30] found that benzidine and betanaphthylamine have the highest carcinogenic power. However, this etiologic factor accounts for only a small percentage of bladder carcinomas.[28] It has been postulated that urinary tryptophan metabolites may be the endogenous counterpart of the carcinogenic dyes.[32, 39] Thorough statistical studies are needed to substantiate the suggestion that smoking is associated with an increased incidence of bladder carcinoma.[33]

About 80% or more of carcinomas of the bladder are of transitional cell type. In spite of the regular and uniform microscopic pattern that these tumors often exhibit, they may recur locally and can easily be implanted in the abdominal wall. Because of their prominent tendency to recur locally and because the microscopic pattern does not always conform with the clinical behavior, we feel that even the benign-appearing papillomatous lesions should be classified as transitional cell carcinomas (Fig. 689). This terminology has been adopted by the Bladder Tumor Registry and by the Armed Forces Institute of Pathology.[29]

The region of the trigone is the most common location (75% of the patients).

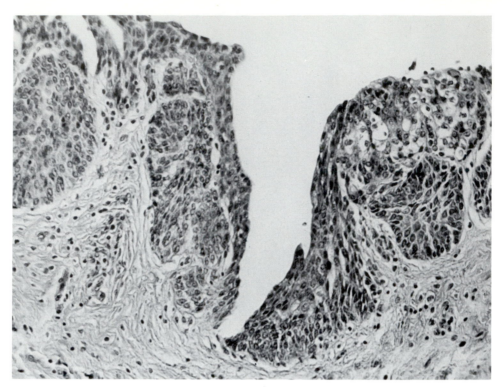

Fig. 690 Apparently normal bladder epithelium taken at distance from invasive carcinoma. These changes represent early carcinoma and suggest multiple foci of origin (×250; WU neg. 52-604.)

Therefore, partial to complete block of one or both ureters is frequent. The resulting hydronephrosis and pyelonephritis may produce serious renal damage and impair the chance of successful bladder resection.

Zones of atypical proliferation, carcinoma in situ, and early invasive carcinomas are often found in areas remote from the main tumor mass, a finding which reinforces the argument for cystectomy[41] (Fig. 690). In some instances, this atypical proliferation extends into the ureters. Thus, Sharma et al.[42] detected ureteral lesions that they interpreted as carcinoma in situ in seventeen (8.5%) of 205 patients undergoing cystectomy for bladder carcinoma. The incidence was highest in patients with multifocal tumors and in those with high-stage and high-grade neoplasms. Schade et al.[40] in a similar study, found ureteral changes varying from mild atypia to early invasive carcinoma in many of the cases. Bladder carcinoma also may extend

into the bladder neck and urethra. This is responsible for the occasional instances of urethral recurrence following cystectomy for carcinoma of the bladder.[34] Most cases of carcinoma in situ of the bladder are associated with invasive carcinoma. However, in some instances the entire lesion is intraepithelial. The microscopic criteria for the diagnosis are essentially the same as for carcinoma in situ of other locations, notably uterine cervix. Of the twenty-five cases so diagnosed by Melamed et al.,[38] eight patients subsequently developed invasive carcinoma after intervals ranging from eight to sixty-seven months.

Transitional cell cancers frequently exhibit foci of glandular metaplasia. In an examination of 340 cases of transitional cell carcinoma of the bladder, Ward[43] found that 25% to 30% had evidence of focal mucin production and a similar number (but not necessarily the same) showed some form of glandular metaplasia. This finding has no prognostic significance. These tumors behave as transitional cell cancers and should be so designated. A clear distinction should be made between them and the pure adenocarcinoma of the bladder. Similarly, many otherwise typical transitional cell cancers (especially Grade III and IV lesions) show small foci of squamous differentiation. These tumors should still be regarded as of transitional origin and clearly separated from pure epidermoid cancers secondary to "leukoplakia" or to *Schistosoma* infestation.

Transitional cell tumors are very rare in children, and usually of a well-differentiated character, noninvasive, and therefore associated with an excellent prognosis.[37]

Grading of carcinoma

The grading of carcinoma of the bladder is of prognostic significance only in large series of cases.[45] The frequency of variations in the grade/prognosis correlation makes grading of little value in the individual case. The differentiation of a given neoplasm may vary from area to area, and biopsies often show a lower degree of malignancy than is present in the surgical specimen. Obviously, if the biopsy shows a very poorly differentiated tumor, the prognosis is poor.[46] If, on the other hand, the lesion is well differentiated, this does not mean that it might not be poorly differentiated in other areas.[49]

Several different systems have been reported for the grading of transitional cell carcinoma based on the *cytologic appearance* of the tumor (Table 30). The one we use is the one postulated by Ash.[44] It designates all transitional cell tumors as carcinomas and divides them in four grades as follows:

Grade I

Grossly Grade I tumors have a soft pink color and delicate frond-like papillary structures which cystoscopically look like ferns suspended by pedicles. The majority are pedunculated, but they may be sessile. Necrosis is exceptionally rare. Microscopically, regular frondlike papillae are present throughout. They are composed of a central fibrovascular core covered by uniform transitional cells practically identical to those in the normal bladder. Mitoses are rare or absent (Fig. 691). Lund and Lundwall[48] followed 183 patients with this lesion (165 of them for an average of six months); 34% of the solitary and 74% of the multiple lesions recurred. The recurrence was of higher cytologic grade in 5% of the solitary and 18% of the multiple lesions. The recurrence rate in the series of 125 patients reported by Lerman et al.[47] was 47% (31% for the solitary and 66% for the multiple lesions). Carcinoma of higher grade developed in twelve patients (9.6%). In eleven of these, the original lesion was multiple. No correlation was found between the size of the original lesion and the later development of cancer.

Grade II

The majority are pedunculated. Necrosis is rare. Grossly, the tumors differ from Grade I by virtue of their more solid appearance and firmer consistency (Fig. 695). Microscopically, the papillary configuration persists, but there is more crowding of cells, enlargement and hyperchromasia of

Table 30 Comparison of three different grading systems

Ash, 1940[44]	Mostofi, 1960[50] (adopted by the American Bladder Tumor Registry)	Bengkvist et al., 1965[45]
Transitional cell carcinoma, Grade I	Papilloma	Transitional cell tumor, Grade 0 Transitional cell tumor, Grade I
Transitional cell carcinoma, Grade II	Transitional cell carcinoma, Grade I	Transitional cell tumor, Grade II
Transitional cell carcinoma, Grade III	Transitional cell carcinoma, Grade II	Transitional cell tumor, Grade III
Transitional cell carcinoma, Grade IV	Transitional cell carcinoma, Grade III	Transitional cell tumor, Grade IV

691 692

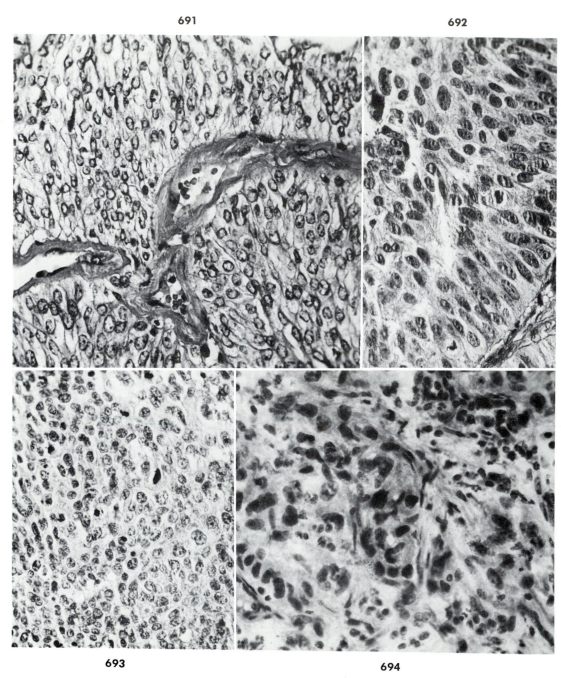

693 694

Fig. 691 Grade I transitional cell carcinoma. Note excellent differentiation of cells, abundant cytoplasm, and few mitotic figures. (×400; WU neg. 49-545.)

Fig. 692 Grade II transitional cell carcinoma. Note variation in cell size, increase in prominence of cell nuclei, and numerous mitotic figures. (×400; WU neg. 49-544.)

Fig. 693 Grade III transitional cell carcinoma. Note loss of any pattern with considerable cell variation. (×400; WU neg. 49-547.)

Fig. 694 Grade IV transitional cell carcinoma. There is complete disorganization with extreme variation in size and shape of cells. (×400; WU neg. 49-549.)

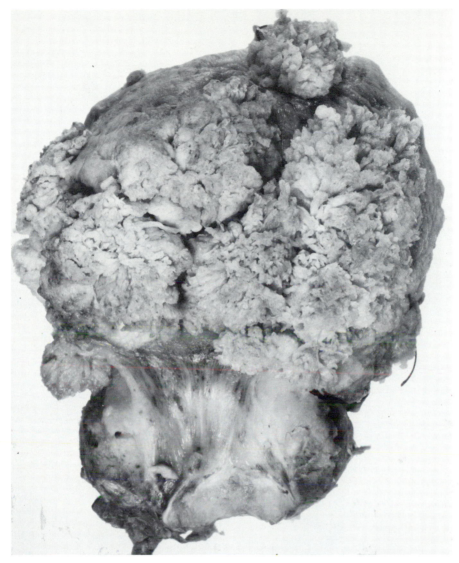

Fig. 695 Grade II transitional cell carcinoma involving large portion of bladder. Papillary configuration persists, but some of nodules are more solid than in Grade I lesions. This was B_1 tumor, according to Jewett's classification. WU neg. 69-10646.)

nuclei, and more than an occasional mitotic figure (Fig. 692).

Grade III

A high percentage of these tumors have a sessile, cauliflower-like appearance. Necrosis and ulceration are frequent. Microscopically, papillary areas may still be present but irregularly distributed. The cell masses are in smaller groups, and mitotic figures are often abundant (Fig. 693).

Grade IV

Most of these lesions are sessile, necrotic, ulcerated, and cauliflower-like (Fig. 696). Micro-scopically, papillary areas are rare. Small nests of tumor cells can be recognized only by their small, homogeneous, deeply blue-staining nuclei. The cytoplasm is small in amount. Mitotic figures are frequent and often atypical (Fig. 694).

Clinicopathologic correlation and prognosis

In our group of 135 patients,[57] Grade I and Grade II carcinomas often were associated with hematuria but not, as a rule, with dysuria. Dysuria usually was associated with the Grade III and Grade IV

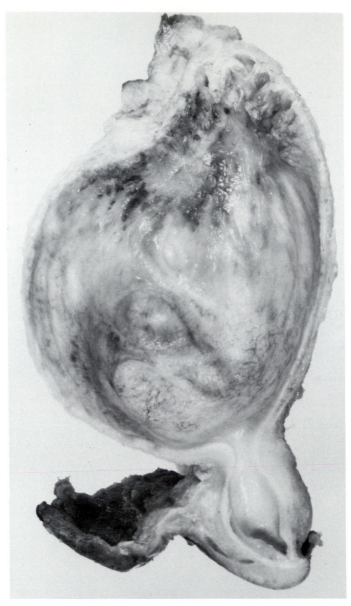

Fig. 696 Grade IV transitional cell carcinoma in dome of bladder. Tumor is ulcerated and deeply invasive. (WU neg. 65-3322.)

carcinomas, very likely the result of infection and involvement of bladder wall.

The more undifferentiated the tumor, the worse the prognosis. In fact, any patient with a Grade III or Grade IV carcinoma has an extremely poor prognosis and for this reason deserves radical therapy. The prognosis of the patients with tumors located on the dome and anterior surface of the bladder is much worse than for tumors located at the base of the bladder. Invasion of the wall of the bladder, possibly because of its rich network of lymphatics, lessens the likelihood of cure (Fig. 697). Using segmental resection and cystectomy specimens, Jewett[54] demonstrated excellent correlation between the depth of invasion and the prognosis (Fig. 698). The prognosis of any group of patients with carcinoma of the bladder reported in

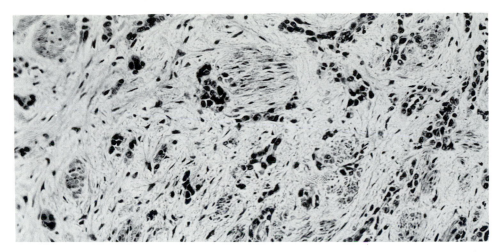

Fig. 697 Extensive growth of bladder carcinoma within lymphatics of bladder musculature. (×97; WU neg. 49-550.)

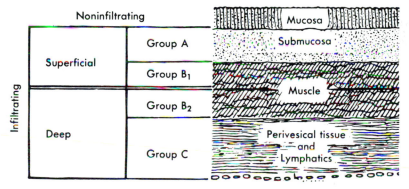

Fig. 698 Schematic representation of depth of invasion of bladder cancer. More superficial the tumor, better the prognosis. (From Jewett, H. J.: Carcinoma of the bladder:
influence of depth of infiltration on the five-year results following complete extirpation
of the primary growth, J. Urol. **67:**672-680, 1952.)

the literature is influenced to a considerable
extent by the number of Grade I carcinomas.

In general, a good correlation exists between the cytologic grading and the topographic staging. Most Grade I and II tumors are superficial, whereas, many Grade
III and IV cancers invade deeply. However, exceptions to both statements occur.
Of the two methods, staging remains as
the single most important therapeutic and
prognostic factor.[51, 55, 56] The presence of
lymphatic and/or blood vessel invasion is
naturally associated with a decreased survival.[52] The presence of regional lymph
node metastases are an ominous prognos-

tic sign. Among eleven patients treated
by total cystectomy in whom this was
demonstrated, there were no five-year survivors.[53] On the other hand, there is some
indication that tumors with pushing margins associated with lymphocytic reaction
have a relatively better prognosis.[58] At
present, operative mortality for a total
cystectomy is low, and pyelonephritis is no
longer a frequent complication if conduit
ureteral diversion is accomplished by implantation of the ureters into an isolated
segment of ileum. In a series of 129 total
cystectomies with ileal loop urinary diversion performed at Barnes Hospital, there
were only six operative deaths.[53] The over-

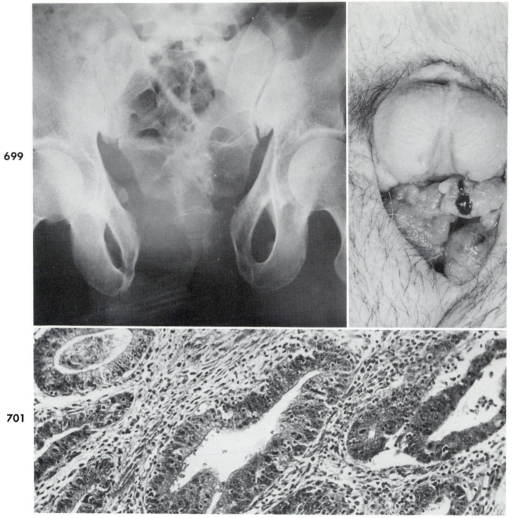

Fig. 699 Pelvis in patient with exstrophy of bladder showing typical separation of symphysis pubis. (WU neg. 49-2468.)
Fig. 700 Exstrophy of bladder with carcinoma arising from it. (WU neg. 48-1807.)
Fig. 701 Same tumor shown in Fig. 700. It is well-differentiated adenocarcinoma. (×200; WU neg. 49-6721.)

all five-year survival rate was 38%. Among the five-year survivors, sixteen were Stage A or B₁, one was Stage B₂ and seven were Stage C.

Adenocarcinoma

Bladder adenocarcinomas develop from sequential changes initiated by chronic inflammation—from Brunn's epithelial island, to cystitis glandularis (cystica), and, finally, to carcinoma that may or may not form mucin. Grossly, fungating masses of tumor

ulcerate the mucosa and invade the bladder wall. The surface in the mucoid type is covered with thick, slimy, gelatinous material.[62] Microscopically, they are usually fairly well differentiated.

Adenocarcinomas arising on the basis of metaplasia of transitional epithelium are most commonly located in the region of the trigone.[60] They may be associated with exstrophy of the bladder (Figs. 699 to 701). This condition consists of absence of the anterior vesicle and lower abdominal wall with eversion of the posterior bladder wall. These changes may be partial or complete and are often associated with other anomalies of the urogenital tract. Malignant change was found in three (7.5%) of forty-two patients with exstrophic bladder reported by Engel and Wilkinson.[59] All three patients had adenocarcinoma, while one also had an epidermoid cancer.

Adenocarcinoma also may arise from the urachus. Seventeen of the forty-four cases of bladder adenocarcinoma reported by Mostofi et al.[60] were thought to arise in this structure. The urachus measures 5 cm to 6 cm in length and can be divided

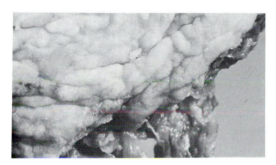

Fig. 702 Prominent squamous metaplasia of bladder. Note plaquelike areas of piled-up epithelium. This is lesion often referred to as "leukoplakia." (WU neg. 49-6452.)

into the extravesical portion lying above the bladder and the intramural area within the wall. The urachal lumen is continuous with the lumen of the bladder in about 33% of the patients.[61] Most neoplasms arise from the intramural portion of the urachus and grow into the wall of the bladder. There may be no evidence of mucosal ulceration.

Epidermoid carcinoma

In practically all instances, marked chronic inflammatory changes with squamous metaplasia of the bladder mucosa (a condition clinically known as *leukoplakia*) coexist with epidermoid carcinoma[64, 65] (Figs. 702 to 704). Epidermoid cancer comprises approximately 5% of all bladder tumors. Grossly, these tumors are ulcerated and necrotic. Microscopically, they are poorly differentiated in most instances (Fig. 705). The prognosis is very poor. Of eighty-four cases reviewed by Newman et al.,[63] 96% were invading muscle at the time of diagnosis. Death within the first year occurred in 59% of the patients.

Other lesions

An apparently benign mucin-secreting *cystadenoma* was reported by Govan.[70]

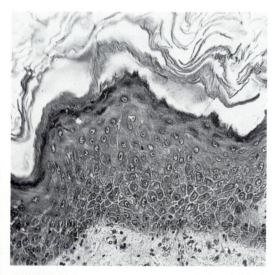

Fig. 703 Extreme squamous metaplasia of bladder. Lining is made of stratified squamous epithelium. (×220; WU neg. 49-2023.)

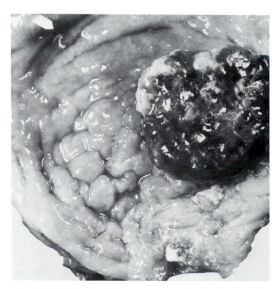

Fig 704 Epidermoid carcinoma of bladder with leukoplakia. (WU neg. 50-4372.)

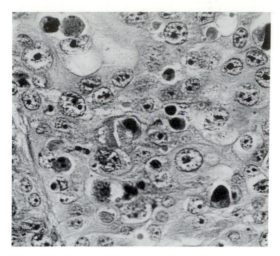

Fig. 705 Poorly differentiated epidermoid carcinoma of bladder. (×400; WU neg. 49-552.)

Five cases of *primary signet ring cell carcinoma* have been reported.[82] The course of the disease was rapidly progressive and fatal in all cases. A case of *malignant teratoma* of the bladder was reported by Pollack.[81] Approximately forty cases of *primary malignant lymphoma* have been described.[86] It may be solitary or multiple. It is covered by normal mucosa and tends to remain localized for a long period of time. The prognosis is favorable. The bladder also can be involved by *leukemia.*[79] The twenty-four reported cases of bladder *pheochromocytoma* were analyzed by Albores-Saavedra et al.[66] These tumors are located within the muscular wall. Approximately one-half of the patients had symptoms produced by the excessive secretion of catecholamines, sometimes associated with voiding. Two tumors were multicentric. Local recurrence was found in two patients and metastases in three. We have also seen *plexiform neurofibromatosis*[69] as well as *malignant bony and cartilaginous tumors* similar to those reported by Pang.[78]

Embryonal rhabdomyosarcoma (sarcoma botryoides) is the most common malignant tumor of the bladder in children.[75] The trigone is the most common location. The tumor has a mucoid, polypoid appearance, stubbornly recurs, infiltrates surrounding tissues, and kills by direct extension rather than by distant metastases[77] (Fig. 706). Microscopically, it shows myxomatous tissue in which small malignant cells are seen (Fig. 707). These are characteristically grouped beneath the epithelium (the so-called "cambium layer"). Cross striations may or may not be present. The prognosis is poor. The greatest chance for cure is radical cystectomy. However, a few cases apparently cured by radiation therapy are now on record.[74] *Hemangiomas* of the bladder usually occur in children and young adults.[71] *Carcinosarcoma* is a rare tumor of elderly individuals associated with rapid growth and poor prognosis.[72] Most cases of *metastatic carcinoma* in the bladder arise in the mammary gland.[80]

Malacoplakia of the bladder is an extremely rare lesion in which there are multiple nodular thickenings of the mucosa and submucosa, usually in the region of the trigone, which may be mistaken for cancer.[67, 83] Microscopically, multiple rounded histiocytes with granular acidophilic cytoplasm accumulate beneath the surface epithelium. In some of these cells, rounded, concentrically layered intracytoplasmic inclusions are seen which stain positively for iron and calcium. They are known as Michaelis-Gutmann bodies or calcospherites.[83] Ultrastructurally, intracellular bacteria are often identified. The presence of transitional forms between them, the lipid inclusions, and the Michaelis-Gutmann bodies suggest that the latter represent the end result of bacterial degradation.[73] Malacoplakia also may involve the renal pelvis and parenchyma, ureter, prostate gland, testis, epididymis, broad ligament, endometrium, retroperitoneal structures, colon, stomach, appendix, lymph nodes, brain, lungs, bones, and skin.[68, 76a, 84, 88]

Bladder calculi (Fig. 708) occur more often in male than in female individuals. In the series reported by Wishard and Nourse,[87] there were 225 male and 17 female patients. In the United States, stones occur most frequently in elderly patients. Usually the stone is single.

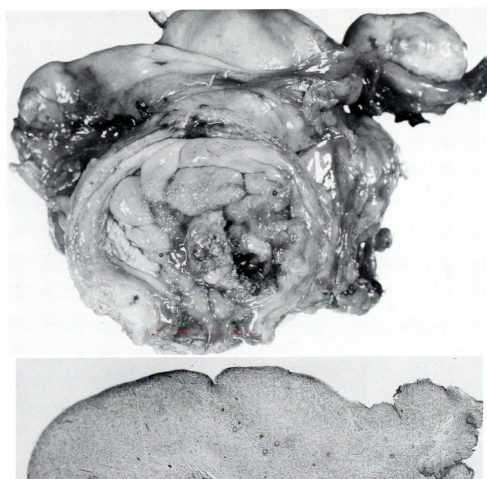

706

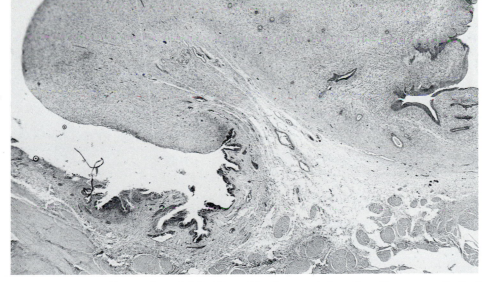

707

Fig. 706 Sarcoma botryoides of bladder with characteristic polypoid masses. Patient, 40-year-old woman, was living and well ten years later. (WU neg. 56-4209.)
Fig. 707 Polypoid mass of tumor in sarcoma botryoides. Lesion occurred in bladder of 4-year-old boy. (Low power; WU neg. 58-1449.)

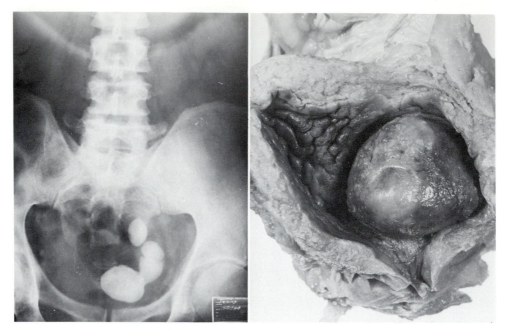

Fig. 708 Several bladder calculi. (WU negs. 49-7082 and 49-7083.)

The most common associated abnormality is hypertrophy of the prostate gland. The stones often consist of phosphate. Urate and oxalate stones are less common.[85] Treatment is removal either via urethra after crushing the stone or by cystotomy. Recurrence appears in about 10% of the patients.

Amyloidosis of the bladder may be the expression of a generalized process or present as a nodular localized mass ("amyloid tumor").[76]

REFERENCES

Cytology

1 Esposti, P. L., Moberger, G., and Zajicek, J.: The cytologic diagnosis of transitional cell tumors of the urinary bladder and its histologic basis, Acta Cytol. (Baltimore) **14**:145-155, 1970.
2 MacFarlane, E. W. E., Ceelen, G. H., and Taylor, J. N.: Urine cytology after treatment of bladder tumors, Acta Cytol. (Baltimore) **8**:288-292, 1964.
2a Melamed, M. D., Voutsa, N. G., and Grabstald, H.: Natural history and clinical behavior of in situ carcinoma of the human urinary bladder, Cancer **17**:1533-1545, 1964.
3 Orell, S. R.: Transitional cell epithelioma of the bladder; correlation of cytologic and histologic diagnosis, Scand. J. Urol. Nephrol. **3**: 93-98, 1969.
4 Papanicolaou, G. N.: Cytology of the urine sediment in neoplasms of the urinary tract, J. Urol. **57**:375-379, 1947.
5 Reichborn-Kjennerud, S., and Hoeg, K.: The value of urine cytology in the diagnosis of recurrent bladder tumors, Acta Cytol. (Baltimore) **16**:269-272, 1972.

Interstitial (Hunner's) cystitis

6 Hunner, G. L.: A rare type of bladder ulcer in women; report of cases, Trans. South. Surg. Gynecol. Assoc. **27**:247-288, 1914.
7 Pool, T. L.: Interstitial cystitis; clinical aspects and treatment, Med. Clin. North Amer. **28**:1008-1015, 1944.
8 Smith, B. H., and Dehner, L. P.: Chronic ulcerating interstitial cystitis (Hunner's ulcer); a study of 28 cases, Arch. Pathol. **93**:76-81, 1972.

Tuberculosis

9 Auerbach, O.: The pathology of urogenital tuberculosis, Int. Clin. **3**:21-61, 1940.

Cystitis glandularis (cystica)

10 Bell, T. E., and Wendel, R. G.: Cystitis glandularis; benign or malignant? J. Urol. **100**: 462-465, 1968.
11 von Brunn, A.: Ueber drüsenähnliche Bildungen in der Schleimhaut des Nierenbeckens des Ureters und der Harnblase beim Menschen, Arch. Mikr. Anat. **41**:294-302, 1893.

12 von Limbeck, R.: Zur Kenntniss der Epithelcysten der Harnblase und der Ureteren, Z. Heilk. **8**:55-66, 1887.

13 Lowry, E. C., Hamm, F. C., and Beard, D. E.: Extensive glandular proliferation of the urinary bladder resembling malignant neoplasm, J. Urol. **52**:133-138, 1944.

14 Patch, F. S.: Pyelitis, ureteritis and cystitis cystica, N. Engl. J. Med. **220**:979-985, 1939.

15 Patch, F. S., and Rhea, L. J.: The genesis and development of Brunn's nests and their relation to cystitis cystica, cystitis glandularis, and primary adenocarcinoma of the bladder, Canad. Med. Assoc. J. **33**:597-606, 1935.

16 Pund, E. R., Yount, H. A., and Blumberg, J. M.: Variations in morphology of urinary bladder epithelium; special reference to cystitis glandularis and carcinoma, J. Urol. **68**:242-251, 1952.

17 Stoerk, O., and Zuckerkandl, O.: Ueber Cystitis glandularis und den Drüsenkrebs der Harnblase, Z. Urol. **1**:133-148, 1907.

18 Ward, A. M.: Glandular neoplasia within the urinary tract; the aetiology of adenocarcinoma of the urothelium with a review of the literature. I. Introduction: the origin of glandular epithelium in the renal pelvis, ureter, and bladder, Virchows Arch. [Pathol. Anat.] **352**:296-311, 1971.

Endometriosis

19 Fein, R. L., and Horton, B. F.: Vesical endometriosis; a case report and review of the literature, J. Urol. **95**:45-50, 1966.

20 Moore, T. D., Herring, A. L., and McCannel, D. A.: Some urologic aspects of endometriosis, J. Urol. **49**:171-177, 1943.

21 O'Conor, V. J., and Greenhill, J. P.: Endometriosis of the bladder and ureter, Surg. Gynecol. Obstet. **80**:113-119, 1945.

Diverticula

22 Abeshouse, B. S., and Goldstein, A. E.: Primary carcinoma in a diverticulum of the bladder; a report of four cases and a review of the literature, J. Urol. **49**:534-557, 1943.

23 Kretschmer, H. L.: Diverticula of the urinary bladder; a clinical study of 236 cases, Surg. Gynecol. Obstet. **71**:491-503, 1940.

24 Kretschmer, H. L., and Barber, K. E.: Carcinoma in a bladder diverticulum; report of a case and review of the literature, J. Urol. **21**:381-394, 1929.

25 Mitchell, R. J., and Hamilton, S. G.: Spontaneous performation of bladder diverticula, Br. J. Surg. **58**:712, 1971.

26 Rathbun, N. P.: Diverticulum of bladder containing large calculus, J. Urol. **12**:181-184, 1924.

27 Spence, H. M., and Baird, S. S.: Vesical diverticula; a clinical study with special reference to treatment, J. Urol. **58**:327-343, 1947.

Carcinoma
Transitional cell carcinoma

28 Anthony, H. M., and Thomas, G. A.: Tumors of the urinary bladder; an analysis of the occupations of 1,030 patients in Leeds, England, J. Natl. Cancer Inst. **45**:879-895, 1970.

29 Ash, J. E.: Epithelial tumors of the bladder, J. Urol. **44**:135-145, 1940.

30 Barsotti, M., and Vigliani, E. C.: Bladder lesions from aromatic amines (Proceedings of the Cancer Prevention Committee), Arch. Indust. Hyg. **5**:50-57, 1952.

31 Bonser, G. M., Faulds, J. S., and Stewart, M. J.: Occupational cancer of the urinary bladder in dyestuffs operatives and of the lung in asbestos textile workers and iron-ore miners, Am. J. Clin. Pathol. **25**:126-134, 1955.

32 Bryan, G. T.: The role of urinary trytophan metabolites in the etiology of bladder cancer, Am. J. Clin. Nutr. **24**:841-847, 1971.

33 Cole, P., Monson, R. R., Haning, H., and Friedell, G. H.: Smoking and cancer of the lower urinary tract, N. Engl. J. Med. **284**:129-134, 1971.

34 Cordonnier, J. J.: Cystectomy for carcinoma of the bladder, J. Urol. **99**:172-173, 1968.

35 Hueper, W. C.: Pathologic aspects of experimental aniline tumors in the bladder of female dogs, Trans. Am. Assoc. Genitourin. Surg. **31**:201-210, 1938.

36 Hueper, W. C.: "Aniline tumors" of the bladder, Arch. Pathol. **25**:856-899, 1938.

37 Javadpour, N., and Mostofi, F. K.: Primary epithelial tumors of the bladder in the first two decades of life, J. Urol. **101**:706-710, 1969.

38 Melamed, M. D., Voutsa, N. G., and Grabstald, H.: Natural history and clinical behavior of in situ carcinoma of the human urinary bladder, Cancer **17**:1533-1545, 1964.

39 Price, J. M., Wear, J. B., Brown, R. R., Satter, E. J., and Olson, C.: Studies on etiology of carcinoma of urinary bladder, J. Urol. **83**:376-382, 1960.

40 Schade, R. O. K., Serck-Hanssen, A., and Swinney, J.: Morphological changes in the ureter in cases of bladder carcinoma, Cancer **27**:1267-1272, 1971.

41 Schade, R. O. K., and Swinney, J.: Pre-cancerous changes in bladder epithelium, Lancet **2**:943-946, 1968.

42 Sharma, T. C., Melamed, M. R., and Whitmore, W. F., Jr.: Carcinoma in situ of the ureter in patients with bladder carcinoma treated by cystectomy, Cancer **26**:583-587, 1970.

43 Ward, A. M.: Glandular metaplasia and mucin production in transitional cell carcinomas of bladder, J. Clin. Pathol. **24**:481, 1971.

Grading of carcinoma

44 Ash, J. E.: Epithelial tumors of the bladder, J. Urol. **44**:135-145, 1940.

45 Bergkvist, A., Ljungqvist, A., and Moberger, G.: Classification of bladder tumours based on the cellular pattern, Acta Chir. Scand. **130**:371-378, 1965.

46 Jewett, H. J., and Blackman, S. S.: Infiltrating carcinoma of the bladder; histologic pattern and degree of cellular differentiation in 97 autopsy cases, J. Urol. **56**:200-210, 1946.

47 Lerman, R. I., Hutter, R. V. P., and Whitmore, W. F., Jr.: Papilloma of the urinary bladder, Cancer **25**:333-342, 1970.

48 Lund, F., and Lundwall, F.: Papillomas of the urinary bladder, Acta Pathol. Microbiol. Scand. **105**(suppl.):118-134, 1955.

49 Melicow, M. M.: The bladder biopsy; an evaluation of the cystoscopic procedure, J. Urol. **56**:339-348, 1946.

50 Mostofi, F. K.: Standardization of nomenclature and criteria for diagnosis of epithelial tumors of urinary bladder, Acta Unio. Intern. Contra Cancr. **16**:310-314, 1960.

Clinicopathologic correlation and prognosis

51 Baker, R.: Pitfalls of clinical versus microscopic staging of cancer of the bladder in relationship to potential curability, Am. Surg. **36**:269-275, 1970.

52 Bell, J. T., Burney, S. W., and Friedell, G. H.: Blood vessel invasion in human bladder cancer, J. Urol. **105**:675-678, 1971.

53 Cordonnier, J. J.: Cystectomy for carcinoma of the bladder, J. Urol. **99**:172-173, 1968.

54 Jewett, H. J.: Carcinoma of the bladder: influence of depth of infiltration on the five-year results following complete extirpation of the primary growth, J. Urol. **67**:672-680, 1952.

55 Jewett, H. J., and Eversole, S. L., Jr.: Carcinoma of the bladder; characteristic modes of local invasion, J. Urol. **83**:383-389, 1960.

56 Jewett, H. J., King, L. R., and Shelley, W. M.: A study of 365 cases of infiltrating bladder cancer; relation of certain pathological characteristics to prognosis after extirpation, J. Urol. **92**:668-678, 1964.

57 Royce, R. K., and Ackerman, L. V.: Carcinoma of the bladder; clinical, therapeutic and pathologic aspects of 135 cases, J. Urol. **65**:66-86, 1951.

58 Sarma, K. P.: The role of lymphoid reaction in bladder cancer, J. Urol. **104**:843-849, 1970.

Adenocarcinoma

59 Engel, R. M., and Wilkinson, H. A.: Bladder extrophy, J. Urol. **104**:699-704, 1970.

60 Mostofi, F. K., Thomson, R. V., and Dean, A. L., Jr.: Mucous adenocarcinoma of the urinary bladder, Cancer **8**:741-758, 1955.

61 Rappoport, A. E., and Nixon, C. E.: Adenocarcinoma of the urachus involving the urinary bladder, Arch. Pathol. **41**:388-397, 1946.

62 Thomas, D. G.: A study of 52 cases of adenocarcinoma of the bladder, Br. J. Urol. **43**:4-15, 1971.

Epidermoid carcinoma

63 Newman, D. M., Brown, J. R., Jay, A. C., and Pontius, E. E.: Squamous cell carcinoma of the bladder, J. Urol. **100**:470-473, 1968.

64 O'Flynn, J. D., and Mullaney, J.: Leukoplakia of the bladder; a report on 20 cases, including 2 cases progressing to squamous cell carcinoma, Br. J. Urol. **39**:461-471, 1967.

65 Royce, R. K., and Ackerman, L. V.: Carcinoma of the bladder, J. Urol. **65**:66-86, 1951.

Other lesions

66 Albores-Saavedra, J., Maldonado, M. E., Ibarra, J., and Rodriguez, H.: Pheochromocytoma of the urinary bladder, Cancer **23**:1110-1118, 1969.

67 Bleisch, V. R., and Konikov, N. F.: Malakoplakia of urinary bladder; report of four cases and discussion of etiology, Arch. Pathol. **54**:388-397, 1952.

68 Brown, R. C., and Smith, B. H.: Malakoplakia of the testis, Am. J. Clin. Pathol. **47**:135-147, 1967.

69 Charron, J. W., and Gariepy, G.: Neurofibromatosis of bladder; case report and review of literature, Can. J. Surg. **13**:303-306, 1970.

70 Govan, A. D. T.: A case of solitary mucus-secreting cystadenoma of the urinary bladder, J. Pathol. Bacteriol. **58**:293-295, 1946.

71 Hendry, W. F., and Vinnicombe, J.: Haemangioma of bladder in children and young adults, Br. J. Urol. **43**:209-216, 1971.

72 Holtz, F., Fox, J. E., and Abell, M. R.: Carcinosarcoma of the urinary bladder, Cancer **29**:294-304, 1972.

73 Lou, T. Y., and Teplitz, C.: Ultrastructural morphogenesis of malakoplakia and so-called Michaelis-Gutmann bodies, Lab. Invest. **28**:390-391, 1973 (abstract).

74 Mackenzie, A. R., Sharma, T. C., Whitmore, W. F., Jr., and Melamed, M. R.: Non-extirpative treatment of myosarcomas of the bladder and prostate, Cancer **28**:329-334, 1971.

75 Mackenzie, A. R., Whitmore, W. F., Jr., and Melamed, M. R.: Myosarcomas of the bladder and prostate, Cancer **22**:833-844, 1968.

76 Malek, R. S., Greene, L. F., and Farrow, G. M.: Amyloidosis of the urinary bladder, Br. J. Urol. **43**:189-200, 1971.

76a Moore, W. M., III, Stokes, T. L., and Cabanas, V. Y.: Malakoplakia of the skin; report of a case, Am. J. Clin. Pathol. **59**:218-221, 1973.

77 Mostofi, F. K., and Morse, W. H.: Polypoid

rhabdomyosarcoma (sarcoma botryoides) of the bladder, J. Urol. **67**:681-687, 1952.

78 Pang, L. S. C.: Bony and cartilaginous tumours of the urinary bladder, J. Pathol. Bacteriol. **76**:357-377, 1958.

79 Pentecost, C. L., and Pizzolato, P.: Involvement of the genitourinary tract in leukemia, J. Urol. **53**:725-731, 1945.

80 Perez-Mesa, C., Pickren, J. W., Woodruff, M. N., and Mohallatee, A.: Metastatic carcinoma of the urinary bladder from primary tumors in the mammary gland of female patients, Surg. Gynecol. Obstet. **121**:813-818, 1965.

81 Pollack, A. D.: Malignant teratoma of the urinary bladder, Am. J. Pathol. **12**:561-568, 1936.

82 Rosas-Uribe, A., and Luna, M. A.: Primary signet ring cell carcinoma of the urinary bladder, Arch. Pathol. **88**:294-297, 1969.

83 Smith, B. H.: Malacoplakia of the urinary tract, Am. J. Clin. Pathol. **43**:409-417, 1965.

84 Terner, J. H., and Lattes, R.: Malakoplakia of the colon and retroperitoneum, Am. J. Clin. Pathol. **44**:20-31, 1965.

85 Twinem, F. P., and Langdon, B. B.: Surgical management of bladder stone, J. Urol. **66**:201-212, 1951.

86 Wang, C. C., Scully, R. E., and Leadbetter, W. F.: Primary malignant lymphoma of the urinary bladder, Cancer **24**:772-776, 1969.

87 Wishard, W. N., and Nourse, M. H.: Vesical calculus with report of a gigantic stone in the female bladder, J. Urol. **63**:794-801, 1950.

88 Yunis, E. J., Estevez, J., Pinzon, G. J., and Moran, T. J.: Malakoplakia; discussion of pathogenesis and report of three cases including one of fatal gastric and colonic involvement, Arch. Pathol. **83**:180-187, 1967.

17 **Male reproductive system**

Prostate and seminal vesicles
Testis
Epididymis and spermatic cord
Penis

Prostate and seminal vesicles

PROSTATE
Introduction

Pathologic study of the prostate generally is made on tissue obtained by needle biopsy, transurethral resection, suprapubic prostatectomy, and, infrequently, radical perineal prostatectomy. When the entire prostate is submitted, large sections should be made of the posterior lobe and adjoining seminal vesicles.

Transurethral biopsy is an inadequate method for the detection of early cases of prostatic carcinoma. Since most cases arise in the periphery of the gland, the material obtained usually will be negative except for advanced cases. Furthermore, it is impractical to section all of the material usually submitted. McHeffey[1] examined ten pieces of tissue from each of fifty patients and then took time to examine all the remaining pieces from the same fifty patients. One additional carcinoma was found.

Nodular hyperplasia

Benign prostatic hypertrophy is the usual name applied to a common benign condition of the prostate occurring in elderly individuals, often resulting in some degree of urinary obstruction and sometimes requiring operative intervention. Moore's *nodular hyperplasia* is a more exact designation.[4] The disease increases in incidence with age until at 80 years about 75% of all men are affected to some degree. As Badenoch[2] put it, nodular hyperplasia of the prostate occurs "in saints and sinners, in fat men and thin, in parsons with large families and monks with none, in postmen and prime ministers."*

*From Badenoch, A.: Benign enlargement of the prostate, Trans. Med. Soc. Lond. **86:**34-40, 1970.

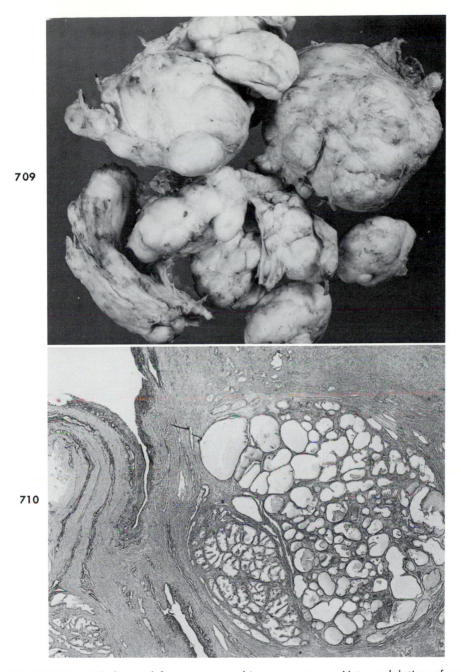

Fig. 709 Material obtained from a suprapubic prostatectomy. Note nodulation of surface. Weight, 360 gm. (WU neg. 50-1685.)

Fig. 710 Early hyperplasia of prostate beginning in suburethral tissues. (Low power; WU neg. 49-5634.)

The involved areas may be excised by suprapubic prostatectomy, transurethral resection, or rarely by perineal prostatectomy.[3] The glands are enlarged, averaging about 100 gm, but extremely large glands (weighing up to 820 gm) have been reported.[5] On cross section, multiple spherical, yellowish nodules project above the cut surface (Fig. 709). The stroma consists of connective tissue and smooth muscle. The early nodule is slightly elevated and gray or grayish yellow with a finely or coarsely granular cut surface.

Suprapubic prostatectomy is the enucleation of *newly formed nodules only*. The prostate itself is not resected. After suprapubic prostatectomy, the compressed posterior and lateral lobes expand by stromal growth to surround the prostatic urethra. Because this operation is not a complete prostatectomy, nodular hyperplasia can recur. Over thirty cases of recurrence have been reported.[4] The microscopic description, according to Moore,[4] is as follows:

> The earliest lesion that has been observed is a proliferation of the perivascular, periductal or intralobular connective tissue in an area bounded medially by the urethra, anteriorly by the capsule and posteriorly and laterally by the sweeping ducts of the lateral lobes, and in the tissues that constitute the middle lobe [Fig. 710]. The type of connective tissue involved depends in large part on the area. Near the urethra, the proliferation is about small sinusoidal spaces while in the glandular parts the periductal or intralobular stroma is hyperplastic.*

With increased growth, the lateral lobes of the prostate are pushed aside and compressed. The hyperplastic nodules most frequently are derived from the stroma and glands about the urethra and the acini anterior and medial to the ducts of the lateral lobes. The true middle lobe is less frequently involved, the anterior lobe rarely, and the posterior lobe very rarely, if at all.

The well-developed nodules are divided into lobules by an interlobular and intralobular stroma. The typical epithelial cell in nodular hyperplasia resembles that of the adult prostate but has little or no secretory activity. The glands are lined by tall epithelium, sometimes with papillary infoldings, and have a well-developed basement membrane. The stroma differs from normal in that there is more smooth muscle and absence of elastic tissue. Periurethral tissues have abundant elastic tis-

sue. In periductal hyperplasia, the proliferation may be concentric or eccentric. In intralobular hyperplasia, there may be a pure stromal reaction or a combined stromal and epithelial hyperplasia. However, nodular hyperplasia usually is associated with the development of masses of glandular tissue. Nodules composed only of smooth muscle arising in periurethral tissue represent a variant in which the stromal hyperplasia does not include glands.

It is evident from histologic studies that the important point is not whether the periurethral or prostatic glands are involved but whether the lesion occurs in a glandular acinus, the duct of which empties into the urethra above or below the caudal extremity of the verumontanum. The earliest nodules may be demonstrated in acini of the middle and lateral lobes of the prostate and about the collicular and subtrigonal periurethral glands, all structures which empty cephalad to the verumontanum. In only one out of 700 patients has a nodule been demonstrated in the posterior lobe of the prostate, which empties caudal to this point.[4]

The only possible conclusion from these morphologic observations is that the stroma of the prostate cephalad to the verumontanum reacts to different stimuli or to a greater extent to the same stimuli as stroma caudal to the verumontanum. The posterior lobe of the prostate may be biologically different from the other lobes. In the senile prostate, atrophy occurs at an earlier age, corpora amylacea are more abundant, and sclerotic atrophy and stromal fibrosis are more marked in the posterior lobe than in the other lobes.

Infarction

Infarction of the prostate has been well described by Abeshouse.[6] It occurs predominantly in large prostates with nodular hyperplasia. Its reported incidence is probably related to the thoroughness of the microscopic examination. In very carefully studied glands, Moore[11] demonstrated in-

---

*From Moore, R. A.: Benign hypertrophy of the prostate; a morphological study, J. Urol. **50:**680-710, 1943.

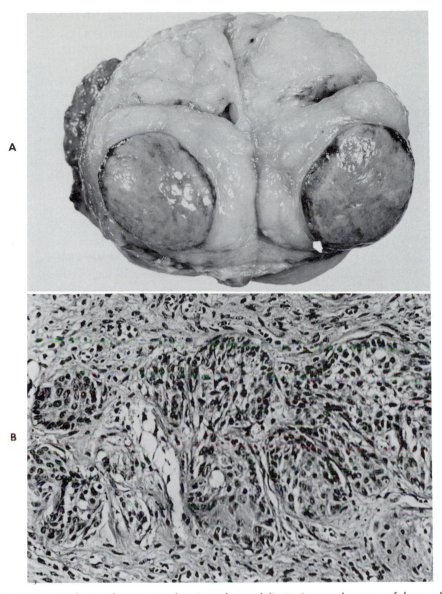

Fig. 711 A, Infarct of prostate showing sharp delimitation and areas of hemorrhage. Nodular hyperplasia is also present. **B,** Margin of infarct shown in **A** demonstrating prominent squamous metaplasia often mistaken for carcinoma. (**A,** WU neg. 48-3984; **B,** ×100; WU neg. 48-4162.)

farction in 25%. Baird et al.[7] found sixty-six instances in 352 surgically enucleated prostates. However, the frequency of clinical manifestations of infarction is much lower. True infarcts occurring on a vascular basis should be distinguished from the areas of necrosis involving the epithelium of a gland or group of glands that are commonly seen in nodular hyperplasia.

The mechanism of infarction is unknown but may be related to the presence of infection, trauma due to an indwelling catheter, cystitis, or prostatitis. The urethral arteries penetrate to the prostatic vesicular junction and then turn distally in a course parallel to the urethral surface, bringing blood to the area of usual hyperplastic growth. Damage or thrombosis of these arteries causes infarction to a major portion of a hyperplastic gland.[8] Baird et al.[7] showed that the size and number of infarctions are related directly to the degree of prostatic hyperplasia.

Grossly, the lesions vary in size from a few millimeters to 4 cm or 5 cm. They are speckled grayish yellow and often contain streaks of blood. The peripheral margins are usually sharp and hemorrhagic and may impinge upon the urethra[7] (Fig. 711, A).

Microscopically, an ischemic infarction shows areas of central coagulation and necrosis with complete destruction of the muscle, epithelium, and connective tissue. The most striking changes are in the periphery. Extremely prominent epithelial metaplasia may occur (Fig. 711, B). True squamous metaplasia is infrequent, and intercellular bridges and keratinization are rare. Mitotic figures are rare, and direct invasion of surrounding prostatic tissue is absent. It is unlikely that metaplasia will be mistaken for squamous carcinoma if the pathologist remembers that metaplasia is normally associated with infection and is confined to the ducts. Epidermoid carcinoma of the prostate is a pathologic rarity.

Clinically, infarction occasionally causes acute urinary retention through rapid prostatic enlargement.[10] Because the infarcts are adjacent to the urethra, gross hematuria may occur. Diffuse oozing of blood from the overlying mucosa may be seen cystoscopically.[12] A certain proportion of prostatic infarcts are accompanied by elevation of the serum acid phosphatase (30% in our experience).[13]

Abscess

In the past, most prostatic abscesses were the result of gonorrhea. The pattern has changed, the majority now having an obstructive etiology representing secondary infection of the prostate from an infected pool of residual urine. *Escherichia coli* is the organism usually responsible. Of the sixty-seven patients reported by Trapnell and Roberts,[15] 36% presented with acute urinary retention and 31% with perineal or suprapubic pain. Transurethral evacuation is the treatment of choice.[14]

Calculi

Prostatic calculi usually are associated with infection. They may occur concomitantly with carcinoma or nodular hyperplasia. The frequency with which they appear with either is approximately 7%.[16]

Young[20] studied 100 cases of prostatic calculi and found stones located in the utricle in one instance and within the prostatic fossa following prostatectomy in five instances. Calculi found in the prostatic urethra may have their origin from the bladder, ureter, or kidney pelvis and are not true prostatic calculi.[18] In Young's group[20] of forty-four operative specimens, infection invariably was present either in the prostatic duct or in acini about the calcification. Calculi may form in the ducts or acini that are blocked by bacterial or epithelial debris.

The corpora amylacea may act as a nucleus for stone formation. Certainly, improper drainage of the prostate due to stricture of the vesicle neck may lead to infection and the formation of calculi. When acini become infected and dilated, small bits of calcium are deposited upon the corpora amylacea and other foreign substances.[18] Calculi usually are present in the line of cleavage between nodular hyperplasia and the posterior prostatic lamella.

The nucleus of a prostatic calculus is composed of corpora amylacea, blood clot, epithelial detritus, bacteria, or tissue. The inorganic elements usually are inorganic salts—calcium phosphate, magnesium phosphate, aminomagnesium phosphate, potassium phosphate, calcium carbonate, and calcium oxalate. Corpora amylacea probably represent inspissated prostatic secretion. Chemically, they are mainly composed of glycoprotein and mucoprotein.[19]

Calculi are diagnosed more frequently by roentgenographic examination than by rectal examination because the stones are

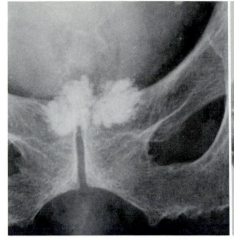
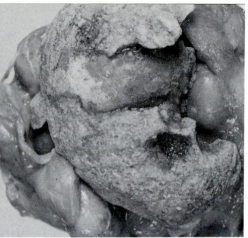

712

713

Fig. 712 Radiopaque calculi in prostate. On palpation, such lesions are often mistaken for carcinoma.
Fig. 713 Large prostate with radiopaque calculus. (WU neg. 48-5595.)

radiopaque (Fig. 712). Because of their hardness, they may be erroneously diagnosed as carcinoma. If the process becomes advanced, prostatectomy is indicated[17] (Fig. 713).

Granulomatous prostatitis

Granulomatous prostatitis is relatively rare.[25] Its pathogenesis is probably related to partial obstruction of the prostatic ducts and urethritis. These changes are accompanied by destruction of the epithelial cells of the ducts and acini plus escape of inflammatory products and altered prostatic secretion into the interstitial tissue.

Grossly, the consistency of the prostate may be firm or stony hard. Invariably, nodular hyperplasia is present. On section, the architecture of the gland may be obliterated. The areas of involvement appear as yellow granular nodules.

Microscopically, granulomatous prostatitis may be confused with neoplasia or tuberculosis. In some areas, the normal acini and ducts are completely destroyed and replaced by an exudate of plasma cells, lymphocytes, and, in part, large, pale-staining mononuclear cells with eosinophilic or vacuolated cytoplasm (Fig. 714). Tubercle-like reaction with foreign body giant cells is seen. At times, collections of poly-morphonuclear leukocytes and detritus are seen within the ducts. The infiltrate has a characteristic lobular distribution. There are no crystals, caseation necrosis, or tubercle bacilli.

Clinically, this lesion usually occurs in patients past 50 years of age. In nine of thirty-two cases reported by Tanner and McDonald,[25] the preoperative diagnosis was probable carcinoma. The firmness of the lesion is caused by replacement of areas of the prostate by dense fibrous tissue.

Of the seventy patients studied by Kelalis et al.,[21] 18% presented with high temperature, followed by symptoms of nonspecific prostatitis and a suggestion of malignancy on rectal palpation. This triad should suggest a diagnosis of granulomatous prostatitis, although microscopic confirmation should be obtained.

Granulomatous prostatitis should be differentiated from the so-called *eosinophilic prostatitis* (or "allergic granuloma" of the prostate), a rare entity characterized microscopically by focal necrosis and massive infiltration by eosinophils.[22, 23] Some of the cases of eosinophilic prostatitis are associated with an allergic history.[26] Others have been found to be the result of parasitic infestation.[24]

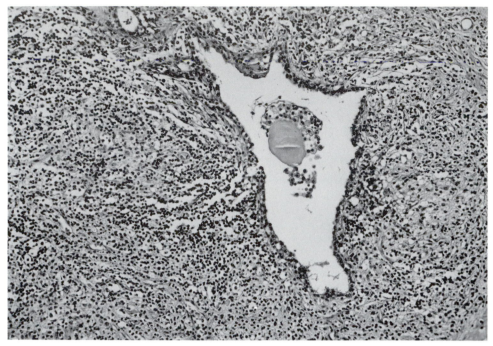

Fig. 714 Granulomatous prostatitis often mistaken for carcinoma by clinical examination. Note inflammatory process around duct. (×130; WU neg. 58-1450.)

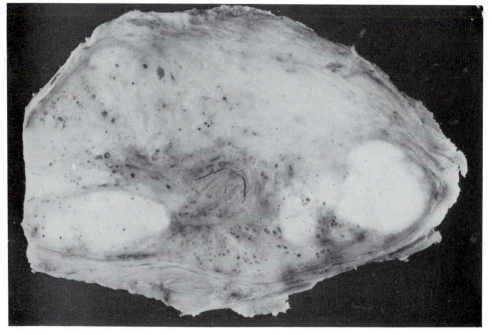

Fig. 715 Caseous tuberculosis of prostate.

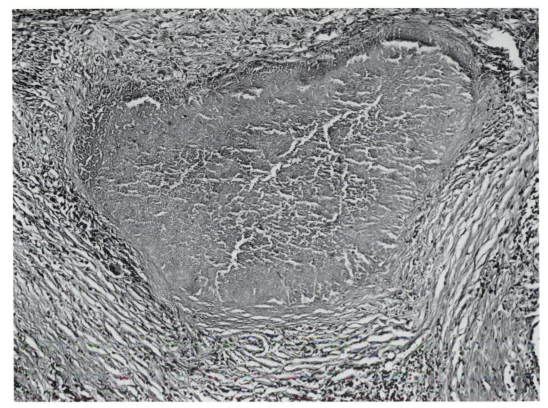

Fig. 716 Tuberculosis of prostate. Large focus of caseation necrosis is surrounded by inflamed and fibrosed stroma containing occasional giant cells. (×80; WU neg. 73-58.)

Tuberculosis

Tuberculosis of the prostate usually follows hematogenous spread from the lungs or, less often, from foci in bones. Autopsy studies show the prostate frequently involved by the infection when tuberculosis of the male genitalia exists. Of 105 cases studied by Auerbach,[27] 100 had prostatic involvement, and in thirty-five the prostate was the only tuberculous organ. Rarely, tuberculosis directly invades the prostate from the urethra. Two of twenty cases of tuberculosis of the prostate described by Moore[28] were infected in this manner.

Grossly, the lesions most frequently appear in the lateral lobes and are bilateral much more often than unilateral. The initial lesion arises in the interstitial tissue but quickly spreads to the acini and forms a caseous mass with a connective tissue wall. Confluent caseous zones occur with liquefaction and cavitation, until finally the pros-

tate becomes an enlarged mass of multiple cavities (Fig. 715). If this tuberculous process becomes secondarily infected, it often perforates into the urethra and involves the urinary bladder. Fourteen of the 105 cases reported by Auerbach[27] showed secondary involvement of the bladder. With still further spread, sinus tracts may form into the rectum, perineum, and peritoneum. At times, healing occurs with calcification which may be seen by radiographic examination. It is only in the late stages that the prostate becomes shrunken, fibrotic, and hard.

Microscopically, tuberculosis of the prostate usually shows extensive caseation with incomplete fibrous encapsulation (Fig. 716). Many of these areas are confluent. There is little tendency for the formation of typical tubercles.

Early lesions in the prostate are seldom discovered on palpation. It is only when the disease is advanced that enlargement occurs and fluctuant, tender zones may be felt. With healing, the hard areas may simulate carcinoma. If tuberculosis of the prostate is suspected, radical perineal prostatectomy is the operation of choice inasmuch as transurethral resection may cause spread.[29]

Other infections

We have had two patients with *blastomycosis* of the prostate. In both, the physical examination suggested carcinoma. Transurethral resections showed granulomatous processes containing double-contoured bodies characteristic of blastomycosis. Most of the bodies were within giant cells. A few presented bud formation. The Schiff stain clearly revealed brilliant pink capsules. In one instance, the patient had an elevated, ulcerated skin lesion which, on biopsy, showed blastomycosis.

Tumors
Biopsy

Many special types of needles and punches have been devised for obtaining prostatic tissue.[32] Carcinoma of the prostate usually arises in the peripheral portions of the gland, so that before a positive diagnosis can be made by transurethral biopsy, the disease is advanced. In most instances, a positive diagnosis can be obtained only by aspiration or Silverman needle biopsy if performed by a surgeon experienced in this method (Fig. 717). The risk of implantation following needle biopsy is extremely low.[30]

An increasing number of transrectal needle biopsies of the prostate have been done for debatable nodules. This procedure has proved to be accurate in needling the nodule and also has been rewarding because of the adequate material that is regularly obtained.[31]

In the interpretation of needle biopsies, it should be remembered that there are normally bundles of striated muscle within the prostate gland. Therefore, the presence of prostatic glands adjacent to a skeletal

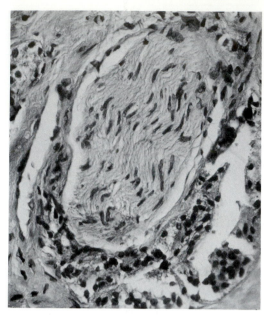

Fig. 717 Needle biopsy demonstrating well-differentiated carcinoma with perineurial invasion in one area. Patient had well-delimited small nodule in prostate. Transurethral resection did not show carcinoma. (×400; WU neg. 52-2874.)

muscle fiber is not necessarily evidence of carcinoma, nor is the presence of skeletal muscle adjacent to a cancer evidence that the tumor has extended outside the gland. The epithelium of the seminal vesicle and ejaculatory ducts, which is occasionally included in prostatic biopsies, has a complex papillary arrangement that may be confused with prostatic carcinoma. A clue to the nature of this epithelium is the presence of abundant lipofuscin granules in the cytoplasm.

Cytology

The use of prostatic cytology as a screening test for cancer in asymptomatic patients is futile.[36-38] Riaboff[39] found only one cancer in 1,738 patients over the age of 50 years. Factors that diminish the practical value of cytologic examination are the large number of false negative diagnoses and the insensitivity of the method for the detection of early cases. Prostatic massage alone yields a 25% to 30% rate of insufficient material. If a voided urine specimen is taken following massage, the rate falls to 3.9%.[36] Clarke and Bamford[33] reviewed the literature in 1960 and found that of 324 patients with prostatic cancer, cytology was positive in 72.8% and suspicious in 10.2%. In over 3,963 patients with benign lesions, cytology was falsely positive in twelve patients (0.3%). Whereas the results of prostatic cytology are comparable to those from other areas of the body, the method has no advantage over direct perineal needle biopsy of suspicious lesions.

Esposti[34] has examined 1,100 patients at the Karolinska Institute with transrectal aspiration biopsy of the prostate. Satisfactory material was obtained in 98% of the cases. Malignant cells were found in 336 cases, 162 of which could be checked by histologic examination. There were no false positives. False negatives, however, amounted to 10%. In a subsequent study,[35] 469 cases of prostatic carcinoma were divided according to cytologic criteria into three grades. It was found that 73% of the 131 patients with Grade I (highly differentiated) cancer, 61% of the 265 with Grade II (moderately differentiated) cancer, and 29% of the seventy-three with Grade III (poorly differentiated) cancer were alive after three years of hormone treatment.

Frozen section

Frozen section of firm areas in the prostate close to the capsule offers the best chances of detecting an adenocarcinoma. The type of perineal exposure advocated by Hudson et al.[42] facilitates frozen section. They obtain a representative section of the entire posterior lobe. If the lesion can be diagnosed as cancer, immediate therapy can be instituted.

Often, adenocarcinoma of the prostate is extremely well differentiated, and a frozen section diagnosis may not be possible. Totten et al.[43] emphasized that normal prostatic glands have a double layer of cells with flattened basal cells against the basement membrane. In cancerous glands, there is a single layer of cells with promi-

nent nucleoli. These findings are particularly helpful in well-differentiated carcinomas in which the diagnosis must be based on the crowding of glands and on cytologic abnormalities. Perineurial invasion is definite evidence of carcinoma. The accuracy of frozen section diagnosis is high. In forty-five frozen sections reported by Culp and McDonald,[41] there were no false positives, and all forty cases diagnosed as cancer were substantiated.

Clinical appraisal of single nodules is extremely difficult. On rectal examination, non-neoplastic process such as tuberculosis, infarct or a calculus can closely mimic carcinoma. In forty-six patients on whom a perineal prostatectomy was done on the basis of a clinical diagnosis of carcinoma, no carcinoma was found in nineteen patients.[40]

Adenocarcinoma

The frequency of cancer of the prostate increases with age. This fact is well substantiated by observations at autopsy. Incidental carcinoma of the prostate often is found at postmortem examination. The frequency varies between 15% and 46%.[54, 58, 59] The more thorough the histologic examination and the older the patient, the higher the frequency.

In sixty-nine occult carcinomas studied by Franks,[54] fifty-two showed invasion of periprostatic tissue and twenty-two showed perineurial invasion. Distant metastases were not present in any case, but direct spread involved the seminal vesicles in four, the base of the bladder in one, and the internal sphincter in one. It is often emphasized that the large majority of prostatic carcinomas arise in the posterior lobe (Fig. 718). Although this statement is basically correct, it is somewhat ambiguous because of the various definitions regarding the boundaries of this lobe.[72, 77] More important than this is the fact that most prostatic cancers arise in the very periphery of the gland, whether posteriorly, laterally, or anteriorly, with sparing of the periurethral region except for the late

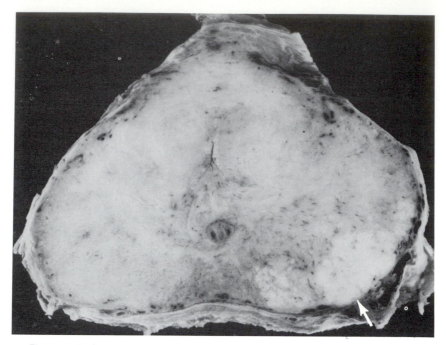

Fig. 718 Early carcinoma of prostate arising in subcapsular area (arrow).

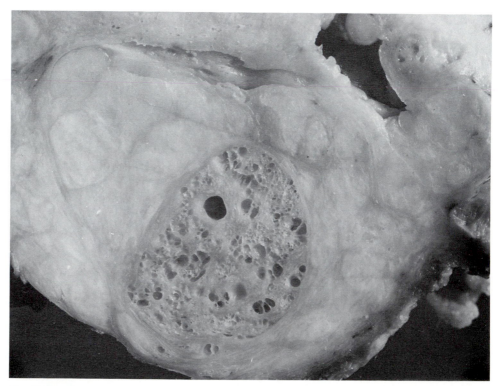

Fig. 719 Large prostatic cancer surrounding well-delimited honeycombed area of nodular hyperplasia. (WU neg. 54-3099.)

stages of the disease. Thus, a division of the prostate into an inner (periurethral) and an outer (cortical) zone correlates better with the pathology of the organ than the time-honored division into anterior, middle, lateral, and posterior lobes.[48] The inner prostate is the primary site for nodular hyperplasia, whereas the outer prostate is the site of predilection for adenocarcinoma.[47, 63]

It is rare for carcinoma to occur in a hyperplastic gland. Franks[55] believes that some adenocarcinomas can arise from zones of postsclerotic hyperplasia.

Grossly, carcinoma of the prostate may be difficult to see but usually can be identified as a gray or yellowish, poorly delineated, firm area (Fig. 719). Minute areas of necrosis may occur within it. When advanced, the tumor extends to surrounding structures such as the seminal vesicles, prostatic urethra, and bladder.

Microscopically, adenocarcinomas of the prostate show variable patterns of growth. Anaplastic tumors are diagnosed easily, but more differentiated ones may closely resemble normal prostate and be diagnosed with difficulty. Totten et al.[74] recognized four major microscopic patterns of carcinoma which may be seen in combination: cribriform, diffuse individual cell infiltration, medium-sized-gland carcinoma and small-gland carcinoma. The first two varieties are easily recognized. In carcinomas composed of medium-sized glands, the most important diagnostic feature is the *architecture* of the lesion: the acini are smaller than normal, have a smooth inner surface, and are closely spaced, with very scanty intervening stroma. Obvious cytologic features of malignancy may or may not be present. On the other hand, small-gland carcinomas are diagnosed mainly on the basis of the *cytologic abnormalities*. The nuclei are enlarged, irregular, and hyperchromatic and have *prominent nucleoli*. Mitoses are significant if present, but they are rarely seen in this type of tumor. The presence of a double cell layer in a given gland is evidence against

carcinoma, but its absence in a small gland is not significant. Something similar can be said in regard to the presence or absence of "basement membrane" around a gland.

Some prostatic cancers are very soft and bright yellow and contain a large amount of cytoplasmic fat. The presence of perineurial invasion by prostatic glands is absolute proof of carcinoma. Rodin et al.[67] have shown that this finding does not represent permeation of perineural lymphatic vessels, but rather spread of the tumor along a plane of lesser tissue resistance.

Azzopardi and Evans[44] noted the presence of argentaffin cells in 80% of normal and hyperplastic prostates and in 10% of the prostatic adenocarcinomas. They believe that these cells are an essential component of the tumor, arising by divergent differentiation. In support of their view, they described a prostatic neoplasm which was in part adenocarcinoma and in part carcinoid tumor. Electron microscopic studies are needed to substantiate this interesting observation.

Microscopic grading of prostatic adenocarcinomas has been found to correlate well with the survival rate and the response to medical and surgical therapy.[61, 65, 75]

Prostatic carcinomas may have multiple foci of origin.[49] Focal metaplastic changes in the prostate may be mistaken for carcinoma (Fig. 720). It is generally believed that prostatic adenocarcinomas do not secrete mucin, this impression being based mainly on the use of the relatively insensitive Mayer's mucicarmine stain. On the contrary, it has been demonstrated that approximately two-thirds of prostatic cancers secrete an acidic mucosubstance of one kind or another, easily demonstrable with Alcian blue or colloidal iron.[57, 60] This pattern of secretion is not found in normal prostatic epithelium, which secretes mucosubstances of neutral character.

It is sometimes very difficult to determine the primary source of advanced cancer in the region of the prostate. The same problem may arise when prostatic carci-

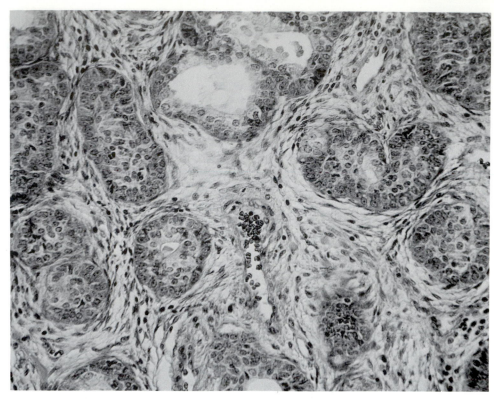

Fig. 720 Focal metaplastic changes in prostate. Such changes do not represent cancer, nor has patient been treated by estrogen. (×275; WU neg. 66-7568; slide contributed by Dr. F. K. Mostofi, Washington, D. C.)

nomas invade the region of the rectum. The prostatic origin of such tumors is definite if tissue from a metastasis or from a locally invasive mass has an acid phosphatase activity exceeding 10 units.[52]

Clinicopathologic correlation

Cancers of the prostate are divided into clinical, latent, and occult types. The *clinical* tumor produces local symptoms and is confirmed by biopsy; the *latent* cancer is unsuspected clinically and found incidentally in specimens of prostatectomy performed for nodular hyperplasia or other benign condition; *occult* cancers result in distant metastases while the primary tumor remains clinically undetected. Staging of prostatic cancer is of greater significance. Stage A tumors correspond to the latent neoplasms of the previous classification; Stage B cancers are clinically detectable but confined within the prostatic capsule;

in Stage C, the disease has spread outside the capsule; in stage D, there are distant metastases.

Carcinoma of the prostate may regress and become soft following estrogen therapy and orchiectomy. Histologically, the tumor cells become pyknotic, show increased staining density, and frequently have naked nuclei (Figs. 721 and 722). Vacuolization of the cytoplasm occurs. The cytoplasmic membrane may rupture, and in some instances only shadows of cells remain. With estrogen therapy, squamous metaplasia may occur in the nonneoplastic glands[45] (Fig. 723). Wattenberg and Rose[76] also found increased stratification with true squamous metaplasia in the urethra and in the verumontanum (Fig. 724). These changes are specific estrogenic effects.

It must be remembered that hormonal sensitivity of prostatic carcinomas is not

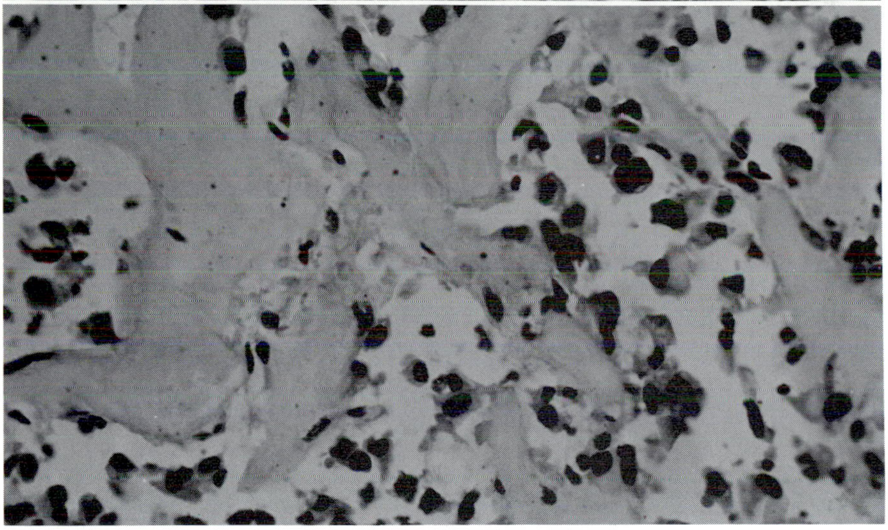

Fig. 721 Fairly well-differentiated adenocarcinoma of prostate before treatment with stilbestrol. (×400; WU neg. 50-956.)
Fig. 722 Same adenocarcinoma shown in Fig. 721 taken after two years of treatment with stilbestrol. Note naked nuclei, prominent nuclear aberrations, and fibrotic stroma. (×400; WU neg. 50-957.)

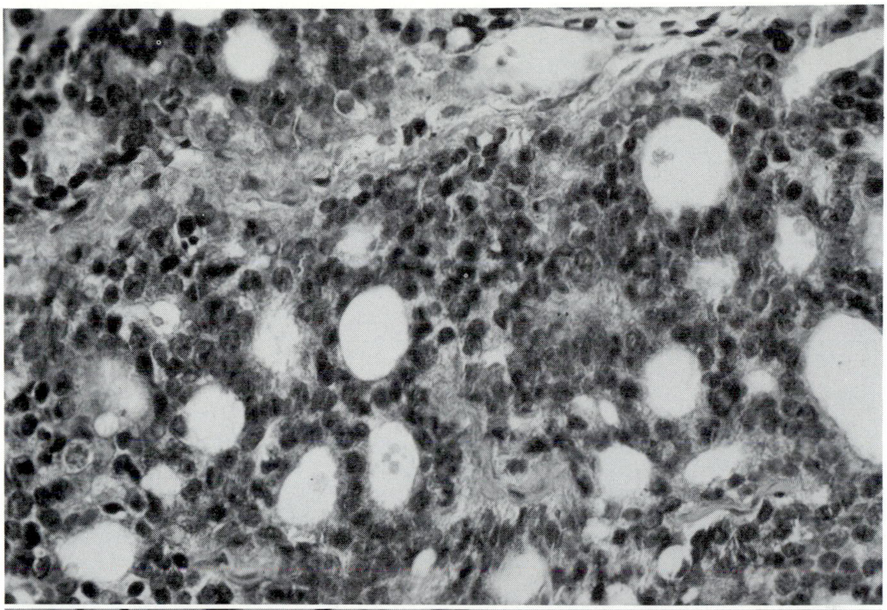

an all-or-none phenomenon but varies in both the primary lesion and its metastases.[56] Intraductal hyperplasia and stromal proliferation in the breast may cause the patient to complain of sore breasts and discharge from the nipples. Rarely, true acinar proliferation and lobule formation may occur.[69] As shown by randomized studies, excessive estrogen therapy may result in an increase of coronary artery disease and myocardial infarction.[51]

Suprapubic prostatectomy and simple perineal prostatectomy do not remove completely the compressed lateral and posterior lobes. Carcinoma may develop in these lobes many years after operation.

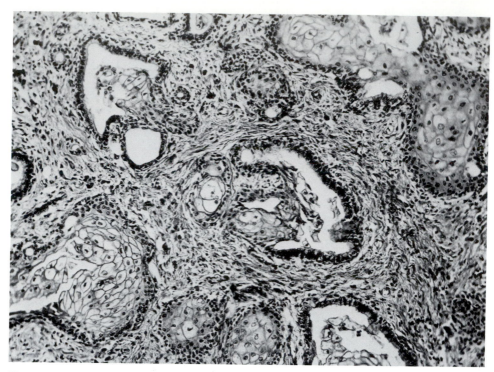

Fig. 723 Extremely prominent squamous metaplasia in prostate following stilbestrol treatment. There is no evidence of carcinoma. (×140; WU neg. 49-347.)

The most common site of metastatic involvement is the skeleton, particularly the pelvis, sacrum, and lower vertebral column. Metastases are usually multiple and osteoblastic, although they may be solitary and osteolytic. They can simulate radiographically Paget's disease and, rarely, osteosarcoma.[64] Sometimes the appearance of a bone metastasis precedes for several years the urologic manifestations. Rarely, metastatic prostatic carcinoma is found unexpectedly in orchiectomy specimens. Prostatic carcinoma also may metastasize to the breast, sometimes bilaterally, particularly in patients taking estrogens.[68] This phenomenon is often confused clinically with gynecomastia and microscopically with primary breast carcinoma. Butler et al.[50] described nineteen patients who presented with supraclavicular lymph node enlargement as the initial manifestation of prostatic cancer: eighteen of the nodes were situated on the left side. Most of the tumors were poorly differentiated and not particularly suggestive of a

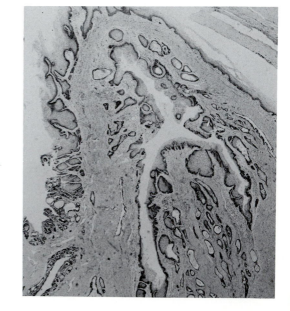

Fig. 724 Microscopic section of verumontanum from patient receiving estrogens. Extreme squamous metaplasia is present. (Low power; WU neg. 50-958.)

prostatic origin on microscopic examination.

When prostatic carcinoma extends to the bones, surrounding soft tissue, or lymph nodes, the serum acid phosphatase level may become elevated. This elevation is evidence of advanced disease, the only exception being transient elevation in a prostatic infarct, after surgery in the area or following a prostatic massage. Removal of an area of infarction promptly returns the acid prosphatase level to normal.[71] Deming and Hovenanian[53] demonstrated by heterologous growth of prostatic cancer that the acid enzyme factor was low in some clinical cases even with extensive metastatic carcinoma.

The clinical detection of carcinoma of the prostate by rectal examination often is difficult because early carcinomas cannot be distinguished from benign prostatic nodules.[62] Some authors advocate more frequent perineal exploration of debatable nodules with frozen section examination, followed by radical perineal prostatectomy if cancer is found. Usually this method is stated to be the only certain method of curing early carcinoma of the prostate. The number of such operations in any given hospital is small. Jewett[61] reported radical perineal prostatectomy in 111 patients with clinically localized and discrete cancer, 103 of whom were followed for a period of at least fifteen years. None of the patients with poorly differentiated cancer or with tumor extending microscopically beyond the prostate survived without recurrence. On the other hand, twenty-eight (33%) of eighty-six patients with limited, well-differentiated, or moderately differentiated cancer lived fifteen years free of disease.

Radical prostatectomy results in impotence in almost 100% of the cases. The incidence of urinary incontinence, once very high, has now been markedly reduced due to technical improvements in the vesicourethral anastomosis.[61] Even discounting this morbidity, the normal long-life history of patients with carcinoma of the prostate

is sufficient argument for many urologists not to pursue perineal prostatectomy enthusiastically. Thirty-five patients with prostatic carcinomas found unexpectedly in the specimens from operations to relieve urinary obstruction were followed eight or more years. None died of carcinoma.[66]

We have found that the pathologist can help the clinician in deciding whether there should be further therapy for patients in whom cancer is found unexpectedly in suprapubic enucleations. Patients with small, well-differentiated cancer, regardless of the use of antiandrogenic therapy, have a ten-year survival rate that is almost the same as that for noncancerous male patients of the same age group. For such patients we favor no further therapy. However, patients with large or less well-differentiated carcinomas do poorly (ten-year survival rate, 14%). The published work on unsuspected carcinoma found in the transurethral resections offers no clear evidence either for or against further surgical therapy.[46] We have found that, contrary to previous statements, the few patients who develop prostatic cancer before the age of 50 years do not have a worse prognosis than the older age group.[70] Prostatic cancer rarely is accompanied by hypofibrinogenemia. Straub et al.[73] believe that this may be secondary to disseminated intravascular coagulation.

Other tumors

Sarcomas of the prostate often occur at an early age. They produce enlargement of the gland, which feels firm and smooth. Extraprostatic extension is the rule. The large majority are *embryonal rhabdomyosarcoma* (Fig. 725). Microscopically, they are extremely cellular, especially around blood vessels. Areas of myxoid or edematous change and foci of necrosis are common. Most of the tumor cells are small, either round or spindle with occasional bizarre forms, with bright acidophilic cytoplasm. The microscopic pattern is distinctive, even in the absence of cross striations. The prognosis is poor, al-

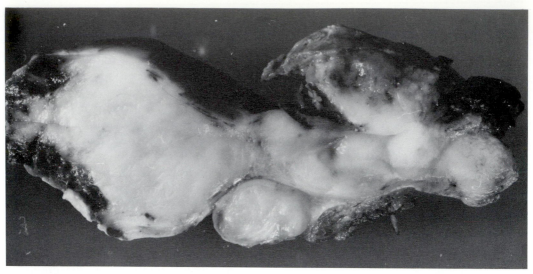

Fig. 725 Rhabdomyosarcoma of prostate in child. Large encephaloid tumor mass replaces gland and extends to surrounding tissue.

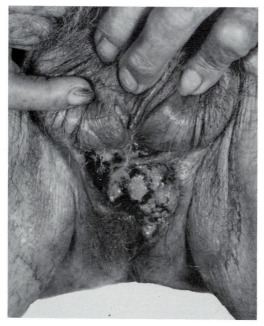

Fig. 726 Adenocarcinoma of Cowper's gland invading scrotum and perineal region. (EFSCH 46-8564.)

though instances of long-term survival after radical surgery as well as after radiation therapy have been reported.[86] *Leiomyosarcoma* is the second most common type of prostatic sarcoma; in contrast to the rhabdomyosarcoma, it occurs frequently

in adults and has a slow growth rate.[91]

We have seen an *adenocarcinoma of Cowper's gland* that ulcerated the skin of the scrotum (Fig. 726), *primary malignant lymphoma* of the prostate,[85] and *leukemia.* The latter two lesions may result in acute urinary obstruction, which is quickly relieved by radiation therapy.[89] *Epidermoid carcinoma* has been reported by Sieracki.[90]

A few cases of *transitional cell carcinoma* of the prostate have been reported.[84] Their microscopic appearance is identical to that of the bladder neoplasms so designated. Before accepting this diagnosis, the possibility of prostatic extension from a primary tumor of the bladder or prostatic urethra should be excluded. The likely origin of these neoplasms are the mucosal and submucosal glands of the prostatic urethra.[79] Ullmann and Ross[92] have described nine instances of hyperplastic changes in these glands, some with atypical features.

Nodular collections of prostatic tissue may protrude in the lumen of the prostatic urethra and appear as a polypoid or papillary mass. Of the sixty-seven cases reported by Butterick et al.,[78] 40% were located in the verumontanum. Most of the patients were young adults. Hematuria was a frequent symptom.

A case of *adenocarcinoma of the prostatic utricle* with a microscopic pattern quite similar to endometrial carcinoma was reported by Melicow and Pachter.[87] The verumontanum and the utricle can exhibit a variety of congenital and acquired abnormalities, the most common being hypertrophy, inflammation, cysts, and the presence of enlarged nodular prostatic glands.[88]

Malacoplakia can involve the prostate, usually in association with bladder disease.[82] *Melanosis* of the prostate has been described in the epithelium[81] as well as in elongated cells within the stroma, resulting in an appearance reminiscent of a blue nevus.[80, 83]

SEMINAL VESICLES

Tuberculosis of the seminal vesicles is usually secondary to infection in the prostate. The greatest amount of involvement is found adjacent to the prostate. Auerbach[93] saw five cases in which only the seminal vesicles were involved. These were probably hematogenous in origin.

Cysts arising from the ducts of the seminal vesicle are rare.[96] Sharma et al.[97] reviewed fifteen reported cases—two were bilateral and four were associated with ipsilateral renal agenesis. They present as a soft cystic mass between the rectum and the base of the bladder.

Primary malignant tumors of the seminal vesicle are pathologic curiosities. Many of the reported cases probably represent invasion from carcinoma originating in other sites, particularly the prostate. In order to make a diagnosis of primary carcinoma of the seminal vesicle, there must be no involvement of the prostate, and the microscopic pattern must be compatible with seminal vesicle origin. After an overall critical review of the literature, Lazarus[95] was of the opinion that there were only seventeen authentic instances of primary cancer of the seminal vesicle. The microscopic type in most instances has been papillary adenocarcinoma.[94]

REFERENCES
PROSTATE
Introduction

1 McHeffey, G. J.: Carcinoma of prostate gland; efficacy of method of examining prostatic tissue removed by transurethral resection to make a pathologic diagnosis of carcinoma, Mayo Clin. Proc. **15**:458-460, 1940.

Nodular hyperplasia

2 Badenoch, A.: Benign enlargement of the prostate, Trans. Med. Soc. Lond. **86**:34-40, 1970.
3 Bennett, A. H., and Harrison, J. H.: A comparison of operative approach for prostatectomy, 1948 and 1968, Surg. Gynecol. Obstet. **128**:969-974, 1969.
4 Moore, R. A.: Benign hypertrophy of the prostate; a morphological study, J. Urol. **50**:680-710, 1943.
5 Ockerblad, N. F.: Giant prostate; the largest recorded, J. Urol. **56**:81-82, 1946.

Infarction

6 Abeshouse, B. S.: Infarct of the prostate, J. Urol. **30**:97-112, 1933.
7 Baird, H. H., McKay, H. W., and Kimmelstiel, P.: Ischemic infarction of the prostate gland, South. Med. J. **43**:234-240, 1950.
8 Flocks, R. H.: The arterial distribution within the prostate gland; its role in transurethral prostatic resection, J. Urol. **37**:524-548, 1937.
9 Hubly, J. W., and Thompson, G. J.: Infarction of the prostate; its clinical significance, Mayo Clin. Proc. **13**:401-403, 1938.
10 Hubly, J. W., and Thompson, G. J.: Infarction of the prostate and volumetric changes produced by the lesion, J. Urol. **43**:459-467, 1940.
11 Moore, R. A.: Benign hypertrophy of the prostate; a morphological study, J. Urol. **50**:680-710, 1943.
12 Roth, R. B.: Prostatic infarction, J. Urol. **62**:474-479, 1949.
13 Silber, I., Rosai, J., and Cordonnier, J. J.: The incidence of elevated acid phosphatase in prostatic infarction, J. Urol. **103**:765-766, 1970.

Abscess

14 Dajani, A. M., and O'Flynn, J. D.: Prostatic abscess; a report of 25 cases, Br. J. Urol. **40**:736-9, 1968.
15 Trapnell, J., and Roberts, M.: Prostatic abscess, Br. J. Surg. **57**:565-9, 1970.

Calculi

16 Cristol, D. S., and Emmett, J. L.: Incidence of coincident prostatic calculi, prostatic hyperplasia and carcinoma of prostate gland, J.A.M.A. **124**:646, 1944.
17 Henline, R. B.: Prostatic calculi; treatment by

subtotal perineal prostatectomy, J. Urol. **44:** 146-168, 1940.

18 Lowsley, O. S., and Hawes, G. A.: True prostatic calculi, Urol. Cutan. Rev. **42:**367-372, 1938.

19 Smith, M. J.: Prostatic corpora amylacea, Monogr. Surg. Sci. **3:**209-265, 1966.

20 Young, H. H.: Prostatic calculi, J. Urol. **32:** 660-709, 1934.

Granulomatous prostatitis

21 Kelalis, P. P., Greene, L. F., and Harrison, E. G., Jr.: Granulomatous prostatitis; a mimic of carcinoma of the prostate, J.A.M.A. **191:**111-113, 1965.

22 Melicow, M. M. J.: Allergic granulomas of the prostate gland, J. Urol. **65:**288-296, 1951.

23 Stewart, M. J., Wray, S., and Hall, M.: Allergic prostatitis in asthmatics, J. Pathol. Bacteriol. **67:**423-430, 1954.

24 Symmers, W. St. C.: Two cases of eosinophilic prostatitis due to metazoan infestation, J. Pathol. Bacteriol. **73:**549-555, 1957.

25 Tanner, F. H., and McDonald, J. R.: Granulomatous prostatitis; a histologic study of a group of granulomatous lesions collected from prostate glands, Arch. Pathol. **36:**358-370, 1943.

26 Towfighi, J., Sadeghee, S., Wheeler, J. E., and Enterline, H. T.: Granulomatous prostatitis with emphasis on the eosinophilic variety, Am. J. Clin. Pathol. **58:**630-641, 1972.

Tuberculosis

27 Auerbach, O.: Tuberculosis of the genital system, Q. Bull., Sea View Hosp. **7:**188-207, 1942.

28 Moore, R. A.: Tuberculosis of the prostate gland, J. Urol. **37:**372-384, 1937.

29 Muchsam, E.: Tuberculosis of the prostate, Q. Bull., Sea View Hosp. **9:**25-29, 1947.

Tumors
Biopsy

30 Labardini, M. M., and Nesbit, R. M.: Perineal extension of adenocarcinoma of the prostate gland after punch biopsy, J. Urol. **97:**891-893, 1967.

31 Pearlman, C. K.: Transrectal biopsy of the prostate, J. Urol. **74:**387-392, 1955.

32 Peirson, E. L., and Nickerson, D. A.: Biopsy of the prostate with the Silverman needle, N. Engl. J. Med. **228:**675-678, 1943.

Cytology

33 Clarke, B. G., and Bamford, S. B.: Cytology of the prostate gland in diagnosis of cancer, J.A.M.A. **172:**1750-1753, 1960.

34 Esposti, P.-L.: Cytologic diagnosis of prostatic tumors with the aid of transrectal aspiration biopsy; a critical review of 1,110 cases and a report of morphologic and cytochemical studies, Acta Cytol. (Baltimore) **10:**182-186, 1966.

35 Esposti, P.-L.: Cytologic malignancy grading of prostatic carcinoma by transrectal aspiration biopsy; a five-year follow-up study of 469 hormone-treated patients, Scand. J. Urol. Nephrol. **5:**199-209, 1971.

36 Fitzgerald, N. W., and Ludbrook, J.: Cytological diagnosis of prostatic cancer; the use of the urinary deposit after prostatic massage, Br. J. Urol. **34:**326-330, 1962.

37 Herbut, P. A., and Lubin, E. N.: Cancer cells in prostatic secretion, J. Urol. **57:**542-551, 1947.

38 Mason, M. K.: The cytological diagnosis of carcinoma of the prostate, Acta Cytol. (Baltimore) **11:**68-71, 1967.

39 Riaboff, P. J.: Detection of early prostatic and urinary tract cancer in asymptomatic patients fifty years of age and over, J. Urol. **72:**62-66, 1954.

Frozen section

40 Colby, F. H.: Cancer of the prostate; results of total prostatectomy, J. Urol. **69:**797-806, 1953.

41 Culp, O. S., and McDonald, J. R.: Importance of frozen section in evaluating prostatic nodules, Trans. Am. Assoc. Genitourin. Surg. **45:**180-186, 1953.

42 Hudson, P. B., Finkle, A. L., Hopkins, J. A., Sproul, E. E., and Stout, A. P.: Prostatic cancer, Cancer **7:**690-703, 1954.

43 Totten, R. S., Heinemann, M. W., Hudson, P. B., Sproul, E. E., and Stout, A. P.: Microscopic differential diagnosis of latent carcinoma of the prostate, Arch. Pathol. **55:**131-141, 1953.

Adenocarcinoma

44 Azzopardi, J. G., and Evans, D. J.: Argentaffin cells in prostatic carcinoma; differentiation from lipofuscin and melanin in prostatic epithelium, J. Pathol. **104:**247-251, 1971.

45 Bainborough, A. R.: Squamous metaplasia of prostate following estrogen therapy, J. Urol. **68:**329-336, 1952.

46 Bauer, W. C., McGavran, M. H., and Carlin, M. R.: Unsuspected carcinoma of the prostate in suprapubic prostatectomy specimens; a clinicopathologic study of fifty-five consecutive cases, Cancer **13:**370-378, 1960.

47 Blennerhassett, J. B., and Vickery, A. L., Jr.: Carcinoma of the prostate gland, Cancer **19:** 980-984, 1966.

48 Brandes, D., Kirchheim, D., and Scott, W. W.: Ultrastructure of the human prostate—normal and neoplastic, Lab. Invest. **13:**1541-1560, 1964.

49 Butler, J., Braunstein, H., Freiman, D. G., and Gall, E. A.: Incidence, distribution and enzymatic activity of carcinoma of the prostate gland, Arch. Pathol. 68:243-251, 1959.

50 Butler, J. J., Howe, C. D., and Johnson, D. E.: Enlargement of the supraclavicular lymph nodes as the initial sign of prostatic carcinoma, Cancer 27:1055-1063, 1971.

51 Byar, D. P.: Treatment of prostatic cancer: studies by the Veterans Administration Cooperative Urological Research Group, Bull. N. Y. Acad. Med. 48:751-766, 1972.

52 Dean, A. L., and Woodard, H. Q.: The differential diagnosis of tumors of the prostate and adjoining areas of the rectum and bladder by chemical analysis, Trans. Am. Assoc. Genitourin. Surg. 38:209-212, 1946; J. Urol. 57:172-174, 1947.

53 Deming, C. L., and Hovenanian, M. S.: The hormonal factor in heterologous growth of human prostatic cancer, J. Urol. 59:215-219, 1948.

54 Franks, L. M.: Latent carcinoma of the prostate, J. Pathol. Bacteriol. 68:603-616, 1954.

55 Franks, L. M.: Atrophy and hyperplasia in the prostate proper, J. Pathol. Bacteriol. 68:617-621, 1954.

56 Franks, L. M.: Estrogen-treated prostatic cancer; the variation in responsiveness, Cancer 13:490-501, 1960.

57 Franks, L. M., O'Shea, J. D., and Thomson, A. E. R.: Mucin in the prostate; a histochemical study in normal glands, latent, clinical, and colloid cancers, Cancer 17:983-991, 1964.

58 Gaynor, E. P.: Zur Frage des Prostatakrebses, Virchows Arch. Pathol. Anat. 301:602-652, 1938.

59 Halpert, B., and Schmalhorst, W. R.: Carcinoma of the prostate in patients 70-79 years old, Cancer 19:695-698, 1966.

60 Hukill, P. B., and Vidone, R. A.: Histochemistry of mucus and other polysaccharides in tumors. II. Carcinoma of the prostate, Lab. Invest. 16:395-406, 1967.

61 Jewett, H. J.: Radical perineal prostatectomy for carcinoma; an analysis of cases at Johns Hopkins Hospital, 1904-1954, J.A.M.A. 156:1039-1041, 1954.

62 Jewett, H. J., Bridge, R. W., Gray, G. F., Jr., and Shelley, W. M.: The palpable nodule of prostatic cancer, J.A.M.A. 203:403-406, 1968.

63 Kirchheim, D., Niles, N. R., Frankus, E., and Hodges, C. V.: Correlative histochemical and histological studies on thirty radical prostatectomy specimens, Cancer 19:1683-1696, 1966.

64 Legier, J. F., and Tauber, L. N.: Solitary metastasis of occult prostatic carcinoma simulating osteogenic sarcoma, Cancer 22:168-172, 1968.

65 Mellinger, G. T., Gleason, D., and Bailar, J., III.: The histology and prognosis of prostatic cancer, J. Urol. 97:331-337, 1967.

66 Montgomery, T. R., Whitlock, G. S., Nohlgren, J. E., and Lewis, A. M.: What becomes of the patient with latent or occult carcinoma of the prostate? J. Urol. 86:655-658, 1961.

67 Rodin, A. E., Larson, D. L., and Roberts, D. K.: Nature of perineural space invaded by prostatic carcinoma, Cancer 20:1772-1779, 1967.

68 Salyer, W. R., and Salyer, D. C.: Metastases of prostatic carcinoma to the breast, Lab. Invest. 26:490, 1972 (abstract).

69 Schwartz, I. S., and Wilens, S. L.: The formation of acinar tissue in gynecomastia, Am. J. Pathol. 43:797-807, 1963.

70 Silber, I., and McGavran, M.: Adenocarcinoma of the prostate in men less than 56 years old; a study of 65 cases, J. Urol. 105:283-285, 1971.

71 Stewart, C. B., Sweetser, T. H., and Delory, G. E.: A case of benign prostatic hypertrophy with recent infarcts and associated high serum acid phosphatase, J. Urol. 63:128-131, 1950.

72 Strahan, R. W.: Carcinoma of the prostate; incidence, origin, pathology, J. Urol. 89:875-880, 1963.

73 Straub, P. W., Reedler, G., and Frick, P. G.: Hypofibrinogenaemia in metastatic carcinoma of prostate: suppression of systemic fibrinolysis with heparin, J. Clin. Pathol. 20:152-157, 1967.

74 Totten, R. S., Heinemann, M. W., Hudson, P. B., Sproul, E. E., and Stout, A. P.: Microscopic differential diagnosis of latent carcinoma of the prostate, Arch. Pathol. 55:131-141, 1953.

75 Utz, D. C., and Farrow, G. M.: Pathologic differentiation and prognosis of prostatic carcinoma, J.A.M.A. 209:1701-1703, 1969.

76 Wattenberg, C. A., and Rose, D. K.: Side effects caused by diethylstilbestrol and correlated with cancer of the prostate gland, J. Urol. 53:135-142, 1945.

77 Weyrauch, H. M.: Surgery of the prostate, Philadelphia, London, 1959, W. B. Saunders Co., p. 47.

Other tumors

78 Butterick, J. D., Schnitzer, B., and Abell, M. R.: Ectopic prostatic tissue in urethra: a clinicopathological entity and a significant cause of hematuria, J. Urol. 105:97-104, 1971.

79 Ende, N., Woods, L. P., and Shelley, H. S.: Carcinoma originating in ducts surrounding the prostatic urethra, Am. J. Clin. Pathol. 40:186-189, 1963.

80 Gardner, W. A., Jr., and Spitz, W. U.: Melanosis of the prostate gland, Am. J. Clin. Pathol. 56:762-764, 1971.

81 Goldman, R. L.: Melanogenic epithelium in the prostate gland, Am. J. Clin. Pathol. 49:75-78, 1968.

82 Hoffman, E., and Garrido, M.: Malakoplakia of the prostate; report of a case, J. Urol. **92**:311-313, 1964.

83 Jao, W., Fretzin, D. F., Christ, M. L., and Prinz, L. M.: Blue nevus of the prostate gland, Arch. Pathol. **91**:187-191, 1971.

84 Johnson, D. E., Hogan, J. M., and Ayala, A. G.: Transitional cell carcinoma of the prostate; a clinical morphological study, Cancer **29**:287-293, 1972.

85 King, L. S., and Cox, T. R.: Lymphosarcoma of the prostate, Am. J. Pathol. **27**:801-823, 1951.

86 Mackenzie, A. R., Whitmore, W. F., Jr., and Melamed, M. R.: Myosarcomas of the bladder and prostate, Cancer **22**:833-844, 1968.

87 Melicow, M. M., and Pachter, M. R.: Endometrial carcinoma of the prostatic utricle (uterus masculinus), Cancer **20**:1715-1722, 1967.

88 Moore, R. A.: Pathology of prostatic utricle, Arch. Pathol. **23**:517-524, 1937.

89 Mitch, W. E., Jr., and Serpick, A. A.: Leukemic infiltration of the prostate: a reversible form of urinary obstruction, Cancer **26**:1361-1365, 1970.

90 Sieracki, J. C.: Epidermoid carcinoma of the human prostate, Lab. Invest. **4**:232-240, 1955.

91 Smith, B. H., and Dehner, L. P.: Sarcoma of the prostate gland, Am. J. Clin. Pathol. **58**:43-50, 1972.

92 Ullmann, A. S., and Ross, O. A.: Hyperplasia, atypism, and carcinoma in situ in prostatic periurethral glands, Am. J. Clin. Pathol. **47**:497-504, 1967.

SEMINAL VESICLES

93 Auerbach, O.: Tuberculosis of the genital system, Q. Bull., Sea View Hosp. **4**:188, 207, 1942.

94 Awadalla, O., Hunt, A. C., and Miller, A.: Primary carcinoma of the seminal vesicle, Br. J. Urol. **40**:574-579, 1968.

95 Lazarus, J. A.: Primary malignant tumors of retrovesical region with special reference to malignant tumors of seminal vesicle; report of case of retrovesical sarcoma, J. Urol. **5**:190-205, 1946.

96 Lund, A. J., and Cummings, M. M.: Cyst of accessory genital tract; case report with review of literature, J. Urol. **56**:383-386, 1946.

97 Sharma, T. C., Dorman, P. S., and Dorman, H. P.: Bilateral seminal vesicular cysts, J. Urol. **102**:741-744, 1969.

Testis

Cryptorchidism

In one out of every ten males, the testis does not descend into the scrotum but remains in the abdomen or inguinal region. The inguinal testis is about four times as common as the abdominal testis.

If, by the age of 6 years, an abdominally retained testis has not spontaneously descended to the scrotum, the administration of gonadotropin may cause its descent. If this therapy is unsuccessful, the testis should be placed in the scrotum by operation. This must be done by the time the child is 6 years of age. Otherwise permanent anatomic alterations occur.[12] Cryptorchid testes in adults are small and brown. The testicular tubules are atrophic and the interstitial cells prominent (Figs. 727 and 728). Not infrequently, foci of hyperplastic Sertoli cells occur. They are usually multiple and may appear grossly as minute white nodules. These never occur in otherwise normal or descended testes.

A cryptorchid testis is thirty to fifty times more likely to develop a malignant germinal tumor than is a normally placed organ. Of 7,000 cases of testicular cancers reviewed by Gilbert and Hamilton,[7] 10.9% occurred in cryptorchid organs. The incidence of cancer is greater in the abdominal than in the inguinal testis.[2] Semi-noma is the most common type, but teratomas also occur. The contralateral testis in patients with unilateral cryptorchidism also has a higher incidence of tumor than does a normal gland.[3] If a cryptorchid testis is surgically placed in the scrotum, it may still develop cancer, especially if the operation has been done at a later age than 6 years.[10] Dow and Mostofi[5] reported fourteen cases of malignant tumors occurring in patients who had had orchiopexy. The ages at which orchiopexy had been performed ranged from 11 to 36 years. It is because of the statistics quoted and the reasons stated that some urologists believe that all unilateral high inguinal or abdominal cryptorchid testes should be excised.[1] Gross and Jewett[8] believe that the risk of cancer in abnormally placed testes is exaggerated and maintain a rather conservative attitude to their removal. They emphasize the great importance of care in doing the operation to avoid damage to the fragile blood supply to the testes. Gross and Replogle[9] reported an incidence of 80% fertility in patients with unilateral cryptorchidism who underwent orchiopexy before or near puberty, and Karcher[11] reported an incidence of 100% fertility in children who underwent surgery before the age of 10 years. Of patients with bilateral cryptorchid testes in whom repair is performed before the age of 5 years, 50% are fertile and 31% are monospermic.[6]

The decision to place a cryptorchid testis in its normal position if it fails to descend before the age of 6 years is based on a careful study of the normal-developing testis and its comparison with the cryptorchid testis. Charny et al.[4] summarized the normal testicular development as follows.

The child testis begins as an organ composed of small seminiferous tubules compactly filled with small undifferentiated cuboidal cells. Increase in

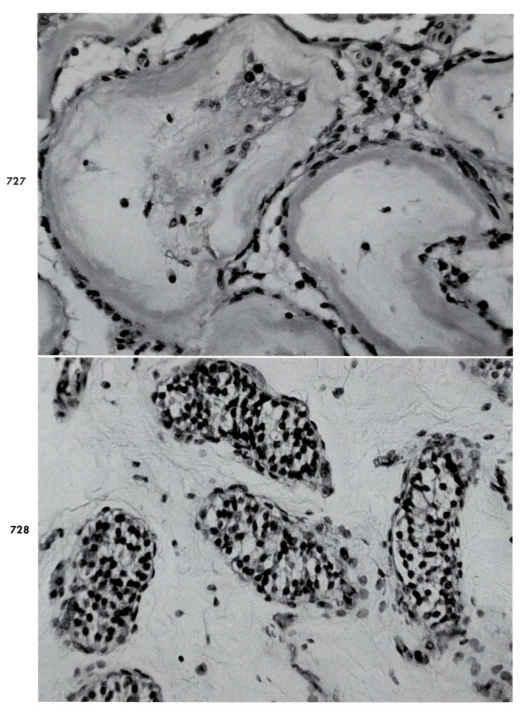

727

728

Fig. 727 Extreme atrophy in cryptorchid testis in 42-year-old man. There is tremendous thickening of walls of tubules, and only scattered Sertoli cells can be seen. (×350; WU neg. 58-1453.)

Fig. 728 Cryptorchid testis in 12-year-old boy. Tubules are of prepubertal type. Note contrast to Fig. 727. (×250; WU neg. 58-1452.)

tubule and cell size is slow and gradual. Tortuosity and lumen formation first appear at age 4 and, with this, a most orderly arrangement of the cells which become identifiable as spermatogonia. Leydig cells cannot be seen except in the newborn. This slow, barely perceptible growth continues up to age 10, at which time a definite spurt is noted. Mitotic figures now appear in the cells of the tubule and Leydig cells are seen in the intertubular spaces. At age 11, mitotic activity is pronounced. Primary and secondary spermatocytes appear. At age 12, spermatids are numerous. Finally, spermatozoa appear. Because of the great variation in the age at which puberty normally occurs, the age of the individual cannot be determined by histologic study of the testis after the twelfth year. The number of maturing tubules with active spermatogenesis increases until the picture seen in the adult is reached. The age of the subject at the final stage of development varies from 11 to 15 years in our series.

It can be seen that although appreciable histologic changes are noted at almost yearly intervals it is possible to divide testicular growth and development into three major phases as follows:

1 Static phase: from birth to age 4
2 Growth phase: from age 4 to age 10
3 Developmental (maturation) phase: from age 10 to puberty

It is interesting to note that the first appearance of tubular development, as differentiated from tubular growth, occurs at age 10, and that this coincides with the age at which gonadotropins and 17-ketosteroids are first found in the urine in any appreciable quantity. Testis maturation may therefore be said to begin at about age 10 and to progress over a period of 2 to 5 years until it is complete.*

Atrophy and infertility

Atrophy of the testis may follow orchitis of mumps or, rarely, some other nonspecific orchitis. Testicular tissue also can be destroyed by local or total body irradiation or radioactive phosphorus.[23] The atrophy associated with cirrhosis of the liver is thought to be caused by circulating endogenous estrogens not detoxified by the diseased liver.[14] The same pathologic changes can occur in the testes of patients who are being given estrogens for carcinoma of the prostate. This therapy causes severe atrophy of the germinal

epithelium. Germ cells may completely disappear, and there may be peritubular sclerosis. Leydig cells may simulate fibroblasts or form hyperplastic clusters[13] but do not develop neoplasms as in some experimental animals. Incisional biopsy of the testis is of great value in the evaluation of the infertile patient, especially of the individual with azoospermia and normal endocrine findings.[17, 21, 27] Punch biopsy is not nearly so satisfactory. The material should be handled with extreme care.[24] Zenker's and Bouin's fixatives are to be preferred over formalin. Biopsy specimens from infertile men with total lack of spermatozoa (azoospermia) usually show one of four well-defined conditions[22]: (1) *germinal cell aplasia* (29%), in which the tubules are populated by Sertoli cells only, (2) *spermatocytic arrest* (26%), characterized by a halt of the maturation sequence at the stage of the primary spermatocyte, (3) *generalized fibrosis* (18%), and (4) *normal spermatogenesis* (27%). The latter is diagnostic of bilateral obstruction or absence of some part of the duct system.

In patients with significant reduction in the number of spermatozoa (oligospermia), five major microscopic patterns are recognizable, often combined (Fig. 729): (1) *sloughing and disorganization* (49%), in which spermatogenesis has a disorderly appearance and the tubular lumina are filled with desquamated immature cells (Fig. 730), (2) *incomplete spermatocytic arrest* (17%), characterized by arrest of spermatogenesis in some of the tubules, (3) *regional or incomplete fibrosis* (15%), (4) *spermatogenic hypoplasia* (13%), marked by tubules with reduced populations of germ cells and a poor order of spermatogenesis, and (5) *normal or essentially normal spermatogenesis* (6%), usually implying a partial occlusion of some part of the duct system.[25, 26]

In the series of over 800 cases of azoospermia studied by testicular biopsy by Girgis et al.,[18] the etiology was obstructive in about 55%. In more than half of these, epididymovasostomy proved bene-

---

*From Charny, C. W., Conston, A. S., and Meranze, D. R.: Development of the testis, Fertil. Steril. 3:461-479, 1952.

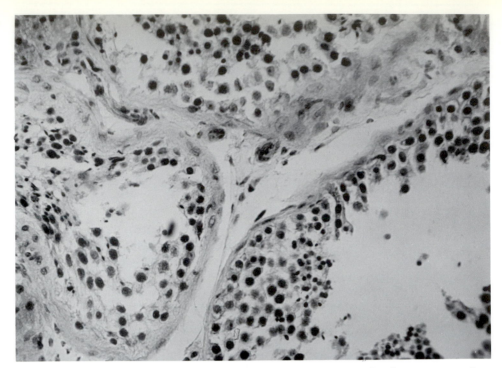

Fig. 729 Testis in sterile male. There apparently has been germinal cell arrest as well as oligospermia. (×350; WU neg. 58-1454.)

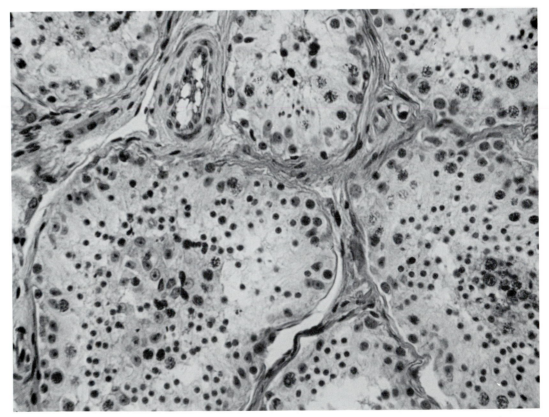

Fig. 730 Sloughing, disorganization, and spermatogenic hypoplasia found in testicular biopsy of young adult with marked oligospermia. (×350; WU neg. 72-6551.)

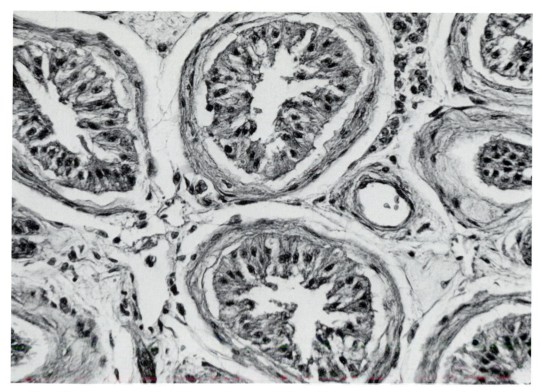

Fig. 731 Extreme atrophy of testis showing thickened basement membranes with Sertoli cells. These changes were caused by cyclophosphamide. (×300; WU neg. 11213.)

ficial. Patients with varicocele are often oligospermic and infertile. The most common patterns at biopsy are those of spermatogenic hypoplasia plus sloughing and disorganization.[15] The azoospermia commonly seen in patients with cystic fibrosis is obstructive in nature, secondary to structural abnormalities of the epididymis and vas deferens.[20]

Biopsies are rarely done in patients with testicular failure involving primarily the endocrine function, since the diagnosis is usually established by hormonal determinations. Failure of puberal maturation is the cardinal symptom. Three different patterns can be seen in testicular biopsies: (1) *hypogonadotrophic eunuchoidism* (60%) accompanied by low gonadotropin levels and characterized by small, infantile tubules with scattered spermatogonia and Sertoli cells but no Leydig cells. (2) *Klinefelter's syndrome* (30%), with fibrosis of tubules and prominent thickening of

the basement membrane, (3) and *testicular aplasia* (10%), characterized by the absence of testicular tissue and elevation of urinary gonadotropins. Patients with Klinefelter's syndrome have an increased incidence of breast carcinoma.[19]

With cyclophosphamide, and other chemotherapeutic agents, sterility and testicular atrophy can occur[16] (Fig. 731).

Tumors

Testicular tumors are best divided into two broad categories: *germinal* (96.5%), arising from the germinal epithelium of the seminiferous tubules, and *nongerminal* (3.5%), originating from Leydig cells, Sertoli cells, or nonspecific cells of the testicular stroma.

Germinal tumors

Testicular germinal tumors make up only a small percentage of all malignant neoplasms but are the most common malig-

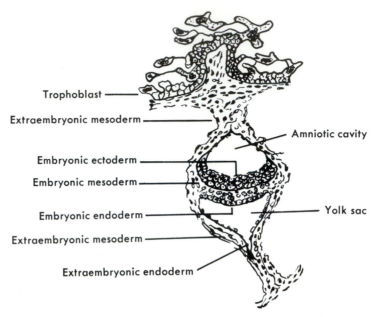

Trophoblast

Extraembryonic mesoderm

Embryonic ectoderm

Embryonic mesoderm

Embryonic endoderm

Extraembryonic mesoderm

Extraembryonic endoderm

Amniotic cavity

Yolk sac

Fig. 732 Scheme of components of normal human embryo. Testicular germ cell tumors other than seminoma attempt to differentiate toward one or more of these structures. (Slightly modified from Marin-Padilla, M.: Histopathology of the embryonal carcinoma of the testes; embryological evaluation, Arch. Pathol. **85:**614-622, 1968; copyright 1968, American Medical Association.)

nant tumors in young men between 25 and 29 years of age. The Armed Forces Institute of Pathology collected almost 1,000 neoplasms of the testes during World War II. The classification of these lesions has undergone so many changes with the passage of time that a state of confusion prevails among pathologists regarding the proper terminology and the interrelation of the different categories. The two major classifications currently used are those of Dixon and Moore[34] and Collins and Pugh,[32] commonly referred to as the American and English classifications, respectively. Although the nomenclature used in the latter is histogenetically more sound, its lengthy, awkward terminology makes it impractical for everyday use. Besides, the terms used by the American authors are already too entrenched in the medical literature to justify a major switch in nomenclature. We will use, therefore, the terms of the American classification with a few necessary changes motivated by recent advances in the field and include under each major heading the

equivalent term of the English classification.

The first and most important concept in the classification of testicular germinal tumors is that they are basically of three morphologic types: *seminoma, teratoma,* or a *combination of both*. **Seminoma** arises from the germinal (seminiferous) epithelium of the mature or maturing testis and has a characteristic homogeneous structure. The histogenesis of **teratoma** is still disputed. Although the bulk of evidence favors a germ cell origin as for seminoma, [42, 50] some observers still adhere to the alternative theory of an origin from embryonic totipotent cells that have escaped the influence of organizers.[32] The important practical point to remember is that tumors of this latter group, all of which can be properly included under the designation of teratoma, recapitulate the normal embryogenesis and their pattern of differentiation is therefore directed toward the formation of one or more of the components of an embryo and related struc-

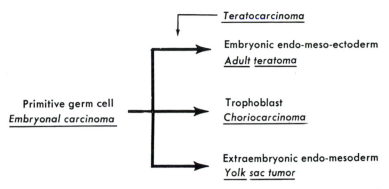

Fig. 733 Possible pathways of differentiation of testicular germ cell tumors of teratoma series.

tures[39, 40, 45] (Fig. 732). The direction of differentiation will determine the morphologic appearance of a given tumor and hence its name (Fig. 733). Four basic patterns are thus seen: *embryonal carcinoma,* wholly composed of primitive cells with minimal or no signs of differentiation; *adult teratoma,* in which the differentiation is toward structures of the embryo proper, usually a combination of endodermic, mesodermic, and ectodermic tissues; *choriocarcinoma,* in which formation of trophoblastic elements is prominent; and *yolk sac tumor,* directed toward the formation of extraembryonic endoderm and mesoderm.

There are two factors complicating this simple scheme. First, differentiation may proceed in two different directions in the same lesion. Second, tumors are often seen in which the differentiation toward a given component is only partial. The result is a bewildering combination of fifteen possible patterns. Fortunately, only one of them is important enough to justify a separation as a special category. This is the combination of embryonal carcinoma and adult teratoma, which is referred to as *teratocarcinoma.* The other combinations can be included, for practical purposes, into one or another of the four major types. The final complication to this scheme is that seminoma can accompany any of these types and combinations of teratomas, a phenomenon for which the generic term of *combined tumor* is applied.

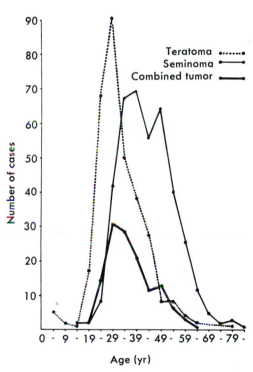

Fig. 734 Age distribution of patients at time of orchidectomy; 400 cases of seminoma, 322 cases of teratoma, and 136 cases of combined tumor. Note how peak age of combined tumors occupies intermediate position between peaks for seminoma and teratoma. (From Collins, D. H., and Pugh, R. C. P.: Classification and frequency of testicular tumours, Br. J. Urol. **36**(suppl.):1-11, 1964.)

Seminoma

Seminomas are distinctive neoplasms, making up 30% to 40% of all testicular tumors (Fig. 734). They can be divided

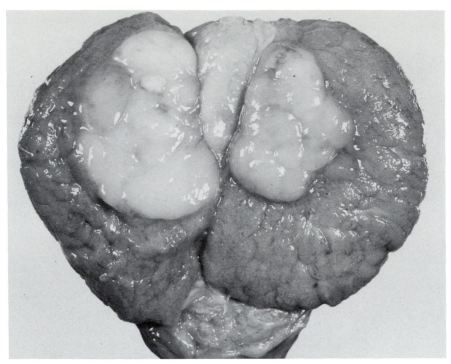

Fig. 735 Typical homogeneous cellular seminoma containing areas of necrosis. (WU neg. 52-1977.)

into two major categories: classical and spermatocytic.

Classical seminomas, which comprise approximately 93% of the cases, have a characteristic gross appearance. They usually are of moderate size, homogeneous, and light yellow and may contain sharply circumscribed zones of necrosis (Fig. 735). Microscopically, the individual cells are uniform, with clear cytoplasm, large nuclei, and prominent nucleoli (Fig. 736). The number of mitoses is highly variable. Cytoplasmic glycogen is usually present. By electron microscopy, some of the cells have an undifferentiated appearance with few cytoplasmic organelles. Others have a more complex arrangement indicating some degree of differentiation.[43] Multinucleated giant tumor cells are seen in 11% to 14% of all seminomas. A tumor should not be called choriocarcinoma because of their presence. Lymphocytic infiltration of the fibrous trabeculae that divide the tumor into lobules is present in about 80% of the cases. It is perhaps an expression of

cellular immunity of the host against the tumor and correlates with a good prognosis.[41] We have seen cases in which the fibrosis was so extensive and the lymphocytic infiltration so heavy that the malignant cells were missed by the pathologist, who diagnosed the condition as chronic orchitis. Areas of peculiar granulomatous reaction with giant cells may be present, as in the ovarian dysgerminoma.

In the English series of 536 cases, 400 were pure and 137 were combined with teratomas of various types.[32] No microscopic differences in the seminomatous component are noticeable between the pure and the combined varieties. In some seminomas, sometimes referred to as "anaplastic," the nuclei are markedly hyperchromatic and the cytoplasm is scanty, resulting in a picture somewhat dissimilar from the usual seminoma. We have seen several of these misdiagnosed as embryonal carcinoma.

Spermatocytic seminomas occur in an older age group than do the classical variety. Grossly, they have a soft gelatinous

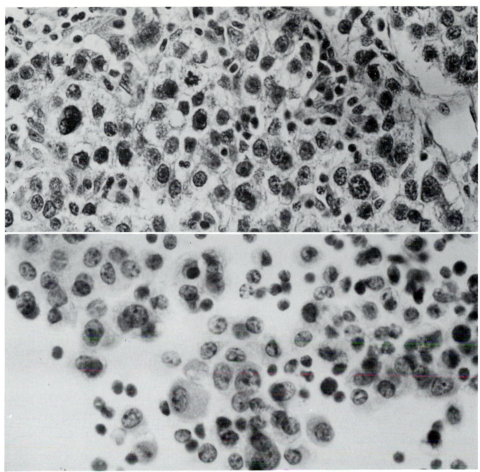

Fig. 736 Routine microscopic section of seminoma and stained smear made from fresh gross specimen. Undistorted seminoma cells have well-defined nuclei and nucleoli. Cytoplasm is abundant. (×520; WU neg. 50-5071; ×750; WU neg. 52-2048.)

appearance. Microscopically, they are composed of cells with *perfectly round* nuclei and prominent variation in size. Bizarre giant forms are common (Fig. 737, *A*). Some of the nuclei have a filamentous appearance consistent with an early stage of meiotic division (Fig. 737, *B*). The cytoplasm is dense and devoid of glycogen. Intratubular growth is often seen at the periphery. Areas of lymphocytic infiltration and granuloma formations are absent.[46] Ultrastructurally, the cells show clear-cut evidence of spermatocytic differentiation[47] (Fig. 737, *C*). In contrast to the classical seminoma, the spermatocytic type occurs *only* in the testicle and is never seen in combination with teratomas.

Seminomas are common in old dogs. Their morphologic features are somewhat intermediate between those of the human classical and spermatocytic variants.[46, 48]

Embryonal carcinoma

Embryonal carcinoma has a grossly more variegated appearance than seminoma. It is mainly solid and gray or white with foci of hemorrhage and necrosis. The latter may be so extensive as to render the diagnosis difficult. Microscopically, it may be composed wholly of solid sheets of undifferentiated cells or show signs of early differentiation toward embryonic structures, trophoblast, or extraembryonic endoderm or mesoderm. However, mature

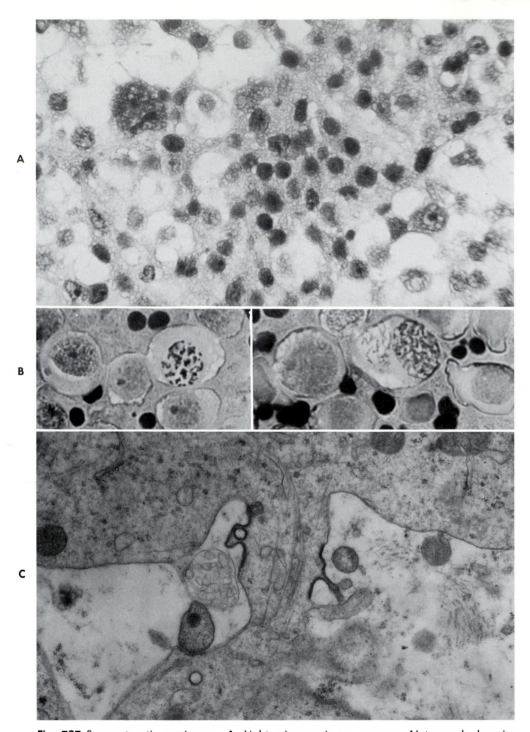

Fig. 737 Spermatocytic seminoma. **A,** Light microscopic appearance. Note marked variations in nuclear size, bizarre nuclear forms, and intercellular edema. **B,** Touch preparation
from same tumor. Two cells are undergoing division, probably of meiotic type. **C,** Electron
micrograph from same tumor. Intercellular bridge joins two tumor cells in manner
analogous to that seen in normal spermatocytes. Note thickening of plasma membrane
and microtubules running across bridge. (**A,** ×600; WU neg. 73-3542; **B,** ×720; WU negs.
73-3410 and 73-3411; **C,** uranyl acetate—lead citrate; ×21,900.)

tissues are by definition absent. In the American classification,[34] all of these morphologic varieties are included under the term of embryonal carcinoma, since the prognosis is determined by the predominant undifferentiated component. In the English classification,[32] the solid undifferentiated type is designated as "malignant teratoma, anaplastic," whereas the variant showing clefts or papillae of epithelial nature indicative of early embryonic differentiation is called "malignant teratoma, intermediate, subgroup B (no differentiated or organoid elements apparent)." In the differential diagnosis with seminoma, it is important to remember that even in the solid, undifferentiated form, the pattern of growth has a carcinomatous appearance. The cells are more anaplastic, with numerous mitoses (often atypical), and exhibit prominent variation in size and shape.[45]

Adult teratoma

The adult teratoma comprises 5% to 10% of all testicular neoplasms. It corresponds to the "pure teratoma" of the American classification[34] and the "teratoma, differentiated" of the English classification.[32] Grossly, the tumors are predominantly cystic and multiloculated (Fig. 738). Foci of cartilage are usually evident, but the presence of bone is infrequent. The type of cystic teratoma full of sebum and hair so commonly seen in the ovary is virtually unknown in the testis.

All types of tissue can be seen microscopically, the most common being nerve, cartilage, and various types of epithelium (Fig. 739). A requisite for the diagnosis of adult teratoma is that all tissues be well differentiated. There is only one exception: otherwise mature neoplasms with small collections of neuroblasts should be included in the category of adult teratomas in view of their generally good prognosis. Naturally this evaluation implies a thorough sampling of the tumor mass.

In adult individuals, even perfectly well-differentiated tumors have been known to metastasize. *This is not the case in microscopically mature teratomas in children.* None of the approximately forty well-documented cases reported in the literature gave rise to distant metastases. There-

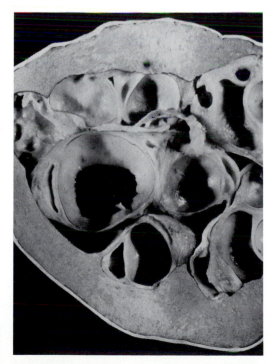

Fig. 738 Large cystic teratoma. (AFIP 539341.)

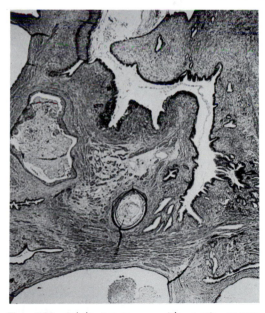

Fig. 739 Adult teratoma with cystic spaces lined by squamous and columnar epithelium. (Low power; WU neg. 49-1519.)

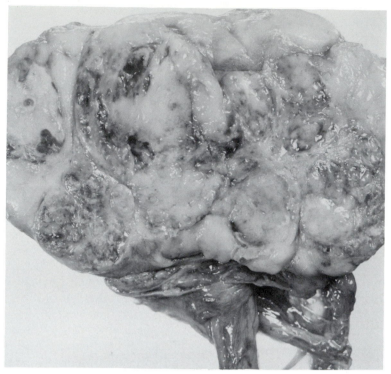

Fig. 740 Large teratocarcinoma containing various tissues. In many areas, tumor was undifferentiated. (WU neg. 49-282.)

fore, orchiectomy is all that is needed under these circumstances.

Teratocarcinoma

Teratocarcinomas have a gross appearance similar to the adult teratomas except for soft areas of cellularity and necrosis (Fig. 740). Microscopically, there are various types of well-differentiated tissue, but in addition focal areas of malignant epithelial and stromal tissue are present. In other words, they represent a combination of the growth pattern of embryonal carcinoma and adult teratoma, the term used in the American classification.[34] In the British classification, they are called "malignant teratoma, intermediate, subgroup A (with differentiated or organoid components)."[32]

Choriocarcinoma

Choriocarcinomas ("teratomas, trophoblastic" of the English classification)[32] are very malignant tumors that account for about 5% of testicular tumors. These neo-plasms are often small. There may be no enlargement of the testis. They are usually hemorrhagic and partially necrotic (Fig. 741). Rarely, the primary tumor may completely regress, leaving only a scar containing hemosiderin pigment.[36] Peculiar hematoxylin deposits may be present within the seminiferous tubules, probably representing remnants of preexisting neo-plasm.[30] Microscopically, these tumors show giant syncytial trophoblastic cells with large, atypical nuclei intermingled with cytotrophoblasts (Fig. 742). As Dixon and Moore[34] remarked, cells with a morphologic appearance suggestive of either syncytiotrophoblast or cytotrophoblast can be seen in several types of testicular tumors. It is only when these cells are prominent and arranged in a villuslike manner that the diagnosis of choriocarcinoma is justified. Something similar can be said of chorionic gonadotropins. Although classically elevated in choriocarcinomas, they also may be increased in any

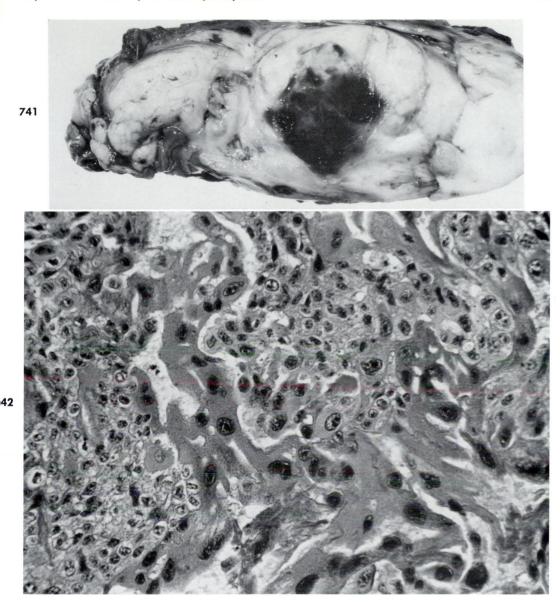

Fig. 741 Hemorrhagic choriocarcinoma in 35-year-old man. Extensive metastases were present when tumor was discovered. (Courtesy Dr. F. Leidler, Houston, Texas.)
Fig. 742 Testicular choriocarcinoma. Close intermingling of cytotrophoblast and syncytiotrophoblast recapitulates that seen in chorionic villi. (×300; WU neg. 3405.)

other type of testicular germinal tumor. This finding, although of important prognostic value, should not influence the morphologic typing of the tumor. The diagnosis of choriocarcinoma should be made on the basis of the microscopic pattern rather than on the basis of the hormone produced. The combination of choriocar-

cinoma and embryonal carcinoma should be included among the choriocarcinomas because of its similar prognosis.

Yolk sac tumor

The term *yolk sac tumor* is probably the best designation for the newest member of the testicular teratoma group.[44] It has an

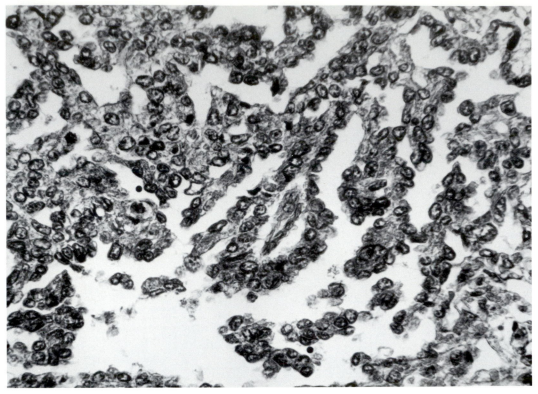

Fig. 743 Typical yolk sac tumor of testis occurring in 1-year-old child. Tumor cells form variety of tubular structures and arrange themselves around blood vessel in manner reminiscent of renal glomerulus. (×340; WU neg. 73-54.)

impressive list of synonyms, including endodermal sinus tumor of Teilum, juvenile embryonal carcinoma, embryonal adenocarcinoma, distinctive adenocarcinoma of the infant testis, testicular adenocarcinoma with clear cells, and orchioblastoma.[32, 37, 51, 52, 54] Although ignored altogether in the original American classification[34] and classified among the "miscellaneous tumors of mainly epithelial type" by the English authors,[32] we believe that it should be included under the category of teratoma.

Grossly, the tumor may be firm or soft. Cystic areas are common. The color varies from yellow to white. Microscopically, epithelial and mesenchymal elements intermingle in a very characteristic organoid fashion. Presence of perivascular rosettelike formations (Schiller-Duval bodies) is the most distinctive feature (Fig. 743). They have been compared to structures seen in the rat placenta[51] and interpreted as an attempt to form yolk sacs. A tumor should be composed of these elements throughout in order to be included in this category. Neoplasms having, in addition, solid undifferentiated areas are better classified as embryonal carcinomas.

Spread

Testicular tumors spread first to iliac and periaortic lymph nodes and later to mediastinal and left supraclavicular nodes. They do not involve the inguinal lymph nodes unless there is invasion of the skin of the scrotum or tumor recurrence in a cutaneous scar. Pulmonary metastases are frequent. Embryonal carcinoma frequently metastasizes early, and choriocarcinoma almost always has widespread metastases by the time the tumor is diagnosed. Of thirteen cases of adult teratoma reviewed

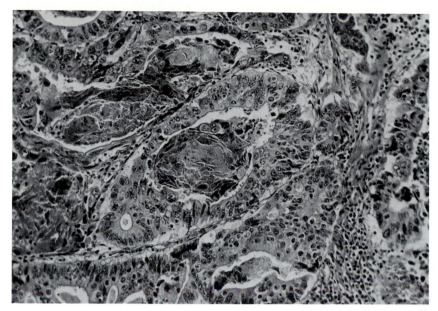

Fig. 744 Area of adenocarcinoma in teratocarcinoma. (Moderate enlargement; WU neg. 47-744.)

by the British Testicular Tumor Panel, two patients died with metastatic disease. Yolk sac tumors only rarely metastasize to periaortic or other lymph node groups.[54]

The microscopic appearance of the metastases is sometimes quite different from that of the primary tumor. Testicular teratocarcinomas may be accompanied by completely mature metastases,[49, 53] whereas mature teratomas may give rise to undifferentiated ones. Friedman and Moore[35] postulated that undifferentiated areas occurring early in the primary tumor might metastasize to distant zones and there undergo maturation so that several years later only adult type of tissue is found. In order to substantiate such a hypothesis, it would be necessary to section serially an adult teratoma having metastases in order to avoid overlooking minute undifferentiated zones (Fig. 744). Crook[33] reported a patient with a pure testicular seminoma (serially sectioned) who died with generalized metastases of choriocarcinoma.

Clinicopathologic correlation

A malignant testicular tumor is accompanied by progressive, painless enlargement of the testis. It may grow slowly or with appalling speed. The choriocarcinoma may not be palpable but may be accompanied by signs of gynecomastia, large amounts of chorionic gonadotropin in the urine,[31] and large mediastinal and/or pulmonary metastases.

There is a good correlation between age and the incidence of the different types of testicular tumors, a fact not well borne out in the work by Dixon and Moore,[34] which was based on material from military personnel. The peak age is 41.9 years for classical seminoma, 65 years for spermatocytic seminoma, 30.4 years for the different types of teratoma, and 35.1 years for the combined tumors.[32] In prepuberal children, seminomas and combined tumors are exceptional. Only teratomas occur with some frequency, notably of the yolk sac tumor type.[28] The majority of yolk sac tumors occur in infants under 2 years of age.[54] In individuals over 60 years of age, teratomas are extremely rare. Seminomas, either classical or spermatocytic, are the most common germinal tumors in this age group, outnumbered only by malignant lymphomas.[29]

The prognosis varies widely according to the tumor type. It is excellent for classical seminoma. Approximately 90% of the patients with disease clinically limited to the testis (Stage 1) or to subdiaphragmatic lymph nodes (Stage 2) can be cured. It is even better for spermatocytic seminoma. Of the fifty cases reviewed by Rosai et al.,[46] only two patients died as a result of the disease. The mortality rate is approximately 23% for adult teratomas, 44% for teratocarcinomas, and 55% for embryonal carcinomas.[32] Choriocarcinoma is practically always a fatal disease. In yolk sac tumors, the prognosis is directly related to the age of the patient at the time of surgery. Pierce et al.[44] reviewed thirty-one cases. Of the twenty-two patients treated surgically under 2 years of age, only two died. In contrast, among the nine patients over 2 years of age, only one survived. The prognosis of the combined tumor is largely determined by the nature of the teratomatous component.

Factors that adversely influence the prognosis of testicular tumors regardless of type are extension of the tumor outside the capsule, gynecomastia, increased urinary gonadotropins, hyperplasia of Leydig cells in the nontumoral testis, vascular invasion, and, in seminomas, absence of lymphoid stroma.

In the evaluation of survival rates of patients with testicular tumors, it is important to remember that the majority of the patients who die of tumor do so in a relatively short period. Dixon and Moore[34] showed that a two-year freedom from recurrence after therapy is evidence of cure in at least 90% of instances.

The initial treatment for all testicular germinal tumors is orchiectomy with high ligation of the spermatic cord. The findings on pathologic examination will determine the course to follow. Patients with classical seminoma receive thorough irradiation of the retroperitoneum whether or not there is clinical or lymphangiographic evidence of metastases. Lymphangiography is helpful in planning the extent and amount of therapy.[38] It is doubtful whether radiation therapy is needed for spermatocytic seminoma, since to our knowledge no case with metastatic retroperitoneal involvement has been documented. The treatment of choice of embryonal carcinoma and teratocarcinoma, whether by orchiectomy followed by radical radiation therapy or by orchiectomy followed by lymphadenectomy combined with preoperative or postoperative irradiation, remains to be determined. The incidence of retroperitoneal spread in yolk sac tumors and adult teratomas of infants and children is too low to justify a lymphadenectomy.

Nongerminal tumors

Interstitial (Leydig) cell tumors are sometimes difficult to differentiate from areas of hyperplasia. They may produce hormonal changes because of increased production of androgens, estrogens, or both. Most of these tumors occur in adults, gynecomastia being the most common symptom. The few that occur in childhood cause precocious pseudopuberty, with growth of pubic hair and penis enlargement. The prefix *pseudo* is used because the spermatogenic function of the testes remains dormant.[62] Removal of the tumor causes regression of these changes.[59] Interstitial cell tumors comprise 1.4% of all testicular tumors.[56] Dalgaard and Hesselberg[57] reviewed ninety-four cases in 1957. They are occasionally bilateral[58] and very rarely malignant. Only eleven of the latter have been described, all with evidence of metastatic disease.[67, 78]

Grossly, these tumors are usually small, reddish brown, and sharply delimited. Microscopically, the tumor cells have well-defined outlines, deeply acidophilic cytoplasm, and round or oval nucleus (Fig. 745). Lipochrome pigment and Reinecke's crystalloids are sometimes present, the latter better demonstrated with Masson's trichrome stain.[76] As in most other endocrine tumors, marked variation in the size and shape of the tumor cells may occur. Bizarre forms with giant nuclei are not

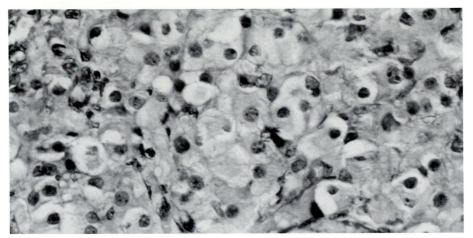

Fig. 745 Interstitial cell tumor of testis in child with precocious puberty. Removal of tumor caused regression of symptoms. Individual cells are uniform with well-defined cytoplasmic outlines and no mitotic figures. (×540; WU neg. 52-4341; slide contributed by Dr. K. B. Fraser, Brisbane, Australia.)

unusual. The remaining testis does not show interstitial cell hyperplasia. It is difficult, if not impossible, to predict on the basis of the morphologic appearance whether a particular tumor is functioning or nonfunctioning or whether it is benign or malignant.

Tumors and tumorlike conditions of Sertoli cells comprise a complex group of lesions which are probably interrelated. First, there is the *Sertoli cell tumor* arising in the descended testis of a normal individual. Of the sixty-six cases reviewed by Hopkins and Parry,[61] nineteen were associated with gynecomastia; seven had given rise to metastases to the iliac and para-aortic lymph nodes.[77] Grossly, the tumors are well circumscribed, white or yellow, and firm, with focal cystic areas. Microscopically, the diagnostic feature is the presence of tubular formations lined by elongated cells having the appearance of Sertoli cells. In other areas, the tumor is solid and can be confused with seminoma. This is the same lesion designated by Mostofi et al.[68] as "tumor of specialized gonadal stroma" and by Teilum[79] as "androblastoma."

The second group of Sertoli cell lesions occurs almost always in cryptorchid testes, whether dysgenetic or not. The changes range from the areas of *Sertoli cell hyperplasia* (also called hypoplastic tubules, dysgenetic zones, and tubular adenomas) often seen in the cryptorchid testis, to the *Sertoli cell adenomas* described by Neubecker and Theiss[69] in patients with the testicular feminization syndrome, to the lesion designated by Scully[73] as *gonadoblastoma.* The first two lesions are composed solely of Sertoli cells, and the difference among them is only of size. Gonadoblastoma has, in addition, a germ cell component. Calcification is a conspicuous feature, but it also may be present in the other lesions. The germ cell proliferation of gonadoblastoma may eventually result in a malignant neoplasm that can totally obliterate the Sertoli cell component. This is usually of the seminoma (or dysgerminoma) type, although adult teratoma, embryonal carcinoma, and yolk sac tumor also have been described. Practically all of the gonadoblastomas so far reported have been in individuals with an underlying gonadal disorder, either pure or mixed gonadal dysgenesis, or male pseudohermaphroditism.[73]

Sohval[74] described foci of Sertoli cell hyperplasia in 50% of cryptorchid testes, a finding that made him regard maldescent as a manifestation of abnormal sexual maturation. He also found them in the

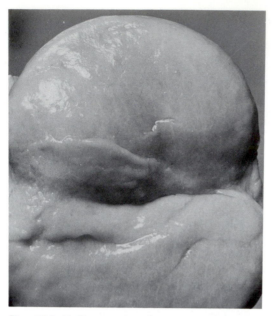

Fig. 746 Malignant lymphoma completely replacing testis. There were no other clinical findings. (WU neg. 52-4426.)

nontumoral testis of 20% of patients with testicular tumors, suggesting that many neoplasms arise in gonads which are already abnormal.[75] The possibility that these hyperplastic stromal lesions are in some instances precursors of the familial types of germ cell tumors by passing through an "in situ" stage currently designated as gonadoblastoma is a very interesting one and should be further explored.

Two cases of **Brenner tumor** in male patients have been reported that were microscopically indistinguishable from the analogous ovarian neoplasm. In both instances, the tumor was small and located between the testis and the head of the epididymis.[72]

Although *malignant lymphoma* comprises only 5% of all testicular cancers, it is the most common testicular tumor in elderly persons (Fig. 746). Approximately 50% of patients with bilateral testicular tumors have lymphoma.[65] The histiocytic type pre-

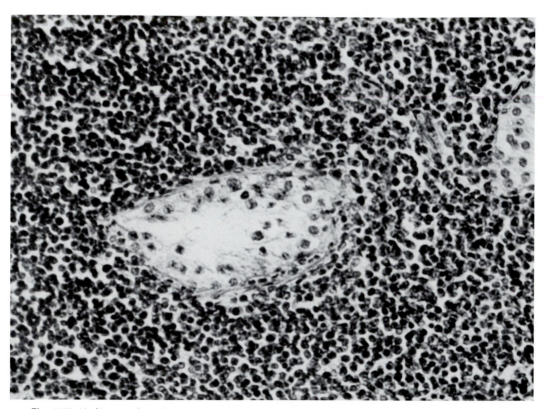

Fig. 747 Malignant lymphoma of testis. Note infiltration of lymphocytes between atrophic tubules. (×225; WU neg. 51-5367.)

dominates over the lymphocytic varieties. The prognosis is generally poor, although long-term cures in cases clinically limited to the testis have been achieved.[55, 65] Microscopically, malignant cells infiltrate the stroma and permeate the seminiferous tubules (Fig. 747). We have seen them confused with spermatocytic seminoma. Levin and Mostofi[66] reported seven cases of testicular *plasmacytoma*, with systemic involvement occurring in all but one of the patients. *Leukemic involvement* of the testis is a common autopsy finding, especially in the acute form, but is rarely of clinical significance.[60]

Carcinoid tumors in the testis may be seen as a component of teratoma, as a primary neoplasm arising from autochthonous argentaffin cells, or as a metastasis from a gastrointestinal tumor.[56, 64]

Most *metastatic tumors* in the testicle arise in the lung or prostate.[70] The latter are usually incidental findings in orchiectomy specimens.[63]

We have seen several examples of *embryonal rhabdomyosarcoma* in children arising in the paratesticular region.[71] The majority had already invaded the substance of the testis at the time of operation.

Other lesions

Granulomatous orchitis is characterized by granulomatous lesions centered in the seminiferous tubules. Epithelioid cells, multinucleated giant cells, lymphocytes, and plasma cells are present. The granulomatous response is probably secondary to the products of disintegrated sperm. A history of trauma is often obtained.[85] We have seen a case in which the diagnosis by various prominent pathologists included undifferentiated carcinoma, seminoma, malignant lymphoma, and Hodgkin's disease. No treatment other than orchiectomy was undertaken. The patient was alive and well ten years later (Fig. 748).

Malacoplakia can involve the testis. It is associated with abscess formation, atrophy of tubules, and the characteristic Michaelis-Guttmann bodies. Thrombosed

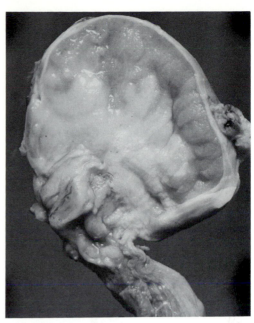

Fig. 748 Granulomatous orchitis in young man. White material of firm consistency and nodular distribution replaces parenchyma. Patient was well ten years later. (WU neg. 52-4639.)

blood vessels were found in seven of the nine patients studied by Brown and Smith.[80] Bacteria (mainly coliform organisms) were found in three of the four cases cultured.

Hourihane[82] reported eighteen cases of *pyogenic epididymoorchitis* complicated by venous thrombosis and septic infarct of the testis. *Escherichia coli* was the organism usually recovered. Microscopically, many similarities were found between this condition and granulomatous orchitis, suggesting a common ischemic background.

Tuberculosis, atypical mycobacteriosis,[81] and *syphilis* can involve the testis (Fig. 749). Clinically, the latter can resemble a neoplasm.

Epidermoid cysts of the testis appear as intraparenchymal lesions filled with keratin and lined by mature squamous epithelium. The absence of adnexal structures and other elements separates them from teratomas.[84]

Ectopic spleen in the scrotum may simulate a malignant neoplasm. Fifty-four

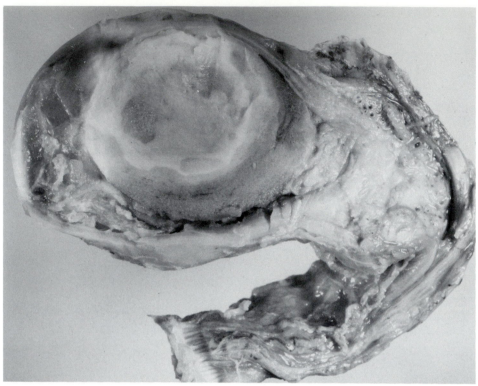

Fig. 749 Gumma of testis, grossly suggesting granuloma. Failure to involve epididymis ruled out tuberculosis. Lesion occurred in 60-year-old white man. (WU neg. 63-1150; case contributed by Dr. S. L. Saltzstein, San Diego, Calif.)

cases have been reported, all on the left side.[83]

REFERENCES
Cryptorchidism

1 Baker, R.: In discussion of Charny, C. W., Coston, A. S., and Meranze, D. R.: Development of the testis; a histologic study from birth to maturity with some notes of abnormal variation, Fertil. Steril. **3**:461-479, 1952.

2 Campbell, H. E.: Incidence of malignant growth of the undescended testicle, Arch. Surg. **44**:353-369, 1942.

3 Campbell, H. E.: The incidence of malignant growth of the undescended testicle: a reply and re-evaluation, J. Urol. **81**:663-668, 1959.

4 Charny, C. W., Conston, A. S., and Meranze, D. R.: Development of the testis, Fertil. Steril. **3**:461-479, 1952.

5 Dow, J. A., and Mostofi, F. K.: Testicular tumors following orchiopexy, South. Med. J. **60**:193-195, 1967.

6 Fonkalsrud, E. W.: Current concepts in the management of the undescended testis, Surg. Clin. N. Am. **50**:847-852, 1970.

7 Gilbert, J. B., and Hamilton, J. B.: Studies in malignant testis tumors, Surg. Gynecol. Obstet. **71**:731-743, 1940.

8 Gross, R. E., and Jewett, T. C., Jr.: Surgical experiences from 1,222 operations for undescended testis, J.A.M.A. **160**:634-641, 1956.

9 Gross, R. E., and Replogle, R. L.: Treatment of the undescended testis, Postgrad. Med. **34**:266-270, 1963.

10 Hinman, F., Jr.: The implications of testicular cytology in the treatment of cryptorchidism, Am. J. Surg. **90**:381-386, 1955.

11 Karcher, G.: Die Fertiliät des behandelten pathologischen Hodenhochstandes (Bauch und Leistenhoden) unter besonderer Berücksichtigung des Zeitpunktes der hormonellen bzw. operativen Therapie, Langenbecks Arch. Klin. Chir. **317**:288-310, 1967.

12 Robinson, J. N., and Engle, E. T.: Some observations on the cryptorchid testis, J. Urol. **71**:726-734, 1954.

Atrophy and infertility

13 de la Balze, F. A., Mancini, R. E., Bur, G. E., and Irazu, J.: Morphologic and histochemical changes produced by estrogens on adult human testes, Fertil. Steril. **5**:421-436, 1954.

14 Bennett, H. S., Baggenstoss, A. H., and Butt, H. R.: The testis and prostate of men who die of cirrhosis of the liver, Am. J. Clin. Path. **20**:814-828, 1950.

15 Durbin, L., and Hotchkiss, R. S.: Testis biopsy in subfertile men with varicocele, Fertil. Steril. **20**:50-57, 1969.

16 Fairley, K. F., Barrie, J. U., and Johnson, W.: Sterility and testicular atrophy related to cyclophosphamide therapy, Lancet **1**:568-569, 1972.

17 Federman, D. D.: The assessment of organ function—the testis, N. Engl. J. Med. **285**:901-904, 1971.

18 Girgis, S. M., Etriby, A., Ibrahim, A. A., and Kahil, S. A.: Testicular biopsy in azoospermia; a review of the last ten years' experience of over 800 cases, Fertil. Steril. **20**:467-477, 1969.

19 Jackson, A. W., Muldal, S., Ockey, C. H., and O'Connor, P. J.: Carcinoma of male breast in association with the Klinefelter syndrome, Br. Med. J. **1**:223-225, 1965.

20 Landing, B. H., Wells, T. R., and Wang, C.-I.: Abnormality of the epididymis and vas deferens in cystic fibrosis, Arch. Pathol. **88**:569-580, 1969.

21 Nelson, W. O.: Interpretation of testicular biopsy, J.A.M.A. **151**:449-454, 1953.

22 Nelson, W. O.: Testicular biopsy. In Tyler, E. T., editor: Sterility—office management of the infertile couple, New York, 1961, McGraw-Hill Book Co.

23 Platt, W. R.: Effects of radioactive phosphorus (P^{32}) on normal tissues; a histologic study of the changes induced in the organs of patients with malignant lymphomas, Arch. Pathol. **43**:1-14, 1947.

24 Rowley, M. J., and Heller, C. G.: The testicular biopsy; surgical procedure, fixation, and staining technics, Fertil. Steril. **17**:177-186, 1966.

25 Sniffen, R. C.: The testis. I. The normal testis, Arch. Pathol. **50**:259-284, 1950.

26 Sniffen, R. C., Howard, R. P., and Simmons, F. A.: The testis. II. Abnormalities of spermatogenesis; atresia of the excretory ducts, Arch. Pathol. **50**:285-295, 1950.

27 Wong, T. W., Straus, F. H., III, and Warner, N.: Testicular biopsy in the study of male infertility, Arch. Pathol. **95**:151-164, 1973.

Tumors

Germinal tumors

28 Abell, M. R., and Holtz, F.: Testicular neoplasms in infants and children. I. Tumors of germ cell origin, Cancer **16**:965-981, 1963.

29 Abell, M. R., and Holtz, F.: Testicular and paratesticular neoplasms in patients 60 years of age and older, Cancer **21**:852-870, 1968.

30 Azzopardi, J. G., Mostofi, F. K., and Theiss, E. A.: Lesions of testes observed in certain patients with widespread choriocarcinoma and related tumors, Am. J. Pathol. **38**:207-225, 1961.

31 Brewer, J. I.: Chorionic gonadotropin in the diagnosis of testicular tumors, Arch. Pathol. **41**:580-591, 1946.

32 Collins, D. H., and Pugh, R. C. P.: Classification and frequency of testicular tumours, Br. J. Urol. 36(suppl.):1-11, 1964.

33 Crook, J. C.: Morphogenesis of testicular tumours, J. Clin. Pathol. **21**:71-74, 1968.

34 Dixon, F. J., and Moore, R. A.: Tumors of the male sex organs. In Atlas of tumor pathology, Sect. VIII, Fasc. 31b and Fasc. 32, Washington, D. C., 1952, Armed Forces Institute of Pathology.

35 Friedman, N. B., and Moore, R. A.: Tumors of the testis; a report on 922 cases, Milit. Surg. **99**:573-593, 1946.

36 Laipply, T. C., and Shipley, R. A.: Extragenital choriocarcinoma in the male, Am. J. Pathol. **21**:921-933, 1945.

37 Magner, D., Campbell, J. S., and Wiglesworth, F. W.: Testicular adenocarcinoma with clear cells occurring in infancy: a distinctive tumour, Can. Med. Assoc. J. **86**:485-488, 1962.

38 Maier, J. G., and Schamber, D. T.: The role of lymphangiography in the diagnosis and treatment of malignant testicular tumors, Am. J. Roentgenol. Radium Ther. Nucl. Med. **114**:481-491, 1972.

39 Marin-Padilla, M.: Origin, nature and significance of the "embryoids" of human teratomas, Virchows Arch. Pathol. Anat. **340**:105-121, 1965.

40 Marin-Padilla, M.: Histopathology of the embryonal carcinoma of the testes; embryological evaluation, Arch. Pathol. **85**:614-622, 1968.

41 Martin, L. S. J., Woodruff, M. W., Webster, J. H., and Pickren, J. W.: Testicular seminoma: a review of 179 patients treated over a 50-year period, Arch. Surg. **90**:306-312, 1965.

42 Pierce, G. B.: Teratocarcinoma: model for a developmental concept of cancer. In Moscona, A. A., and Monroy, A., editors: Current topics in developmental biopsy, New York, 1967, Academic Press, Inc., pp. 223-246.

43 Pierce, G. B., Jr.: Ultrastructure of human testicular tumors, Cancer **19**:1963-1983, 1966.

44 Pierce, G. B., Jr., Bullock, W. K., and Huntington, R. W., Jr.: Yolk sac tumors of the testis, Cancer **25**:644-658, 1970.

45 Pierce, G. B., and Abell, M. R.: Embryonal carcinoma of the testis. In Pathology annual, 1970, New York, 1970, Appleton-Century-Crofts, pp. 27-60.

46 Rosai, J., Silber, I., and Khodadoust, K.:

Spermatocytic seminoma. I. Clinicopathologic study of six cases and review of the literature, Cancer 24:92-102, 1969.

47 Rosai, J., Khodadoust, K., and Silber, I.: Spermatocytic seminoma. II. Ultrastructural study, Cancer 24:103-106, 1969.

48 Scully, R. E., and Coffin, D. L.: Canine testicular tumors; with special reference to their histogenesis, comparative morphology, and endocrinology, Cancer 5:592-605, 1952.

49 Snyder, R. N.: Completely mature pulmonary metastasis from testicular teratocarcinoma; case report and review of the literature, Cancer 24:810-819, 1969.

50 Stevens, L. C.: Experimental production of testicular teratomas in mice, Proc. Nat. Acad. Sci. 52:654-661, 1964.

51 Teilum, G.: Endodermal sinus tumor of the ovary and testis: comparative morphogenesis of the so-called mesonephroma ovarii (Schiller) and of extraembryonic (yolk sac–allantoic) structures of the rat's placenta, Cancer 12:1092-1105, 1959.

52 Teoh, T. B., Steward, J. K., and Willis, R. A.: The distinctive adenocarcinoma of the infant's testis: an account of 15 cases, J. Pathol. Bacteriol. 80:147-156, 1960.

53 Willis, G. W., and Hajdu, S. I.: Histologically benign teratoid metastasis of testicular embryonal carcinoma; report of five cases, Am. J. Clin. Pathol. 59:338-343, 1973.

54 Young, P. G., Mount, B. M., Foote, F. W., Jr., and Whitmore, W. F., Jr.: Embryonal adenocarcinoma in the prepubertal testis; a clinicopathologic study of 18 cases, Cancer 26:1065-1075, 1970.

Nongerminal tumors

55 Abell, M. R., and Holtz, F.: Testicular and paratesticular neoplasms in patients 60 years of age and older, Cancer 21:852-870, 1968.

56 Collins, D. H., and Pugh, R. C. P.: Classification and frequency of testicular tumours, Br. J. Urol. 36(suppl.):1-11, 1964.

57 Dalgaard, J. B., and Hesselberg, F.: Interstitial cell tumours of the testis; two cases and survey, Acta Pathol. Microbiol. Scand. 41:219-234, 1957.

58 Flynn, P. T., and Severance, A. O.: Bilateral interstitial-cell tumors of the testis, Cancer 4:817-822, 1951.

59 Fraser, K. B.: Interstitial cell tumours of the testis, the male sex hormone, Aust. N. Z. J. Surg. 19:48-57, 1949.

60 Givler, R. L.: Testicular involvement in leukemia and lymphoma, Cancer 23:1290-1295, 1969.

61 Hopkins, G. B., and Parry, H. D.: Metastasizing Sertoli-cell tumor (androblastoma), Cancer 23:463-467, 1969.

62 Jungck, E. C., Thrash, A. M., Ohlmacher, A. P., Knight, A. M., Jr., and Dyrenforth, L. Y.: Sexual precocity due to interstitial-cell tumor of the testis: report of 2 cases, J. Clin. Endocrinol. Metab. 17:291-295, 1957.

63 Kay, S., Hennigar, G. R., and Hooper, J. W., Jr.: Carcinoma of the testes metastatic from carcinoma of the prostate, Arch. Pathol. 57:121-129, 1954.

64 Kemble, J. V.: Argentaffin carcinomata of the testicle, Br. J. Urol. 40:580-584, 1968.

65 Kiely, J. M., Massey, B. D., Jr., Harrison, E. G., Jr., and Utz, D. C.: Lymphoma of the testis, Cancer 26:847-852, 1970.

66 Levin, H. S., and Mostofi, F. K.: Symptomatic plasmacytoma of the testis, Cancer 25:1193-1203, 1970.

67 Mahon, F. B., Jr., Gosset, F., Trinity, R. G., and Madsen, P. O.: Malignant interstitial cell testicular tumor, Cancer 31:1208-1212, 1973.

68 Mostofi, F. K., Theiss, E. A., and Ashley, D. J. B.: Tumors of specialized gonadal stroma in human male patients; androblastoma, Sertoli cell tumor, granulosa-theca cell tumor of the testis, and gonadal stromal tumor, Cancer 12:944-957, 1959.

69 Neubecker, R. D., and Theiss, E. A.: Sertoli cell adenomas in patients with testicular feminization, Am. J. Clin. Pathol. 38:52-59, 1962.

70 Price, E. B., Jr., and Mostofi, F. K.: Secondary carcinoma of the testis, Cancer 10:592-595, 1957.

71 Rosas-Uribe, A., Luna, M. A., and Guinn, G. A.: Paratesticular rhabdomyosarcoma; a clinicopathologic study of seven cases, Am. J. Surg. 120:787-791, 1970.

72 Ross, L.: Paratesticular Brenner-like tumor, Cancer 21:722-726, 1968.

73 Scully, R. E.: Gonadoblastoma; a review of 74 cases, Cancer 25:1340-1356, 1970.

74 Sohval, A. R.: Testicular dysgenesis as an etiologic factor in cryptorchidism, J. Urol. 72:693-704, 1954.

75 Sohval, A. R.: Testicular dysgenesis in relation to neoplasm of the testicle, J. Urol. 75:285-291, 1956.

76 Sternberg, W. H.: The morphology, androgenic function, hyperplasia and tumors of the human ovarian hilus cells, Am. J. Pathol. 25:493-521, 1949.

77 Talerman, A.: Malignant Sertoli cell tumor of the testis, Cancer 28:446-455, 1971.

78 Tamoney, H. J., Jr., and Noriega, A.: Malignant interstitial cell tumor of the testis, Cancer 24:547-551, 1969.

79 Teilum, G.: Classification of testicular and ovarian androblastoma and Sertoli cell tumors, Cancer 11:769-782, 1958.

Other lesions

80 Brown, R. C., and Smith, B. H.: Malacoplakia of the testis, Am. J. Clin. Pathol. **47**:135-147, 1967.

81 Hepper, N. G. G., Karlson, A. G., Leary, F. J., and Soule, E. H.: Genitourinary infection due to *Mycobacterium kansasii,* Mayo Clin. Proc. **46**:387-390, 1971.

82 Hourihane, D. O'B.: Infected infarcts of the testis: a study of 18 cases preceded by pyogenic epididymoorchitis, J. Clin. Pathol. **23**:668-675, 1970.

83 Mendez, R., and Morrow, J. W.: Ectopic spleen simulating testicular tumor, J. Urol. **102**:598-601, 1969.

84 Price, E. B., Jr.: Epidermoid cysts of the testis: a clinical and pathologic analysis of 69 cases from the testicular tumor registry, J. Urol. **102**:708-713, 1969.

85 Spjut, H. J., and Thorpe, J. D.: "Granulomatous orchitis," Am. J. Clin. Pathol. **26**:136-145, 1956.

Epididymis and spermatic cord

EPIDIDYMIS
Granulomatous lesions

Tuberculosis of the epididymis is hematogenous in most instances, with the process beginning in the interstitial tissue.[1, 2] Confluent caseation eventually involves the entire epididymis, from which the testis may be secondarily infected (Fig. 750). When the epididymis is infected through the bloodstream, the ductus deferens is usually not involved, whereas the head of the epididymis is extensively involved. Conversely, infection originating from the prostate causes extensive involvement of the ductus deferens and the tail of the epididymis.[1, 2]

Spermatic granulomas of the epididymis are probably due to damage to the epithelium and the basement membrane by inflammation or trauma[4] (Fig. 751). The granulomatous reaction may be related to an acid-fast fraction of lipid from the sperm since this material can provoke a granulomatous reaction if injected subcutaneously in hamsters.[3] The most frequent site of these lesions is the superior pole. They measure up to 3 cm in diameter. Caseation necrosis is absent.

True *spermatoceles* arise most often from the efferent ducts. Epididymal ducts are filled with masses of sperm. These ducts are embedded in loose connective tissue rather than in smooth muscle. Such spermatoceles are lined with ciliated tall columnar cells similar to those in the ducts. Granulomatous inflammation, foreign body giant cell reaction, and cholesterol clefts are common in such lesions. It should be added that removal of hernial sacs is unfortunately sometimes accompanied by the removal of portions of the vas deferens, and indeed even portions of the epididymis.

Tumors
Adenomatoid tumor

A tumor of the epididymis designated as mesothelioma by Evans[5] and by Masson et al.[13] has been called adenomatoid tumor by Golden and Ash.[7] In the past, it had numerous other names such as lymphangioma, adenoma, and adenocarcinoma, Grade I.

This distinctive neoplasm has been described in the epididymis, testicular tunics, serosal surface of the fallopian tube, and uterus.[10] It usually causes no symptoms when it arises from the salpingeal serous surface but produces mass and pain in the region of the testis.

These neoplasms most frequently occur in the third or fourth decade of life. Grossly, they appear encapsulated, firm, and grayish white, rarely contain small cysts, and have an average diameter of 2 cm (Figs. 752 and 753).

Microscopically, these tumors have diverse patterns and contain a variable amount of stroma. They may form solid cords of cells that suggest an epithelial neoplasm. In other instances, they show cystic spaces lined by flattened cells simulating lymph channels[13] (Fig. 754). These cells frequently contain vacuoles that do not stain for fat[7] but that may stain faintly or strongly for mucicarmine.[13] Evans[5] demonstrated that the lining of the serous surface of the peritoneum may be continuous with the cells lining glandular structures in the tumors arising in the region of the fallopian tube. Microscopically, such tumors do not

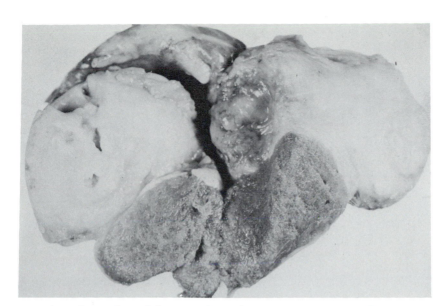

Fig. 750 Tuberculosis of epididymis with confluent caseous masses. Testis is atrophic. (WU neg. 49-6173.)

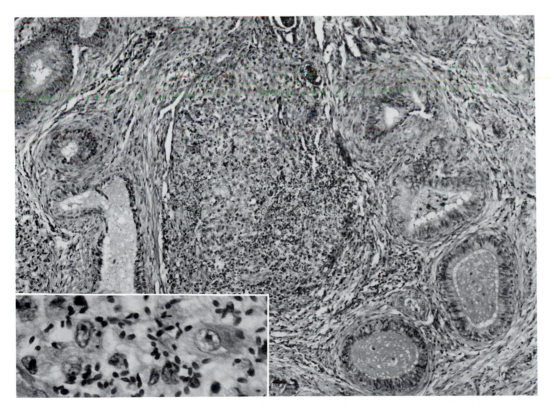

Fig. 751 Spermatic granuloma of epididymis. It is probably result of rupture of epididymal tubules, with subsequent histiocytic reaction to extravasated secretion. **Inset,** Numerous spermatozoa alternate with histiocytes with abundant cytoplasm and large vesicular nuclei. (×90; WU neg. 73-4266; **inset,** ×600; WU neg. 73-4269.)

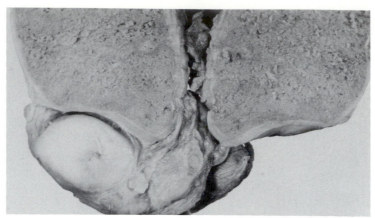

Fig. 752 Typical adenomatoid tumor of epididymis. It is white, encapsulated, and about 2 cm in its greatest diameter. (WU neg. 49-6449.)

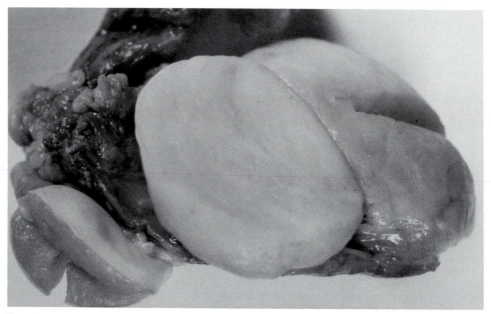

Fig. 753 Firm, encapsulated, rather large adenomatoid tumor with homogeneous grayish white surface.

have a true capsule, but, so far as is known, they do not recur locally or metastasize distantly.

The histogenesis of this neoplasm has long been debated. The cells of origin that have been considered include endothelial, mesonephric, müllerian, and mesothelial. The finding of a combined papillary mesothelioma and adenomatoid tumor in the omentum[8] and the electron microscopic observations on this neoplasm[6, 11, 12] strongly support the hypothesis of a meso-

thelial origin. Two malignant mesotheliomas of the tunica vaginalis testis reported by Kasdon[9] could be interpreted as the malignant counterpart of the adenomatoid tumor.

Other tumors

Papillary cystadenoma of the epididymis arises from the efferent ducts. It may be unilateral or bilateral. Grossly, the size ranges from 1 cm to 5 cm in maximum diameter. It is well circumscribed, either

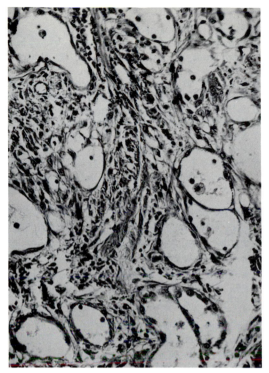

Fig. 754 Typical adenomatoid tumor with cystic spaces lined by flattened cells. (Moderate enlargement; WU neg. 49-1518.)

cystic or solid. Microscopically, papillary infoldings lined by columnar cells with abundant clear cytoplasm is the distinctive feature. Price[15] believes that papillary cystadenoma is the epididymal component of Lindau's disease. Four of his five patients with bilateral cystadenoma had other components of the syndrome.

Primary carcinoma of the epididymis is extremely rare. Salm[16] found thirteen acceptable cases in the literature and added one more. The prognosis was invariably poor. Microscopically, most of the tumors were either undifferentiated or adenocarcinomas.

Leiomyomas present as small, firm nodules. Twenty-five cases were analyzed by Spark.[17] We have seen a *pigmented neuroectodermal tumor of infancy (melanotic progonoma)* involving the epididymis.[14] The patient remains well five years after excision.

Most *secondary tumors* represent direct extension from testicular lesions. Prostate,

lung, and kidney account for most of the other primary sources.[18]

SPERMATIC CORD

Torsion of the spermatic cord, if not treated promptly, may result in testicular infarct. Most cases occur in the first year of life, with a second peak toward puberty.[24] In 64% of the cases, the torsion is located in the intravaginal portion of the cord.[21] The treatment varies from untwisting of the torsion and fixation of the testis to orchiectomy according to the viability of the testis as determined at operation. Whatever procedure is carried out, the opposite testis should be fixed to the dartos musculature as a preventive measure.

Torsion of a testicular appendage results in a dramatic clinical picture out of proportion with the minute size and significance of this structure. The appendix testis, a vestigial structure of Müllerian derivation, is the most often involved (92%). It is a small (1 mm to 10 mm in diameter) round or oval structure, usually pedunculated, attached to the tunica albuginea of the upper pole of the testis.[22, 23]

We have seen several lesions resembling *spermatic granulomas* in the vas deferens following vasectomy or herniorrhaphy.

Most benign tumors of the spermatic cord are *lipomas.* They are surrounded by the tunica vaginalis and derive their blood supply from the vessels of the cord.[25] The collections of mature fatty tissue often seen in association with hernia sacs are not true lipomas. The most common malignant tumor of the spermatic cord in childhood is *embryonal rhabdomyosarcoma.* In adults, *fibrosarcoma, leiomyosarcoma,* pleomorphic *rhabdomyosarcoma,* and *liposarcoma* predominate.[19, 20]

REFERENCES
EPIDIDYMIS
Granulomatous lesions

1 Auerbach, O.: The pathology of urogenital tuberculosis, Int. Clin. 3:21-61, 1940.
2 Auerbach, O.: Tuberculosis of the genital system, Q. Bull., Sea View Hosp. 7:188-207, 1942.

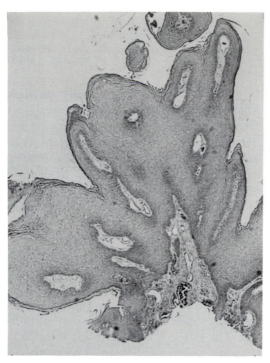

Fig. 755 Condyloma acuminatum with complicated papillary infolding of well-differentiated squamous epithelium. Basement membrane is intact. (Low power; WU neg. 50-477.)

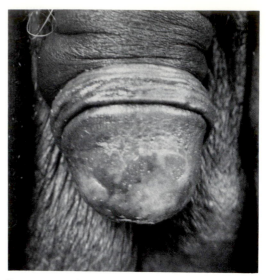

Fig. 756 Erythroplasia of Queyrat (epidermoid carcinoma in situ) of penis. Lesion had been present for considerable period of time. Changes seen microscopically in all sections did not violate basement membrane. (WU neg. 51-2073.)

Carcinoma

Carcinoma of the penis is relatively infrequent in this country but is common in Asia and Paraguay.[5, 19] In some countries, such as Ceylon and Viet Nam, it may constitute 10% of all the cancers.

If circumcision is done shortly after birth, carcinoma practically never develops. If it is delayed until the age of 10 years, as is the Moslem custom, carcinoma is more likely to develop. Carcinoma of the penis is conspicuously frequent in young black men.[12] It is possible that carcinoma is related to personal hygiene and the carcinogenic effect of the smegma bacillus. These factors would be enhanced by failure to circumcise.

Grossly, carcinoma of the penis has primarily two forms. It may develop as a papillary verrucous mass or as an ulcerating lesion. Lesions of the prepuce tend to infiltrate, whereas those of the glans fungate.[2]

The **verrucous** type grows to be a large polypoid tumor that may replace the penis. It rarely metastasizes in spite of its large size (Fig. 757). Microscopically, it is an extremely well-differentiated papillary squamous tumor having the same pattern as verrucous squamous carcinoma of the buccal mucosa. Local excision is the only treatment necessary.

We believe that the lesion known as giant condyloma acuminatum of Buschke-Lowenstein is in reality a verrucous carcinoma.[3, 6] Kraus and Perez-Mesa[11] reported eight verrucous carcinomas of the glans penis. It is important to emphasize that not all tumors with an exophytic gross appearance are verrucous carcinomas. Only those with an extremely well-differentiated cytologic appearance on the surface *as well as* in the deep portions qualify for this diagnosis.

The **ulcerating** variety begins on the glans and eventually destroys it (Fig. 758). It may metastasize to the inguinal lymph nodes, invade the urethra, and involve distant lymph nodes. It is rather poorly differentiated. If the tumor has invaded the

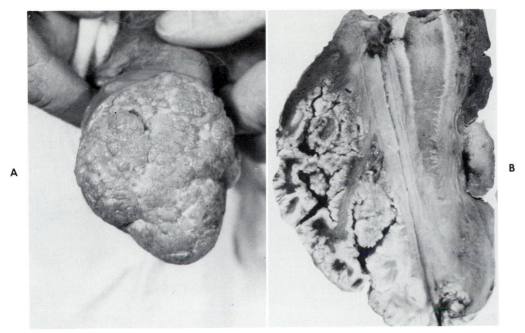

Fig. 757 A, Extensive verrucous squamous carcinoma in 79-year-old man. There were no metastases. **B,** Cross section of tumor shown in **A** demonstrating its failure to involve urethra. (**A** and **B,** Courtesy Dr. R. Johnson, Columbia, Mo.)

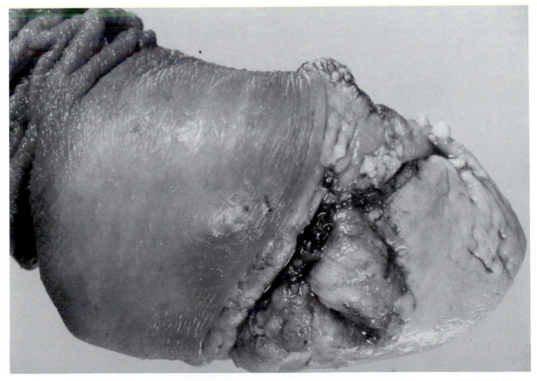

Fig. 758 Ulcerating, undifferentiated carcinoma of glans penis. (WU neg. 62-4745.)

corpora cavernosa or the urethra, distant metastases are more probable.

Carcinoma, either squamous or transitional, may arise primarily in the male urethra. It may follow stricture produced by trauma or gonorrhea. It is most common in the bulbomembranous portion.[26]

Carcinoma of the penis can be treated by local resection or partial or total penectomy, according to size and location of the lesion and microscopic type.[10] Local recurrence is rare. This tumor mestastasizes to the inguinal lymph nodes. Because of infection associated with the carcinoma, enlargement of these nodes almost invariably occurs, so that the clinical appraisal is extremely inaccurate. If metastases are present, practically no cases are cured.[2]

Metastatic carcinoma of the penis is rare.[16] The most common primary tumors occur in the prostate, bladder, rectum, kidney, and testis, in that order of frequency.[13, 17]

Other tumors

Fronstin and Hutcheson[8] described two cases of **malignant melanoma** and reviewed the twenty-five previously reported. Dehner and Smith[7] analyzed forty-six primary **soft tissue tumors** of the penis. Twenty-four were benign, mainly of vascular, neurogenic, and smooth muscle origin. Among the twenty-two malignant lesions, there were three angiosarcomas, four Kaposi's sarcomas, three leiomyosarcomas, three fibrosarcomas, two malignant schwannomas, and two malignant lymphomas.

REFERENCES

1 Andersson, L., Jonsson, G., and Brehmer-Andersson, E.: Erythroplasia of Queyrat—carcinoma in situ, Scand. J. Urol. Nephrol. 1: 303-306, 1967.
2 Bassett, J. W.: Carcinoma of the penis, Cancer 5:530-538, 1952 (extensive bibliography).
3 Bulkley, G., Wendel, R., and Graynack, J.: Buschke-Lowenstein tumor of the penis, J. Urol. 94:731-737, 1967.
4 Campbell, M.: Clinical pediatric urology, Philadelphia, 1951, W. B. Saunders Co., p. 285.
5 Chu, N. X., and Tam, P. B.: Le cancer de la verge chez les vietnamiens, Presse Méd. 62: 125-126, 1954.
6 Dawson, D. F., Duckworth, J. K., Bernhardt, H., and Young, J. M.: Giant condyloma and

verrucous carcinoma of the genital area, Arch. Pathol. 79:225-231, 1965.
7 Dehner, L. P., and Smith, B. H.: Soft tissue tumors of the penis; a clinicopathologic study of 46 cases, Cancer 25:1431-1447, 1970.
8 Fronstin, M. H., and Hutcheson, J. B.: Malignant melanoma of the penis; a report of two cases, Br. J. Urol. 41:324-326, 1969.
9 Graham, J. H., and Helwig, E. B.: Erythroplasia of Queyrat: a clinicopathologic and histochemical study, Cancer (in press).
10 Hanash, K. A., Furlow, W. L., Utz, D. C., and Harrison, E. G., Jr.: Carcinoma of the penis: a clinicopathologic study, J. Urol. 104: 291-297, 1970.
11 Kraus, F. T., and Perez-Mesa, C.: Verrucous carcinoma; clinical and pathologic study of 105 cases involving oral cavity, larynx and genitalia, Cancer 19:26-38, 1966.
12 Lenowitz, H., and Graham, A. P.: Carcinoma of the penis, J. Urol. 56:458-484, 1946.
13 McCrea, L. E., and Tobias, G. L.: Metastatic carcinoma of the penis, J. Urol. 80:489-500, 1958.
14 McRoberts, J. W.: Peyronie's disease, Surg. Gynecol. Obstet. 129:1291-1294, 1969.
15 Marcial-Rojas, R. A., Colon, J. E., and Figueroa, J. J.: Sclerosing lipogranulomas of the male genitalia: report of one case and review of the literature, J. Urol. 75:334-338, 1956.
16 Paquin, A. J., Jr., and Roland, S. I.: Secondary carcinoma of the penis; a review of the literature and a report of nine new cases, Cancer 9:626-632, 1956.
17 Pond, H. S., and Wade, J. C.: Urinary obstruction secondary to metastatic carcinoma of the penis: a case report and review of the literature, J. Urol. 102:333-335, 1969.
18 Queyrat: Erythroplasia de gland, Bull. Soc. Fr. Dermatol. Syphiligr. 22:378, 1911.
19 Riveros, M., and Lebron, R. F.: Geographical pathology of cancer of the penis, Cancer 16: 798-811, 1963 (excellent bibliography).
20 Savatard, L.: Psoriasiform carcinoma of the penis, Br. J. Dermatol. 52:87-93, 1940.
21 Smetana, H. F., and Bernhard, W.: Sclerosing lipogranuloma, Arch. Pathol. 50:296-325, 1950.
22 Smith, B, H.: Peyronie's disease, Am. J. Clin. Pathol. 45:670-678, 1966.
23 Smith, B. H.: Subclinical Peyronie's disease, Am. J. Clin. Pathol. 52:385-390, 1969.
24 Sulzberger, M. B., and Garbe, W.: Nine cases of a distinctive exudative discoid and lichenoid chronic dermatosis, Arch. Dermatol. 36:247-272, 1937.
25 Sulzberger, M. B., Witten, V. H., and Hunt, J. A.: Puzzling persistent penile plaques, Arch. Dermatol. 73:101-109, 1956.
26 Vernon, H. K., and Wilkins, R. D.: Primary carcinoma of the male urethra, Br. J. Urol. 21:232-236, 1950.

18 Female reproductive system

Vulva

Inflammation

Cyst and abscess of Bartholin's gland

Cysts and abscesses of Bartholin's gland are the result of chronic bacterial inflammation, especially gonorrhea. The cyst may be excised or marsupialized. The lining, which is usually of squamous type, can be destroyed partially or totally by the inflammatory infiltrate. The nature of the cyst can be established by the presence of residual mucinous glands in the fibrotic inflammatory connective tissue that forms the cyst wall. Friedrich and Wilkinson[3] reported twenty cases of mucous cysts of the vulva. They were usually solitary and invariably located within the vestibular area.

Granuloma inguinale

Granuloma inguinale begins as a soft elevated granulomatous area that enlarges very slowly by peripheral extension and ulcerates (Fig. 521). Microscopically, there is a dense dermal inflammatory infiltrate composed of histiocytes and plasma cells, with a scattering of small abscesses throughout the lesion.[5] The diagnosis rests upon the demonstration of the Donovan bodies, which are seen as small round encapsulated bodies inside the cytoplasm of the histiocytes. They can be seen in hematoxylin-eosin sections but are best demonstrated with the Giemsa or the Wright stain[2] (Fig. 522). The pronounced pseudoepitheliomatous hyperplasia of squamous epithelium that accompanies chronic lesions should be differentiated from the very rare epidermoid carcinoma that arises in areas of granuloma inguinale.[1]

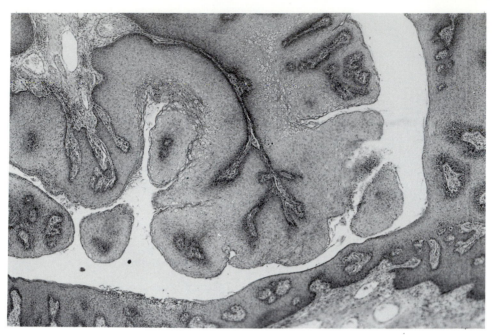

Fig. 759 Condyloma acuminatum with complicated papillary arrangement of well-differentiated squamous cells with intact basement membrane. (Low power; WU neg. 52-2478.)

Lymphogranuloma venereum

Lymphogranuloma venereum is a viral disease affecting primarily lymphatics and lymphoid tissue. The initial small ulcer at a site of venereal contact is often unnoticed. The first clinical manifestation is swelling of inguinal lymph nodes caused by "stellate" abscesses surrounded by pale epithelioid cells[4] (Fig. 943). There is extensive scarring as the disease progresses, often leading to fistulas and strictures of the urethra, vagina, and rectum (Fig. 523). The Frei test has been replaced by a complement fixation test in endemic areas.[2] Rainey[6] reported eleven cases of epidermoid carcinoma or adenocarcinoma engrafted on lymphogranulomatous strictures. Most of the tumors were located in the anorectal area.

Condyloma acuminatum

Condyloma acuminatum is a viral-induced papilloma. Multiple soft elevated masses are commonly present. Microscopic examination shows a complicated papillary arrangement of well-differentiated squamous epithelium supported by delicate vascular connective tissue stalks (Fig. 759). Focal vacuolization of the malpighian epithelium and lymphocytic infiltration of the stroma are regular features.

Chronic vulvar dystrophies

The skin and subcutaneous tissues of the vulva may atrophy after menopause. When associated with irregular patchy areas of thickened white skin, the clinically descriptive term "leukoplakia" has been used. Another clinical term, "kraurosis," implies that severe shrinkage has occurred. Because of the variable connotations of these inexact terms, it has proved desirable to lump these lesions under the designation of *chronic vulvar dystrophies*, emphasizing the lack of specificity of the clinical appearance.

Pruritus is often severe. Large areas may be red and excoriated. These symptoms and physical findings are not specific. Biopsy is necessary to establish the diagnosis.

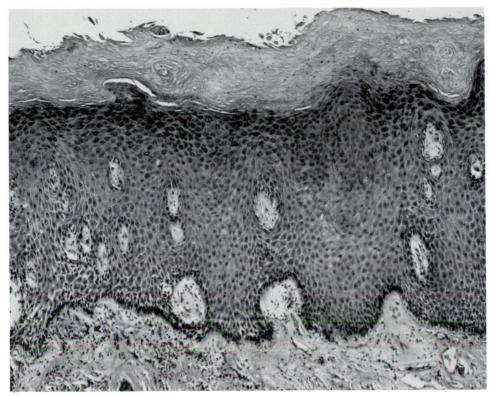

Fig. 760 Hyperkeratosis and chronic inflammation. Note especially acanthosis and lack of dermal homogenization in contrast to pattern of lichen sclerosus et atrophicus. (×85; WU neg. 63-9612.)

Keratosis and chronic inflammation

Keratosis and chronic inflammation together form the lesion usually meant when the clinical term "leukoplakia" is used. The vulvar skin may be white and scaling, or red, or a mixture of both. It often feels thickened but may be thin and easily traumatized. The vulvar soft tissues may be normal but are often atrophied and shrunken.

The microscopic features of thick keratinized layer, prominent stratum granulosum, acanthosis, and dermal chronic inflammatory infiltrate are encountered in variable proportions (Fig. 760). Foci of dysplastic epithelium similar to changes seen in actinic keratoses are sometimes found. This has been partially responsible for the concept that hyperkeratosis is premalignant.

An association of vulvar dystrophies with vulvar carcinoma is undeniable.[12]

However, gynecologists admit that rarely have they seen carcinoma develop in a patient under observation for "leukoplakia."[10]

There is no place for the term "leukoplakia" in the pathologic diagnosis. The physician can see for himself that a white plaque is white, and his confidence will hardly be stimulated by a pathologist's use of this word if the lesion he saw was actually red. It is better to designate the lesion as keratosis, followed by an evaluation of the degree of atypia present, if any.

Lichen sclerosus et atrophicus

Lichen sclerosus et atrophicus is a specific dermatosis that may occur anywhere on the skin.[8] The large majority of cases occur in adults, but a few cases have been reported in children. The vulvar region was the most common location, and

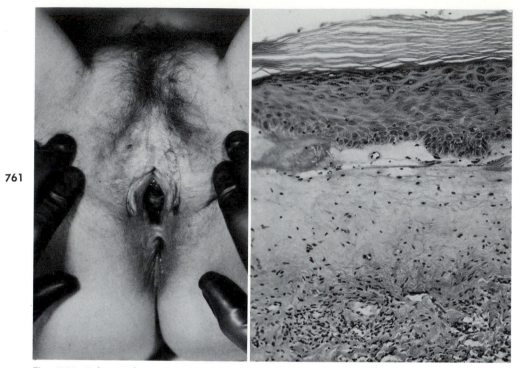

761

762

Fig. 761 Lichen sclerosus et atrophicus of vulva. Note shrinkage and atrophy. (EFSCH 8550.)

Fig. 762 Lichen sclerosus et atrophicus of vulva with hyperkeratosis, atrophy, and homogeneous band of edema in dermis. (×125; WU neg. 50-3746.)

there was a high incidence of spontaneous involution at the time of puberty.[11] When the associated atrophy and shrinkage are pronounced, as they may be in older people, the clinically descriptive but pathologically inexact term "kraurosis" has been used. The distinctive pathologic features (Figs. 761 and 762) were discussed previously (Chapter 3).

Clinicopathologic correlation

Chronic vulvar dystrophies are uncomfortable and are difficult to eradicate by any form of treatment, including vulvectomy. The cause or causes are unknown. Evolution into a carcinoma is possible but unlikely, and vulvectomy does not preclude such a development.[9]

The clinical appearance of carcinoma in situ or Paget's disease may be indistinguishable from that of a dystrophy. The presence of a systemic disease such as diabetes or a specific dermatosis amenable to medi-

cation, such as psoriasis or lichen planus, should be excluded in every case. Biopsy is indispensable. Multiple biopsies are necessary if the lesion is large or varies in appearance from place to place.[7]

Benign tumors
Hidradenoma papilliferum

Hidradenoma papilliferum is a small, nodular, well-circumscribed lump that apparently originates from apocrine sweat glands of the vulva and perianal region and clinically may suggest epidermal inclusion cyst.[13] Rarely, it may ulcerate through the skin, simulating carcinoma.

A papillary or complex glandular pattern is apparent. The epithelial cells occur in two layers and some hidradenomas resemble papillomas of the breast (Fig. 763). Cellular stratification and pleomorphism may occur in predominantly papillary lesions.

All acceptable examples of this lesion

have been benign. The sixty-one patients studied by Meeker et al.[15] and the sixty-nine reported by Woodworth et al.[17] were all white women.

Fibroadenoma

Fibroadenomas may originate in accessory breast tissue in the vulva. Swelling and lactation in such breast tissue may oc-

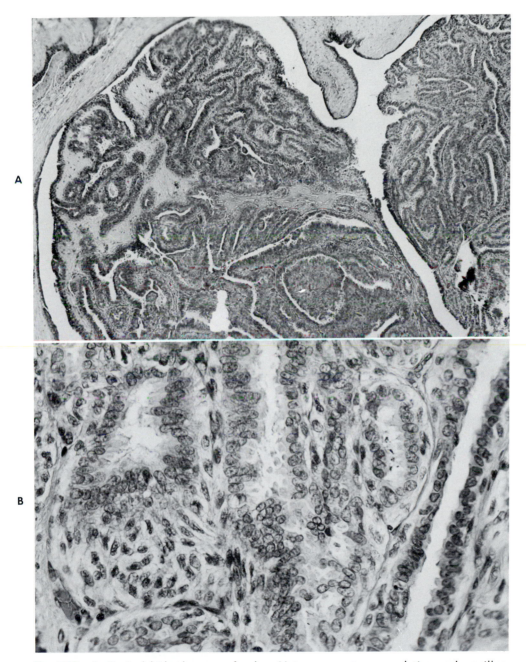

Fig. 763   A, Typical hidradenoma of vulva. Note apparent encapsulation and papillary pattern. **B,** Same specimen shown in **A** at higher magnification. Double layer of cells and characteristic cellular pattern can be seen. Note evidence of active secretion substantiating origin from apocrine-type glands. (**A,** Low power; WU neg. 52-2045; **B,** ×440; WU neg. 52-2047.)

cur in pregnancy.[16] The gross and microscopic appearance resembles that of mammary fibroadenoma with some variations.[14]

Malignant tumors
Carcinoma in situ

Epidermoid carcinoma in situ is an uncommon, slightly elevated, plaquelike le-

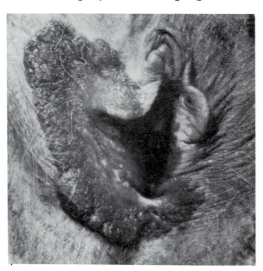

sion of the vulvar mucous membranes (Fig. 764). It is probably identical with penile erythroplasia of Queyrat (Fig. 765).

A very similar lesion of the outer vulvar skin is probably equivalent to Bowen's disease of the skin.[18] The distinction between the two should be attempted because of the slower evolution and association with other carcinomas encountered in Bowen's disease (Chapter 3). Carcinoma in situ, on the other hand, may harbor unexpected foci of invasion[29] and may be multifocal with similar lesions in the vagina and cervix.[19]

Paget's disease

Paget's disease of the vulva presents as a crusting, elevated scaling erythematous rash (Fig. 766). The epidermis contains

Fig. 764 Carcinoma in situ involving wide area of vulva as elevated plaque (WU neg. 52-2102; from Gonin, R.: Maladie de Bowen—Erythroplasie des muqueuses, Dermatologica 92:74-79, 1946.)

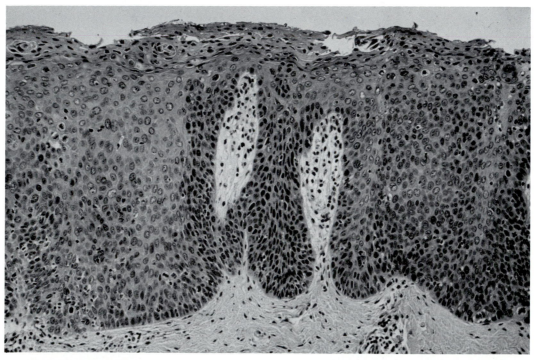

Fig. 765 Epidermoid carcinoma in situ. There is disorganization of all layers with prominent variation in size and shape of cells, but basement membrane is intact. (×140; WU neg. 64-344.)

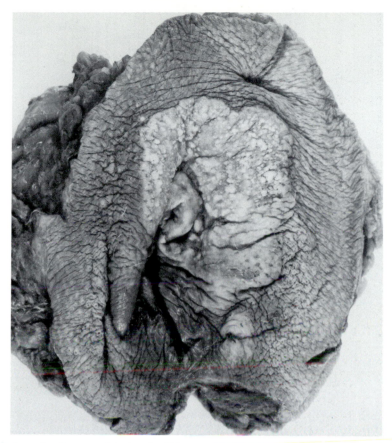

Fig. 766 Paget's disease of vulva in 87-year-old woman. Disease involves labia majora and labia minora. Note clinical similarity to leukoplakia. (From Fenn, M. E., Morley, G. W., and Abell, M. R.: Paget's disease of vulva, Obstet. Gynecol. **38:**660-670, 1971.)

large pale adenocarcinoma cells that give positive reactions with mucicarmine and aldehyde fuchsin[36] (Fig. 767). The tumor cells may form solid nests or glandular spaces. We have seen several cases confused with malignant melanoma. The presence of occasional melanin granules in some tumor cells *does not* rule out the diagnosis of Paget's disease.

Paget's disease of the vulva differs in several respects from Paget's disease of the breast. The latter is *always* associated with an underlying carcinoma that may be intraductal or invasive. The intraepidermal malignant cells may or may not contain mucin. In contrast, the majority of the cases of vulvar Paget's disease are not associated with an invasive underlying carcinoma and are practically always positive

for mucin stains.[32] Of seven cases reported by Fenn et al,[28] the labius majus was involved in all seven, the labium minus in three, and the perineal skin in three. Paget's cells were present in the epidermis and in the pilosebaceous structures of all patients and in the sweat ducts of two. Invasive cancer was not found in any of these patients and only in two of the twenty-six studied by Taylor.[41] Paget's disease of the vulva probably represents a sweat gland carcinoma arising primarily from the intraepidermal component of the glands.

Paget cells may be found in the apparently normal skin at the margins of the rash. If no invasive component is found in the resected specimen, the prognosis is good. Metastases do not occur under these

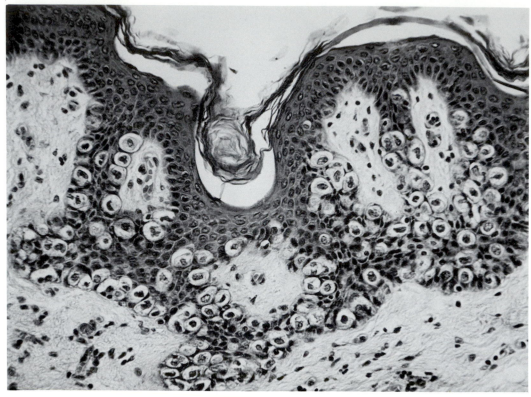

Fig. 767 Paget's disease of vulva in 60-year-old woman. Paget cells are shown with clarity and stain positively for epithelial mucin. (WU neg. 65-347.)

circumstances, although local recurrence may supervene. Therefore, excision should include a margin of normal skin and the subcutaneous tissue to incorporate all sweat glands.

Invasive epidermoid carcinoma

Invasive epidermoid carcinoma of the vulva frequently is associated with hyperkeratosis. It begins usually on the labia majora but may arise on the labia minora or even in the region of the clitoris. This tumor grows rather slowly, ulcerates, and eventually spreads widely[42] (Fig. 768). Microscopically, it usually is a well-differentiated squamous carcinoma. It may have multiple foci of origin[33] and is not infrequently associated with malignant tumors elsewhere in the lower genital tract, notably the uterine cervix.[34] This has led to the hypothesis that the epithelium of the entire lower genital tract (cervix, vagina, vulva, and perianal area) reacts as a single tissue field to a given carcinogenic stimulus.

Epidermoid carcinoma in situ occurs frequently at the margins of invasive carcinoma. The presence of hyperkeratotic dysplastic skin at the edge of the cancer is associated with a significantly better prognosis.[30] In the region of the clitoris, the tumor may be undifferentiated. Carcinoma that arises from the labium spreads to inguinal lymph nodes. Since this tumor is invariably infected, the regional nodes enlarge. It is impossible to predict whether the nodes are enlarged because of cancer or infection. If the carcinoma is in the region of the clitoris, it may spread directly to deep nodes.

The treatment of choice is radical vulvectomy followed by bilateral inguinal lymph node dissection. Iliac lymphadenectomy should probably be reserved for selected cases.

Verrucous carcinoma is a special type of epidermoid carcinoma of the vulva, often confused with condyloma accuminatum. Cytologically, it is an extremely well-differentiated tumor. It infiltrates locally but practically never metastasizes.[35]

In our experience, *metastatic carcinoma* in the vulva is usually an expression of

School of Medicine, only six showed junctional activity, and all of these were compound in type (Chapter 3).

Malignant melanoma is the second most common malignant tumor of the vulva, although it is much less frequent than epidermoid carcinoma. Malignant change in a mole is accompanied by deepening pigmentation, increased growth rate, and ulceration. The microscopic pattern is sim-

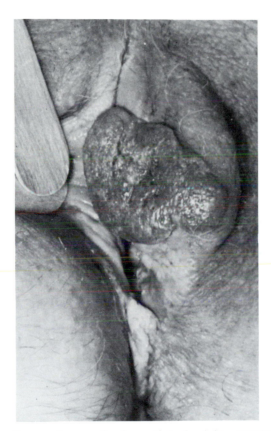

Fig. 768 Large ulcerating carcinoma of vulva with leukoplakia. (EFSCH 11929; courtesy Dr. R. Johnson, Columbia, Mo.)

far-advanced disease. The most common location is the labius major, and the most common sources are the uterine cervix, endometrium, urethra, and kidney.[26]

Malignant melanoma

Malignant melanomas of the vulva may arise from a preexisting junctional nevus. In twenty-seven consecutive moles of the vulva seen at Washington University

ilar to malignant melanoma of the skin (Chapter 3). The treatment of choice is radical vulvectomy with bilateral inguinal lymph node dissection. Practically no cases are cured.[25]

Clinicopathologic correlation

The aggressive treatment of lymphopathia venereum of the vulva may prevent some carcinomas. The surgical treatment of carcinoma is radical vulvectomy with bilateral radical inguinal lymph node dissection.[27] In thirty-six patients with lymph node metastases who had this form of therapy, twenty-nine survived without evidence of disease from three and one-half years to five or more years—there were seventeen who survived five or more years.[31]

Prophylactic removal of moles from the vulva may prevent malignant melanoma. When malignant melanoma is obvious clinically, no cures are likely to be obtained. The absolute five-year survival rate in patients treated for vulvar epidermoid carcinoma has been in the 50% to 60% range in most large series.[21, 23, 39, 42] Collins et al.[24] obtained a five-year survival rate of 20.8% in ninety-eight patients with lymph node metastases.

Carcinoma of female urethra

Carcinomas of the female urethra are included with the vulva by some authors because many of these lesions occur at the meatus, at the junction of transitional and stratified squamous epithelium. The commonest symptom is bleeding or dysuria in an elderly woman.[40] The majority are epidermoid carcinomas. Rarely, they may be adenocarcinomas or transitional cell carcinomas.[20] Of thirty-five tumors examined by Rogers and Burns,[38] nineteen were anterior (vulvourethral), four were posterior (vesicourethral), and twelve involved the entire urethra. Of the twenty-four patients who were followed for five years or longer, only seven were alive and well (29%). Seventeen of the twenty-five patients reported by Skjaerassen[40] died of spread of the urethral cancer. The prognosis was worse for those with posterior lesions than for those with vulvourethral tumors.

The **urethral caruncle** occurs exclusively in the female urethra and is not a true neoplasm. It has the appearance of a small raspberry, bleeds easily, and may become infected. Microscopically, extreme vascularity and complicated small nests of epithelium may cause it to be incorrectly diagnosed as malignant. Caruncles often recur after excision.[37] *Prolapse* of the urethral mucosa in childhood may simulate a vulvovaginal neoplasm.[22]

Other lesions

Palladino et al.[46] accepted sixty-one reported cases of **basal cell carcinoma** and added four new ones. There was not a single instance of metastatic spread. The usual presentation was an ulcerated mass in the labius majus in an elderly patient. These neoplasms should be treated by local excision. It is important to distinguish between basal cell carcinoma of the vulvar skin which does not metastasize and **adenoid cystic carcinoma** of the vestibular glands which does.[43] The former looks and behaves like basal cell carcinoma elsewhere in the skin. The appearance of the latter is undistinguishable from its more common counterpart in the salivary glands.

Leiomyomas, hemangiomas, endometriosis, and **granular cell tumors** have been reported.[47] Kempson and Sherman[44] reported a case of **sclerosing lipogranuloma** quite similar to the lesion more commonly seen in the skin of the penis and scrotum. A case of **benign lymphoid hyperplasia** located in the labium minus was studied by Kernen and Morgan.[45]

REFERENCES
Inflammation

1 Alexander, L. J., and Shields, T. L.: Squamous cell carcinoma of the vulva secondary to granuloma inguinale, Arch. Dermatol. **67:**395-402, 1953.

2 Douglas, C. P.: Lymphogranuloma venereum and granuloma inguinale of the vulva, J. Obstet. Gynaecol. Br. Commonw. **69:**871-880, 1962.

3 Friedrich, E. G., Jr., and Wilkinson, E. J.: Mucous cysts of the vulvar vestibule, Obstet. Gynecol. **42:**407-414, 1973.

4 Koteen, H.: Lymphogranuloma venereum, Medicine (Baltimore) **24:**1-69, 1945.

5 Pund, E. R., and Greenblatt, R. B.: Specific histology of granuloma inguinale, Arch. Pathol. **23:**224-229, 1937.

6 Rainey, R.: The association of lymphogranu-

loma inguinale and cancer, Surgery **35**:221-235, 1954.

Chronic vulvar dystrophies

7 Clark, W. H., Jr.: A histological study of kraurosis vulvae, lichen sclerosus et atrophicus, and leukoplakia of the vulva—a preliminary report, Bull. Tulane Med. Fac. **16**:123-128, 1957.

8 Janovski, N. A., and Ames, S.: Lichen sclerosus et atrophicus of the vulva; a poorly understood disease entity, Obstet. Gynecol. **22**:697-708, 1963.

9 Jeffcoate, T. N. A.: Chronic vulval dystrophies, Am. J. Obstet. Gynecol. **95**:61-74, 1966.

10 Jeffcoate, T. N. A., and Woodcock, A. S.: Premalignant conditions of the vulva with particular reference to chronic epithelial dystrophies, Br. Med. J. **5245**:127-134, 1961.

11 Lascano, E. F., Montes, L. F., and Mazzini, M. A.: Lichen sclerosus et atrophicus in childhood; report of 6 cases, Obstet. Gynecol. **24**:872-877, 1964.

12 Macafee, C. H. G.: Some aspects of vulvar cancer, J. Obstet. Gynaecol. Br. Commonw. **69**:177-195, 1962.

Benign tumors

13 Anderson, N. P.: Hidradenoma of the vulva, Arch. Dermatol. **62**:873-891, 1950 (extensive bibliography).

14 Burger, R. A., and Marcuse, P. M.: Fibroadenoma of the vulva, Am. J. Clin. Pathol. **24**:965-968, 1954.

15 Meeker, J. H., Neubecker, R. D., and Helwig, E. B.: Hidradenoma papilliferum, Am. J. Clin. Pathol. **37**:182-195, 1962.

16 Tow, S. H., and Shanmugaratnam, K.: Supernumerary mammary gland in the vulva, Br. Med. J. **5314**:1234-1236, 1962.

17 Woodworth, H., Jr., Dockerty, M. B., Wilson, R. B., and Pratt, J. H.: Papillary hidradenoma of the vulva; a clinicopathologic study of 69 cases, Am. J. Obstet. Gynecol. **110**:501-508, 1971.

Malignant tumors

18 Abell, M. R., and Gosling, J. R. G.: Intraepithelial and infiltrating carcinoma of the vulva; Bowen's type, Cancer **14**:318-329, 1961.

19 Barclay, D. L., and Collins, C. G.: Intraepithelial cancer of the vulva, Am. J. Obstet. Gynecol. **86**:95-106, 1963.

20 Brack, C. B., and Farber, G. J.: Carcinoma of the female urethra, J. Urol. **64**:710-715, 1950.

21 Brunschwig, A., and Brockunier, A., Jr.: Surgical treatment of squamous cell carcinoma of the vulva, Obstet. Gynecol. **29**:362-368, 1967.

22 Capraro, V. J., Bayonet-Rivera, N. P., and Magoss, I.: Vulvar tumor in children due to prolapse of urethral mucosa, Am. J. Obstet. Gynecol. **108**:572-575, 1970.

23 Collins, C. G., Collins, J. H., Barclay, D. L., and Nelson, E. W.: Cancer involving the vulva, Am. J. Obstet. Gynecol. **87**:762-772, 1963.

24 Collins, C. G., Lee, F. Y. L., and Roman-Lopez, J. J.: Invasive carcinoma of the vulva with lymph node metastasis, Am. J. Obstet. Gynecol. **109**:446-452, 1971.

25 Das Gupta, T., and D'Urso, J.: Melanoma of female genitalia, Surg. Gynecol. Obstet. **119**:1074-1078, 1964.

26 Dehner, L. P.: Metastatic and secondary tumors of the vulva, Obstet. Gynecol. **42**:47-57, 1973.

27 Edsmyr, F.: Carcinoma of the vulva; an analysis of 560 patients with histologically verified squamous cell carcinoma, Acta Radiol. [Diagn.] (Stockh.) **217**(suppl.):1-135, 1962.

28 Fenn, M. E., Morley, G. W., and Abell, M. R.: Paget's disease of vulva, Obstet. Gynecol. **38**:660-670, 1971.

29 Gardiner, S. H., Stout, F. E., Arbogast, J. L., and Huber, C. P.: Intraepithelial carcinoma of the vulva, Am. J. Obstet. Gynecol. **65**:539-549, 1953.

30 Gosling, J. R. G., Abell, M. R., Prolette, B. M., and Loughrin, T. D.: Infiltrative squamous cell (epidermoid) carcinoma of vulva, Cancer **14**:330-343, 1961.

31 Green, T. H., Jr., Ulfelder, H., and Meigs, J. V.: Epidermoid carcinoma of the vulva; an analysis of 238 cases. Part I. Etiology and diagnosis. Part II. Therapy and end results, Am. J. Obstet. Gynecol. **75**:834-864, 1958.

32 Helwig, E. B., and Graham, J. H.: Anogenital (extramammary) Paget's disease: a clinicopathological study, Cancer **16**:387-403, 1963.

33 Jeffcoate, T. N. A.: The dermatology of the vulva, J. Obstet. Gynaecol. Br. Commonw. **69**:888-890, 1962.

34 Jimerson, G. K., and Merrill, J. A.: Multicentric squamous malignancy involving both cervix and vulva, Cancer **26**:150-153, 1970.

35 Kraus, F. T., and Perez-Mesa, C.: Verrucous carcinoma; clinical and pathologic study of 105 cases involving oral cavity, larynx and genitalia, Cancer **19**:26-38, 1966.

36 Paget, G. E., Rowley, A., and Woodcock, A. S.: Paget's disease of the vulva, J. Pathol. Bacteriol. **67**:256-258, 1954.

37 Palmer, J. K., Emmett, J. L., and McDonald, J. R.: Urethral caruncle, Surg. Gynecol. Obstet. **87**:611-620, 1948.

38 Rogers, R. E., and Burns, B.: Carcinoma of the female urethra, Obstet. Gynecol. **33**:54-57, 1969.

39 Rutledge, F., Smith, J. P., and Franklin, E. W.: Carcinoma of the vulva, Am. J. Obstet. Gynecol. **106**:1117-1130, 1970.

40 Skjaeraasen, E.: Cancer of the female urethra; a clinical study of 25 cases, Acta Obstet. Gynecol. Scand. **48**:589-597, 1969.

41 Taylor, H. B.: Personal communication, 1967.

42 Way, S.: Carcinoma of the vulva, Am. J. Obstet. Gynecol. **79**:692-697, 1960.

Other lesions

43 Abell, M. R.: Adenocystic (pseudoadenomatous) basal cell carcinoma of vestibular glands of vulva, Am. J. Obstet. Gynecol. **86**:470-482, 1963.

44 Kempson, R. L., and Sherman, A. I.: Sclerosing lipogranuloma of the vulva, Am. J. Obstet. Gynecol. **101**:854-856, 1968.

45 Kernen, J. A., and Morgan, M. L: Benign lymphoid hamartoma of the vulva; report of a case, Obstet. Gynecol. **35**:290-292, 1970.

46 Palladino, V. S., Duffy, J. L., and Bures, G. J.: Basal cell carcinoma of the vulva, Cancer **24**:460-470, 1969.

47 Weinshel, L. R.: Benign tumors of vulva, Am. J. Surg. **71**:210-215, 1946.

Vagina

Benign lesions

The adult vagina is impervious to most bacterial infections. Indolent infections caused by *Trichomonas vaginalis* and *Candida albicans* are relatively common, especially during pregnancy. *Lymphogranuloma venereum* can involve the vagina during the late stage of the disease and result in stricture.

Benign tumors of the vagina are rare. We have seen **squamous papillomas, hemangiomas,** and **leiomyomas.** Occasionally, following vaginal hysterectomy, the *tubal fimbria* may become entrapped in the healing vaginal apex, a finding that must not be confused with neoplastic change.

Endometriosis of the vagina is rare.[4] Its most common occurrence is in episiotomy scars, presumably by implantation. **Adenosis** of the vagina represents a partial or complete conversion of the vaginal mucosa from squamous to glandular epithelium of endocervical type.[21] Excess mucus discharge is the most common complaint. Sandberg[20] found occult vaginal adenosis in nine (41%) of twenty-two vaginas from postpuberal patients obtained at autopsy. In contrast, glands were not found in the vagina of any of the thirteen prepuberal patients.

Gartner's duct cysts are fairly common. They are located in the anterolateral or lateral vaginal wall. Gartner's duct is the vestigial remnant of the wolffian duct. The cysts are lined by low cuboidal epithelial cells with or without cilia. We have seen two carcinomas arising within such cysts. They have a distinctive microscopic pattern and, unlike cervical adenocarcinomas, do not form mucin. Another cyst of common occurrence is the one resulting from inclusion of squamous epithelium, either spontaneously or secondary to surgery or trauma.[3]

Vaginal **polyps** may have a disturbing histologic appearance and be incorrectly diagnosed as sarcoma botryoides. Norris and Taylor[14] reported twenty-four cases, twenty-two from adults (five of them pregnant) and two from newborn infants. Twelve contained atypical cells within the stroma (Fig. 769). Local excision was curative in every case, with only one instance of local recurrence. The age of the patients and the absence of rapid growth, "cambium layer," invasion of epithelium, and cross striations are the main features that differentiate this lesion from sarcoma botryoides. We have seen a few benign vaginal polyps in infants and children with a prominent papillary configuration and lined by a single layer of cuboidal epithelial cells. They are sometimes referred to as **mesonephric papillomas,** although convincing evidence of a mesonephric origin is lacking. A case of a pedunculated **rhabdomyoma** of the vagina in a 34-year-old patient was reported by Ceremsak.[1]

Malignant tumors

Epidermoid carcinoma arising primarily in the vagina is a rare neoplasm[24] (Fig. 770). Most of the tumors represent extension from cervical cancers. By convention, only vaginal tumors that spare the uterine cervix are regarded as primary. Those involving both areas are classified as cervical carcinomas with vaginal extension, regardless of the relative proportion of involvement. The majority are grossly nodular or ulcerative. The upper third and the anterior or lateral walls are the most common sites of origin.[18]

Carcinoma in situ of the vagina is often

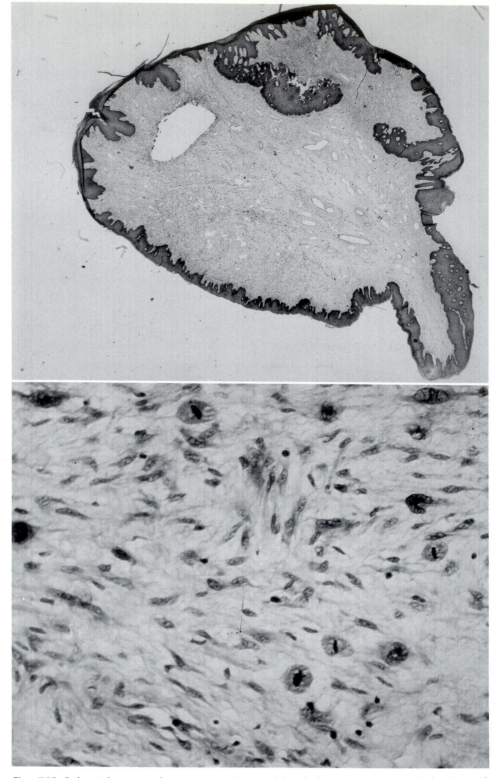

Fig. 769 Polypoid tumor of vagina in 15-year-old girl demonstrating atypical cells with numerous mitotic figures that easily could be mistaken for sarcoma botryoides. (×300; WU negs. 65-383 and 67-1171.)

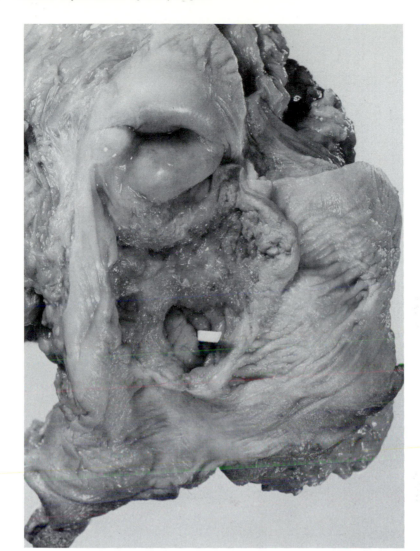

Fig. 770 Ulcerating carcinoma of vagina that had infiltrated rectovaginal septum. It was removed by pelvic evisceration. (WU neg. 50-2111.)

multifocal and frequently associated with similar lesions of the cervix and vulva.[11] Small lesions can be treated satisfactorily by local excision, followed by careful periodic clinical and cytologic examinations. Extensive lesions may necessitate the performance of a vaginectomy.[5]

Most primary *vaginal adenocarcinomas* are mucus secreting and have an appearance indistinguishable from those arising in the endocervix (Fig. 771). They occur in middle-aged or elderly patients. The remaining cases fall into one or two well-defined categories. The first and most com-

mon is designated as *clear cell carcinoma* (or adenocarcinoma, mesonephric type). It is characterized microscopically by the presence of tubules and cysts lined by clear cells, some of which have a "hobnail" appearance (Fig. 772). The clear cytoplasm usually contains a significant amount of glycogen and fat. Vaginal adenosis was seen in four of six cases reported by Herbst and Scully.[7] This tumor characteristically occurs in the anterior or lateral vaginal wall of adolescents and is associated with a relatively good prognosis. Herbst et al.[9] made the startling observa-

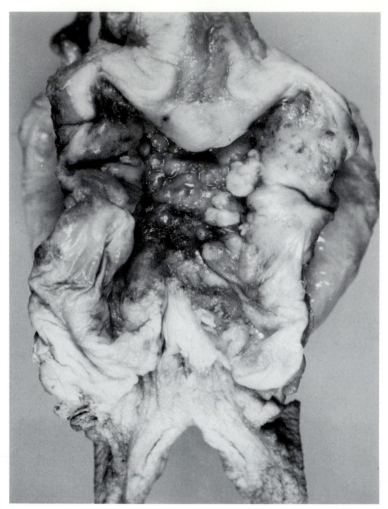

Fig. 771 Primary mucus-secreting adenocarcinoma of vagina in 45-year-old patient. Vaginal adenosis was identified in nontumoral vagina. (MU neg. 70-3126.)

tion that seven of the eight mothers of patients with this type of vaginal adenocarcinoma had been treated with diethylstilbestrol during the first trimester of their pregnancy. This was also true of the mothers of all five patients reported by Greenwald et al.[6] In a more recent report, history of maternal estrogen therapy was obtained in forty-nine of ninety-one cases.[8]

The second type of vaginal adenocarcinoma is an extremely rare neoplasm, which has been repeatedly confused with the one previously described. Its microscopic appearance is remarkably similar to that of the gonadal *yolk sac tumor* (Chapter 17 under Testis). In contrast to the clear cell carcinoma, it typically affects infants under 2 years of age and is more commonly located in either the posterior wall or the fornices. Clinically, it simulates sarcoma botryoides. Four of the six patients reported by Norris et al.[16] died with generalized metastases.

Botryoid rhabdomyosarcoma (sarcoma botryoides) is a rare polypoid invasive tumor usually occurring in infants and arising from the anterior vaginal wall (Fig. 773). Approximately 90% of the cases occur in girls under 5 years of age, with close to two-thirds appearing during the first two years. Grossly, it presents as a conglomerate of soft polypoid masses resembling

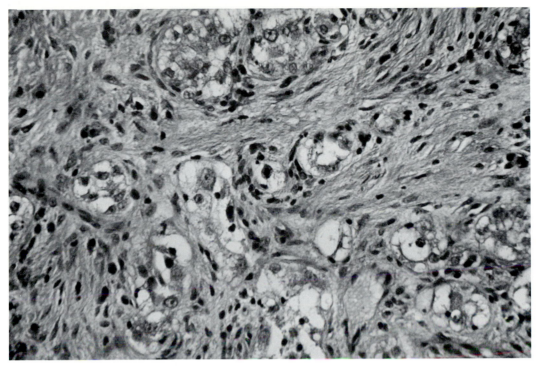

Fig. 772 Vaginal carcinoma occurring in young girl whose mother had received stilbestrol during pregnancy. (×300; WU neg. 72-5400.)

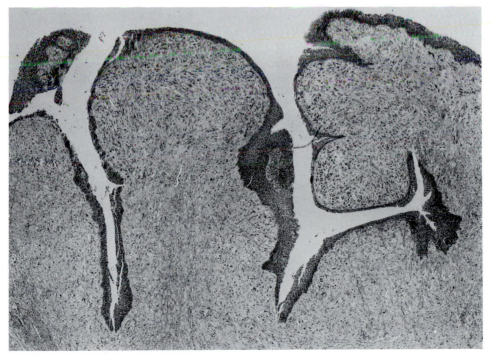

Fig. 773 Botryoid sarcoma of vagina with polypoid configuration and intact overlying epithelium. (Low power; WU neg. 51-154; slide contributed by Dr. H. Ulfelder, Boston, Mass.)

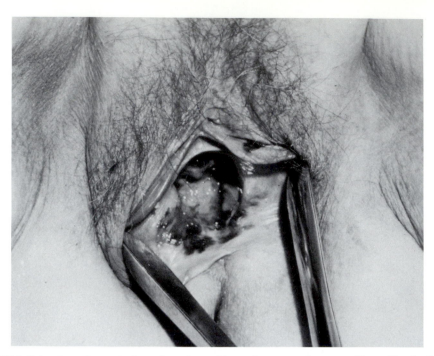

Fig. 774 Extensive pigmentation of vagina with malignant melanoma. (From Norris, H. J., and Taylor, H. B.: Melanomas of the vagina, Am. J. Clin. Pathol. **46:**420-426, 1966.)

a bunch of grapes—hence its name.

Microscopically, a myxomatous stroma is seen containing undifferentiated round or spindle cells, some of which may be seen invading the overlying epithelium. Some of the tumor cells contain a bright eosinophilic granular cytoplasm and are regarded as rhabdomyoblasts. Their racquet or strap-shaped form mimics that of the cells seen during normal muscle embryogenesis. Cross striations may or may not be present. They are not indispensable for the diagnosis. An important diagnostic feature is the crowding of the tumor cells around blood vessels and, most important, beneath the squamous epithelium. The latter results in a distinctive subepithelial dense zone (the "cambium layer" of Nicholson). These tumors probably represent a variant of growth pattern of embryonal rhabdomyosarcoma, as a result of their location immediately beneath an expansile epithelial or mesothelial lining. They cause death more often by direct extension than by distant metastases.[2] Of the fifteen autopsied cases reviewed by Hilgers et al.,[10] the tu-

mor was confined to the pelvis in about half.

The prognosis is poor. Nine of the ten patients studied by Hilgers et al.[10] died of their disease. Of the nine long-term survivors reported in the literature, five were treated by hysterovaginectomy, three by pelvic exenteration, and one by radiation therapy. However, there is some doubt if all of these cases were bona fide examples of sarcoma botryoides. The treatment of choice at the present time seems to be radical pelvic surgery, which implies either an anterior or a total pelvic exenteration,[19] supplemented by radiation therapy and/or chemotherapy.

The most common sources of **metastatic carcinoma** to the vagina are the uterine cervix and endometrium, followed by ovary, rectum, and kidney.[12] Some of them represent direct extension, and others are instances of distant metastases. The metastases from endometrial adenocarcinoma are often submucosal and located in the upper third of the organ. The routine practice of preoperative radiation therapy has reduced them to a minimum.

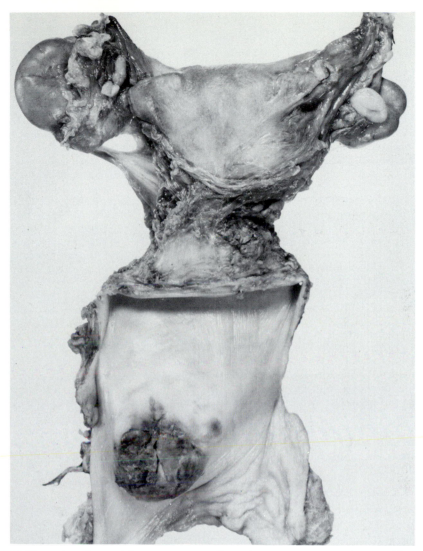

Fig. 775 Ulcerating large leiomyosarcoma of vagina occurring in 62-year-old woman. (WU neg. 64-10451.)

It is likely that most reported cases of primary adenocarcinomas of the rectovaginal septum (without mucosal involvement of either vagina or rectum) arise on the basis of endometriosis.[25]

Malignant melanoma can occur as a primary vaginal tumor.[15] It presents as a soft polypoid mass, blue or black, frequently ulcerated (Fig. 774). Microscopically, the appearance is the same as in the cutaneous melanomas. Intraepithelial spread (so-called junctional activity) should be identified in order to substantiate a local origin. The prognosis is extremely poor. The melanocytes that have been identified in 3% of normal vaginas[13] most likely represent the cell of origin of this neoplasm.

We have seen a large ulcerated *leiomyosarcoma* arising from the lower vagina (Fig. 775).

REFERENCES

1 Ceremsak, R. J.: Benign rhabdomyoma of the vagina, Am. J. Clin. Pathol. **52:**604-606, 1969.
2 Daniel, W. W., Koss, L. G., and Brunschwig, A.: Sarcoma botryoides of the vagina, Cancer **12:**74-84, 1959.
3 Evans, D. M. D., and Hughes, H.: Cysts of the

vaginal wall, J. Obstet. Gynaecol. Br. Commonw. 68:247-253, 1961.

4 Gardner, H. L.: Cervical and vaginal endometriosis, Clin. Obstet. Gynecol. 9:358-372, 1966.

5 Gray, L. A., and Christopherson, W. M.: Insitu and early invasive carcinoma of the vagina, Obstet. Gynecol. 34:226-230, 1969.

6 Greenwald, P., Barlow, J. J., Nasca, P. C., and Burnett, W. S.: Vaginal cancer after maternal treatment with synthetic estrogens, N. Engl. J. Med. 285:390-392, 1971.

7 Herbst, A. L., and Scully, R. E.: Adenocarcinoma of the vagina in adolescence; a report of 7 cases including 6 clear-cell carcinomas (so-called mesonephromas), Cancer 25:745-757, 1970.

8 Herbst, A. L., Kurman, R. J., Scully, R. E., and Poskanzer, D. C.: Clear-cell adenocarcinoma of the genital tract in young females; Registry report, N. Engl. J. Med. 287:1259-1264, 1972.

9 Herbst, A. L., Ulfelder, H., and Poskanzer, D. C.: Adenocarcinoma of the vagina; association of maternal stilbestrol therapy with tumor appearance in young women, N. Engl. J. Med. 284:878-881, 1971.

10 Hilgers, R., Malkasian, G. D., Jr., and Soule, E. H.: Embryonal rhabdomyosarcoma (botryoid type) of the vagina; a clinicopathologic review, Am. J. Obstet. Gynecol. 107:484-502, 1970.

11 Marcus, S. L.: Multiple squamous cell carcinomas involving cervix, vagina, and vulva: theory of multicentric origin, Am. J. Obstet. Gynecol. 80:802-812, 1960.

12 Nerdrum, T. A.: Vaginal metastasis of hypernephroma; report of three cases, Acta Obstet. Gynecol. Scand. 45:515-524, 1966.

13 Nigogosyan, G., De La Pava, S., and Pickren, J. W.: Melanoblasts in the vaginal mucosa: origin for primary malignant melanoma, Cancer 17:912-913, 1964.

14 Norris, H. J., and Taylor, H. B.: Polyps of the vagina, Cancer 19:227-232, 1966.

15 Norris, H. J., and Taylor, H. B.: Melanomas of the vagina, Am. J. Clin. Pathol. 46:420-426, 1966.

16 Norris, H. J., Bagley, G. P., and Taylor, H. B.: Carcinoma of the infant vagina; a distinctive tumor, Arch. Pathol. 90:473-479, 1970.

17 Ober, W.: Personal communication, 1953.

18 Rutledge, F.: Cancer of the vagina, Am. J. Obstet. Gynecol. 97:635-655, 1967.

19 Rutledge, F., and Sullivan, M. P.: Sarcoma botryoides, Ann. N. Y. Acad. Sci. 142:694-708, 1967.

20 Sandberg, E. C.: The incidence and distribution of occult vaginal adenosis, Trans. Pac. Coast Obstet. Gynecol. Soc. 35:36-48, 1967.

21 Siders, D. B., Parrott, M. H., and Abell, M. R.: Gland cell prosoplasia (adenosis) of vagina, Am. J. Obstet. Gynecol. 91:190-203, 1965.

22 Silverberg, S. G., and DeGiorgi, L. S.: Clear cell carcinoma of the vagina, Cancer 29:262-272, 1972.

23 Ulfelder, H., and Quan, S. H.: Sarcoma botryoides vaginae; complete excision of the tumor in an infant by the combined abdominal and perineal approach, Surg. Clin. North Am. 27:1240-1245, 1947.

24 Whelton, J., and Kottmeier, H. L.: Primary carcinoma of the vagina; a study of a Radium-hemmet series of 145 cases, Acta Obstet. Gynecol. Scand. 41:22-40, 1962.

25 Young, E. E., and Gamble, C. H.: Primary adenocarcinoma of the rectovaginal septum arising from endometriosis; report of a case, Cancer 24:597-601, 1969.

Uterus—cervix

Chronic cervicitis, cysts, and polyps

Chronic cervicitis, cysts, and polyps of the cervix are expressions of inflammation. The biopsies of cervices of adults all show some degree of chronic inflammation. Bilharziasis (schistosomiasis), common in Africa, can involve any portion of the gynecologic tract[2] (Fig. 776). Primary lesions of syphilis can occur in the uterine cervix.

Herpes simplex infection of the cervix is now recognized as a relatively common occurrence. The microscopic appearance at the time of biopsy is usually that of an intense nonspecific inflammation with ulceration. Only rarely are the diagnostic multinucleated squamous cells with intranuclear inclusions encountered.[5]

Retention nabothian cysts develop with block of the cervical glands. They appear grossly as cystic spaces filled with mucoid material.

The cervical polyp may be small or several centimeters in diameter. On cut surface, cystic spaces exist. Microscopically, dilated endocervical glands are seen in an edematous and inflamed stroma. The surface epithelium often shows extensive foci of squamous metaplasia. Such polyps are not true neoplasms. We have not seen carcinoma develop in a cervical polyp. Hertig[3] found five carcinomas in situ in 1,600 polyps, thus demonstrating that polyps are no more or no less potentially malignant than the cervix as a whole.

Vestiges of the mesonephric ducts are sometimes demonstrable in the lateral muscular walls of the cervix. Occasionally, they may form sizable cysts.[7] A rare benign polypoid tumor of the cervix and vagina of young children has been described by Selzer and Nelson[6] and Janovski and Kasdon.[4] It is a papilloma composed of delicate connective tissue stalks covered by a layer of cuboidal cells. It often has been referred to as mesonephric papilloma, although its relationship with mesonephric remnants is far from established.

Abell[1] designated as *papillary adenofibroma* a peculiar benign polypoid cervical lesion occurring in adults that microscopically resembles the pattern of a mammary fibroadenoma or even that of a cystosarcoma phylloides (Fig. 777).

Hormonal reactions and endometriosis

Decidual reaction in the cervix during pregnancy may be confused with carcinoma. The lesions are multiple small yellowish or red elevations of the cervical mucosa. They are soft and friable and bleed easily with trauma. Rarely, these processes may be transformed into fungating masses difficult to distinguish from carcinoma.[9] Microscopically, the diagnosis should not be difficult (Fig. 778).

Microglandular hyperplasia of the endocervical epithelium occurs in women using oral contraceptive drugs, and, less frequently, during pregnancy.[10, 11] It is important to avoid the misdiagnosis of cancer since this reaction is invariably benign (Fig. 779). Microscopically, this lesion is characterized by a complex proliferation of small glands lined by *flat* epithelial cells with little or no atypia. The intervening

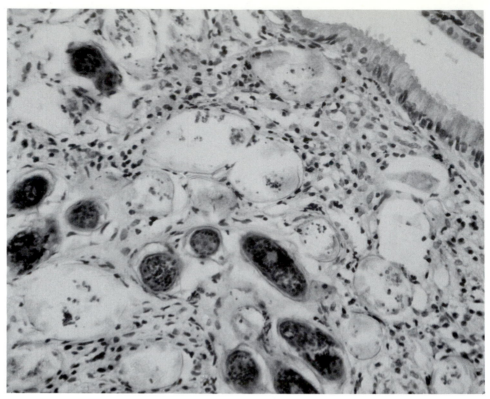

Fig. 776 Cervical polyp from African woman. Calcified rounded areas are diagnostic of bilharziasis (schistosomiasis). (×275; WU neg. 66-7570; slide contributed by Dr. A. Schmamann, Johannesburg, South Africa.)

stroma invariably shows chronic inflammation.

Endometriosis of the cervix may appear as blue or hemorrhagic nodules. It is one of the less common of the many causes of abnormal uterine bleeding. Both endometrial glands and stroma are present.

Squamous metaplasia

The term *squamous metaplasia* is used to designate the focal or extensive replacement of the mucus-secreting glandular epithelium of the endocervix by stratified squamous epithelium which, in its late stage, is morphologically indistinguishable from the epithelium normally lining the exocervical portion. The pathogenesis of this process has been a subject of a heated controversy. It is now generally agreed that it most commonly arises on the basis of proliferation and metaplasia of a row of normally inconspicuous cells located be-

neath the endocervical epithelium known as reserve or subcylindrical cells. It is possible that in other instances it results from the healing of a cervical erosion by an overglide of squamous epithelium from the exocervix.[12] Some degree of squamous metaplasia is present in almost every uterine cervix during the child-bearing age. Most commonly, the process involves only the superficial epithelium and is recognized by the presence of squamous epithelium overlying stroma containing endocervical glands (thus forming the so-called transitional zone). In other instances, it affects the glandular component as well, resulting in a complex microscopic appearance that can be confused with invasive carcinoma by the inexperienced (Fig. 780). Although most cervical cancers probably arise in areas of the cervix which sometime in the past had been involved by squamous metaplasia, the latter process has no premalig-

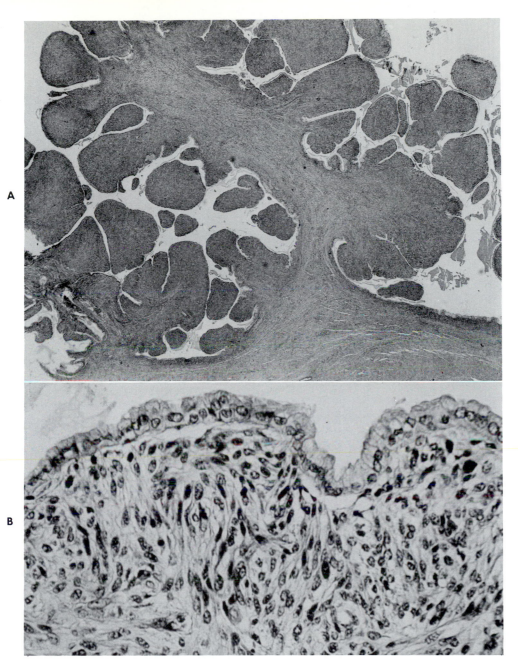

Fig. 777   A, Papillary adenofibroma of uterine cervix of adult. Stout ramifying connective tissue core is covered by endocervical epithelium. **B,** High power of same lesion shown in **A.** Because of cellularity of stroma, these lesions are sometimes misinterpreted as botryoid sarcomas or carcinosarcomas. (**A,** ×10; WU neg. 73-2071; **B,** ×350; WU neg. 73-2077.)

nant connotations. Actually, it is so common and insignificant that, unless quite extensive and/or involving the glandular component, we tend to ignore it altogether in our pathology reports.

A somewhat different appearance is seen often in the cervix of prolapsed uteri. The clinical appearance is usually referred to as "leukoplakic." Microscopically, the process involves mainly the exocervical

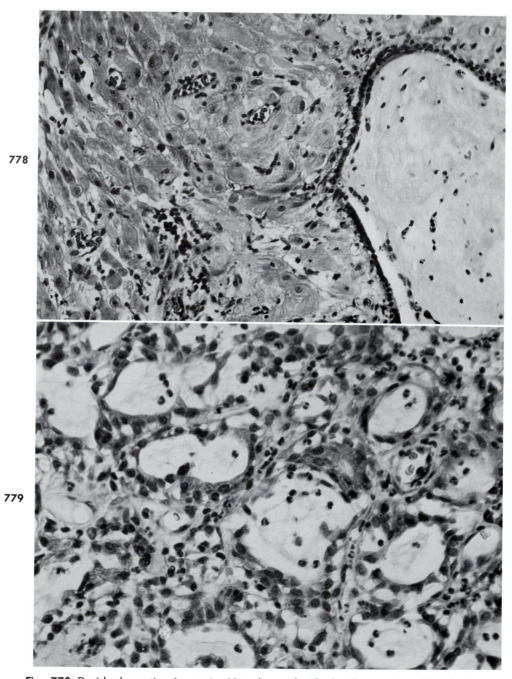

778

779

Fig. 778 Decidual reaction in cervix. Note large decidual cells growing diffusely through cervix. Clinically, patient was thought to have early carcinoma of cervix. (×220; WU neg. 50-2839.)

Fig. 779 Microglandular hyperplasia of endocervical epithelium, benign change associated with use of cyclic artificial progestogens. These changes may be mistaken for cancer. (×300; WU neg. 67-8213.)

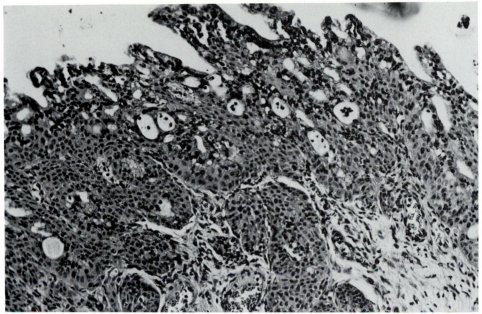

Fig. 780 Extensive squamous metaplasia of cervix. Individual cells are uniform, and there is considerable inflammation. This type of lesion often is incorrectly diagnosed as carcinoma. (×180; WU neg. 50-3947.)

portion and is characterized by the appearance of granular and horny layers. This process, which is also unrelated to carcinoma, is best designated as *hyperkeratosis*.

Tumors
Dysplasia

In current gynecologic terminology, dysplasia is the preferred term to designate the presence of *atypical cytologic features* in the cervical *squamous epithelium*. In the large majority of cases, this process involves not the squamous epithelium of the exocervix but rather areas of squamous metaplasia of the endocervical portion. The zone of junction between both epithelia is where the most severe changes tend to occur. In contrast to what is seen in squamous metaplasia, the nuclei of the dysplastic cells are enlarged, irregular, and hyperchromatic. However, the maturation pattern is maintained throughout the section. Cervical dysplasias are graded as *slight, moderate,* or *severe,* according to the degree of nuclear abnormalities seen.

Approximately 23% of patients with invasive epidermoid carcinoma of the cervix treated by radiation therapy develop changes known as *postirradiation dysplasia*. There are some features suggesting that this is not merely a reaction of a previously normal epithelium to the radiation but rather the expression of a basically abnormal mucosa. Wentz and Reagan[13] found that postirradiation dyplasia appearing within three years after treatment was associated with poor prognosis.

Carcinoma in situ

Kraus[21] defines carcinoma in situ of the cervix as "a change in the surface squamous epithelial cells to an anaplastic pattern with no differentiation at any level. Although surface cells may be flattened, they retain their fundamentally anaplastic appearance"* (Fig. 781). Disorganization of the basal layer is an important characteristic.[20] Cytoplasmic glycogen is markedly diminished or absent, this being the

---

*From Kraus, F. T.: Gynecologic pathology, St. Louis, 1967, The C. V. Mosby Co.

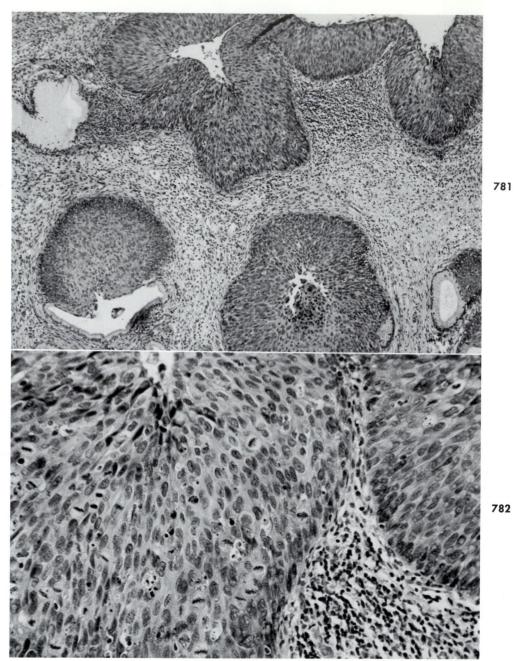

Fig. 781 Epidermoid carcinoma in situ. Lesion has extended into glands and partially or completely replaced them. This is not evidence of invasion. (×150; WU neg. 73-64.)

Fig. 782 This demonstrates complete disorganization throughout all layers of this carcinoma in situ with innumerable normal and atypical mitotic figures. (×300; WU neg. 73-63.)

reason for the lack of staining in the Schiller's (iodine) test. The microscopic features of carcinoma in situ were well described by Schottlaender and Ker-

mauner[25] in 1912. Tweeddale and Roddick[28] have subdivided carcinoma in situ into four histologic types. The process practically always involves the surface

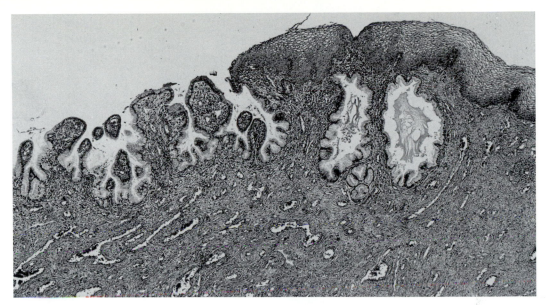

Fig. 783 Squamocolumnar junction of uterine cervix. It is in this area that most dysplasias and carcinomas in situ arise. (×30; WU neg. 73-183.)

epithelium as well as the glandular elements but by definition shows no stromal invasion (Fig. 782). It arises predominantly in the endocervical side of the squamocolumnar junction[19] (Fig. 783). The microscopic changes often occur abruptly.[27] The extension of the lesion is highly variable. Occasionally it seems to consist of only a minute focus removable by a simple biopsy. More commonly, it involves large areas of the endocervix and exocervix. Extension to the upper vagina is not uncommon.[14] We have seen cervical carcinoma in situ extending into the vagina to the introitus and into the endometrial cavity and even the fallopian tubes.[24] Extension up the endocervical canal is much more common than down on the portio.[16] In many instances, carcinoma in situ as seen in a cervical biopsy represents the peripheral manifestation of an invasive carcinoma that is diagnosed only by endocervical curettement. True carcinoma in situ of the cervix usually occurs at an earlier age (average, 36.6 years) than does invasive carcinoma (48.6 years).[22, 23]

The incidence of carcinoma in situ is influenced greatly by the liberality of the pathologist in diagnosing it.[18] With the passing of the years, the criteria have become more and more stringent.[15] An extensive review of our own material showed that 11% of the lesions originally diagnosed as carcinoma in situ would now be classified as either dysplasia or squamous metaplasia with inflammation (Fig. 780). The cervical changes occurring in pregnancy are particularly confusing. They include a combination of squamous metaplasia, chronic inflammation, decidual reaction, and sometimes dysplasia. The microscopic criteria for the diagnosis of carcinoma in situ in the pregnant woman should be the same as in the absence of pregnancy. Bona fide carcinoma in situ, diagnosed using the criteria just described, *does not regress postpartum.*[17, 26]

Clinicopathologic correlation

There is now general agreement that the large majority of invasive epidermoid carcinomas of the cervix arise from the endocervical portion close to the squamocolumnar junction, preceded by the sequence squamous metaplasia–dysplasia–carcinoma in situ.[30] This by no means implies that all cases along this sequence will develop invasive cancer. The pre-

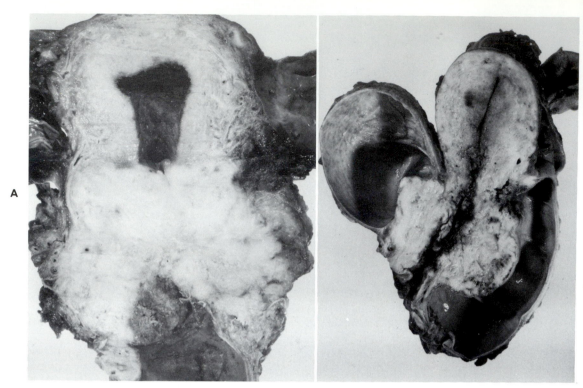

Fig. 784 Advanced epidermoid carcinoma of uterine cervix. **A,** Tumor replaces whole circumference of cervix and invades both parametria. **B,** Extensive neoplasm has invaded vagina, urinary bladder, and posterior rectal wall. (**A** and **B,** Courtesy Dr. H. Rodriguez, Mexico City, Mexico.)

malignant potential of squamous meta-plasia can be disregarded altogether. Dysplasia of mild or moderate degree is an unstable process.[33] In one series of 278 patients in whom the diagnosis was made by cytology and who had no therapy, follow-up over an eleven-year period revealed that the condition regressed in eighty-six, persisted unchanged in twenty-five, and progressed to either severe dysplasia and/or carcinoma in situ in 167.[29] The latter two conditions rarely regress and may persist for long periods. Petersen[32] studied the course of 127 untreated patients with "precancerous lesions" of the cervix. Invasive carcinoma had developed in 11% at the end of three years, in 22% at the end of five years, and in 33% at the end of nine years. The assumption that carcinoma in situ will *inevitably* lead to invasive cancer if left untreated is unproved and unprovable. Nevertheless, the proportion is

high enough to fully justify the removal of the diseased area. The choice of terms is somewhat unfortunate in the sense that it implies a significant biologic difference between severe dysplasia and carcinoma in situ which probably does not exist. To many surgeons, the diagnosis of dysplasia is an indication for follow-up cytologic study, whereas that of carcinoma in situ is an indication for a hysterectomy. This need not be the case. If a proper cytologic follow-up can be assured, carcinoma in situ may be safely treated by conization. In the experience of Kreiger and McCormack,[31] conization resulted in control of cervical carcinoma in situ in 90% of the patients. In the final decision regarding the timing and type of therapy for this group of lesions, the microscopic diagnosis is only one of the factors to be considered, albeit a very important one. The extension of the lesion, age of the patient, parity,

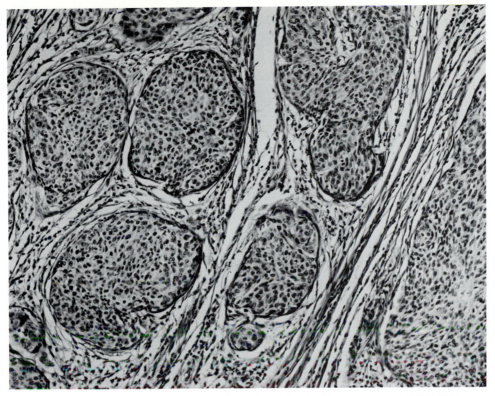

Fig. 785 Typical squamous carcinoma of cervix with plexiform masses. (×127; WU neg. 65-4297.)

and the desire to have more children all have to be considered.

Once the pathologist has made the diagnosis of severe dysplasia or carcinoma in situ in a cervical biopsy, it is the responsibility of the gynecologist to determine the presence or absence of invasive cancer. Cold knife cervical conization and the proper sectioning of tissue should establish whether or not invasive carcinoma exists. If the latter is found, conventional methods of therapy may be instituted.

Epidermoid carcinoma

Invasive epidermoid carcinoma of the cervix is the most common malignant tumor of the gynecologic tract. It appears most often in the older age groups but is also common in patients under 40 years of age. There is a low incidence in Jewish women. Evidence exists supporting the association of early marriage, multiparity, low economic level, and possibly syph-

ilis with a high incidence of cervical carcinoma. Carcinoma of the cervix has an extremely low incidence in nuns.[35] The single most important factor is probably age at first intercourse.[40]

Grossly, carcinoma may grow out of, or may infiltrate, the cervix (Fig. 784). The bulky carcinomas that grow out of the cervix are less likely to invade surrounding structures than are the infiltrating ones. Carcinoma of the cervix is usually a poorly differentiated epidermoid carcinoma forming plexiform masses (Fig. 785). Only rarely is it highly keratinized or so poorly differentiated that tumor giant cells are prominent.

Epidermoid carcinomas in which the depth of stromal invasion is minimal (5 mm or less) are segregated from the others by some authors and designated as "microinvasive carcinomas" or "carcinomas with early stromal invasion."[36, 38] Regardless of the terminology used, there is justification

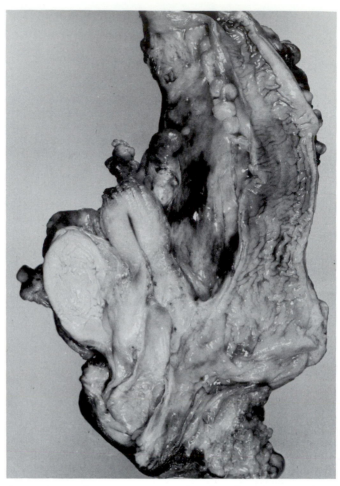

Fig. 786 Specimen from pelvic exenteration that has been sectioned so that intimate relation between bladder, cervix, vagina, and large bowel can be seen. There was persistent carcinoma in cervix with invasion of right parametrium. There were no involved lymph nodes of thirty examined. (WU neg. 51-699; pelvic exenteration done by Dr. E. Bricker, St. Louis, Mo.)

for this segregation since the natural history of this lesion is quite different from that of the ordinary invasive cancer and more akin to that of carcinoma in situ.[34a] Ng and Reagan[38] diagnosed as microinvasive carcinomas sixty-six (8.4%) of the cervical epidermal carcinomas they reviewed. The area of microinvasion originated practically always from a focus of carcinoma in situ and/or dysplasia. The majority of the tumors were located in the anterior lip of the cervix. They emphasized the common occurrence of pleomorphism, cellular differentiation, presence of conspicuous nucleoli, and individual cell keratinization.

Since these features are rarely seen together in carcinoma in situ, their presence in an apparently intraepidermal cervical lesion should stimulate for the search of areas of incipient invasion. None of the patients in Ng and Reagan's series[38] and only two of the ninety-one patients reported by Mussey et al.[37] had evidence of lymph node metastases.

The primary treatment of invasive carcinoma of the cervix is radium implantation and external pelvic irradiation. This treatment cures the majority of patients with the earlier stages of cervical cancer. When carcinoma is found to persist locally after

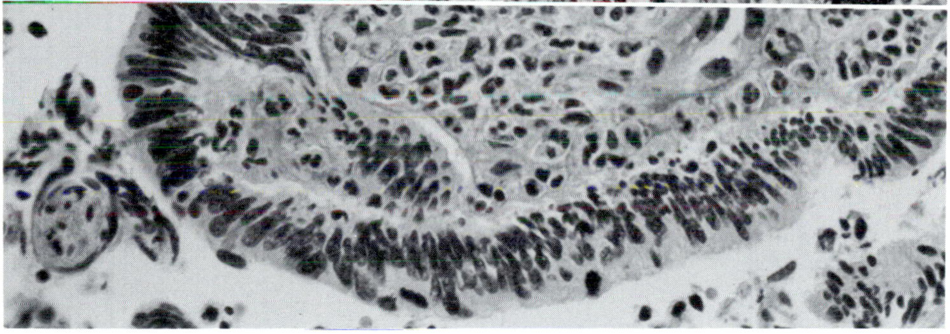

Fig. 787 Well-differentiated mucin-secreting adenocarcinoma of cervix. (×360; WU neg. 50-5074.)

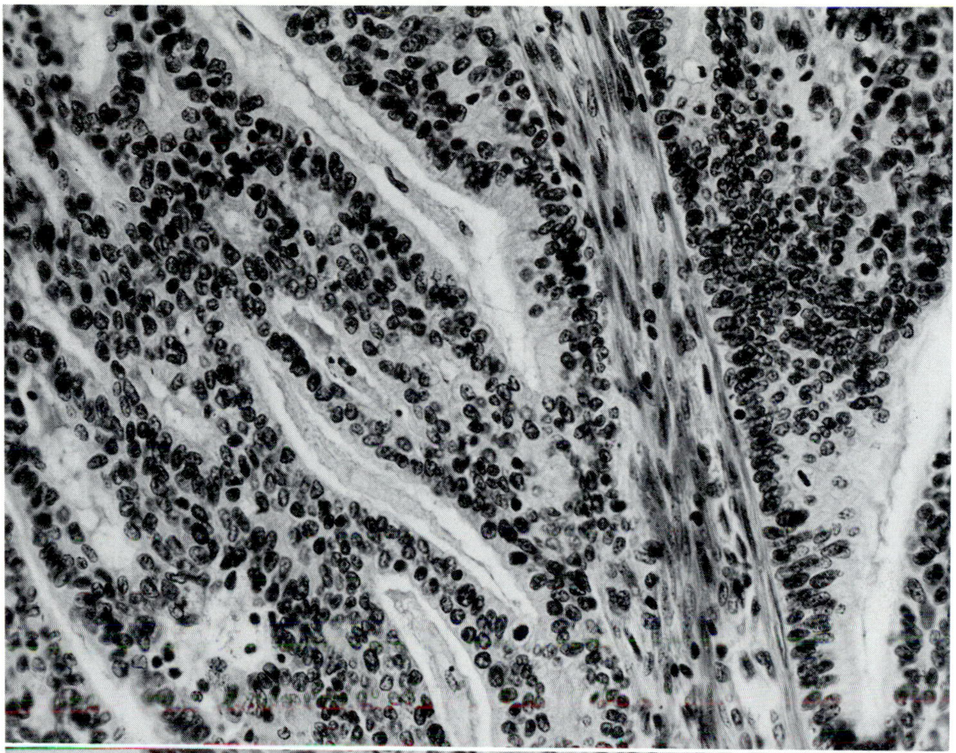

Fig. 788 Extremely well-differentiated adenocarcinoma of cervix. Note stratification of cells with loss of nuclear polarity. (×440; WU neg. 52-1832.)

irradiation therapy, pelvic exenteration should be seriously considered because a considerable number of the patients will have the persistent tumor confined to the pelvis. This operation removes all pelvic viscera and lateral pelvic lymph node-bearing tissue (Fig. 786).

At laparotomy, the surgeon should examine the upper abdomen carefully, particularly the periaortic area, for evidence of spread outside the pelvis. Any suspicious lymph nodes or liver nodules should be submitted to the pathologist for frozen section before the operative procedure is begun. Gross appraisal of enlarged extrapelvic nodes is unreliable. The study of the surgical specimen should include a careful examination of the lymph nodes, the lateral edges of the resection, and the local extent of the tumor. Microscopically, the nodes, vessels, and adjacent organs should be examined for evidence of tumor. The finding of greater prognostic relevance in the pathologic evaluation of pelvic exenteration specimens is the presence or absence of lymph node metastases.[39]

Other indications for pelvic exenteration are locally invasive carcinoma of the rectum, severe pelvic irradiation necrosis, and recurrent carcinoma of the endometrium. The five-year survival rate for patients undergoing this formidable procedure for postirradiation-persistent carcinoma of the cervix is approximately 25%.[34, 35a]

Verrucous carcinoma is a highly differentiated variant of epidermoid carcinoma. The gross and microscopic features of this tumor have been described in Chapter 4.

Adenocarcinoma

Primary adenocarcinomas make up about 5% of all carcinomas of the cervix. This percentage is higher in Jewish women.[44] The tumor presents no differentiating gross characteristics. Microscopically, the most common pattern is that of a well-differentiated adenocarcinoma (Fig. 787). Mucin secretion is invariably present.[49] We have seen several tumors in which excellent differentiation made the diagnosis difficult (Fig. 788). Endocervical adenocarcinoma can also be poorly differentiated, papillary, or have an appearance indistinguishable from endometrial adenocarcinoma.[48] A significant proportion of tumors have a squamous component. When the latter is prominent, the tumor is designated as *adenosquamous carcinoma.* This pattern seems to be particularly common during pregnancy.[43] A glandular form of carcinoma in situ has been described by Helper et al.[47] In six of the eight cases reviewed by Weisbrot et al.,[50] there was coexisting epidermoid carcinoma in situ.

Gallager et al.[42] reported four cases of *adenoid cystic carcinoma* and reviewed the six previously published. Most of the patients were elderly multigravid black women and the prognosis was poor.

Clear cell carcinoma (adenocarcinoma, mesonephric type) of the cervix is probably of müllerian rather than of mesonephric origin. Glands lined by large cells with abundant clear cytoplasm are characteristic.[41] "Hobnail" cells are common, as well as intraglandular papillary projections. Grossly, the tumor is usually exophytic. This tumor is the most common cervical carcinoma in young females, although it occurs in all age groups.[45] The prognosis is relatively good. In the thirteen cases studied by Hart and Norris,[46] the actuarial survival rate was 55% at five years and 40% at ten years.

Metastatic carcinoma

Carcinomas of the endometrium and ovary and even those of the gallbladder and breast may metastasize to the cervix and be called primary. The clinical findings may make this mistake avoidable. Carcinomas of the endometrium usually produce no mucin and resemble endometrial glands. Carcinomas of the ovary often have secondary papillary projections. On this basis, we have diagnosed carcinoma of the ovary invading the cervix in two patients.

Cytology

Michael Kyriakos, M.D.

The broadest and most successful application of clinical cytology has been in the diagnosis of carcinoma of the uterine cervix.[62] Mass cytologic screening has shifted the presentation of cervical cancer from the clinical to the preclinical stage.[56, 57] This is an established fact, the argument that the incidence of cervical cancer was already declining prior to the introduction of this diagnostic method notwithstanding. Incidentally, the accuracy of this argument has been disputed.[51, 55] Following mass screening, there has been a reduction of 38% to 57% in the overall incidence of invasive carcinoma and a reduction of 67% in the incidence of clinically evident carcinoma (Stages 1B to IV).[52-54, 65] Whereas in the prescreening era invasive cancer contributed approximately 80% of all diagnosed cases, at the present time it makes only 16% to 35% of the cases, the remaining being carcinomas in situ.[53, 55] This has resulted in an increased cure rate for the screened population and in an increase in the survival times for the patients with invasive carcinoma.[55, 55a, 64]

It is important that an endocervical sample be examined in addition to the ordinary specimen from exocervix and vaginal pool. The former, which is essential for the detection of early carcinomas, can be obtained by aspiration or by the use of special wooden spatulas.

We have abandoned the time-honored numerical division of smears into "classes" because of the vague and sometimes misleading information they may convey. A "Class III" smear, for instance, may represent anything from a moderate dysplasia to an invasive carcinoma. Instead, we have chosen to use the same terms employed for the evaluation of cervical biopsies—i.e., negative, benign atypia, dysplasia (of mild, moderate, or severe degree), carcinoma in situ, and invasive carcinoma (epidermoid or adenocarcinoma).[61, 66, 66a]

The diagnostic accuracy of cervical cytology is high. In a series reviewed by Patten,[63] it was 97% for dysplasia, 96% for carcinoma in situ, and 94% for invasive carcinoma. Wied et al.[67] reported practically identical findings. Careful attention to technical factors is essential in order to achieve these results. An endocervical sample should be regularly obtained. The smear should be promptly fixed and carefully stained. Air-dried smears are grossly inadequate in this regard. Even if squamous cells can be rehydrated, they never exhibit the fine structural details of wet-fixed material; glandular cells are even more distorted. If due to some catastrophy the usual cytologic fixatives are unavailable, a commercial hair spray can be used as a substitute.[58] It is also important that the specimen be secured by a trained individual. Self-made samples, obtained with a pipette, are not so effective in this regard. Invasive carcinoma is detected in almost the same rate as with the material obtained by the physician, but the accuracy for dysplasia or carcinoma in situ is considerably lower. Furthermore, the percentage of unsatisfactory specimens approaches 20%.[54, 59]

In the evaluation of some remarkably high figures on the accuracy of vaginal cytology, one cannot escape from the suspicion that they might have been influenced by the fact that the same person diagnoses the cytology specimen and the cervical biopsy. To avoid subconscious bias, we have separated these two functions in our department.[61] Seybolt[66] also demonstrated this by distributing twenty-five problem cases to eight authorities in cytopathology, requesting them to interpret the cytology slides independently of the histology. There was no universal agreement in any case, and in some instances the disagreements were quite disparate. The conclusion from this survey was that it is not always possible to determine the exact histologic change in the cervix on the basis of the cytology smear. However, a more important demonstration was that if a cervical abnormality was present, this was detected by cytologic examination in the large majority of the cases.

Cytology is also useful in the follow-up of patients with cervical carcinoma treated by either conservative surgery or irradiation.[60]

Other lesions

Epidermoid carcinomas, adenocarcinomas, and the variants of these two main types comprise about 99% of all primary cervical tumors. The remaining 1% is made up of a wide variety of neoplasms, including botryoid rhabdomyosarcoma, malignant mixed müllerian tumor,[68] benign and malignant smooth muscle tumors, teratoma, carcinoid tumor,[69] ganglioneuroma, blue nevus, cellular blue nevus,[71] malignant melanoma, malignant lymphoma, hemangioma, and angiosarcoma.[70] We have seen a case clinically presenting as a large pigmented spot in the exocervix in which the microscopic sections showed extensive melanin pigmentation of the basal layer of the squamous epithelium. Islands of mature cartilage can rarely be found in the cervix.[72] It is important not to confuse this lesion of probable metaplastic nature with a malignant mixed müllerian tumor.

REFERENCES
Chronic cervicitis, cysts, and polyps

1 Abell, M. R.: Papillary adenofibroma of the uterine cervix, Am. J. Obstet. Gynecol. **110:** 991-993, 1971.
2 Berry, A.: A cytopathological and histopathological study of bilharziasis of the female genital tract, J. Pathol. Bacteriol. **91:**325-338, 1966.
3 Hertig, A.: Proceedings of Eighteenth Seminar of the American Society of Clinical Pathologists, October, 1952, Chicago, Ill.
4 Janovski, N. A., and Kasdon, E. J.: Benign mesonephric papillary and polypoid tumors of the cervix in childhood, J. Pediatr. **63:**211-216, 1963.
5 Naib, Z. M., Nahmias, A. J., and Josey, W. E.: Cytology and histopathology of cervical herpes simplex infection, Cancer **19:**1026-1031, 1966.
6 Selzer, I., and Nelson, H. M.: Benign papilloma (polypoid tumor) of the cervix uteri in children; report of 2 cases, Am. J. Obstet. Gynecol. **84:**165-169, 1962.
7 Sherrick, J. C., and Vega, J. G.: Congenital intramural cysts of uterus, Obstet. Gynecol. **19:**486-493, 1962.
8 Tchertkoff, V., and Ober, W. B.: Primary chancre of cervix uteri, N. Y. State J. Med. **66:** 1921-1924, 1966.

Hormonal reactions and endometriosis

9 Bausch, R. G., Kaump, D. H., and Alles, R. W.: Observations on the decidual reaction of the cervix during pregnancy, Am. J. Obstet. Gynecol. **58:**777-783, 1949.
10 Kyriakos, M., Kempson, R. L., and Konikov, N. F.: A clinical and pathologic study of endocervical lesions associated with oral contraceptives, Cancer **22:**99-110, 1968.
11 Taylor, H. B., Irey, N. S., and Norris, H. J.: Atypical endocervical hyperplasia in women taking oral contraceptives, J.A.M.A. **202:**637-639, 1967.

Squamous metaplasia

12 Johnson, L. D., Easterday, C. L., Gore, H., and Hertig, A. T.: Histogenesis of carcinoma in situ of the uterine cervix; a preliminary report of the origin of carcinoma in situ in subcylindrical cell anaplasia, Cancer **17:**213-229, 1964.

Tumors
Dysplasia

13 Wentz, W. B., and Reagan, J. W.: Clinical significance of post-irradiation dysplasia of the uterine cervix, Am. J. Obstet. Gynecol. **106:** 812-817, 1970.

Carcinoma in situ

14 Foote, F. W., Jr., and Stewart, F. W.: The anatomical distribution of intraepithelial epidermoid carcinomas of the cervix, Cancer **1:** 431-440, 1948.
15 Govan, A. D. T., Haines, R. M., Langley, F. A,. Taylor, C. W., and Woodcock, A. S.: Changes in the epithelium of the cervix uteri, J. Obstet. Gynaecol. Br. Commonw. **73:**883-896, 1968.
16 Gusberg, S. B., and Moore, D. B.: The clinical pattern of intraepithelial carcinoma of the cervix and its pathologic background, Obstet. Gynecol. **2:**1-14, 1953.
17 Hamperl, H., Kaufmann, C., and Ober, K. G.: Histologische Untersuchungen an der Cervix schwangerer Frauen, Arch. Gynäk. **184:**181-280, 1954.
18 Holmquist, N. D., McMahan, C. A., and Williams, O. D.: Variability in classification of carcinoma in situ of the uterine cervix, Arch. Pathol. **84:**334-345, 1967.
19 Howard, L., Erickson, C. C., and Stoddard, L. D.: A study of the incidence and histogenesis of endocervical metaplasia and intraepithelial carcinoma, Cancer **4:**1210-1223, 1951.
20 Klavins, J. V.: Intra-epithelial carcinoma with differentiated surface cells and dysplasia; definition and separation of these lesions, Acta Cytol. (Baltimore) **7:**351-356, 1963.
21 Kraus, F. T.: Gynecologic pathology, St. Louis, 1967, The C. V. Mosby Co., p. 174.
22 Pund, E. R., and Auerbach, S. H.: Preinvasive carcinoma of the cervix uteri, J.A.M.A. **131:** 960-963, 1946.
23 Pund, E. R., Nieburgs, H. E., Nettles, J. B., and Caldwell, J. D.: Preinvasive carcinoma of the cervix: seven cases in which it was detected by examination of routine endocervical smears, Arch. Pathol. **44:**571-577, 1947.
24 Salm, R.: Superficial intra-uterine spread of intra-epithelial cervical carcinoma, J. Pathol. **97:**719-723, 1969.
25 Schottlaender, J., and Kermauner, F.: Uterus Karzinomas, Berlin, 1912, S. Karger.
26 Spjut, H. J., Ruch, W. A., Jr., Martin, P. A., and Hobbs, J. E.: Exfoliative cytology during pregnancy for detection of carcinoma of the cervix, Obstet. Gynecol. **15:**19-27, 1960.
27 Te Linde, R. W., and Galvin, G.: The minimal histological changes in biopsies to justify a diagnosis of cervical cancer, Am. J. Obstet. Gynecol. **48:**774-797, 1944.

28 Tweeddale, D. N., and Roddick, J. W.: Histo-logic types of squamous-cell carcinoma in situ of the cervix, Obstet. Gynecol. 33:35-40, 1969.

Clinicopathologic correlation

29 Fox, C. H.: Biologic behavior of dysplasia and carcinoma in situ, Am. J. Obstet. Gynecol. 99: 960-974, 1967.
30 Johnson, L. D., Nickerson, R. J., Easterday, C. L., Stuart, R. S., and Hertig, A. T.: Epi-demiologic evidence for the spectrum of change from dysplasia through carcinoma in situ to invasive cancer, Cancer 22:901-914, 1968.
31 Kreiger, J. S., and McCormack, L. J.: Graded treatment for in situ carcinoma of the uterine cervix, Am. J. Obstet. Gynecol. 101:171-182, 1968.
32 Petersen, O.: Spontaneous course of cervical precancerous conditions, Am. J. Obstet. Gyne-col. 72:1063-1071, 1956.
33 Richart, R. M., and Barron, B. A.: A follow-up study of patients with cervical dysplasia, Am. J. Obstet. Gynecol. 105:386-393, 1969.

Epidermoid carcinoma

34 Bricker, E. M., Butcher, H. R., Jr., Lawler, W. H., Jr., and McAfee, C. A.: Surgical treatment of advanced and recurrent cancer of the pelvic viscera: an evaluation of ten years' experience, Ann. Surg. 152:388-402, 1960.
34a Brudenell, M., Cox, B. S., and Taylor, C. W.: The management of dysplasia, carcinoma in situ and microcarcinoma of the cervix, J. Obstet. Gynaecol. Br. Commonw. 80:673-679, 1973.
35 Gagnon, F.: Contribution to the study of the etiology and prevention of cancer of the cervix of the uterus, Am. J. Obstet. Gynecol. 60:516-522, 1950.
35a Kiselow, M., Butcher, H. R., and Bricker, E. M.: Results of the radical surgical treatment of advanced pelvic cancer, Ann. Surg. 166:428-437, 1967.
36 Margulis, R. R., Ely, C. W., Jr., and Ladd, J. E.: Diagnosis and management of stage IA (microinvasive) carcinoma of cervix, Obstet. Gynecol. 29:529-538, 1967.
37 Mussey, E., Soule, E. H., and Welch, J. S.: Microinvasive carcinoma of the cervix, Am. J. Obstet. Gynecol. 104:738-744, 1969.
38 Ng, A. B. P., and Reagan, J. W.: Microinva-sive carcinoma of the uterine cervix, Am. J. Clin. Pathol. 52:511-529, 1969.
39 Perez-Mesa, C., and Spjut, H. J.: Persistent postirradiation carcinoma of cervix uteri; a pathologic study of 83 pelvic exenteration specimens, Arch. Pathol. 75:462-474, 1963.
40 Rotkin, I. D., and Cameron, J. R.: Clusters of variables influencing risk of cervical cancer, Cancer 21:663-671, 1968.

Adenocarcinoma

41 Fawcett, K. J., Dockerty, M. B., and Hunt, A. B.: Mesonephric carcinoma of the cervix uteri; clinical and pathologic study, Am. J. Ob-stet. Gynecol. 95:1068-1079, 1966.
42 Gallager, H. S., Simpson, C. B., and Ayala, A. G.: Adenoid cystic carcinoma of the uterine cervix; report of 4 cases, Cancer 27:1398-1402, 1971.
43 Glücksmann, A.: Relationships between hor-monal changes in pregnancy and the develop-ment of "mixed carcinoma" of the uterine cervix, Cancer 10:831-837, 1957.
44 Gusberg, S. B., and Corscaden, J. A.: The pa-thology and treatment of adenocarcinoma of the cervix, Cancer 4:1066-1072, 1951.
45 Hameed, K.: Clear-cell carcinoma of the uter-ine cervix, Am. J. Obstet. Gynecol. 101:954-958, 1968.
46 Hart, W. R., and Norris, H. J.: Mesonephric adenocarcinomas of the cervix, Cancer 29: 106-113, 1972.
47 Helper, T. K., Dockerty, M. B., and Randall, L. M.: Primary adenocarcinoma of the cervix, Am. J. Obstet. Gynecol. 63:800-808, 1952.
48 Rombaut, R. P., Charles, D., and Murphy, A.: Adenocarcinoma of the cervix; a clinicopatho-logic study of 47 cases, Cancer 19:891-900, 1966.
49 Sorvari, T. E.: A histochemical study of epi-thelial muco-substances in endometrial and cervical adenocarcinomas; with reference to normal endometrium and cervical mucosa, Acta Pathol. Microbiol. Scand. 207 (Suppl):1-85, 1969.
50 Weisbrot, I. M., Stabinsky, C., and Davis, A. M.: Adenocarcinoma in situ of the uterine cervix, Cancer 29:225-233, 1972.

Cytology

51 Boyes, D. A.: The British Columbia screening program, Obstet. Gynecol. Surv. 24:1005-1011, 1969.
52 Bryans, F. E., Boyes, D. A., and Fidler, H. K.: The influence of a cytological screening pro-gram upon the incidence of invasive squa-mous cell carcinoma of the cervix in British Columbia, Am. J. Obstet. Gynecol. 88:898-906, 1964.
53 Christopherson, W. M., Mendez, W. M., Ahuja, E. M., Lundin, F. E., and Barker, J. E.: Cervix cancer control in Louisville, Kentucky, Cancer 26:29-38, 1970.
54 Coleman, S. A., Rube, I. F., Kashgarian, M., and Erickson, C. C.: An appraisal of the irrigation cytology method for uterine cancer

detection, Acta Cytol. (Baltimore) **14**:502-506, 1970.

55 Dickinson, L., Mussey, M. E., and Kurland, L. T.: Evaluation of the effectiveness of cytologic screening for cervical cancer. II. Survival parameters before and after inception of screening, Mayo Clin. Proc. **47**:545-549, 1972.

55a Dickinson, L., Mussey, M. E., Soule, E. H., and Kurland, L. T.: Evaluation of the effectiveness of cytologic screening for cervical cancer. I. Incidence and mortality trends in relation to screening, Mayo Clin. Proc. **47**:534-544, 1972.

56 Erickson, C. C., Everett, B. E., Jr., Graves, L. M., Kaiser, R. F., Malmgren, R. A., Rube, I., Schreier, P. C., Cutler, S. J., and Sprunt, D. H.: Population screening for uterine cancer by vaginal cytology, J.A.M.A. **162**:167-173, 1956.

57 Fidler, H. K., Boyes, D. A., and Worth, A. J.: Cervical cancer detection in British Columbia, J. Obstet. Gynaecol. Br. Commonw. **75**:392-404, 1968.

58 Freeman, J. A.: Hair-spray: an inexpensive aerosol fixative for cytodiagnosis, Acta Cytol. (Baltimore) **13**:416-419, 1969.

59 Klinken, L., Koch, F., and Albrechtsen, R.: Comparison of pipette and smear methods in population screenings for carcinoma of the uterine cervix, Dan. Med. Bull. **19**:138-140, 1972.

60 Kohn, G.: The postradiation vaginal smear: its usefulness as a routine procedure, Acta Obstet. Gynecol. Scand. **33**:264-282, 1953.

61 Konikov, N. F., Kempson, R. L., and Piskie, V.: Cytohistologic correlation of dysplasia, carcinoma-in-situ, and invasive carcinoma of the uterine cervix, Am. J. Clin. Pathol. **51**:463-469, 1969.

62 Koss, L. G.: Diagnostic cytology and its histopathologic bases, ed. 2, Philadelphia, 1968, J. B. Lippincott Co.

63 Patten, S. F.: Diagnostic cytology of the uterine cervix, Baltimore, 1969, The Williams & Williams Co.

64 Petersen, O.: Spontaneous course of cervical precancerous conditions, Am. J. Obstet. Gynecol. **72**:1063-1071, 1956.

65 Ruch, R. M., Blake, C., Abou, A., Lado, M., and Ruch, W. A., Jr.: The changing incidence of cervical carcinoma, Am. J. Obstet. Gynecol. **89**:727-731, 1964.

66 Seybolt, J. F.: Thoughts on "the numbers game," Acta Cytol. (Baltimore) **12**:271-273, 1968.

66a Seybolt, J. F., and Johnson, W. D.: Cervical cytodiagnostic problems; a survey, Am. J. Obstet. Gynecol. **109**:1089-1103, 1971.

67 Wied, G. L., Legorreta, G., Mohr, D., and Rauzy, A.: Cytology of invasive cervical carcinoma and carcinoma in situ, Ann. N. Y. Acad. Sci. **97**:759-766, 1962.

Other lesions

68 Abell, M. R., and Ramirez, J. A.: Sarcomas and carcinosarcomas of the uterine cervix, Cancer **31**:1176-1192, 1973.

69 Albores-Saavedra, J., Poucell, S., and Rodriguez-Martinez, H. A.: Primary carcinoid of the uterine cervix, Patología (Mexico) **10**:185-193, 1973.

70 Benitez, E., Rodriguez, H. A., Rodriguez-Cuevas, H., and Chavez, G. B.: Adenoid cystic carcinoma of the uterine cervix; report of a case and review of 4 cases, Obstet. Gynecol. **33**:757-762, 1969.

71 Goldman, R. L., and Friedman, N. B.: Blue nevus of the uterine cervix, Cancer **20**:210-214, 1967.

72 Roth, E., and Taylor, H. B.: Heterotopic cartilage in the uterus, Obstet. Gynecol. **27**:838-844, 1966.

Uterus—endometrium

Curettage and biopsy

Tissue from the endometrial cavity taken for diagnostic purposes is usually obtained by dilatation and curettage. As a sampling technique, it is unsurpassed. If properly performed, very few lesions (perhaps those located in a cornua) should escape detection. It is the method of choice for the evaluation of lesions presumed to be localized, such as polyps and carcinoma. Information about endocervical extension of an endometrial neoplasm can be obtained by performing a *fractional curettage,* a useful method too often neglected. Naturally, the endocervical specimen should be obtained first so as to minimize contamination from the endometrium. Even with this precaution taken, small isolated tumor fragments may be found in endocervical specimens in cases without actual infiltration of the cervix. Therefore, it is our policy to document the presence of endocervical extension of a tumor *only* if cancer and normal endocervical glands are seen in the same fragment. Otherwise, we simply record the presence of cancer in the material submitted as "endocervical scrapings" and

let the clinician decide whether this is significant on the basis of his findings at the time of curettage.

Regeneration of the endometrium proceeds very rapidly after curettage. Complete restoration occurs in two or three days in most instances.[4] Exceptionally, intrauterine adhesions develop, resulting in amenorrhea and other menstrual abnormalities. This condition, designated by some as Asherman's syndrome, is seen most often after postpartum or postabortal curettages and is thought to be the result of a subclinical uterine infection.[1, 2]

Endometrial biopsy is a safe alternative to dilatation and curettage for the evaluation of infertile or dysmenorrheic patients. Kahler et al.,[3] in their study of 160 patients, demonstrated that when the endometrial biopsy was performed successfully (137 patients), the tissue obtained was truly representative of the endometrium in all but six, as proved by subsequent dilatation and curettage and hysterectomy. Furthermore, no endometrial cancer was missed when sufficient tissue was obtained.

Cytology

Michael Kyriakos, M.D.

Carcinoma of the endometrium is rising in incidence in the United States.[10] The success of mass screening in reducing invasive cervical cancer has not had the same effect on endometrial cancer.[6] The routine "Pap" smear is not adequate for the detection of this tumor. Cervical scraping yields a positive rate of approximately 50% to 60%; vaginal pool material, about 75%; and direct suction curettage, approximately 90%.[11, 12] To remedy these deficiencies, Gravlee[8] has developed a technique which uses endometrial lavage done under negative pressure. The technique can be done as an office procedure without

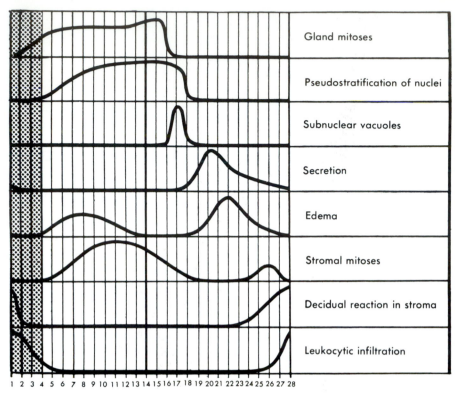

Fig. 789 Cyclic changes in endometrium. Approximate relationship of useful microscopic changes. (After Latour; from Noyes, R. W., Hertig, A. T., and Rock, J.: Dating the endometrial biopsy, Fertil. Steril. **1:**3-25, 1950.)

anesthesia. The accuracy of recent reports has been from 93% to 100% for patients with endometrial carcinoma.[5, 7, 9] Whether the method will prove successful in mass screening in patients with high risk factors for developing endometrial carcinoma awaits clinical trials.

Cyclic changes

The ovulatory cycle is accompanied by changes in the endometrium that prepare it to receive the ovum. If the ovum is not fertilized, the proliferative endometrium is cast off by menstruation and the cycle repeats itself. A normal endometrial cycle is associated with changes in both endometrial glands and stroma which allow the pathologist to diagnose microscopically the phase of the menstrual cycle. Noyes et al.[21] set forth specific criteria by which a more accurate dating of the endometrium was made possible (Figs. 789 and 790).

They divided the endometrial cycle into two phases:

Proliferative phase
Early (4th to 7th day)—thin regenerating surface epithelium; straight, short, narrow glands; compact stroma, with some mitotic activity and large nuclei

Mid (8th to 10th day)—columnar surface epithelium; longer, curving glands; variable amount of stromal edema; numerous mitoses in naked nuclei of stroma

Late (11th to 14th day)—undulant surface; tortuous glands showing active growth and pseudostratification; moderately dense, actively growing stroma

Secretory phase
36 to 48 hours after ovulation—no microscopic changes apparent

16th day—subnuclear vacuolation of epithelium appears

17th day—orderly row of nuclei with homogeneous cytoplasm above them and large vacuoles below

18th day—vacuoles decrease in size; nuclei approach base of cell

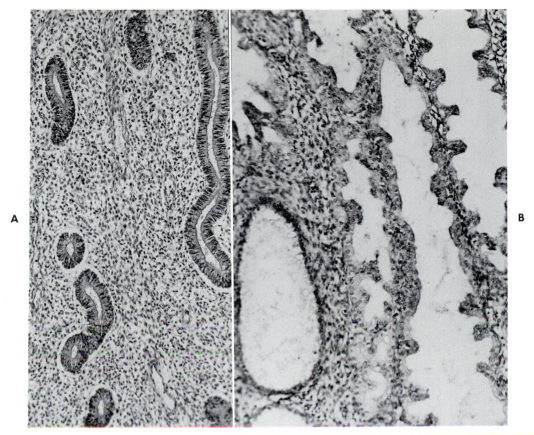

Fig. 790 Sequential endometrial changes during normal menstrual cycle. **A**, Late proliferative endometrium. Note straight elongated glands and lack of vascularity. **B**, Late secretory endometrium. Note sawtooth epithelium and intraluminal secretion, edematous stroma, and congested blood vessels. (**A**, ×115; WU neg. 52-3608; **B**, ×115; WU neg. 52-3609.)

19th day—few vacuoles; appearance of intraluminal secretion

20th day—peak of acidophilic intraluminal secretion

21st day—tissue edema appears rather abruptly

22nd day—edema reaches its peak

23rd day—spiral arterioles become prominent

24th day—collections of predecidual cells appear around arterioles

25th day—predecidua appears under surface epithelium

26th day—predecidua appears as solid sheet of well-developed cells; polynuclear cell infiltration appears

27th day—polynuclear infiltration becomes prominent; areas of focal necrosis and hemorrhage begin to appear

28th day—necrosis and hemorrhage prominent.

In general, the changes are quite uniform throughout the functional endometrium.[19]

When this is not the case, the dating should be based on the most advanced area rather than on the average morphologic picture. The surface epithelium is less responsive to the hormonal influences than the glandular epithelium. In order for subnuclear vacuolation to be regarded as evidence of ovulation, it should be present in at least 50% of the functional glands present in the section. A markedly compact stroma may simulate predecidua. One of the earlier signs of the menstrual phase (and of pathologic crumbling of the stroma) is the presence of nuclear fragments beneath the glandular epithelium.[17] The nuclear crowding seen in menstrual endometrium may simulate a malignant neoplasm.

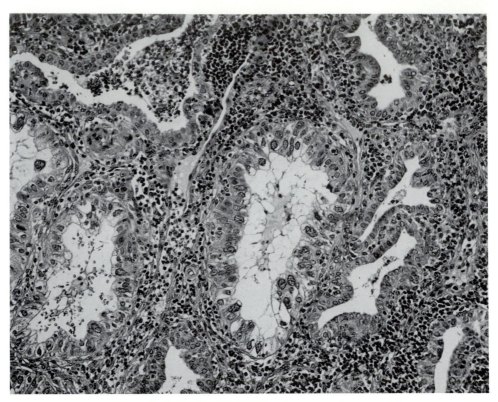

Fig. 791 Gestational hyperplasia (Arias-Stella reaction) of endometrium occurring in early pregnancy. Slight nuclear dysplasia is characteristic of this normal anatomic variation. (×250; WU neg. 65-175; from Kraus, F. T.: Gynecologic pathology, St. Louis, 1967, The C. V. Mosby Co.)

The basal layer of the endometrium is not subject to the influence of progesterone. Therefore, if biopsies are taken in the premenstrual phase for evidence of secretory activity (ovulation) and contain only the basal layer, the diagnosis cannot be made. Similarly, the mucosa of the lower uterine segment responds only sluggishly to the hormonal stimulations and should be disregarded for dating purposes. Biopsies to determine anovulatory cycles are most informative when performed about two days before the expected onset of menstruation.

A physiologic hyperplastic change of endometrial glands known as Arias-Stella reaction occurs in early pregnancy and is frequently encountered in curettings after abortion[13, 14] (Fig. 791). A similar endometrial reaction may be produced in ectopic pregnancy, hydatidiform mole, and chorio-carcinoma and following the administration of contraceptive agents.[15, 16] According to Hertig,[18] the reappearance of glandular secretion and stromal edema, once that predecidual reaction is established, is evidence that a fertilized ovum has implanted.

Iatrogenic changes

The use of intrauterine contraceptive devices can result in focal or extensive chronic inflammatory changes of the endometrial mucosa.[28] In a series of 200 cases reported by Ober et al.,[32] only 29% of symptomatic patients and 40% of asymptomatic patients with a polyethylene intrauterine device had a normal endometrial biopsy. The biologic effects of various intrauterine devices in man and animals have been extensively reviewed by Corfman and Segal.[24]

Endometrial biopsies taken in patients

receiving estrogen therapy may range from a normal proliferative pattern to a highly atypical growth that may be confused with carcinoma. The most common finding is a mild to moderate degree of hyperplasia. Whether prolonged estrogen administration has ever been directly responsible for the development of endometrial carcinoma in human beings has yet to be demonstrated.

Owing to the widespread use of progestin agents for therapeutic and contraceptive purposes, a new endometrial morphology has emerged. The pathologist should be thoroughly familiar with the variety of changes that the "pill" may induce in the endometrium in order not to confuse them with pathologic conditions. The effect of the progestin agents is exerted upon the glands and stroma and differs more according to the regimen used than to the actual drug employed.[31, 34] In the *combined program,* pills of the same mixture, representing a combination of progestogen and estrogen, are taken on consecutive days. They can be administered *continuously* for therapeutic purposes or *cyclically* (for twenty to twenty-one days with seven-day to eight-day intervals) for contraception or therapy. In the *sequential program,* also used for both purposes, predominantly estrogenic pills are taken for fourteen to sixteen days followed by progestin-dominant pills for five or six days. The changes to be described are those to be expected in a previously normal endometrium.

Combined program—continuous

The glands are small, straight, and inactive with no mitoses or secretion. The stroma is very prominent and edematous, is infiltrated by some neutrophils, and shows striking pseudodecidual changes[22] (Fig. 792). The latter, which may appear as fragments of frankly necrotic decidua, are distinguished from the decidua of pregnancy by the completely atrophic glandular pattern. The stromal reaction may be so florid as to simulate a sarcoma.[25] Foci

of endometriosis respond in a similar manner. This must be kept in mind whenever masses of any pelvic organ are being evaluated microscopically, especially by frozen section (Fig. 793).

Combined program—cyclic

The glands show little or no evidence of proliferation. There is a short, poorly developed stage of secretory activity, reaching a peak about the fourteenth or fifteenth day, followed by regression of the glands.[30, 33] Pseudodecidual changes appear in the stroma about the twentieth day of the cycle (fifteenth day of treatment). Development of spiral arterioles is inhibited. After prolonged therapy, glandular secretion and stromal pseudodecidual changes become inconspicuous or recede altogether. The stroma acquires an atrophic, fibroblast-like appearance and may form characteristic small polypoid projections covered by atrophic surface epithelium[23] (Fig. 794). On very rare occasions, we have seen focal glandular changes of the Arias-Stella type in patients taking contraceptive pills. In most cases, discontinuation of therapy results in a restoration of a normal endometrial pattern in a matter of weeks.[26]

Sequential program

The sequential program method more nearly parallels the normal cycle and results in a somewhat similar endometrial morphology.[29] The glands show signs of proliferation, followed by tortuosity and the appearance of well-developed secretory changes. The stroma shows inconspicuous pseudodecidual changes. Thus, the endometrial morphology on the twenty-sixth day of a cycle induced by sequential therapy (the day after treatment is completed) is roughly analogous to that of the eighteenth or nineteenth day of a normal menstrual cycle. Regressive changes and crumbling of stroma, resulting in withdrawal bleeding, occur soon thereafter.

There is now agreement that the use of contraceptive pills is not free of complica-

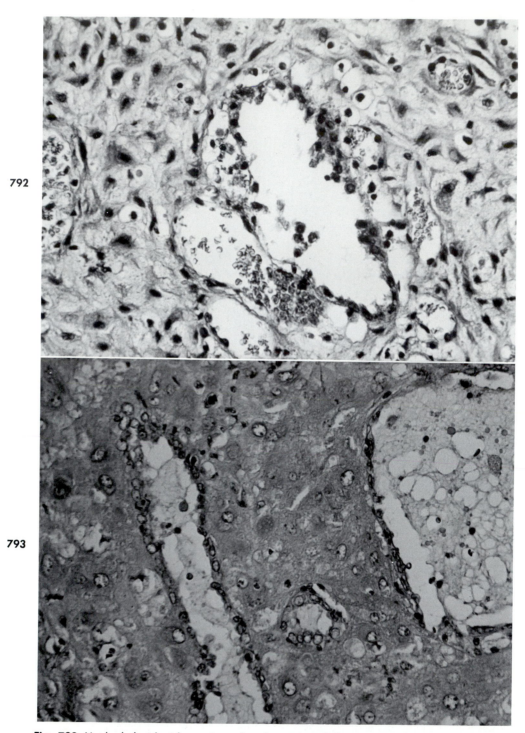

Fig. 792 Marked deciduoid reaction of endometrium following "combined" contraceptive program. Glandular epithelium is inactive and stromal vessels are markedly dilated. (×350; WU neg. 73-370.)
Fig. 793 Biopsy of endometriosis of rectosigmoid area in patient who had been receiving Enovid. Note marked deciduoid proliferation. (WU neg. 62-4550A.)

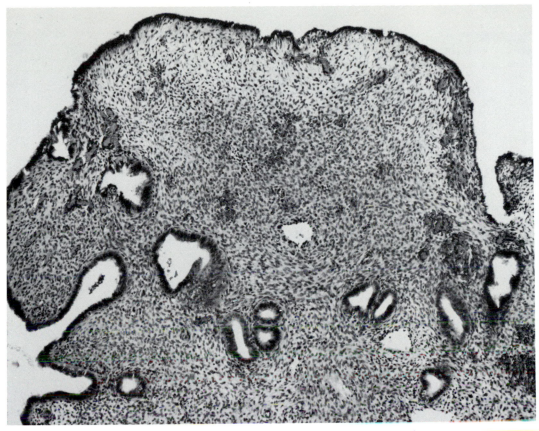

Fig. 794 Typical polypoid appearance of endometrium in patient taking contraceptive pill. Note proliferation of spindle stromal cells and scanty number of glandular structures. (Low power; WU neg. 73-371.)

tions. Studies in England and in the United States have shown an increased incidence of thrombophlebitis and pulmonary embolism in those using oral contraceptives.[35, 36] Morphologically, the vascular changes are widely distributed and involve arteries and veins. They include thrombi and intimal thickening with endothelial proliferation.[27]

Inflammation and metaplasia

Chronic endometritis, characterized by an infiltrate of lymphocytes and plasma cells, may follow pregnancy or abortion in association with abnormal uterine bleeding.[38] It should be emphasized that lymphoid follicles, with or without germinal centers, are a normal occurrence in the endometrial mucosa and therefore should not be considered as evidence of chronic endometritis. Actually, they are seen more commonly in normal than in abnormal endometria.[43]

The term *pyometra* refers to the accumulation of pus within the endometrial cavity. It is the consequence of the combined effect of obstruction and infection. Whiteley and Hamlett[44] reviewed thirty-five cases in postmenopausal patients. Only five were secondary to carcinoma. The remaining thirty were the result of benign cervical stricture originating from senile atresia, surgery, or cauterization.

Endometrial tuberculosis is rare in the United States but common in many European and South American countries.[42] Menstrual disturbances are common. The microscopic diagnosis is based upon the demonstration of acid-fast bacilli in tubercles or culture. The presence of plasma

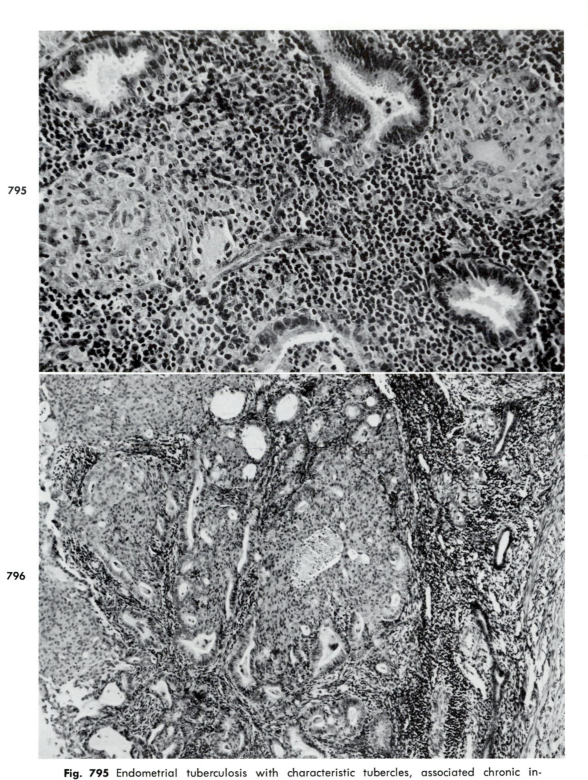

Fig. 795 Endometrial tuberculosis with characteristic tubercles, associated chronic inflammation, and irregular glands. (×250; WU neg. 65-3336A.)
Fig. 796 Squamous metaplasia composed of ill-defined masses of pale cells that blend with glandular epithelium. (×90; WU neg. 66-11888A.)

cells and leukocytes probably results from secondary infection.[41] Tubercles may be missed unless multiple levels of curettings are examined (Fig. 795).

Small circumscribed solid nests of round pale cells occasionally seen within endometrial glands (Fig. 796) were designated as *intraglandular morules* by Dutra.[39] They are generally considered to represent foci of squamous metaplasia, although clearcut evidence for this is lacking in most instances. An electron microscopic study of this curious lesion is needed. The etiology is not known. Similar lesions occur in experimental animals after castration.[40] Associated findings in the group of thirty specimens studied by Bomze and Friedman[37] included leiomyomas, polyps, and adenomatous hyperplasia.

Endometriosis and adenomyosis

The theories of the production of *endometriosis* are numerous. Probably endometriosis results from a combination of factors rather than from a single cause. Such factors would include myometrial extension, implantation, and lymphatic or hematogenous metastases. Javert[50] outlined the main theories of the spread of endometrial tissue and listed the authorities who supported them*:

1 Direct myometrial extension	Schatz (1884)
	Baraban (1891)
	Pilliet (1894)
	Cullen (1896)
2 Congenital theories	
a Müllerian	Cullen (1908)
b Wolffian cell rests	von Recklinghausen (1896)
3 Serosal metaplasia	Iwanoff (1896)
	Meyer (1903)
	Novak (1931)
4 Implantation theory	Sampson (1922)
5 Lymphatic metastasis	Sampson (1922)
	Halban (1924)
	Javert (1948)
6 Hematogenous metastasis	Sampson (1924)
7 Analogy to endometrial carcinoma	Sampson (1925)

*From Javert, C. J.: Pathogenesis of endometriosis based on endometrial homeoplasia, direct extension, exfoliation and implantation, lymphatic and hematogenous metastasis, Cancer **2**:399-410, 1949.

Endometrium can directly invade the myometrium and grow along lymph and blood vessels.[56] Coelomic metaplasia also occurs.[54] Corner et al.[46] reported nine cases suggesting origin of endometriosis from germinal epithelial elements. Implantation certainly occurs. Sampson[56] explained this on the basis of regurgitation and implantation of menstrual endometrium.

Misplaced endometrium has been seen in the vagina, pelvic peritoneum, vulva, bladder, large bowel, small bowel, appendix, abdominal incisions, kidney, lung, and groin and even in various skeletal muscles.[50] Spontaneous cutaneous endometriosis is limited to the umbilicus and inguinal area.[57] In other locations, such as lower abdominal wall, perineum, and vulva, it practically always arises in surgical scars.[59] Scars from cesarean sections are particularly susceptible. Hysterosalpingography can cause some cases of ovarian and peritoneal endometriosis.[58]

By definition, *adenomyosis* is the heterotopic occurrence of islands of endometrial glands and stroma in the myometrium.[45] The term endometriosis should be reserved for heterotopic endometrium situated outside the uterus. Endometriosis may occur without adenomyosis. This supports the theory of coelomic metaplasia. The typical uterus with adenomyosis is enlarged and globular.[47] The diagnosis may be made on cut section because of depressed brown cystic lesions in obvious but ill-defined bulging zones of muscle hypertrophy (Fig. 797). In elderly women, the uterus with extensive adenomyosis may be atrophic. Leiomyomas in uteri with adenomyosis may contain endometrial foci.[52]

Microscopically, the diagnosis of adenomyosis depends on the criteria used by the pathologist. There is no submucosa in the endometrium. The endometrium lies directly on the myometrium. It is not rare to see slight endometrial invagination. This should not be diagnosed as adenomyosis. With deep muscular penetration, the diagnosis becomes more certain. By convention, the diagnosis of adenomyosis is reserved to those cases in which endometrial glands

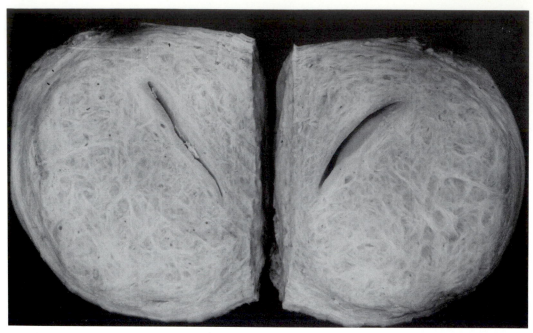

Fig. 797 Typical gross appearance of uterine adenomyosis. Ill-defined whorled pro-liferation of myometrial muscle results in thickening of wall. Circumscription of leiomyoma is lacking. (Courtesy Dr. E. F. Lascano, Buenos Aires, Argentina.)

and stroma are seen in the myometrium at a distance of at least one low-power field from the endometrial-myometrial junction.

Hypertrophy of the muscle is often seen in areas of adenomyosis. In endometriosis both glands and stroma often reflect the hormonal changes of the menstrual cycle and respond to therapeutically administered hormones.[55] The glands of adenomyosis are less responsive, perhaps due to their basal nature. Molitor[53] found that when the surface endometrium was secretory, the ectopic glands were secretory in only 26.6% of the cases.

Hyperplasia and carcinoma in situ may occur in foci of adenomyosis in association with similar lesions of the endometrium proper.[60] Rupture of the pregnant uterus can occur because of adenomyosis.[49] Although well-authenticated cases of endometriosis of lymph nodes exist, most cases so designated represent müllerian glandular inclusions analogous to the so-called germinal inclusion cysts of the ovary.[48] Endometrial stroma is absent. Microscopically, glands lined by ciliated or nonciliated

cuboidal epithelium are seen in the capsule or in the cortical portion of the node. Karp and Czernobilsky[51] found these inclusions at autopsy in 14% of fifty females but in none of fifty males.

Dysfunctional uterine bleeding and hyperplasia

A *normal menstruation* can be defined as the bleeding from secretory endometrium associated with an ovulatory cycle not exceeding a length of five days. A bleeding not fulfilling these criteria is referred to as an ***abnormal uterine bleeding.*** Some of these are the result of an organic lesion, such as endometriosis, submucous myoma, endometrial polyp, or cancer, particularly in the postmenopausal patient. In most series, approximately 15% to 20% of the cases of postmenopausal bleeding are due to endometrial carcinoma and about the same proportion to endometrial polyps.[64, 70] The only finding on dilatation and curettage in about 20% of postmenopausal bleeders is an atrophic endometrium. Vascular degenerative changes in the uterine blood vessels have been suggested as a possible etiology in these cases.[67]

Bleeding not associated with an organic cause in women of child-bearing age belongs to the large and somewhat nebulous category known as *dysfunctional uterine bleeding.* Examination of specimens obtained on dilatation and curettage or endometrial biopsy is a continuous source of frustration for the pathologist. Sometimes provided with minimal clinical information or bound to examine material taken at an inappropriate moment of the menstrual cycle, he is often unable to recognize any abnormality in the material examined. At the most, he can detect changes that only confirm what the gynecologist already knows—i.e., that the patient has an abnormal bleeding. These include the presence of fibrin clumps in the endometrial stroma (a finding not usually present in the normal menstrual endometrium)[71] or the appearance of fragmented portions with dense stromal cellularity (a process known as *stromal crumbling*).

On the other hand, if a thorough clinical study is available, examination of a correctly timed biopsy can be quite informative. Cases of dysfunctional uterine bleeding can be divided in two large categories: those associated with ovulation and the more numerous ones in which ovulation has not occurred. A hybrid group in which ovulatory and anovulatory cycles alternate is not infrequently seen in premenopausal patients.

In the ovulatory group, bleeding may occur because of an *inadequate proliferative phase.* This is recognized by a disparity between the endometrial pattern observed and that expected from the time of the cycle (i.e., a fourteenth-day endometrium with an appearance suggestive of one on the sixth or seventh day) or by the inconspicuousness of morphologic signs of proliferation, such as pseudostratification of nuclei or mitotic activity. Bleeding due to an *inadequate secretory phase* (underdeveloped secretory endometrium; luteal phase inadequacy) is recognized by analogous criteria. The curetting or biopsy should be preferably obtained on the twelfth postovulatory day or two days prior to the expected menstruation.[68] According to Noyes,[69] biopsies should be taken of at least two menstrual cycles, and both the basal temperature shift and the onset of succeeding menses should be used as points of reference to time the length of the secretory phase. The "date" obtained from the endometrial biopsy should be more than two days retarded before the diagnosis of underdeveloped secretory endometrium is entertained. Hormone administration often corrects this defect.[62, 68] Another type of defect seen in the ovulatory group of bleeders is known as *irregular shedding of the endometrium.* The term refers to a regularly recurring menorrhagia in which the bleeding phase of the cycle requires seven days or more for completion, without subsequent prolongation of the cycle.[65] This is due to a lag in the shedding of the secretory endometrium, which is normally completed by the fourth day of menstruation.[66] The tissue should be obtained five or more days after the onset of menstrual bleeding, and the diagnosis is made by detecting in this material retained secretory endometrium in addition to fragmented menstual and/or early proliferative endometrium. It has been estimated that between 10% and 17% of cases of functional bleeding belong to this category.[72]

An *anovulatory cycle* can be recognized, at its earliest stage, by finding a proliferative endometrium at a time of the cycle when a secretory pattern would be expected. Most commonly, the prolonged unremitting estrogen stimulation results in *endometrial hyperplasia.* All grades of this phenomenon occur, ranging from the one distinguished only with difficulty from an exuberant proliferative endometrium to the atypical one that can simulate adenocarcinoma. Accordingly, we grade our cases of endometrial hyperplasia as *mild, moderate,* or *severe* (Fig. 798). We dis-

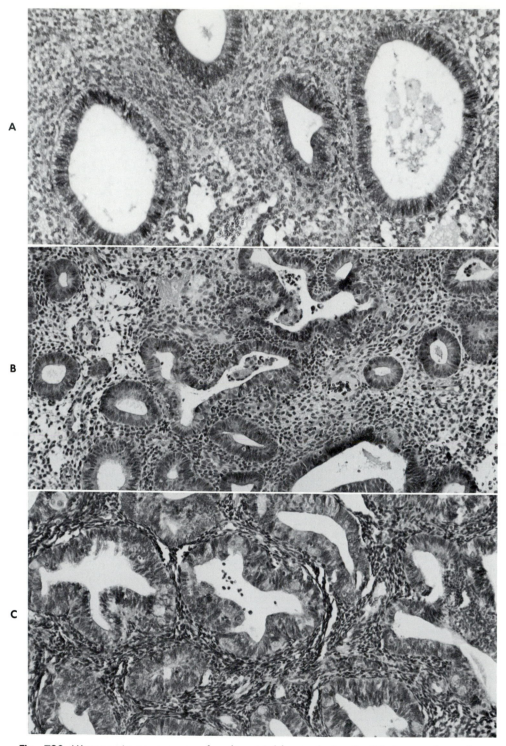

Fig. 798 Microscopic appearance of endometrial hyperplasia of mild degree, **A,** moderate degree, **B,** and severe degree, **C.** With increasing severity of disease, cystic changes in glands and amount of stroma diminish, whereas epithelial proliferation becomes more intense. (**A** to **C,** ×175; **A,** WU neg. 73-367; **B,** WU neg. 73-368; **C,** WU neg. 73-369.)

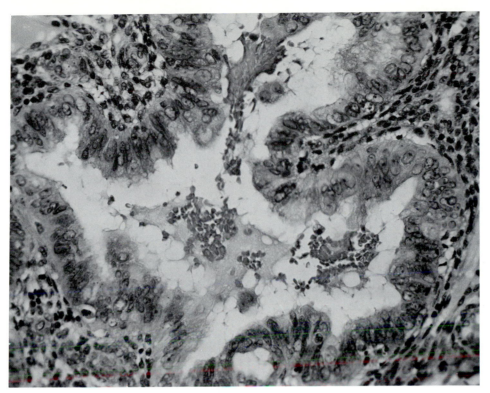

Fig. 799 Endometrial hyperplasia of type sometimes designated as carcinoma in situ of endometrium. Cells are large with abundant clear eosinophilic cytoplasm and some disorientation. These changes were focal in nature in curettage specimen. No invasive carcinoma was found in hysterectomy specimen. Patient remained free of disease thirteen years later. (×320; WU neg. 52-2873.)

regard for this purpose the presence or absence of cystic changes, since they are only a secondary feature of the process and can be found in the absence of hyperplasia. Hyperplastic changes entirely analogous to those described here occur often after exogenous estrogenic stimulation, in the Stein-Leventhal syndrome, and with estrogen-secreting ovarian neoplasms.

A great deal of experience is needed to differentiate an extreme case of hyperplasia from an adenocarcinoma. Microscopic features favoring the latter include marked pleomorphism, loss of polarity, complex ramification of the glands, disorderly arrangement, and intraglandular budding—i.e., the formation within a gland of a group of smaller glandular structures without stroma in between.

Gore and Hertig[63] have designated an endometrial pattern characterized by en-dometrial glands composed of large cells with abundant eosinophilic cytoplasm as *carcinoma in situ of the endometrium* (Fig. 799). Since the assumption that this change inevitably progresses to invasive adenocarcinoma has never been proved and has, on occasion, been reversed by hormone manipulations,[73] we prefer to regard it as a morphologic variant of endometrial hyperplasia.

The relationship between hyperplasia and carcinoma has been a hotly debated subject. Undoubtedly, most cases of endometrial carcinoma are preceded by a stage of hyperplasia. On the other hand, relatively few patients with hyperplasia (approximately 2%) will subsequently develop cancer. Therefore, the mere presence of hyperplasia is not a basis for hysterectomy. In general, the more severe the hyperplasia, the more likely it is to be followed

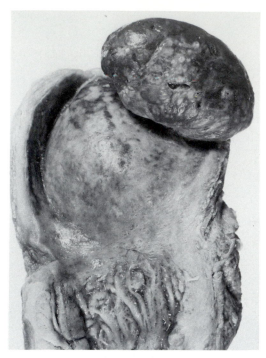

Fig. 800 Large benign endometrial polyp distending endometrial cavity. (WU neg. 52-766.)

by invasive carcinoma. In the series reported by Chamlian and Taylor,[61] a long-term follow-up study of ninety-seven young women with *severe ("adenomatous or atypical") hyperplasia,* 14% subsequently developed endometrial adenocarcinoma.

Tumors
Endometrial polyps

The large majority of endometrial polyps are not true neoplasms but rather represent circumscribed foci of hyperplasia (Fig. 800). The glands usually show some degree of cystic change. They may be lined by an active pseudostratified epithelium containing mitotic figures or, in the postmenopausal patient, by a flat, inactive epithelium.

The glands and stroma of the polyp are unresponsive to progesterone stimulation and retain their integrity throughout the menstrual cycle. In material obtained from curettage, where usually only fragments of the polyp are obtained, the differentiation with endometrial hyperplasia is made by examining the stroma. In the

latter condition, the stromal cells are quite active, with large vesicular nuclei and occasional mitotic figures, whereas the stroma of a polyp is composed of spindle, fibroblast-like cells, contains abundant extracellular connective tissue, and has large blood vessels with thick walls. Not infrequently, both conditions coexist.

Rarely, polyps made of functional endometrium are encountered. The diagnosis is made on the gross features of the lesion rather than on the microscopic pattern of glands and stroma and is, therefore, difficult or even impossible to make on a curettage specimen.

Endometrial polyps having smooth muscle fibers (not connected with blood vessel walls) in addition to the customary glands and stroma are designated as **adenomyomatous polyps.** They have a characteristic hard consistency and a grayish color.

Carcinoma

The large majority of endometrial cancers are adenocarcinomas. They typically occur in elderly patients: approximately 80% are postmenopausal at the time of the diagnosis. A large proportion of the patients have a particular body build, are obese, and have a high incidence of diabetes and hypertension.[88, 89] Premenopausal patients with endometrial cancer have a similar constitutional background.[77] Kempson and Pokorny[87] showed that young patients (40 years of age or younger) with well-differentiated endometrial adenocarcinomas have an excellent prognosis (Fig. 801). They pointed out the difficulties in differentiating hyperplasia from carcinoma and emphasized that the borderline cases should be treated conservatively.

It is generally accepted that excess estrogenic stimulation is causally related to endometrial cancer.[82] This tumor is extremely rare after castration. Prolonged estrogen therapy can result in a complicated proliferative pattern of difficult interpretation. Gusberg and Hall[80] reported twenty-three patients with a lesion they interpreted as carcinoma following estro-

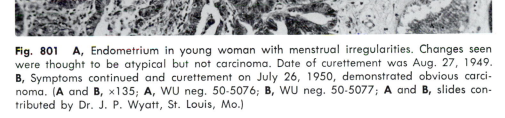

Fig. 801   A, Endometrium in young woman with menstrual irregularities. Changes seen were thought to be atypical but not carcinoma. Date of curettement was Aug. 27, 1949. **B,** Symptoms continued and curettement on July 26, 1950, demonstrated obvious carcinoma. (**A** and **B,** ×135; **A,** WU neg. 50-5076; **B,** WU neg. 50-5077; **A** and **B,** slides contributed by Dr. J. P. Wyatt, St. Louis, Mo.)

gen therapy. Tumor dissemination occurred in only two patients. It requires considerable judgment and experience to evaluate and treat these borderline lesions.

Patients with Stein-Leventhal syndrome may show extremely atypical endometrial changes. In the majority of the cases, these changes represent hyperplasia and will regress with medical therapy.[79, 85] However, a few well-documented cases of carcinomas have been reported.[75] Similar findings can

be encountered in patients with functioning theca and granulosa cell tumors. In most instances, the endometrial proliferation will regress after excision of the tumor, thus proving its hyperplastic nature.

Hertig and Sommers[82] have provided convincing evidence that endometrial adenocarcinoma rarely, if ever, develops from a completely normal endometrium. In almost every instance in which proper documentation is available, the changes have been preceded by those of hyperplasia. In their series, all patients who had adequate material from curettage examined fifteen years or less prior to the development of adenocarcinoma had an abnormal endometrial pattern. This does not imply by any means that all hyperplasias will progress to carcinoma, the situation being analogous to the relationship between cervical dysplasia and cervical carcinoma.

Grossly, carcinoma of the endometrium may form broad-based polypoid masses or grow diffusely into the myometrium. In general, extensive myometrial invasion is accompanied by clinically detectable uterine enlargement. However, notable exceptions occur. At times, the tumor begins in a cornu and is missed by curettement. Microscopically, most tumors are well-differentiated or moderately differentiated adenocarcinomas. Mucin secretion is seen not infrequently and is not necessarily an indication of endocervical origin.[93, 97] The tumor may grow in a papillary fashion reminiscent of ovarian serous carcinoma and it may exceptionally contain psammoma bodies.[81] Collections of foamy macrophages, seen in the stroma of some cases, are probably the result of tumor necrosis. They are not pathognomic of cancer. We have seen them on several occasions accompanying hyperplastic endometria but only once in a normal mucosa.[84]

Approximately 25% of endometrial adenocarcinomas contain well-differentiated squamous elements arisen by metaplasia of the tumor glands. These tumors are known as *adenoacanthomas.* Contrary to previous statements, recent studies have indicated that the natural history of these neoplasms closely parallels that of the ordinary adenocarcinoma.[74, 91] Ng[90] separated from this group those adenocarcinomas having *malignant-appearing* squamous elements and designated them as *mixed carcinomas.* Patients with this tumor type were older and had a worse prognosis than those with adenocarcinoma or adenocanthoma. The incidence of mixed carcinomas in his series is notably high: almost 7% and on the

rise, quite at variance with our experience.

Pure *epidermoid carcinomas* are extremely rare. Most cases have occurred in elderly patients with pyometra, presumably on the basis of a preexisting endometrial squamous metaplasia.[83]

Occasionally, adenocarcinomas are composed of large clear cells with distinct cellular margins and containing a greater or lesser amount of glycogen (Fig. 802). Papillary formations and "hobnail" cells present in this variant of adenocarcinoma resemble those seen in the ovarian, cervical, and vaginal tumors formerly called "mesonephric carcinomas."[86, 92] However, their presence in superficial endometrial cancers and even in nonneoplastic endometrium[76] is evidence against a relationship with mesonephric remnants. Although the number of published cases is too small to draw definite conclusions, it seems that the behavior of these tumors is similar to that of the ordinary adenocarcinoma.[95]

Gospel[78] has done an excellent electron microscopic study of endometrial cancer.

Morphologic parameters bearing on the prognosis of endometrial cancer are the grade of differentiation of the tumor and level of infiltration of the myometrial wall.[91]

The treatment of endometrial cancer is total abdominal hysterectomy with bilateral salpingo-oophorectomy, usually preceded by a course of radiation therapy. The routine application of the latter has significantly improved the survival rate and markedly decreased the incidence of recurrences in the vaginal cuff.[94] Progestin agents, although not curative, can induce striking temporary regressions in the primary tumor as well as in the metastases. Well-differentiated lesions are more likely to respond[96] (Figs. 803 and 804).

Endometrial stromal tumors

Norris and Taylor[102] have clarified the nature and behavior of the rare tumors arising from the endometrial stroma. They have divided these tumors according to the nature of their margins into a benign type ("stromal nodule") having pushing mar-

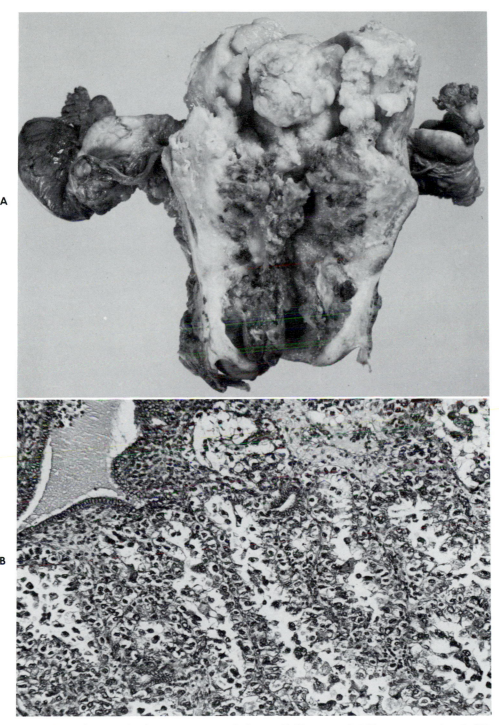

Fig. 802 Endometrial adenocarcinoma of clear cell ("mesonephric") type occurring in 71-year-old woman. **A,** Gross appearance of tissue. Large polypoid masses fill endometrial cavity. Extension into myometrium and endocervix is evident. **B,** Microscopic appearance of same tumor. Neoplastic glands are lined by large cells with abundant clear cytoplasm and well-defined cytoplasmic margins. (**A,** WU neg. 61-7994; **B,** ×150; WU neg. 73-454.)

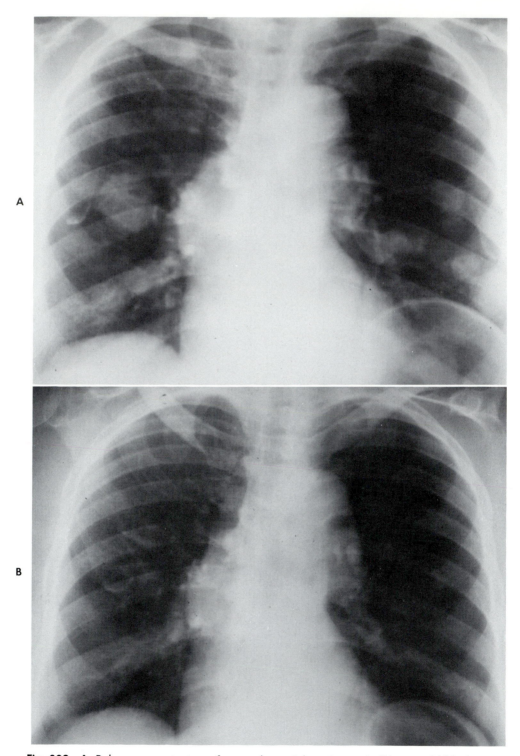

Fig. 803 A, Pulmonary metastases from endometrial carcinoma in 74-year-old black woman. **B,** Following progesterone therapy, metastases completely disappeared. Patient also was given full course of radiotherapy to pelvis. She remained in remission for several months.

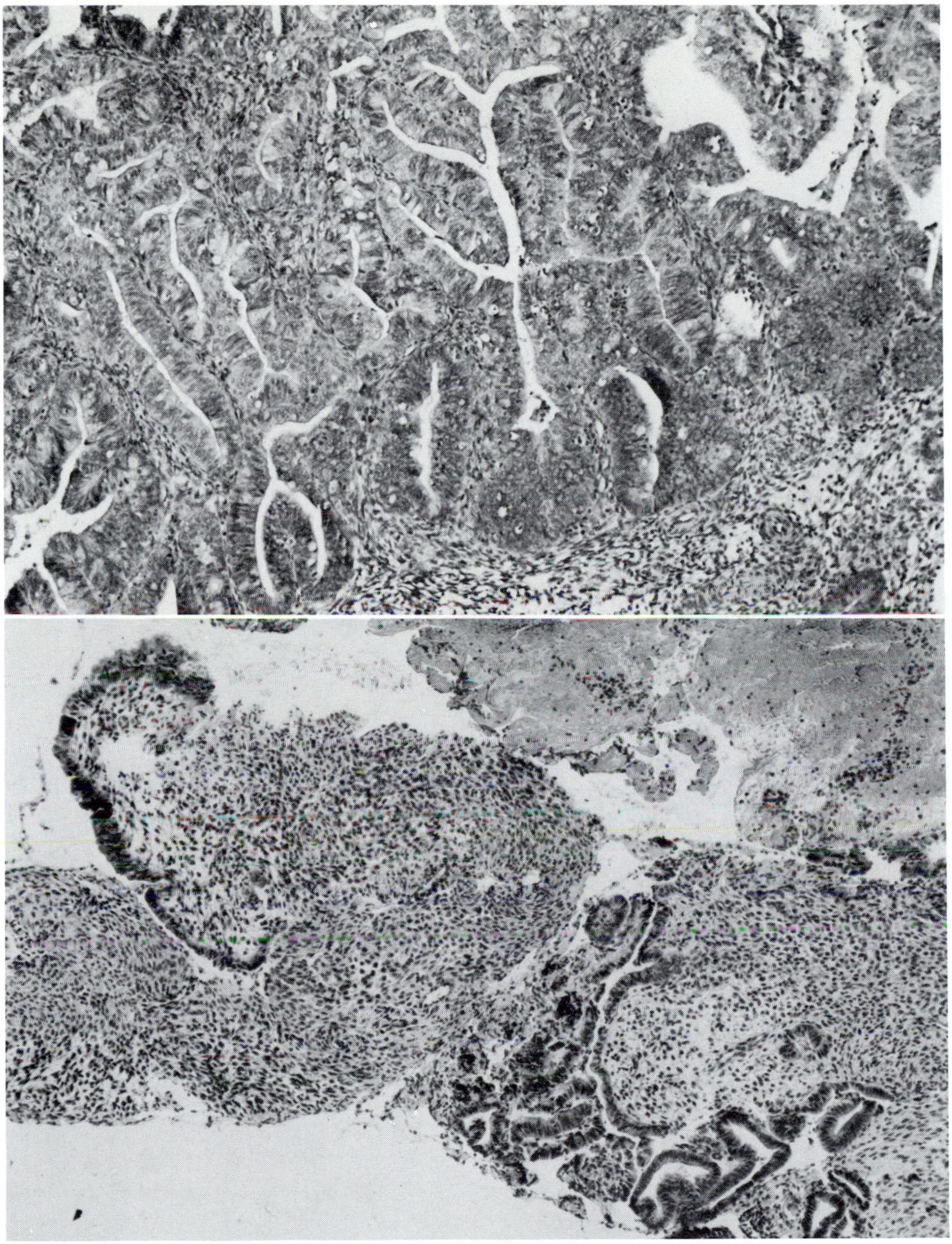

Fig. 804   A, Adenocarcinoma of endometrium invading stroma. Patient was treated for three weeks with progestogens and curettage repeated twice. **B,** Repeat curettage. Endometrium shows progestogen effect without evidence of carcinoma. Patient was well seven years after last curettage and had been pregnant twice. (**A** and **B,** ×90; **A,** WU neg. 67-3366; **B,** WU neg. 67-3367; **A** and **B,** from Kempson, R. L., and Pokorny, G. E.: Adenocarcinoma of the endometrium in women aged forty and younger, Cancer **21:**650-662, 1968.)

gins and a malignant type characterized by infiltrating margins. The latter was further subdivided on the basis of the mitotic count into a low-grade ("endolymphatic stromal myosis") variety and a high-grade ("stromal sarcoma") variety.

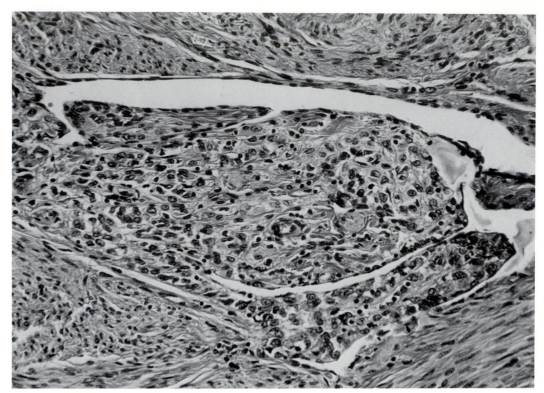

Fig. 805 Low-grade endometrial stromal sarcoma ("endolymphatic stromal myosis"). This was incidental finding in 43-year-old patient whose uterus had been removed for myoma. (×300; WU neg. 65-2431.)

Features common to the benign type and both varieties of the malignant types include a soft, yellow to orange gross appearance and a microscopic pattern characterized by uniform small cells closely resembling those of the endometrial stroma, individually enveloped by reticulin fibers, and the presence within the tumor of glandular formations more or less resembling those of endometrium in approximately one-third of the cases. Clinically, the tumors often present with uterine bleeding and enlargement. Abdominal or pelvic pain is less common.

Stromal nodules present grossly as solitary sharply circumscribed masses. They do not invade veins, lymphatics, or the myometrium. The prognosis is excellent. None of the eighteen patients studied by Norris and Taylor[102] had recurrence after surgery.

Low-grade stromal sarcomas, which Nor-

ris and Taylor[102] prefer to call endolymphatic stromal myosis, infiltrate the myometrium and vascular spaces, usually lymphatic vessels (Fig. 805). The latter feature sometimes can be detected grossly by the presence of yellowish ropy or ball-like masses filling dilated channels.[105] The local invasion may extend into the broad ligament, tubes, and ovaries[99, 100] (Fig. 806). Microscopically, the tumors should contain fewer than ten mitoses per ten high-power fields in the most active areas in order to qualify for this category. Their natural history is characterized by slow clinical progression, repeated local recurrences, and relatively favorable prognosis. Of the twenty patients reported by Norris and Taylor,[102] only one had died of the tumor, but 31% had persistent or recurrent tumor at the time of last follow-up.

High-grade stromal sarcomas show the same propensity for local and vascular in-

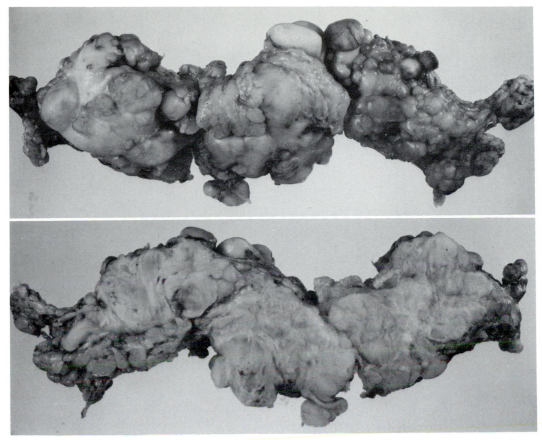

Fig. 806 External view and cross section of peritoneal implant of low-grade endometrial stromal sarcoma (so-called endolymphatic stromal myosis). Primary tumor had been removed two years previously from 53-year-old patient. (WU negs. 68-8609 and 68-8610.)

vasion as the low-grade variety. They are differentiated from the latter only by virtue of their high mitotic count (ten or more mitoses per ten high-power fields). Grossly, they often are a diffuse growth involving the entire endometrial surface (Fig. 807). Their prognosis is poor. Of the fifteen patients reviewed by Norris and Taylor,[102] four were free of disease, seven had died, and another four were living with tumor. An even more striking difference in prognosis between these two types of stromal sarcoma was reported by Kempson and Bari.[101]

Size of the tumor and presence or absence of extrauterine extension are important prognostic features. Stromal neoplasms less than 4 cm in diameter practically never recur, and tumors confined to the

uterus at the time of the initial surgery very rarely do so, regardless of the variety to which they may belong.

The marked vascularity that these tumors possess can be responsible for a misdiagnosis of vascular neoplasm. Although a few well-documented uterine hemangiopericytomas are on record,[104] we feel that most of the lesions so reported are in actuality examples of stromal neoplasms. Confusion also may arise with malignant lymphoma and undifferentiated carcinoma. Reticulin stain can be useful in the differential diagnosis with the latter.[103]

Tumors with the appearance of endometrial stromal neoplasms may exceptionally arise outside the uterus. We have seen one case in the pelvis, and Gerber and Toker[98] have reported another example.

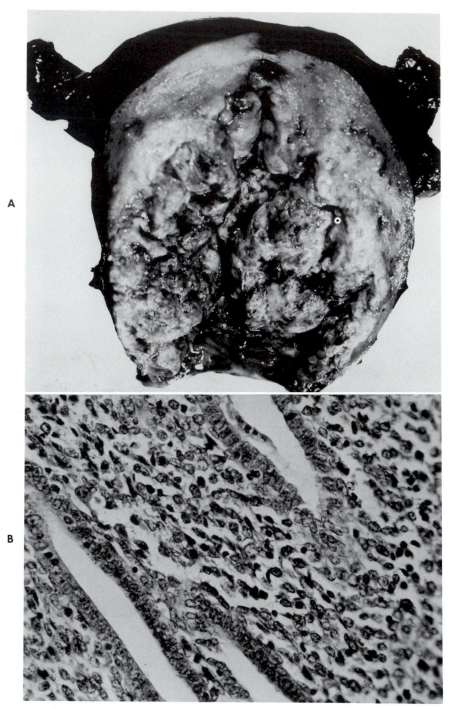

Fig. 807 A, High-grade endometrial stromal sarcoma replacing entire endometrial cavity. **B,** Same lesion shown in **A.** Note uniform cells, vesicular nuclei, and fine nucleoli. Mitotic figures, not seen here, were numerous in other areas of neoplasm. Patient died with pelvic recurrence and distant metastases four months after surgery. (**A,** EFSCH 50-658; courtesy Dr. R. Johnson, Columbia, Mo.; **B,** ×400; WU neg. 50-3554.)

Malignant mixed müllerian tumors (mixed mesodermal tumors)

Malignant mixed müllerian tumors are rare uterine neoplasms that are seen practically always in postmenopausal patients, in whom they present with uterine bleeding and enlargement. They arise in the uterine body, the most common site being the posterior wall in the region of the fundus.[114] Grossly, they present as large, soft, polypoid growths involving the endometrium and myometrium, sometimes protruding from the cervix (Fig. 808).

Foci of necrosis and hemorrhage are common. Microscopically, the characteristic feature is the *admixture of carcinomatous and sarcomatous elements.* The carcinomatous component is usually adenocarcinoma, often well differentiated, although epidermoid and undifferentiated patterns also may occur. The nature of the sarcomatous component is the basis for the division of these neoplasms into a homologous and a heterologous variety. In the former, the malignant stroma is "nonspecific," formed by either round cells

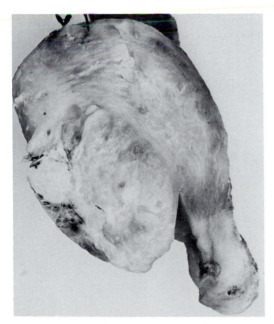

Fig. 808 Polypoid malignant mixed müllerian tumor of uterus. Metastases in peritoneal cavity appeared one year following surgery. (WU neg. 49-4401.)

resembling those of the endometrial stroma or by spindle cells resembling leiomyosarcoma or fibrosarcoma. In the latter, specific heterologous mesenchymal elements (such as skeletal muscle, cartilage, bone, or fat) also are present (Fig. 809). Cross striations are required to categorize a tissue as rhabdomyosarcoma (Fig. 810). The distinction between these two varieties may require the study of numerous sections and, therefore, may not be possible on material obtained by curettage. Actually, the malignant stroma may be so inconspicuous in such a specimen as to be missed altogether, the lesion being misdiagnosed as an ordinary adenocarcinoma.

Malignant mixed müllerian tumors are easily separated from teratomas by the absence of skin appendages, glia, and thyroid.[107] They should also be clearly separated from botryoid rhadomyosarcoma (sarcoma botryoides). The latter term should be reserved to the tumor of childhood arising from the cervix or vagina and lacking a carcinomatous component.

Extension into the pelvis, lymphatic and vascular permeation, and distant lymphborne and blood-borne metastases are common. If the tumor has extended to the serosa of the uterus or beyond at the time of surgery, the prognosis is hopeless.[108] The only patients with some chance of cure are those in whom the tumor is restricted to the inner half of the myometrium at the time of surgery. This determination implies a thorough sampling of the hysterectomy specimen by the pathologist.

In most series, tumors having only homologous stromal elements (called "carcinosarcomas" by Norris and Taylor[110]) have been found to have a slightly better prognosis than those with heterologous elements, a fact that probably justifies their separation.[108, 110, 111, 113] In other series, no differences were found.[106] The claim that the presence of cartilage in heterologous tumors is associated with a relatively better prognosis, the reverse being true for skeletal muscle, has not been substantiated by subsequent studies.

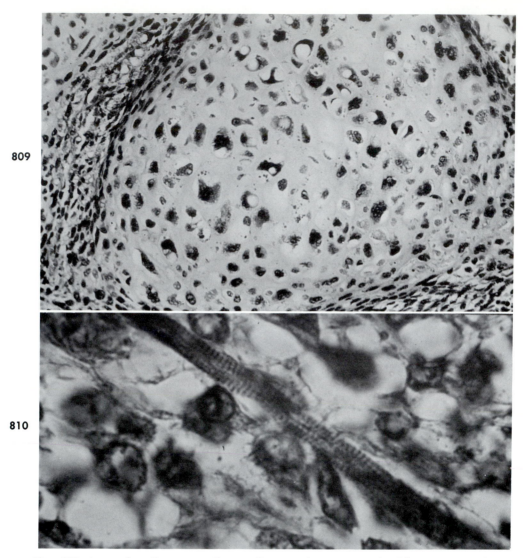

Fig. 809 Area of malignant cartilage cells in malignant mixed müllerian tumor shown in Fig. 808. (×210; WU neg. 50-5070.)
Fig. 810 Striated muscle cells in malignant mixed müllerian tumor. (×2,000; AFIP 29-2563.)

Response to radiation therapy and chemotherapy has been uniformly poor. Total abdominal hysterectomy with bilateral salpingo-oophorectomy and pelvic lymphadenectomy is the treatment of choice.

Norris and Taylor[109] made the disturbing observation that 30% of the patients with heterologous malignant mixed müllerian tumors and 13% of those with homologous tumors that they studied had a history of previous irradiation to the pelvic area, usually given for some benign disorder. The median interval between irradiation and the time of diagnosis of the tumor was 16.4 years in their series and 11.8 years in the patients reported by Thomas et al.[115]

Malignant mixed müllerian tumors can arise in extrauterine locations, the most common sites being ovary and pelvic structures.[112]

Metastatic tumors

Occasionally, metastatic carcinoma from extrapelvic sites may cause uterine bleeding as the presenting symptoms.[116] The breast and colon have been the most frequent primary sites in our experience.

REFERENCES
Curettage and biopsy

1 Carmichael, D. E.: Asherman's syndrome, Obstet. Gynecol. **36**:922-928, 1970.
2 Foix, A., Bruno, R. O., Davison, T., and Lema, B.: The pathology of postcurettage intrauterine adhesions, Am. J. Obstet. Gynecol. **96**:1027-1033, 1966.
3 Kahler, V. L., Creasy, R. K., and Morris, J. A.: Value of the endometrial biopsy, Obstet. Gynecol. **34**:91-95, 1969.
4 McLennan, C. E.: Endometrial regeneration after curettage, Am. J. Obstet. Gynecol. **104**:185-194, 1969.

Cytology

5 Bibbo, M., Shanklin, D. R., and Wied, G. L.: Endometrial cytology on jet wash material, J. Reprod. Med. **8**:90-96, 1972.
6 Christopherson, W. M., Mendez, W. M., Ahuja, E. M., Lundin, F. E., and Parker, J. E.: Cervix cancer control in Louisville, Kentucky, Cancer **26**:29-38, 1970.
7 Dowling, E. A., Gravlee, L. C., and Hutchins, K. E.: A new technique for the detection of adenocarcinoma of the endometrium, Acta Cytol. (Baltimore) **13**:496-501, 1969.
8 Gravlee, L. C.: Jet-irrigation method for the diagnosis of endometrial adenocarcinoma, Obstet. Gynecol. **34**:168-173, 1969.
9 Hibbard, L. T., and Schwinn, C. P.: Diagnosis of endometrial jet washings, Am. J. Obstet. Gynecol. **111**:1039-1042, 1971.
10 Reagan, J. W.: In Endometrial cancer. I. Rising incidence, Kalamazoo, Mich., 1972, The Upjohn Co.
11 Reagan, J. W., and Ng, A. B. P.: The cells of uterine adenocarcinoma, Baltimore, 1965, The Williams & Wilkins Co.
12 Wied, G. L.: In Endometrial cancer. II. Detection, Kalamazoo, Mich., 1972, The Upjohn Co.

Cyclic changes

13 Arias-Stella, J.: A topographic study of uterine epithelia atypia associated with chorionic tissue; demonstration of alteration in the endocervix, Cancer **12**:782-790, 1959.
14 Arias-Stella, J.: Atypical endometrial changes produced by chorionic tissue, Hum. Pathol. **3**:450-453, 1972.

15 Azzopardi, J. C., and Zayid, I.: Synthetic progestogen-oestrogen therapy and uterine changes, J. Clin. Pathol. **20**:731-738, 1967.
16 Dallenbach-Hellweg, G.: Histopathology of the endometrium (English translation by F. D. Dallenbach), New York, 1971, Springer-Verlag.
17 Ehrmann, R. L.: In Histologic dating of the endometrium (an invitational symposium), J. Reprod. Med. **3**:179-200, 1969.
18 Hertig, A. T.: Gestational hyperplasia of the endometrium; a morphologic correlation of ova, endometrium, and corpora lutea during early pregnancy, Lab. Invest. **13**:1153-1191, 1964.
19 Noyes, R. W.: Uniformity of secretory endometrium; study of multiple sections from 100 uteri removed at operation, Fertil. Steril. **7**:103-109, 1956.
20 Noyes, R. W., and Haman, J. O.: Accuracy of endometrial dating, Fertil. Steril. **4**:504-517, 1954.
21 Noyes, R. W., Hertig, A. T., and Rock, J.: Dating the endometrial biopsy, Fertil. Steril. **1**:3-25, 1950.

Iatrogenic changes

22 Azzopardi, J. G., and Zayid, I.: Synthetic progestogen-oestrogen therapy and uterine changes, J. Clin. Pathol. **20**:731-738, 1967.
23 Charles, D.: Iatrogenic endometrial patterns, J. Clin. Pathol. **17**:205-212, 1964.
24 Corfman, P. A., and Segal, S. J.: Biologic effects of intrauterine devices, Am. J. Obstet. Gynecol. **100**:448-459, 1968.
25 Dockerty, M. B., Smith, R. A., and Symmonds, R. E.: Pseudomalignant endometrial changes induced by administration of new synthetic progestins, Mayo Clin. Proc. **34**:321-328, 1959.
26 Goldzieher, J. W., Rice-Wray, E., Schulz-Contreras, M., and Aranda-Rosell, A.: Fertility following termination of contraception with norethindrone, Am. J. Obstet. Gynecol. **84**:1474-1477, 1962.
27 Irey, N. S., Manion, W. C., and Taylor, H. B.: Vascular lesions in women taking oral contraceptives, Arch. Pathol. **89**:1-8, 1970.
28 Jessen, D. A., Lane, R. E., and Greene, R. R.: Intrauterine foreign body; a clinical and histopathologic study on use of Graefenberg ring, Am. J. Obstet. Gynecol. **85**:1023-1032, 1963.
29 Maqueo, M., Becerra, C., Munguia, H., and Goldzieher, J. W.: Endometrial histology and vaginal cytology during oral contraception with sequential estrogen and progestin, Am. J. Obstet. Gynecol. **90**:396-400, 1964.
30 Martinez-Manautou, J., Maqueo, M., Gilbert, R. A., and Goldzieher, J. W.: Human endometrial activity of several new derivatives of

17-acetoxyprogesterone, Fertil. Steril. 13:169-183, 1962.

31 Ober, W. B.: Synthetic progestogen-oestrogen preparations and endometrial morphology, J. Clin. Pathol. 19:138-147, 1966.

32 Ober, W. B., Sobrero, A. J., Kurman, R., and Gold, S.: Endometrial morphology and polyethylene intrauterine devices; a study of 200 endometrial biopsies, Obstet. Gynecol. 32:782-793, 1968.

33 Rice-Wray, E., Aranda-Rosell, A., Maqueo, M., and Goldzieher, J. W.: Comparison of the long-term endometrial effects of synthetic progestins used in fertility control. Am. J. Obstet. Gynecol. 87:429-433, 1963.

34 Roland, M., Clyman, M. J., Decker, A., and Ober, W. B.: Classification of endometrial response to synthetic progestogen-estrogen compounds, J. Clin. Pathol. 15:143-163, 1964.

35 Sartwell, P. E., Masi, A. T., Arthes, F. G., Greene, G. R., and Smith, H. E.: Thromboembolism and oral contraceptives: an epidemiological case-control study, Am. J. Epidemiol. 90:365-380, 1969.

36 Vessey, M. P., and Doll, R.: Investigation of relation between use of oral contraceptives and thromboembolic disease; a further report, Br. Med. J. 2:651-657, 1969.

Inflammation and metaplasia

37 Bomze, E. J., and Friedman, N. B.: Squamous metaplasia and adenoacanthosis of the endometrium, Obstet. Gynecol. 30:619-625, 1967.

38 Dumoulin, J. G., and Hughesdon, P. E.: Chronic endometritis, J. Obstet. Gynaecol. Br. Commonw. 58:222-235, 1951.

39 Dutra, F. R.: Intraglandular morules of the endometrium, Am. J. Clin. Pathol. 31:60-65, 1959.

40 Fluhmann, C. F.: The histogenesis of squamous metaplasia in the cervix and endometrium, Surg. Gynecol. Obstet. 97:45-58, 1953.

41 Govan, A. D. T.: Tuberculous endometritis, J. Pathol. Bacteriol. 83:363-372, 1962.

42 Israel, S. L., Roitman, H. B., and Clancy, E.: Infrequency of unsuspected endometrial tuberculosis; histologic and bacteriologic study, J.A.M.A. 183:63-65, 1963.

43 Sen, D. K., and Fox, H.: The lymphoid tissue of the endometrium, Gynaecologia (Basel) 163:371-378, 1967.

44 Whiteley, P. F., and Hamlett, J. D.: Pyometra—a reappraisal, Am. J. Obstet. Gynecol. 109:108-112, 1971.

Endometriosis and adenomyosis

45 Brines, O. A.: Adenomyosis of the uterus, Surg. Gynecol. Obstet. 76:197-203, 1943.

46 Corner, G. W., Jr., Hu, C. Y., and Hertig, A. T.: Ovarian carcinoma arising in endometriosis, Am. J. Obstet. Gynecol. 59:760-774, 1950.

47 Emge, L. A.: The elusive adenomyosis of the uterus; its historical past and its present state of recognition, Am. J. Obstet. Gynecol. 83:1541-1563, 1962.

48 Ferguson, B. R., Bennington, J. L., and Haber, S. L.: Histochemistry of mucosubstances and histology of mixed müllerian pelvic lymph node glandular inclusions; evidence for histogenesis by müllerian metaplasia of coelomic epithelium, Obstet. Gynecol. 33:617-625, 1969.

49 Hertig, A.: Proceedings of Eighteenth Seminar of the American Society of Clinical Pathologists, October, 1952, Chicago, Ill.

50 Javert, C. J.: Pathogenesis of endometriosis based on endometrial homeoplasia, direct extension, exfoliation and implantation, lymphatic and hematogenous metastasis, Cancer 2:399-410, 1949 (extensive bibliography).

51 Karp, L. A., and Czernobilsky, B.: Glandular inclusions in pelvic and abdominal para-aortic lymph nodes, Am. J. Clin. Pathol. 52:212-218, 1969.

52 Mathur, B. B. L., Shah, B. S., and Bhende, Y. M.: Adenomyosis uteri, Am. J. Obstet, Gynecol. 84:1820-1829, 1962.

53 Molitor, J. J.: Adenomyosis: a clinical and pathological appraisal, Am. J. Obstet. Gynecol. 110:275-284, 1971.

54 Novak, E., and Te Linde, R. W.: The endometrium of the menstruating uterus, J.A.M.A. 83:900-906, 1924.

55 Sampson, J. A.: The life history of ovarian hematomas (hemorrhagic cysts) of endometrial (müllerian) type, Am. J. Obstet. Gynecol. 4:451-512, 1922.

56 Sampson, J. A.: Metastatic or embolic endometriosis, due to menstrual dissemination of endometrial tissue into the venous circulation, Am. J. Pathol. 3:93-110, 1927.

57 Steck, W. D., and Helwig, E. B.: Cutaneous endometriosis, J.A.M.A. 191:167-170, 1965.

58 Teilum, G., and Madsen, V.: Endometriosis ovarii et peritonaei caused by hysterosalpingography (contribution to the pathogenesis of endometriosis), J. Obstet. Gynaecol. Br. Emp. 57:10-17, 1950.

59 Tornquist, B.: Endometriosis in vaginal, vulvar and perineal scars, Acta Obstet. Gynecol. Scand. 29:485-489, 1949.

60 Winkelman, J., and Robinson, R.: Adenocarcinoma of endometrium involving adenomyosis; report of an unusual case and review of the literature, Cancer 19:901-908, 1966.

Dysfunctional uterine bleeding and hyperplasia

61 Chamlian, L. D., and Taylor, H. B.: Endometrial hyperplasia in young women, Obstet. Gynecol. 36:659-666, 1970.

62 Gillam, J. S.: Study of the inadequate secretion phase endometrium, Fertil. Steril. **6**:18-36, 1955.

63 Gore, H., and Hertig, A. T.: Carcinoma in situ of the endometrium, Am. J. Obstet. Gynecol. **94**:134-155, 1966.

64 McElin, T. W., Bird, C. C., Reeves, B. D., and Scott, R. C.: Diagnostic dilation and curettage; a 20-year survey, Obstet. Gynecol. **33**:807-812, 1969.

65 McLennan, C. E.: Current concepts of prolonged or irregular endometrial shedding, Am. J. Obstet. Gynecol. **64**:988-998, 1952.

66 McLennan, C. E., and Rydell, A. H.: Extent of endometrial shedding during normal menstruation, Obstet. Gynecol. **26**:605-621, 1965.

67 Meyer, W. C., Malkasian, G. D., Dockerty, M. B., and Decker, D. G.: Postmenopausal bleeding from atrophic endometrium, Obstet. Gynecol. **38**:731-738, 1971.

68 Moszkowski, E., Woodruff, J. D., and Jones, G. E. S.: The inadequate luteal phase, Am. J. Obstet. Gynecol. **83**:363-372, 1962.

69 Noyes, R. W.: The underdeveloped secretory endometrium, Am. J. Obstet. Gynecol. **83**:363-372, 1962.

70 Pacheco, J. C., and Kempers, R. D.: Etiology of postmenopausal bleeding, Obstet. Gynecol. **32**:40-46, 1968.

71 Picoff, R. C., and Luginbuhl, W. H.: Fibrin in the endometrial stroma; its relation to uterine bleeding, Am. J. Obstet. Gynecol. **88**:642-646, 1964.

72 Sinykin, M. B., Goodlin, R. C., and Barr, M. M.: Irregular shedding of the endometrium, Am. J. Obstet. Gynecol. **71**:990-1000, 1956.

73 Steiner, G., Kistner, R. W., and Craig, J. M.: Histological effects of progestins on hyperplasia and carcinoma in situ of the endometrium—further observations, Metabolism **14**:356-386, 1965.

Tumors

Carcinoma

74 Badib, A. O., Kurohara, S. S., Vongtama, V. Y., Selim, M. A., and Webster, J. H.: Biologic behavior of adenoacanthoma of endometrium, Am. J. Obstet. Gynecol. **106**:205-209, 1970.

75 Baker, W. H., and Scully, R. E.: Case records of the Massachusetts General Hospital, N. Engl. J. Med. **267**:1311-1317, 1962.

76 Fechner, R. E.: Endometrium with pattern of mesonephroma; report of a case, Obstet. Gynecol. **31**:485-490, 1968.

77 Geisler, H. E., Huber, C. P., and Rogers, S.: Carcinoma of the endometrium in premenopausal women, Am. J. Obstet. Gynecol. **104**:657-663, 1969.

78 Gospel, C.: Ultrastructure of endometrial carcinoma; review of fourteen cases, Cancer **28**:745-754, 1971.

79 Grattarola, R.: Misdiagnosis of endometrial adenocarcinoma in young women with polycystic ovarian disease; report of a case with an endocrine study, Am. J. Obstet. Gynecol. **105**:498-502, 1969.

80 Gusberg, S. B., and Hall, R. E.: Precursors of corpus cancer. III. The appearance of cancer of the endometrium in estrogenically conditioned patients, Obstet. Gynecol. **17**:397-412 1961.

81 Hameed, K., and Morgan, D. A.: Papillary adenocarcinoma of endometrium with psammoma bodies, Cancer **29**:1326-1335, 1972.

82 Hertig, A. T., and Sommers, S. C.: Genesis of endometrial carcinoma. I. Study of prior biopsies, Cancer **2**:946-956, 1949.

83 Hopkin, I. D., Harlow, R. A., and Stevens, P. J.: Squamous carcinoma of the body of the uterus, Br. J. Cancer **24**:71-76, 1970.

84 Isaacson, P. G., Pilot, L. M. J. R., and Gooselaw, J. G.: Foam cells in the stroma in carcinoma of the endometrium, Obstet. Gynecol. **23**:9-11, 1964.

85 Kaufman, R. H., Abbott, J. P., and Wall, J. A.: The endometrium before and after wedge resection of the ovaries in the Stein-Leventhal syndrome, Am. J. Obstet. Gynecol. **77**:1271-1285, 1959.

86 Kay, S.: Clear-cell carcinoma of the endometrium, Cancer **10**:124-130, 1957.

87 Kempson, R. L., and Pokorny, G. E.: Adenocarcinoma of the endometrium in women aged forty and younger, Cancer **21**:650-662, 1968.

88 Lynch, H. T., Krush, A. J., and Larsen, A. L.: Endometrial carcinoma; multiple primary malignancies, constitutional factors and heredity, Am. J. Med. Sci. **252**:381-390, 1966.

89 Moss, W. T.: Common peculiarities of patients with adenocarcinoma of the endometrium; with special reference to obesity, body build, diabetes, and hypertension, Am. J. Roentgenol. Radium Ther. Nucl. Med. **58**:203-210, 1947.

90 Ng, A. B. P.: Mixed carcinoma of the endometrium, Am. J. Obstet. Gynecol. **102**:506-515, 1968.

91 Ng, A. B. P., and Reagan, J. W.: Incidence and prognosis of endometrial carcinoma by histologic grade and extent, Obstet. Gynecol. **35**:437-443, 1970.

92 Rutledge, F., Kotz, H. L., and Chang, S. C.: Mesonephric adenocarcinoma of the endometrium; report of a case and a review of the literature, Obstet. Gynecol. **25**:362-370, 1965.

93 Salm, R.: Mucin production of abnormal endometrium, Arch. Pathol. **73**:30-39, 1962.

94 Schultz, A. E., Peckham, B. M., Herzog, P. A., and Kiekhofer, W.: Isolated vaginal cuff

recurrence following therapy of endometrial adenocarcinoma, Am. J. Obstet. Gynecol. **104:** 679-686, 1969.

95 Silverberg, S. G., and DeGiorgi, L. S.: Clear cell carcinoma of the endometrium, Cancer **31:**1127-1140, 1973.

96 Smith, J. P., Rutledge, F., and Soffar, S. W.: Progestins in the treatment of patients with endometrial adenocarcinoma, Am. J. Obstet. Gynecol. **94:**977-984, 1966.

97 Sorvari, T. E.: A histochemical study of epithelial muco-substances in endometrial and cervical adenocarcinomas; with reference to normal endometrium and cervical mucosa, Acta Pathol. Microbiol. Scand. **207**(suppl.): 56-60, 1969.

Endometrial stromal tumors

98 Gerber, M. A., and Toker, C.: Primary extrauterine endometrial stromal sarcoma, Arch. Pathol. **89:**477-480, 1970.

99 Hunter, W. C.: Benign and malignant (sarcoma) stromal endometriosis, Surgery **34:**258-278, 1953.

100 Hunter, W. C.: Uterine stromal endometriosis (stromatosis), Am. J. Obstet. Gynecol. **83:** 1564-1573, 1962.

101 Kempson, R. L., and Bari, W.: Uterine sarcomas; classification, diagnosis, and prognosis, Hum. Pathol. **1:**331-349, 1970.

102 Norris, H. J., and Taylor, H. B.: Mesenchymal tumors of the uterus. I. A clinical and pathological study of 53 endometrial stromal tumors, Cancer **19:**755-766, 1966.

103 Ober, W. B., and Jason, R. S.: Sarcoma of the endometrial stroma, Arch. Pathol. **56:** 301-311, 1953.

104 Silverberg, S. G., Willson, M. A., and Board, J. A.: Hemangiopericytoma of the uterus; an ultrastructural study, Am. J. Obstet. Gynecol. **110:**397-404, 1971.

105 Symmonds, R. E., Dockerty, M. B., and Pratt, J. H.: Sarcoma and sarcoma-like proliferations of the endometrial stroma. III. Stromal hyperplasia and stromatosis (stromal endometriosis), Am. J. Obstet. Gynecol. **73:** 1054-1069, 1957.

Malignant mixed müllerian tumors (mixed mesodermal tumors)

106 Chuang, J. T., Van Velden, D. J. J., and Graham, J. B.: Carcinosarcoma and mixed mesodermal tumor of the uterine corpus; review of 49 cases, Obstet. Gynecol. **35:**769-780, 1970.

107 Clark, W. H., Jr., Sternberg, W. H., and Smith, R. C.: Histogenesis of malignant mixed tumors of müllerian origin (mixed mesodermal tumor of the uterus), Am. J. Pathol. **28:**563, 1952.

108 Kempson, R. L., and Bari, W.: Uterine sarcomas; classification, diagnosis, and prognosis, Hum. Pathol. **1:**331-349, 1970.

109 Norris, H. J., and Taylor, H. B.: Postirradiation sarcomas of the uterus, Obstet. Gynecol. **26:**689-694, 1965.

110 Norris, H. J., and Taylor, H. B.: Mesenchymal tumors of the uterus. III. A clinical and pathologic study of 31 carcinosarcomas, Cancer **19:**1459-1465, 1966.

111 Norris, H. J., Roth, E., and Taylor, H. B.: Mesenchymal tumors of the uterus. II. A clinical and pathologic study of 31 mixed mesodermal tumors, Obstet. Gynecol. **28:**57-63, 1966.

112 Palladino, V. S., and Trousdell, M.: Extrauterine müllerian tumors; a review of the literature and the report of a case, Cancer **23:**1413-1422, 1969.

113 Schaepman-van Geuns, E. J.: Mixed tumors and carcinosarcomas of the uterus evaluated five years after treatment, Cancer **25:**72-77, 1970.

114 Sternberg, W. H., Clark, W. H., and Smith, R. C.: Malignant mixed müllerian tumor (mixed mesodermal tumor of the uterus); study of 21 cases, Cancer **7:**704-724, 1954.

115 Thomas, W. O., Jr., Harris, H. H., and Enden, J. A.: Postirradiation malignant neoplasms of the uterine fundus, Am. J. Obstet. Gynecol. **104:**209-219, 1969.

Metastatic tumors

116 Stemmermann, G. N.: Extrapelvic carcinoma metastatic to the uterus, Am. J. Obstet. Gynecol. **82:**1261-1266, 1961.

Uterus—myometrium

Leiomyoma
Leiomyosarcoma
Other lesions

Leiomyoma

Leiomyomas of the uterus are extremely common neoplasms. About 40% of women over the age of 50 years have one or more of them. The incidence in the general female population varies between 4% and 11%. They are much more common in blacks, in whom they have a tendency to be large in number (Fig. 811). These tumors occur subserosally, intramurally, or directly beneath the endometrium (Figs. 811 to 813) and produce symptoms referable to their size and location. They may become large enough to block the ureters, interfere with pregnancy, or cause inflammatory complications.

Submucosal tumors often result in secondary endometrial changes that range from gland distortion to atrophy and ulceration. These neoplasms may fill the endometrial cavity and emerge from the cervical canal as polypoid growths (Fig. 814). Under these circumstances, their surface is usually ulcerated and infected, the gross appearance thus simulating that of a malignant neoplasm.

We often have difficulty in making a diagnosis of leiomyoma when only a few small fragments of smooth muscle are present in a curettage specimen. Unless these fragments show an obvious increase in cellularity or definite hyaline changes, we are unable in most instances to decide whether they originated in a submucosal leiomyoma or whether they represent normal superficial myometrium curetted out by a vigorous operator. In rare instances, uterine leiomyomas have been associated with polycythemia, which regressed after the tumor was excised.[4]

The cut surface of a typical leiomyoma has a raw silk appearance. In approximately 65% of the cases, secondary changes occur. These include hyaline degeneration (63%), mucoid or myxomatous degeneration (19%), calcification (8%), cystic changes (4%), fatty metamorphosis (3%), and red degeneration (3%).[5] There is no relationship between symptomatology and the presence of secondary changes, except in the case of red degeneration. The latter, which is often associated with pregnancy, can result in abdominal pain, vomiting, and fever.

Rarely, leiomyomas become separated from the uterus and acquire vascular connections with the omentum; they are designated as parasitic. We have seen one

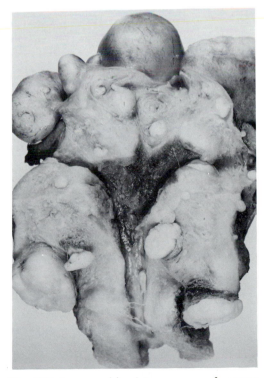

Fig. 811 Innumerable leiomyomas of uterus. (WU neg. 50-1877.)

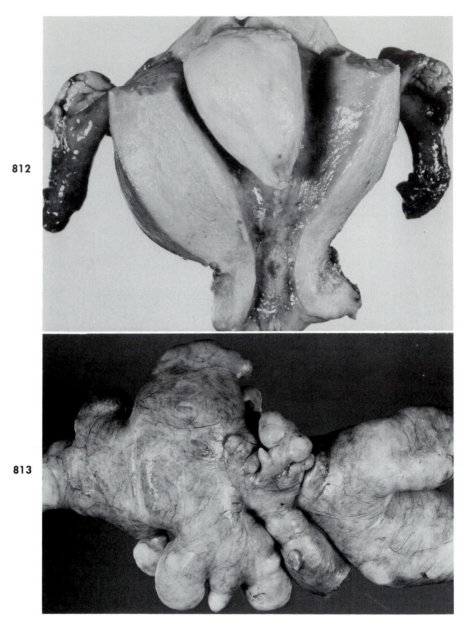

Fig. 812 Single leiomyoma growing within endometrial cavity and causing prominent signs and symptoms because of its location. (WU neg. 49-4651.)

Fig. 813 Huge leiomyoma weighing over 1,500 gm growing mainly within peritoneal cavity. (WU neg. 50-3396.)

attached to the cecum that was mistaken for carcinoma of the cecum.

Microscopically, leiomyomas are formed by interlacing bundles of smooth muscle cells separated by a greater or lesser amount of connective tissue and are usually well vascularized. The term *cellular* *leiomyoma* is reserved for those tumors having increased cellularity but no atypical features nor an excessive number of mitotic figures. Their natural history seems to be the same as for the ordinary leiomyoma. Tumors having bizarre tumor cells with variation in size and shape, hyperchromatic

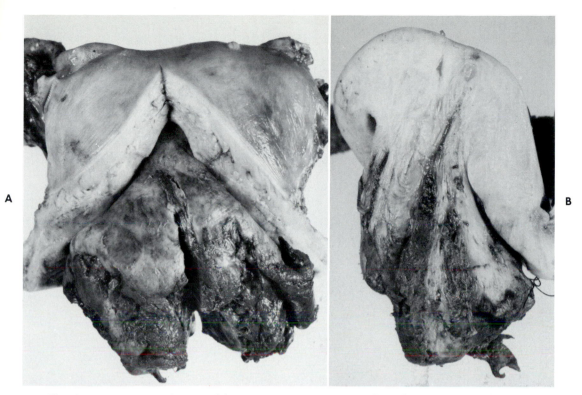

Fig. 814 **A,** Large submucosal leiomyoma presenting as polypoid mass in cervical canal and upper vagina. Note necrotic ulcerated surface. **B,** Gross section shows that tumor is implanted in fundus and has, in deep portion, typical appearance of leiomyoma. (**A,** WU neg. 71-10979; **B,** WU neg. 71-10980.)

nuclei, and multinucleated forms, but no increased mitotic activity, are designated as *atypical leiomyomas* (Fig. 815). They may occur spontaneously but are often seen in patients taking progestin compounds.[2, 6] Rywlin et al.[7] have described uterine leiomyomas partially or totally composed of clear cells, thus approaching the morphology of the leiomyoblastomas of the gastrointestinal tract. Infrequently, leiomyomas have an admixture of mature adipose tissue; they are designated as *leiomyolipomas.* Pure *lipomas* of the myometrium are exceptional.[3]

Most asymptomatic leiomyomas need not be excised. Malignant transformation, if it happens at all, is such a rare event in these tumors that it should not be considered in this regard. Symptomatic neoplasms can be treated by hysterectomy or, in the case of patients who desire to have children, by myomectomy.[1]

Leiomyosarcoma

The time-honored assumption that most leiomyosarcomas arise from preexisting leiomyomas has never been proved. The fact that 67% of the leiomyosarcomas are solitary militates against this possibility.[12] Some leiomyosarcomas are grossly indistinguishable from ordinary leiomyomas, but the majority are soft or fleshy, with necrotic or hemorrhagic areas (Fig. 816).[9] The most important microscopic criterion in the differentiation between uterine leiomyomas and leiomyosarcomas *is the number of mitotic figures.* Tumors with fewer than five mitoses per high-power field ($\times 675$) in the most active areas behave practically always as benign tumors, even in the presence of atypical cells, hyperchromatic nuclei, and multinucleated forms (Fig. 815). Tumors with ten or more mitoses per high-power field behave as malignant neoplasms, regardless of how bland their

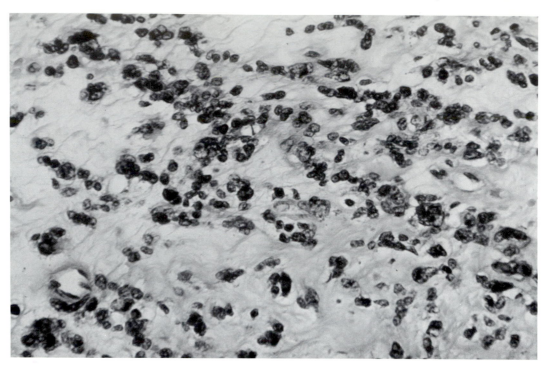

Fig. 815 Atypical uterine leiomyoma in 54-year-old patient. Note large hyperchromatic nuclei and numerous multinucleated cells. However, mitotic figures were not identified. (WU neg. 71-8659.)

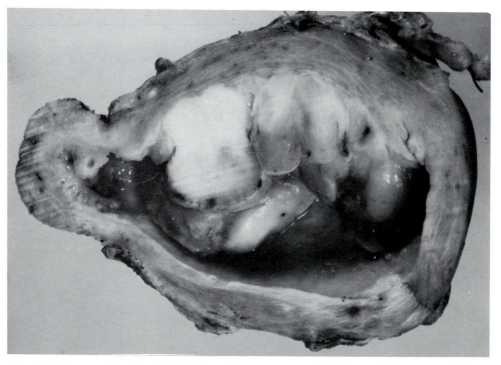

Fig. 816 Large polypoid soft bleeding leiomyosarcoma in 69-year-old woman. Patient died two years later with metastatic disease. (WU neg. 65-4311.)

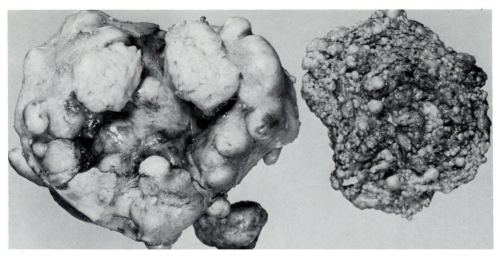

Fig. 817 Multiple leiomyomas of uterus and omentum. This is an example of condition known as leiomyomatosis peritonealis disseminata. Patient was 45 years old at time of operation. She remains well twenty years later. (WU neg. 52-3541; specimen contributed by Dr. J. Hobbs, St. Louis, Mo.)

microscopic appearance may be otherwise. The behavior of tumors having from five to nine mitoses per high-power field is less certain, but a certain number will metastasize.[10] Fortunately, only a small minority of uterine smooth muscle tumors belong to this gray zone. Exceptions to this rule sometimes occur. Occasional tumors have been reported to produce distant metastases in the presence of few or no mitotic figures.[11]

Extension outside the confines of the uterus is a finding of ominous prognosis in leiomyosarcoma. Of twenty patients studied by Bartsich et al.[8] in whom this occurred, no survivors were recorded beyond twenty-nine months.

Other lesions

Intravenous leiomyomatosis is an extremely rare condition characterized by the growth of mature smooth muscle inside the lumen of uterine and pelvic veins.[13] It is often associated with typical uterine leiomyomas. The clinical and gross features are quite similar to those of endolymphatic stromal myosis (discussed previously in this chapter under Uterus—endometrium). The distinction is microscopic—

intravenous leiomyomatosis is composed of elongated smooth muscle cells, whereas the former condition is made up of round or oval endometrial stromal cells. The vessel permeation can proceed along the vena cava and even reach the right atrium. However, distant metastases have not been reported in this disease.

Leiomyomatosis peritonealis disseminata is a rare benign condition in which typical uterine leiomyomas are associated with multiple small nodules of mature smooth muscle distributed throughout the omentum and both visceral and parietal layers of the peritoneum (Fig. 817). Taubert et al.[15] reported three cases of this phenomenon, which could be easily confused with metastatic leiomyosarcoma. An eliciting hormonal factor was suggested by the fact that two of their three patients were pregnant.

Rarely, *adenomatoid tumors* identical to those more commonly seen in the fallopian tube are found in the uterine wall, usually beneath the serosa and close to the cornua. They are often accompanied by smooth muscle hypertrophy and can be confused with leiomyomas.[16]

Arteriovenous fistula in the wall of the uterus may produce large pulsating masses.

The vascular connections are demonstrated by angiography.[14]

REFERENCES

Leiomyoma

1 Brown, J. M., Malkasian, G. D., Jr., and Symmonds, R. E.: Abdominal myomectomy, Am. J. Obstet. Gynecol. **99:**126-129, 1967.

2 Fechner, R. E.: Atypical leiomyomas and synthetic progestin therapy, Am. J. Clin. Pathol. **49:**697-703, 1968.

3 Jacobs, D. S., Cohen, H., and Johnson, J. S.: Lipoleiomyomas of the uterus, Am. J. Clin. Pathol. **44:**45-51, 1965.

4 Nedwich, A., Frumin, A., and Meranze, D. R.: Erythrocytosis associated with uterine myomas, Am. J. Obstet. Gynecol. **84:**174-178, 1962.

5 Persaud, V., and Arjoon, P. D.: Uterine leiomyoma; incidence of degenerative change and a correlation of associated symptoms, Obstet. Gynecol. **35:**432-436, 1970.

6 Prakash, S., and Scully, R. E.: Sarcoma-like pseudopregnancy; changes in uterine leiomyomas; report of a case resulting from prolonged norethindrone therapy, Obstet. Gynecol. **24:** 106-110, 1964.

7 Rywlin, A. M., Recher, L., and Benson, J.: Clear cell leiomyoma of the uterus; report of 2 cases of a previously underscribed entity, Cancer **17:**100-104, 1964.

Leiomyosarcoma

8 Bartsich, E. G., Bowe, E. T., and Moore, J. G.: Leiomyosarcoma of the uterus; a 50-year review of 42 cases, Obstet. Gynecol. **32:** 101-106, 1968.

9 Christopherson, W. M., Williamson, E. O., and Gray, L. A.: Leiomyosarcoma of the uterus, Cancer **29:**70-75, 1972.

10 Kempson, R. L., and Bari, W.: Uterine sarcomas; classification, diagnosis, and prognosis, Hum. Pathol. **1:**331-349, 1970.

11 Spiro, R. H., and McPeak, C. J.: On the so-called metastasizing leiomyoma, Cancer **19:** 544-548, 1966.

12 Taylor, H. B., and Norris, H. J.: Mesenchymal tumors of the uterus. IV. Diagnosis and prognosis of leiomyosarcomas, Arch. Pathol. **82:** 40-44, 1966.

Other lesions

13 Harper, R. S., and Scully, R. E.: Intravenous leiomyomatosis of the uterus, Am. J. Clin. Pathol. **4:**45-51, 1965.

14 Liggins, G. C.: Uterine arteriovenous fistula, Obstet. Gynecol. **23:**214-217, 1964.

15 Taubert, H.-D., Wissner, S. E., and Haskins, A. L.: Leiomyomatosis peritonealis disseminata; an unusual complication of genital leiomyomata, Obstet. Gynecol. **25:**561-574, 1965.

16 Youngs, L. A., and Taylor, H. B.: Adenomatoid tumors of the uterus and fallopian tube, Am. J. Clin. Pathol. **48:**537-545, 1967.

Fallopian tubes

Infection
Metaplasias and nonneoplastic nodules
Pregnancy
Carcinoma
Other lesions

Infection

Bacterial infection of the fallopian tubes is a common disease which causes luminal obliteration by progressive destruction of epithelium. Microscopically, there is acute and chronic inflammation with fusion of the tubal plicae. The ostium becomes obliterated. Collections of secretions or pus distend the tube (Fig. 818). The trapped epithelial spaces produce a gland-like pattern (Fig. 819). Tubo-ovarian abscesses obliterate the pelvic anatomic relationships. The most common agents recovered from these abscesses are *coliform* organisms. *Neisseria gonorrhoeae* was isolated only once in a series of ninety-three patients studied by Mickal et al.,[18] although this finding does not rule out its role as a possible initiating factor.

Hydrosalpinx is generally regarded as the end-stage of a purulent salpingitis in which pus has been reabsorbed and replaced by a transudate of plasma.[4] The wall is thin and fibrotic, with atrophy or even disappearance of the smooth muscle wall. The epithelium is flat and focally absent. The rupture of a tubo-ovarian abscess is an emergency that requires prompt surgical intervention.[18, 21] It should be remembered that at the time of menstruation, as well as a few days postpartum, the tube may be *normally* infiltrated by neutrophils. This is probably a reaction to blood and necrotic debris. It is accompanied by negative cultures and, therefore, should not be confused with a bacterial salpingitis.[20, 23]

Tuberculous tubal infection is hematogenous. Both tubes frequently are replaced by caseous tuberculous masses that may be mistaken for cancer both grossly and microscopically. There is often extreme adenomatous proliferation of the tubal mucosa in association with the mucosal tuberculosis (Fig. 820). Most patients with pelvic tuberculosis are young. Infertility is common.[8, 13]

We have seen *granulomatous inflammation* of the tubes produced by *Schistosoma* and by *Oxyuris vermicularis*. Foreign bodies introduced for diagnostic or therapeutic measures can induce a bizarre granulomatous response.

Reaction to Lipiodol following the Rubin test may be so proliferative that it resembles neoplasm. The push of a uterine sound may drive lubricant into the tube, causing *lipoid granulomas*.[6]

Metaplasias and nonneoplastic nodules

Pelvic endometriosis frequently involves the tube. The most common manifestation is the focal replacement of tubal epithelium by uterine mucosa.[24] The ectopic endometrium can also involve the wall in a typical fashion or present as nodular formations on the tubal serosa.[28]

Walthard cell nests are small glistening round collections of serosal cells on the tubal serosa. They probably are the result of focal serosal hyperplasia or metaplasia.[29] They should not be mistaken for serosal implants in patients with ovarian neoplasms.

Salpingitis isthmica nodosa is usually a bilateral lesion. The tubes show a well-delimited whitish nodular enlargement of the isthmic portion. Microscopically, there is an outpouching of the tubal mucosa and focal myohypertrophy (Fig. 821). Sections

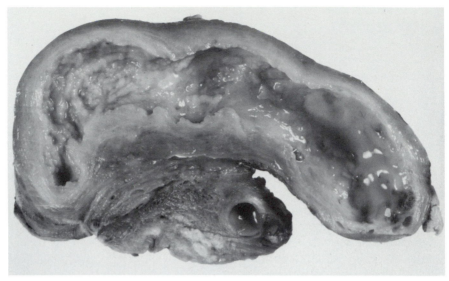

Fig. 818 Large dilated fallopian tube with shaggy lining and thick scarred wall, end result of chronic inflammation. (WU neg. 64-2680.)

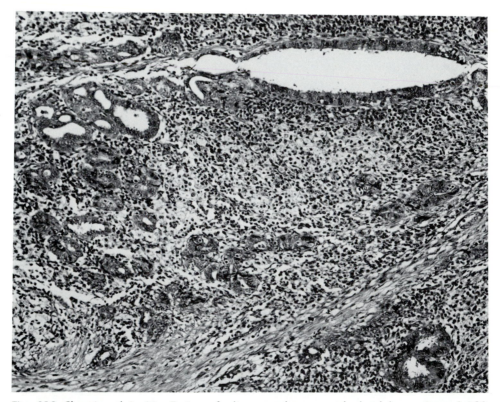

Fig. 819 Chronic salpingitis. Fusion of plicae produces pseudoglandular pattern. (×130; WU neg. 63-7315.)

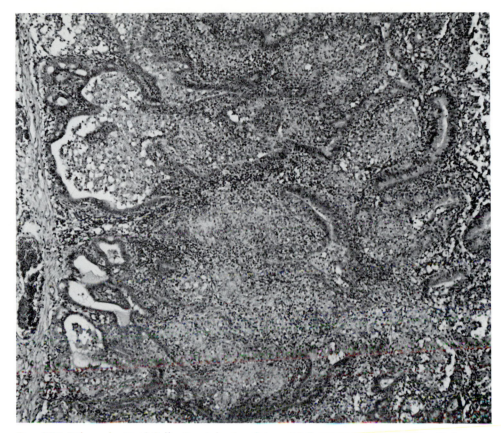

Fig. 820 Tuberculosis of fallopian tube involving chiefly mucosal layers. Glands become hyperplastic, and their borders may be indistinct as result of inflammatory reaction in which characteristic tubercles are often inconspicuous. (×85; WU neg. 62-8859.)

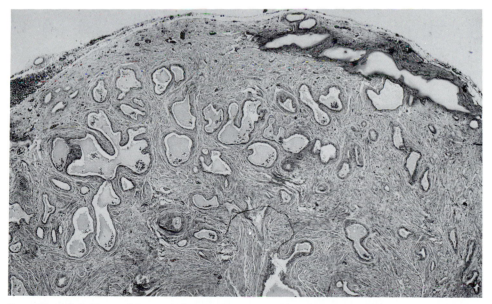

Fig. 821 Salpingitis isthmica nodosa with outpouching of tubal mucosa and prominent myohypertrophy. (×250; WU negs. 58-2715 and 58-2716.)

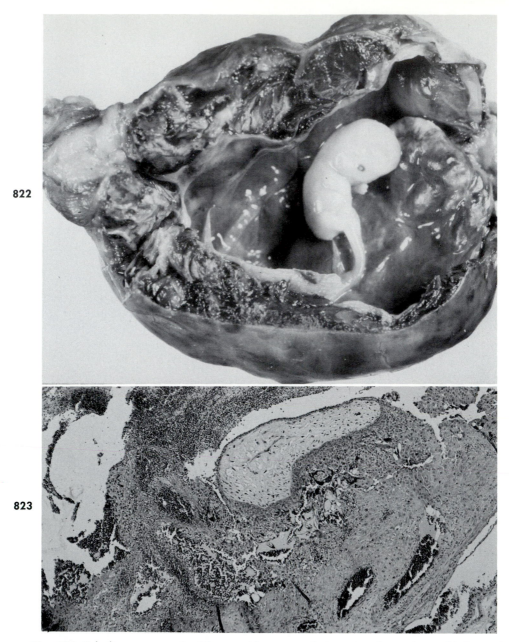

Fig. 822 Tubal pregnancy in 34-year-old woman that ruptured at about third month. (WU neg. 63-199.)

Fig. 823 Implantation site of placenta in fallopian tube. Chorionic villus can be seen. Placenta is firmly attached to edematous wall of tube, which was filled with blood. (Low power; WU neg. 52-194.)

of the wall show isolated glands surrounded by muscle. However, if Thorotrast is given under pressure, with x-ray and reconstruction, these tubal spaces are seen to be connected to the lumen of the tube.[25] This lesion generally has been considered to be the result of inflammation. Benjamin and Beaver[1] have presented a convincing argument for a pathogenesis analogous to that of adenomyosis. Approximately one-half of the patients affected by this disease are infertile.

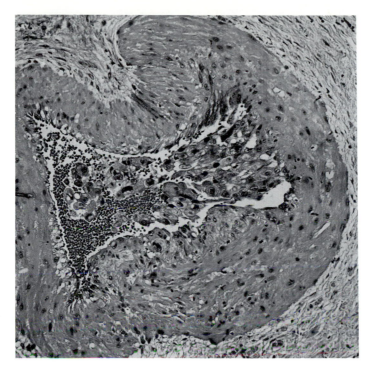

Fig. 824 Trophoblastic vascular invasion in tubal pregnancy, common finding of no clinical significance. (×130; WU neg. 67-796A.)

Endosalpingiosis refers to the presence of tubal epithelium outside the tube proper, a process somewhat analogous to endometriosis. The most common location is the ovarian surface close to the fimbria, suggesting that it may be secondary to inflammatory adhesions and overgrowth of tubal epithelium. Burmeister et al.[3] have reported two cases in the pelvic peritoneum.

Pregnancy

The development of tubal pregnancy follows chronic inflammation. Because of inflammatory destruction and fibrosis of lining folds, the ovum is retained. Congenital abnormalities may be responsible also for retention of the ovum. The curettings from the enlarged uterus in the presence of a viable tubal pregnancy show decidual cells without chorionic villi, sometimes associated with the Arias-Stella reaction. If these changes are associated with a tubal mass, a presumptive diagnosis of tubal pregnancy is justified, and operation is indicated. On the other hand, death of the embryo or fetus often results in expulsion of the decidual cast, regeneration of the epithelium, and reestablishment of the cyclic pattern. Therefore, the presence of a proliferative, secretory, or menstrual endometrium in a patient with an adnexal mass *does not* rule out the possibility of an ectopic pregnancy. With implantation of the placenta in the tube, the chorionic villi penetrate deeply in the wall.

A tubal pregnancy terminates in several ways. Rupture may occur near the end of the second month due to the destruction of the wall of the tube by trophoblast, resulting in severe intra-abdominal hemorrhage. Abortion is the common method of termination. The maternal vessels rupture into the gestation sac and cause hematosalpinx (Figs. 822 and 823).

Blaustein and Shenker[2] have demonstrated changes resembling atherosclerosis in tubal arteries at the place of implantation. These changes are analogous to those seen in the uterine vessels following normal implantation.

In the presence of a large hematosalpinx, it may be quite difficult to identify the products of gestation. Numerous blocks from the intratubal blood clot should be taken. Trophoblastic invasion of muscle and vessels is a common and expected finding of no clinical significance (Fig. 824).

A few cases have been reported in which tubal pregnancies went to term. It is possible to conserve the ovary at operation in 80% of the patients.

Carcinoma

Carcinoma may invade the fallopian tube by direct extension from the endometrium or ovary or can involve it through lymphatic channels. The neoplasm most commonly involving the fallopian tube secondarily is ovarian carcinoma.[14]

Primary carcinoma of the fallopian tube is rare.[27] Approximately eighty cases have been reported. Infection is secondary and not causally related. Tubal carcinoma is rarely bilateral, and usually the contralateral tube is normal.[7] The classical triad of the disease, present in approximately 50% of the patients, includes pain, vaginal discharge, and a palpable adnexal mass. In our experience, vaginal cytologic examination has been of no value for the diagnosis.[16] Grossly, the tube is always enlarged. The external appearance may be indistinguishable from that of chronic salpingitis. Fibrous adhesions are invariably found. On cross section, a solid or papillary tumor is seen filling the lumen (Fig. 825, A). Microscopically, the tumor is usually an adenocarcinoma, with or without papillary formations. Undifferentiated variants are rare (Fig. 825, B).

In most reported series, the prognosis has been poor. In the series of twenty-seven patients reported by Hanton et al.[12] the five-year survival rate was 44%. The lesions of all five of the survivors studied by Green and Scully[10] were confined to a tube with fimbriated end sealed by previous inflammatory disease. In our experience the prognosis has been remarkably good.[19] Involvement of tubal serosa, ovary, or corpus uteri

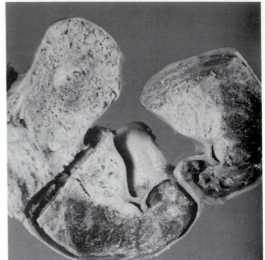

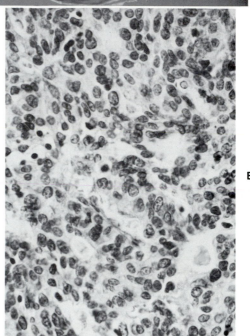

Fig. 825 **A,** Carcinoma of fallopian tube with extensive replacement of organ. Uterus and ovaries were normal. **B,** Same tumor shown in **A.** It is poorly differentiated adenocarcinoma. (**A,** WU neg. 50-1684; **B,** ×400; WU neg. 52-3600.)

or of other pelvic and abdominal structures is a sign of poor prognosis.[26]

The criteria for the diagnosis of primary carcinoma of the fallopian tube should be highly critical. They have been well outlined by Finn and Javert.[7] The uterus and ovaries should be either grossly normal or affected by a lesion other than cancer. By convention, a cancer extensively involving both endometrium and tube is classified as a uterine tumor, and one involving both ovary and tube is regarded as an ovarian neoplasm. Microscopically, if the endometrium and/or ovaries contain a malignant lesion, this should appear metastatic by its small size, distribution, and microscopic characteristics.

gross and microscopic features are identical to those of adenomatoid tumors of the epididymis (Chapter 17). Contrasting theories of histogenesis have been reviewed by Jackson.[15] A mesothelial origin is presently favored.[17] These tumors should never be confused with carcinoma. The presence of an infiltrating margin is not evidence of aggressive behavior.[31]

Other rare tumors include *cystic teratoma*[9] (Fig. 826), *leiomyoma, hemangio-*

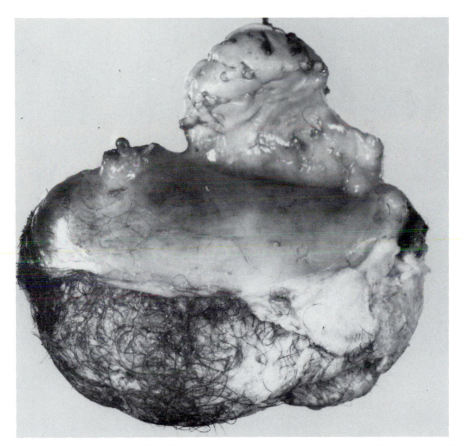

Fig. 826 Benign teratoma of fallopian tube in 41-year-old woman. (WU neg. 66-4385.)

Foci of epithelial atypia may appear in the fallopian tube in cases of ovarian tumors.[30] We have seen them most commonly associated with serous neoplasms.

Other lesions

Adenomatoid tumors are benign neoplasms that rarely arise on the tube or beneath the uterine serosa near a cornua. The

ma, malignant mixed müllerian tumor[5] (Fig. 827), *leiomyosarcoma,* and *primary trophoblastic tumors.*[22]

Torsion of the fallopian tube is usually secondary to inflammation or tumor, but occasionally it occurs in a previously normal organ. The latter presents grossly as a hemorrhagic infarct and occurs most often in the reproductive years.[11]

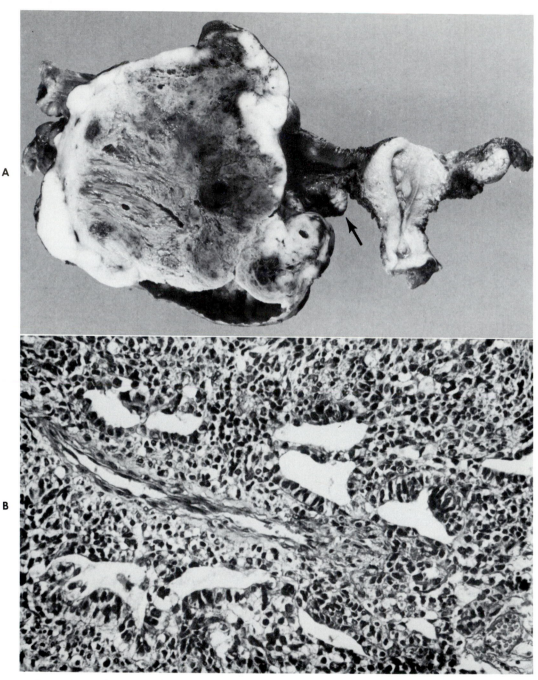

Fig. 827 Malignant mixed müllerian mesodermal tumor of fallopian tube. **A,** Large tumor, partially necrotic and hemorrhagic, totally obliterates salpinx. Ovary is not involved (arrow). **B,** Photomicrograph showing areas of adenocarcinoma and undifferentiated stromal sarcoma. There were also areas of osteosarcoma. (**A** and **B,** Courtesy Dr. H. Rodriguez, Mexico City, Mexico.)

REFERENCES

1 Benjamin, C. L., and Beaver, D. C.: Pathogenesis of salpingitis isthmica nodosa, Am. J. Clin. Pathol. **21**:212-222, 1951.

2 Blaustein, A., and Shenker, L.: Vascular lesions of the uterine tube in ectopic pregnancy, Obstet. Gynecol. **30**:551-555, 1967.

3 Burmeister, R. E., Fechner, R. E., and Franklin, R. R.: Endosalpingiosis of the peritoneum, Obstet. Gynecol. **34**:310-318, 1969.

4 David, A., Garcia, C.-S., and Czernobilsky, B.: Human hydrosalpinx; histologic study and chemical composition of fluid, Am. J. Obstet. Gynecol. **105**:400-411, 1969.

5 DeQueiroz, A. C., and Roth, L. M.: Malignant mixed müllerian tumor of the fallopian tube; report of a case, Obstet. Gynecol. **36**:554-557, 1970.

6 Elliott, G. B., Brody, H., and Elliott, K. A.: Implications of "lipoid salpingitis," Fertil. Steril. **16**:541-548, 1965.

7 Finn, W. F., and Javert, C. T.: Primary and metastatic cancer of the fallopian tube, Cancer **2**:803-814, 1949.

8 Francis, W. A. J.: Female genital tuberculosis; a review of 135 cases, J. Obstet. Gynaecol. Br. Commonw. **71**:418-428, 1964.

9 Gray, D. H., and Hitchcock, G. C.: Benign cystic teratoma of the fallopian tube, Br. J. Surg. **56**:475-476, 1969.

10 Green, T. H., and Scully, R. E.: Tumors of the fallopian tube, Clin. Obstet. Gynecol. **5**:886-906, 1962.

11 Hansen, O. H.: Isolated torsion of the fallopian tube, Acta Obstet. Gynecol. Scand. **49**:3-6, 1970.

12 Hanton, E. M., Malkasian, G. D., Jr., Dahlin, D. C., and Pratt, J. H.: Primary carcinoma of the fallopian tube, Am. J. Obstet. Gynecol. **94**:832-839, 1966.

13 Henderson, D. N., Harkins, J. L., and Stitt, J. F.: Pelvic tuberculosis, Am. J. Obstet. Gynecol. **94**:630-633, 1966.

14 Hertig, A. T., and Gore, H.: Tumors of the female sex organs. Part 3. Tumors of the ovary and fallopian tube. In Atlas of tumor pathology, Sect. IX, Fasc. 33, Washington, D. C., 1961, Armed Forces Institute of Pathology.

15 Jackson, J. R.: The histogenesis of the "adenomatoid" tumor of the genital tract, Cancer **11**:337-350, 1958.

16 Lehto, L.: Cytology of the human fallopian tube, Acta Obstet. Gynecol. Scand. **42**(suppl. 14):1-95, 1963.

17 Mackay, B., Bennington, J. L., and Skoglund, R. W.: The adenomatoid tumor: fine structural evidence for a mesothelial origin, Cancer **27**:109-115, 1971.

18 Mickal, A., Sellmann, A. H., and Beebe, J. L.: Ruptured tuboovarian abscess, Am. J. Obstet. Gynecol. **100**:432-436, 1968.

19 Momtazee, S., and Kempson, R. L.: Primary adenocarcinoma of the fallopian tube, Obstet. Gynecol. **32**:649-656, 1968.

20 Nassberg, S., McKay, D. G., and Hertig, A. T.: Physiologic salpingitis, Am. J. Obstet. Gynecol. **67**:130-137, 1954.

21 Pedowitz, R., and Bloomfield, R. D.: Ruptured adnexal abscess (tuboovarian) with generalized peritonitis, Am. J. Obstet. Gynecol. **88**:721-729, 1964.

22 Riggs, J. A., Wainer, A. S., Hahn, G. A., and Farell, M. D.: Extrauterine tubal choriocarcinoma, Am. J. Obstet. Gynecol. **88**:637-641, 1964.

23 Rubin, A., and Czernobilsky, B.: Tubal ligation; a bacteriologic, histologic and clinical study, Obstet. Gynecol. **36**:199-203, 1970.

24 Rubin, I. C., Lisa, J. R., and Trinidad, S.: Further observations of ectopic endometrium of fallopian tube, Surg. Gynecol. Obstet. **103**:469-474, 1956.

25 Schencken, J. R., and Burns, E. L.: A study and classification of nodular lesions of the fallopian tube, Am. J. Obstet. Gynecol. **45**:624-636, 1943.

26 Schiller, H. M., and Silverberg, S. G.: Staging and prognosis in primary carcinoma of the fallopian tube, Cancer **28**:389-395, 1971.

27 Sedlis, A.: Primary carcinoma of the fallopian tube, Obstet. Gynecol. Survey **16**:209-226, 1961.

28 Sheldon, R. S., Wilson, R. B., and Dockerty, M. B.: Serosal endometriosis of fallopian tubes, Am. J. Obstet. Gynecol. **99**:882-884, 1967.

29 Teoh, T. B.: The structure and development of Walthard nests, J. Pathol. Bacteriol. **66**:433-439, 1953.

30 Woodruff, J. D., and Pauerstein, C. J.: The fallopian tube; structure, function, pathology, and management, Baltimore, 1969, The Williams & Wilkins Co.

31 Youngs, L. A., and Taylor, H. B.: Adenomatoid tumors of the uterus and fallopian tube, Am. J. Clin. Pathol. **48**:537-545, 1967.

Ovary

Introduction

Ovarian diseases of surgical importance can be broadly divided into nonneoplastic cysts, inflammations, endometriosis, and neoplasms. Nonneoplastic cysts are unfortunately too commonly seen as surgical specimens. In Miller and Willson's series[2] of surgically removed ovarian masses measuring 5 cm or less in diameter, 97% were follicular or corpus luteum cysts. Of 461 small ovarian cysts, only 3% were neoplastic and only three cases were malignant. The symptoms associated with small cysts disappeared without excision in over 80% of the patients. Carpenter[1] analyzed 1,137 separate gynecologic specimens, 314 of which were ovarian. The high percentage without significant pathologic changes is indicated in Table 31. It has been said that if the ovaries were placed externally, their removal would be undertaken with more hesitation. The general surgeon exploring the abdomen may find a mildly cystic or nodular ovary in an otherwise normal abdominal cavity and remove it with the hope that a pathologic process will be found to justify the patient's symptoms and the operation. More often than not, the microscopic diagnosis will be that of "cystic follicle" or "mature corpus luteum," but it will be too late to replace the organ. The risk of carcinoma developing is much less than has been assumed. The common belief that ovarian substitutes will do almost everything for a woman except have her baby is false.[2]

Table 31 Analysis of 314 ovarian specimens*

Findings	Number	%
Follicular cyst	179	57.0 ⎫
Simple cyst	36	11.1 ⎬ —78.9
Corpus luteum cyst	33	10.8 ⎭
Chronic oophoritis	32	10.3
Hemorrhagic cyst	16	5.1
Pseudomucinous cyst	6	1.9
Serous cystadenoma	3	1.0
Carcinoma	2	0.6
Krukenberg tumor	2	0.6
Fibroma	2	0.6
Dermoid cyst	2	0.6
Granulosa cell tumor	1	0.3

*From Carpenter, C. C.: Consideration of physiology and pathology in gynecology; analysis of 2,933 surgical specimens, Trans. Med. Soc. North Carolina 83:236-242, 1936.

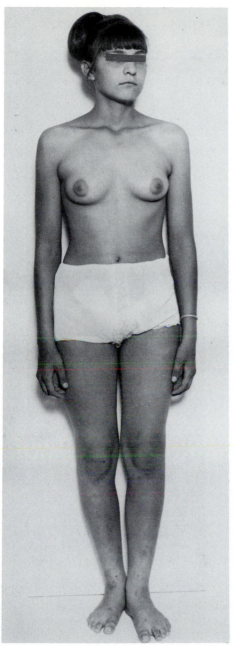

Fig. 828 Testicular feminization. Note female development of secondary sex characteristics and absence of axillary hair. Patient had no uterus and short vagina. There were testes in each inguinal area. (Courtesy Dr. W. J. Pepler, Pretoria, South Africa.)

Embryonal remnants

The vestigial mesonephros is represented by the wolffian body at the ovarian hilus.

Small ductlike structures are almost constant in this area between the fallopian tube and the ovary. The wolffian duct passes distally and medially along the lateral wall of the uterus, cervix, and vagina, where it is called Gartner's duct. Cystic dilatations of these duct remnants are called *hydatids of Morgagni* when they occur at the fimbriated end of the salpinx, *parovarian* and *paratubal cysts* in the tubovarian ligament, and *Gartner's duct cysts* in the vaginal wall.

Gonadal dysgenesis

Occasionally, gonadal tissue is biopsied in the course of evaluation of genital tract malformations. In patients with *gonadal dysgenesis, either "pure" or associated with the somatic features of Turner's syndrome,* both gonads are represented by a streak of fibrous tissue that vaguely resembles ovarian stroma.[5, 10] These patients do not seem to have an increased incidence of gonadal tumors.[11] In *mixed gonadal dysgenesis,* one gonad is represented by a streak and the other by a testis. Individuals with this condition are particularly prone to the development of gonadoblastomas.[7] The tumors may totally obliterate the testicular elements and thus lead to an incorrect typing of the dysgenesis. True hermaphrodites may have ovotestes containing both ova and immature seminiferous tubules or other combinations of ovary and testis.[3, 6]

The familial syndrome of *testicular feminization* is a type of male pseudohermaphroditism occurring in genetic males with well-develoved female secondary sex characteristics (Fig. 828). These patients consult a gynecologist because of amenorrhea or sterility. They prove to have a vagina, no uterus, and bilateral cryptorchid testes. The latter often contain nodular masses of immature tubules that should not be confused with arrhenoblastoma[4, 9] (Fig. 829). The syndrome is of further clinical importance because of the eventual occurrence of malignant tumors in the cryptorchid testes of about 9% of these pa-

Table 32 Disorders of sexual development*†

Syndrome	Gonad	Ducts	External genitalia	Puberty
Klinefelter's	Testis with hyalinized sclerotic tubules and clumped Leydig cells	Male	Male	Normal penis with small testes; pa[r]tial androgen lo[ss]
Turner's	Streak gonad with whorled stroma	Female	Female	No pubertal development; rare cases show mild viriliz[a]tion
True hermaphrodite	Ovary and testis	All have uterus, most have tubes too, a few have vasa	Ambiguous but 80% favor the male	80% have gynecomastia, 50% menstruate
Mixed gonadal dysgenesis	Streak plus testis or tumor	Female; vas found occasionally	Vary from female (often with clitoromegaly) to male with hypospadias to normal male	Virilization, sometimes complete; breast development only with tumors
Dysgenetic male pseudohermaphroditism	Dysgenetic testis	Mixed male and/or female	Variably virilized	Rarely patients m[ay] be fertile
Familial male pseudohermaphroditism—ranges from testicular feminization to	Immature infertile testis	No uterus, ± rudimentary vas	Female with short, blind vagina	Breasts develop b[ut] sexual hair is missing
Reifenstein's syndrome	Infertile testis	Male	Male with hypospadias, ± cleft scrotum	Androgen lack is e[vi]dent in incompl[ete] virilization
Female pseudohermaphroditism				
1. Congenital adrenal hyperplasia	Ovary	Female	Variably virilized	Amenorrhea with virilization
2. Nonadrenal	Ovary	Female	Variably virilized	Normal

*The summaries under the several headings are necessarily brief; the text should be consulted for details, qualifications, and cru[de]

†From Federman, D. D.: Abnormal sexual development; a genetic and endocrine approach to differential diagnosis, Philadelph[ia]

tients.[8] For this reason, the testes should be removed after puberty and supplemental estrogen therapy given.

The current classification of disorders of sexual development is presented in Table 32.

Nonneoplastic cysts and stromal hyperplasia

Follicular cysts of the ovary form by distention of developing atretic follicles. They may occur at any age from infancy to menopause and are asymptomatic in the majority of cases. Occasionally, twisting of the pedicle occurs with the resulting hemorrhagic infarct. In children, the cysts are rarely associated with precocious puberty. During reproductive life, they may be associated at times with endometrial hyperplasia and metrorrhagia.[20]

The cyst wall is lined by theca with or without an inner granulosa layer. The theca layer is frequently luteinized. The granulosa layer may be luteinized after puberty but not before. The cyst fluid may contain estrogenic hormone. Follicular cysts usually do not exceed 10 cm in diameter.

Barr	Chromosomes	Hormones			Remarks
		FSH	17-KS	Estrogen	
ue" are chromatin positive, a few are 2+ or 3+	All chromatin positive have 2 X's and a Y in at least some cells. Chromatin negative are 46/XY	↑ ↑	N or ↓	N	Affects 1:400 newborn males
% chromatin negative	2nd sex chromosome missing or abnormal in some or all of the cells	↑ ↑	↓	↓	1:7000 newborns, commoner in abortuses; short stature
% chromatin positive	~60% are 46/XX in blood cells only; Y present in most of the others	N	N	N	
romatin negative	Almost all are mosaics including XO stem; many have Y-bearing stem as well	↑	N	?	
romatin negative	Some are XO/XY	↑	N	?	
romatin negative	46/XY	↑ or N	↑ or N	N	Sex-linked recessive or sex-limited autosomal dominant
romatin negative	46/XY	↑ or N	↑ or N	?	
romatin positive	46/XX	N	↑ ↑	N	Autosomal recessive
romatin positive	46/XX	N	N	N	Consider maternal exposure to progestins or androgens

ceptions. ↑ = increased; ↑↑ = markedly increased; N = normal.
67, W. B. Saunders Co.

Polycystic ovaries are composed of multiple follicular cysts with varying degrees of luteinization of the theca interna. Ordinarily, such ovaries are enlarged and are covered by a dense fibrous capsule (Fig. 830). Various clinical syndromes may develop in patients with polycystic ovaries, including amenorrhea and sterility (Stein-Leventhal syndrome), metropathia hemorrhagica (with endometrial hyperplasia), and frank virilism. The clinical syndromes tend to overlap considerably, as do the actual pathologic findings.

The clinical, biochemical, and histologic findings of various authors have been reviewed by Goldzieher and Green.[14] In general, the ovaries of patients with the Stein-Leventhal syndrome tend to have multiple subcapsular cystic follicles each surrounded by a luteinized theca[17] (Figs. 830 and 831). Corpora lutea and albicantia are almost always absent. The latter should not be confused with residua of atretic follicles. We have seen more pronounced virilism associated with stromal hyperplasia and focal stromal luteinization (Fig. 832). The etiology of these strange syndromes is not known. Rarely, typical poly-

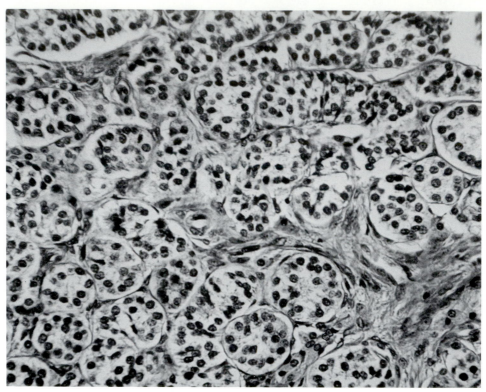

Fig. 829 Nodular masses of immature tubules in cryptorchid testis in patient with testicular feminization. Both testes were removed. Patient was given replacement therapy and is now a happily married housewife. (×340; WU neg. 67-527; slide contributed by Dr. D. W. Frazier, Jacksonville, Fla.)

cystic ovaries associated with the clinical features of the Stein-Leventhal syndrome have been found associated with (and perhaps the results of) congenital adrenal hyperplasia and ovarian neoplasms.[18, 26]

Most patients will respond favorably with restoration of the menstrual cycle after wedge resection of the ovary. Endometrial carcinoma has been reported as a late complication in a small percentage of patients with the Stein-Leventhal syndrome if restoration of the normal cycle is not effected.[16] If this indeed happens, it must be extremely rare. We have never seen such a complication in our institution. On the other hand, we have often seen patients with Stein-Leventhal syndrome in whom a florid endometrial hyperplasia was present, of a degree that could have been easily mistaken for carcinoma.

Stromal hyperplasia is usually seen in the absence of cysts. The stromal cells become plump and form nodular masses that encroach upon the medulla. Occasionally, small clusters of stromal lutein cells are encountered. The endocrine significance of these changes is debatable.

Cysts of the corpus luteum are single and usually less than 6 cm in diameter. They may develop at the end of the menstrual cycle or may occur in pregnancy (Fig. 833). The cyst wall is composed of a luteinized granulosa. The fluid content often is bloody. If the cyst ruptures, hemorrhage into the peritoneal cavity occurs, and an erroneous diagnosis of ruptured ectopic pregnancy may be made. The bleeding may be severe (500 ml or more).[15]

Ectopic decidual reaction in the absence of current or recent pregnancy can occur. In fourteen of sixteen patients reported by Ober et al.,[22] a functioning corpus luteum

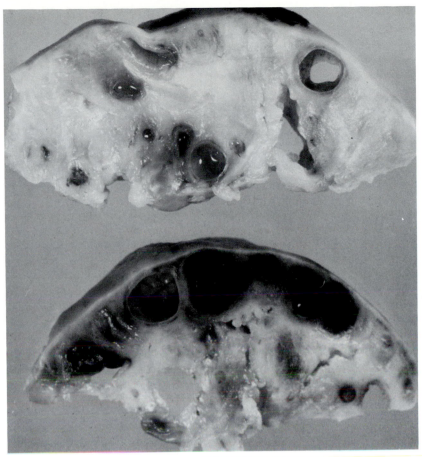

Fig. 830 Wedges of ovarian tissue resected from 21-year-old woman with Stein-Leventhal syndrome. Multiple cystic follicles, dense outer capsule, and abundant pale gray stroma are characteristic features. (WU neg. 62-8124.)

that had undergone destruction was present.

So-called *luteomas of pregnancy* are yellow or orange solid nodules that may reach sizable proportions (Fig. 834). They have been typically encountered during cesarean section in multiparous women. If left undisturbed, they will regress after delivery.[24] A mild degree of virilization was noted in four of the fifteen patients reported by Norris and Taylor.[21] Microscopically, the lesions are composed of masses of uniform theca-lutein cells (Fig. 835). All have been benign. It is reasonable to regard them as nodular hyperplasias of theca-lutein cells.[21] If pregnancy luteoma is correctly identified by frozen section biopsy, no further surgery is necessary.

Multiple theca-lutein cysts are common in cases of hydatidiform mole and choriocarcinoma but also have been seen in twin pregnancies and, exceptionally, in uncomplicated single pregnancies (Fig. 836).

The hili of 80% of adult human ovaries contain nests of cells morphologically identical to testicular Leydig cells.[23] Variations in the size of these nests occur at different ages. Larger clusters are found more frequently in older women.[13] Individual cells measure 14μ to 25μ in diameter and have a vesicular nucleus with acidophilic granular cytoplasm. The cytoplasm contains neutral lipids, a small amount of gold-brown lipochrome pigment, and may contain acidophilic rodlike structures known as crystalloids of Reinke. These

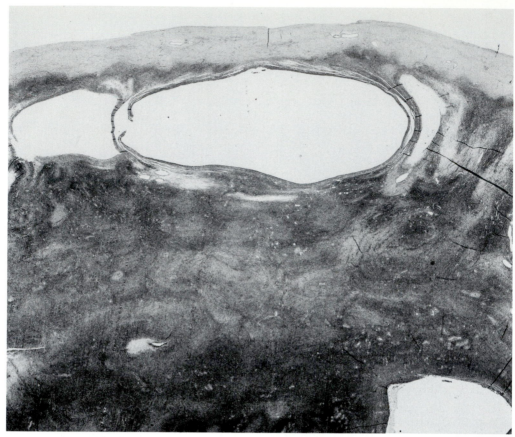

Fig. 831 Ovary from patient with Stein-Leventhal syndrome showing dense outer fibrous coat, multiple follicular cysts and atretic follicles, and abundant cortical stroma. Theca interna is well developed. (×15; WU neg. 63-3244; slide contributed by Dr. H. B. Taylor, St. Louis, Mo.)

cells probably secrete androgen. They have been called sympathicotropic cells by Berger[12] because of their intimate association with nerves. Hyperplasia or neoplasia of these cells results in the formation of nodular masses in or adjacent to the ovarian hilus (Fig. 837). They may cause masculinization and occasionally estrinism.[20] Such lesions are extremely rare. Sternberg[23] reported four instances of masculinization, two of which were due to hyperplasia and two to benign neoplasms of extraglandular Leydig cells. Furthermore, hyperplasia of these hilar cells is found following the administration of chorionic gonadotropin, in pregnancy, and in the presence of choriocarcinoma. Such occurrences are further evidence relating these cells to the Leydig cells of the testis.[25] Variations in the clinical features and microscopic patterns of hilus cell nests, hyperplasia, and neoplasms have been described by Merrill.[19]

Inflammation

Nonspecific inflammation of the ovary usually spreads from the endometrium and is practically always associated with tubal involvement. A large, loculated cystic mass filled with pus or secretion is often the end result, the ovarian stroma forming part of the cystic wall. Specific infections such as tuberculosis occur in the ovary. Invariably this is hematogenous in origin and often also involves tube and endometrium. In time, the infection may subside and leave a large tubal ovarian cystic mass.

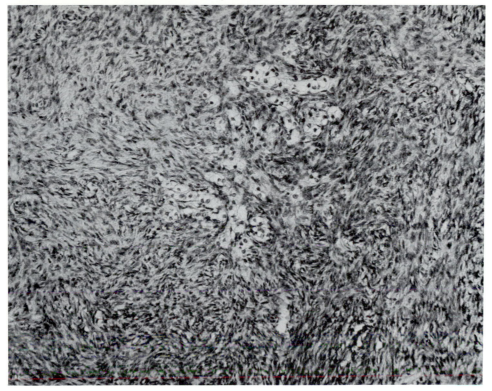

Fig. 832 Focal stromal luteinization and ovarian stromal hyperplasia associated with amenorrhea, hypertension, and virilization syndrome in 40-year-old woman. Ovaries were symmetrically enlarged and solid. There was no improvement following wedge resection. (×150; WU neg. 67-2404A.)

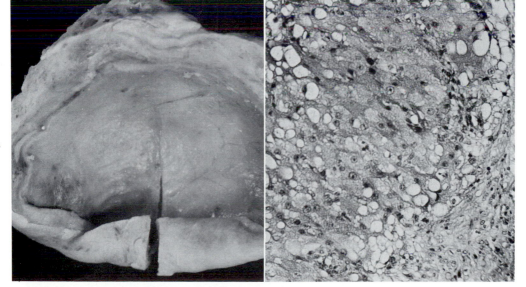

Fig. 833 A, Cyst of corpus luteum. Cyst was found at time of exploration for another condition, and surgeon incorrectly removed ovary. **B,** Wall of cyst shown in **A** composed of luteinized granulosa. (**A,** WU neg. 52-1978; **B,** ×170; WU neg. 52-2041.)

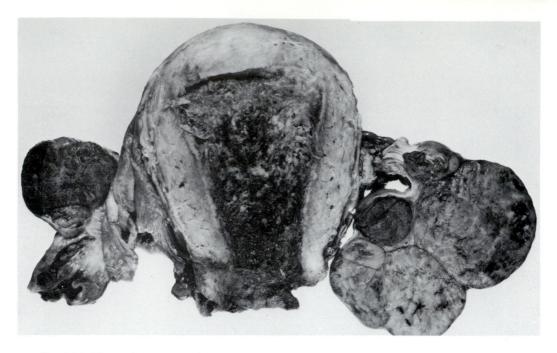

Fig. 834 Bilateral pregnancy luteomas in 29-year-old black woman that were discovered incidentally at time of cesarean section performed for cord prolapse. Tumors bled excessively on manipulation by surgeon and had to be removed. (WU neg. 73-8106.)

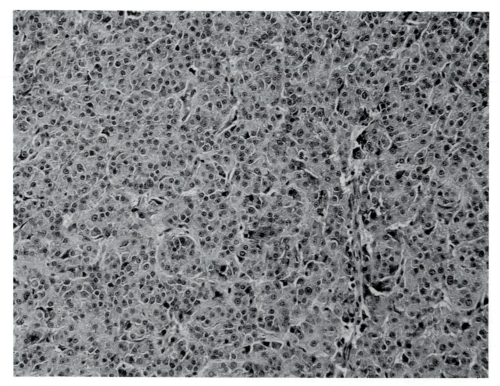

Fig. 835 Luteoma of pregnancy showing small clusters and masses of uniform luteinized theca cells. (×150; WU neg. 66-10346A.)

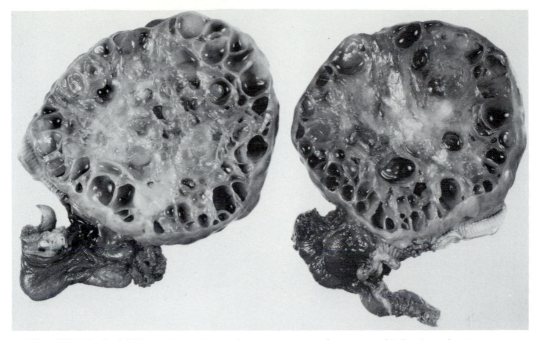

Fig. 836 Marked bilateral ovarian enlargement secondary to multiple theca-lutein cysts associated with normal pregnancy. Changes were misinterpreted as representing neoplasms and both ovaries were excised. (WU neg. 72-7260.)

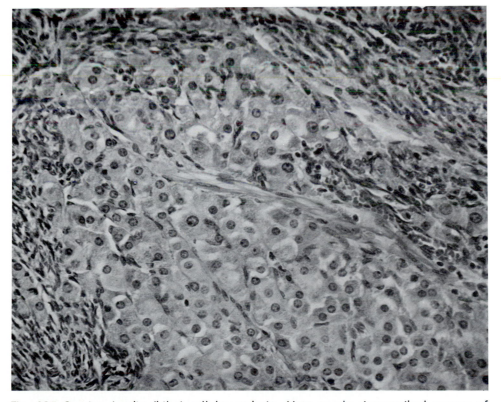

Fig. 837 Ovarian Leydig (hilus) cell hyperplasia. Note poorly circumscribed masses of large cells separated by ovarian stroma. (×300; WU neg. 62-7600.)

Endometriosis

Ovarian endometriosis usually occurs in childless women.[27] The process often is active for many years. At operation, small blueberry-like spots may be seen on the surface of the peritoneum and ovary. These blue areas are slightly raised and surrounded by fibrosis.[28] The entire ovary may be converted to a chocolate cyst as a result of repeated hemorrhage within it (Fig. 838). Infrequently, such cysts perforate.[29] The ovary involved by endometriosis often is fixed by fibrous adhesions.

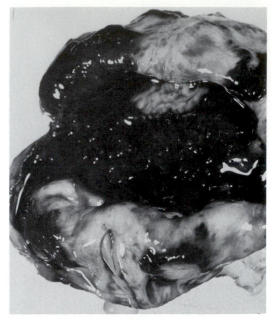

Fig. 838 Chocolate cyst of ovary due to endometriosis. There were also endometrial implants on peritoneal surface. (WU neg. 52-3832; specimen contributed by Dr. W. M. Allen, Baltimore, Md.)

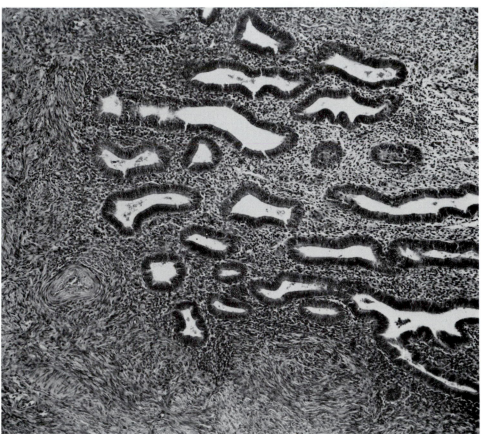

Fig. 839 Ovarian endometriosis composed of narrow proliferative glands surrounded by endometrial stroma which contrasts sharply with ovarian stoma at lower left. (×85; WU neg. 62-8861.)

Microscopically, typical endometriosis may be seen, although in chocolate cysts multiple sections are frequently necessary to prove the diagnosis (Fig. 839). The more advanced the endometrial lesion, the more difficult the diagnosis. To be absolutely certain, the pathologist should find endometrial glands, stroma, and hemorrhage. The endometrial stroma is responsible for the bleeding and may have typical "naked nucleus" cells surrounded by reticulin and a typical spiral arteriole in conjunction with old and recent hemorrhage. Unfortunately, this combination of findings is not always present. Not infrequently, the repeated hemorrhages have totally destroyed the endometrial tissue, the cyst being lined by several layers of hemosiderin-laden macrophages.

Biopsy

Examination of an ovarian biopsy obtained by either laparotomy or surgical culdoscopy can be useful in the evaluation of selected patients with amenorrhea and sterility resulting from anovulation. The specimen, which corresponds to about one-fifth of the organ, is evaluated for the presence and quantity of follicles, evidence of ovulation (corpora lutea and albicantia), and the character of the stroma. In a series of twenty-eight patients reported by Steele et al.,[31] the diagnosis was that of normal or potentially normal ovary in nineteen, gonadal dysgenesis (streaks) in four, polycystic ovaries in two, and ovarian failure with premature menopause in three. In the latter condition, the ovaries were small but still recognizable. Microscopically, there was total absence of germ cells, the appearance thus resembling that of the atrophic postmenopausal state. In a series of eighty-one patients, Stevenson[32] found eleven instances of endometriosis, thirteen of polycystic ovaries, forty-four of "microcystic ovaries," and eight of "small, hard and pale dysgenetic ovaries." Although the significance of some of these changes could be argued, it is interesting to note that thirty-six (44%) of the pa-

tients carried one or more pregnancies to successful termination following laparotomy.

Mori[30] attempted to correlate the morphologic findings in the ovarian biopsy with a series of endocrinologic analyses. He found that the ovaries of patients with hypergonadotropic ovarian failure contained no follicles, whereas in those of patients with normogonadotropic or hypogonadotropic ovarian failure, many developing follicles were present.

Frozen section

When patients undergo operation for ovarian tumor, the pathologist should be present. He can be of help in the gross diagnosis and can use frozen section as indicated. The decisions involve these questions. Should only the involved ovary or ovaries be removed? Should a hysterectomy be performed? Most ovarian tumors are relatively simple to recognize—at least it can be decided whether they are benign or malignant. The age of the patient influences the extent of the operation if the lesion is benign, but if the tumor is malignant, age must not be allowed to limit its adequate removal. The pathologist and the surgeon should remember:

1 *To remove only the involved ovary in benign tumors.* Normal ovarian tissue of this ovary at times can be preserved. These tumors include fibromas, thecomas, Brenner tumors, and cystic teratomas (dermoid cysts).

2 *That certain malignant neoplasms tend to be unilateral.* These tumors include mucinous cystadenocarcinomas (about 15% bilateral), dysgerminomas, granulosa cell tumors, Sertoli-Leydig cell tumors, and lipoid cell tumors. In most cases, ovariectomy alone may be adequate. In other instances, hysterectomy and bilateral salpingo-ovariectomy are required because of the size of the neoplasm and the possibility of its extension.

3 *That certain malignant tumors tend to be bilateral.* These include serous cyst-

adenocarcinomas (about 40%) and undifferentiated carcinomas. For these, bilateral salpingo-ovariectomy with total abdominal hysterectomy is the operation of choice.

Tumors
Embryology

The classification of ovarian tumors is based on the developmental morphology of the ovary. The gonadal anlage is an accumulation of cells beneath the coelomic epithelium on the anterior ventral surface of the wolffian body. In this indifferent phase, it is impossible to determine histologically whether the sex gland is ovary or testis.

At the beginning of sex differentiation, sex cords or medullary tubules develop and converge in a zigzag fashion toward the hilus of the gland.[33] The germ cells originate in the yolk sac endoderm near the allantoic evagination.[35] Their subsequent path and maturation in the developing ovary have been traced with the aid of a variety of histochemical stains.[34] Cells that become disassociated from germinal function may, in later life, give rise to tumors such as dysgerminoma. These tumors have no endocrine function. In the testes, they are known as seminoma.

It is probable that tumors composed of cells resembling granulosa, theca, Sertoli, and Leydig cells originate from the same ovarian stroma that produces the normal structures composed of these cells (Figs. 840 to 842). The common serous, mucinous, and endometrioid tumors of the ovary originate from its outer coat of müllerian epithelium. This is the same epithelium that invaginates to form the lining of the müllerian ducts and, eventually, the mucosa of tube, endometrium, and endocervix.

Classification

The classification of tumors of the ovary is intended to reflect the present concepts of histogenesis in as uncomplicated a manner as possible.[36, 37, 61] Since the embryogenesis of this intricate organ is still debated, the ultimate origin of its many tumors will probably remain a controversy for some time. Some alternate concepts are presented in the text.

A Tumors of surface (müllerian) epithelial origin with or without a stromal component
  1 Serous cystadenoma and cystadenocarcinoma
  2 Mucinous cystadenoma and cystadenocarcinoma
  3 Endometrioid cystadenoma and cystadenocarcinoma
  4 Clear cell ("mesonephric") adenocarcinoma
  5 Brenner tumor
  6 Malignant mixed müllerian tumor
  7 Mixed types
B Tumors of germ cell origin
  1 Dysgerminoma
  2 Yolk sac tumor (endodermal sinus tumor; embryonal carcinoma)
  3 Choriocarcinoma
  4 Embryonal teratoma
  5 Adult solid teratoma
  6 Adult cystic teratoma, benign and with malignant change
  7 Struma ovarii
  8 Carcinoid tumor
  9 Mixed types
C Tumors of stromal origin
  1 Granulosa cell tumor
  2 Thecoma-fibroma
  3 Sertoli-Leydig cell tumor (arrhenoblastoma; androblastoma)
  4 Lipid cell tumors
  5 Mixed and indeterminate types
D Tumors of germ cell and stromal origin
  1 Gonadoblastoma, without or with dysgerminoma or other germ cell tumors
E Tumors of undeterminate origin
  1 Adenocarcinomas and undifferentiated carcinomas not otherwise specified
F Tumors of metastatic origin

Tumors of surface (müllerian) epithelial origin with or without stromal component
Serous, mucinous, and endometrioid tumors

Serous neoplasms make up about one-fourth of all ovarian tumors. Most cases occur in adults, but many cases in children also have been reported.[38] Their pathologic evaluation is extremely important in prognosis. A high percentage of them are bilateral (30% to 50%).

Grossly, the tumors consist of rather large

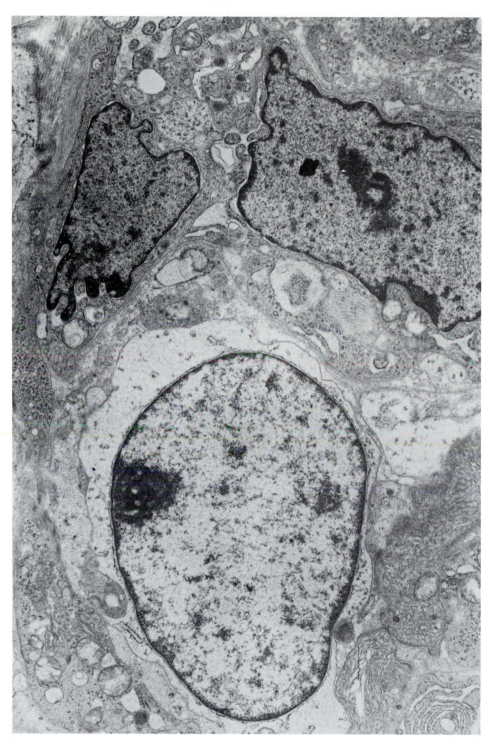

Fig. 840 Normal ovarian stroma has both dark spindle cells and pale polygonal cells. Nuclei of two spindle cells at top are irregular, and cytoplasm is filled with ribosomes. Polygonal cell at bottom center has paucity of cytoplasmic organelles and regular ovoid nucleus. (Approximately ×10,500.)

masses that usually contain serous fluid. Rarely, the fluid is viscous. In the better-differentiated tumors, papillary projections protrude inside the cavity and occasionally on the outer surface (Fig. 843). The more malignant tumors commonly are

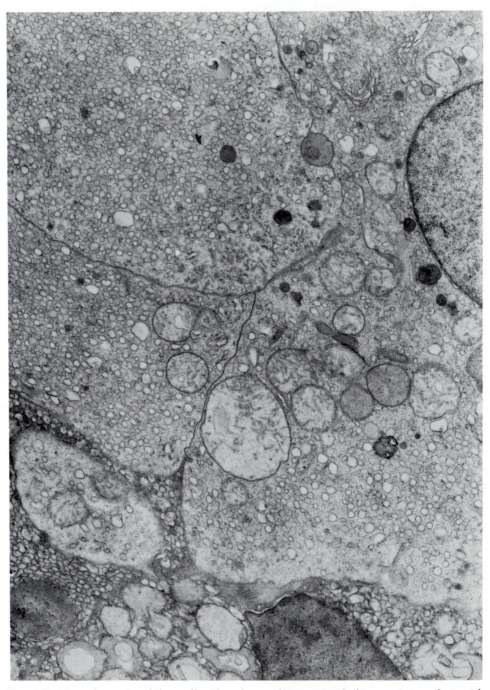

Fig. 841 Normal ovarian hilus cells. They have ultrastructural characteristics of steroid-producing cells such as those of adrenal cortex, Leydig cells of testis, and cells of corpus luteum. Cells have cytoplasm filled with microtubular forms of smooth endoplasmic reticulum and mitochondria with tubular cristae. (Approximately ×10,500.)

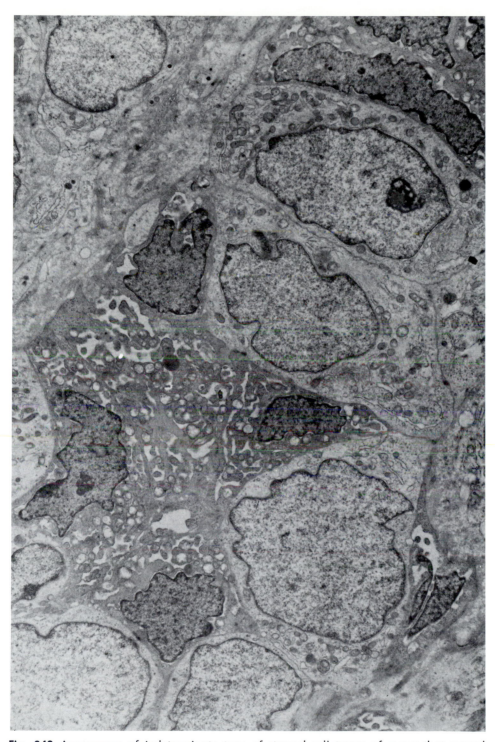

Fig. 842 Appearance of indeterminate type of stromal cell tumor of ovary that caused masculinization. Such tumors are often classified as arrhenoblastomas or Sertoli–Leydig cell tumors. Tumors are formed, however, by cells similar to ovarian stromal cells (see Fig. 840). (Approximately ×6,000.)

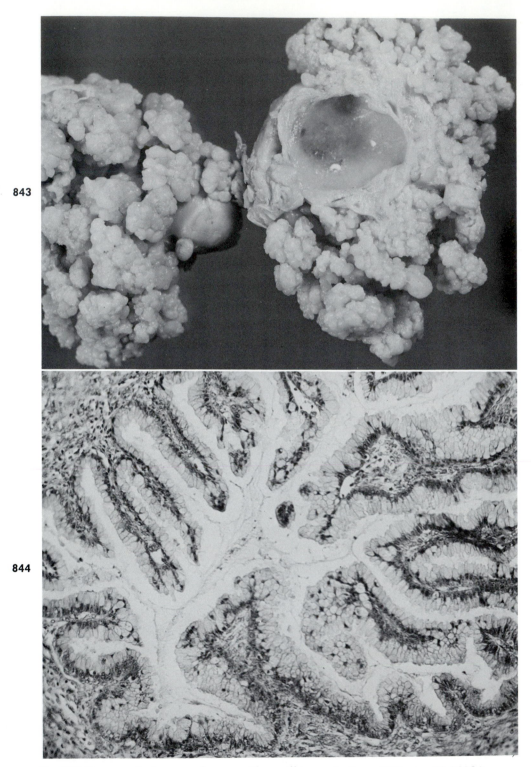

Fig. 843 Serous cystadenoma of ovary with papillary projections. (WU neg. 50-1682.)
Fig. 844 Ovarian mucinous cystadenoma composed of well-differentiated mucinous glands resembling endocervix. (×180; WU neg. 53-2997.)

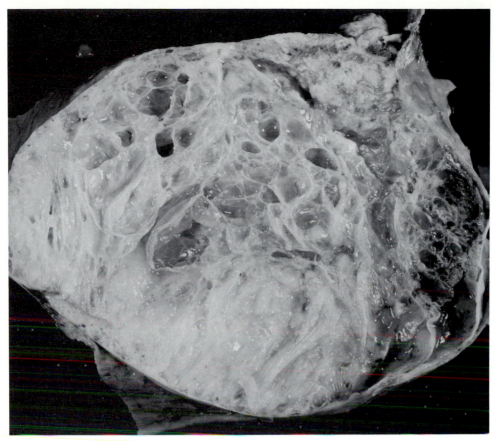

Fig. 845 Huge mucinous cystadenoma in 59-year-old woman. Note characteristic cystic spaces. (WU neg. 54-2877.)

solid, show areas of necrosis, and invade the ovary. Serous tumors with a prominent stromal fibroblastic component are subclassified as *cystadenofibromas* and *cystadenofibrocarcinomas*.[43] The stroma element appears grossly as a solid, white, nodular mass in an otherwise typical cystic neoplasm. The benign variant predominates greatly over the malignant.

Until recently, *mucinous neoplasms* of the ovary have been designated as pseudomucinous. The epithelium and cyst contents contain, for the most part, acid mucopolysaccharides. Mucins are chemically characterized as mucopolysaccharides. Therefore, the term pseudomucinous is incorrect.[42, 48] Mucinous neoplasms of the ovary are about as frequent as serous neoplasms, but they are not bilateral so often (5% to 15%).[62] Hertig[48] believes that the surface epithelium of the ovary is potential müllerian epithelium. From the müllerian system is formed tubal mucosa, endometrium, endocervix, and a portion of vagina. He believes that mucinous tumors of the ovary resemble cervical epithelium (Fig. 844) and that the serous type of neoplasm resembles fallopian tube epithelium. Roberts et al.[55] examined twenty-eight serous cystadenocarcinomas by electron microscopy. The tumors were composed of several cell types, some of which were quite reminiscent of tubal epithelium. It is probable that some mucinous neoplasms arise from a teratoma. They may have obvious intestinal mucosa and may contain intestinal enzymes such as lipase, trypsin, amylase, and sucrase.[42] The mucinous tumor contains a viscid fluid and tends to grow larger than the serous type (Fig.

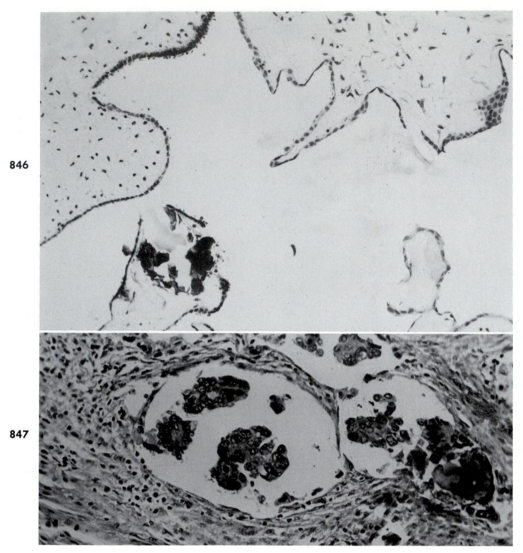

846

847

Fig. 846 Serous cystadenoma lined by flat or cuboidal layer of epithelial cells. (×200; WU neg. 50-3848.)
Fig. 847 Serous cystadenoma with "psammoma" bodies. (×110; WU neg. 48-4714.)

845). They may have papillary projections and, if malignant, develop solid areas that invade the remainder of the ovary.

There is a good correlation between prognosis and microscopic appearance.[60] The five-year survival rate will be greater if the pathologist is not conservative.[47] There is little difficulty in the diagnosis of benign tumors which are predominantly fibrous with a single layer of lining cells and without invasive tendencies (Fig. 846). In approximately 30% of the well-differen-

tiated neoplasms, whether benign or malignant, calcific spherules called psammoma bodies may be present (Fig. 847). Aure et al.[39] concluded that their presence is a favorable prognostic sign. However, even in the apparently microscopically benign variant, there have been exceptional instances of metastases. In a group of thirteen patients with such tumors reported by Marchetti,[52] there was one death.

Similarly, there is little doubt as to the

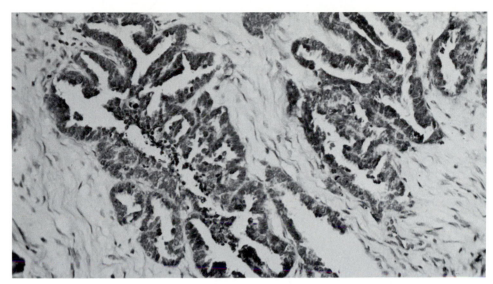

Fig. 848 Obviously malignant serous cystadenocarcinoma of ovary. (×200; WU neg. 50-3847.)

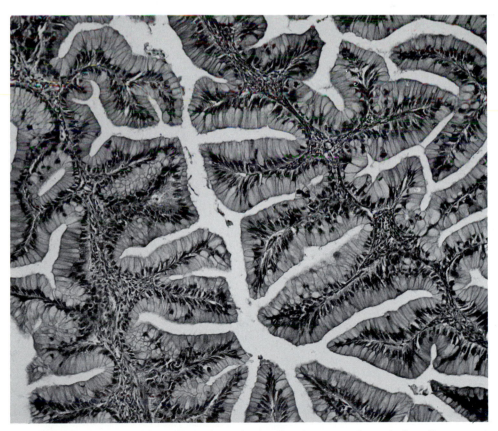

Fig. 849 Mucinous cystadenoma composed of tall columnar cells with basally situated nuclei supported on delicate fibrous septa. (×130; WU 62-5212.)

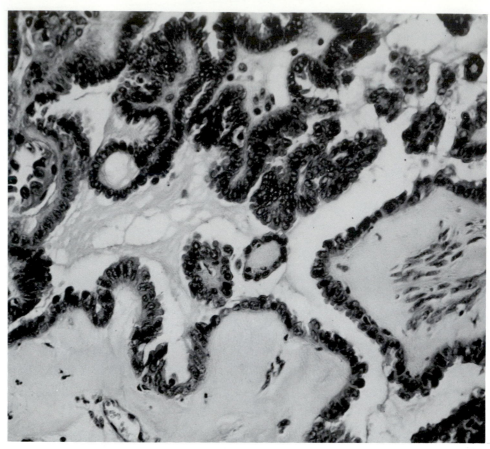

Fig. 850 Serous tumor of intermediate type. Epithelial pattern is somewhat more complicated occasionally with stratification of cells. (×300; WU neg. 62-5214.)

malignancy of the cellular tumor that shows layering of cells, prominent variation in the size and shape, numerous mitotic figures, and invasion of the stroma (Fig. 848). It is the interpretation of the borderline group of tumors that is most difficult. The tumor showing more complex branching with beginning layering of lining cells has an increased tendency to invade.[40] These tumors tend to implant upon the peritoneal surface, but they also metastasize to regional lymph nodes, liver, and more distant organs.

The benign variants of mucinous neoplasms are lined by tall, columnar, non-ciliated cells with basally situated nuclei (Fig. 849). Goblet cells and argentaffin cells may be present.[53, 54] Evidences of malignancy are increased layering of cells, anaplasia, and invasion of the stroma in

the areas of papillary branching. This tumor tends to implant upon and locally invade surrounding tissues such as the bowel, abdominal wall, and bladder. At times, gelatinous masses of tumor within the distended abdomen cause intestinal obstruction, and peritonitis frequently supervenes. Ovarian mucinous cystadenocarcinoma is the most common cause of the condition called *pseudomyxoma peritonei.* Metastases to distant areas are infrequent.

Santesson[57] separated the intermediate group of suspicious serous and mucinous tumors as "possibly malignant." These tumors have a more complicated pattern microscopically but do not invade beyond the stroma of the tumor itself (Fig. 850). It is not possible to predict which of such tumors will behave aggressively. The prognosis in eighty-seven patients with "pos-

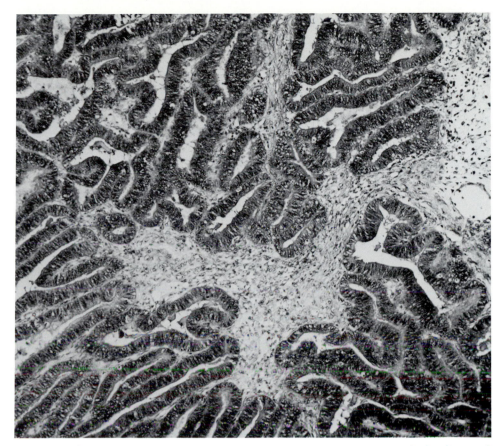

Fig. 851 Classic example of endometrioid carcinoma of ovary. Pattern of glands exactly resembles that of usual endometrial carcinoma. (×130; WU neg. 62-5213.)

sibly malignant" serous cystadenomas was the same whether they were treated by simple excision or by radical extirpation. It would seem logical to limit therapy to adequate local excision of all such tumors except those showing unquestionable features of malignancy.

Endometrioid carcinoma of the ovary is morphologically indistinguishable from primary carcinoma of the endometrium (Fig. 851). Grossly, it is often cystic, large, and hemorrhagic and may contain papillae. Gross distinction with the other tumors of surface epithelium is difficult. Microscopically, most tumors are well differentiated. Psammoma bodies are exceptional. Approximately 50% of the cases have foci of squamous metaplasia. Thus, the current term endometrioid carcinoma encompasses the type of ovarian tumor

formerly called adenoacanthoma.[49, 50] Coexistent endometriosis can be demonstrated in 10% to 20% of the cases, but this finding is not necessary for the diagnosis of endometrioid carcinoma. Admixture with serous cystadenocarcinoma can occur.[45]

Samson[56] was the first to report an adenocarcinoma of the ovary arising from an endometrial cyst. He proposed the following criteria:

1 Coexistence of benign and malignant tissue in the same ovary with the same histologic relationship to each other as in carcinoma of the body of the uterus

2 Carcinoma must actually appear to be arising in the tissue, not invading it

Additional supporting evidence includes the presence of tissue resembling endo-

Table 33 Differential characteristics of serous, mucinous, and endometrioid cystadenocarcinomas

Characteristic	Serous	Mucinous	Endometrioid
Relative frequency	65%-80%	10%	10%-25%
Size	Moderate	Often huge	Moderate
Usual character of fluid	Clear	Slimy, viscid	Hemorrhagic
Coexistent endometriosis	Less than 1%	Less than 1%	10%-20%
Papillary areas	Common	Rare	Rare
Coexistent endometrial hy-perplasia or carcinoma	Exceptional	Exceptional	27%
Epithelium	Cuboidal	Columnar, with basally located nucleus	Columnar, with central-ly located nucleus
Mucin	Only in luminar border	Often abundant, intra-cytoplasmic	Only in luminal border
Squamous metaplasia	Exceptional	Exceptional	50%
Cilia	Frequent	Absent	Rare
Psammoma bodies	Frequent	Exceptional	Exceptional
Survival rate (for well-differentiated tumors)	35.7%	39%	61.8%

metrial stroma around characteristic epithelial glands and the finding of old rather than fresh hemorrhage.[44, 46, 59]

Reanalysis of the histology of two series of ovarian tumors has shown a higher incidence of endometrioid carcinoma than hitherto realized, ranging from 10% to almost 25% of all primary ovarian adenocarcinomas.[41, 51, 58] The prognosis in patients with endometrioid carcinoma of the ovary is apparently twice as good as that expected in patients with serous and mucinous ovarian cystadenocarcinomas. Coexistent endometrial adenocarcinoma or adenoacanthoma was found in 14.6% of the seventy-five cases reviewed by Czernobilsky et al.[45] They most likely represent independent primary tumors. In the same series, endometrial hyperplasia was encountered in 12% of the patients. Perhaps related to the latter was the finding of luteinized cells in the stroma of the ovarian tumor in 12% of the cases.

The important differences between serous, mucinous, and endometrioid tumors are given in Table 33.

Clear cell ("mesonephric") adenocarcinoma

A distinctive ovarian tumor characterized by large clear cell in a glandular and papillary arrangement was included in Schiller's original description[65] of "mesonephroma" and since then it has been regarded as a tumor arising from mesonephric rests. Grossly, it often presents a spongy, partially cystic appearance. The tumor cells usually contain glycogen, mucin, and fat. Some of the nuclei protrude into the glandular lumen, resulting in hobnail-shaped cells (Fig. 852).

Scully et al.[66] have provided convincing evidence that this tumor has no relationship with mesonephric structures but arises instead from the surface epithelium. They regard this neoplasm as a variant of endometrioid carcinoma. In support of this theory, they report a high incidence of pelvic endometriosis, frequent admixture with typical endometrioid carcinoma, and origin in some cases from endometriotic cysts.

The incidence of bilaterality is less than 10%. Patients in the fifth and sixth decades are more commonly affected. The five-year survival rate ranges from 37% to 47%.[63, 64] Benign clear cell tumors are exceptional. They are often included under the designation of adenofibroma.

Brenner tumor

Brenner tumors constitute a little more than 1% of all ovarian neoplasms.[69, 73, 81] The average age in a series of ninety patients was slightly less than 50 years, and

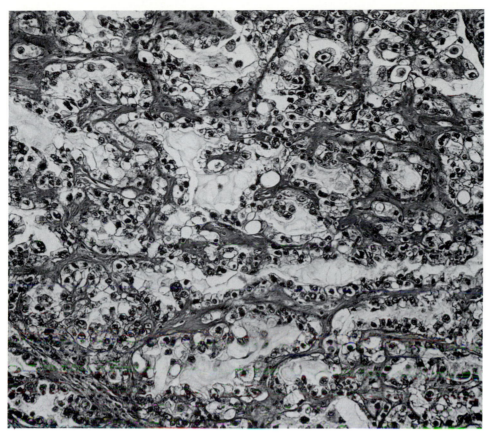

Fig. 852 Clear cell ("mesonephric") adenocarcinoma showing characteristic peg cells supported by delicate fibrous trabeculae forming small cystic spaces. (High power; WU neg. 62-5071.)

71% were over 40 years of age.[83] Grossly, these tumors vary greatly in size and are almost always unilateral. Invariably they are firm and white or yellowish white. They can be easily confused with fibromas or thecomas on gross inspection, except for the presence of small cystic areas filled with opaque, viscous, yellow-brown fluid. Meyer[75] suggested an origin from Walthard cell rests on the basis of the morphologic similarities between both lesions. Walthard found these sexually indifferent cell complexes in ovaries of newborn babies and infants, sometimes accompanied by epithelial cysts. Muller[78] found these nests within the ovarian parenchyma in 2.8% of 251 operative specimens. This same type of epithelial formation has been found more frequently beneath the serosa of the tubes and in the mesosalpinx. Solid

Brenner tumors theoretically might originate from the latter.[78] However, tumors from this area have not as yet been reported.

Arey[68] has shown continuity between the epithelial nests of Brenner tumor and surface epithelium, a finding which supports his concept of histogenesis from surface (müllerian) epithelium. The association with benign mucinous cysts, also of müllerian epithelial origin, is consistent with this concept (Fig. 853).

Other concepts of histogenesis, including origin from follicular granulosa cells,[82] have been advanced. These theories have been concisely reviewed by Hertig and Gore.[72]

Brenner tumor consist of nests of closely packed epithelial cells, closely resembling by light and electron microscopy the

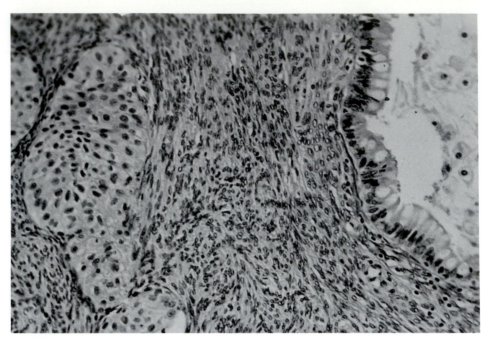

Fig. 853 Mucinous cystadenoma and Brenner tumor. Mucinous tumor with typical lining epithelium is at right, and Brenner tumor with its characteristic collection of cells is at left. (WU neg. 50-6473; slide contributed by Dr. R. Johnson, Columbia, Mo.)

transitional epithelium of the urinary tract.[79] They have a clear cytoplasm, oval nucleus, and distinct nucleolus (Fig. 854). A longitudinal groove is present in many of the nuclei, identical in appearance to that seen in granulosa–theca cell tumors. The stromal component is abundant and of dense fibroblastic nature. Cystic degeneration occasionally produces cavities lined by flattened, cuboidal, or cylindrical cells in the centers of the epithelial areas. The epithelial cells may secrete mucin.

This tumor is sometimes associated with mucinous cystadenoma (Fig. 853) and exceptionally with struma ovarii.[74] Stromal lipid is usually demonstrable in those tumors associated with clinical evidence of hyperestrinism. It may be found in epithelial cells as well.[77] Brenner tumors contain glycogen, whereas granulosa cell tumors do not.[70]

On occasion, the epithelial component of Brenner tumor can proliferate to such a degree as to form a large intracystic papillary mass quite reminiscent of a low-grade transitional cell carcinoma of the urinary bladder. The behavior of this lesion, which Roth and Sternberg[80] refer to as *proliferating Brenner tumor,* has been benign in the cases so far reported.[76] A high proportion of Brenner tumors occur in patients over 50 years of age. They are apparently associated with evidence of hyperestrinism such as endometrial hyperplasia and uterine bleeding in the postmenopausal woman more often than has been appreciated in the past.[77, 83] The growth rate is slow, and ascites is rare. Malignant Brenner tumors are exceedingly rare, but undoubted instances have been described.[67, 71, 76]

Malignant mixed müllerian tumor

The gross and microscopic features of malignant mixed müllerian tumor parallel in every respect those of the more common counterpart in the uterine corpus. Thus, a *homologous* variety (with nonspecific malignant stroma; also called carcinosarcoma) and a *heterologous* variety (with malignant heterologous elements) occur. The prognosis is extremely poor, especially

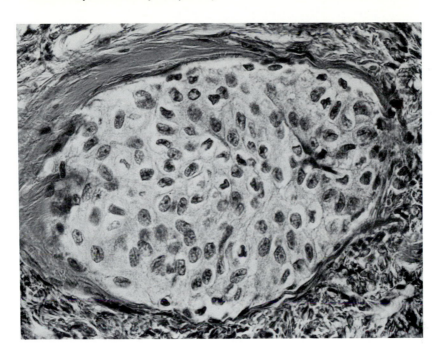

Fig. 854 Characteristic collection of closely packed cells with clear cytoplasm and deeply staining nuclei seen in Brenner tumor. Longitudinal groove is seen in several nuclei. (High power; WU neg. 49-6946.)

with the latter.[84] Most tumors have already extended outside the ovary at the time of surgery.[85] The most important differential diagnosis is with embryonal teratoma. Clinically, almost all malignant mixed müllerian tumors are seen in postmenopausal patients, whereas embryonal teratomas are typically tumors of children and adolescents. Furthermore, the former lack the neural and other germ cell elements as well as the organoid arrangement of teratomas.

Tumors of germ cell origin
Dysgerminoma

Dysgerminoma constitutes somewhat less than 1% of ovarian tumors or about 5% of malignant ovarian tumors. There have been about 540 cases reported in the literature.[93] Abell et al.[86] encountered eleven dysgerminomas in a series of 188 ovarian neoplasms in children (6%). Santesson[96] collected 299 cases, in which 81% of the patients were under 30 years of age and 44% were under 20 years of age. This tumor is often large (over 1,000 gm) and

occurs most frequently on the right side, although approximately 15% are bilateral.[90]

The dysgerminoma has a smooth, often convoluted surface that may resemble cerebral cortex[95] (Fig. 855). Frequently there is a well-defined fibrous capsule. The cut surface is gray and cellular and frequently contains yellow and brown areas of hemorrhage and necrosis.

The nuclear sex of a group of twenty dysgerminomas examined by Theiss et al.[97] was female. This has been cited as evidence that dysgerminomas originate from diploid female germ cells prior to the stage of reduction division.

The tumor cells may have a pseudotubular or cordlike arrangement. Individual cells are uniform and have large nuclei, one or two nucleoli, and poorly defined cytoplasmic outlines (Fig. 856). Glycogen and sometimes fine droplets of fat are present in the cytoplasm. The stromal contents vary. There may be hyaline change in vessels, lymphocytic infiltration, focal necrosis, and areas of granulomatous reaction. The presence of a heavy lymphocytic

855

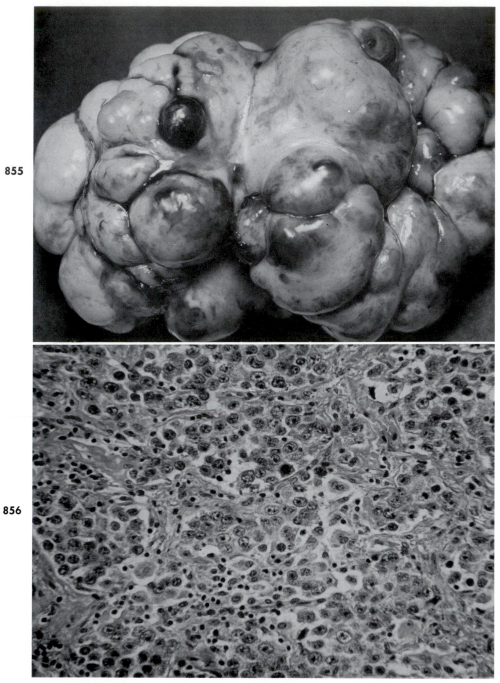

856

Fig. 855 Large dysgerminoma with external surface suggesting convolutions of cerebral cortex. (From Potter, E. B.: Dysgerminoma of the ovary, Am. J. Pathol. **22:**551-563, 1946).
Fig. 856 Dysgerminoma composed of irregular masses of anaplastic germ cells separated by fibrous tissue septa containing lymphocytes. Microscopic pattern is identical to that of testicular seminoma. (×275; WU neg. 62-7603.)

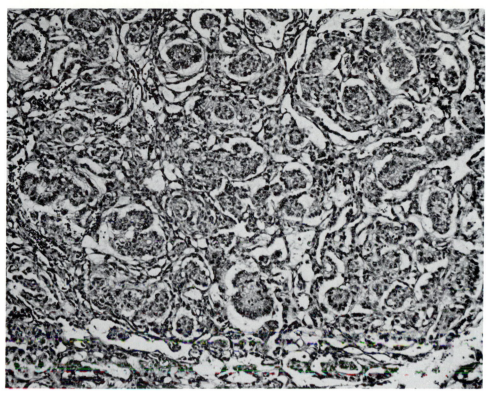

Fig. 857 Yolk sac tumor of ovary. Loose reticular pattern and rounded papillary processes with central capillary are typical. These do not resemble glomeruli at any stage of development. (×90; WU neg. 64-339.)

infiltration has a favorable influence in prognosis, as in the case of testicular seminoma.

Dysgerminoma has exactly the same origin, microscopic pattern, ultrastructural appearance, and clinical behavior as seminoma of the testes.[90]

Dysgerminoma is reputedly more common in disorders of sexual differentiation. Many tumors reported as ovarian dysgerminoma are probably more accurately regarded as seminomas arising in the cryptorchid testes of patients with testicular feminization. Similarly, seminoma is the most common testicular tumor in otherwise normal men with cryptorchidism. However, over one-half of dysgerminomas occur in normal women. Hypoplasia of the genitalia and hirsutism may occur. Removal of these tumors has no effect on such sex changes.[94]

Dysgerminomas are radiosensitive and radiocurable, even in the presence of metastases.[92] Survival in sixty patients with dysgerminoma studied at the Radium-hemmet by Brody[89] was closely related to the clinical findings. The five-year survival rate when the tumor was encapsulated and movable was 95%. With ascites, adhesions, or rupture it was 78%, and with metastases it was 33%. Areas of embryonal carcinoma, teratocarcinoma, or choriocarcinoma are found in approximately 10% of all dysgerminomas and are of distinctly unfavorable prognosis. In a series of fifty-six patients with follow-up, five of the six deaths occurred in patients whose tumors contained such an association.[88]

A conservative approach is justified in the management of the young woman with dysgerminoma confined to one ovary.[87] Even those patients who develop a recurrence after unilateral oophorectomy have a good prognosis with properly directed radiation therapy, and many of these may have successful pregnancy in the meantime.[89, 91] Infrequently, the Friedman test is positive.

Yolk sac tumor (endodermal sinus tumor; embryonal carcinoma)

A rare but distinctive neoplasm, yolk sac tumor was included in Schiller's original description of mesonephroma,[100] together with the ovarian tumor presently designated as clear cell adenocarcinoma.[101] Grossly, it usually presents an admixture of solid and cystic areas. It has a soft consistency and large areas of necrosis. The characteristic microscopic features include papillary and glandular formations, "glomeruloid bodies" (Fig. 857), perivascular pseudorosettes, and PAS-positive intracellular and extracellular hyaline bodies. This is a tumor of children and young adults.[98] In contrast to its testicular counterpart, the prognosis is poor. Of twenty-one patients with follow-up studied by Neubecker and Breen,[99] eighteen died, and the remaining three were known to have metastases. The average survival time was 13.5 months.

Choriocarcinoma

Most choriocarcinomas of the ovary represent metastases from uterine tumors. Exceptionally, a primary choriocarcinoma can develop from either an ovarian pregnancy or de novo, as a form of teratoma. The prognosis is exceedingly poor.[102]

Embryonal teratoma

Scully[103] prefers the term embryonal teratoma for the malignant ovarian teratoma composed of a mixture of embryonal and adult tissues derived from all three germ layers, regardless of its gross appearance. The tumor may be solid throughout, solid with multiple minute cysts, or predominantly cystic. It is a tumor of children and adolescents. The prognosis, generally poor, depends a great deal on the nature of the embryonal component. It is best when the latter is predominantly made up of neural tissue.

Adult solid teratoma

Adult solid teratoma has a predominantly solid gross appearance, although multi-

Table 34 Incidence of ovarian tumors*†

	Benign		Malignant		Benign and malignant	
	Number	% of type	Number	% of type	Number	% of all cases
Serous tumors	406	65.5	214	34.5	620	24.5
Mucinous tumors	420	88.0	57	12.0	478	18.9
Teratomas	438	98.9	5	1.2	443	17.5
Unclassified cystadenomas	42	—	—	—	42	1.7
Granulosa cell tumors	29	66.0	15	34.0	44	1.7
Fibromas	739	99.9	1	0.1	740	29.2
Brenner tumors	31	100.0	—	—	31	1.2
Thecomas	56	100.0	—	—	56	2.2
Sertoli–Leydig cell tumors	1	—	1	—	2	0.1
Miscellaneous benign tumors‡	19	100.0	—	—	19	0.8
Undifferentiated carcinomas	—	—	30	—	30	1.5
Clear cell ("mesonephric") carcinomas	—	—	9	—	9	0.4
Endometrioid carcinomas	—	—	13	—	13	0.5
Dysgerminomas	—	—	2	—	2	0.1
Malignant mixed müllerian tumors	—	—	2	—	2	0.1
Total	2,181		349	(13.8)	2,531	100.0

*From Kent, S. W., and McKay, D. G.: Primary cancer of the ovary, Am. J. Obstet. Gynecol. 80:430-438, 1960.
†Terms slightly modified to conform to classification.
‡Includes leiomyomas, adenomas, adenomatoid tumors, adenomyomas, and paragangliomas.

ple small cystic areas also are present. Because of this, some authors prefer the designation of polycystic. By definition, it should be *composed entirely of adult tissues* derived from all three germ layers.[105, 106] It occurs in young women, predominantly in the second decade. The prognosis is generally excellent, although exceptionally metastases have developed.[104]

Adult cystic teratoma, benign and with malignant change

Cystic teratomas make up almost 20% of the entire group of ovarian neoplasms. They constitute the most common ovarian tumor in children.[110]

Most *cystic teratomas* of the ovary are benign. In the series reported by Kent and McKay,[114] 438 were benign and five were malignant (1%) (Table 34). Peterson[115] found 147 carcinomas in a group of 8,038 reported dermoid cysts (1.8%).

Grossly, these tumors are usually unilateral (12% bilateral) and provoke only symptoms relating to mass. The greasy material within them is liquid at body temperature. If a teratoma ruptures into the peritoneal cavity, the greasy fluid provokes a prominant fibroblastic peritonitis resulting in nodules exactly simulating metastatic cancer. The diagnosis is resolved by frozen section.[107]

Usually, cystic teratomas are multiloculated and contain a well-defined nipplelike structure covered with hair (known as Rokitansky's protuberance). Teratomas often contain teeth or an imperfectly formed mandible. Other well-organized structures are rare (Fig. 858). Microscopically, they are lined by well-differentiated stratified squamous epithelium. Skin appendages are extremely common, brain and nerve tissue occur frequently, and thyroid tissue is found in about 10% of them. Kidney and liver tissue occur rarely, if at all. The number of different tissues found depends on the number of sections studied. The most rewarding sections are those from the nipplelike structure, even if it contains bone. In a thorough study of 225 teratomas by Blackwell et al.,[108] ectodermal derivatives were present in 100%, mesodermal structures in 93%, and entodermal derivatives in 71%.

A female nuclear sex chromatin pattern

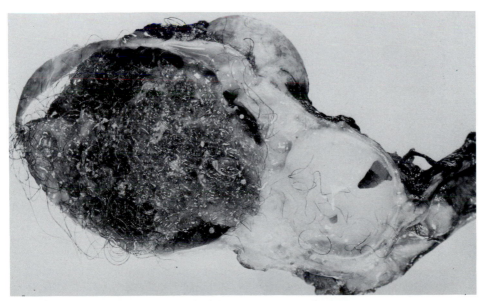

Fig. 858 Adult cystic teratoma (dermoid cyst) of ovary showing greasy contents and hair. (WU neg. 50-1876.)

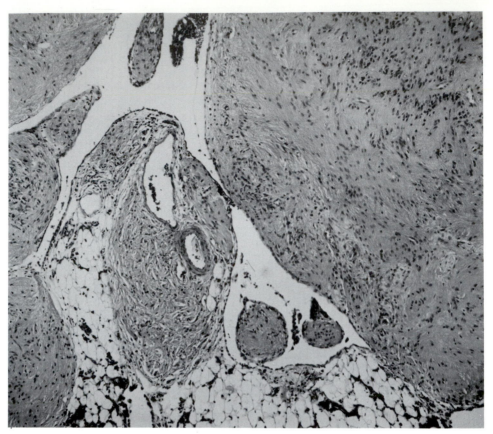

Fig. 859 Omental implants composed of glial tissue in child. Multiple tumor masses were removed from peritoneal cavity eighteen months following ovariectomy for rather well-differentiated solid teratoma in which all three germ layers were represented. Maturation of tissues had apparently recurred in intervening time. Child was living and well twelve years following original ovariectomy. (Low power; WU neg. 62-7608.)

is present in all cases.[119] Chromosomal analyses have shown a 46 XX pattern.[117]

The most common malignant change in cystic teratoma is epidermoid carcinoma, followed by carcinoid tumor and adenocarcinoma.[109, 113] We have seen a case of sweat gland carcinoma.

Adult teratomas of both the cystic and solid variety (especially the latter) are occasionally accompanied by peritoneal implants. If the latter are exclusively composed of mature glial tissue, the prognosis is excellent[112, 118] (Fig. 859). We have seen a case in which a "second-look" operation some months later showed regression and fibrosis of the glial implants. Conversely, if other tissues are present, such as epithelium, the prognosis is poor.

Struma ovarii

Thyroid tissue is probably the most interesting tissue occurring in cystic teratoma of the ovary (Fig. 860). This entity represents dominant growth of a single tissue in a teratoma. About 150 cases have been reported. This thyroid tissue may show all pathologic changes seen in a normally placed thyroid gland, including diffuse or nodular hyperplasia, inflammation, and tumors.[111] There is no doubt that this tissue is true thyroid tissue, a concept further substantiated by biologic tests.[116]

Struma ovarii can occur in the absence of any other component of cystic teratoma, either pure or combined with mucinous cystadenoma, Brenner tumor, or carcinoid tumor.[120, 121]

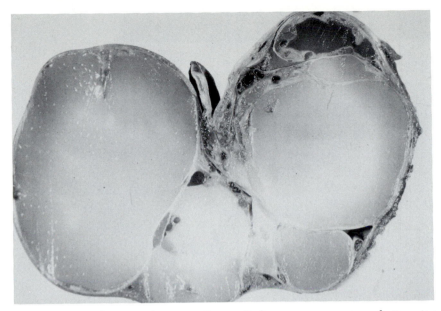

Fig. 860 Teratoma of ovary demonstrating typical gross appearance of struma ovarii. Tumor was composed almost entirely of thyroid tissue. (EFSCH 51-2608; contributed by Dr. R. Johnson, Columbia, Mo.)

Carcinoid tumor

The large majority of ovarian carcinoid tumors arise within a cystic teratoma.[122] Many of them are predominantly formed by ribbons and festoons, thus corresponding to the type of carcinoid tumor arising from hindgut derivatives. Sometimes they are seen in the absence of teratoma.[123] In the past, they have been frequently confused with granulosa cell tumors. A curious combination, only recently emphasized, is that of carcinoid tumor and struma ovarii, referred to as *strumal carcinoid*.[125] Many cases of this entity are probably mistakenly reported in the literature as struma ovarii with malignant change. Finally, some ovarian carcinoid tumors represent metastases from gastrointestinal neoplasms.

The prognosis of primary ovarian carcinoid tumor, whether pure or as a component of cystic teratoma, is good. Only one of the thirty odd cases reported in the literature has given rise to metastases.[124]

Ovarian carcinoid tumors may give rise to the carcinoid syndrome in the absence of liver metastases.

Tumors of stromal origin

The stromal cells of the ovary include the follicular granulosa cells, the surrounding theca cells, and large masses of morphologically unspecialized stromal cells that form the bulk of the tissue surrounding the ova and follicles. A variety of tumors occurring in the ovary resemble the patterns produced by the stroma during embryogenesis of both ovary and testis.[126, 129] Whether granulosa–theca cell tumors arise from the ovarian stroma or from the theca and granulosa cells that have differentiated from it is debatable.

It is reasonable to believe that Sertoli–Leydig cell tumors (arrhenoblastomas) arise from more primitive stromal cells. These male-appearing tumors are composed of cells with female sex chromatin pattern.[127] The terms Sertoli–Leydig and arrhenoblastoma are descriptive and not meant to imply that a tumor is composed of actual male Sertoli and Leydig cells that somehow have persisted or crept into the ovary. Most lipid cell tumors probably originate from ovarian stromal cells in a manner comparable to the focal luteiniza-

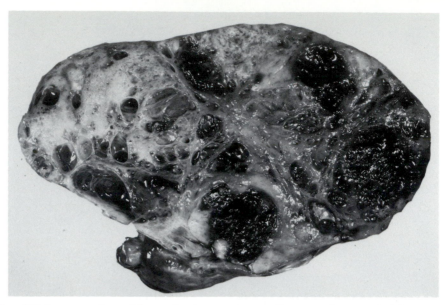

Fig. 861 Large cystic and hemorrhagic granulosa cell tumor of ovary. (EFSCH 48-28.)

tion of these cells seen in some virilizing states.

In view of the common origin of these tumors, it is not surprising that mixtures of the main types can occur or that a few will not fit easily into this classification.

Most granulosa–theca cell tumors produce hyperestrinism. A majority of Sertoli–Leydig cell tumors (arrhenoblastomas) and lipid cell tumors have a masculinizing effect. There may be no demonstrable endocrine effect, and rare examples of hormonal effects opposite to what should be expected from the morphology of the tumor have been described in both groups.[128, 129] The entire group comprises about 4% of ovarian tumors.

Granulosa cell tumor

Granulosa cell tumors account for approximately 10% of all solid ovarian tumors. About 10% are bilateral. They are often partially cystic and hemorrhagic and vary in size from microscopic masses to tumors filling the abdomen (Fig. 861). Nine unusually cystic granulosa cell tumors, grossly resembling cystadenomas, were reported by Norris and Taylor.[134] Two of the cases were associated with

signs of masculinization. Approximately 5% of granulosa cell tumors occur before puberty and 40% after menopause. We have seen several cases of granulosa cell tumor in patients who had endometrial hyperplasia without palpable tumor. Both ovaries appeared normal, but in one there was a microscopic granulosa cell tumor.

These tumors are encapsulated and have a smooth, lobulated surface. The cysts contain straw-colored or mucoid fluid. The solid portions of tumor frequently are gray but may show focal yellow areas caused by luteinization of the tumor. Three of the sixty-two cases reported by Hodgson et al.[130] showed luteinization.

The microscopic pattern of the granulosa cell tumor is extremely variable. Different parts of the same tumor may show dissimilar patterns.[135] The folliculoid type of cell arrangement is the most common. It may suggest a normal follicle of the ovary (macrofollicular pattern) or be composed of small masses of cells interspersed with tiny round spaces, designated Call-Exner bodies (microfollicular pattern) (Fig. 862). A nuclear fold or groove is often present.

The tumor may have a cylindroid pattern with cystic areas and rarely may have a

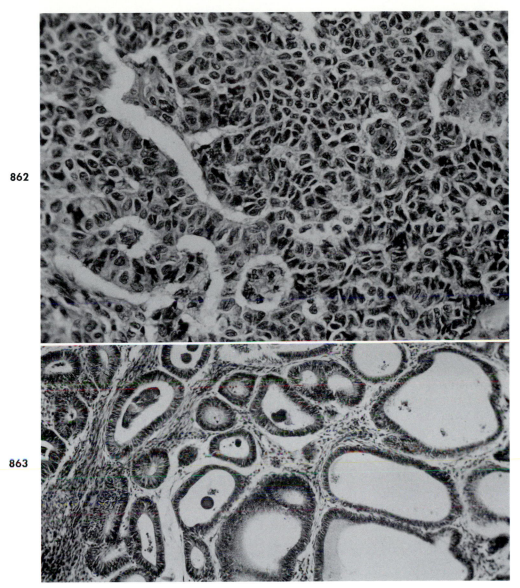

Fig. 862 Typical granulosa cell tumor of ovary with folliculoid pattern. (×400; WU neg. 50-3555.)

Fig. 863 Prominent endometrial hyperplasia occurring in association with tumor shown in Fig. 862. (×115; WU neg. 50-3556.)

sarcomatoid or even adenomatoid appearance.[138, 139] In a study of 125 patients with granulosa cell tumor, recurrence after excision was more frequent when the tumor had a sarcomatoid pattern (70%) than when it had a follicular or trabecular pattern (18.5%).[132] On the other hand, Norris and Taylor[133] found no distinctive histologic criteria by which an aggressive

tumor could be identified. Twelve of 187 patients in their study with follow-up information had persistent tumor after surgery. Only ten of the 187 patients died as a result of the neoplasm. In most other series, the prognosis has not been so favorable, probably because of less strict morphologic criteria and the use of crude rather than actuarial survival rates.[135] Un-

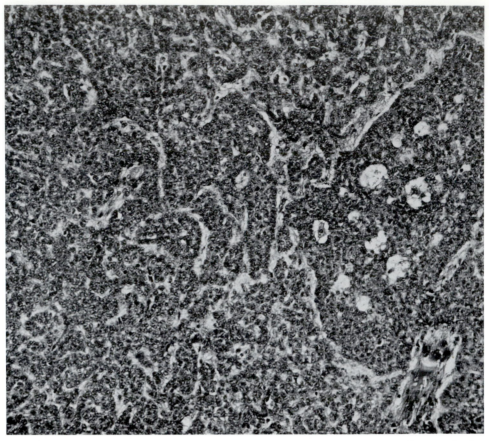

Fig. 864 Granulosa cell tumor of less well-differentiated pattern. Note Call-Exner bodies in small mass of cells on right. (×150; WU neg. 62-5070.)

differentiated or poorly differentiated carcinomas which superficially resemble granulosa cell tumors should not be included in this group. Most deaths occurred more than five years after original diagnosis and treatment. A five-year follow-up is not sufficient because recurrences may appear ten or more years after operation. A single granulosa cell tumor may show the typical granulosa cell pattern blending with the typical pattern of a thecoma. Scully[136] has emphasized the resemblance between metastatic carcinoid tumors and the pattern of granulosa cell tumor with Call-Exner bodies (Fig. 864).

The possible relationship of granulosa cell tumors with endometrial carcinoma is discussed below.[131] Granulosa cell tumors are not uncommon in the mouse.[137]

Thecoma-fibroma

In about 65% of patients, the **thecoma** appears after menopause[145] and is unilateral, usually benign, and at times partially cystic. Rare instances of a malignant variant have been reported.[143] The thecoma varies considerably in size, has a well-defined capsule, and cuts with increased resistence (Fig. 865). The small yellow areas in thecomas are the most helpful positive finding in differentiating these tumors from fibromas. Microscopically, these yellow areas contain clumps of spindle cells with centrally placed nuclei and lipid-rich cytoplasm (Fig. 866). The intervening tissue may show considerable hyalinization and may contain focal hyaline plaques. The epithelial cells in this connective tissue network may have vacuolated or acid-

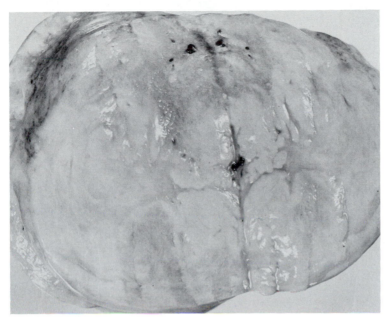

Fig. 865 Large thecoma that has small yellow areas. (WU neg. 49-5296.)

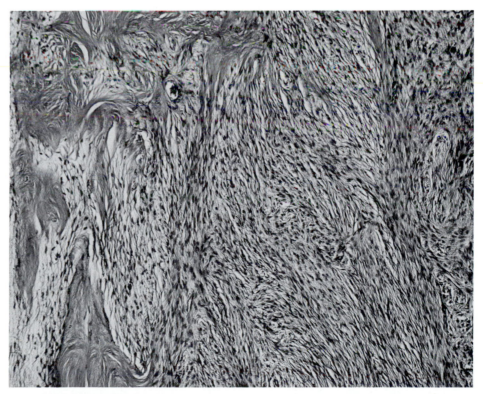

Fig. 866 Thecoma composed of spindle-shaped cells intermixed with dense hyaline plaques. Fat stains showed cytoplasmic lipid. Patient, 59-year-old woman, had endometrial hyperplasia. (×130; WU neg. 63-4799.)

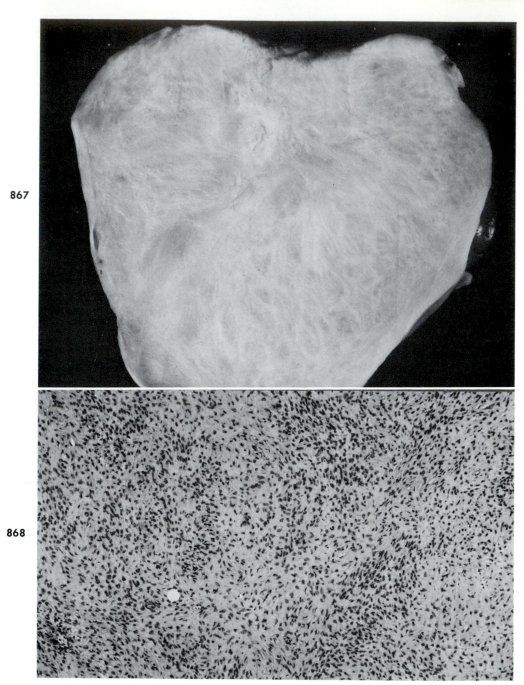

Fig. 867 Typical cut surface of ovarian fibroma showing interlacing bands of dense fibrous tissue. (WU neg. 63-6414.)
Fig. 868 Fibroma with well-differentiated fibroblasts separated by hyaline stroma. (×85; WU neg. 66-4697; from Kraus, F. T.: Gynecologic pathology, St. Louis, 1967, The C. V. Mosby Co.)

ophilic cytoplasm and clearly defined poly-hedral cell boundaries, giving the cells a luteinlike appearance.[142]

Thecomas of the ovary may be associated with prominent stromal hyperplasia. This is uncommon in patients under 40 years of age and is of greatest frequency in the sixth decade. These findings suggested to Sternberg and Gaskill[150] that stromal hyperplasia is the soil in which theca cell tumors are likely to develop. They believe that transition can be traced from stromal hyperplasia through diffuse thecomatosis to theca cell tumors.

Granulosa cells are reticulin free, and theca cells are individually surrounded by reticulin. However, in a theca cell tumor there are invariably islands of reticulin-free cells. Luteinized cells when found in a thecoma are almost invariably reticulin free.[142]

Fibromas of the ovary are common and occur almost invariably after puberty. They are solid, lobulated, encapsulated, and firm and usually are not accompanied by adhesions (Fig. 867). The average diameter of 312 tumors in Dockerty and Masson's series[141] was 6 cm. The tumor is grayish white and may contain focal yellow areas of fatty degeneration. These areas may become cystic. About 90% of these tumors are unilateral. They are not malignant.

Differentiation from thecoma may be impossible inasmuch as some fibromas are undoubtedly inactive thecomas, a point of view supported by electron microscopic observations.[140] Krukenberg tumors also superficially resemble thecomas but almost invariably are bilateral. Microscopically, fibromas appear to be an overgrowth of ovarian stroma. These connective tissue cells are often closely packed and arranged in a "feather-stitched" pattern (Fig. 868). There may be hyaline bands such as seen in thecomas, and considerable edema between tumor cells may be present.

In Dockerty and Masson's group,[141] fifty-one of the 283 patients with fibroma had ascites. Ascitic fluid usually is a transudate. Infrequently, the ascites may be associated with pleural effusion, usually right-sided. This combination is known as Meigs' syndrome. Samanth and Black[149] found that all the ovarian fibromas associated with Meigs' syndrome they examined

were 10 cm or more in diameter and had areas of myxoid degeneration. When both ascites and pleural effusion are present, a diagnosis of inoperable ovarian neoplasm often is made, but after removal of the tumor both of these complications disappear.

The mechanism of pleural effusion has been demonstrated by Meigs et al.[147, 148] The intrathoracic negative pressures are thought to account for the transdiaphragmatic passage of fluid through pleural peritoneal "pores" or lymphatics. Flow from the pleural cavity into the abdomen apparently does not take place. Other tumors also may cause this syndrome.[146] Kalstone et al.[144] have described four patients with *massive edema of the ovary* grossly simulating fibroma. One case was associated with lutein cell hyperplasia. They postulated partial torsion of the mesovarium as the probable pathogenesis.

Effects of hyperestrogenism in granulosa cell tumors and thecoma

Both granulosa cell tumor and thecoma may produce clinical signs of hyperestrogenism, particularly in prepubertal and postmenopausal patients. Precocious puberty occurs in the former and prominent menstrual abnormalities in the latter. These tumors frequently produce enlargement of the uterus characterized by muscle hypertrophy and prominent endometrial hyperplasia (Fig. 863). However, not all thecomas and granulosa cell tumors function. We have seen patients with atrophic endometrium. Norris and Taylor[159] found endometrial hyperplasia in 22% of seventy-seven patients with granulosa–theca cell tumors in whom material from endometrial curettage was examined.

Histochemically, Dempsey and Bassett[152] and McKay et al.[157, 158] found that the graafian follicles of both the rat and human ovaries have steroid substances confined to the thecal layer. None was present in the granulosa layer. McKay et al.[158] demonstrated that histochemical studies helped differentiate thecomas from fibromas, and they demonstrated the functional state of the tumor. Estrogens come from thecal cells of the thecoma and from thecalike cells in granulosa cell tumors. In the granulosa cell tumors, it may be the thecal component rather than the tumor cells which produces the hormones. Histochemical agents cannot differentiate inactive thecoma from fibroma.

Occurrence of carcinoma of endometrium with granulosa cell tumors and thecomas

Functioning granulosa cell tumors and thecomas cause endometrial hyperplasia with such extreme atypical changes that a mistaken diagnosis of carcinoma is often made. The fact that complete regression of these changes frequently occurs after simple removal of the functioning ovarian tumor is evidence that the atypical changes are not truly cancer. Stohr[162] reported a case diagnosed as endometrial adenocarcinoma before removal of a granulosa cell tumor. A repeat curetting of the endometrium five weeks postoperatively showed normal early typical secretory epithelium coinciding with the clinical phase of the menstrual cycle.

Henderson[155] reported two endometrial carcinomas among twenty-one patients with granulosa cell tumors and three others among nine patients with thecomas. In all instances, the endometrium was diffusely involved, but the myometrium was only superficially invaded. Glandular epithelium was of the secretory type. It is interesting that none of these patients suffered recurrence or died from cancer. Greene et al.[153] found no evidence to support an etiologic relationship between granulosa cell tumor and endometrial carcinoma. Seven of the 203 patients with granulosa–theca cell tumors studied by Norris and Taylor[159] were judged to have endometrial carcinoma. How extensive or aggressive these lesions may have been is uncertain.

In eighty-two granulosa cell tumors and in sixteen thecomas reported by Kottmeier,[156] there were four carcinomas of the endometrium. In nine of the same group,

the endometrium showed atypical changes which were not considered carcinoma but could easily have been confused with it. Novak and Rutledge[160] reported atypical endometrial hyperplasia simulating adenocarcinoma in patients who received estrogens. The incidence of cancer of the body of the uterus in a group of 157 patients with granulosa cell tumor studied by Sjöstedt and Wahlen[161] was no greater than the expected incidence if each disease had been considered separately.

In a series of 115 patients with granulosa cell tumors and thecomas studied by Gusberg and Kardon,[154] the diagnosis of adenocarcinoma was made in 21%. The myometrium was invaded in none of the premenopausal patients and in only five of the postmenopausal patients. No mention is made whether any of these patients suffered from tumor recurrence or metastases. There is certainly a striking disparity between the alleged high frequency of endometrial carcinomas in these patients and the almost total absence of well-documented cases in which the tumor resulted in recurrence or metastases. We must conclude that either these lesions in reality are extreme examples of hyperplasia masquerading as cancer or, if they are cancers, they are endowed with a very limited biologic malignant potential.

Sertoli–Leydig cell tumor (arrhenoblastoma; androblastoma)

As the name indicates, Sertoli–Leydig cell tumors, which are usually masculinizing neoplasms, are composed of a mixture in variable proportions of cells resembling (at a light microscopic level) male Sertoli and Leydig cells. This has led to the concept, championed by Meyer,[166] that male-directed cells persisting from the primitive testislike structure that develops during embryogenesis in the ovarian medulla near the hilus are the origin of this tumor. However, by electron microscopy, the Sertolilike cells resemble ovarian granulosa cells more than they do male Sertoli cells.[165] Furthermore, both tumor cell types con-

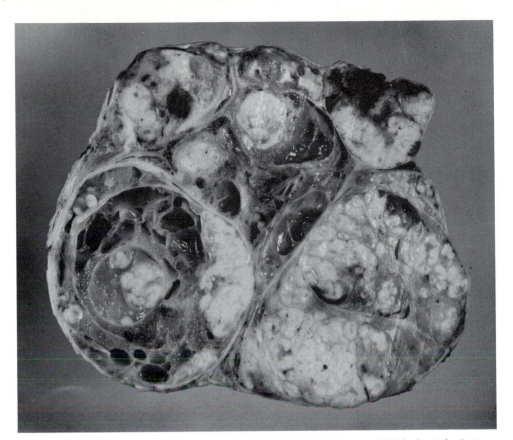

Fig. 869 Large Sertoli–Leydig cell tumor appearing in 17-year-old black girl. Patient had amenorrhea and increased body and facial hair. (WU neg. 69-7643.)

tain female sex chromatin.[168] It is perhaps more logical to think of these tumors as derived directly from specialized ovarian stromal cells through different stages of differentiation.[171] They are uncommon, comprising less than 0.1% of ovarian neoplasms. About 240 cases have been reported.[169] Those without demonstrable endocrine effect or accompanied by signs of hyperestrinism are often misdiagnosed. It is opportune to mention here that the diagnosis of stromal ovarian tumors should be made on the basis of their morphologic appearance rather than on the nature of their secretions. Terms such as "feminizing mesenchymoma" should be discarded.

Grossly, Sertoli–Leydig cell tumors are usually solid and composed of nodules of soft, gray tissue. There may be foci of hemorrhage and cyst formation (Fig. 869).

The microscopic pattern is extremely variable. The well-differentiated tubular pattern (type I of Meyer) is composed of tubules lined by Sertoli-like cells. Leydig-like cells may be found between the tubules (Fig. 870). The immediate form (type II) may vary widely from solid masses to anastomosing cords of Sertoli-like cells at times interspersed with small clusters and rows of Leydig-like cells (Fig. 871). The undifferentiated form is composed of masses of spindle-shaped cells in a "sarcomatoid" pattern (type III). Wide variations and admixtures of these patterns may appear in the same tumor. Unusual types of associated tissue such as cartilage have been described, and we have seen glandular areas composed of mucin-secreting cells.

Sertoli–Leydig cell tumors frequently occur in women 20 to 30 years of age.[167] They are relatively rare after menopause.

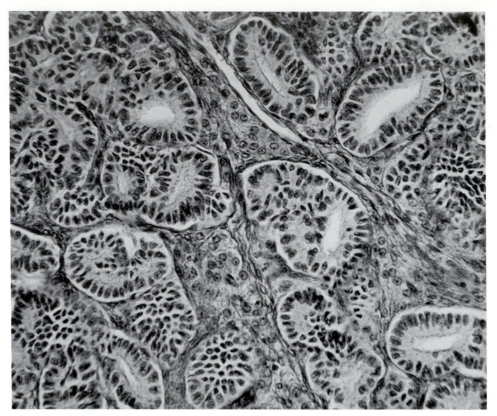

Fig. 870 Well-differentiated tubular type of Sertoli–Leydig cell tumor (Type I). This pattern is usually not associated with masculinization. Note clusters of Leydig cells in trabeculae between tubules. (×300; WU neg. 62-4716; slide contributed by Dr. W. Ober, New York, N. Y.)

Clinically, *defeminization* manifested by amenorrhea, atrophy of the breasts, and loss of subcutaneous fatty deposits is often the first expression of the disease. This is followed by signs of *masculinization*, such as hypertrophy of the clitoris and deepening of the voice. Usually prompt return of feminine characteristics follows excision of the tumor, but the manifestations of masculinization disappear more slowly.

Bilateral involvement of the ovaries is seen in fewer than 5% of the cases. The more differentiated tumors often produce no masculinizing effect, probably because they are almost exclusively composed of Sertoli-like cells. The main secretory activity of these tumors most likely resides in the Leydig-like cell. Urinary 17-keto-steroids are frequently normal even in the presence of masculinization, but elevations have been recorded. Tumor tissue incubated with progesterone caused a synthesis of androstenedione and 17-hydroxy-progesterone,[172] as well as testosterone.[170] The final aromatizing reaction to estrogens did not occur.

The prognosis is good in the large majority of the cases. Of twenty-nine patients with follow-up data studied by O'Hern and Neubecker,[168] only one had died of the tumor. Conservative surgery is indicated for the tumor grossly confined to one ovary.[163, 164]

Lipid cell tumors

A small group of ovarian tumors is composed of large, fat-containing cells. They are usually associated with a virilizing syndrome. A significant percentage of patients meet some of the criteria for

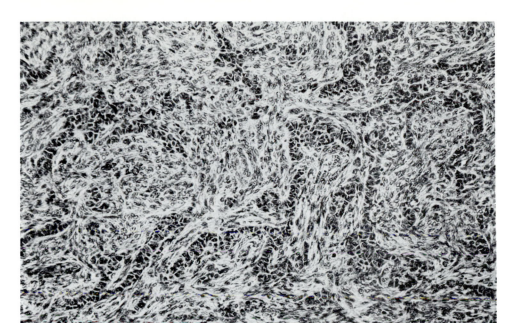

Fig. 871 Ovarian Sertoli–Leydig cell tumor (arrhenoblastoma, Type II of Meyer). This pattern of irregular branching rows of Sertoli cells mimics sex cord formation in embryonic testis prior to formation of lumina. Virilization syndrome occurs most frequently in this group, which is also most common. (×150; WU neg. 65-7788.)

Cushing's syndrome. [175, 177] The occasional demonstration of adrenal cortical rests around the ovary and broad ligament[176] has suggested a possible heterotopic source for adrenal tumors in this area. However, the existence of adrenal rest tumors in the ovary is questionable because the adrenal rests occur near, but never within, the ovary and because ovarian stromal cells have the biosynthetic capabilities to do everything claimed for the "adrenal" adenomas of the ovary.[178] As shown in Fig. 832, nonneoplastic ovarian stromal cells are capable of differentiating into large round cells with clear or foamy cytoplasm indistinguishable from cells of the adrenal cortex or the ovarian hilus. Theoretically, these tumors could arise from luteinized theca cells, luteinized stromal cells, or from hilus cells, in addition to the unlikely possibility of adrenal rests. With the excep-

tion of the few cases in which Reinke's crystalloids can be found (and the corresponding tumor thus categorized as hilus cell tumor), the exact origin usually remains undetermined.

The clinical findings will depend on how the pathways of hormone production have been altered in the neoplastic lipoid cells, not upon the histogenetic source of the cells. For this reason, the descriptive term *lipid cell tumor,*[180] together with a description of its effect, is preferable to "luteoma," "hypernephroma," "masculinovoblastoma," or adrenal cortical tumor. Enzymatic conversion studies performed on freshly excised tumors have demonstrated that a variety of androgenic hormones are produced by these tumors in vitro,[174, 179] and rarely large amounts of adrenal corticoids have been found.[173]

Lipid cell tumors are usually unilateral

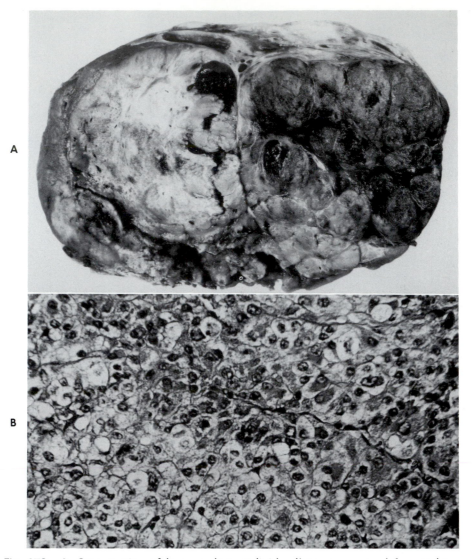

Fig. 872 **A,** Cross section of large malignant lipid cell tumor removed from right ovary of 75-year-old woman with mild hirsutism and marked elevation of blood testosterone level. Bright yellow areas alternate with darker foci. Ragged edge at lower margin corresponds to site of attachment to pelvic wall. **B,** Microscopic appearance of same tumor. Large cells with abundant lipid-containing cytoplasm alternate with smaller cells of deeply acidophilic cytoplasm. (**A,** WU neg. 73-1474; **B,** ×300; WU neg. 73-2074.)

and are composed of yellow or yellow-brown nodules separated by fibrous trabeculae (Fig. 872, A). Microscopically, they are characterized by masses of large rounded or polyhedral cells having abundant clear or pink cytoplasm and a small nucleus near the center (Fig. 872, B). Abundant cytoplasmic fat is readily demonstrable by specific stains.

In the series of thirty cases reported by

Taylor and Norris,[180] all age groups were represented. Although generally associated with defeminization and amenorrhea, a few tumors were apparently biologically inert. Ten percent of their cases met some of the criteria for Cushing's disease. The incidence of malignant change in this group was 20%. Malignant tumors tended to be larger than 8 cm in diameter, to be associated with peritoneal implants, and to have a more pleomorphic microscopic pattern. All of the tumors with Reinke's crystalloids followed a benign clinical course.

Mixed and indeterminate types

Rarely, a stromal tumor may be composed of a mixture of clearly identifiable granulosa–theca cell and Sertoli–Leydig cell elements. These tumors which are sometimes referred to as *gynandroblastomas,* may have androgenic, estrogenic, or no hormonal effects upon the patient.[181, 182]

In some tumors, the uniform pattern and nuclear grooving identify its stromal origin, but assignment to granulosa-theca or Sertoli–Leydig category is not possible on morphologic grounds. The indeterminate designation of "stromal tumor" is justified in such a case.

Within this category of stromal tumors not clearly classifiable into one of the types previously discussed is the benign neoplasm designated by Scully[183] as *sex cord tumor with annular tubules.* At least six of the thirteen cases he reviewed occurred in patients with the Peutz-Jeghers syndrome. Topographically, the lesion seems to arise from granulosa cells but grows in a pattern reminiscent of Sertoli cells. The most characteristic feature is the presence of simple and complex annular tubules containing eosinophilic hyaline bodies, often calcified. The appearance is remarkably similar to that seen in gonadoblastoma. The differential diagnosis is made on the basis of the clinical background and the presence in the latter of a germ cell component.

Tumors of germ cell and stromal origin

The most distinctive member of the group of tumors composed of both germ cells and stromal cells is the *gonadoblastoma.* This term is preferable to the formerly used dysgenetic gonadoma. It is a hormonally active gonadal tumor composed of a mixture of germ cells, stromal cells resembling granulosa cells, Sertoli cells, and, occasionally, cells resembling lutein

or Leydig cells. This tumor occurs practically always in sexually abnormal individuals, most commonly affected by mixed gonadal dysgenesis. The sex chromatin is usually negative, although exceptions have been recorded. It is often impossible to determine the nature of the gonad bearing the tumor. In some cases it has been identified as a streak and in others as a cryptorchid testis but never as a normal ovary. About 36% of the tumors are bilateral. They are usually quite small.

In Scully's series,[184] twenty-four became apparent only after microscopic study of the gonad. The clue to the microscopic diagnosis is the presence of areas in which primitive germ cells are mixed with stromal cells resembling immature Sertoli and granulosa cells. Leydig-like and luteinlike cells also may be present, especially after puberty. Hyalinization and calcification are common. The latter can become obvious on plain abdominal roentgenograms. The germ cell component may overgrow the stromal elements and result in the formation of a dysgerminoma or, exceptionally, other germ cell tumors. Only under these circumstances the tumor is endowed with a malignant potential.

In Teter's elaborate classification,[185] gonadoblastomas are divided in two types designated as gonocytomas type 2 and type 3 on the basis of rather questionable criteria. The ordinary dysgerminoma is called gonocytoma type 1 when pure and type 4 when associated with stromal luteinization.

Tumors of metastatic origin

The most common sources of ovarian metastases are the gastrointestinal tract and the breasts. Stone[189] reviewed 133 cases of secondary ovarian carcinoma and found 102 to be primary in the stomach or intestine. Young women with carcinoma of the breast undergoing surgical castration often are found to have ovarian metastases. Scully and Richardson[188] described hormonal changes (usually masculinizing) in patients with metastatic

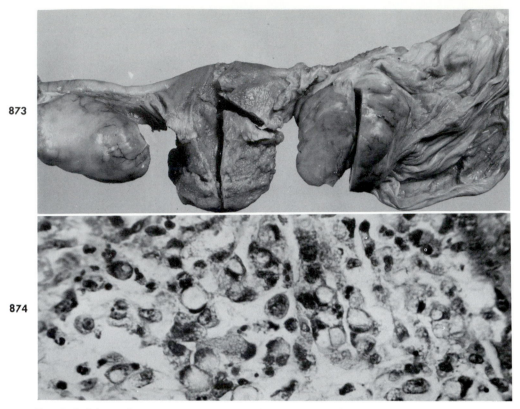

873

874

Fig. 873 Bilateral metastatic carcinoma of ovary (Krukenberg tumor) appearing in young woman. Primary tumor was in stomach. (WU neg. 52-563.)
Fig. 874 Signet ring cells in metastatic carcinoma (Krukenberg tumor) of ovary. (×540; WU neg. 52-140.)

ovarian cancer associated with—and probably due to—stromal luteinization. This curious effect was most often seen with metastases from large bowel tumors.

The eponym Krukenberg tumor is used to designate a bilateral ovarian neoplasm, practically always of metastatic origin, characterized grossly by moderate multinodular enlargement of the ovaries and microscopically by a diffuse infiltration by signet-ring cells containing abundant mucin[187] (Figs. 873 and 874). Marked stromal proliferation is common and may obscure the diagnosis.[191] Although most examples of Krukenberg tumors occur in women after the age of 40 years, we have seen several cases in much younger patients. The latter were often confused with granulosa cell tumors and lipoid cell tumors. The primary source is usually the

gastrointestinal tract, particularly the stomach. Retroperitoneal lymph node metastases are usually present. Tumor cells probably travel in a retrograde fashion to the ovary via these lymph nodes and ovarian lymphatics. Peritoneal implantation may coexist. In the series of forty-one Krukenberg tumors reported by Warren and Macomber,[190] carcinoma of the breast was as frequent a source as gastrointestinal carcinoma.

Exceptionally, a primary tumor cannot be found at autopsy in patients with Krukenberg's tumor. These are assumed to be primary in the ovary.[186] Before accepting such an occurrence, a meticulous gross and microscopic study of every organ should be carried out. In the only case that we were almost ready to accept as primary Krukenberg tumor of the ovaries, a ran-

Table 35 Relative malignant potential of ovarian neoplasms

Negligible	Low	High
Serous, mucinous, and endometrioid cystadenomas	Serous, mucinous, and endometrioid tumors of indeterminate type	Serous, mucinous, and endometrioid cystadenocarcinomas
Brenner tumor	Dysgerminoma	Clear cell ("mesonephric") adenocarcinoma
Adult teratoma, cystic and solid Struma ovarii	Carcinoid tumor	Malignant mixed müllerian tumor Yolk sac tumor
Thecoma-fibroma	Granulosa cell tumor Sertoli–Leydig cell tumor	Choriocarcinoma Embryonal teratoma
Gonadoblastoma (without germ cell tumor)	Lipid cell tumor	Adenocarcinoma and undifferentiated carcinoma

dom section through a grossly unremarkable gastric antrum revealed diffuse infiltration by signet-ring cells.

Prognosis

Unfortunately, the overall five-year survival rate of patients with malignant ovarian tumors is extremely poor. Munnell and Taylor[194] reviewed 200 primary tumors of the ovary seen at the Sloane Hospital for Women. They emphasized that 60% of the patients had a hopeless prognosis and died within eighteen months. After eighteen months, the rate of dying slowed so that during the next five years only 10% or 12% died. This mortality probably is related to the lack of symptoms during the early stages of these tumors and to their rather rapid growth rate.

The most important signs and symptoms of malignant ovarian tumors include lower abdominal pain, abdominal enlargement, and signs of increased pressure on neighboring organs. The prognosis is influenced by the type of tumor (Table 35). Dysgerminomas, granulosa cell tumors, and Sertoli–Leydig cell tumors have a low malignant potential and often the patients are cured. Unfortunately, these tumors make up but a small proportion of ovarian tumors.[193, 195]

There is a direct correlation between the differentiation of the serous tumors and the prognosis. Similarly, some correlation also exists with grading of mucinous tumors. The most important pathologic

finding is spread of tumor beyond the ovary. This spread frequently is associated with ascites, which makes the prognosis more unfavorable. The solid tumors generally are more malignant than the cystic ones.

REFERENCES

Introduction

1 Carpenter, C. C.: Consideration of physiology and pathology in gynecology; analysis of 2,933 surgical specimens, Trans. Med. Soc. North Carolina 83:236-242, 1936.

2 Miller, N. F., and Willson, J. R.: Surgery of the ovary; the small ovarian cysts, N. Y. State J. Med. 42:1851-1855, 1942.

Gonadal dysgenesis

3 Federman, D. D.: Abnormal sexual development; a genetic and endocrine approach to differential diagnosis, Philadelphia, 1967, W. B. Saunders Co.

4 Ferenczy, A., and Richart, R. M.: The fine structure of the gonads in the complete form of testicular feminization syndrome, Am. J. Obstet. Gynecol. 113:399-409, 1972.

5 Jones, H. W., Ferguson-Smith, M. A., and Heller, R. H.: The pathology and cytogenetics of gonadal agenesis, Am. J. Obstet. Gynecol. 87:578-600, 1963.

6 Jones, H. W., Ferguson-Smith, M. A., and Heller, R. H.: Pathologic and cytogenetic findings in true hermaphroditism; report of 6 cases and review of 23 cases from the literature, Obstet. Gynecol. 25:435-447, 1965.

7 Melicow, M. M., and Uson, A. C.: Dysgenetic gonadomas and other gonadal neoplasms in intersexes, Cancer 12:552-572, 1959.

8 Morris, J. M.: The syndrome of testicular feminization in male pseudohermaphrodites, Am. J. Obstet. Gynecol. 65:1192-1211, 1953.

9 Neubecker, R. D., and Theiss, E. A.: Sertoli

cell adenomas in patients with testicular feminization, Am. J. Clin. Pathol. 38:52-59, 1962.

10 Sohval, A. R.: The syndrome of pure gonadal dysgenesis, Am. J. Med. 38:615-625, 1965.

11 Taylor, H., Barter, R. H., and Jacobson, C. B.: Neoplasms of dysgenetic gonads, Am. J. Obstet. Gynecol. 96:816-823, 1966.

**Nonneoplastic cysts
and stromal hyperplasia**

12 Berger, L.: Tumeur des cellules sympathicotropes de l'ovaire avec virilisation, Rev. Canad. Biol. 1:539-566, 1942.

13 Dhom, G.: Morphologische, quantitative und histochemische Studien zur Function der Hiluszellen des Ovars, Z. Geburtshilfe Gynaekol. 142:183-228, 1954.

14 Goldzieher, J. W., and Green, J. A.: The polycystic ovary. I. Clinical and histologic features, J. Clin. Endocrinol. 22:325-338, 1962.

15 Hoyt, W. F., and Meigs, J. V.: Rupture of the graafian follicle and corpus luteum, Surg. Gynecol. Obstet. 62:114-117, 1936.

16 Jackson, R. L., and Dockerty, M. B.: The Stein-Leventhal syndrome: analysis of 43 cases with special reference to association with endometrial carcinoma, Am. J. Obstet. Gynecol. 73:161-173, 1957.

17 Leventhal, M. L.: Functional and morphologic studies of the ovaries and suprarenal glands in the Stein-Leventhal syndrome, Am. J. Obstet. Gynecol. 84:154-164, 1962.

18 Lucis, O. J., Hobkirk, R., Hollenberg, C. H., MacDonald, S. A., and Blahey, P.: Polycystic ovaries associated with congenital adrenal hyperplasia, Can. Med. Assoc. J. 94: 1-7, 1966.

19 Merrill, J. A.: Ovarian hilus cells, Am. J. Obstet. Gynecol. 78:1258-1271, 1959.

20 Morris, J. M., and Scully, R. E.: Endocrine pathology of the ovary, St. Louis, 1958, The C. V. Mosby Co.

21 Norris, H. J., and Taylor, H. B.: Nodular thecalutein hyperplasia of pregnancy (so-called "pregnancy luteoma"), Am. J. Clin. Pathol. 47:557-566, 1967.

22 Ober, W. B., Grady, H. G., and Schoenbucher, A. K.: Ectopic ovarian decidua without pregnancy, Am. J. Pathol. 33:199-217, 1957.

23 Sternberg, W. H.: The morphology, androgenic function, hyperplasia and tumors of the human ovarian hilus cells, Am. J. Pathol. 25:493-521, 1949.

24 Sternberg, W. H., and Barclay, D. L.: Luteoma of pregnancy, Am. J. Obstet. Gynecol. 95:165-184, 1966.

25 Sternberg, W. H., Segaloff, A., and Gaskill, C. J.: Influence of chorionic gonadotrophin on human ovarian hilus cells (Leydig-like

cells), J. Clin. Endocrinol. 13:139-153, 1953.

26 Zourlas, P. A., and Jones, H. W., Jr.: Stein-Leventhal syndrome with masculinizing ovarian tumors; report of 3 cases, Obstet. Gynecol. 34:861-866, 1969.

Endometriosis

27 Devereux, W. P.: Endometriosis; long-term observation with particular reference to incidence of pregnancy, Obstet. Gynecol. 22: 444-450, 1963.

28 Fallon, J., Brosnan, J. T., and Moran, W. G.: Endometriosis, N. Engl. J. Med. 235:669-673, 1946.

29 Pratt, J. H., and Shamblin, W. R.: Spontaneous rupture of endometrial cysts of the ovary presenting as an acute abdominal emergency, Am. J. Obstet. Gynecol. 108:56-62, 1970.

Biopsy

30 Mori, T.: Histological and histochemical studies of human anovulatory ovaries correlated with endocrinological analysis, Acta Obstet. Gynaecol. Jap. 16:156-164, 1969.

31 Steele, S. J., Beilbui, J. O. W., and Papadaki, L.: Visualization and biopsy of the ovary in the investigation of amenorrhea, Obstet. Gynecol. 36:899-902, 1970.

32 Stevenson, C. S.: The ovaries in infertile women: a clinical and pathologic study of 81 women having ovarian surgery at laparotomy, Fertil. Steril. 21:411-425, 1970.

Tumors
Embryology

33 Gillman, J.: The development of the gonads in man, with a consideration of the role of fetal endocrines and the histogenesis of ovarian tumors, Contrib. Embryol. 32:83-131, 1948 (Carnegie Institute of Washington).

34 Pinkerton, J. H. M., McKay, D. G., Adams, E. L., and Hertig, A. T.: Development of the human ovary—a study using histochemical technics, Obstet. Gynecol. 18:152-181, 1961.

35 Witschi, E.: Migration of the germ cells of human embryos from the yolk sac to the primitive gonadal folds, Contrib. Embryol. 32: 69-80, 1948 (Carnegie Institute of Washington).

Classification

36 Hertig, A. T., and Gore, H.: Tumors of the female sex organs. Part 3. Tumors of the ovary and fallopian tube. In Atlas of tumor pathology, Sect. IX, Fasc. 33, Washington, D. C., 1961, Armed Forces Institute of Pathology.

37 Scully, R. E.: Recent progress in ovarian cancer, Hum. Pathol. 1:73-98, 1970.

Tumors of surface (müllerian) epithelial origin
with or without stromal component
  Serous, mucinous, and endometrioid tumors

38 Abell, M. R., and Holtz, F.: Ovarian neo-plasms in childhood and adolescence. II. Tumors of non-germ cell origin, Am. J. Obstet. Gynecol. **93**:850-866, 1965.

39 Aure, J. C., Høeg, K., and Kolstad, P.: Psammoma bodies in serous carcinoma of the ovary; a prognostic study, Am. J. Obstet. Gynecol. **109**:113-118, 1971.

40 Brakemann, O.: Zur Histologie und Klinik der papillären ovarialtumoren, Arch. Gynaekol. **164**:69-87, 1937.

41 Campbell, J. S., Magner, D., and Fournier, P.: Adenoacanthomas of ovary and uterus occurring as coexistent or sequential primary neoplasms, Cancer **14**:817-826, 1961.

42 Cariker, M., and Dockerty, M.: Mucinous cystadenoma and mucinous cystadenocarcinoma of the ovary, Cancer **7**:302-310, 1954.

43 Compton, H. L., and Finck, F. M.: Serous adenofibroma and cystadenofibroma of the ovary, Obstet. Gynecol. **36**:636-645, 1970.

44 Corner, G. W., Jr., Hu, C. Y., and Hertig, A. T.: Ovarian carcinoma arising in endometriosis, Am. J. Obstet. Gynecol. **59**:760-774, 1950.

45 Czernobilsky, B., Silverman, B. B., and Mikuta, J. J.: Endometrioid carcinoma of the ovary; a clinicopathologic study of 75 cases, Cancer **26**:1141-1152, 1970.

46 Greene, J. W., and Enterline, H. T.: Carcinoma arising in endometriosis, Obstet. Gynecol. **9**:417-421, 1957.

47 Hart, W. R., and Norris, H. J.: Borderline and malignant mucinous tumors of the ovary, Cancer **31**:1031-1045, 1973.

48 Hertig, A. T.: Proceedings of Eighteenth Seminar of the American Society of Clinical Pathologists, October, 1952, Chicago, Ill.

49 Kay, S.: Carcinoma with squamous metaplasia of the ovary (so-called adenoacanthoma), Am. J. Obstet. Gynecol. **81**:763-772, 1961.

50 Kistner, R. W., and Hertig, A. T.: Primary adenoacanthoma of the ovary, Cancer **5**:1134-1145, 1952.

51 Long, M. E., and Taylor, H. C., Jr.: Endometrioid carcinoma of the ovary, Am. J. Obstet. Gynecol. **90**:936-950, 1964.

52 Marchetti, A. A.: Ovarian cancer: clinicopathologic evaluation, N. Y. State J. Med. **41**:2324-2331, 1941.

53 Masson, P.: Sur la présence de cellules argentaffines des les kystes pseudomucineux de l'ovarie, Un. Méd. Canada **67**:2-5, 1938.

54 Reagan, J. W.: Histopathology of ovarian pseudomucinous cystadenoma, Am. J. Pathol. **25**:689-708, 1949.

55 Roberts, D. K., Marshall, R. B., and Wharton, J. T.: Ultrastructure of ovarian tumors.

I. Papillary serous cystadenocarcinoma, Cancer **25**:947-958, 1970.

56 Samson, J. A.: Endometrial carcinoma of the ovary arising in endometrial tissue in that organ, Arch. Surg. **10**:1-72, 1925.

57 Santesson, L.: Proposal for the classification of the common epithelial ovarian tumors. Cancer Committee of the International Federation of Gynecology, Aug. 7, 1961.

58 Schueller, E. F., and Kirol, P. M.: Prognosis in endometrioid carcinoma of the ovary, Obstet. Gynecol. **27**:850-858, 1966.

59 Scully, R. E., Richardson, G. S., and Barlow, J. F.: The development of malignancy in endometriosis, Clin. Obstet. Gynecol. **9**:384-411, 1966.

60 Taylor, H. C., Jr., and Greeley, A. V.: Factors influencing the end-results in carcinoma of the ovary, Surg. Gynecol. Obstet. **74**:928-934, 1942.

61 Teilum, G.: Classification of ovarian tumours, Acta Obstet. Gynecol. Scand. **31**:292-312, 1952.

62 Woodruff, J. D., Bie, L. S., and Sherman, R. J.: Mucinous tumors of the ovary, Obstet. Gynecol. **16**:699-711, 1960.

Clear cell ("mesonephric") adenocarcinoma

63 Czernobilsky, B., Silverman, B. B., and Enterline, H. T.: Clear-cell carcinoma of the ovary; a clinicopathologic analysis of pure and mixed forms and comparison with endometrioid carcinoma, Cancer **25**:762-772, 1970.

64 Norris, H. J., and Robinowitz, M.: Ovarian adenocarcinoma of mesonephric type, Cancer **28**:1074-1081, 1971.

65 Schiller, W.: Mesonephroma ovarii, Am. J. Cancer **35**:1-21, 1939.

66 Scully, R. E., and Barlow, J. F.: Mesonephroma of the ovary; tumor of müllerian nature related to the endometrioid carcinoma, Cancer **20**:1405-1417, 1967.

Brenner tumor

67 Abell, M. R.: Malignant Brenner tumors of the ovary, Cancer **10**:1263-1274, 1957.

68 Arey, L. B.: Origin and form of Brenner tumor, Am. J. Obstet. Gynecol. **81**:743-751, 1961.

69 Ehrlich, C. E., and Roth, L. M.: The Brenner tumor; a clinicopathologic study of 75 cases, Cancer **27**:332-342, 1971.

70 Fox, R. A.: Brenner tumors of the ovary, Am. J. Pathol. **18**:223-235, 1942 (extensive bibliography).

71 Hallgrimsson, J., and Scully, R. E.: Borderline and malignant Brenner tumours of the ovary; a report of 15 cases, Acta Pathol. Microbiol. Scand. **233**(suppl.):56-66, 1972.

72 Hertig, A. T., and Gore, H.: Tumors of female sex organs. Part 3. Tumors of the ovary

and fallopian tube. In Atlas of tumor Pathology, Sect. IX, Fasc. 33, Washington, D. C., 1961, Armed Forces Institute of Pathology.

73 Kent, S. W., and McKay, D. G.: Primary cancer of the ovary, Am. J. Obstet. Gynecol. 80:430-438, 1960.

74 Klein, H. Z., Strauss, S. H., and Unger, A. M.: Coexisting Brenner tumor and struma ovarii (mature gonadoblastoma); report of a case, Obstet. Gynecol. 31:779-784, 1968.

75 Meyer, R.: Der Tumor ovarii Brenner eine besondere Art von Geschwulst und ihre Stellung unter den Geschwulsten des Eierstocks, Z. Geburtshilfe Gynaekol. 101:800-802, 1932.

76 Miles, P. A., and Norris, H. J.: Proliferative and malignant Brenner tumors of the ovary, Cancer 30:174-186, 1972.

77 Ming, S. C., and Goldman, H.: Hormonal activity of Brenner tumors in postmenopausal women, Am. J. Obstet. Gynecol. 83:666-673, 1962.

78 Muller, J. H.: Les nodules et kystes paramalpighiens à la surface de l'ovaire, de la trompe et du ligament large, Ann. Anat. Pathol. (Paris) 11:483-498, 1934.

79 Roth, L. M.: Fine structure of the Brenner tumor, Cancer 27:1482-1488, 1971.

80 Roth, L. M., and Sternberg, W. H.: Proliferating Brenner tumors, Cancer 27:687-693, 1971.

81 Silverberg, S. G.: Brenner tumor of the ovary; a clinicopathologic study of 60 tumors in 54 women, Cancer 28:588-596, 1971.

82 Teoh, T. B.: Further observations on the histogenesis of minute and small Brenner tumours, J. Pathol. Bacteriol. 78:145-150, 1959.

83 Woodruff, J. D., and Acosta, A. A.: Variations in the Brenner tumor, Am. J. Obstet. Gynecol. 83:657-665, 1962.

Malignant mixed müllerian tumor

84 Dehner, L. P., Norris, H. J., and Taylor, H. B.: Carcinosarcomas and mixed mesodermal tumors of the ovary, Cancer 27:207-216, 1971.

85 Fenn, M. E., and Abell, M. R.: Carcinosarcoma of the ovary, Am. J. Obstet. Gynecol. 110:1066-1074, 1971.

Tumors of germ cell origin
  Dysgerminoma

86 Abell, M. R., Johnson, V. J., and Holtz, F.: Ovarian neoplasms in childhood and adolescence, Am. J. Obstet. Gynecol. 92:1059-1081, 1965.

87 Asadourian, L. A., and Taylor, H. B.: Dysgerminoma; an analysis of 105 cases, Obstet. Gynecol. 33:370-379, 1969.

88 Breen, J. L., and Neubecker, R. D.: Dysgerminoma of the ovary; an analysis of 68

cases (presented at the tenth annual clinical meeting of the American College of Obstetricians & Gynecologists, April 1-4, 1962, Chicago, Ill.).

89 Brody, S.: Clinical aspects of dysgerminoma of the ovary, Acta Radiol. (Stockh.) 56:209-230, 1961.

90 Kay, S., Silverberg, S. G., and Schatzki, P. F.: Ultrastructure of an ovarian dysgerminoma, Am. J. Clin. Pathol. 58:458-468, 1972.

91 Malkasian, G. D., and Symmonds, R. E.: Treatment of the unilateral encapsulated ovarian germinoma, Am. J. Obstet. Gynecol. 90:379-382, 1964.

92 Moreton, R. D., and Desjardins, A.: Dysgerminoma of the ovary; a review of 11 cases of proved tumor with special reference to radiosensitivity, Am. J. Roentgenol. Radium Ther. Nucl. Med. 57:84-90, 1947.

93 Morris, J. M., and Scully, R. E.: Endocrine pathology of the ovary, St. Louis, 1958, The C. V. Mosby Co.

94 Novak, E., and Gray, L. A.: Dysgerminoma of the ovary, Am. J. Obstet. Gynecol. 35:925-937, 1938.

95 Potter, E. B.: Dysgerminoma of the ovary, Am. J. Pathol. 22:551-563, 1946.

96 Santesson, L.: Clinical and pathological survey of ovarian tumors treated at the Radiumhemmet, Acta Radiol. (Stockh.) 28:643-668, 1947.

97 Theiss, E. A., Ashley, D. J. B., and Mostofi, F. K.: Nuclear sex of testicular tumors and some related ovarian and extragonadal neoplasms, Cancer 13:323-327, 1959.

Yolk sac tumor (endodermal sinus tumor; embryonal carcinoma)

98 Huntington, R. W., and Bullock, W. K.: Yolk sac tumors of the ovary, Cancer 25:1357-1367, 1970.

99 Neubecker, R. D., and Breen, J. L.: Embryonal carcinoma of the ovary, Cancer 15:546-556, 1962.

100 Schiller, W.: Mesonephroma ovarii, Am. J. Cancer 35:1-21, 1939.

101 Teilum, G.: Endodermal sinus tumors of the ovary and testis; comparative morphogenesis of the so-called mesonephroma ovarii (Schiller) and extraembryonic (yolk-sac-allantoic) structures of the rat's placenta, Cancer 12:1092-1105, 1959.

Choriocarcinoma

102 Marrubini, G.: Primary chorionepithelioma of the ovary, Am. J. Obstet. Gynecol. Scand. 28:251-284, 1949.

Embryonal teratoma

103 Scully, R. E.: Recent progress in ovarian cancer, Hum. Pathol. 1:73-98, 1970.

Adult solid teratoma

104 Benirschke, K., Easterday, C., and Abramson, D.: Malignant solid teratoma of the ovary: report of three cases, Obstet. Gynecol. **15:** 512-521, 1960.

105 Peterson, W. F.: Solid, histologically benign teratomas of the ovary: a report of four cases and review of the literature, Am. J. Obstet. Gynecol. **72:**1094-1102, 1956.

106 Thurlbeck, W. M., and Scully, R. E.: Solid teratoma of the ovary; a clinicopathological analysis of 9 cases, Cancer **13:**804-811, 1960.

Adult cystic teratoma, benign and with malignant change

107 Auer, E. A., Dockerty, M. B., and Mayo, C. W.: Ruptured dermoid cyst of the ovary simulating abdominal carcinomatosis, Mayo Clin. Proc. **26:**489-497, 1951.

108 Blackwell, W. J., Dockerty, M. B., Masson, J. C., and Mussey, R. D.: Dermoid cysts of the ovary: their clinical and pathologic significance, Am. J. Obstet. Gynecol. **51:** 151-172, 1946.

109 Climie, A. R. W., and Heath, L. P.: Malignant degeneration of benign cystic teratomas of the ovary; review of the literature and report of a chondrosarcoma and carcinoid tumor, Cancer **22:**824-832, 1968.

110 Ein, S. H., Darte, J. M. M., and Stephens, C. A.: Cystic and solid ovarian tumors in children: a 44-year review, J. Pediatr. Surg. **5:**148-156, 1970.

111 Emge, L. A.: Functional and growth characteristics of struma ovarii, Am. J. Obstet. Gynecol. **40:**738-750, 1940.

112 Fortt, R. W., and Mathie, I. K.: Gliomatosis peritonei caused by ovarian teratoma, J. Clin. Pathol. **22:**348-353, 1969.

113 Kelley, R. R., and Scully, R. E.: Cancer developing in dermoid cysts of the ovary, Cancer **14:**989-1000, 1961.

114 Kent, S. W., and McKay, D. G.: Primary cancer of the ovary, Am. J. Obstet. Gynecol. **80:**430-438, 1960.

115 Peterson, W. F.: Malignant degeneration of benign cystic teratomas of the ovary; a collective review of the literature, Obstet. Gynecol. Survey **12:**793-830, 1957.

116 Plaut, A.: Ovarian struma: a morphologic, pharmacologic, and biologic examination, Am. J. Obstet. Gynecol. **25:**351-360, 1933.

117 Rashad, M. H., Fathalla, M. F., and Kerr, M. G.: Sex chromatin and chromosome analysis in ovarian teratomas, Am. J. Obstet. Gynecol. **96:**461-465, 1966.

118 Robboy, S. J., and Scully, R. E.: Ovarian teratoma with glial implants on the peritoneum; an analysis of 12 cases, Hum. Pathol. **1:**644-653, 1970.

119 Theiss, E. A., Ashley, D. J. B., and Mostofi, F. K.: Nuclear sex of testicular tumors and some related ovarian and extragonadal neoplasms, Cancer **13:**323-327, 1959.

Struma ovarii

120 Emge, L. A.: Functional and growth characteristics of struma ovarii, Am. J. Obstet. Gynecol. **40:**738-750, 1940.

121 Plaut, A.: Ovarian struma: a morphologic, pharmacologic, and biologic examination, Am. J. Obstet. Gynecol. **25:**351-360, 1933.

Carcinoid tumor

122 Blackwell, W. J., and Dockerty, M. B.: Argentaffin carcinoma (carcinoid tumor) arising in an ovarian dermoid cyst, Am. J. Obstet. Gynecol. **51:**575-577, 1946.

123 Doucette, J. W., and Estes, W. B.: Primary ovarian carcinoid tumors; case report and review of the literature, Obstet. Gynecol. **25:** 94-101, 1965.

124 Saunders, A. M., and Hertman, V. O.: Malignant carcinoid teratoma of the ovary, Can. Med. Assoc. J. **83:**602-605, 1960.

125 Scully, R. E.: Recent progress in ovarian cancer, Hum. Pathol. **1:**73-98, 1970.

Tumors of stromal origin

126 Mostofi, F. K., Theiss, E. A., and Ashley, D. J. B.: Tumors of specialized gonadal stroma in human male patients; androblastoma, Sertoli cell tumor, granulosa-theca cell tumor of the testis, and gonadal stroma tumor, Cancer **12:**944-957, 1959.

127 O'Hern, T. M., and Neubecker, R. D.: Arrhenoblastoma of the ovary, Obstet. Gynecol. **19:**758-770, 1962.

128 Scully, R. E., and Morris, J. McL.: Functioning ovarian tumors. In Meigs, J. V., and Sturgis, S. H.: Progress in gynecology, vol. 3, New York, 1957, Grune & Stratton, Inc., p. 20.

129 Teilum, G.: Estrogen-producing Sertoli cell tumors (androblastoma tubulare lipoides) of the human testis and ovary; homologous ovarian and testicular tumors, J. Clin. Endocrinol. **9:**301-318, 1949.

Granulosa cell tumor

130 Hodgson, J. E., Dockerty, M. B., and Mussey, R. D.: Granulosa cell tumor of the ovary, Surg. Gynecol. Obstet. **81:**631-642, 1945.

131 Ingraham, C. B., Black, W. C., and Rutledge, E. K.: The relationship of granulosa cell tumors of the ovary to endometrial carcinoma, Am. J. Obstet. Gynecol. **48:**760-773, 1944.

132 Kottmeier, H. L.: Personal communication.

133 Norris, H. J., and Taylor, H. B.: Prognosis of granulosa-theca tumors of the ovary, Cancer **21:**255-263, 1968.

134 Norris, H. J., and Taylor, H. B.: Virilization

associated with cystic granulosa tumors, Obstet. Gynecol. **34**:629-635, 1969.

135 Novak, E. R., Kutchmeshgi, J., Mupas, R. S., and Woodruff, J. D.: Feminizing gonadal stromal tumors; analysis of the granulosa-theca cell tumors of the ovarian tumor registry, Obstet. Gynecol. **38**:701-713, 1971.

136 Scully, R. E.: Recent progress in ovarian cancer, Hum. Pathol. **1**:73-98, 1970.

137 Traut, H. F., and Butterworth, M. M.: The theca, granulosa, lutein cell tumors of the human ovary and similar tumors of the mouse's ovary, Am. J. Obstet. Gynecol. **34**:987-1003, 1937.

138 Traut, H. F., Kuder, A., and Cadden, J. S.: A study of the reticulum and of luteinization in granulosa and theca cell tumors of the ovary, Am. J. Obstet. Gynecol. **38**:798-814, 1939.

139 Varangot, J.: Les tumeurs de la granulosa (folliculomes de l'ovaire), J. Chir. (Paris) **51**:651-681, 1938.

Thecoma-fibroma

140 Amin, H. K., Okagaki, T., and Richart, R. M.: Classification of fibroma and thecoma of the ovary; an ultrastructural study, Cancer **27**:438-446, 1971.

141 Dockerty, M. B., and Masson, J. C.: Ovarian fibromas: a clinical and pathologic study of two hundred and eighty-three cases, Am. J. Obstet. Gynecol. **47**:741-752, 1944.

142 Henderson, D. N.: Granulosa and theca cell tumors of the ovary, Trans. Am. Assoc. Obstet. Gynecol. Abd. Surg. **54**:86-103, 1941.

143 Jew, E. W., Jr., and Gross, P.: Malignant thecoma with metastases, Am. J. Obstet. Gynecol. **69**:857-860, 1955.

144 Kalstone, C. E., Jaffe, R. B., and Abell, M. R.: Massive edema of the ovary simulating fibroma, Obstet. Gynecol. **34**:564-571, 1969.

145 McGoldrick, J. L., and Lapp, W. A.: Theca cell tumors of the ovary, Am. J. Obstet. Gynecol. **48**:409-416, 1944.

146 Meigs, J. V.: Pelvic tumors other than fibromas of the ovary with ascites and hydrothorax, Obstet. Gynecol. **3**:471-486, 1954.

147 Meigs, J. V., and Cass, J. W.: Fibroma of the ovary with ascites and hydrothorax, Am. J. Obstet. Gynecol. **33**:249-266, 1937.

148 Meigs, J. V., Armstrong, S. H., and Hamilton, H. H.: A further contribution to the syndrome of fibroma of the ovary with fluid in the abdomen and chest, Meigs' syndrome, Am. J. Obstet. Gynecol. **46**:19-37, 1943.

149 Samanth, K. K., and Black, W. C., III.: Benign ovarian stromal tumors associated with free peritoneal fluid, Am. J. Obstet. Gynecol. **107**:538-545, 1970.

150 Sternberg, W. H., and Gaskill, C. J.: Theca-

cell tumors, Am. J. Obstet. Gynecol. **59**:575-587, 1950.

151 Wolfe, S. A., and Neigus, I.: Theca cell tumors of the ovary, Am. J. Obstet. Gynecol. **42**:218-228, 1941.

Effects of hyperestrogenism in granulosa cell tumors and thecoma/Occurrence of carcinoma of endometrium with granulosa cell tumors and thecomas

152 Dempsey, E. W., and Bassett, D. L.: Observations on the fluorescence, birefringence and histochemistry of the rat ovary during the reproduction cycle, Endocrinology **33**:384-401, 1943.

153 Greene, R. R., Roddick, J. W., Jr., and Milligan, M.: Estrogens, endometrial hyperplasia, and endometrial carcinoma, Ann. N. Y. Acad. Sci. **75**:586-600, 1959.

154 Gusberg, S. B., and Kardon, P.: Proliferative endometrial response to theca-granulosa cell tumors, Am. J. Obstet. Gynecol. **111**:633-643, 1971.

155 Henderson, D. N.: Granulosa and theca cell tumors of the ovary, Trans. Am. Assoc. Obstet. Gynecol. Abd. Surg. **54**:86-103, 1941.

156 Kottmeier, H. L.: Ueber Blutungen in der Menopause, Acta Obstet. Gynecol. Scand. **27** (suppl. 6):1-227, 1947.

157 McKay, D. G., and Robinson, D.: Observations on the fluorescence, birefringence and histochemistry of the human ovary during the menstrual cycle, Endocrinology **41**:378-394, 1947.

158 McKay, D. G., Robinson, D., and Hertig, A. T.: Histochemical observations on granulosa cell tumors, thecomas and fibromas of the ovary, Am. J. Obstet. Gynecol. **58**:625-639, 1949.

159 Norris, H. J., and Taylor, H. B.: Prognosis of granulosa-theca tumors of the ovary, Cancer **21**:255-263, 1968.

160 Novak, E., and Rutledge, F.: Atypical endometrial hyperplasia simulating adenocarcinoma, Am. J. Obstet. Gynecol. **55**:46-61, 1948.

161 Sjöstedt, S., and Wahlen, T.: Prognosis of granulosa cell tumors, Acta Obstet. Gynecol. Scand. **40**(suppl. 6):1-26, 1961.

162 Stohr, G.: Granuloma cell tumor of the ovary and coincident carcinoma of the uterus, Am. J. Obstet. Gynecol. **43**:586-599, 1942.

Sertoli–Leydig cell tumor (arrhenoblastoma; androblastoma)

163 Dockerty, M. B.: Arrhenoblastoma, Mayo Clin. Proc. **14**:369-374, 1939.

164 Hughesdon, P. E., and Fraser, I. T.: Arrhenoblastoma of ovary, Acta Obstet. Gynecol. Scand. **32**:1-78, 1953.

165 Jenson, A. B., and Fechner, R. E.: Ultra-

structure of an intermediate Sertoli-Leydig cell tumor; a histogenetic misnomer, Lab. Invest. **21**:527-535, 1969.

166 Meyer, R.: Tubuläre (testikuläre) und solide Foramen des Andreiblastoma ovarii und ihre Beziehung zur Vermännlickung, Beitr. Pathol. Anat. **84**:485-520, 1930.

167 Novak, E.: Masculinizing tumors of the ovary, Am. J. Obstet. Gynecol. **36**:840-858, 1938.

168 O'Hern, T. M., and Neubecker, R. D.: Arrhenoblastoma of the ovary, Obstet. Gynecol. **19**:758-770, 1962.

169 Pedowitz, P., and O'Brien, F. B.: Arrhenoblastoma of the ovary; review of the literature and report of 2 cases, Obstet. Gynecol. **16**:62-77, 1960.

170 Savard, K., Gut, M., Dorfman, R. I., Gabrilove, J. L., and Soffer, L. J.: Formation of androgens by human arrhenoblastoma tissue *in vitro*, J. Clin. Endocrinol. **21**:165-174, 1961.

171 Taylor, H. B.: Functioning ovarian tumors and related conditions. In Sommers, S. C., editor: Pathology annual, vol. 1, New York, 1966, Appleton-Century-Crofts, pp. 127-147.

172 Wiest, W. G., Zander, J., and Holmstrom, E. G.: Metabolism of progesterone-4-C[14] by an arrhenoblastoma, J. Clin. Endocrinol. **19**:297-305, 1959.

Lipid cell tumors

173 Bauer, J., and Karl, J.: Der chemische und krystalline Nachweiss von androgenen und corticoiden Wirkstoffen aus Urin und Geschwulstgewebe bei virilisierendem Ovarialtumor, Z. Gesamte Exp. Med. **118**:425-452, 1952.

174 Bryson, M. J., Dominguez, O. V., Kaiser, I. H., Samuels, L. T., and Sweat, M. L.: Enzymatic steroid conversions in masculinovoblastoma, J. Clin. Endocrinol. **22**:773-783, 1962.

175 Kepler, E. J., Dockerty, M. B., and Priestley, J. T.: Adrenal-like ovarian tumor associated with Cushing's syndrome (so-called masculinovoblastoma, luteoma, hypernephroma, adrenal cortical carcinoma of the ovary), Am. J. Obstet. Gynecol. **47**:43-62, 1944.

176 Nelson, A. A.: Accessory adrenal cortical tissue, Arch. Pathol. **27**:955-965, 1939.

177 Pedowitz, P., and Pomerance, W.: Adrenal-like tumors of the ovary; review of the literature and report of two new cases, Obstet. Gynecol. **19**:183-194, 1962.

178 Ryan, K. J.: Synthesis of hormones in the ovary. In Grady, H. G., and Smith, D. E., editors: The ovary, Baltimore, 1963, The Williams & Wilkins Co.

179 Sandberg, A. A., Slaunwhite, W. R., Jackson, J. E., and Frawley, T. F.: Androgen biosynthesis by an ovarian lipoid cell tumor, J. Clin. Endocrinol. **22**:929-934, 1962.

180 Taylor, H. B., and Norris, H. J.: Lipid cell tumors of the ovary, Cancer **20**:1953-1962, 1967.

Mixed and indeterminate types

181 Neubecker, R. D., and Breen, J. L.: Gynandroblastoma; a report of five cases, with a discussion of the histogenesis and classification of ovarian tumors, Am. J. Clin. Pathol. **38**:60-69, 1962.

182 Novak, E. R.: Gynandroblastoma of the ovary; review of 8 cases from the Ovarian Tumor Registry, Obstet. Gynecol. **30**:709-715, 1967.

183 Scully, R. E.: Sex cord tumor with annular tubules; a distinctive ovarian tumor of the Peutz-Jeghers syndrome, Cancer **25**:1107-1121, 1970.

Tumors of germ cell and stromal origin

184 Scully, R. E.: Gonadoblastoma; a review of 74 cases, Cancer **25**:1340-1356, 1970.

185 Teter, J.: The mixed germ tumours with hormonal activity, Acta Pathol. Microbiol. Scand. **58**:306-320, 1963.

Tumors of metastatic origin

186 Joshi, V. V.: Primary Krukenberg tumor of ovary; review of literature and case report, Cancer **22**:1199-1207, 1968.

187 Leffel, J. M., Masson, J. C., and Dockerty, M. B.: Krukenberg's tumors, Ann. Surg. **115**:102-113, 1942.

188 Scully, R. E., and Richardson, G. S.: Luteinization of the stroma of metastatic cancer involving the ovary and its endocrine significance, Cancer **14**:827-840, 1961.

189 Stone, W. S.: Metastatic carcinoma of the ovaries, Surg. Gynecol. Obstet. **22**:407-423, 1916.

190 Warren, S., and Macomber, W. B.: Tumor metastasis. IV. Ovarian metastasis of carcinoma, Arch. Pathol. **19**:75-82, 1935.

191 Woodruff, J. D., and Novak, E. R.: The Krukenberg tumor; study of 48 cases from the Ovarian Tumor Registry, Obstet. Gynecol. **15**:351-360, 1960.

Prognosis

192 Allan, M. S., and Hertig, A. T.: Carcinoma of the ovary, Am. J. Obstet. Gynecol. **58**:640-653, 1949.

193 Brody, S.: Clinical aspects of dysgerminoma of the ovary, Acta Radiol. (Stockh.) **56**:209-230, 1961.

194 Munnell, E. W., and Taylor, H. C., Jr.: Ovarian carcinoma, Am. J. Obstet. Gynecol. **58**:943-955, 1949.

195 Sjöstedt, S., and Wahlen, T.: Prognosis of granulosa cell tumors, Acta Obstet. Gynecol. Scand. **40**(suppl. 6):1-26, 1961.

Placenta

Abortion

The morphologic confirmation of the occurrence of a pregnancy is one of the most common determinations performed by the pathologist.[26] It is a very easy task when viable chorionic villi are identified, although this may require the examination of numerous blocks. Necrotic ("ghost") villi are more difficult to recognize, since clumps of fibrin may closely simulate them. The overall configuration and the presence of shadows of stromal cells and the trophoblast are the main identifying criteria.

In the absence of chorionic villi, a search should be made for trophoblastic cells, isolated or in clumps. Care should be exercised not to confuse multinucleated decidua cells with the syncytiotrophoblast. In the absence of these features, the diagnosis of pregnancy cannot be made with certainty. However, certain patterns of endometrial response are strongly suggestive. The Arias-Stella reaction (discussed earlier in this chapter under Uterus—endometrium) had long been regarded as pathognomonic of pregnancy, but it has now been reported following the use of contraceptive pills. The endometrial pattern designated by Hertig[1] as *gestational hyperplasia* is not always easily recognized. It is characterized by the *simultaneous* presence in an endometrial biopsy of glandular secretion, stromal edema, and deciduoid reaction. The appearance of the decidua of pregnancy can be closely simulated by the pseudodecidual changes secondary to the use of contraceptive pills. The latter usually lacks the dilated vascular channels of true decidua and has a more inactive glandular pattern.

Septic abortion is most often seen as a complication or criminal abortion and is usually caused by coliform organisms or anaerobic streptococci. The pathologist should identify the microorganisms in the tissue sections before making a diagnosis of septic abortion. The presence of polymorphonuclear neutrophils, even in large numbers, is not necessarily an indication of infection, since it may simply represent an inflammatory reaction to the necrotic decidua and fetal tissues.

Examination of term placenta

The normal term placenta measures 15 cm to 20 cm in diameter and 1.5 cm to 3 cm in thickness. It weighs (together with the umbilical cord and the membranes) from 450 gm to 600 gm.[3, 7] Much information of practical value can be gained from examination of the fresh placenta immediately after delivery.[2, 8, 35, 54] An *enlarged* placenta may be the result of polyhydramnios, erythroblastosis fetalis, syphilis, toxoplasmosis, cytomegalic inclusion disease, and renal vein thrombosis. *Small* placentas are found in premature birth, intrauterine growth, retarded ("small-for-dates") infants, diabetic mothers with chronic renal disease, and infants with 17-18 trisomy.[20, 25]

Placenta accreta refers to a condition in which placental villi adhere to, invade, or penetrate through the myometrium.[16]

Placenta circumvallata and *placenta circummarginata* are two morphologic variants of extrachorial placenta. Wentworth[23] examined 895 placentas and found 6.5% to be circumvallate and 25.5% circummarginate. He considered these two malforma-

Possible combinations of fetal membranes in monozygotic twin
placenta (identical twins)

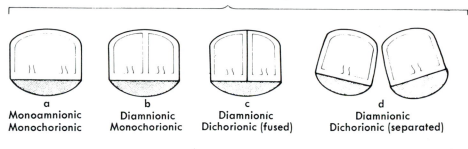

a	b	c	d
Monoamnionic	Diamnionic	Diamnionic	Diamnionic
Monochorionic	Monochorionic	Dichorionic (fused)	Dichorionic (separated)

Possible combinations of fetal membrane in dizygotic twin
placenta (fraternal twins)

Fig. 875 Diagrammatic representation of common variations possible in monochorionic and dichorionic twin placentation. Types **a** and **b** of monochorionic twin placenta are seen only with identical twins. Variations **c** and **d** are common to both identical and fraternal twins. Hence, identification of dichorionic twin placenta does not distinguish between identical and fraternal twins. (From Kraus, F. T.: Gynecologic pathology, St. Louis, 1967, The C. V. Mosby Co.)

tions of no clinical significance. Others have reported an increased incidence of antepartum bleeding.[4]

Amnion nodosum is the result of fetal renal agenesis and is associated with oligohydramnios. It presents as small plaques on the amniotic surface, formed by squamous cells and fibrin.

Gross inspection of a *twin placenta* provides significant information in regard to the type of twinning (Fig. 875). A monochorionic placenta (whether monoamnionic or diamnionic) is indicative of monozygotic twins. On the other hand, dichorionic placentas (whether fused or separated) are compatible with either monozygotic or dizygotic twinning. In a monochorionic placenta, stripping of the amnion reveals a continuous chorionic plate beneath the septum and major arterial anastomoses between the two cords. In contrast, dichorionic fused placentas have a rough chorionic ridge at the base of the septum and lack vascular anastomoses.[6]

Two important malformations of the umbilical cord are **velamentous insertion** and **absence of one umbilical artery.** The former is seen in 1% of all placentas and may result in massive hemorrhage if located at the cervical opening. The latter, also pres-

ent in approximately 1% of all cords, is associated with congenital abnormalities of the infant in almost 30% of the cases.[18] The abnormalities may involve the cardiac, renal, skeletal, or other systems. The absence of one umbilical artery can be detected by gross inspection of the cross section of the cord, but it should always be confirmed microscopically.

Infection of the placenta and cord may be grossly evident by virtue of a cloudy amniotic fluid and a dull fetal surface but is usually detected only after microscopic examination. Fox and Langley[17] found leukocytic infiltration of the placenta or membranes in 24.4% of 1,000 consecutive cases. This process was directly related to prolonged rupture of the membranes, whether or not evidence of fetal hypoxia was obtained. They postulated that prolonged membrane rupture led to infection through intrauterine (or intra-amniotic) spread of bacteria. In support of this hypothesis is the finding of Blanc[5] that placental leukocytic infiltration is invariably associated with the presence of microorganisms. Overbach et al.[21] noted a fivefold increase in clinically diagnosed perinatal infection and an eightfold increase in bacteriologically proved infection in neonates in the presence of leukocytic in-filtration of the umbilical cord.

A *placental infarct* is a focus of villous necrosis secondary to a local obstruction to the maternal uteroplacental circulation. When fresh, grossly it is dark red and of firmer consistency than the surrounding tissue. Microscopically it is characterized by crowding of villi, virtual obliteration of the intervillous space, and marked congestion of the villous vessels. When old, grossly it appears a hard white mass of granular appearance and microscopically as a mass of crowded "ghost" villi. True infarcts should be clearly separated from hematomas, subchorionic fibrin plaques, foci of intervillous fibrin deposition, and intervillous laminated thrombi.[22] Wigglesworth[24] demonstrated by injection studies that infarcts and hematomas have a lobular distribution, thrombi occur in either arterial or venous regions of the intervillous space, and perivillous fibrin deposits are predominantly a venous lesion.

Minor degrees of infarction are seen in about 25% of placentas from uncomplicated full-term pregnancies and can therefore be regarded as an almost physiologic phenomenon. On the other hand, Fox[10] found a significant increase in the incidence and severity of infarcts in pregnancies associated with preeclamptic toxemia, essential hypertension, Rh incompatibility, and nontoxic antepartum hemorrhage. However, the fact that over half the placentas from pregnancies associated with pre-eclamptic toxemia showed no infarcts indicates that the infarct per se is not necessarily the cause of the clinical manifestations of this disease. In most instances, the infarcts were the result of a retro-placental hematoma or a thrombosed maternal vessel. Extensive degrees of placental infarcts were associated with a high incidence of neonatal asphyxia, low birth weight, and intrauterine death.

Placental infarcts, which are always secondary to abnormalities of the placental circulation, also should be differentiated from the focal changes resulting from *thrombosis of fetal arteries.* They are seen grossly as roughly triangular or hemispheric pale areas, otherwise indistinguishable from the surrounding normal placenta. They are better seen after formalin fixation. Microscopically, the villi are fibrosed and avascular, except for occasional small thickened vessels. A thrombosed fetal artery is present at the apex of the lesion. Fox[9] found this lesion in 3.6% of 715 placentas examined. It was particularly frequent in diabetic women, and it did not seem to result in any deleterious effect on the fetus.

In addition to fetal artery thrombosis, other lesions seen with increased frequency in placentas of diabetic women include an increased number of syncytial knots, fibrotic villi, Langhans cells, and foci of villous fibrinoid necrosis.[12, 13, 15]

Table 36 Correlation between morphologic changes in placenta and variety of clinical situations*

	Normal pregnancy	Prolonged pregnancy	Premature onset of labor	Rh incompatibility	Diabetes	Essential hypertension	Toxemia
Infarct	±	±	±	±	+	++	++
Thrombosis of fetal arteries	±	±	±	±	++	±	±
Fibrinoid necrosis of villi	±	−	++	++	++	±	+
Immaturity of villi	±	±	±	++	++	±	±
Senescence of villi[11]	±	++	±	±	±	±	+
Basement membrane thickening in villi[14]	±	+	±	+	+	++	+++
Fibrosis of villi	±	+++	±	±	++	±	±

*Based almost entirely on the gross and microscopic examination of placentas by Fox.[9-17]

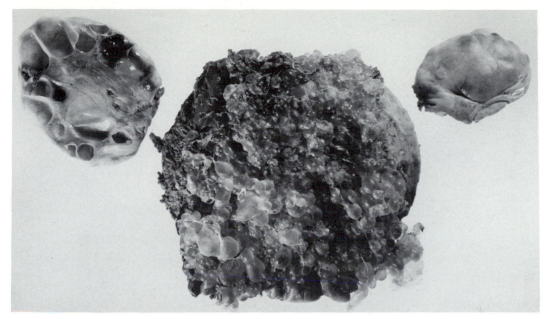

Fig. 876 Classic example of hydatidiform mole almost obscuring wall of uterus. Note multiple theca-lutein cysts in ovaries. (Courtesy Dr. M. Carter, Houston, Texas.)

The diagnosis of red blood cell sickling can often be made by examination of the placenta, as a result of the hypoxia created by the separation of the placenta from the uterine wall. Fujikura and Froehlich[19] found this change in 9.4% of 2,117 placentas from black women.

Table 36 shows the correlation between morphologic changes in the placenta and a variety of clinical situations.

Tumors and tumorlike conditions
Hydatidiform mole

Hydatidiform mole is an abnormality of the placenta characterized by vesicular swelling of many or all villi. The large, bizarre mass fills and distends the uterus (Fig. 876). The pathogenesis is still debated. According to Hertig and Mansell,[58] it represents a pathologic gestation that does not abort as soon as the embryo dies. In support of this theory is mentioned the fact that hydropic changes in the villi resembling a "miniature" mole can be found in 17% to 41% of spontaneous abortions.[26] The percentage is even higher if only the abortions containing a pathologic ovum are considered. All transitions can be found between this common phenomenon and the rare (at least in the United States) full-blown hydatidiform mole. As a result, it is not always easy to separate these two processes, which, although perhaps related, have markedly different connotations for the patient and the clinician. The use of the term "transitional mole" is not too helpful in this regard, because it only tends to obscure this desirable distinction.

We make the diagnosis of hydatidiform mole when hydropic swelling of the villi, whether gross or microscopic, is accompanied by trophoblastic hyperplasia and designate as "hydropic abortions" those specimens lacking the hyperplasia of the trophoblast.[69]

Park[69] has advanced the theory that hydatidiform mole represents a primary abnormality of the trophoblast, whether dysplastic, hyperplastic, or neoplastic, and that the hydropic swelling of the villi is only a secondary phenomenon caused by the altered physiology of the trophoblast.

None of the foregoing theories gives an explanation for the recently made obser-

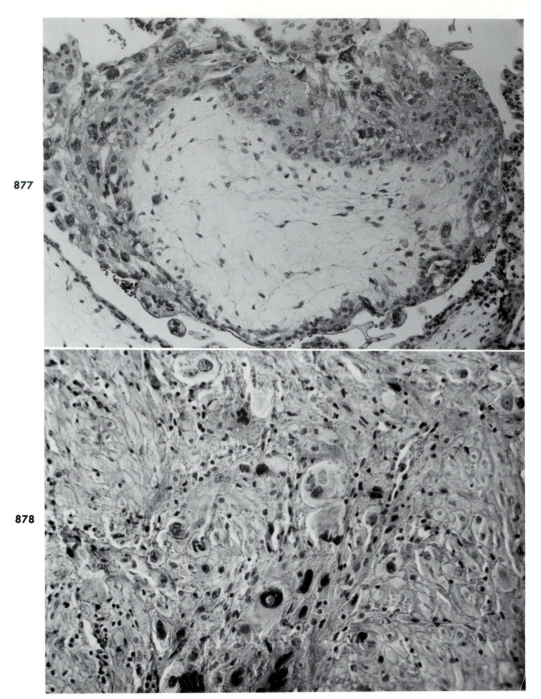

877

878

Fig. 877 Rather hyperplastic villus in hydatidiform mole. This should not be interpreted as sign of malignancy. (×220; WU neg. 50-3843.)
Fig. 878 Normal trophoblastic invasion of uterine wall at implantation site in pregnancy. These changes should not be misinterpreted as choriocarcinoma. (×310; WU neg. 58-4206.)

vation that the large majority of moles are of female sex, as determined by nuclear sex chromatin and karyotyping.[31, 63]

There is a surprising variation in the frequency of hydatidiform mole in different parts of the world. The incidence of

1 in 2,000 deliveries reported by Hertig and Mansell[58] represents an average for young healthy women in the United States. In Southeast Asia, various writers report an incidence at least four to five times as great as that in the United States.[28, 42, 60, 75] The highest incidences have been reported from Mexico City (1:200), the Philippines (1:173), India (1:160), Taiwan (1:125), and Indonesia (1:82).[64, 70] Marquez-Monter et al.[66] suggest that poor nutrition may increase the risk of hydatidiform mole and choriocarcinoma. The possibility that a genetic factor is involved is unlikely in view of the fact that Asian immigrants to the United States have the same incidence as Caucasians.[61]

In the presence of a hydatidiform mole, the uterus is disproportionately large for this stage of pregnancy. Serum chorionic gonadotropin levels continue to rise after the fourteenth week, when they should have begun to diminish in the course of normal gestation. Evidence of toxemia of pregnancy (hypertension, edema, albuminuria) is frequently present and appears earlier in the course of pregnancy than usual. Exceptionally, hyperthyroidism develops as a result of a thyroid stimulator secreted by the molar tissue.[57] The mole may begin to abort spontaneously. Evacuation of the uterus is usually completed by curettage.

The microscopic appearance of the copious material produced in this manner is variable. Molar villi are usually surrounded by an attenuated layer of degenerating trophoblast. Occasionally, the trophoblast forms large hyperplastic sheets of cells[52] (Fig. 877). The distended core of the villus is traversed by widely separated, broken strands of fibrillar material. Vessels are usually absent or are demonstrated with difficulty. Some degree of hyperplasia of the trophoblast is the rule, and curettings from the implantation site show a bizarre pattern. Ultrastructurally, the molar trophoblast resembles quite closely that seen during the first trimester of a normal pregnancy.[68]

Histologic grading of moles according to the apparent degree of anaplastic change has not proved to be helpful in predicting the subsequent course of the patient. It is true than the more pronounced the trophoblastic hyperplasia, the higher the chance of the development of a choriocarcinoma. However, the number of exceptions is such as to render this evaluation of little practical value. The plexiform pattern of intermixed syncytiotrophoblast and cytotrophoblast seen in choriocarcinoma does not occur.[74]

Invasion of the myometrium by individual syncytiotrophoblastic masses occurs beneath the implantation site in all gestations, including abortions and hydatidiform mole (Fig. 878). The undesirable term *syncytial endometritis* has been applied to this normal anatomic event. It should never lead to overdiagnosis of malignancy. The demonstration of choriocarcinoma in curettings of molar tissue has occurred rarely, if at all, and would be a most unusual and unexpected finding.[58] The production of chorionic gonadotropin is a specific and invariable characteristic of the trophoblast, whether it be normal, abnormal, or neoplastic. This important manifestation makes it possible to demonstrate the presence of living trophoblast even in the absence of symptoms or radiographic changes.[51]

Sequential quantitative chorionic gonadotropin determinations are the most important requirement in the evaluation of a patient after evacuation of a hydatidiform mole. Normal levels are reached by sixty days after evacuation in about 80% of the cases and by the 250th day in 90% to 95% of the cases.[33]

Brewer et al.[41] recommend serial determination of chorionic gonadotropin at 10, 20, 30, 45, and 60 days after termination of the molar gestation. About 21% of their patients were treated with chemotherapy in view of a rising titer between day 45 and day 60 or the presence of a low but still elevated level by day 60. Delfs[45] found rising or persistently elevated gonadotropin titers, between eight and thirty-five weeks after evacuation of a mole, in eleven of 129 patients studied. Six of these eleven proved to have destructive moles, and five had choriocarcinoma.

Sensitive and accurate methods for chorionic gonadotropin determination are essential. Mouse uterine weight bioassay and radioimmunoassay are far superior to the commercially available test methods. The latter are often inadequate in detecting the low levels of hormone seen in the early stages of recurrent trophoblastic disease following evacuation of a mole or chemotherapy. This may result in a delay of grave consequence to the patient.[39]

Invasive mole (chorioadenoma destruens)

Vascular invasion is a necessary property of human trophoblast. Trophoblastic emboli were demonstrable in normal pregnancy in 43.6% of the patients studied by Attwood and Park.[30] Vaginal nodules of placental villi after normal pregnancy have been observed by Haines.[55] The patients remain well after excision of the nodule.

Vessel invasion with embolization also occur in patients with hydatidiform mole.[72] Myometrial invasion by molar villi may occur in a manner probably analogous to placenta accreta. When extrauterine nodules of molar trophoblast survive and grow, their existence is detectable by the chorionic gonadotropin they produce. The radiographic appearance may be characteristic.[32, 49] Cockshott et al.[44] demonstrated arteriographic differences between molar emboli and choriocarcinoma.

Invasive masses of hydatidiform mole in the uterine wall cause persistent hemorrhage. Deported masses of molar trophoblast are also hemorrhagic. The symptoms depend upon the site involved. A sizable mass in the lung may regress spontaneously without ever causing significant symptoms. A hemorrhagic nodule in the brain could be as fatal as choriocarcinoma.

Invasive mole is distinguished from choriocarcinoma on pathologic examination primarily by the presence of villi. The trophoblast may be extremely hyperplastic (Figs. 879 and 880). Villous stroma is never produced by choriocarcinoma.[36] It is clear that the deported masses of destructive mole eventually regress in the great majority of instances.[53, 65, 77] Their clinical importance derives from the fact that a strategically located lesion may kill the patient before it regresses. For this reason, chemotherapy has been advantageously employed in carefully selected patients.[59, 73]

A change in nomenclature has recently been suggested by Tow[76] and already adopted by several Asian investigators. Invasive mole and choriocarcinoma are regarded as two variants of the same basic process, differing morphologically by the presence of villi in invasive mole and clinically by the more aggressive features of choriocarcinoma. The term of "villous choriocarcinoma" is proposed for the former and that of "avillous choriocarcinoma" for the latter. The main objection we have to this classification is that it fails to emphasize the striking differences in the natural history and survival rates (at least among the untreated cases) between these two entities.

Choriocarcinoma

Choriocarcinoma is a rare, highly malignant neoplasm composed entirely of syncytiotrophoblast and cytotrophoblast. It usually follows a gestation and is much more likely to occur after hydatidiform mole and other abnormal gestations. In cases of choriocarcinomas appearing after nonmolar abortion, review of the microscopic sections obtained at the time of abortion will often show an increased trophoblastic proliferation. The latent period between the abortion, either molar or not, and the development of choriocarcinoma is almost always less than one year. However, notable exceptions have been reported.[46]

Bagshawe et al.[34] have shown a striking relationship between the incidence and prognosis of choriocarcinoma and the

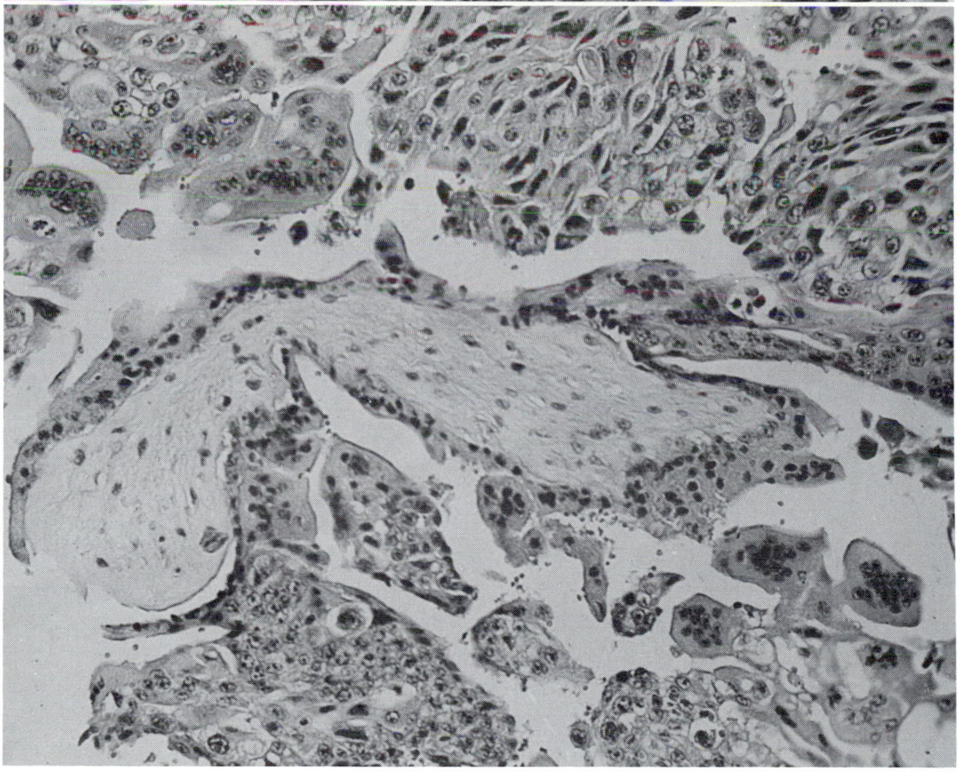

Fig. 879 Large syncytial trophoblast in lung of patient with invasive mole. Lesion was biopsied two months after hysterectomy because of nodulation of lung. Patient remains well. (×600; WU neg. 63-997; slide contributed by Dr. B. D. Canlas, Manila, Philippine Islands.)

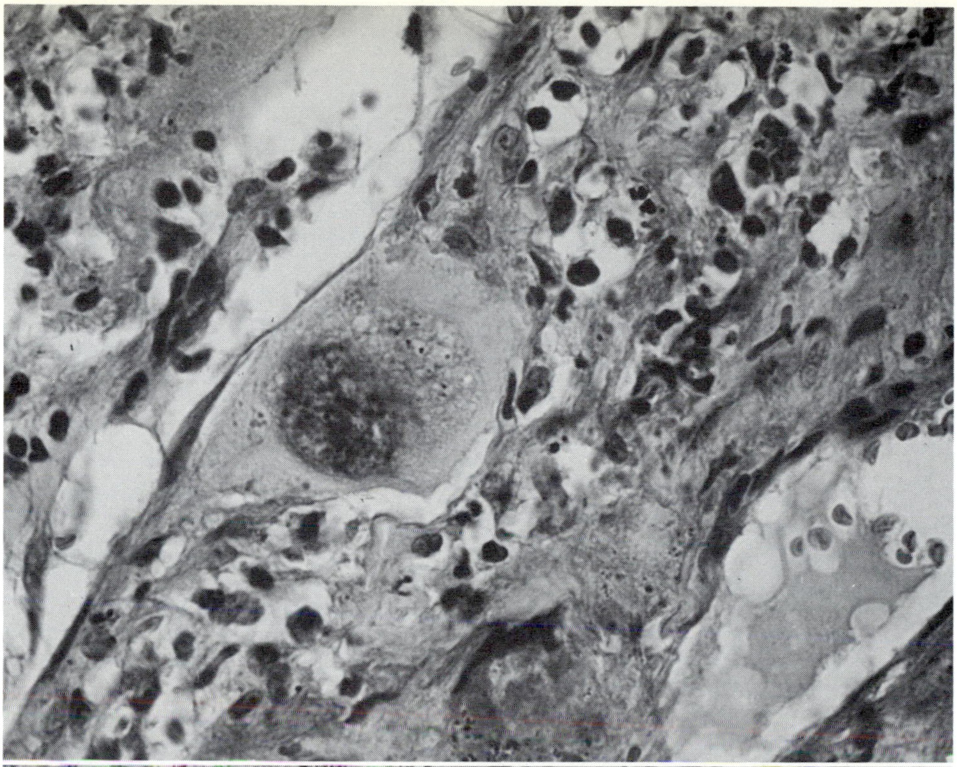

Fig. 880 Chorionic villus that prompted diagnosis of invasive mole. Patient died. There were also chorionic villi in metastases. (×190; WU neg. 54-5842; Case 61147; slide contributed by Dr. S. Tjokronegoro, Jakarta, Indonesia.)

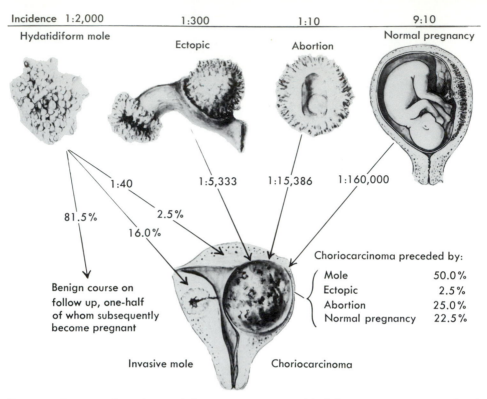

Incidence 1:2,000   1:300   1:10   9:10

Hydatidiform mole   Ectopic   Abortion   Normal pregnancy

1:40   1:5,333   1:15,386   1:160,000

81.5%   2.5%   16.0%

Benign course on follow up, one-half of whom subsequently become pregnant

Choriocarcinoma preceded by:

Mole	50.0%
Ectopic	2.5%
Abortion	25.0%
Normal pregnancy	22.5%

Invasive mole   Choriocarcinoma

Fig. 881 Origin and incidence of choriocarcinoma. (Modified from Hertig, A. T.: Hydatidiform mole and chorionepithelioma. In Meigs, J. V., and Sturgis, S. H., editors: Progress in gynecology, New York, 1950, Grune & Stratton, Inc.)

ABO groups of both the woman and her husband. The highest risk is for women of Group A married to men of the same group. The relative risk of these two extreme groups was 10.4:1. Women mated to men of their own ABO group had the highest incidence of spontaneous regression of trophoblast after evacuation of a hydatidiform mole.

Choriocarcinoma is not a rare disease in those parts of the world in which hydatidiform mole is common. The exact incidence in the United States is difficult to estimate because the largest series reported are from medical centers or individual authorities to whom patients are referred from great distances. The incidence figures computed by Hertig[58] are shown in Fig. 881. A consensus of other reports summarized by Benirschke and Driscoll[36] suggests that 1 in 100 moles is followed by choriocarcinoma, which is still much higher than the inci-

dence after other abortions or normal pregnancy. Small choriocarcinomas arising in two otherwise normal placentas have been described by Brewer and Gerbie.[37] Both patients died with metastases.

Choriocarcinoma characteristically forms soft, dark red, hemorrhagic, round nodular tumor masses (Fig. 882). Metastases occur early. Residual tumor in the uterus may be inconspicuous and is frequently absent.[67]

The microscopic pattern, although variable, always shows syncytiotrophoblast and cytotrophoblast (Fig. 883) and no other component. Villous stroma is not produced. It is important not to overdiagnose the hyperplastic trophoblast around the villi of an early abortion, especially on the basis of the normal finding of trophoblast involving decidual blood vessels.[48] The typical choriocarcinoma is composed of clusters of cytotrophoblast cells separated by streaming masses of **syncytiotrophoblast**

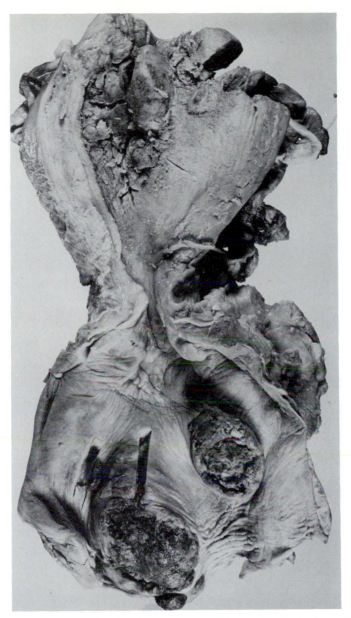

Fig. 882 Uterus and vagina showing large masses of hemorrhagic choriocarcinoma within uterus and metastatic to vagina. (WU neg. 49-3585.)

(Fig. 884). Anaplastic-appearing nuclei are a common but not necessarily diagnostic feature and also may be found in the curettings of molar tissue. No reliable method of histologic grading has been developed. Hemorrhage and necrosis are usually present but have no real diagnostic significance since they are invariably found in spontaneous abortions also. A cellular infiltrate composed of lymphocytes, histiocytes, and plasma cells is often seen at the interphase between tumor and stroma. According to Elston,[47] cases in which this infiltrate is intense are associated with a better survival rate.

Many of the morphologic changes seen in patients with choriocarcinoma are the result of increased gonadotropin secretion.

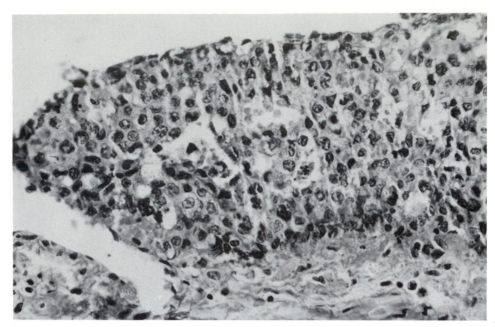

Fig. 883 Choriocarcinoma in large vein within uterus. Cytotrophoblasts predominate. Patient died with pulmonary metastases. (×420; WU neg. 52-2573.)

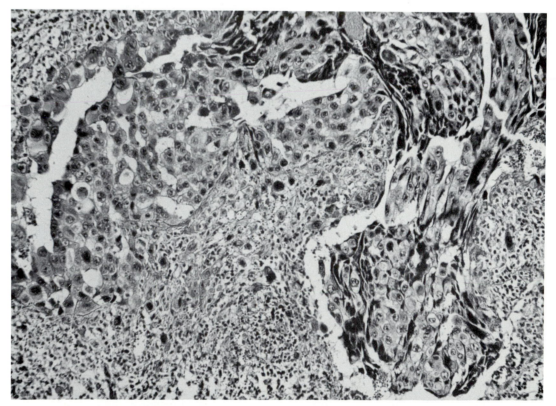

Fig. 884 Choriocarcinoma invading myometrial wall, accompanied by extensive inflammatory response. Cytotrophoblastic and syncytiotrophoblastic elements can easily be identified. Chorionic villi are absent. (×150; WU neg. 73-3400.)

These include hyperplasia of endocervical glands, decidual reaction (endometrial and ectopic), Arias-Stella phenomenon, bilateral enlargement of the ovaries by theca-lutein cysts, and hyperplasia of mammary lobules. Ober et al.[67] remarked that in the endometrial decidual reaction of patients with choriocarcinoma, the spiral arterioles fail to develop as they do in the normal cycle, the appearance thus approaching that seen after the administration of progestogens.

When treated by surgery alone, choriocarcinoma was attended by a dismal prognosis. Brewer et al.[40] found that fewer than 20% of patients with metastases survived prior to the success of chemotherapy.

The development of effective drugs has transformed the entire outlook for patients with gestational choriocarcinoma. Approximately 75% of all patients treated at the National Institute of Health have undergone remission after treatment with methotrexate and actinomycin D.[73] Surgery, in the sense of hysterectomy, does not add to the effectiveness of chemotherapy in the primary treatment of choriocarcinoma.[38, 40, 73] Surgery remains useful in controlling life-threatening hemorrhage from metastatic lesions.[62] Ross et al.[73] emphasize the importance of early diagnosis, prompt institution of therapy, and monitoring of the effects of treatment with sensitive, and sequential, quantitative determination of chorionic gonadotropin production. Under the most favorable conditions, thirteen of fourteen patients with choriocarcinoma had remissions.

Hammond et al.[56] emphasize the necessity of using the most sensitive methods of quantitating chorionic gonadotropin in following patients because clinically significant titers may be missed by commercial test methods.

Gonadotropin secretion is by no means restricted to gestational choriocarcinomas. It also has been found in extrauterine choriocarcinomas, in other ovarian and testicular germ cell tumors, lung carcinomas, **gastric** adenocarcinomas, hepatoblastomas,

and several other types of malignant neoplasms. A feature common to many of these tumors is the presence of tumor giant cells. The latter have been shown to contain chorionic gonadotropin by immunofluorescent techniques.[43]

Other tumors

Hemangiomas can be found in approximately one of every 100 placentas if a careful gross examination is performed.[50] They may protrude on the fetal surface or be located entirely in the placental substance. Grossly, they are well circumscribed and purplish red. Microscopically, they are composed of a network of proliferating capillaries. Mitoses can be found in some cases. Degenerative changes are common. The majority are asymptomatic, but the larger ones may be associated with hydramnios, hemorrhage, premature delivery, premature placental separation, and placenta previa.[29] There is apparently no relationship with toxemia.

Metastatic tumors of maternal origin can rarely lodge in the placenta and form distinct nodules. This phenomenon has been seen most often with malignant melanoma.[71] Metastases to the fetus may or may not be present. The knowledge of this dramatic event should not obscure the fact that in the large majority of pregnant women with widespread metastatic disease, the placenta and fetus are totally spared from the effects of the neoplasia.

REFERENCES
Abortion

1 Hertig, A. T.: Gestational hyperplasia of endometrium; a morphologic correlation of ova, endometrium, and corpora lutea during pregnancy, Lab. Invest. **13:**1153-1191, 1964.

Examination of term placenta

2 Benirschke, K.: Examination of the placenta, Obstet. Gynecol. **18:**309-333, 1961.
3 Benirschke, K., and Driscoll, S. G.: The pathology of the human placenta, New York, 1967, Springer-Verlag New York Inc.
4 Benson, R. C., and Fujikura, T.: Circumvallate and circummarginate placenta; unimportant clinical entities, Obstet. Gynecol. **34:**799-804, 1969.

5 Blanc, W. A.: Pathways of fetal and early neonatal infection; viral placentitis, bacterial and fungal chorioamnionitis, J. Pediatr. **59:** 473-496, 1961.

6 Bleisch, V. R.: Diagnosis of monochorionic twin placentation, Am. J. Clin. Pathol. **42:** 277-284, 1964.

7 Boyd, J. D., and Hamilton, W. J.: The human placenta, Cambridge, 1970, W. Heffer & Sons, Ltd.

8 Bradford, W. D.: The case for careful examination of the placenta; helpful information from the delivery room, Clin. Pediatr. (Phila.) **7:** 716-719, 1968.

9 Fox, H.: Thrombosis of foetal arteries in the human placenta, J. Obstet. Gynaecol. Br. Commonw. **73:**961-965, 1966.

10 Fox, H.: The significance of placental infarction in perinatal morbidity and mortality, Biol. Neonate **11:**87-105, 1967.

11 Fox, H.: Senescence of placental villi, J. Obstet. Gynaecol. Br. Commonw. **74:**881-885, 1967.

12 Fox, H.: Fibrinoid necrosis of placental villi, J. Obstet. Gynaecol. Br. Commonw. **75:**448-452, 1968.

13 Fox, H.: Fibrosis of placental villi, J. Pathol. Bacteriol. **95:**573-579, 1968.

14 Fox, H.: Basement membrane changes in the villi of the human placenta, J. Obstet. Gynaecol. Br. Commonw. **75:**302-306, 1968.

15 Fox, H.: Pathology of the placenta in maternal diabetes mellitus, Obstet. Gynecol. **34:** 792-798, 1969.

16 Fox, H.: Placenta accreta, 1945-1969, Obstet. Gynecol. Survey **27:**475-490, 1972.

17 Fox, H., and Langley, F. A.: Leukocytic infiltration of the placenta and umbilical cord; a clinico-pathologic study, Obstet. Gynecol. **37:**451-458, 1971.

18 Froehlich, L. A., and Fujikura, L. A.: Significance of single umbilical artery; report from collaborative study of cerebral palsy, Am. J. Obstet. Gynecol. **94:**274-279, 1966.

19 Fujikura, T., and Froehlich, L. A.: Diagnosis of sickling by placental examination; geographic differences in incidence, Am. J. Obstet. Gynecol. **100:**1122-1124, 1968.

20 Morris, E. D.: Placental insufficiency, Br. Med. Bull. **24:**76-79, 1968.

21 Overbach, A. M., Daniel, S. J., and Cassady, G.: The value of umbilical cord histology in the management of potential perinatal infection, J. Pediatr. **76:**22-31, 1970.

22 Wentworth, P.: Placental infarction and toxemia of pregnancy, Am. J. Obstet. Gynecol. **99:**318-326, 1967.

23 Wentworth, P.: Circumvallate and circummarginate placentas; their incidence and clinical significance, Am. J. Obstet. Gynecol. **102:** 44-47, 1968.

24 Wigglesworth, J. S.: Vascular anatomy of the human placenta and its significance for placental pathology, Obstet. Gynaecol. Br. Commonw. **76:**979-989, 1969.

25 Younoszai, M. K., and Haworth, J. C.: Placental dimensions and relations in preterm, term, and growth-retarded infants, Am. J. Obstet. Gynecol. **103:**265-271, 1969.

Tumors and tumorlike conditions

26 Abaci, F., and Aterman, K.: Changes of the placenta and embryo in early spontaneous abortion, Am. J. Obstet. Gynecol. **102:**252-263, 1968.

27 Acosta-Sison, H.: Studies on choriocarcinoma from 88 patients admitted to the Philippine General Hospital from 1950-1961, Philipp. J. Cancer **4:**197-203, 1962.

28 Acosta-Sison, H.: Changing attitudes in the management of hydatidiform mole; a report on 196 patients admitted to the Philippine General Hospital from April 10, 1959, to March 27, 1963, Am. J. Obstet. Gynecol. **88:** 634-636, 1964.

29 Asadourian, L. A., and Taylor, H. B.: Clinical significance of placental hemangiomas, Obstet. Gynecol. **31:**551-555, 1968.

30 Attwood, H. D., and Park, W. W.: Embolism to the lungs by trophoblast, J. Obstet. Gynaecol. Br. Commonw. **68:**611-617, 1961.

31 Baggish, M. S., Woodruff, J. D., Tow, S. H., and Jones, H. W.: Sex chromatin pattern in hydatidiform mole, Am. J. Obstet. Gynecol. **102:**362-370, 1968.

32 Bagshawe, K. D., and Garnett, E. S.: Radiological changes in the lungs of patients with trophoblastic tumours, Br. J. Radiol. **36:**673-679, 1963.

33 Bagshawe, K. D., Golding, P. R., and Orr, A. H.: Choriocarcinoma after hydatidiform mole; studies related to effectiveness of follow-up practice after hydatidiform mole, Br. Med. J. **3:**733-737, 1969.

34 Bagshawe, K. D., Rawlins, G., Pike, M. C., and Lawler, S. D.: ABO blood groups in trophoblastic neoplasia, Lancet **1:**553-557, 1971.

35 Benirschke, K.: A review of the pathologic anatomy of the human placenta, Am. J. Obstet. Gynecol. **84:**1595-1622, 1962.

36 Benirschke, K., and Driscoll, S. G.: The pathology of the human placenta, New York, 1967, Springer-Verlag New York Inc.

37 Brewer, J. I., and Gerbie, A. B.: Early development of choriocarcinoma, Am. J. Obstet. Gynecol. **94:**692-705, 1966.

38 Brewer, J. I., Gerbie, A. B., Dolkart, R. E., Skom, J. H., Nagle, R. G., and Torok, E. E.: Chemotherapy in trophoblastic diseases, Am. J. Obstet. Gynecol. **90:**566-578, 1964.

39 Brewer, J. I., Eckman, T. R., Dolkart, R. E.,

Torok, E. E., and Webster, A.: Gestational trophoblastic disease; a comparative study of the results of therapy in patients with invasive mole and with choriocarcinoma, Am. J. Obstet. Gynecol. **109:**335-340, 1971.

40 Brewer, J. I., Smith, R. T., and Pratt, G. B.: Choriocarcinoma: absolute 5-year survival rates of 122 patients treated by hysterectomy, Am. J. Obstet. Gynecol. **85:**841-843, 1963.

41 Brewer, J. I., Torok, E. E., Webster, A., and Dolkart, R. E.: Hydatidiform mole: a follow-up regimen for identification of invasive mole and choriocarcinoma and for selection of patients for treatment, Am. J. Obstet. Gynecol. **101:**557-563, 1968.

42 Chun, D., Braga, C., Chow, C., and Lok, L.: Treatment of hydatidiform mole, J. Obstet. Gynaecol. Br. Commonw. **71:**185-197, 1964.

43 Civantos, F., and Rywlin, A. M.: Carcinomas with trophoblastic differentiation and secretion of chorionic gonadotrophins, Cancer **29:** 789-798, 1972.

44 Cockshott, W. P., Evans, K. T., and Hendrickse, J. P.: Arteriography of trophoblastic tumours, Clin. Radiol. **15:**1-8, 1964.

45 Delfs, E.: Chorionic gonadotropin determinations in patients with hydatidiform mole and choriocarcinoma, Ann. N. Y. Acad. Sci. **80:** 125-139, 1959.

46 Dyke, P. C., and Fink, L. M.: Latent choriocarcinoma, Cancer, **20:**150-154, 1967.

47 Elston, C. W.: Cellular reaction to choriocarcinoma, J. Pathol. **97:**261-268, 1969.

48 Elston, C. W., and Bagshawe, K. D.: The diagnosis of trophoblastic tumours from uterine curettings, J. Clin. Pathol. **25:**111-118, 1972.

49 Evans, K. T., Cockshott, W. P., and Hendrickse, P. de V.: Pulmonary changes in malignant trophoblastic disease, Br. J. Radiol. **38:** 161-171, 1965.

50 Fox, H.: Vascular tumors of the placenta, Obstet. Gynecol. Survey **22:**697-711, 1967.

51 Fox, F. J., and Tow, W. S. H.: Immunologically determined chorionic gonadotropin titers in Singapore women with hydatidiform mole, choriocarcinoma, and normal intrauterine pregnancy, Am. J. Obstet. Gynecol. **95:**239-248, 1966.

52 Gore, H., and Hertig, A. T.: Problems in the histologic interpretation of the trophoblast, Clin. Obstet. Gynecol. **10:**269-289, 1967.

53 Greene, R. R.: Chorioadenoma destruens, Ann. N. Y. Acad. Sci. **80:**143-148, 1959.

54 Gruenwald, P.: Examination of the placenta by the pathologist, Arch. Pathol. **77:**41-46, 1964.

55 Haines, M.: Hydatidiform mole and vaginal nodules, J. Obstet. Gynaecol. Br. Emp. **62:** 6-11, 1955.

56 Hammond, C. B., Hertz, R., Ross, G. T., Lipsett, M. B., and O'Dell, W. D.: Diagnostic problems of choriocarcinoma and related trophoblastic neoplasms, Obstet. Gynecol. **29:**224-229, 1967.

57 Hershman, J. M., and Higgins, H. P.: Hydatidiform mole—a cause of clinical hyperthyroidism; report of two cases with evidence that the molar tissue secreted a thyroid stimulator, N. Engl. J. Med. **284:**573-577, 1971.

58 Hertig, A. T.: Hydatidiform mole and chorionepithelioma. In Meigs, J. V., and Sturgis, S. H., editors: Progress in gynecology, New York, 1950, Grune & Stratton, Inc.

59 Hertz, R., Ross, G. T., and Lipsett, M. B.: Chemotherapy in women with trophoblastic disease; choriocarcinoma, chorioadenoma destruens, and complicated hydatidiform mole, Ann. N. Y. Acad. Sci. **114:**881-885, 1964.

60 Hsu, C. T., Chen, T. Y., Chiu, W. H., et al.: Some aspects of trophoblastic diseases peculiar to Taiwan, Am. J. Obstet. Gynecol. **90:** 308-316, 1964.

61 Joint Project for Study of Choriocarcinoma and Hydatidiform Mole in Asia: Geographic variation in the occurrence of hydatidiform mole and choriocarcinoma, Ann. N. Y. Acad. Sci. **80:**178-195, 1959.

62 Lewis, J., Ketcham, A. S., and Hertz, R.: Surgical intervention during chemotherapy of gestational trophoblastic neoplasms, Cancer **19:** 1517-1522, 1966.

63 Loke, Y. W.: Sex chromatin of hydatidiform moles, J. Med. Genet. **6:**22-25, 1969.

64 McGregor, C., Ontiveros, E., Vargas, L. E., and Valenzuela, L. S.: Hydatidiform mole; analysis of 145 patients, Obstet. Gynecol. **33:** 343-351, 1969.

65 McKay, D. G.: The significance of mola destruens. In Park, W. W., editor: The early conceptus, normal and abnormal (papers and discussions presented at a symposium held at Queen's College, Dundee, September, 1964), Edinburgh, 1965, E. & S. Livingstone, Ltd., pp. 118-120.

66 Marquez-Monter, H., Alfaro de la Vega, G., Robles, M., and Bolio-Cicero, A.: Epidemiology and pathology of hydatidiform mole in the General Hospital of Mexico: study of 104 cases, Am. J. Obstet. Gynecol. **85:**856-864, 1963.

67 Ober, W. B., Edgcomb, J. H., and Price, E. B., Jr.: The pathology of choriocarcinoma, Ann. N. Y. Acad. Sci. **172:**299-321, 1971.

68 Okudaira, Y., and Strauss, L.: Ultrastructure of molar trophoblast; observations on hydatidiform mole and chorioadenoma destruens, Obstet. Gynecol. **30:**172-187, 1967.

69 Park, W. W.: Choriocarcinoma; a study of its pathology, Philadelphia, 1971, F. A. Davis Co.

70 Park, W. W., and Lees, J. C.: Choriocarcinoma, a general review with an analysis of 516 cases, Arch. Pathol. **49:**73-104, 1950.

71 Potter, J. F., and Schoeneman, M.: Metastasis of maternal cancer to the placenta and fetus, Cancer **25**:380-388, 1970.

72 Ring, A. M.: The concept of benign metastasizing hydatidiform moles, Am. J. Clin. Pathol. **58**:111-117, 1972.

73 Ross, G. T., Goldstein, D. P., Hertz, R., Lipsett, M. B., and Odell, W. D.: Sequential use of methotrexate and actinomycin D in the treatment of metastatic choriocarcinoma and related trophoblastic diseases in women, Am. J. Obstet. Gynecol. **93**:223-229, 1965.

74 Smalbraak, J.: Problems in the classification of hydatidiform moles, Ann. N. Y. Acad. Sci. **80**: 105-120, 1959.

75 Tjokronegoro, S.: Choriocarcinoma in Indonesia, Schweiz. Z. Allg. Pathol. **18**:791-803, 1955.

76 Tow, W. S. H.: The classification of malignant growths of the chorion, J. Obstet. Gynaecol. Br. Commonw. **73**:1000-1001, 1966.

77 Wilson, R. B.: Hunter, J. S., Jr., and Dockerty, M. B.: Chorioadenoma destruens, Am. J. Obstet. Gynecol. **81**:546-559, 1961.

19 Breast

Introduction

The breast is the most important organ from the standpoint of surgical pathology because of the frequency of both benign and malignant mammary lesions. Breast cancer is the most common malignant tumor of women. Since 1947, in the United States it has replaced the uterus as the leading cause of death from cancer. Whether a lesion is benign or malignant is usually the problem faced by both the pathologist and the surgeon. This decision may be quite difficult but must be resolved before therapy is instituted.

Method of pathologic examination

The examination of a radical mastectomy specimen should be thorough. Much information may be gained by meticulous study. The specimens submitted by different surgeons in large general hospitals may vary widely.

A radical mastectomy must include adequate skin, all breast parenchyma, the underlying and surrounding fat, the pectoralis major and minor muscles, and the axillary contents in continuity and en bloc. Specimens that do not contain the pectoral muscles or that include only halfhearted dissections of the axillary contents are not radical mastectomies and should not be so designated by the pathologist. At operation, the surgeon should tag the high point of the axillary contents as he removes it from about the medial end of the axillary vein. This allows the pathologist to orient the specimen. Evidence of edema and ulceration of the skin should be noted. If a mass is felt, its borders should be measured. At least three sections should be taken from the tumor with an attempt to include underlying muscle, fascia, and overlying skin if they appear involved. It is our custom to section all breast quadrants, particularly the most prominent parenchymal areas, for such sections may show unexpected extension of the tumor, multiple foci of origin, or various proliferative and possible precancerous lesions.

The most complete method of examining the axillary contents is to clear the axilla and to section each node serially. Such a study is obviously too time consuming and financially extravagant to be used routinely. Saphir and Amromin[6] studied thirty carcinomas of the breast with apparently negative axillary lymph nodes. By serially sectioning the nodes, they discovered that ten of the thirty patients actually had axillary metastases. However, the number of nodes found in this series totaled only 149, an average of less than five nodes per specimen. In other words, the thirty patients had not had adequate initial nodal examination. The necessity for serially sectioning the nodes is obviated by thorough search of the axillary contents for nodes with single sections of each node. An average of at least twenty-five axillary nodes can thus be examined (Table 37).

We divide the axillary contents arbitrarily into high, mid, and low areas according to their relation to the pectoralis minor muscle. By studying the fresh material in a strong light, one can see and feel the small gray nodes even 0.2 cm in diameter against the glistening yellow fat. Small nodes missed by superficial study may contain carcinoma. The number and distribution of involved nodes in the axilla bear a relationship to prognosis.

In Monroe's study of eighty-seven radical mastectomy specimens,[2] the axilla was cleared and all nodes sectioned. The variable numbers of nodes per specimen were thought to be related to the different surgical techniques used. He found an average of 30.4 lymph nodes per specimen and as many as sixty-five in a single case. Eleven of the most radical dissections contained an average of 46.3 lymph nodes. We do not believe that the extra time necessary to clear a specimen is justified by the information gained.

Pickren[3] reported a group of fifty-one patients in whom the lymph nodes were negative initially but which, after subserial sectioning, showed metastases in 22%. However, in this group of radical mastectomies, the survival rate for patients with occult metastases was similar to that of patients with no metastases.

The final step in the examination of the specimen is to place sections of the main tumor, the three other quadrants, and the lymph nodes from the high, mid, and low areas of the axilla into seven separate bottles. While this procedure is time consuming to both pathologist and technician, the information gained is worthwhile, particularly from the standpoint of prognosis.

The widespread use of mammography has resulted in the discovery of extremely small carcinomas (1 mm or 2 mm in diameter). The proper handling of these lesions requires a close cooperation between radiologist, surgeon, and pathologist.[4, 7] Once the radiologist identifies the abnormal area on mammography, he should provide the surgeon with a "map" showing the relative position of the suspicious area within the breast. Once the appropriate area is excised, the cephalad and lateral margins should be marked by sutures and a roentgenogram should be taken of the specimen. If no lesion is seen, the surgeon should obtain additional tissue. If the abnormal area is present in the specimen, this can be accurately located by

Table 37 Number of lymph nodes found in axilla

Year	Number of nodes found	Number of cases	Average number of nodes
1944	833	41	21.5
1945	900	32	28.1
1946	1,192	51	23.4
1947	1,103	41	26.9
Total	4,028	165	25.4

slicing the specimen, identifying the slices with a lead number, taking another roentgenogram, and selecting for frozen sections the slice (and the specific area within the slice) containing the abnormal area. The whole procedure takes no more than fifteen minutes and is well worth the small delay. Otherwise, small carcinomas can be entirely missed.[1, 5]

Cytology

On occasion, an unexpected intraductal cancer may be diagnosed by the examination of nipple secretions. However, the number of times that this is possible is so small that there is little justification for the routine use of this technique.

In some institutions, it is common practice to diagnose breast lesions by cytology from material obtained with aspiration biopsy.[8, 9] We find this technique of little practical value. If the cytology is interpreted as "benign," the lesion still has to be excised. If it is interpreted as "negative," open biopsy with frozen section needs to be done to determine the nature of the lesion. Finally, if the cytology is diagnosed as "positive," the type of cancer still has to be determined, since this greatly influences the type of therapy. The saving of operative time is not enough of an objective to warrant the routine use of this method.

Frozen section

In our institution, radical mastectomy is practically never done without a histologic diagnosis. Needle biopsy is permissible in order to avoid the necessity of frozen section in those instances in which the mass in the breast is large and the operability of the lesion has been determined. In these cases, the needle biopsy is usually diagnostic.[10]

In most instances, the surgeon requests a frozen section at the time of operation. If the lesion is small (2.5 cm or less), it is entirely excised. If it is larger, then careful incisional biopsy is the best procedure. Incisional biopsy is preferable for large lesions because it disturbs the tumor bed the least. Frozen section diagnosis is accurate. In 679 consecutive frozen sections, there were no false positives and three (0.4%) false negatives. The diagnosis was deferred for the permanent sections in six (0.9%) instances. The use of the cryostat has reduced substantially the need to delay diagnosis.

There is no evidence that waiting for the results of the permanent sections (twenty-four hours) causes harm. The greatest difficulty is encountered with papillary lesions, intraductal carcinomas, and sclerosing adenosis (Figs. 885 and 886). Both the surgeon and the pathologist should take great precaution to avoid an erroneous diagnosis of cancer that will result in an unnecessary radical mastectomy.

Inflammatory lesions
Abscess

With the advent of chemotherapy, suppurative mastitis during lactation is no longer frequent. Grossly, in the breast parenchyma near the abscess, chronic inflammation with duct stasis and obliteration of lobular pattern is usually present. Microscopically, all signs of inflammation are present. Plasma cells usually are abundant. A localized abscess may simulate cancer.[14]

Tuberculosis

Tuberculosis of the breast is rare and invariably is secondary to bloodstream dissemination or invasion from an adjacent tuberculous process. Grossly, in advanced tuberculosis of the breast, there are suppurating multiple sinuses and areas of necrosis and caseation. This lesion may be mistaken clinically for advanced breast cancer. The regional nodes are quite often involved in caseating forms of tuberculosis. In these instances, radical mastectomy may be necessary. Usually, however, simple mastectomy is adequate.

Plasma cell mastitis

Plasma cell mastitis is a vanishingly rare lesion.[11] We have not seen a single case during the past ten years. It has been described most often in patients between

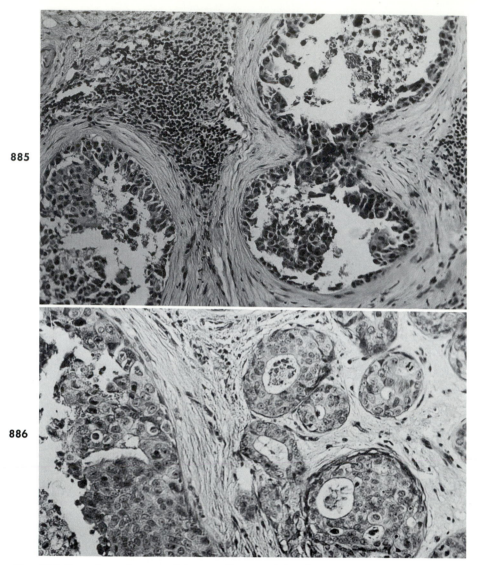

885

886

Fig. 885 Ductal carcinoma of breast diagnosed by frozen section. Patient was young woman with single nodule clinically thought to be benign. (×165; WU neg. 49-4436.)
Fig. 886 Radical mastectomy demonstrated carcinoma in other quadrants and in one axillary lymph node. Tumor in this section is from quadrant remote from primary tumor shown in Fig. 885. (×195; WU neg. 49-4437.)

35 and 40 years of age.[12] It probably does not represent an entity but rather a pattern of reaction to the ductal changes of fibrocystic disease or to fat necrosis. A history of trauma is sometimes present. Clinically, the edema, firmness, and tenderness frequently suggest a diagnosis of carcinoma. The regional lymph nodes also may be enlarged by inflammatory infiltration. Rarely, the disease is bilateral. It may be associated with underlying cancer.[13] Grossly, extensive edema, duct stasis, and interstitial induration are present. Areas of fat necrosis also may be evident. Microscopically, there is duct stasis, focal fat necrosis, and an intense inflammatory infiltrate composed almost exclusively of plasma cells. Local excision is all that is needed, provided the possibility of an underlying carcinoma has been ruled out.

Fat necrosis

Fat necrosis of the breast usually occurs in obese patients with pendulous breasts. The lesion was described well by Lee and Adair in a number of articles dating from 1920.[19, 20] Adair and Munzer[15] reported its incidence to be 2.76% of the patients with primary operable carcinoma.

The pathogenesis varies from lesion to lesion. In most instances, it is probably a secondary event following the rupture of a dilated duct (or a cyst) in an area of fibrocystic disease, perhaps precipitated by minor trauma.

Severe trauma in a previously normal breast is the causative agent in most other instances. Such a history was given by thirty-eight of 110 patients reported by Adair and Munzer.[15]

An increased incidence of mammary fat necrosis has been noted after surgical excision of breast nodules. Rarely, fat necrosis of the subcutaneous tissue overlying the breast is a local manifestation of Weber-Christian disease.[16]

Grossly, the lesion may be in the subcutaneous tissue or in the breast. When it is located within the breast, it measures from 1 cm to 8 cm, in diameter, is firm but not stony hard, is rather sharply defined, and at times occurs as multiple masses. The gross appearance is sufficiently characteristic to differentiate it from carcinoma. Early fat necrosis is confined to several well-defined fat lobules. Later, the lesion may become cystic. The cysts may be small or large. They contain yellow granular material and pools of fat. The firmer areas may be opaque, yellowish brown, and greasy. There is considerable surrounding fibrous induration. Calcareous masses may eventually develop in the cystic areas.

Fat necrosis is nonbacterial. It is caused by slow aseptic saponification of nodular fat by blood and tissue lipase.[18] Microscopically, there are fat-filled cystic spaces surrounded by foreign body giant cells, collections of fat-filled macrophages, and interstitial infiltration by plasma cells. Duct stasis is often present, a finding probably related to the pathogenesis of some of these lesions.[17] Interstitial tissues may also show an increased number of plasma cells. The prominent proliferation of the connective tissue around the lesion may cause it to be confused with a malignant neoplasm.

Clinicopathologic correlation

The firm lesions of fat necrosis closely mimic carcinoma. Over one-half of the lesions are attached to the overlying skin. The nipple seldom is retracted, and deep attachment is rare (Fig. 887). Breast pain and axillary lymph node enlargement are usually absent. The close clinical resemblance of this lesion to carcinoma was emphasized by Hadfield.[18] In a review of forty-five cases, he found that twelve patients had a radical mastectomy for supposed cancer. Of twelve consecutive cases of fat necrosis at Barnes Hospital seen before 1948, five were thought to be carcinoma and two of the patients had a radical mastectomy.

Mammary duct ectasia

Haagensen[21] gave the name of **mammary duct ectasia** to a lesion previously described under designations such as varicocele tumor, comedomastitis, and mastitis obliterans.[22] In this process, there are dilatation of the ducts, fibrous thickening of the walls, and ductal accumulation of fatty detritus (Fig. 888). When this material escapes from the ducts, it causes inflammation. Ductal thickening and shortening may be associated with retraction of the skin and nipple, resulting in a clinical diagnosis of carcinoma.

We have been impressed by the similarity among plasma cell mastitis, fat necrosis, and mammary duct ectasia. We believe that in most instances they represent different stages of the same process. Duct stasis is the common denominator in all of them. If the material escapes from the ducts, fat necrosis and inflammation may result. The inflammatory component invari-

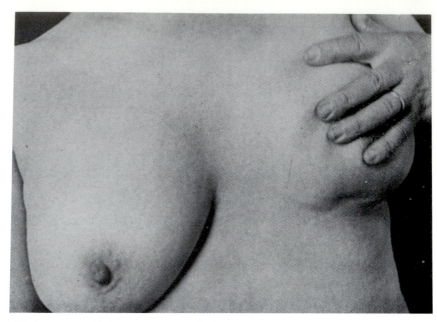

Fig. 887 Retraction of skin in patient with fat necrosis. (WU neg. 50-2035; from Lee, B. J., and Adair, F.: Traumatic fat necrosis of the female breast and its differentiation from carcinoma, Ann. Surg. **80:**670-691, 1924.)

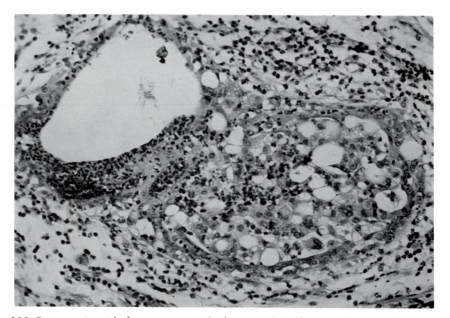

Fig. 888 Duct stasis with fat necrosis and plasma cell infiltration. Patient had retraction of nipple and indefinite mass. There was no carcinoma. (×225; WU neg. 51-4212.)

ably contains a larger number of plasma cells.

Fibrocystic disease

Two questions are frequently asked concerning fibrocystic disease. Does fibrocystic disease predispose to carcinoma? Does carcinoma arise from areas of fibrocystic disease? It is very difficult to answer these questions dogmatically. Frantz et al.[24] studied the incidence of fibrocystic disease in 225 women at postmortem examination.

Table 38 The relationship of gross cystic disease in 1693 patients to the subsequent development of carcinoma of the breast, 1930-1968*

Age	Person years	Observed breast carcinomas	Expected breast carcinomas
25–29	88.50		.004
30–34	586.75		.098
35–39	1552.50	2	.594
40–44	2999.50	8	2.138
45–49	3946.50	12	4.185
50–54	3377.00	23	3.963
55–59	2125.00	14	2.977
60–64	1107.25	5	1.835
65–69	492.25	7	.987
70 +	207.00	1	.569
Total	16482.25	72	17.35

Observed incidence   72
Expected incidence   17.35

The observed incidence is four times the expected incidence.

Note: 23 carcinomas were found concomitantly with cysts and are excluded.

*From Haagensen, C. D.: Diseases of the breast, ed. 2, Philadelphia, 1971, W. B. Saunders Co.

The incidence of fibrocystic disease compared to that occurring in surgical specimens was exceedingly low. In fact, they found only one instance of a cyst large enough (2 cm in diameter) to have constituted a dominant lump. The incidence of fibrocystic disease found in these breasts was significantly lower than that in cancerous breasts.

By contrast, florid and atypical proliferative changes are frequently found by careful examination of breasts containing carcinoma and in the previous breast biopsies from women who later developed carcinoma.[26, 30] In some instances, histologic transition to carcinoma can be traced from proliferative lesions, from areas of hyperplasia in acinar epithelium, from epithelial proliferation within a cyst, and from apocrine epithelium. In the noncancerous breast, areas of atypical intraductal epithelial proliferation may represent the first detectable microscopic evidence of intraductal cancer. It is in such rare cases that

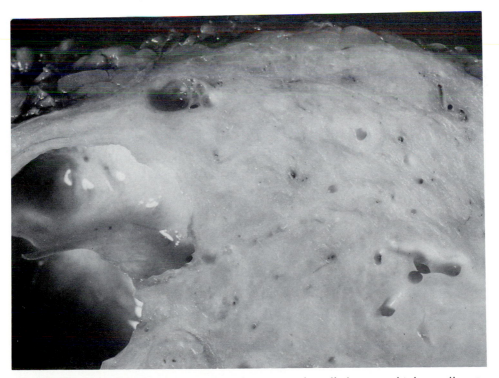

Fig. 889 Fibrocystic disease demonstrating large smooth-walled cyst, multiple small cysts, and increased stromal tissue. (WU neg. 52-3540.)

simple mastectomy should be considered. Haagensen's study[25] showed that in a group of patients with fibrocystic disease the risk of developing cancer was four times greater than in a group of similarly aged women without it (Table 38). Kiaer,[27] in an exhaustive study, also showed that there was an increased risk of the development of breast cancer in women with mammary fibrocystic disease. This risk was at about the same level as indicated by Haagensen.[25]

Foote and Stewart[23] demonstrated that a patient with fibrocystic disease primarily in one breast has just as much chance of developing cancer in the oppo-

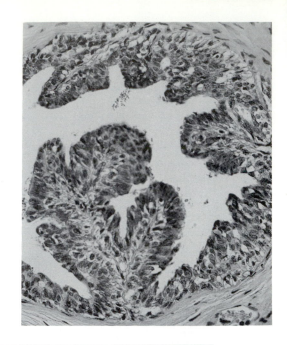

Fig. 890 Intraductal papillomatosis. This lesion is an expression of fibrocystic disease. (×240; WU neg. 51-931.)

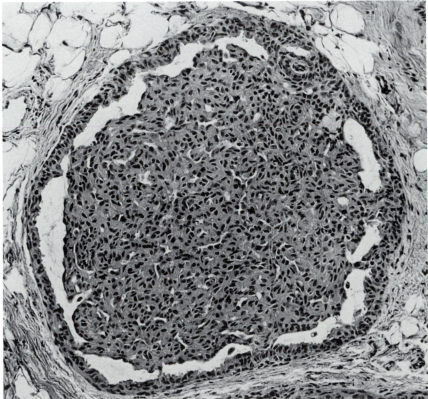

Fig. 891 Photomicrograph demonstrating marked epithelial hyperplasia within dilated duct. There is no evidence of necrosis, and individual cells are well supported by their stroma. Lesion is completely benign. Prominent cleft has formed between solid intraluminal proliferation and outer epithelial row. In our experience, this is usually indicative of benign condition. (×160; WU neg. 72-9814.)

site breast. Therefore, the only rational form of prophylactic treatment would be to remove both breasts. The only procedure indicated for the slightly increased frequency of carcinoma in fibrocystic disease is a close follow-up, particularly of premenopausal women.

Fibrocystic disease is extremely important in surgical pathology. Because it is proliferative, it often is confused with carcinoma. Its incidence is difficult to estimate because the diagnosis depends upon the liberality of the individual pathologist.[23] It is most frequent in women between 25 and 45 years of age.

Fibrocystic disease has all gradations of severity. The cysts have a bluish cast (blue dome cyst of Bloodgood) and contain cloudy yellow or clear fluid. The breast parenchyma between the larger cysts is yellowish gray and may contain numerous small thin-walled cysts (Fig. 889). Large cysts are relatively infrequent. The process is most often bilateral, but one breast may be much more diseased than the other and appear clinically to be the only one involved. At times, no cysts are present. There is only diffuse, fibrous thickening of the parenchyma.

Microscopically, the proliferative changes vary. The walls of the cysts may be lined by flattened epithelium. This epithelium often is absent, the cyst having only thick, fibrous walls. The breast parenchyma in patients with cystic disease invariably contains patches of apocrine epithelium that may have a papillary pattern. The individual cells are large and contain medium-sized nuclei and bright pink cytoplasm. Multiple areas of microscopic intraductal hyperplasia and papillomatosis are frequent (Figs. 890 and 891). There

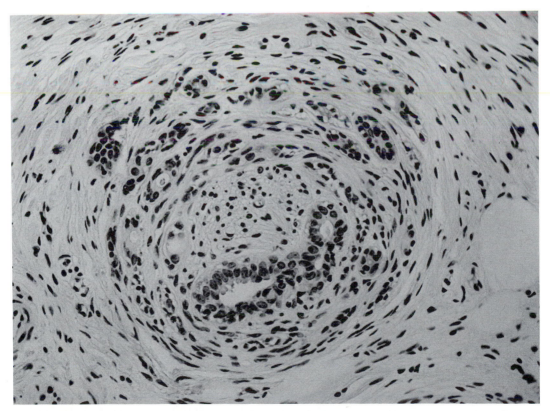

Fig. 892 Perineurial involvement in patient with fibrocystic disease. Nests of well-differentiated glands are present. This is not evidence of malignancy. (×335; AFIP 55-22047.)

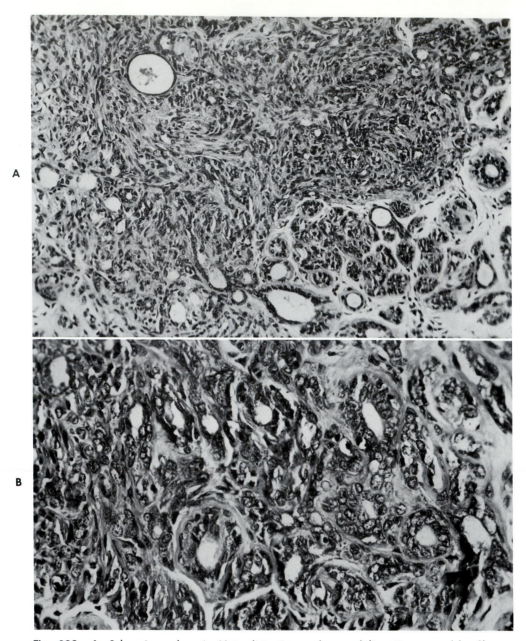

Fig. 893 A, Sclerosing adenosis. Note distortion and poor delineation caused by fibrous tissue proliferation. **B,** Same lesion illustrated in **A** showing absence of necrosis, uniformity of cells, and lack of mitotic activity. (**A,** ×200; WU neg. 49-4500; **B,** ×400; WU neg. 49-4501.)

also is considerable proliferation of the acinar epithelium, the pattern being modified by the accompanying connective tissue proliferation. In time, the proliferative connective tissue may become acellular and hyalinized. With this change, individual breast lobules invariably are dis-torted. This distortion may be sufficient to be misdiagnosed as invasive carcinoma. The ducts may proliferate and end blindly. This change has been designated by Foote and Stewart[23] as blunt-duct adenosis. It is this melange that constitutes the entity fibrocystic disease.

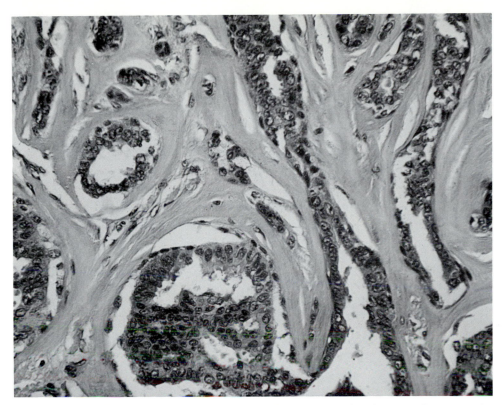

Fig. 894 Well-differentiated glands growing in dense stroma. This distortion by stroma is one reason why adenoma of nipple is incorrectly called carcinoma. Note double layering, which helps to indicate that lesion is benign. (×275; WU neg. 66-7569.)

Rarely, benign glands of florid fibrocystic disease may be seen growing within perineurial spaces (Fig. 892). This is not an indication of malignancy but rather an expression of increased rate of growth along planes of lesser resistance.[31]

Sclerosing adenosis

Sclerosing adenosis is merely a rather uncommon, highly proliferative form of fibrocystic disease. It is found about once in every 100 benign breast lesions. In a large series reported by Urban and Adair,[33] the average age of the patient was 31 years (20 to 50 years). The process usually occurs in the upper outer quadrant (which is also the most common site of carcinoma of the breast) has a disclike configuration, and cuts with increased resistance.

The most important identifying feature is the architecture of the lesion seen at very low magnification. A fibrohyaline center with scattered entrapped glands is seen completely surrounded by an extremely cellular glandular proliferation *that retains a lobular pattern*. There is no cytologic atypia and no necrosis. If the characteristic configuration of sclerosing adenosis is recognized, then the cellularity of the lesion, the distortion of the epithelial component by proliferating connective tissue, and the presence of an occasional mitotic figure will not result in a mistaken diagnosis of carcinoma (Fig. 893).

Adenoma of nipple

Adenoma of the nipple (papillomatosis of the nipple ducts) is a form of fibrocystic disease with distinct clinical and pathologic findings. Taylor and Robertson[32] have reported twenty-nine cases from 26 women and 3 men. The majority occurred in the fourth and fifth decades. The

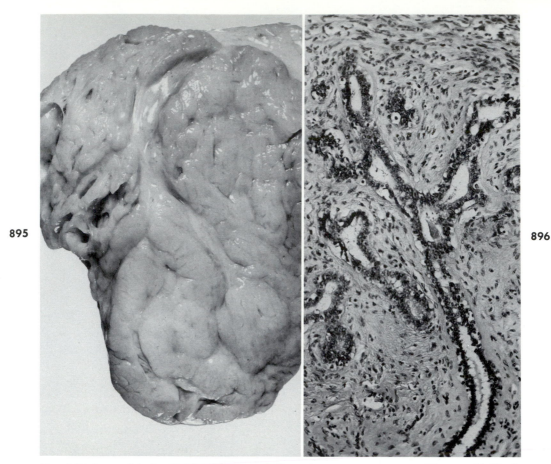

895

896

Fig. 895 Large lobulated "fetal" type of fibroadenoma occurring in 37-year-old black woman. Note absence of necrosis. (WU neg. 51-5002.)

Fig. 896 "Fetal" type of fibroadenoma with cellular stroma and well-defined glands. (×150; WU neg. 49-5941.)

nipple may become eroded.[28] For this reason, it has been mistaken clinically for Paget's disease. The most common complaint is that of serous or bloody discharge from the nipple. It is practically always unilateral.

Microscopically, the lesion shows marked proliferative changes and distortion of ductal elements by dense stroma that may be mistaken for invasive cancer (Fig. 894).

Presence of a two-cell layer in most ducts, uniformity of the cells, and lack of atypia and necrosis identify the lesion as benign, despite the occasional presence of mitoses and the presence of solid nests of cells. In the series reported by Taylor and Norris,[31] ten of the patients had been erroneously treated by mastectomy. Local excision is curative.[29]

Benign tumors
Fibroadenoma

Fibroadenomas of the breast are frequent in women between 20 and 35 years of age. These tumors increase in size during pregnancy and tend to regress as the age of the patient increases. Grossly, they are usually single but may be multiple in the same breast or in both breasts. In the younger age group, a type of fibroadenoma sometimes designated as giant, fetal, or juvenile, may weigh as much as 1,000 gm (Figs. 895 and 896). The usual fibroadenoma, however, is a sharply demarcated,

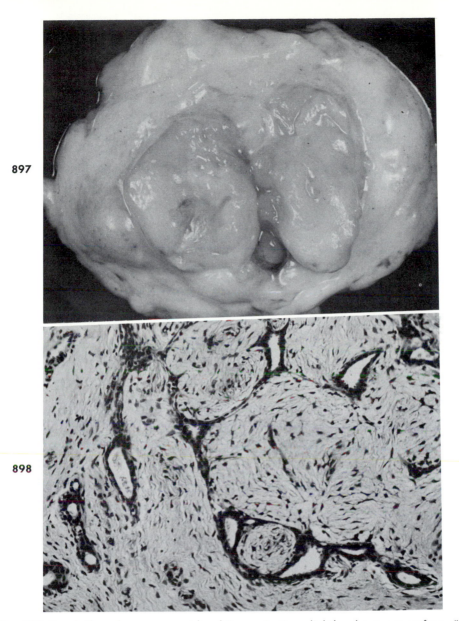

897

898

Fig. 897 Usual fibroadenoma, grayish white, projecting slightly above cut surface. (WU neg. 48-4541.)
Fig. 898 Intracanalicular fibroadenoma with rather cellular stroma. (Low power; WU neg. 47-102.)

firm tumor, usually no more than 3 cm in diameter. In time, it may calcify or ossify and become extremely hard. Rarely, in the younger woman a fibroadenoma may undergo partial or complete mucoid degeneration. The cut surface is grayish white with a whorllike pattern in which poorly defined nodules project slightly above the cut surface (Fig. 897). Slitlike spaces are often present. The absence of necrosis is valuable diagnostically. The type of breast cancer that is occasionally mistaken for fibroadenoma is the medullary type. It is softer, more opaque, and frequently contains minute areas of necrosis.

Microscopically, the pattern of the fibroadenoma varies greatly because of different amounts of the epithelial and connective tissue components. Fibroadenomas are labeled *intracanalicular* when the growth of connective tissue is so rapid that it invaginates the ducts into slitlike spaces (Fig. 898) and *pericanalicular* when the regular round configuration of the glands is maintained. Often, both types of growth are seen in the same lesion. The distinction has no practical connotations.

The well-defined ducts of a fibroadenoma are composed of cuboidal or cylindrical cells with round uniform nuclei. The stroma is made of loose connective tissue rich in acid mucopolysaccharides, although in ancient lesions it may undergo hyaline, calcific, or osseous metaplasia. The cellularity varies a great deal from case to case. Exceptionally, mature adipose tissue is seen intermingled with the fibrous stroma.[45]

Malignant transformation of a fibroadenoma is exceptional and for practical purposes can be disregarded in the management of this lesion. However, we have seen a few unquestionable cases in which part of the epithelial component of a fibroadenoma had the microscopic appearance of carcinoma.[37] In some cases the malignant tumor was entirely within the confines of the fibroadenoma and in others involved the surrounding breast as well. The latter may simply represent invasion of the fibroadenoma by a cancer originated elsewhere in the breast. McDivitt et al.[43] collected twenty-six cases of cancers arising in fibroadenomas. Of the sixteen lobular tumors, nine were limited to the fibroadenoma (seven being in situ and two infiltra-

tive) and seven were also present in the surrounding breast (six in situ and one infiltrative). Of the ten ductal carcinomas, eight were present only in the fibroadenoma (six in situ and two infiltrative) and two (both infiltrative) also involved the neighboring gland. The prognosis of the tumors limited to the fibroadenoma was excellent.

Sarcomatous transformation of the stroma of a fibroadenoma is an even rarer phenomenon, if it happens at all. We have seen only one suggestive case in which a well-circumscribed small nodule had in some areas the appearance of an osteosarcoma, whereas in others it was composed of hyaline stroma enclosing slitlike glandular spaces, a configuration strongly reminiscent of an ancient fibroadenoma.[35]

Lactating adenoma

The term lactating adenoma refers to a localized focus of hyperplasia in the lactating breast. Grossly, the lesion is well-circumscribed and lobulated. The cut surface is gray or tan, in contrast to the white color of fibroadenoma. Necrotic changes are frequent.[41] Microscopically, proliferated glands are seen lined by actively secreting cuboidal cells. This lesion should be differentiated from proliferative and secretory changes brought upon by pregnancy on a preexisting fibroadenoma.

Intraductal papilloma

The intraductal papilloma is one of the most important lesions arising from the ducts of the breast. The management of these lesions in the past has included no

Table 39 Follow-up of seventy-six patients with intraductal papilloma treated by local excision (Presbyterian Hospital, New York, N. Y., 1916-1941)*

Site in breast	Total patients treated by local excision	Recurrence of papilloma		Developed carcinoma	% follow-up
		Under 5 years	After 5 years		
Central	56	2	0	0	94.6
Peripheral	20	0	1	0	95.0
All sites	76	2	1	0	94.7

*Compiled from Haagensen, C. D., Stout, A. P., and Phillips, J. S.: The papillary neoplasms of the breast, Ann. Surg. 133:18-36, 1951.

treatment, local excision, simple mastectomy, and radical mastectomy. The inexperienced pathologist frequently diagnoses them incorrectly as carcinoma. Evidence of their benign character, their distribution, and the results of treatment are indicated in Table 39.

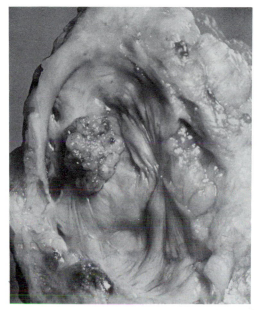

Fig. 899 Soft, rather large intraductal papilloma. (WU neg. 47-3569.)

These lesions can usually be palpated when they are in the region of the nipple. They are often small but may become 4 cm or 5 cm in diameter (Fig. 899). They usually are quite soft and fragile, being supported only by filamentous fibrous tissue trabeculae. Areas of hemorrhage are common. The larger ones appear to lie inside a cystic dilatation of the duct. The multiplicity and the danger of malignant change of these lesions have been markedly exaggerated.[42] Haagensen et al.[39] reported recurrences in only three out of 108 instances. These recurrences may have represented new lesions, but, in any event, the disease did not progress.

Microscopically, frozen section diagnosis of the intraductal papilloma often is difficult because of the extreme cellularity of the lesion (Fig. 900). The papillary projections may be trapped in the wall of the cyst, suggesting invasion and malignancy. Infarction and squamous metaplasia may be confusing.

The difficulty in diagnosis increases with the size and complexity of the papilloma. Kraus and Neubecker[40] summarized the various criteria by which an intraductal papilloma can be differentiated from a

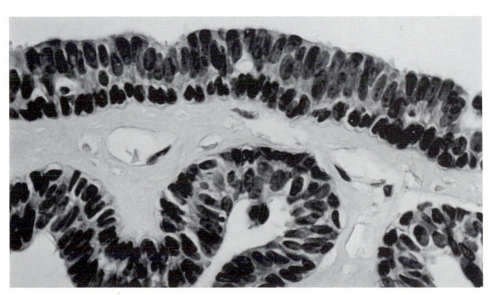

Fig. 900 Intraductal papilloma showing clearly defined double layer. (High power; WU neg. 61-6991.)

papillary cancer, a common diagnostic dilemma for the pathologist (Table 40). Of the last 100 consecutive breast cases sent to us in consultation, forty-four were intraductal papillary lesions. Double layer-

Table 40 Differential diagnosis between intraductal papilloma and papillary carcinoma*

Papilloma	Papillary carcinoma
Two types of epithelial cells	Single type of epithelial cell
Nuclei normochromatic	Nuclei hyperchromatic
Aprocrine metaplasia present	Apocrine metaplasia absent
Complex glandular pattern	Cribriform pattern
Prominent connective tissue stroma	Delicate or absent connective tissue stroma
Periductal fibrosis with epithelial entrapment	Epithelial invasion of stroma
Intraductal hyperplasia in adjacent ducts	Intraductal carcinoma in adjacent ducts
Sclerosing adenosis sometimes present in adjacent breast tissue	Sclerosing adenosis generally absent in adjacent breast tissue

*From Kraus, F. T., and Neubecker, R. D.: The differential diagnosis of papillary tumors of the breast, Cancer **15**:444-455, 1962.

ing of the cells in papillomas and cribriform pattern and cytologic atypia in carcinomas have been the main distinguishing features in our experience (Fig. 900).

If a major duct contains a papilloma, local excision is adequate therapy. Long-term follow-up without the development of further difficulty emphasizes the wisdom of conservative treatment.[44, 47] Simple mastectomy is not indicated.

Gynecomastia

Gynecomastia may result from innumerable causes.[46, 49] In a report of 160 cases, Wheeler et al.[48] emphasized that enlargement of the male breast before 25 years of age is usually related to hormonal pubertal changes, but after 25 years of age it is often a manifestation of a serious underlying disease. In a series of 351 cases reported by Bannayan and Hajdu,[34] fifty were classified as juvenile, 103 as idiopathic, and thirty-eight as drug-induced (digitalis, reserpine, Dilantin, etc.). The remaining were secondary to a large variety of causes. The

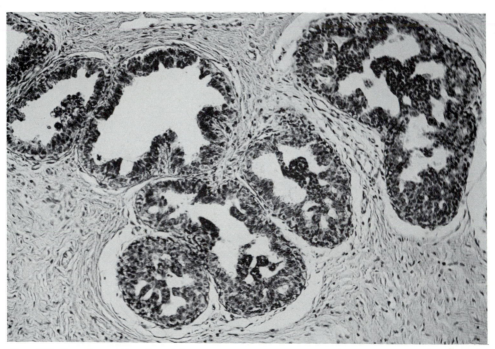

Fig. 901 Prominent intraductal hyperplasia and stromal edema in gynecomastia. (×145; WU neg. 56-4822.)

disease was unilateral (the left breast being involved more often than the right) in 244 patients and was bilateral in 107. Gynecomastia was centrally located in 311 patients and eccentrically located in the remaining. The authors concluded that pubertal and hormone-induced gynecomastias tend to be bilateral, whereas idiopathic and nonhor-

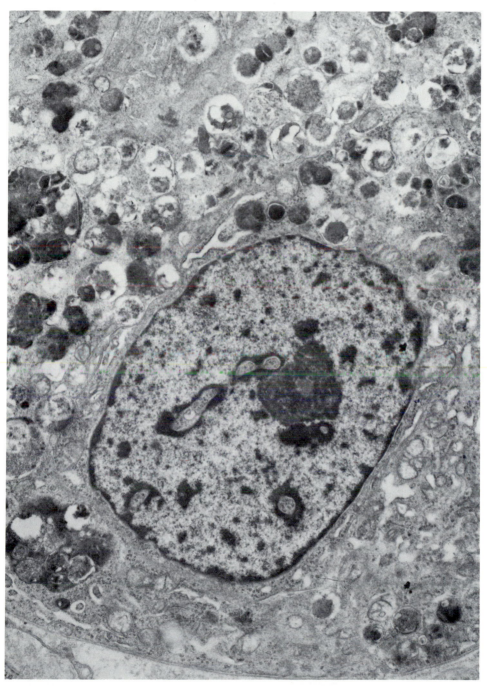

Fig. 902 Cells from cutaneous granular cell tumor containing numerous osmiophilic cytoplasmic granules. Some contain myelin figures. Myofilaments are not present. (Approximately ×12,000.)

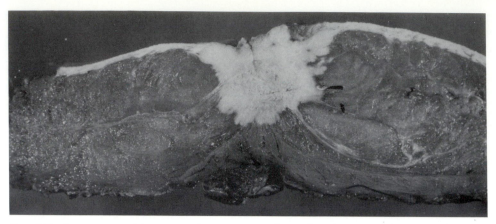

Fig. 903 Carcinoma of breast with retraction of nipple. There are fine grayish white streaks of tumor ramifying into fat. (Courtesy Dr. R. Johnson, Columbia, Mo.)

monal drug-induced gynecomastias are usually unilateral.

Gynecomastia is characterized by considerable epithelial intraductal hyperplasia and stromal edema (Fig. 901). This swollen stroma around ducts produces a characteristic "halo" effect. It is mainly composed of acid mucopolysaccharides (particularly hyaluronic acid) and remarkably similar to that found in fibroadenoma of the female breast.[36]

In rare cases, the intraductal epithelial hyperplasia is so extreme as to simulate carcinoma. The microscopic changes are related to the duration of the gynecomastia. Cases of short duration tend to have a prominent hyperplastic epithelial component and stromal edema, whereas in those of long duration stromal fibrosis is prominent. Formation of lobules was observed in twenty-one of the 351 patients reviewed by Bannayan and Hajdu.[34]

Granular cell tumor

Granular cell tumor (a better designation than the misleading granular cell myoblastoma) is a rare but important lesion because no other benign lesion so closely mimics mammary carcinoma. On section, it is firm, homogeneous, and usually white or grayish yellow. As a rule, it is not attached to the overlying skin. Occasionally, it is fixed to the underlying fascia. It may be as large as 10 cm in diameter.

Microscopically, the tumor cells are uniform and large, with vesicular nuclei, abundant granular cytoplasm, and well-defined cytoplasmic outlines. Mitotic figures usually are absent. Necrosis may occur at times. Sudanophilic material seldom is present in the tumor cells. The cytoplasmic granules are PAS positive, contain abundant acid phosphatase and other hydrolytic enzymes, and have an heterogeneous appearance under the electron microscope (Fig. 902). They represent markedly increased, bizarre lysosomes. Only frozen section will differentiate granular cell tumor from carcinoma.[38]

Malignant tumors
Carcinoma

The overwhelming number of malignant tumors of breast parenchyma are carcinomas (95% or more). These tumors can arise from the duct as well as from the lobular epithelium. Their gross and microscopic features are influenced by their growth within the ducts and lobules, the amount of connective tissue and mucin which they form, their cellular type, and their degree of invasiveness, if any. Extraneous adjectives that have no significance are often applied to breast carcinomas: scirrhous means hard, encephaloid means soft, and carcinoma simplex means a simple carcinoma. These titles are of no prognostic value and should be discarded.

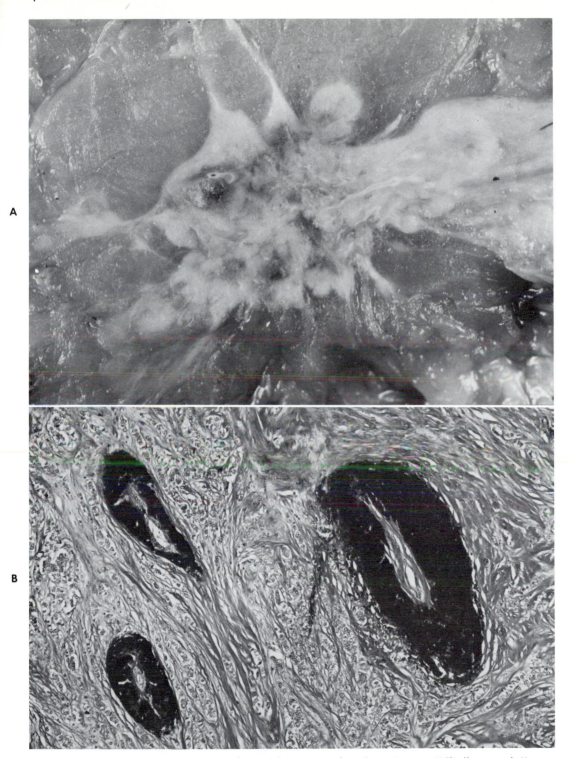

Fig. 904   A, Gross appearance of typical invasive ductal carcinoma. "Chalky streaks" can be seen throughout tumor. Central space can be identified in some of them. **B,** Elastic tissue stain of lesion illustrated in **A** showing that "chalky streaks" correspond to grossly thickened elastic layer in wall of nonneoplastic ducts crossing tumor. (**A,** WU neg. 72-10775; **B,** Verhoeff–van Gieson; ×90; WU neg. 72-6052.)

Invasive ductal carcinoma

Grossly, the usual carcinoma of the breast arising from duct epithelium is a poorly defined mass, the hardness of which depends upon the amount of connective tissue present. The tumor cuts with a resistant gritty sensation (unripe pear), is usually yellowish gray, and has fibrous trabeculae radiating through the bright yellow fat of the breast parenchyma (Fig. 903). It is not rare for these fibrous strands to connect with other nodules of carcinoma at some distance from the primary tumor. The characteristic "chalky streaks" fre-

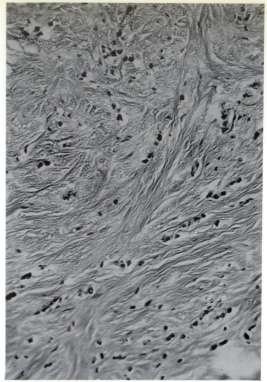

Fig. 905 Carcinoma of breast (small cell type) with extreme production of fibrous tissue. Individual tumor cells are arranged in "Indian file." This probably represents invasive lobular carcinoma. (×200; WU neg. 49-5467.)

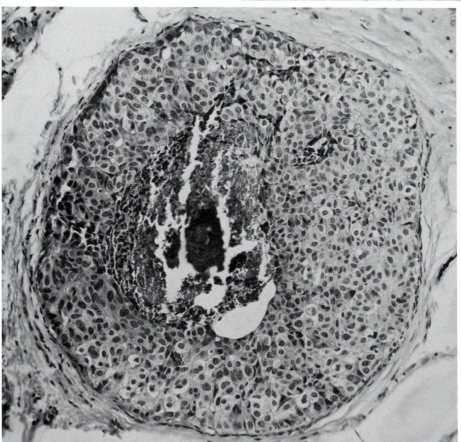

Fig. 906 Intraductal carcinoma of breast confined to duct with central necrosis and calcification. (×180; WU neg. 50-687.)

quently seen in the cut surface do not represent foci of tumor necrosis, as generally believed, but rather bulky masses of elastic tissue surrounding large mammary ducts[51] (Fig. 904). This change also can be seen in benign conditions.[49a] Predominantly cellular tumors are much softer and often contain larger areas of necrosis. The tumor may invade the underlying fascia or muscle.

Microscopically, the tumor cells vary in size and shape and may or may not form glandular spaces. The individual cells of a cellular tumor have prominent nucleoli and many mitotic figures. Areas of necrosis are frequent. It may be difficult to identify tumor cells if the connective tissue is greatly increased. They may occur in groups of only five or six cells containing very little cytoplasm and surrounded by hyalinized connective tissue. Under low power,

this infrequent variant of breast carcinoma (small cell type) may be completely missed (Fig. 905).

Multiple foci of origin are common, especially in younger women. They have been clearly demonstrated by whole organ preparations examined by radiography and light microscopy.[50, 52]

Intraductal carcinoma with or without invasion

The intraductal carcinoma is a relatively infrequent form of breast cancer that grows predominantly within ducts. The duct wall becomes greatly thickened largely because of increase in elastic tissue.

Grossly, the tumor contains thick-walled ducts with normal breast parenchyma between them. When the ducts are compressed, wormlike masses of necrotic tumor sometimes extrude from them—thus

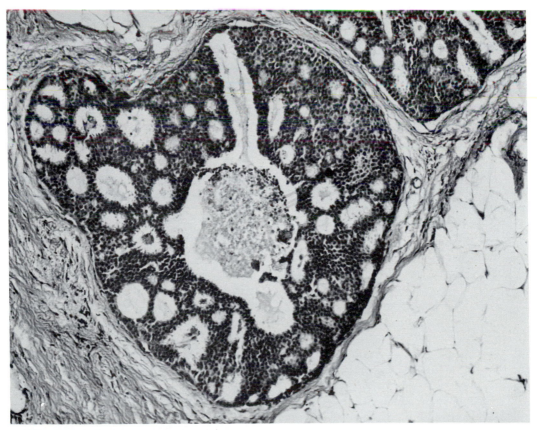

Fig. 907 Intraductal carcinoma. There is cribriform pattern and central necrosis. Compare with Fig. 891. (×160; WU neg. 72-9813.)

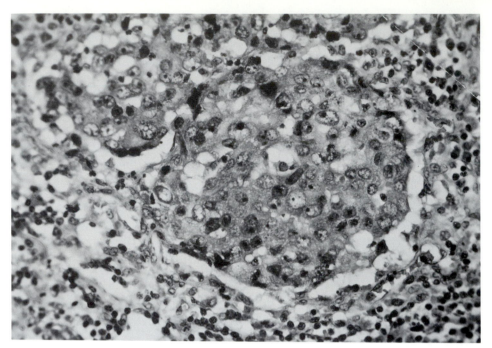

Fig. 908 Medullary carcinoma with considerable lymphoid stroma. Note poor differentiation of tumor cells. (×400; WU neg. 50-1419.)

the name comedocarcinoma given to this variety. If the tumor is contained within the duct lumina and the duct walls are not too greatly thickened, tumor may not be recognized grossly.

Microscopically, the tumor cells resemble those of the usual breast carcinoma. In this instance, however, the cells are confined to the ducts and are apparently noninvasive. Individual tumor cells have nuclei of variable size and shape with numerous mitotic figures. There is very little supporting connective tissue, and areas of central necrosis in the ducts are common (Figs. 906 and 907). Calcium salts frequently are deposited in these necrotic areas and can be identified by mammography.

Some ductal carcinomas, both in situ and invasive, are formed by cells with abundant acidophilic cytoplasm resembling apocrine epithelium. There is no need to separate these "apocrine carcinomas" from the rest, since there are no differences in their natural history.[53]

If a frozen section shows tumor confined to the ducts and there is no definitive mass palpable in the breast, invasion outside of the ducts in other levels may still be present, with the resulting possibility of low axillary lymph node metastases. Therefore, simple mastectomy is inadequate as definitive treatment. The usual type of invasive ductal carcinoma may have occasional areas of tumor growing intraductally. Such growth is not sufficient to justify a diagnosis of intraductal carcinoma.

Medullary carcinoma

The so-called medullary carcinoma of the breast has been well described by Moore and Foote.[55] The lesion has a distinctive gross and microscopic pattern. Patients often are under 50 years of age. The tumor is very well circumscribed and may be mistaken clinically and grossly for fibroadenoma. It may become large, usually has a homogeneously gray color, and contains small focal areas of necrosis.

Microscopically, the cells of medullary carcinoma are rather uniform and have large nuclei with numerous mitotic figures.

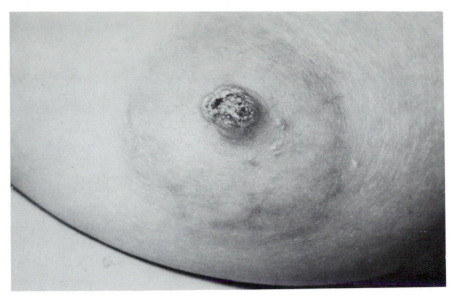

Fig. 909 Early Paget's disease of nipple. There was underlying carcinoma. (WU neg. 48-1456.)

The borders are always well circumscribed. An important part of the picture is a prominent lymphoid infiltrate (Fig. 908), which may represent a reaction of the host tissues to the neoplasm. If unduly prominent, it can be mistaken microscopically for malignant lymphoma.

Of the last twenty-three cases of medullary carcinoma seen at our institution, thirteen had axillary lymph node metastases. However, in nine of the thirteen cases, only one node was involved, always in the low group. The prognosis of this tumor type is excellent.[54, 56]

Paget's disease

Paget's disease of the breast is a name given to the crusted lesion of the nipple caused by cancer.[59] It is merely a peripheral manifestation of an underlying carcinoma of the breast (Fig. 909). A malignant intraductal component is always present, with or without associated stromal invasion. In this regard, the presence of Paget's disease is only a secondary, albeit dramatic feature of the tumor. The management and prognosis depend largely on the intraductal versus invasive nature of the underlying carcinoma rather than on the presence or appearance of the intraepithelial component.

Grossly, these weeping, eczematoid lesions appear to start on the nipple but later involve the areola and surrounding epidermis. They rarely extend more than a few centimeters. If a definite mass can be palpated beneath the diseased nipple, the underlying tumor will almost always be invasive. This was true in 106 of the 113 cases reviewed by Ashikari et al.[57] On the other hand, absence of a palpable mass is most often than not an indication that the carcinoma is purely intraductal. In the same series, this was found to be the case in sixty-three of ninety-six patients.

Microscopically, these tumors have the general characteristics of the usual ductal carcinoma. Invariably, if enough sections are studied, a connection between the carcinoma within the duct and carcinoma in the overlying nipple can be demonstrated. The large tumor cells lying within the epithelium are identical to the tumor cells lying within the ducts (Fig. 910).

The heated controversies held in the past regarding the histogenesis of Paget's disease of the breast have largely subsided.

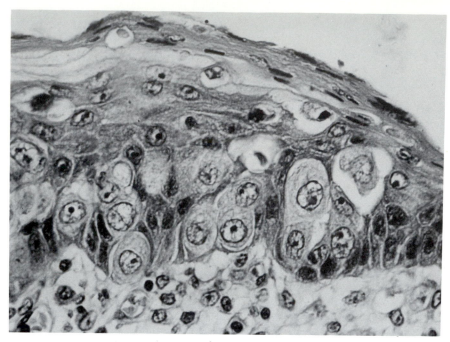

Fig. 910 Large Paget cells involving epidermis. (×450.)

Careful histochemical and electron microscopic studies have demonstrated that the intraepidermal Paget's cells are of mammary ductal origin and not keratinocytes or melanocytes.[58] The melanin granules that they occasionally contain in their cytoplasm have been, in all likelihood, transferred from neighboring melanocytes rather than manufactured by the tumor cells. The minor controversial point still unsettled is whether the intraepidermal carcinoma cells originate in deeper structures and gradually work their way upward or whether they represent a simultaneous malignant transformation of the intraepidermal portion of the mammary ducts.[60]

Inflammatory carcinoma

The term inflammatory carcinoma was originally used in a clinical sense for a type of breast cancer in which the entire breast was reddened and warm, with widespread edema of the skin, thus simulating the appearance of mastitis. Pathologic studies in some of these cases revealed the

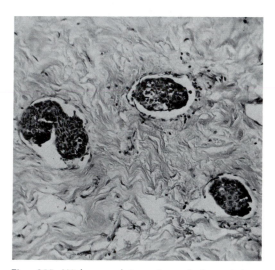

Fig. 911 Widespread invasion of dermal lymphatics in inflammatory carcinoma. (×140; WU neg. 49-5372.)

lesion to be an undifferentiated carcinoma with widespread carcinomatosis of the dermal lymphatic vessels (Fig. 911). This led to the belief that an "inflammatory" clinical appearance always corresponded pathologically to dermal lymphatic permeation and vice versa. This assumption is

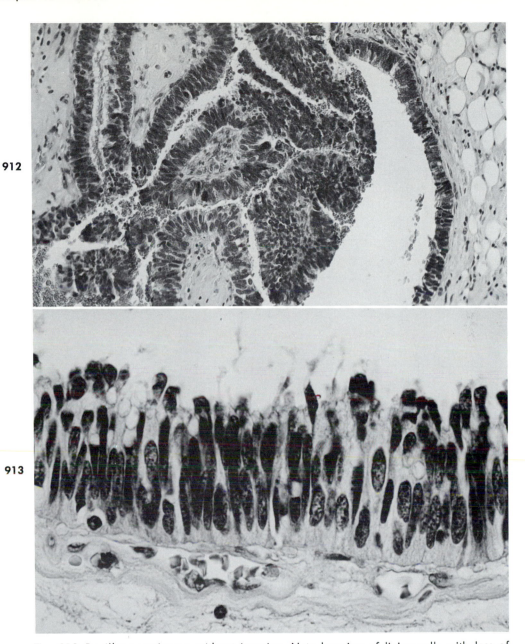

Fig. 912 Papillary carcinoma without invasion. Note layering of lining cells with loss of nuclear polarity. (×180; WU neg. 52-5317.)
Fig. 913 Papillary carcinoma demonstrating extreme layering of cells with loss of nuclear polarity. (×775; WU neg. 55-2816.)

false. Patients may have inflammatory carcinoma clinically in the absence of dermal invasion; conversely, widespread permeation of dermal lymphatics can be seen in the absence of the clinical features of inflammatory carcinoma. From a prognostic standpoint, the important finding is the presence of dermal lymphatic permeation on microscopic examination (a sign of ominous prognosis and of inoperability) and not the clinical appearance of the breast. It would probably be better to discard the term inflammatory carcinoma altogether.[60a]

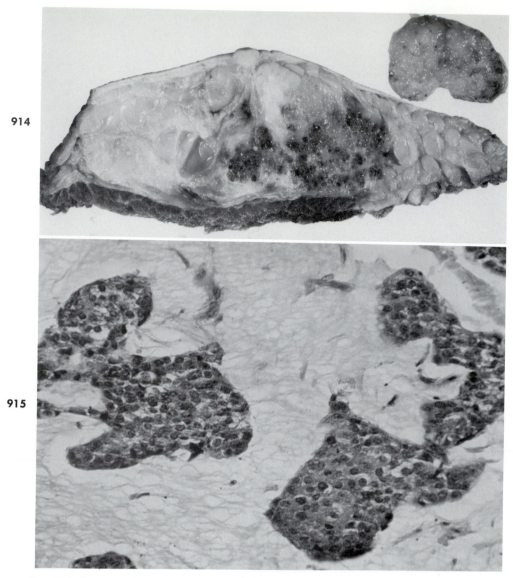

914

915

Fig. 914 Pure mucinous carcinoma of breast in 55-year-old woman. Note typical gelatinous appearance. Tumor measured 7 cm in greatest diameter and was associated with axillary metastases (right upper corner). (WU neg. 66-7609.)

Fig. 915 Typical appearance of mucinous carcinoma. Note well-differentiated character of cells floating in sea of mucin. (×310; WU neg. 62-9046.)

Papillary carcinoma with or without invasion

Papillary carcinomas of the breast are rare in our experience. They tend to ramify within ducts and to involve an entire breast segment. Microscopically, they show papillary projections within the ducts, layering of epithelium, loss of nuclear polarity, and occasional zones of necrosis (Figs. 912 and 913).

Frequently, these tumors are inadequately excised. Recurrence may not appear for many years (five or more are not rare). Such recurrence may be local or be accompanied by lymph node metastases.[61] This is the tumor that has often been diagnosed as benign intraductal papilloma undergoing malignant change. In truth, however, it was malignant from the start.

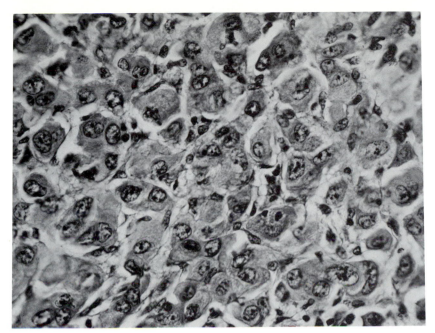

Fig. 916 Extremely undifferentiated carcinoma of breast that contains large amounts of cytoplasmic mucin. (×400; WU neg. 50-959.)

Mucinous carcinoma

If multiple sections of the breast are stained for mucin, small amounts nearly always will be found within the cytoplasm of the ductal epithelial cells. The diagnosis of mucinous carcinoma of the breast is justified only when the changes due to mucin are dominant. These tumors are well circumscribed, are palpably crepitant, and consist grossly of a currant jellylike mass often held together by delicate connective tissue septa (Fig. 914). Hemorrhage within the mass is frequent. Microscopically, tumor cells, often few in number, are seen floating in a sea of mucin (Fig. 915). The individual cells usually form well-defined acini.

The patient with a tumor with these gross and microscopic characteristics has a good prognosis.[62] The pure form of mucinous carcinoma occurs most often in older women as a solitary circumscribed lesion which rarely, if ever, metastasizes when the tumor is less than 5 cm in maximal dimension. In such selected instances, this lesion may be treated by wide local excision or by simple mastectomy. Conversely, if areas of mucinous carcinoma alternate with others of ordinary infiltrating ductal carcinoma, the incidence of metastases and ultimate prognosis are dependent on the latter. Mucinous carcinoma as just described should be clearly separated from the tumor consisting primarily of cells with large amounts of intracellular mucin (the rare signet ring type). The prognosis of this variety is extremely poor if not hopeless[63] (Fig. 916).

Epidermoid carcinoma

Epidermoid carcinomas of the breast are seldom seen. Tumors of epidermal origin and those in which the squamous component is a portion of an otherwise typical cystosarcoma phylloides should be excluded. The gross appearance of epidermoid carcinoma differs little from the usual breast carcinomas. Sometimes a large central cyst filled with keratin can be identified. Microscopically, most cases seem to represent instances of squamous metaplasia in ductal adenocarcinoma.[65] The squamous foci are often seen lining the wall of cystic formations. Intercellular bridges can usually be identified. The stroma can be quite prominent and cellu-

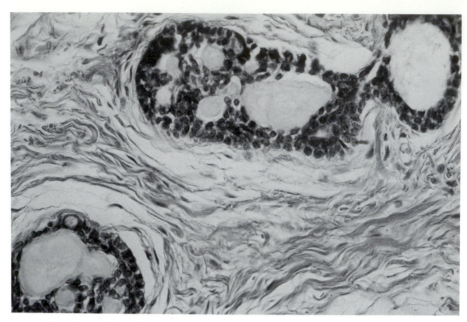

Fig. 917 Adenoid cystic carcinoma of breast. (×200; WU neg. 52-3872.)

lar. Epidermoid carcinoma is a tumor of elderly women and carries a similar prognosis to that of the ordinary ductal adenocarcinoma.[64]

Adenoid cystic carcinoma

The adenoid cystic type of carcinoma is an exceedingly rare variant of breast cancer. Microscopically, it resembles the homonymous tumor of salivary gland origin (Fig. 917). The similarity is maintained at the electron microscopic level.[68] Perineurial infiltration is prominent. Lymph node metastases practically never occur. Nayer[69] reported a patient with this type of carcinoma who had no lymph node metastases at the time of radical mastectomy but who died thirteen years later of pulmonary metastases. We have had seven patients, none of whom had axillary metastases. One patient developed pulmonary metastases six years after mastectomy.[67] Of the twenty-one patients reported by Cavanzo and Taylor,[66] none had evidence of axillary metastases and none died of the tumor. Two patients had local recurrence after simple excision but remained well after mastectomy. It is important not to confuse adenoid cystic carcinoma with intraductal carcinoma with a prominent cribriform pattern.

Well-differentiated (tubular) carcinoma

A microscopically deceptive neoplasm, well-differentiated (tubular) carcinoma is often confused with sclerosing adenosis. Grossly, it suggests carcinoma by virtue of its poorly circumscribed margins and hard consistency, but microscopically it simulates a benign condition because of the well-differentiated nature of the glands and the absence of necrosis, mitoses, and cytologic atypia. The striking ductal differentiation of this malignant neoplasm is also maintained at the electron microscopic level.[70] The clues to the diagnosis are the haphazard arrangement of the glands in the stroma, the resulting complete lack of lobular configuration, and the frequent occurrence of typical intraductal carcinoma in large ducts situated within the lesion (Fig. 918).

Metastases to axillary lymph nodes were documented in ten of thirty-three cases

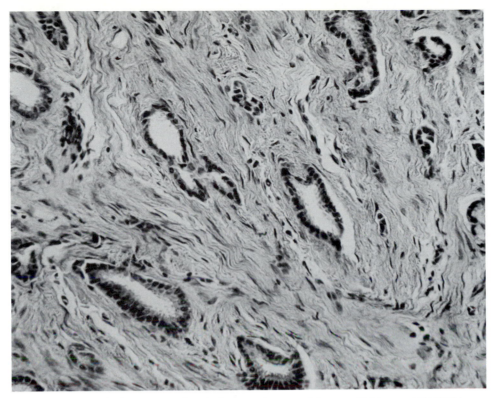

Fig. 918 Well-differentiated (tubular) carcinoma of breast. (WU neg. 59-7303.)

reviewed by Taylor and Norris.[71] The involved nodes were usually few and situated low in the axilla. Only one patient was known to have died as a result of the mammary tumor.

Lobular carcinoma, in situ and invasive

Lobular carcinoma arises in lobules and terminal ducts and comprises 6% to 10% of all breast cancers.[75] Three stages of evolution are recognized: lobular carcinoma *in situ*, lobular carcinoma *in situ* with infiltration, and infiltrative lobular carcinoma without an identifiable *in situ* component. The *in situ* form tends to occur in younger women. It has no gross distinguishing features and is usually found incidentally in breasts removed for other reasons. The disease, which is often multicentric and bilateral, concentrates within 5 cm of the nipple from the skin surface in the outer and inner upper quadrants.[78, 79] Residual foci of tumor are found regularly in breasts removed following a diagnosis of lobular carcinoma in situ made on a biopsy specimen.

Microscopically, the lobules are greatly enlarged and filled with closely packed cells having few mitotic figures and practically no necrosis (Fig. 919). The cells are quite uniform. Their nuclei are round and normochromatic, with minimal atypical features. Examination of the neighboring terminal ducts often reveals proliferation of similar cells, in some cases forming a continuous row beneath the secretory epithelium and in others resulting in a solid intraluminal growth.[81] Fechner[73] found these ductular changes in thirty-four of forty-five breasts with lobular carcinoma and remarked that their presence should stimulate a careful search for more diagnostic areas. We use the term lobular carcinoma in situ only for those cases in which the cellular proliferation has resulted in the formation of large solid nests

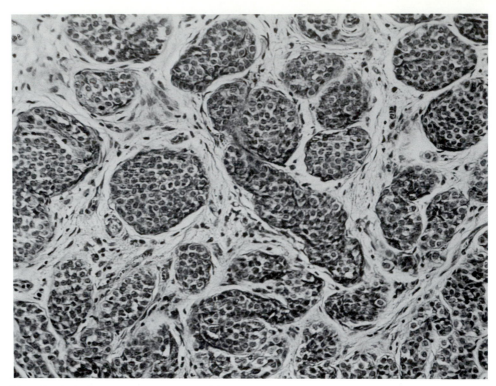

Fig. 919 Lobular carcinoma in situ of breast. Note lobular pattern, small cells, and lack of necrosis. (×200; WU neg. 52-3452.)

and prefer to designate as lobular hyperplasia those lesions having normal-sized lobules and ducts and preserving a central lumen (Fig. 920). Lobular carcinoma in situ should be differentiated from ductal carcinoma with secondary invasion of the lobules. The latter event, which occurs in about 20% of ductal cancers, is identified by the presence of necrosis, cellular pleomorphism, obviously atypical nuclear configuration, formation of small lumina, and the presence of typical changes of ductal carcinoma in the surrounding large ducts.[72]

The infiltrative component of lobular carcinoma is characterized by a haphazard cell growth without tendency to gland formation. The cells are arranged in "Indian files" in a dense fibrous stroma, quite often in a concentric manner around lobules involved by *in situ* tumor (Fig. 921). Once the pathologist has learned to recognize the architectural features of invasive lobular carcinoma by careful examination of lesions associated with an *in situ* component, he will be able to suggest a diagnosis of lobular carcinoma even in the absence of the noninvasive element.[74] It is probable that most of the tumors designated as "small cell" cancers represent infiltrative lobular carcinomas (Fig. 905). Mammography can detect approximately one-half of the cases of lobular carcinoma in situ. The positive mammograph shows finely stippled calcification, different from that seen in ductal carcinoma. Microscopically, the calcification is not in the cancer itself but in the surrounding normal lobules.[76, 77] The cell of origin of lobular carcinoma is still disputed. It is quite clear that the tumor arises from a cell normally situated beneath the layer of secretory epithelium, but whether this cell represents a myoepithelial element or an undifferentiated ("reserve") epithelial cell has not yet been established.[80]

Classification and grading

It is important to divide breast carcinomas into different types in order to be able to make some predictions regarding the

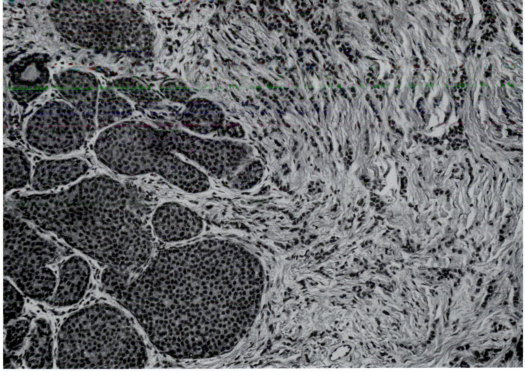

Fig. 920 Lobular hyperplasia. This is not lobular carcinoma in situ. Individual lobules are not solidly filled with cells, and lesion is confined to lobules. (×145; WU neg. 72-9812.)
Fig. 921 Lobular carcinoma in situ with areas of invasive small cell cancer. In situ areas demonstrate complete packing of individual lobules by uniform cells. These same cells have invaded surrounding tissue and have typical pattern of small cell cancer. (×150; WU neg. 73-60.)

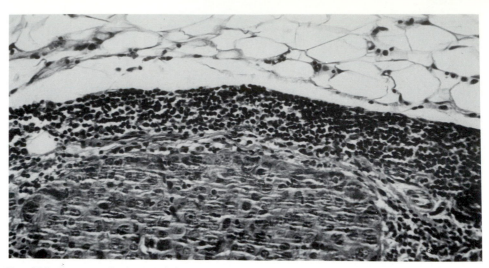

Fig. 922 Circumscribed, pushing border of medullary carcinoma of breast. There is also mantle of lymphocytes present. (×250; WU neg. 62-9048.)

presence and extent of lymph node metastases and thereby the prognosis and treatment. Some of the criteria used for such division are common to those employed for the grading of breast cancer.[83] The value of the latter practice in estimating prognosis has been demonstrated repeatedly.[82] Certain features, such as "pushing" peripheral margins, lymphocytic infiltration, and good microscopic differentiation correlate with a good prognosis regardless of tumor type[84-86] (Fig. 922). By applying these general criteria to the common classification by tumor type, we have divided breast cancers into four well-defined categories:

Type I—Not invasive

This type includes all *in situ* neoplasms, whether arising from ductal or lobular epithelium. The members of this group are (1) intraductal carcinoma (with or without Paget's disease), (2) intraductal papillary carcinoma, and (3) lobular carcinoma in situ. Numerous blocks should be obtained in all tumors of the Type I group in order to rule out the presence of invasion. If no invasion can be demonstrated, the incidence of metastases is practically zero and the prognosis after mastectomy is excellent.

Type II—Invasive, well circumscribed

This group is composed of five microscopically unrelated neoplasms, having in common invasive features, well-delineated margins, and good prog-

nosis after surgical therapy. Metastases to the axillary nodes are either absent or, when present, usually limited to the low group. The five tumors are (1) pure mucinous carcinoma, (2) medullary carcinoma, (3) well-differentiated (tubular) carcinoma, (4) invasive papillary carcinoma, and (5) adenoid cystic carcinoma.

Type III—Invasive, moderately metastasizing

This group, which is the most numerous, includes (1) the ordinary invasive ductal carcinoma, (2) intraductal carcinoma with invasion (with or without Paget's disease), (3) invasive lobular carcinoma, and (4) the rare epidermoid carcinoma. Actually, all carcinomas not definitely classified as Type I, II, or IV constitute Type III. Some recent reports suggest that invasive lobular carcinomas might have a worse prognosis than the other three varieties.

Type IV—Invasive, highly metastasizing

This group is composed of the undifferentiated carcinomas composed of cells without ductal or lobular arrangement, including the rare signet ring type of carcinoma. Tumors indisputably invading blood vessels, regardless of type, also belong to this category.

Effects of irradiation

Well-planned irradiation of breast carcinoma always causes skin changes, but its effect on the tumor is unpredictable. There is no doubt that focal areas of the tumor may be sterilized. Sometimes the tumor completely disappears or is replaced by fibrosis. Lumb[89] found that in tissue doses between 3,000 and 3,500 R, complete sterilization of the breast carcinomas occurred in only a few patients, (only one of thirteen), but that with doses of 3,500 to 4,000 R, the percentage was higher (four of eleven patients).

Tumors prominently affected by irradiation contain giant cells with atypical nuclei, naked nuclei, and abnormal mitotic figures. The viability of these tumor cells is difficult to assess. In spite of large amounts of axillary irradiation, tumors often are unaffected in some of the regional lymph nodes. Occasionally, tumor appears to have been sterilized in one portion of a lymph node yet unaffected in another area of the same node. Because of these findings we have been unable to assess objectively the value of irradiation to involved axillary lymph nodes.[87, 90] Undoubtedly, irradiation can wall off carcinoma for variable periods by partially sterilizing the tumor and by creating fibrosis. Such a palliative effect is well justified. Guttman[88] showed that it is possible to achieve a five-year survival rate of approximately 50% by means of roentgentherapy of mammary carcinomas which have been shown to be locally inoperable by biopsy.

Effects of steroid hormones

Estrogens, androgens, and steroids have been tried in different dosages for variable periods to relieve extensive inoperable carcinoma of the breast.[93] Older patients with soft tissue lesions are best treated with stilbestrol or other estrogenic preparations. Testosterone may cause regression of bone metastases in all age groups. Of course, regression of either the primary tumor or its metastases is only temporary. The majority have no objective regression at all—only progression despite treatment.

Microscopically, the changes produced by any steroid hormone are comparable. There may be prominent collagen hyalinization, increase in the amount of collagen, increase in the prominence of the elastic tissue, necrosis, and even complete disappearance of tumor cells. The changes in tumor cells often are scattered. One group of cells may disappear completely, another partially, and still another may be morphologically unaffected. The microscopic pattern of affected tumors does not show why there was a response to therapy. Cytoplasmic vacuolation, nuclear aberrations, and cell wall ruptures are present. These changes are roughly analogous to those caused by irradiation.

Rarely, prominent regressive changes, including complete disappearance of tumor cells, have been demonstrated in both the primary lesion and in the axillary lymph nodes[92] (Fig. 923). These morphologic changes also are seen infrequently after adrenalectomy for carcinoma of the breast. They are most likely to occur when adrenalectomy has been performed for inflammatory carcinoma of the breast.[91] It is impossible to predict by histologic examination which cancer of the breast will respond to hormonal or endocrine ablative therapy.

Sarcoma
Cystosarcoma phyllodes

The most common sarcoma of the breast is cystosarcoma phyllodes.[103] It occurs in the same age group as breast carcinoma. In the series of ninety-four cases reported by Norris and Taylor,[101] the median age at the time of diagnosis was 45 years. Only three patients were younger than 20 years of age, in striking contrast with the age distribution of patients with ordinary fibroadenoma. Although cystosarcoma phyllodes is well known for its propensity to reach giant proportions, it is well to remember that more than one-half of these tumors measure less than 5 cm in diameter.[100] It follows, then, that the diagnosis of cystosarcoma phyllodes can neither be made nor ruled out by size alone.[109, 110] A lesion with the microscopic appearance of fibroadenoma should still be diagnosed as such even if it reaches 5 cm or more in diameter (a rare event, predominantly seen in young black females).

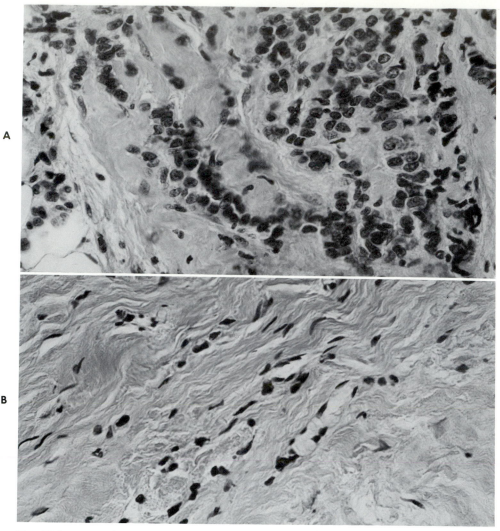

Fig. 923 **A,** Undifferentiated carcinoma of breast before treatment with testosterone. **B,** Same tumor shown in **A** after treatment with testosterone demonstrating prominent regression. Note naked nuclei and increased fibrosis. (**A** and **B,** ×400; **A,** WU neg. 50-2970; **B,** WU neg. 50-2971; slides contributed by Dr. R. Johnson, Columbia, Mo.)

Grossly, the typical cystosarcoma presents a teardrop appearance to the breast. The nipple may be flattened, but the overlying skin is almost never attached. On the other hand, attachment of the tumor to the underlying fascia is not infrequent. Cystosarcomas are usually well circumscribed, gray-white, and firm (Fig. 924). Areas of necrosis, cystic degeneration, and hemorrhage are seen in the larger tumors. Cleftlike spaces may be present. Infection may develop secondary to ulceration. We

have seen four cases in which the entire neoplasm had undergone massive hemorrhagic infarct.

The microscopic main points for the diagnosis of cystosarcoma are the prominent stromal cellularity and the presence of benign ductal elements as an integral component of the neoplasm.[103] Although the distinction between benign and malignant cystosarcoma can be very difficult to make in a given case, sufficient information is now available on the natural history

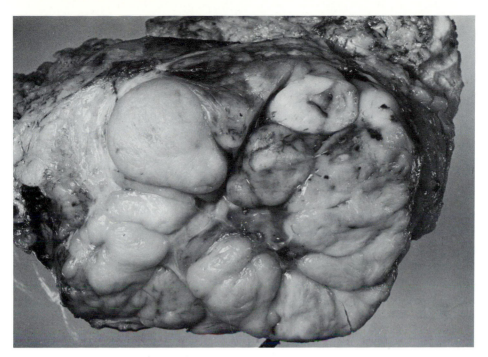

Fig. 924 Large cystosarcoma phyllodes of breast showing pseudoencapsulation and nodularity. (WU neg. 52-3814.)

of this neoplasm as to allow a statement to be made about the likelihood of metastases and proper management on the basis of the pathologic features. Tumors with the configuration of fibroadenomas having a cellular stroma without atypical features concentrated in the periductal areas generally lack the capacity to metastasize but have an increased incidence of local recurrence (Fig. 925, *A*). If an enucleation has been done under the clinical impression of fibroadenoma, the patient can be safely followed for the possibility of recurrence. If the latter develops, or if this type of cystosarcoma is recognized at the time of initial surgery, local excision with a wide margin of normal tissue is the treatment of choice. Recurrent cystosarcoma may still be cured by wide local excision even if resection of the chest wall is required. Recurrence is the consequence of inadequate excision.[99]

On the other hand, obvious sarcomatous tumors with marked nuclear atypia, large number of mitoses, and loss of the relationship between glands and stroma are poten-

tially metastasizing neoplasms and should be treated accordingly (Fig. 925, *B*). Simple mastectomy is sufficient in most instances, but if there is any question of invasion of the fascia, it should be removed together with the underlying muscle. Metastases of cystosarcoma to axillary nodes are exceptional. They were documented only once in the ninety-four cases reported by Norris and Taylor.[101] Therefore, there is hardly any justification for routine axillary dissection. For those cystosarcomas that do not fall easily into one of these two extreme categories, the decision has to be made on the basis of size, pushing versus peripheral margins, cellular atypia, and mitotic count.[101]

In the benign neoplasms, the stromal component has almost always a fibrous appearance, with occasional admixture of mature adipose foci. In the malignant variant, the stroma may have the appearance of fibrosarcoma, liposarcoma, chondrosarcoma, or osteosarcoma. The epithelial element is practically always benign. Norris and Taylor[101] identified a carcinomatous

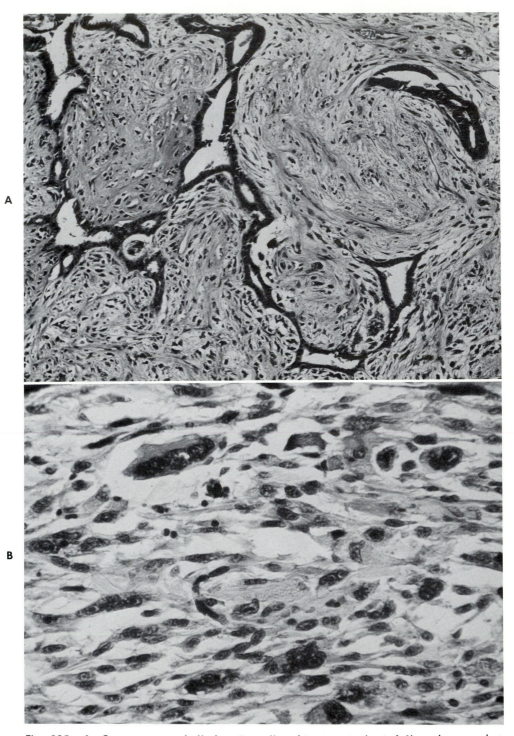

Fig. 925 **A,** Cystosarcoma phyllodes. Overall architecture is that of fibroadenoma, but there is marked stromal cellularity. **B,** Another area of tumor shown in **A.** Stroma is highly atypical and grows independently from epithelial components, two signs indicative of malignancy. (**A,** ×130; WU neg. 73-3408; **B,** ×300; WU neg. 73-3407.)

element in only two of their ninety-four cases.

Other sarcomas and related stromal lesions

Fibrosarcomas of breast stroma are usually large and firm and often circumscribed. Grossly, the tumors appear grayish white and homogeneous. Necrosis may be present. Microscopically, they have the characteristics of a fibrosarcoma (Chapter 23). These lesions may be distinguished clinically from carcinomas by their large size and by their failure to become attached to the skin. Microscopically, they are differentiated from cystosarcoma phyllodes by the lack of an epithelial component. Infiltrative margins and severe atypia indicate a greater tendency for local recurrence and distant metastases.[102]

We have seen a few cases of *fibromatosis* of the breast and one of *nodular fasciitis.* Haggitt and Booth[96] reported a case of bilateral fibromatosis of the breast associated with Gardner's syndrome.

We have also seen primary *liposarcomas, rhabdomyosarcomas, malignant pleomorphic fibrous histiocytomas (fibroxanthosarcomas),* and *osteosarcomas.*[97] The latter should be differentiated from intraductal papillomas with osseous or cartilaginous metaplasia, from cystosarcomas phyllodes in which the bone is part of the neoplastic stroma, and from carcinomas with osseous or cartilaginous metaplasia.[106]

Hemangiosarcoma is a distinctive breast neoplasm with an ominous prognosis. Forty-two cases have been reported.[95] Grossly, the tumor is soft, spongy, and hemorrhagic. Microscopically, the diagnostic areas are characterized by anastomosing vascular channels lined by atypical endothelial cells. The appearance may vary in the same tumor from that of a highly undifferentiated solid neoplasm to one indistinguishable from a hemangioma. Metastases occur early through the bloodstream.[107]

One hundred sixty-two examples of *lymphangiosarcoma* of the upper extremity following radical mastectomy have been reported. This sarcoma usually follows long-standing edema but may occur after mastectomy without edema.[108] The tumor appears at an average of ten years after radical mastectomy. In most patients, lymphedema had appeared within one year after mastectomy.

Clinically, the early lesions appear as bluish or purple papules in an edematous skin. They are often multiple and accompanied by deeper independent foci, the latter accounting for the failure of local excision to control the disease. The region most affected at first is the arm, followed by the forearm and elbow. Microscopically, dilated lymphatic channels lined by atypical cells alternate with solid tumor masses. The microscopic diagnosis of this lesion may be difficult in its early phases, for only a small nodule of innocuous-appearing collections of vessels lined by a single layer of endothelium may exist. We agree with Sternby et al.[108] that if such apparent benign vascular proliferation occurs in areas of chronic lymphedema, it has to be regarded and treated as a lymphangiosarcoma.

The prognosis is poor. Approximately 50% of the patients die within two years of the onset, with recurrence in the chest wall and pulmonary metastases. Of the eleven patients known to have survived for more than five years, nine had been treated by radical surgery (wide excision, forequarter amputation, or shoulder disarticulation).[112]

Malignant lymphoma

Malignant lymphoma can present as a primary mammary neoplasm or involve the breast as part of a generalized process.[94] Grossly, it is soft and grayish-white. It grows rapidly and is not accompanied by skin retraction or nipple discharge. For some peculiar reason, the right breast is involved more commonly than the left. Multiple nodules are sometimes encountered. The involvement is bilateral in one of every four patients. Wiseman and Liao[111] reviewed sixteen cases of primary

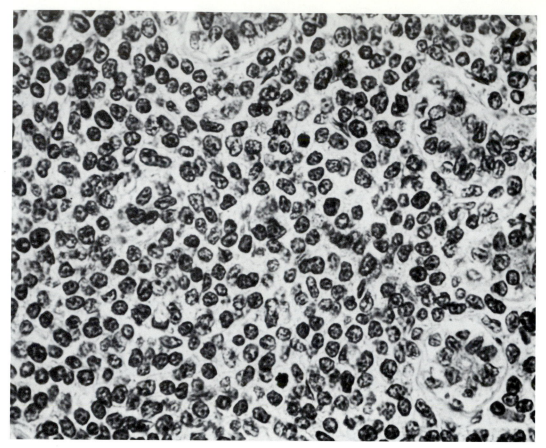

Fig. 926 Involvement of breast by myelocytic leukemia. It would be extremely difficult to differentiate this lesion from histiocytic lymphoma on hematoxylin-eosin sections. (×720; WU neg. 68-7080.)

malignant lymphoma of the breast from our institution. Nine were classified as histiocytic, five as poorly differentiated lymphocytic, and two as well-differentiated lymphocytic neoplasms. The prognosis was poor. Only two patients had a documented long-term survival; in both, the tumor was of lymphocytic type.

We have never seen Hodgkin's disease presenting as a primary breast tumor, although we have seen several cases of breast involvement in Stage IV disease. Oberman[104] reported two cases of pseudolymphoma of the breast.

Acute and chronic myelocytic leukemia can present as a localized mass in the breast and be microscopically confused with histiocytic lymphoma[105] (Fig. 926). The most important clue to the diagnosis

of "granulocytic sarcoma" in hematoxylin-eosin sections is the presence of eosinophilic myelocytes or metamyelocytes, identified as cells with a round or slightly indented nucleus and bright eosinophilic cytoplasmic granules. We have found the von Leder stain very useful in the confirmation of this diagnosis. This is an esterase reaction that can be easily performed in formalin-fixed, paraffin-embedded material and which stains the specific lysosomal granules of the cells belonging to the granulocytic series a bright red color.[98]

Other lesions

Skin lesions such as *basal cell carcinoma, epidermoid carcinoma, keratinous cysts,* and *sweat gland tumors* may arise in the skin of the breast and should not be considered as primary breast neoplasms. Finck et al.[115] described six examples of a benign breast tumor having the general configuration of an intraductal papilloma but being composed of cells with abundant clear cytoplasm. They considered this neoplasm as the mammary counterpart of the cutaneous sweat gland tumor known as clear cell hydradenoma (eccrine acrospiroma).

Hemangioma and *hemangiopericytoma* may occur within the breast parenchyma. *Metastatic carcinomas* rarely affect the breast except in widely disseminated tumors. They typically appear as superficial, well-defined multinodular masses. In the series reported by Hajdu and Urban,[116] there were fourteen malignant melanomas and six lung carcinomas.

Fungal disease (coccidioidomycosis, actinomycosis) may occur and form multiple sinus tracts. We have seen several instances of *foreign body reaction* to polyvinyl plastic (Ivalon). This spongy plastic material is used for mammoplasty. It becomes impregnated with granulation and fibrous tissue. Instead of enhancing beauty, the plastic contracts, hardens, becomes fixed, and may even result in the formation of sinus tracts.[117] A similar foreign body reaction has been described following silicone injections.[121]

A unique case of *Wegener's granulomatosis* with breast involvement was reported by Elsner and Harper.[113] *Hemorrhagic necrosis* of the breast can result from anticoagulant therapy.[120]

The eponym *Mondor's disease* is given to a peculiar thrombophlebitis involving breast and the contiguous thoracicoabdominal wall.[114] The condition, which may simulate a malignant neoplasm, has often a sudden onset and appears as a firm slightly nodular cord beneath the skin. Ecchymosis may or may not be present. Microscopically, the process is one of phlebitis wtih thrombosis.[119] With time, the thrombus recanalizes completely. The condition is self-limited and practically never recurs. It may be related to mechanical injury. In eight of the fifteen cases reported by Herrmann,[118] the disease appeared a few months following a radical mastectomy.

Oral contraceptive therapy and breast

Painful engorgement of the breasts occurs not infrequently during the first cycles of contraceptive therapy. This is usually a mild and transient symptom. Pathologically, the only definite mammary change that can be ascribed to the "contraceptive pill" on the basis of the presently available evidence is the development of true acini resembling lactating breast.[125] Hyperplastic epithelial changes in fibroadenomas have been described,[126] but whether they are indeed the result of the therapy is not yet established. Fechner[122] found no differences in the incidence, gross appearance, and microscopic configuration of fifty-four fibroadenomas removed in patients who were receiving oral contraceptives and fifty-four control cases, except for the occasional formation of acini in the former. He obtained similar results when comparing twenty-five cases of fibrocystic disease in patients receiving progestogens with twenty-five control cases.[123]

Nothing definite can be said at the present time about a possible relationship between contraceptive agents and breast carcinoma. Naturally, several cases of breast cancers occurring in patients on progestogen therapy have already been reported. With an estimated 8,500,000 women taking these drugs in the United States, this is hardly surprising. Pathologically, these cancers do not seem to differ from those seen in control cases.[124, 125] Obviously, only a carefully designed epidemiologic study will answer the question whether oral contraceptive therapy results in an increased risk of mammary carcinoma or whether it exerts any influence on an existing neoplasm.

Breast diseases in children and adolescents

Infant breast tissue may undergo *focal intraductal hyperplasia* associated with

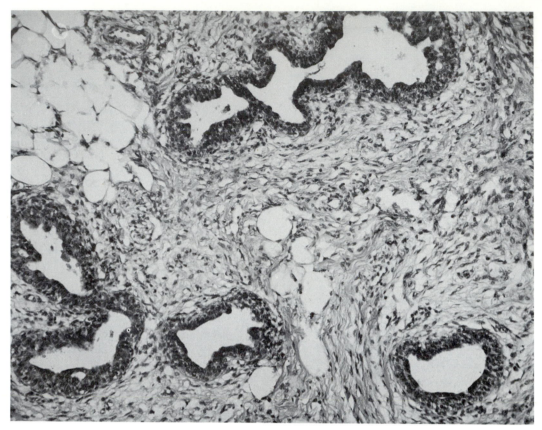

Fig. 927 Nodule of developing breast removed from 8-year-old girl with clinical diagnosis of fibroadenoma. (WU neg. 70-4685.)

stromal alterations.[131] This may result in the formation of a unilateral mass beneath the nipple. Also, at the time of puberty, the physiologic development may be initially unilateral, simulatinig a breast neoplasm (Fig. 927). Should such nodules be removed by mistake, no development of the breast will occur.

Fibroadenomas are exceptional before the age of puberty but are the most common pathologic condition seen between puberty and 20 years of age.[127,130] So-called *virginal hypertrophy* may result in massive unilateral or bilateral enlargement. Microscopically, it is characterized by a combined proliferation of ducts and stroma with little, if any, lobular participation. Farrow and Ashikari[127] encountered thirteen *intraductal papillomas* in patients between the ages of 15 and 19 years.

Most cases of **breast carcinoma** in children fall into one of two well-defined categories. Some are infiltrative ductal tumors with a microscopic appearance quite similar to that seen in carcinoma of adults, except for a tendency of the tumor cells to have a clear cytoplasm with evidence of secretory activity[128] (Fig. 928). The prognosis in this tumor type is excellent. In the series of seven cases reported by McDivitt and Stewart[128] there was not a single instance of metastatic spread, and the five-year survival rate was 100%, despite the fact that three of the patients were treated only by local excision. The other type of carcinoma is a highly undifferentiated solid neoplasm formed by medium-sized round cells without ductular or acinar formation. The prognosis of this variety is extremely poor. Extensive lymphatic and blood-borne metastases develop early in the course of the disease.[129]

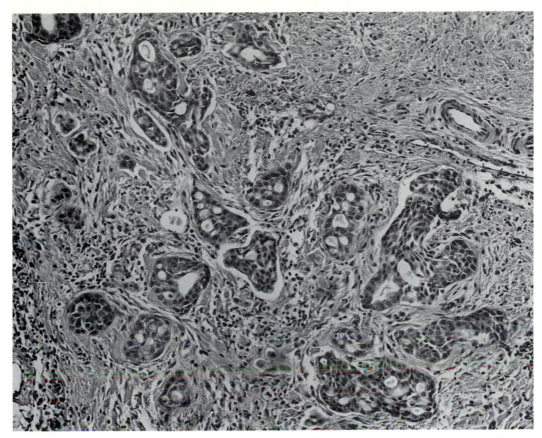

Fig. 928 Breast carcinoma in 10-year-old girl. Small glands composed of atypical cells infiltrate mammary stroma. Total mastectomy was performed. Patient is alive and well six years later. (×150; WU neg. 72-9816; courtesy Dr. W. S. Medart, Savannah, Ga.)

Carcinoma of male breast

In the United States, only 1% of all breast cancer occurs in males, but in Egypt and certain other tropical regions, the incidence rises to nearly 10%.[133] There is no documented association between pubertal gynecomastia and cancer. There are some reports of mammary carcinoma appearing in breasts with estrogen-induced gynecomastia in patients treated for prostatic carcinoma. Although a few unquestionable cases are on record,[136] it is likely that most of these represent instead metastatic foci from the prostatic cancer.[132] An increased incidence of breast cancer is seen in patients with Klinefelter's disease.[134]

Clinically, most tumors present in elderly individuals as breast nodules, with or without associated nipple abnormalities. Nipple discharge in an adult male, especially if bloody, should arouse a strong suspicion of carcinoma.[137] Grossly and microscopically, cancers of the male breast are remarkably similar to those seen in females (Fig. 929). All of the microscopic types identified in the female breast have been encountered in males with the only exception of lobular carcinoma. Skin involvement by fixation and Paget's disease are much more common in males. The incidence of axillary metastasis is the same in men as in women, but the prognosis is slightly worse in the former.[135] We have never seen a fibroadenoma nor a cystosarcoma phyllodes occurring in a male breast.

Clinicopathologic correlation

It is imperative that the clinician be skilled in accurate palpation of the breast

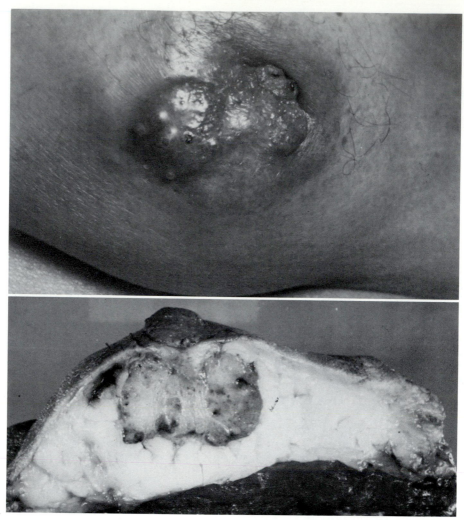

Fig. 929 Right breast of 65-year-old man showing marked nipple deformity and ulceration with nodularity of areolar skin secondary to infiltrating duct carcinoma. (Courtesy Dr. J. C. Ashhurst, Tuskegee, Ala.)

and axilla when examining a patient with a lump in the breast. We have demonstrated that the benign or malignant nature of a dominant mass can be diagnosed correctly by fourth-year medical students in 55% of instances (5% better than tossing a coin). The experienced clinician can diagnose only 70% correctly. Therefore, a policy of look and see must replace that of wait and see. Once lumps are exposed and sectioned, the surgeon proficient in surgical pathology can grossly identify their benign or malignant nature in over 85% of the patients. The fallacy of attempting to determine the presence or absence of axillary nodal metastases by palpation is illustrated by the following findings:

Clinically negative and microscopically negative—84 cases
Clinically negative and microscopically positive—71 cases
} Examiner correct in 54%

Clinically positive and microscopically positive—124 cases
Clinically positive and microscopically negative—22 cases
} Examiner correct in 85%

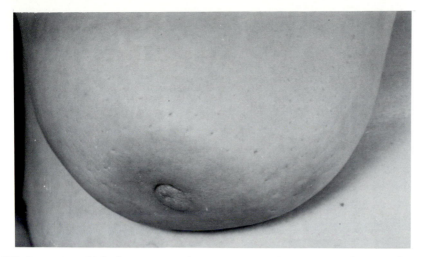

Fig. 930 Breast in which there was rather prominent edema surrounding nipple. This is an ominous finding. (WU neg. 50-3770.)

The error in saying that an axilla is negative when an involved node is present approaches 50%. Conversely, the error is only about 15% when the axilla is thought to contain disease because of the presence of enlarged nodes. Usually these nodes are associated with ulceration or infection. The overall error in axillary palpation is 30%.

When the axillary lymph nodes contain metastatic cancer in the presence of a clinically and radiographically normal breast, the management becomes a difficult problem. The differential diagnosis is usually between breast carcinoma and amelanotic malignant melanoma. Dopa or tyrosinase reaction and electron microscopic examination can be helpful in this regard.[147, 156, 157] If a metastatic tumor in an axillary node is compatible with breast carcinoma and the possibility of melanoma has been reasonably ruled out, removal of the homolateral breast is justified even in the absence of positive findings. A primary malignant tumor, which can be extremely small, will be found in practically every instance.[146]

The examining physician must be well aware of certain ominous clinical findings of breast carcinoma. The clinical signs indicating inoperability have been listed by Haagensen and Stout.[148] Extensive edema of the breast usually means that tumor has permeated and blocked cutaneous lymphatics and is a sign of an advanced stage of the disease (Fig. 930).

Handley et al.[150, 151] routinely explored the second and third intercostal spaces at the time of radical mastectomy. With thorough pathologic study of the axillary lymph nodes after radical mastectomy, the probability of internal mammary lymph node metastases can be estimated. If the axillary lymph nodes are *negative* and the tumor is located in the outer half, the internal mammary lymph nodes will practically never contain tumor. If the tumor is located in the inner half, no more than 20% of the internal mammary lymph nodes will contain cancer. However, if the axillary lymph nodes are *positive* and the tumor arises in the outer half, at least 30% of the internal mammary nodes will be involved. If the axillary nodes contain metastases and the tumor arises in the inner half, over 50% of the internal mammary nodes will contain tumor. Approximately one-third of the patients with operable breast cancer will have involvement of the internal mammary chain. These nodes may be extremely small.

The sign of most diagnostic significance in a radical mastectomy specimen is the presence or absence of involved axillary lymph nodes. The most important single

Table 41 Relationship of size of breast cancers to frequency of nodal metastases and aeath after radical mastectomy*

Diameter of cancer (cm)	Number of patients in whom cancers measured	Number of cancers associated with axillary nodal metastases	Number of patients dying within 60 months after radical mastectomy
1	63	7 (11%)	6 (9%)
1-2	151	60 (40%)	43 (28%)
2-3	190	99 (52%)	72 (38%)
3-4	136	102 (75%)	70 (51%)
4-5	75	56 (74%)	47 (63%)
5-6	37	29 (78%)	30 (81%)
6-7	24	21 (87%)	19 (79%)
7-10	30	25 (83%)	24 (80%)
10+	11	8 (73%)	7 (64%)
Total	717	407 (57%)	318 (44%)

*From Butcher, H. R., Jr.: Effectiveness of radical mastectomy for mammary cancer: an analysis of mortalities by the method of probits, Ann. Surg. **154**:383-396, 1961.

clinical factor relating to whether or not these nodes are involved is the size of the primary tumor[145] (Table 41). If the pectoralis muscle is invaded, tumor is probably in distant areas such as the anterior mediastinal lymph nodes. Blood vessel invasion is a bad prognostic sign especially if associated with lymph node metastases.[153]

All patients must be followed indefinitely. Local recurrence may take place many years after the original operation (Fig. 931). Local recrudescence after operation is more a function of the extent of the disease and its biologic characteristics than it is of the kind of operative therapy.[138] All instances of supraclavicular lymph node enlargement must be proved to be cancer by biopsy. The enlargement may be only the result of a chronic inflammatory process such as tuberculosis. The presence of satellite skin nodules and parasternal nodules means that the tumor has escaped blocked lymphatics and formed subcutaneous masses.

During the last decade, there has been dissatisfaction with the survival rates of patients treated for carcinoma of the breast. Urban[158] and Handley et al.[151] extended the conventional radical mastectomy.

Urban's operation[158] had practically no operative mortality and little morbidity and included only the internal mammary chain with radical mastectomy. He stated that twenty-one out of fifty-eight patients with involved internal mammary lymph nodes survived over five years.[159] However, the patients that had the extended operation were selected for it. In addition, some of these patients had postoperative radiation therapy. The group constituted approximately one-third of the mammary cancers seen by him.

Butcher et al.[144] reported that five out of twenty-three patients who had internal mammary nodal metastases proved by biopsy at the end of a standard radical mastectomy survived five years or more. McWhirter[155] reported a large series of patients treated by simple mastectomy and postoperative irradiation therapy. His results have been comparable to those reported by competent surgeons. In his group, it is hard to determine what the radiation therapy contributed since no one as yet knows the effects of irradiation on involved lymph nodes.

Auchincloss[139] has made a provocative argument in favor of a conservative approach. His operation consists in removal of the breast and of low and mid axillary lymph nodes, with preservation of the pectoralis muscle. It seems certain that this operation is perfectly adequate for at least the Types I and II carcinomas.

Wise et al.[160] found that patients with clinical Stage I and Stage II breast carcinoma treated by local excision and post-

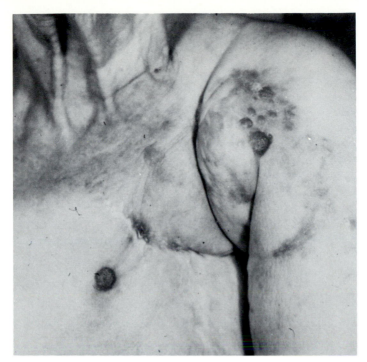

Fig. 931 Patient with local recurrence of carcinoma twenty-seven years after original operation. (WU neg. 50-1781.)

operative radiation therapy had survival rates comparable to those obtained with radical mastectomy. Bruce and Tough[141] feel that the outcome in breast cancer depends more on the biologic nature of the individual tumor than on therapeutic efforts. There is certainly a striking similarity in survival rates from different centers employing widely disparate therapeutic approaches.[154] Bloom et al.[140] provided the baseline on which to base the effectiveness of a given therapy. In their series of 250 cases of *untreated* breast cancer, the five-year survival rate after diagnosis was 18%. Patients with tumors of low-grade malignancy had an average survival of forty-seven months, whereas those with highly malignant tumors survived for an average of only twenty-two months.

In patients with disease beyond the axilla, postoperative irradiation, hormone therapy, adrenalectomy, hypophysectomy, and, at times, elective oophorectomy are successful in producing palliation. Vari-

ations in the natural life history of this disease make it extremely difficult to analyze critically the end results of treatment by any method.

The factors that basically are responsible for our inability to assess the relative effectiveness of the various methods of treating mammary cancer are as follows:

1 The marked variation of the disease
2 The lack of carefully randomized and controlled clinical studies
3 The failure of investigators to remove from their population samples those cases of cancer of the breast in which the methods of treatment being compared cannot possibly influence survival[142, 143]

The problem is well illustrated by the data presented in a cooperative international study published by Haagensen et al.[149] As Butcher[143] remarked, "The time has come for controlled prospective clinical trials which will permit us to scientifically assess the effectiveness of the many variously proposed methods of treating mammary carcinoma relative to the effectiveness of the standard radical mastectomy."[*]

Such clinical trials are being carried out at the present time.[144a] In one of them, a comparison is being made on the relative effectiveness of standard radical mastectomy and modified mastectomy in the control of Stage I and Stage II breast carcinomas. Another trial will compare the results obtained with local excision followed by radiation therapy, local excision alone, and standard radical mastectomy. Until the results of these studies are available, no dogmatic statements about the ideal treatment of breast carcinoma are justified.

---

[*]From Butcher, H. R., Jr.: Mammary carcinoma; a discussion of therapeutic methods, Cancer **24:** 1272-1279, 1969.

REFERENCES
Method of pathologic examination

1 Koehl, R. H., Snyder, R. E., Hutter, R. V. P., and Foote, F. W., Jr.: The incidence and significance of calcifications within operative breast specimens, Am. J. Clin. Pathol. **53:** 3-14, 1970.
2 Monroe, C. W.: Lymphatic spread of carcinoma of the breast, Arch. Surg. **57:**479-486, 1948.
3 Pickren, J. W.: Significance of occult metastases; a study of breast cancer, Cancer **14:** 1266-1273, 1961.
4 Rogers, J. V., Jr., and Powell, R. W.: Mammographic indications for biopsy of clinically normal breasts; correlation with pathologic findings in 72 cases, Am. J. Roentgenol. Radium Ther. Nucl. Med. **115:**794-800, 1972.
5 Rosen, P., Snyder, R. E., Foote, F. W., and Wallace, T.: Detection of occult carcinoma in the apparently benign breast biopsy through specimen radiography, Cancer **26:** 944-952, 1970.
6 Saphir, O., and Amromin, G. D.: Obscure axillary lymph node metastasis in carcinoma of the breast, Cancer **1:**238-241, 1948.
7 Stevens, G. M., and Jamplis, R. W.: Mammographically directed biopsy of nonpalpable breast lesions, Arch. Surg. **102:**292-295, 1971.

Cytology

8 Franzén, S., and Zajicek, J.: Aspiration biopsy in diagnosis of palpable lesions of the breast, Acta Radiol. (Stockh.) **7:**241-262, 1968.
9 Rosen, P., Najdu, S. I., Robbins, G., and Foote, F. W.: Diagnosis of carcinoma of the breast by aspiration biopsy, Surg. Gynecol. Obstet. **134:**837-838, 1972.

Frozen section

10 Saltzstein, S. L.: Histologic diagnosis of breast carcinoma with the Silverman needle biopsy, Surgery **48:**366-374, 1960.

Inflammatory lesions

11 Adair, F. E.: Plasma cell mastitis; a lesion simulating mammary carcinoma, Arch. Surg. **26:**735-749, 1933.
12 Cutler, M.: Plasma-cell mastitis; report of a case with bilateral involvement, Br. Med. J. **1:**94-96, 1949.
13 Halpert, B., Parker, J. M., and Thuringer, J. M.: Plasma cell mastitis, Arch. Pathol. **46:** 313-319, 1948.
14 Tuttle, H. K., and Kean, B. H.: Circumscribed chronic suppurative mastitis simulating cancer, Surg. Gynecol. Obstet. **84:**933-938, 1947.

Fat necrosis

15 Adair, F. E., and Munzer, J. T.: Fat necrosis of the female breast, Am. J. Surg. **74:**117-128, 1947.
16 Binkley, J. S.: Relapsing nodular nonsuppurative panniculitis, J.A.M.A. **113:**113-116, 1939.
17 Foote, F. W., and Stewart, F. W.: Comparative studies of cancerous vs. noncancerous breasts, Ann. Surg. **121:**6-79, 1945.
18 Hadfield, G.: Fat necrosis of the breast, Br. J. Surg. **17:**673-682, 1930.
19 Lee, B. J., and Adair, F. E.: Traumatic fat necrosis of the female breast and its differentiation from carcinoma, Ann. Surg. **72:**188-195, 1920.
20 Lee, B. J., and Adair, F. E.: Traumatic fat necrosis of the female breast and its differentiation from carcinoma, Ann. Surg. **80:**670-691, 1924.

Mammary duct ectasia

21 Haagensen, C. D.: Mammary-duct ectasia; a disease that may simulate carcinoma, Cancer **4:**749-761, 1951.
22 Lepper, E. H., and Weaver, M. O.: Generalized distention of the ducts of the breast by fatty secretion, J. Pathol. Bacteriol. **45:** 465-467, 1937.

Fibrocystic disease

23 Foote, F. W., and Stewart, F. W.: Comparative studies of cancerous vs. noncancerous breasts, Ann. Surg. **121:**6-79, 1945.
24 Frantz, V. K., Pickren, J. W., Melcher, G. W., and Auchincloss, H., Jr.: Incidence of chronic cystic disease in so-called "normal breast," Cancer **4:**762-783, 1951.

25 Haagensen, C. D.: Diseases of the breast, ed. 2, Philadelphia, 1971, W. B. Saunders Co.

26 Kern, W. H., and Brooks, R. N.: Atypical epithelial hyperplasia associated with breast cancer and fibrocystic disease, Cancer **24**:668-675, 1969.

27 Kiaer, W.: Relation of fibroadenomatosis ("chronic mastitis") to cancer of the breast, Copenhagen, 1954, Ejnar Munksgaard.

28 Le Gal, Y., Gros, C. M., and Bader, P.: L'adenomatose erosive du mamelon, Ann. Acad. Path. (Paris) **4**:292-304, 1959.

29 Perzin, K. H., and Lattes, R.: Papillary adenoma of the nipple (florid papillomatosis, adenoma, adenomatosis); a clinicopathologic study, Cancer **29**:996-1009, 1972.

30 Steinhoff, N. G., and Black, W. C.: Florid cystic disease preceding mammary cancer, Ann. Surg. **171**:501-508, 1970.

31 Taylor, H. B., and Norris, H. J.: Epithelial invasion of nerves in benign diseases of the breast, Cancer **20**:2245-2249, 1967.

32 Taylor, H. B., and Robertson, A. G.: Adenomas of the nipple, Cancer **18**:995-1002, 1966.

33 Urban, J. A., and Adair, F. E.: Sclerosing adenosis, Cancer **2**:625-634, 1949.

Benign tumors

34 Bannayan, G. A., and Hajdu, S. I.: Gynecomastia: clinicopathologic study of 351 cases, Am. J. Clin. Pathol. **57**:431-437, 1972.

35 Curran, R. C., and Dodge, O. G.: Sarcoma of breast, with particular reference to its origin from fibroadenoma, J. Clin. Pathol. **15**:1-16, 1962.

36 Fisher, E. R., and Creed, D. L.: Nature of the periductal stroma in gynecomastia, Lab. Invest. **5**:267-275, 1956.

37 Goldman, R. C., and Friedman, N. B.: Carcinoma of the breast arising in fibroadenomas with emphasis on lobular carcinoma; a clinicopathologic study, Cancer **23**:544-550, 1969.

38 Haagensen, C. D., and Stout, A. P.: Granular cell myoblastoma of the mammary gland, Ann. Surg. **124**:218-227, 1946.

39 Haagensen, C. D., Stout, A. P., and Phillips, J. S.: The papillary neoplasms of the breast, Ann. Surg. **133**:18-36, 1951.

40 Kraus, F. T., and Neubecker, R. D.: The differential diagnosis of papillary tumors of the breast, Cancer **15**:444-455, 1962.

41 Le Gal, Y.: Adenomas of the breast: relationship of adenofibromas to pregnancy and lactation, Am. Surg. **27**:14-22, 1961.

42 McDivitt, R. W., Holleb, A. I., and Foote, F. W.: Prior breast disease in patients treated for papillary carcinoma, Arch. Pathol. **85**:117-124, 1968.

43 McDivitt, R. W., Stewart, F. W., and Farrow, J. H.: Breast carcinoma arising in solitary fibroadenomas, Surg. Gynecol. Obstet. **125**:572-576, 1967.

44 Madalin, H. E., Clagett, O. T., and McDonald, J. R.: Lesions of the breast associated with discharge from the nipple, Ann. Surg. **146**:751-763, 1957.

45 Oberman, H. A., Nosanchuk, J. S., and Finger, J. E.: Periductal stromal tumors of breast with adipose metaplasia, Arch. Surg. **98**:384-387, 1969.

46 Sirtori, C., and Veronesi, U.: Gynecomastia; a review of 218 cases, Cancer **10**:645-654, 1957.

47 Snyder, W. H., and Chaffin, L.: Main duct papilloma of the breast, Arch. Surg. **70**:680-685, 1955.

48 Wheeler, C. E., Cawley, E. P., and Curtis, A. C.: Gynecomastia: a review and an analysis of 160 cases, Ann. Intern. Med. **40**:985-1004, 1954.

49 Williams, M. J.: Gynecomastia: its incidence, recognition and host characterization in 447 autopsy cases, Am. J. Med. **34**:103-112, 1963.

Malignant tumors
Carcinoma
Invasive ductal carcinoma

49a Davies, J. D.: Hyperelastosis, obliteration and fibrous plaques in major ducts of the human breast, J. Pathol. **110**:13-26, 1973.

50 Hutter, R. V. P., and Kim, D. U.: The problem of multiple lesions of the breast, Cancer **28**:1591-1607, 1971.

51 Jackson, J. G., and Orr, J. W.: The ducts of carcinomatous breasts, with particular reference to connective-tissue changes, J. Pathol. Bacteriol. **74**:265-273, 1957.

52 Qualheim, R. E., and Gall, E. A.: Breast carcinoma with multiple sites of origin, Cancer **10**:460-468, 1957.

Intraductal carcinoma with or without invasion

53 Frable, W. J., and Kay, S.: Carcinoma of the breast; histologic and clinical features of apocrine tumors, Cancer **21**:756-763, 1968.

Medullary carcinoma

54 Bloom, H. J. G., Richardson, W. W., and Fields, J. R.: Host resistance and survival in carcinoma of breast; a study of 104 cases of medullary carcinoma in a series of 1,411 cases of breast cancer followed for 20 years, Br. Med. J. **3**:181-188, 1970.

55 Moore, O. S., Jr., and Foote, F. W., Jr.: The relatively favorable prognosis of medullary carcinoma of the breast, Cancer **2**:635-642, 1949.

56 Richardson, W. W.: Medullary carcinoma of the breast; a distinctive tumour type with a

relatively good prognosis following radical mastectomy, Br. J. Cancer 10:415-423, 1956.

Paget's disease

57 Ashikari, R., Park, K., Huvos, A. G., and Urban, J. A.: Paget's disease of the breast, Cancer 26:680-685, 1970.
58 Neubecker, R. D., and Bradshaw, R. P.: Mucin, melanin, and glycogen in Paget's disease of the breast, Am. J. Clin. Pathol. 36:40-53, 1961.
59 Paget, J.: On disease of the mammary areola preceding cancer of the mammary gland, St. Barth. Hosp. Rep. 10:87-89, 1874.
60 Sagebiel, R. W.: Ultrastructural observations on epidermal cells in Paget's disease of the breast, Am. J. Pathol. 57:49-64, 1969.

Inflammatory carcinoma

60a Ellis, D. L., and Teitelbaum, S. L.: Inflammatory carcinoma of the breast; a pathological definition, Cancer (in press).

Papillary carcinoma with or without invasion

61 Kraus, F. T., and Neubecker, R. D.: The differential diagnosis of papillary tumors of the breast, Cancer 15:444-455, 1962.

Mucinous carcinoma

62 Norris, H. J., and Taylor, H. B.: Prognosis of mucinous (gelatinous) carcinoma of the breast, Cancer 18:879-885, 1965.
63 Saphir, O.: Mucinous carcinoma of the breast, Surg. Gynecol. Obstet. 72:908-914, 1941.

Epidermoid carcinoma

64 Cornog, J. L., Mobini, J., Steiger, E., and Enterline, H. T.: Squamous carcinoma of the breast, Am. J. Clin. Pathol. 55:410-417, 1971.
65 McDivitt, R. W., Stewart, F. W., and Berg, J. W.: Tumors of the breast. In Atlas of tumor pathology, 2nd series, Fasc. 2, Washington, D. C., 1968, Armed Forces Institute of Pathology.

Adenoid cystic carcinoma

66 Cavanzo, F. J., and Taylor, H. B.: Adenoid cystic carcinoma of the breast; an analysis of 21 cases, Cancer 24:740-745, 1969.
67 Elsner, B.: Adenoid cystic carcinoma of the breast; review of the literature and clinicopathologic study of seven patients, Pathol. Eur. 5:357-364, 1970.
68 Koss, L. G., Brannan, C. D., and Ashikari, R.: Histologic and ultrastructural features of adenoid cystic carcinoma of the breast, Cancer 26:1271-1279, 1970.
69 Nayer, H. R.: Cylindroma of the breast with pulmonary metastases, Dis. Chest. 31:324-327, 1957.

Well-differentiated (tubular) carcinoma

70 Erlandson, R. A., and Carstens, P. H. B.: Ultrastructure of tubular carcinoma of the breast, Cancer 29:987-995, 1972.
71 Taylor, H. B., and Norris, H. J.: Well-differentiated carcinoma of the breast, Cancer 25:687-692, 1970.

Lobular carcinoma, in situ and invasive

72 Fechner, R. E.: Ductal carcinoma involving the lobule of the breast: a source of confusion with lobular carcinoma in situ, Cancer 28:274-281, 1971.
73 Fechner, R. E.: Epithelial alterations in the extralobular ducts of breasts with lobular carcinoma, Arch. Pathol. 93:164-171, 1972.
74 Fechner, R. E.: Infiltrating lobular carcinoma without lobular carcinoma in situ, Cancer 29:1539-1545, 1972.
75 Foote, F. W., and Stewart, F. W.: Lobular carcinoma in situ, Am. J. Pathol. 17:491-496, 1941.
76 Hassler, O.: Microradiographic investigations of calcifications of the female breast, Cancer 23:1103-1109, 1969.
77 Hutter, R. V. P., Snyder, R. E., Lucas, J. C., Foote, F. W., Jr., and Farrow, J. H.: Clinical and pathologic correlation with mammographic findings in lobular carcinoma in situ, Cancer 23:826-839, 1969.
78 Lambird, P. A., and Shelley, W. M.: The spatial distribution of lobular in situ mammary carcinoma; implications for size and site of breast biopsy, J.A.M.A. 210:689-693, 1969.
79 Newman, W.: Lobular carcinoma of the female breast, Ann. Surg. 164:305-314, 1966.
80 Tobon, H., and Price, H. M.: Lobular carcinoma in situ; some ultrastructural observations, Cancer 30:1082-1091, 1972.
81 Warner, N. E.: Lobular carcinoma of the breast, Cancer 23:840-846, 1969.

Classification and grading

82 Bloom, H. J. G., and Richardson, W. W.: Histological grading and prognosis in breast cancer; a study of 1409 cases of which 359 have been followed for 15 years, Br. J. Cancer 11:359-377, 1957.
83 Gricouroff, G.: Du pronostic histologique dans le cancer du sein, Extrait Bull. Cancer 35:275-290, 1948.
84 Hultborn, K. A., and Tornberg, B.: Mammary carcinoma; the biologic character of mammary carcinoma studied in 517 cases by a new form of malignancy grading, Acta Radiol. [Suppl.] (Stockh.) 196:1-143, 1960.
85 Kouchoukos, N. T., Ackerman, L. V., and Butcher, H. R., Jr.: Prediction of axillary nodal metastases from the morphology of pri-

mary mammary carcinomas—a guide to operative therapy, Cancer 20:948-960, 1967.

86 Lane, N., Boksel, H., Salerno, R. A., and Haagensen, C. D.: Clinico-pathologic analysis of the surgical curability of breast cancers: a minimum ten-year study of a personal series, Ann. Surg. 153:483-498, 1961.

Effects of irradiation

87 Ackerman, L. V.: An evaluation of the treatment of cancer of the breast at the University of Edinburgh (Scotland), under the direction of Dr. Robert McWhirter, Cancer 8:883-887, 1955.

88 Guttman, R.: Survival and results after 2-million volt irradiation in the treatment of primary operable carcinoma of the breast with proved internal mammary and/or highest axillary node metastases, Cancer 15:383, 1962.

89 Lumb, G.: Changes in carcinoma of the breast following irradiation, Br. J. Surg. 38:82-94, 1950.

90 McWhirter, R.: The treatment of carcinoma of the breast, Irish J. Med. Sci., 6th series, pp. 475-483, 1956.

Effects of steroid hormones

91 Eckert, C., Aikman, W., Weichselbaum, T. E., Elman, R., and Ackerman, L. V.: Surgical oophorectomy and adrenalectomy in the management of advanced breast cancer: clinical indications and results, South. Med. J. 49:437-443, 1956.

92 Emerson, W. J., Kennedy, B. J., Graham, J. N., and Nathanson, I. T.: Pathology of primary and recurrent carcinoma of the human breast after administration of steroid hormones, Cancer 6:641-670, 1953.

93 Lemon, H. M.: Medical treatment of cancer of the breast and prostate, Disease-a-Month, May, 1959.

Sarcoma

94 De Cosse, J. J., Berg, J. W., Fracchia, A. A., and Farrow, J. H.: Primary lymphosarcoma of the breast: a review of 14 cases, Cancer 15:1264-1268, 1962.

95 Gulesserian, H. P., and Lawton, R. L.: Angiosarcoma of the breast, Cancer 24:1021-1026, 1969.

96 Haggitt, R. C., and Booth, J. L.: Bilateral fibromatosis of the breast in Gardner's syndrome, Cancer 25:161-166, 1970.

97 Hill, R. P., and Stout, A. P.: Sarcoma of the breast, Arch. Surg. 44:723-759, 1942.

98 Leder, L. D.: Über die selektive fermentcytochemische Darstellung von neutrophilen myeloischen Zellen und Gewebsmastzellen in Paraffinschnitt, Klin. Wochenschr. 42:553, 1964.

99 Lester, J., and Stout, A. P.: Cystosarcoma phyllodes, Cancer 7:335-353, 1954.

100 McDivitt, R. W., Urban, J. A., and Farrow, J. H.: Cystosarcoma phyllodes, Johns Hopkins Med. J. 120:33-45, 1967.

101 Norris, H. J., and Taylor, H. B.: Relationship of histologic features to behavior of cystosarcoma phyllodes; analysis of ninety-four cases, Cancer 20:2090-2099, 1967.

102 Norris, H. J., and Taylor, H. B.: Sarcomas and related mesenchymal tumors of the breast, Cancer 22:22-28, 1968.

103 Oberman, H. A.: Cystosarcoma phyllodes of the breast, Cancer 18:697-710, 1965.

104 Oberman, H. A.: Primary lymphoreticular neoplasms of the breast, Surg. Gynecol. Obstet. 123:1047-1051, 1966.

105 Pascoe, H. R.: Tumors composed of immature granulocytes occurring in the breast in chronic granulocytic leukemia, Cancer 25:697-704, 1970.

106 Smith, B. H., and Taylor, H. B.: The occurrence of bone and cartilage in mammary tumors, Am. J. Clin. Pathol. 51:610-618, 1969.

107 Steingaszner, L. C., Enzinger, F. M., and Taylor, H. B.: Hemangiosarcoma of the breast, Cancer 18:352-361, 1965.

108 Sternby, N. H., Gynning, I., and Hogeman, K. E.: Postmastectomy angiosarcoma, Acta Chir. Scand. 121:420-432, 1961.

109 Treves, N.: A study of cystosarcoma phyllodes, Ann. N. Y. Acad. Sci. 114:922-936, 1964.

110 Treves, N., and Sunderland, D. A.: Cystosarcoma phyllodes of the breast, Cancer 4:1286-1332, 1951 (extensive bibliography and beautiful illustrations).

111 Wiseman, C., and Liao, K. T.: Primary lymphoma of the breast, Cancer 29:1705-1712, 1972.

112 Woodward, A. H., Ivins, J. C., and Soule, E. H.: Lymphangiosarcoma arising in chronic lymphedematous extremities, Cancer 30:562-572, 1972.

Other lesions

113 Elsner, B., and Harper, F. B.: Disseminated Wegener's granulomatosis with breast involvement; report of a case, Arch. Pathol. 87:544-547, 1969.

114 Farrow, J. H.: Thrombophlebitis of the superficial veins of the breast and anterior chest wall (Mondor's disease), Surg. Gynecol. Obstet. 101:63-68, 1955.

115 Finck, F. M., Schwinn, C. P., and Keasby, L. E.: Clear cell hidradenoma of the breast, Cancer, 22:125-135, 1968.

116 Hajdu, S. I., and Urban, J. A.: Cancers metastatic to the breast, Cancer 22:1691-1696, 1968.

117 Hamit, H. F.: Implantation of plastics in the breast, Arch. Surg. **75**:224-229, 1957.

118 Herrmann, J. B.: Thrombophlebitis of breast and contiguous thoracicoabdominal wall (Mondor's disease), N. Y. State J. Med. **66**: 3146-3152, 1966.

119 Johnson, W. C., Wallrich, R., and Helwig, E. B.: Superficial thrombophlebitis of the chest wall, J.A.M.A. **180**:103-108, 1962.

120 Nudelman, H. L., and Kempson, R. L.: Necrosis of the breast; a rare complication of anticoagulant therapy, Am. J. Surg. **111**:728-733, 1966.

121 Symmers, W. St. C.: Silicone mastitis in "topless" waitress and some other varieties of foreign-body mastitis, Br. Med. J. **3**:19-22, 1968.

Oral contraceptive therapy and breast

122 Fechner, R. E.: Fibroadenomas in patients receiving oral contraceptives: a clinical and pathologic study, Am. J. Clin. Pathol. **53**:857-864, 1970.

123 Fechner, R. E.: Fibrocystic disease in women receiving oral contraceptive hormones, Cancer **25**:1332-1339, 1970.

124 Fechner, R. E.: Breast cancer during oral contraceptive therapy, Cancer **26**:1204-1211, 1970.

125 Fechner, R. E.: The surgical pathology of the reproductive system and breast during oral contraceptive therapy, Pathol. Annu. **6**: 299-319, 1971.

126 Goldenberg, V. E., Wiegenstein, L., and Mottet, N. K.: Florid breast fibroadenomas in patients taking hormonal oral contraceptives, Am. J. Clin. Pathol. **49**:52-59, 1968.

Breast diseases in children and adolescents

127 Farrow, J. H., and Ashikari, H.: Breast lesions in young girls, Surg. Clin. North Am. **49**:261-269, 1969.

128 McDivitt, R. W., and Stewart, F. W.: Breast carcinoma in children, J.A.M.A. **195**:388-390, 1966.

129 Ramirez, G., and Ansfield, F. J.: Carcinoma of the breast in children, Arch. Surg. **96**: 222-225, 1968.

130 Sandison, A. T., and Walker, J. C.: Diseases of the adolescent female breast, Br. J. Surg. **55**:443-448, 1968.

131 Steiner, M. W.: Enlargement of the breast during childhood, Pediatr. Clin. North Am. **2**:575-593, 1955.

Carcinoma of male breast

132 Benson, W. R.: Carcinoma of the prostate with metastases to breast and testis, Cancer **10**:1235-1245, 1957.

133 El-Gazayerli, M., and Abdel-Aziz, A. S.: On

bilharziasis and male breast cancer in Egypt—a preliminary report and review of the literature, Br. J. Cancer **17**:566-571, 1963.

134 Jackson, A. W., Muldal, S., Ockey, C. H., and O'Connor, P. J.: Carcinoma of male breast in association with the Klinefelter syndrome, Br. Med. J. **1**:223-225, 1965.

135 Norris, H. J., and Taylor, H. B.: Carcinoma of the male breast, Cancer **23**:1428-1435, 1969.

136 O'Grady, W. P., and McDivitt, R. W.: Breast cancer in a man treated with diethylstilbestrol, Arch. Pathol. **88**:162-165, 1969.

137 Treves, N., and Holleb, A. I.: Cancer of the male breast; a report of 146 cases, Cancer **8**: 1239-1250, 1955.

Clinicopathologic correlation

138 Auchincloss, H., Jr.: The nature of local recurrence following radical mastectomy, Cancer **11**:611-619, 1958.

139 Auchincloss, H., Jr.: Significance of location and number of axillary metastases in carcinoma of the breast; a justification for a conservative operation, Ann. Surg. **158**:37-46, 1963.

140 Bloom, H. J. G., Richardson, W. W., and Harries, E. D.: Natural history of untreated breast cancer; comparison of untreated cases according to histological grade of malignancy, Br. Med. J. **2**:213-221, 1962.

141 Bruce, J., and Tough, I.: Early cancer of the breast, West. J. Surg. **72**:60-63, 1964.

142 Butcher, H. R., Jr.: Effectiveness of radical mastectomy for mammary cancer: an analysis of mortalities by the method of probits, Ann. Surg. **154**:383-396, 1961.

143 Butcher, H. R., Jr.: Mammary carcinoma; a discussion of therapeutic methods, Cancer **24**: 1272-1279, 1969.

144 Butcher, H. R., Jr., Seaman, W. B., Eckert, C., and Saltzstein, S.: An assessment of radical mastectomy and postoperative irradiation therapy in the treatment of mammary cancer, Cancer **17**:480-485, 1964.

144a Fisher, B.: Cooperative clinical trials in primary breast cancer: a critical appraisal, Cancer **31**:1271-1286, 1973.

145 Fisher, B., Slack, N. H., and Bross, I. D. J.: Cancer of the breast: size of neoplasm and prognosis, Cancer **24**:1071-1080, 1969.

146 Fitts, W. T., Jr., Steiner, G. C., and Enterline, H. T.: Prognosis of occult carcinoma of the breast, Am. J. Surg. **106**:460-463, 1963.

147 Fitzpatrick, T. B.: Human melanogenesis; tyrosinase reaction in pigment cell neoplasms, with particular reference to the malignant melanoma: preliminary report, Arch. Dermatol. Syphilol. **65**:379-391, 1952.

148 Haagensen, C. D., and Stout, A. P.: Carci-

noma of the breast, Ann. Surg. 116:801-815, 1942.

149 Haagensen, C. D., Cooley, E., Kennedy, C. S., Miller, E., Butcher, H. R., Jr., Dahl-Iversen, E., Tobiassen, T., Williams, I. G., Curwen, M. P., Kaae, S., and Johansen, H.: The treatment of early mammary carcinoma, Ann. Surg. 157:157-179, 1963.

150 Handley, R. S., and Thackray, A. C.: Internal mammary lymph chain in carcinoma of the breast, Lancet 2:276-278, 1949.

151 Handley, R. S., Patey D. H., and Hand, B. H.: Excision of the internal mammary chain in radical mastectomy, Lancet 1:457-461, 1956.

152 Johnson, R. E.: A rational basis for extending the radical mastectomy, Missouri Med. J. 59: 1174-1178, 1962.

153 Kister, S. J., Sommers, S. C., Haagensen, C. D., and Cooley, E.: Re-evaluation of blood vessel invasion as a prognostic factor in carcinoma of the breast, Cancer 19:1213-1216, 1966.

154 Lewison, E. F., Montague, A. C. W., and Kuller, L.: Breast cancer treated at The Johns Hopkins Hospital, 1951-1956; review of international ten-year survival rates, Cancer 19: 1359-1368, 1966.

155 McWhirter, R.: The treatment of carcinoma of the breast, Irish J. Med. Sci., 6th series, pp. 475-483, 1956.

156 Rodriguez, H. A., and McGavran, M. H.: A modified dopa reaction for the diagnosis and investigation of pigment cells, Am. J. Clin. Pathol. 52:219-227, 1969.

157 Rosai, J., and Rodriguez, H. A.: Application of electron microscopy to the differential diagnosis of tumors, Am. J. Clin. Pathol. 50:555-562, 1968.

158 Urban, J. A.: Clinical experience and results of excision of the internal mammary lymph node chain in primary operable breast cancer, Cancer 12:14-22, 1959.

159 Urban, J. A.: Personal communication, 1966.

160 Wise, L., Mason, A. Y., and Ackerman, L. V.: Local excision and irradiation: an alternative method for the treatment of early mammary cancer, Ann. Surg. 174:392-401, 1971.

20 Lymph nodes

Biopsy

The microscopic interpretation of abnormal lymph nodes is extremely difficult. Probably more diagnostic errors are made on lymph nodes than on any other organ of the body. The most common mistake is the diagnosis of a benign node as malignant lymphoma. Thus, Symmers[5, 6] found that of 600 cases submitted with an initial histologic diagnosis of Hodgkin's disease, the diagnosis was mistaken in 47%. The condition most commonly confused with Hodgkin's disease was chronic nonspecific lymphadenitis. Of 226 cases initially diagnosed as reticulum cell sarcoma (histiocytic lymphoma), the error was 27%. Although in our experience the percentage of diagnostic errors is appreciably lower, these figures clearly indicate the need for a review of the pathologic material whenever a patient is admitted to the hospital because a lymph node biopsy done elsewhere was interpreted as malignant lymphoma.

There are several ways to mishandle a patient with lymphadenopathy. The internist requests lymph node biopsy in a patient with generalized lymphadenopathy. The surgeon, tempted by its accessibility, biopsies an inguinal node. Unfortunately, inguinal lymph nodes invariably show chronic inflammatory changes and fibrosis which obscure the presence of other pathologic processes. The surgeon should biopsy the more elusive axillary or deep cervical node rather than superficial or inguinal nodes when generalized lymphadenopathy exists. A superficial cervical lymph node may show only hyperplasia, yet a deeper node of the same group may contain metastatic carcinoma or Hodgkin's disease.[4] Similarly, the most accessible enlarged lymph node found at laparotomy may not show the pathologic process causing the intra-abdominal lymphadenopathy. Whenever possible, the largest lymph node of the region should be the one biopsied.[2]

The surgeon biopsying intra-abdominal nodes or large cervical or axillary masses should have frozen section performed to be certain that the tissue is representative. This may save a second biopsy. The biopsy of a lymph node in the cervical or axillary area should be performed only by a surgeon. An inexperienced physician trying to biopsy an apparently easily accessible node may be unable to find the node or may encounter hemorrhage from adjacent large vessels.

If there is any question that the node contains something other than a tumor, an adequate sample of the biopsied lymph node must be sent directly for bacteriologic study or must be placed in a sterile Petri dish in the refrigerator. We recommend and follow the latter procedure. If permanent sections show an inflammatory process, the material can then be taken from the refrigerator and studied bacteriologically. Furthermore, the microscopic pattern of the permanent sections may be helpful in suggesting the diagnosis to the bacteriologist. In numerous instances, the bacteriologic study is more rewarding than the microscopic study.[8] The search for acid-fast bacilli or fungi in the paraffin section often is fruitless. A technique which complements the study of tissue sections and which is too often neglected is the examination of touch preparations from the cut surface of the fresh lymph node stained with Giemsa or Wright's solution.[3, 7] This is particularly useful in the evaluation of lymphoma and leukemia. Granulocytic leukemia can closely simulate histocytic lymphoma in an hematoxylin-eosin section, but an imprint will readily differentiate the two conditions.

The most frequent reason for an incorrect diagnosis of a lymph node is improper preparation of the biopsied tissue. A poorly prepared slide may be produced in the following ways:

1 Fragmenting or crushing the lymph node at time of excision
2 Carefully delaying placing the node in fixative
3 Leaving the node in a strong light where it will be subjected to heat and drying and then incompletely fixing it
4 Running the node too quickly through various solutions and then having the technician cut the sections with a dull knife at about 20μ or 30μ and overstain them with hematoxylin (Fig. 932, A and B).

We make it our policy never to make a diagnosis on any poorly prepared lymph node that is sent to us. We are often amazed at the confident diagnoses that others make on such sections. We recommend that the lymph node be placed in 10% buffered formalin and thereafter carefully passed through the various solutions and cut with a sharp knife without distortion at 5μ or less. As a routine, satisfactory results can be attained with hematoxylin-eosin staining[1] (Fig. 932, C).

Needle biopsy of a lymph node can be very useful to confirm a diagnosis of metastatic carcinoma. On the other hand, whenever a diagnosis of lymphoma is seriously considered clinically, we strongly recommend removal of the entire node, in one piece, with the capsule intact.

Microscopic examination

In the histologic evaluation of a lymph node, more than in any other tissue, it is important that a systematic approach be used. The critical features to be assessed are as follows:

1 Capsular and pericapsular infiltration
2 Sinusoidal, follicular, interfollicular, or diffuse pattern of the proliferation
3 If the proliferation is follicular, distribution, size, shape, and cell composition of the follicles
4 Preservation or effacement of the nodal architecture
5 Phagocytosis by histiocytes
6 Vascular proliferation
7 Granulomas
8 Necrosis
9 Cell composition of the infiltrate

Whereas none of these features can be

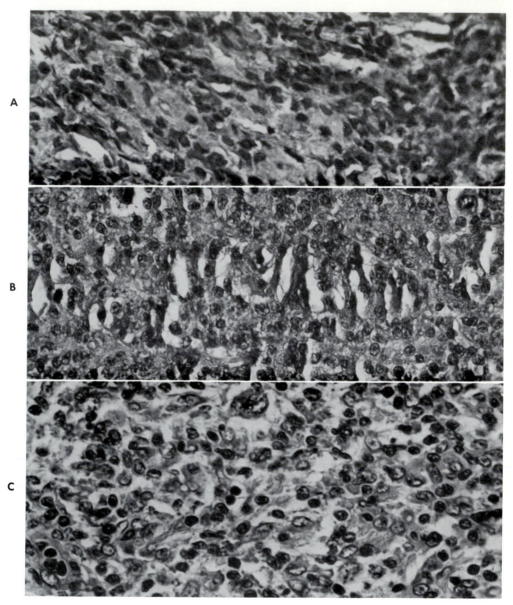

Fig. 932 A, Hodgkin's disease. Lymph node was poorly fixed and somewhat dry before being stained. No diagnosis is possible. **B,** Section of node shown in **A** cut with dull knife. Note distortion. Diagnosis is difficult. **C,** Same node shown in **A** and **B** well fixed and stained. There is no cytologic distortion, and nuclear details are clear. (**A** to **C,** ×600; **A,** WU neg. 51-1662; **B,** WU neg. 51-1664; **C,** WU neg. 51-1661.)

regarded as pathognomonic for a given entity, they usually allow a distinction between a benign and a malignant process to be made when all are taken into consideration.

A new dimension to the microscopic in-

terpretation of lymph node biopsies has been added by the recently acquired knowledge of lymph node structure in relation to immunologic function. Important information about the immunologic status of a patient can be gained by examination of a routinely processed lymph node bi-opsy.[8a] Changes in both architectural features and cell composition are important. The three major regions of a lymph node are the cortex, paracortex, and medulla. The cortex is situated beneath the capsule and contains the largest number of reactive centers. The medulla, close to the hilum, is rich in lymphatic sinuses, arteries, and veins but contains only a minor lymphocytic component. Both cortex and medulla are associated with humoral types of immune response. Proliferated reactive centers are always indicative of humoral antibody production. They are usually located in the cortical portion, but under conditions of intense antigenic stimulation, they can also appear within the medullary cords. The paracortex, situated between the cortex and the medulla, is in close relation to the postcapillary venules. It contains the mobile pool of lymphocytes, which are mainly responsible for cell-mediated immune responses. Its expansion is therefore suggestive of a cell-mediated immunologic reaction. The number of lymphocytes within the lumen and wall of postcapillary venules gives a rough indication of the degree of lymphocyte recirculation. Some cell types are always associated with a specific type of immune response. Proliferation of plasma cells, usually within the medullary cords, indicates the production of immunoglobulins and therefore of a humoral response. Epithelioid cells are usually an expression of a cell-mediated reaction. On the other hand, the function of small lymphocytes and of large lymphoid cells, whether related to humoral or cell-mediated immunity, cannot be determined by microscopic examination. The terms "reticulum cells," "immunoblast," and "hemocytoblast" are confusing and should not be employed in the microscopic description of a lymph node.

Immunodeficiencies

The many varieties of primary immunodeficiencies, most of which remain unclassified at the present time, can be broadly divided in three major categories according to the type of the immunologic deficit: humoral, cell-mediated, and combined.[11, 15a] The diagnosis of these is based on a variety of laboratory tests, including qualitative and quantitative immunoglobulin determinations, delayed-type skin reactions, and *in vitro* stimulation of lymphocytes. Sometimes lymph nodes are biopsied in order to assess the amount and composition of the lymphoid tissue. In immune diseases of the humoral type, cortical reactive centers and medullary plasma cells are scanty or absent. In diseases of cell-mediated immunity, the thickness of the paracortical area is greatly diminished. When both humoral and cell-mediated types of immunities are defective, the lymphocyte and plasma cell content of the node is practically nil. The lymph node is reduced to a mass of connective tissue and blood vessels. If an antigen such as diphtheria or tetanus toxoid is injected into the medial aspect of the thigh and an ipsilateral inguinal node is biopsied five to seven days later, its capacity to react to the antigenic stimulus can be evaluated.[12]

There is an increased incidence of malignant tumors, particularly lymphomas, in patients with primary immunodeficiencies. Those with ataxia-telangiectasia and the Wiskott-Aldrich syndrome are particularly prone to this complication, about 10% of the reported patients having died from it. The microscopic diagnosis in the early stages can be extremely difficult. This complication should be seriously considered whenever a patient with one of the immunodeficiency diseases develops lymphadenopathy and the node biopsy shows proliferation of histiocytes or large lymphoid cells in an interfollicular distribution.

Chronic granulomatous disease is not a disorder of either cellular or humoral immunity but rather the result of an intracellular (probably enzymatic) defect of granulocytes and monocytes. These cells ingest microorganisms but are unable to destroy them. The leukocytic abnormality can be detected by the nitro blue tetra-zolium test.[9] The original description was that of a familial disease in male children, but what seems to be a closely related condition has now been observed in females.[13] The main clinical features are recurrent lymphadenitis, hepatosplenomegaly, skin rash, pulmonary infiltrates, anemia, leukocytosis, and hypergammaglobulinemia.[10] Microscopically, granulomas with necrotic purulent centers are seen in lymph nodes and other organs. They closely simulate the appearance of cat-scratch disease and lymphopathia venereum.[14] Collections of histiocytes containing a lipofuscin-like pigment also are commonly observed.[15]

Hyperplasia

Lymph nodes respond to infection by enlarging. A carcinoma of the large bowel or lung may be associated with inflammation which alone may cause regional lymph node enlargement. Regardless of the skill of the surgeon, he cannot determine by palpation whether an enlarged, firm lymph node does or does not contain cancer. On many occasions, we have been handed inflamed lymph nodes by surgeons who have told us with confidence that they were simply "checking" those nodes which they knew contained cancer. If the surgeon relies on palpation, he may be denying his patient a curative operation.

It is not generally realized how large hyperplastic nodes may be. We have seen them reaching a size of 10 cm. Probably one of the largest hyperplastic nodes on record is the one mentioned by Gall and Rappaport,[22] which measured 17 cm × 12 cm × 8 cm. A hyperplastic lymph node often is firm and its cut surface homogeneously gray. Frozen section of such nodes is not difficult to interpret.

Microscopically, the hyperplasia may be primarily located in the reactive centers, in the intervening lymphoid tissue, or within the sinuses. In the first case, the hyperplasia may simulate nodular lymphoma; in the second, diffuse lymphoma; and in the latter, metastatic carcinoma or

malignant histiocytosis. Although a combination of these three patterns is not uncommon, it is useful to evaluate them separately, since the predominance of one over another may provide the clue to the specific agent involved.

Dermatopathic lymphadenitis (lipomelanosis reticularis of Pautrier)

Dermatopathic lymphadenitis is merely advanced hyperplasia associated with chronic dermatitis. It may occur in any skin condition in which itching, scratching, and infection are prominent. Rarely, it may occur in the absence of clinical skin disease. In the series reported by Cooper et al.,[17] the disease was associated with malignant lymphoma in nearly 25% of the cases. The authors found no distinguishing features between this group and the rest. The lymph node may be quite large, the cut surface bulging, and the color pale yellow. Sometimes, black linear areas are seen in the periphery, representing clumps of melanin pigment and simulating the appearance of malignant melanoma.

Microscopically, the nodal architecture is preserved. The main change is nodular histiocytic hyperplasia of the sinuses, particularly pronounced in the subcapsular region. Many of the histiocytes contain phagocytosed melanin and neutral fat in their cytoplasm. Plasma cell infiltration and follicular hyperplasia are often present (Fig. 933). A scattering of eosinophils also may be seen. These nodes may be confused with Hodgkin's disease or monocytic leukemia.[29]

Infectious mononucleosis

It is rare for the pathologist to see a lymph node from a patient with a typical clinical picture of infectious mononucleosis, for in most instances the presumptive clinical diagnosis is confirmed by finding the characteristic cells in blood smears and an elevated heterophil antibody titer. It is in the atypical case, presenting with lymphadenopathy without fever, sore throat, or splenomegaly, that the clinician will

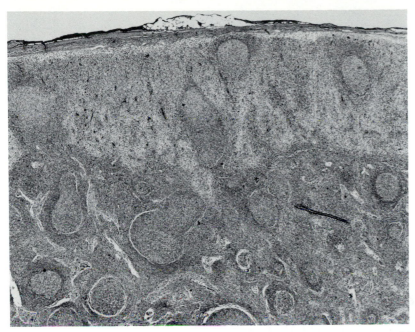

Fig. 933 Dermatopathic lymph node. Note excessive *subcapsular* histiocytic proliferation. There is also marked follicular hyperplasia. Lesion often contains melanin pigment. (Low power; WU neg. 49-4548.)

perform a lymph node biopsy to rule out the possibility of malignant lymphoma.

Microscopically, nodes affected by infectious mononucleosis can be confused with malignant lymphoma because of the effacement of the architecture, infiltration of the trabeculae, capsule, and perinodal fat, and the marked proliferation of large lymphoid cells.[18] Features of importance in the differential diagnosis with lymphoma include predominantly sinusal distribution of the large lymphoid cells, follicular hyperplasia with marked mitotic activity and phagocytosis, increase in the number of plasma cells, and vascular proliferation[40] (Fig. 934, *A*). Sieracki and Fisher[42] describe as a quite characteristic feature of this disease the presence in the sinuses of clusters or colonies of lymphocytes in graduated sizes, from the small lymphocyte to the large lymphoid cell. The latter cell usually has only one large vesicular nucleus with a thin nuclear membrane and one or two prominent amphophilic nucleoli. When binucleated, it may closely resemble a Sternberg-Reed cell.[31] Under the electron

microscope, the large lymphoid cell bears a striking similarity to a lymphocyte transformed *in vitro* under the influence of phytohemagglutinin.[16]

Postvaccinial hyperplasia

Lymph nodes draining an area of the skin subjected to smallpox vaccination can enlarge and become painful. If removed and examined microscopically, they can be easily confused with lymphoma, especially if the history of vaccination is overlooked. Of twenty cases reported by Hartsock,[24] thirteen were located in the supraclavicular region on the side of the vaccination. The largest node measured 6 cm in diameter. The interval between the vaccination and the biopsy varied between one week and three months.

Microscopically, the changes are those of a diffuse or nodular hyperplasia, with mixed cellular proliferation, consisting of eosinophils, plasma cells, and a large number of large lymphoid cells, accompanied by vascular and sinusoidal changes (Fig. 934, *B*). According to Hartsock,[24] the most

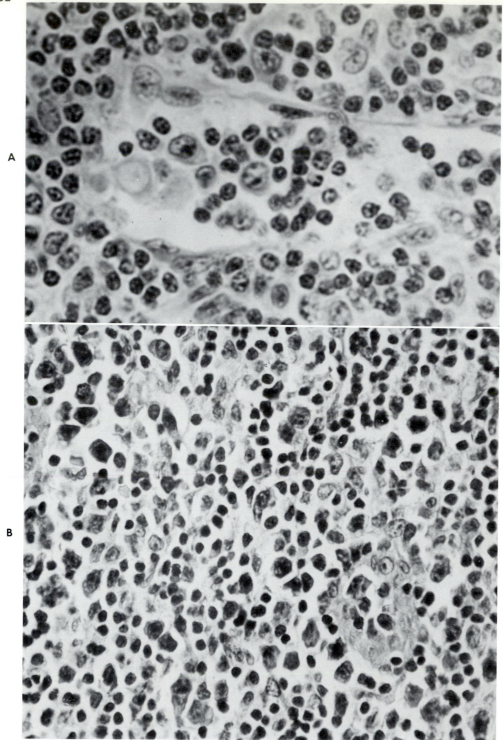

Fig. 934 Two examples of lymph node hyperplasia due to viruses. **A,** Lymph node from patient with infectious mononucleosis. Medullary cord contains lymphocytes of graduated sizes, large lymphoid cells, and hyperplastic lining cells. **B,** Lymph node draining vaccination site. Note pleomorphism, loss of architecture, and large lymphoid cells. (**A,** ×1,000; AFIP 94401; from Custer, R. P., and Smith, E. B.: The pathology of infectious mononucleosis, Blood **3:**830-857, 1948; **B,** ×720; WU neg. 67-438.)

important histologic feature of postvaccinial hyperplasia is the presence of numerous large lymphoid cells (which he calls "reticular lymphoblasts") scattered among the lymphocytes and imparting to the lymphoid tissue a mottled appearance. He noted that follicular hyperplasia was present only in those nodes removed more than fifteen days after the vaccination. The lymph node changes of postvaccinial hyperplasia, which have been reproduced experimentally,[24] are indistinguishable from those of herpes zoster and quite similar to those of infectious mononucleosis. It is likely that similar morphologic changes occurring in the absence of these three clinical conditions are, in most cases, the result of some unidentified viral infection.

Significant regional lymphadenopathy also may follow the administration of live attenuated measles virus vaccine. Microscopically, the typical multinucleated giant cell of Warthin-Finkeldey may be found[20] (Fig. 455).

Rheumatoid arthritis

Most patients with rheumatoid arthritis have generalized lymphadenopathy at some time during their illness.[33, 36] The lymph node enlargement may precede the arthritis and raise the clinical suspicion of lymphoma.

Microscopically, the most important changes are follicular hyperplasia and plasma cell proliferation, with formation of Russell bodies.[34] Vascular proliferation is also a consistent finding. Small foci of necrosis and clumps of neutrophils are seen in some instances. The capsule is often infiltrated by lymphocytes. For a differential diagnosis between reactive follicular hyperplasia and nodular lymphoma, see Table 42. Other "collagen diseases," such as lupus erythematosus, polyarteritis nodosa, and scleroderma, are usually not associated with this type of lymph node abnormality.

Syphilis

Generalized lymphadenopathy is a common finding in secondary syphilis, whereas localized node enlargement can be seen in the primary and tertiary stages of the disease. The former is the one more likely to be confused with malignant lymphoma.

Microscopically, the most striking changes occur in the inguinal nodes. They include capsular and pericapsular inflammation and extensive fibrosis, diffuse plasma cell proliferation, proliferation of blood vessels, with endothelium swelling and inflammatory infiltration of their wall (phlebitis and endarteritis), and follicular hyperplasia.[25] Rarely, noncaseating granulomas and abscesses are present. Spirochetes can be identified in most cases by the Warthin-Starry or Levaditi techniques. They are most frequently found in the wall of blood vessels. Other lymph node groups show only nonspecific follicular hyperplasia.[21]

Anticonvulsant therapy

Antiepileptic drugs derived from hydantoin, such as diphenylhydantoin (Dilantin) and mephenytoin (Mesantoin), can result in a hypersensitivity reaction manifested by skin rash, fever, generalized lymphadenopathy (mainly cervical), and peripheral eosinophilia. The reaction, which is quite uncommon, tends to occur within the first few months of therapy. The changes disappear if the drug is discontinued. The nodal enlargement can occur in the absence of some of the other manifestations of the drug reaction.

Microscopically, partial effacement of the architecture by a *pleomorphic* cellular infiltration is seen. Histiocytes, eosinophils, neutrophils, and plasma cells are all present. Some of the histiocytes have atypical nuclear features, but Sternberg-Reed cells are absent. Foci of necrosis are common[39] (Fig. 935).

Angiofollicular lymph node hyperplasia

We believe that angiofollicular lymph node hyperplasia, also known as lymph nodal hamartoma and Castleman's disease, represents a peculiar type of lymph node

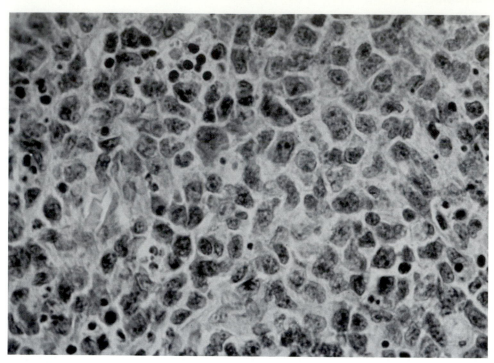

Fig. 935 Lymph node with profound hyperplasia of large lymphoid cells, eosinophilia, and nuclear debris. Patient was child with generalized lymphadenopathy and spleno-megaly and had been taking Peganone, an anticonvulsant drug. Clinically and patho-logically, he was first thought to have malignant lymphoma. With discontinuance of drug, symptoms and clinical findings completely disappeared, and child recovered. (×750; WU neg. 58-1456.)

hyperplasia rather than a neoplasm or a hamartoma. The mediastinum is by far the most common location, but this lesion also has been found in the neck, lung, axilla, mesentery, retroperitoneum, and soft tissues of the extremities.[44] It may reach a size of 16 cm. Grossly, it is round, well-circumscribed and has a solid gray cut surface.

Microscopically, large follicles are seen scattered in a mass of lymphoid tissue. Prominent vascular proliferation and hyalin-ization are the most characteristic features. The well-vascularized follicles have been confused with Hassall's corpuscles and with splenic red pulp, prompting in the first case a mistaken diagnosis of thymoma and in the second of ectopic spleen. Plasma cells, eosinophils, and large lymphoid cells are present in variable numbers. Remnants of normal lymph node structures or early changes of similar nature in adjacent nodes

are sometimes observed. Seven of the eighty-one cases reviewed by Keller et al.[27] differed from the rest by virtue of a diffuse plasma cell proliferation in the interfollicu-lar tissue, sometimes accompanied by nu-merous Russell bodies. This latter group was often found associated with anemia, elevated erythrosedimentation rate, hyper-gammaglobulinemia, and hypoalbumine-mia, whereas the usual variety (desig-nated by Keller et al.[27] as "vascular-hyaline") was in most instances asympto-matic. Surgical excision is the treatment of choice.

Sinus histiocytosis with massive lymphadenopathy

A newly recognized disease, sinus histio-cytosis with massive lymphadenopathy is characterized by fever, leukocytosis, ele-vated erythrosedimentation rate, hyper-gammaglobulinemia, and massive lymph

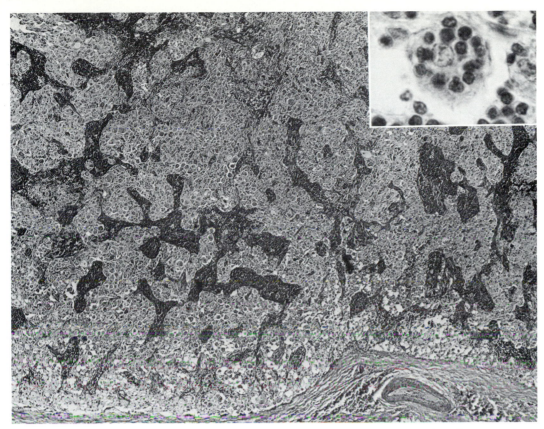

Fig. 936 Sinus histiocytosis with massive lymphadenopathy. Note capsular fibrosis and extreme dilatation of sinuses. **Inset** illustrates phenomenon of lymphophagocytosis by sinus histiocytes. (×39; WU neg. 71-9685; **inset,** ×720; WU neg. 71-9690.)

node enlargement, mainly in the cervical region. The large majority of cases occur during the first decade of life. Blacks are affected more than whites. A significant proportion of cases has originated in Africa and the West Indies.

Microscopically, the striking abnormality is a pronounced dilatation of the lymphatic sinuses, resulting in almost complete architectural effacement (Fig. 936). The sinuses are occupied, among other inflammatory cells, by numerous histiocytes with large vesicular nucleus and abundant clear cytoplasm. The latter often contain within their cytoplasm numerous phagocytosed lymphocytes, a feature of diagnostic significance[37] (Fig. 936, *inset*). Plasma cells are numerous in the intersinusal tissue. Capsular and pericapsular inflammation and fibrosis are common. The disease is unaffected by medical therapy and follows a protracted course leading eventually to complete recovery in the majority of the cases. The etiology is unknown.

Hyperplasia and malignant lymphoma

Unfortunately, there is not a single microscopic feature than can be used as an absolute criterion in the differential diagnosis between hyperplasia and malignant lymphoma.[19] Infiltration of the capsule and perinodal fat, effacement of the architecture, atypical lymphoid cells, and (exceptionally) even elements indistinguishable from Sternberg-Reed cells can all appear, alone or in combination, in a hyperplastic node. The final diagnosis should be based on a thorough evaluation of the microscopic features having a full knowledge of the clinical picture. Features favoring a diagnosis of hyperplasia include pleomorphic nature of the infiltrate in the absence of Sternberg-Reed cells, presence of plasma cells, vascular proliferation, and preservation of the lymphatic sinuses. In the presence of a follicular (nodular) pattern of growth, we have found the criteria laid out by Rappaport et al.[35] extremely useful (see Table 42). In case of doubt, the pathologist must be conservative. A false positive diagnosis results in mental anguish to the patient and in treatment that usually consists of irradiation therapy, often combined with some form of chemotherapy. We know of several instances in which the incorrect diagnosis of lymphoma was made and the patients died of complications of the therapy.

In some patients with apparently abnormal and even normal-appearing lymph nodes, the clinical signs and symptoms may strongly support a diagnosis of lymphoma. Further biopsies are indicated during the following months in order to establish the diagnosis. No evidence exists to suggest that a short delay in diagnosis will shorten the useful life of the patient if he is treated.[28] Of fifty-six patients in whom a nonspecific diagnosis was made initially by lymph node biopsy, the diagnosis was established in fifty-one within six months.[38] Treatment should not be instituted until the diagnosis is established.

The clinical information is extremely important but, like everything else, should be viewed with an open mind. We have seen unquestionable cases of malignant lymphoma in patients receiving anticonvulsivant drugs[26] and in individuals affected by rheumatoid arthritis. We also have seen lymphoma and hyperplasia coexisting in the same patient and even in the same lymph node. In the majority of the cases of lymphoma associated with a history of arthritis, anticonvulsivant therapy, or vaccination, the association is probably coincidental. There is obviously no reason why a patient with malignant lymphoma could not receive a smallpox vaccination or be also affected by rheumatoid arthritis

or epilepsy. On the other hand, there is some suggestion that in exceptional instances the group of diseases resulting in nodal hyperplasia may actually induce the appearance of a malignant lymphoma, perhaps as a result of persistent immunologic stimulation. The oncogenic effect of such stimulation has been demonstrated in experimental conditions.[32, 41] As increased incidence of lymphoma has been reported in rheumatoid arthritis.[23] Hyman and Sommers[26] found six cases of malignant lymphoma in patients on anticonvulsivant therapy and suggested a possible relationship. At one institution, twenty-nine cases have been collected of infectious mononucleosis preceding Hodgkin's disease, the interval being less than one year in eight.[30, 43]

Granulomatous inflammation

The pathologist is often asked to make a definite diagnosis of a lymph node containing chronic granulomatous inflammation. Sometimes he may make such a diagnosis with fair accuracy. However, the reaction of the lymph nodes to the presence of various bacteria and fungi may be quite similar. In fact, some disease entities cause identical microscopic alterations. Often, definite diagnosis of a lymph node lesion can be made only by careful bacteriologic study.

The surgical pathologist should know the results of prior bacteriologic studies and of serologic and skin tests before attempting to interpret a granulomatous lymph node lesion. The clinical history and physical findings also may be quite helpful. Fluorescent antibody techniques may provide a specific diagnosis. This can be made even from formalin-fixed and paraffin-embedded tissues for such lesions as tularemia.[83]

It is not rare for a lymph node containing a chronic granulomatous process to remain undiagnosed despite careful and extensive bacteriologic and pathologic study. It should be remembered that noncaseating granulomas in a lymph node may simply be the secondary manifestation of an

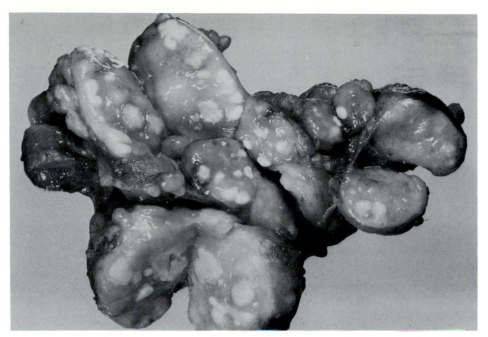

Fig. 937 Large adherent tuberculous lymph nodes containing large zones of caseation necrosis. (WU neg. 50-3030.)

underlying malignant disorder. We have seen them in lymph nodes draining carcinoma,[56, 66] and in nodes involved by Hodgkin's disease and other lymphomas.[59]

Tuberculosis

Tuberculous lymph nodes show caseation, epithelioid cells, and Langhans' giant cells. They may be adherent to each other and may form a large multinodular mass (Fig. 937). Large, firm, tuberculous cervical nodes in the adult may be confused with metastatic cancer. We have seen radical neck dissection mistakenly performed under this circumstance. With evidence of pulmonary tuberculosis and draining sinuses in the neck, the diagnosis becomes almost certain. However, we still do not make this diagnosis unless acid-fast organisms are found. These are best demonstrated by culture.

Atypical mycobacteriosis

Atypical mycobacteria are a common cause of granulomatous lymphadenitis. A caseating granulomatous disease in a cervical lymph node of a child unaccompanied by pulmonary involvement is more likely to be caused by an atypical organism than by *Mycobacterium tuberculosis*.[62] Microscopically, the host reaction may be indistinguishable from that of tuberculosis, but often the granulomatous response is overshadowed by necrotic and suppurative changes.[64, 72] An acid-fast stain should be performed in every granulomatous and suppurative lymphadenitis of unknown etiology, especially if the patient is a child. The final identification of the organism rests on the cultural characteristics.

Sarcoidosis

The diagnosis of sarcoidosis is always one of exclusion. A noncaseating granulomatous inflammation in the lymph nodes or skin microscopically indistinguishable from sarcoidosis can be seen in tuberculosis, atypical mycobacteriosis (including swimming pool granuloma), fungal diseases, leprosy, syphilis, leishmaniasis, brucellosis, tularemia, chalazion, zirconium granuloma, berylliosis, Crohn's disease, Hodgkin's disease, in nodes draining a carcinoma, and in several other condi-

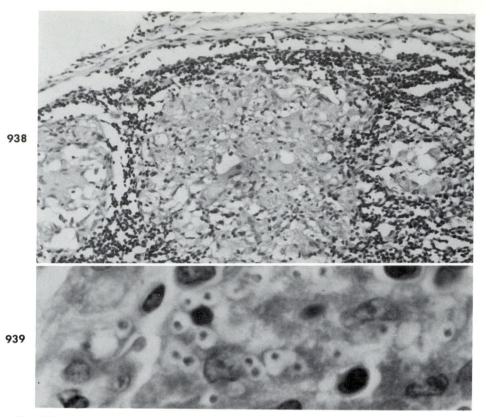

Fig. 938 Noncaseating lesion in axillary lymph node. No organisms could be identified. At postmorten examination it was discovered that patient had disseminated histoplasmosis. (×200; WU neg. 50-2057.)

Fig. 939 Histoplasmosis. Note well-defined bodies surrounded by clear area. (High power; WU neg. 47-394.)

tions[45, 51] (Figs. 938 and 939). If all these possibilities have been excluded and the clinical picture is characteristic, there is justification in labeling a case as sarcoidosis for clinical purposes. Whether this is a specific disease or a peculiar granulomatous reaction to a variety of agents is unknown at the present time. Scandinavian countries are particularly affected.[76] In the United States, the disease is ten to fifteen times more common in blacks than in whites. Practically every organ can be involved, but the ones most commonly affected are the lung, lymph nodes, eyes, and skin. Erythema nodosum often precedes or accompanies the disease. Functional hypoparathyroidism is the rule, although a few cases of sarcoidosis coexisting with primary hyperparathyroidism have been reported.[52, 84]

Microscopically, the basic lesion is a small granuloma mainly composed of epithelioid cells, with scattered Langhans' giant cells and lymphocytes (Figs. 940 and 941). Necrosis is either absent or limited to a small central fibrinoid focus. Schaumann bodies, asteroid bodies, and calcium oxalate crystals are sometimes found in the cytoplasm of the giant cells (Fig. 942). None of these inclusions are specific for sarcoidosis. Schaumann bodies are round, have concentric laminations, and contain iron and calcium. Azar and Lunardelli[46] have shown by electron microscopy that asteroid bodies are made of crisscrossing bundles of collagen fibrils. Peculiar Schiff-positive inclusions, recently designated as Wesenberg-Hamazaki bodies, have been claimed to be specific for sarcoidosis.[49, 82] Histochemical and electron

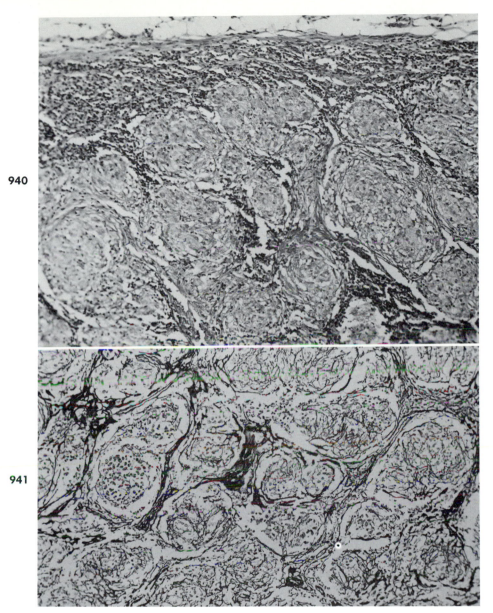

Fig. 940 Lymph node involved by sarcoidosis demonstrating noncaseating granulomatous lesions. (Moderate enlargement; WU neg. 49-6723.)

Fig. 941 Even distribution of reticulin in sarcoidosis. (Moderate enlargement; WU neg. 49-6724.)

microscopic studies by Sieracki and Fisher[74] have shown instead that they have no etiologic or pathogenetic significance. They probably represent large lysosomes containing hemolipofuscin material.

The Kveim skin test is positive in 60% to 85% of patients with sarcoidosis. False positive results are rare. The skin should be biopsied four to six weeks after injec-

tion and examined microscopically. If positive, a granulomatous inflammation identical to that of the original disease is encountered.[65] An international Kveim trial employing a single test suspension has been completed among 2,400 subjects in thirty-seven countries on six continents.[75] The level of Kveim reactivity was similar from country to country, and the excised

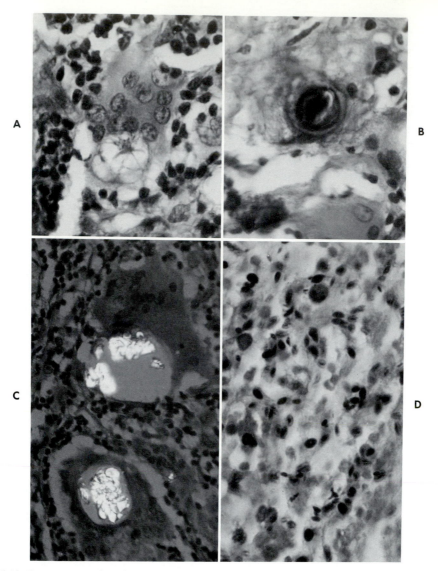

Fig. 942 Four types of inclusions that can be found in sarcoidosis. None of them is specific for this condition. **A,** Asteroid body within cytoplasm of multinucleated giant cell. **B,** Schaumann body. Note round shape and concentric lamination. **C,** Calcium oxalate crystals seen under polarized light. **D,** So-called Wesenberg–Hamasaki bodies concentrated in perivascular location. They are of small size and have oval or needlelike configuration. All sections are from same case and originated in lymph node involved by disease. (**A,** ×600; WU neg. 73-564; **B,** ×600; WU neg. 73-563; **C,** ×350; WU neg. 73-562; **D,** acid-fast stain; ×600; WU neg. 73-681; **A** to **D,** AFIP; slides contributed by Dr. F. B. Johnson, Washington, D. C.)

Kveim papules were histologically indistinguishable from one country to another, supporting the concept that sarcoidosis is the same disease the world over. Although the etiology remains elusive, mycobacterial organisms are the prime suspects. Substances like α, ε-diaminopimelic acid and mycolic acid, which occur in mycobacteria but are foreign to human tissue, have been identified in sarcoid lesions.[68] In several careful microscopic and cultural studies performed on supposedly typical cases of

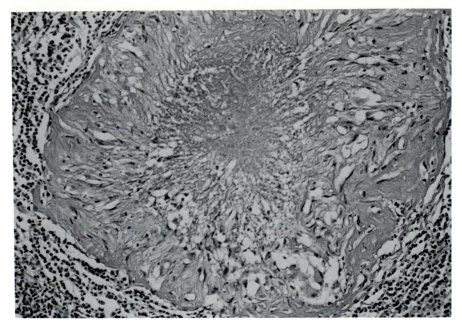

Fig. 943 Classic example of stellate abscess in lymphopathia venereum. (×520; WU neg. 52-4494; slide contributed by Armed Forces Institute of Pathology.)

sarcoidosis, acid-fast organisms have been identified in a significant number.[63, 79]

Tularemia

Tularemia causes caseation necrosis with less epithelioid cell production than in tuberculosis. Axillary lymph nodes may be enlarged. A history of handling or cleaning rabbits suggests the diagnosis. The organism may pass through the intact skin. In practically all cases, the agglutination titer is elevated.

Brucellosis

Brucellosis causes a chronic granulomatous reaction that is indistinguishable from tuberculosis. It may even suggest Hodgkin's disease. A definite diagnosis can be made only by bacteriologic isolation of the organism and a high agglutination titer.[81]

Fungal diseases

Fungal diseases cause a chronic granulomatous process that may or may not be associated with caseation necrosis. We have seen several cases of generalized histoplasmosis producing striking hyperplasia of the sinus histiocytes without granuloma formation. In one instance, this resulted in a mistaken diagnosis of reticuloendotheliosis. The Gomori methenamine-silver (GMS) and PAS-Gridley stains are extremely helpful in identifying organisms such as *Histoplasma capsulatum, Coccidioides,* and *Blastomyces.* In some instances, however, the number of organisms in a given section may be so few that they are not seen by the use of these stains. In such cases, only bacteriologic study can be diagnostic.

Lymphopathia venereum

The diagnosis of lymphopathia venereum usually is possible with a positive Frei test if the node involved is inguinal and the microscopic pattern is characteristic.

The earliest change in a lymph node is focal accumulation of neutrophilic leukocytes in tiny necrotic foci. These coalesce to form the classic stellate abscess (Fig. 943). A marginal zone of epithelioid cells and fibroblasts appears with aging. This process may become confluent and be associated with cutaneous sinus tracts. In

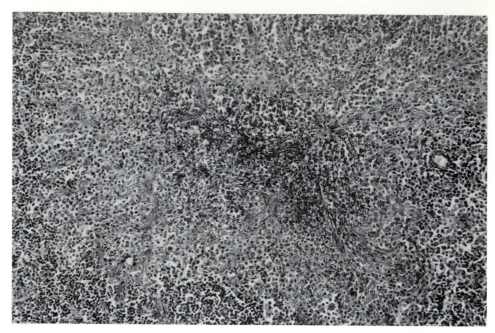

Fig. 944 Classic area of stellate necrosis in proved case of cat-scratch disease. (×115; WU neg. 62-7610.)

healing stages, a dense fibrous wall surrounds amorphous material.[77] This microscopic pattern is highly suggestive of this disease. However, we have seen it with chronic tuberculosis. Smith and Custer[77] reported it with chronic tularemia.

Cat-scratch disease

Cat-scratch disease is characterized by a primary cutaneous lesion and enlargement of regional lymph nodes, usually axillary or cervical. The changes in the nodes vary with time. Early lesions have histiocytic proliferation and follicular hyperplasia, intermediate lesions have granulomatous changes, and late lesions have microscopic and macroscopic abscesses.[67, 85] These abscesses are very suggestive of the diagnosis (Fig. 944). Suppuration was present in forty-seven of 160 cases reported by Daniels and MacMurray.[53]

The primary lesion is a red papule in the skin at the site of inoculation, usually appearing between seven and twelve days following contact. It may become pustular or crusted. Microscopically, there are foci of necrosis in the dermis surrounded by

a mantle of histiocytes. Multinucleated giant cells, lymphocytes, and eosinophils are also present.[58] The etiology of this condition is unknown, but the most likely agent is thought to be a microorganism of the psittacosis-lymphogranuloma group. The diagnosis can be confirmed by skin testing. Rare complications of the disease include granulomatous conjunctivitis ("oculoglandular syndrome of Parinaud"), thrombocytopenic purpura, and central nervous system manifestations.[48]

Toxoplasmosis

Toxoplasmosis is not the rare disease it was once thought to be.[78] There are benign forms of this entity. The patient is often a woman, and the nodes involved are frequently the cervical.[73] These nodes feel firm, and their microscopic appearance, to those experienced with the disease, is highly suggestive, if not diagnostic. Certainly, the cases of Saxen et al.,[73] which we have reviewed, had a distinctive pattern. The architecture of the lymph node is rather well preserved, and there is follicular hyperplasia. Characteristically, collections of numerous enlarged epithelioid-like histio-

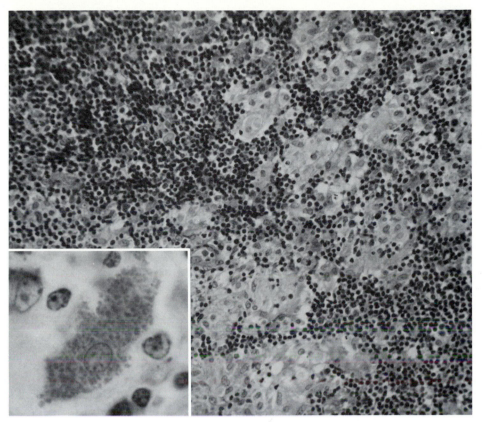

Fig. 945 Typical collection of proliferating histiocytes in cervical lymph node of patient with proved toxoplasmosis. **Inset** shows innumerable PAS-positive organisms within single cell. (×275; WU neg. 62-7377; **inset,** ×1,225; WU neg. 62-7378; slide contributed by Dr. E. Saxen, Helsinki, Finland.)

cytes, often in groups, are seen in the medulla and sinuses and *within lymphoid follicles*[70] (Fig. 945). Frequently, there is phagocytosis of nuclear debris. It is rare to find *Toxoplasma* organisms (Fig. 945, *inset*). Such nodes may be mistaken for Hodgkin's disease. Some of the apparent cures of Hodgkin's paragranuloma type fall in this group. If the diagnosis is suspected from the microscopic pattern, it can be confirmed serologically or by mouse inoculation. However, serologic tests may be normal early in the process.

Allergic granulomatosis

We have seen only three examples of allergic granulomatosis, a rare condition which simulates Hodgkin's disease. It is characterized by nodular infiltration of the lymph node by mature histiocytes and eosinophils. Multiple foci of necrosis are

seen, many of them apparently arising in a cluster of eosinophilic leukocytes. Sternberg-Reed cells are absent.[55]

Lipophagic granulomas

There are several conditions that result in the accumulation of phagocytosed fat within foamy histiocytes and multinucleated giant cells in the lymph node sinuses. The most common is the type seen in periportal and mesenteric nodes in asymptomatic individuals, probably the result of mineral oil ingestion.[60] Boitnott and Margolis[47] found this change in 78% of a series of forty-nine autopsied adults. Their chemical and histochemical studies showed that the oil droplets represented deposits of liquid-saturated hydrocarbons. Mineral oil is extensively used in the food processing industry, as a release agent and lubricant in capsules, tablets, bakery prod-

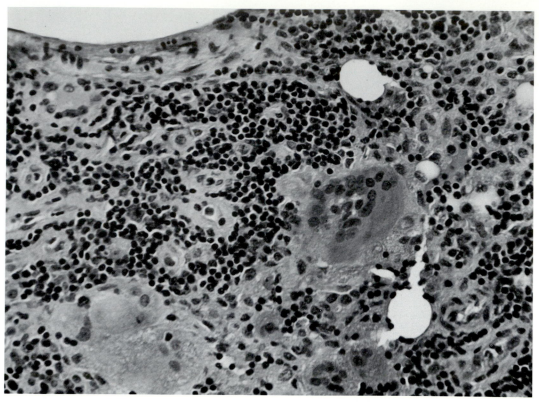

Fig. 946 Lipophagic granuloma of lymph node following lymphangiography. Foamy histiocytes and multinucleated giant cells fill dilated sinuses. (×350; WU neg. 72-1301.)

ucts, and dehydrated fruits and vegetables.

In *Whipple's disease*, the lipophagic granulomas are accompanied by collections of histiocytes containing a PAS-positive glycoprotein.[54] Under oil immersion, and with electron microscopy, characteristic bacillary bodies may be identified.[80] The glycoprotein-containing histiocytes also can be seen in the peripheral nodes,[50] and this may be the first clue to the diagnosis in a patient with gradual weight loss, weakness, and polyarthritis. Steatorrhea, the other classical symptom of the disease, may appear only in a later stage. Unfortunately, the peripheral lymph node changes are not pathognomonic unless bacillary bodies can be demonstrated. All that the pathologist can do is to suggest the possibility and request a small bowel biopsy.

Lymphangiography, an increasingly popular technique, induces a lipophagic granulomatous reaction that may persist for several months. This is preceded by a predominantly neutrophilic infiltration[71] (Fig. 946).

Mesenteric lymphadenitis

The diagnosis of mesenteric lymphadenitis is too often made on normal or mildly hyperplastic nodes in an attempt to explain why a patient with the clinical picture of acute appendicitis has a normal appendix. This is not to say that mesenteric lymphadenitis is a myth. Cases having histiocytic hyperplasia, granuloma formation, and abscesses have been reported, sometimes accompanied by inflammation of the terminal ileum and cecum. *Yersinia pseudotuberculosis* and *Yersinia enterocolitica*, two gram-negative polymorphic coccoid or ovoid motile organisms, have been isolated from many of these lesions.[57, 69] Knapp[61] identified 115 cases of mesenteric lymphadenitis due to *Yersinia pseudotuberculosis* in a five-year period. The disease is benign and self-limited.

Malignant lymphoma

The current microscopic classification of malignant lymphomas is based on three main criteria: (1) cell type, (2) degree of differentiation, and (3) pattern of growth, whether nodular or diffuse. Diffuse lymphomas are slightly more common (56%) than nodular lymphomas (44%). The latter type is more prevalent in females but is distinctly rare in children and blacks. Rappaport et al.[104] believe that a nodular configuration is not restricted to a specific lymphoma but rather that it is a type of proliferation that any of the malignant lymphomas can exhibit at some point of their evolution. These authors also maintain that the natural history of the disease is primarily related to the cell type, that within a given cell type a nodular pattern indicates a slower evolution and a better prognosis than a diffuse one, and that most nodular lymphomas change later to a diffuse pattern but maintaining the same cell composition.

Other pathologists believe instead that nodular lymphoma is a specific tumor arising from the cells of the lymphoid follicle. The ultrastructural demonstration of dendritic cells with well-developed desmosomes (as normally present in the lymphoid follicle) between the tumor cells of nodular lymphoma but not between those of diffuse lymphomas would seem to favor the latter hypothesis.[95a]

Grossly, the nodules of nodular lymphoma present as small gray areas protruding on the surface. The main features that differentiate nodular lymphoma from reactive follicular hyperplasia are described in Table 42 (Figs. 947 and 948). Features of little help in this regard are increase in number or size of the follicles, compression of sinuses, cracking artifact,

Table 42 Architectural and cytologic features of nodular lymphoma and of reactive follicular hyperplasia*

Nodular lymphoma	Reactive follicular hyperplasia
Architectural features	
Complete effacement of normal architecture	Preservation of nodal architecture
Even distribution of "follicles" throughout cortex and medulla	Follicles more prominent in cortical portion of lymph node
Slight or moderate variations in size and shape of "follicles"	Marked variations in size and shape of follicles with presence of elongated, angulated, and dumbbell-shaped forms
Fading of "follicles"	Sharply demarcated reaction centers
Massive infiltration of capsule and pericapsular fat with or without formation of neoplastic follicles outside capsule	No, or only moderate, infiltration of capsule and pericapsular fat tissue with inflammatory cells that may be arranged in perivascular focal aggregates (when associated with lymphadenitis)
Condensation of reticulin fibers at periphery of "follicles"	Little or no alteration of reticular framework
Cytologic features	
"Follicles" composed of neoplastic cells exhibiting cellular pleomorphism with nuclear irregularities	Centers of follicles (reaction centers) composed of reticulum cells and their histiocytic derivatives, with few or no cellular and nuclear irregularities
Lack of phagocytosis	Active phagocytosis in reaction centers
Relative paucity of mitotic figures usually without significant difference in their number inside and outside the "follicles"; occurrence of atypical mitoses	Moderate to pronounced mitotic activity in reaction centers; rare or no mitoses outside reaction centers; no atypical mitoses
Similarity of cell type inside and outside "follicles"	Infiltration of tissue between reaction centers with inflammatory cells (when associated with lymphadenitis)

*From Rappaport, H., Winter, W. J., and Hicks, E. B.: Follicular lymphoma; a re-evaluation of its position in the scheme of malignant lymphoma, based on a survey of 253 cases, Cancer 9:792-821, 1956.

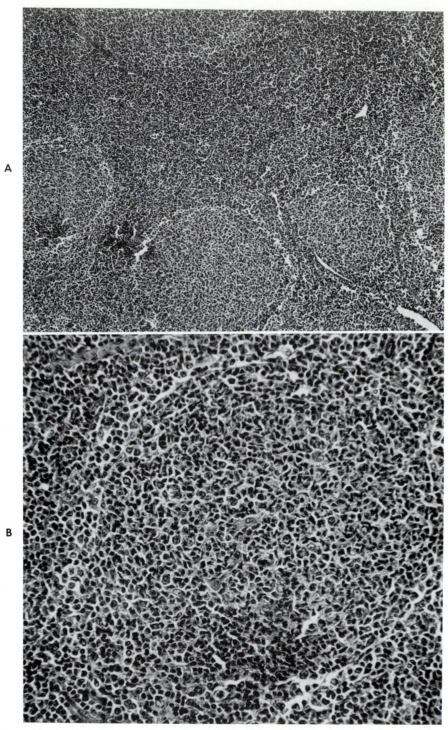

Fig. 947 Nodular lymphoma of poorly differentiated lymphocytic type occurring in 51-year-old man with generalized lymphadenopathy. **A,** Large nodules scattered throughout. **B,** Large nodule in which cells inside are streaming outside follicle. There is no evidence of phagocytosis. (**A,** ×87; WU neg. 62-8265; **B,** ×285; WU neg. 62-8264.)

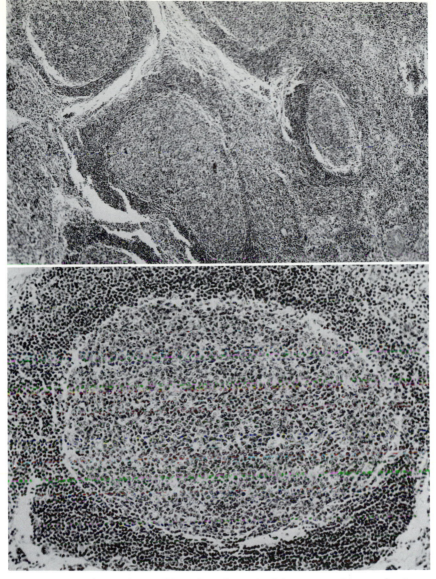

Fig. 948 Prominent hyperplasia of lymph node. Note delimitation of hyperplastic germinal centers surrounded by mantle of lymphocytes. Germinal center has syncytial pattern with prominent phagocytes. (WU negs. 48-5750 and 48-5746.)

packing of lymphocytes around follicles, and fusion of follicles.[104]

It should be remarked that in nodular lymphoma there is lymphoid tissue within as well as around the nodules. In contrast, in the nodular sclerosing variants of Hodgkin's disease and lymphocytic lymphoma, the lymphoid nodules are surrounded by (and probably the result of) thick bands of dense fibrous tissue.

The classification we currently use, based on the classifications of Rappaport et al.[104]

and of Lukes et al.,[99] is as follows:

1 Malignant lymphoma, undifferentiated type
2 Malignant lymphoma, histiocytic type
3 Malignant lymphoma, lymphocytic type, poorly differentiated
4 Malignant lymphoma, lymphocytic type, well differentiated
5 Malignant lymphoma, mixed (histiocytic-lymphocytic) type
6 Malignant lymphoma, Hodgkin's type
  a Lymphocytic predominance
  b Nodular sclerosis
  c Mixed cellularity
  d Lymphocytic depletion

Malignant lymphomas with a nodular pattern are designated by the addition of the word "nodular" preceding the cytologically appropriate term.

It is likely that this classification will eventually be superseded by one that will take into account the new body of information that is emerging from basic immunologic studies, such as the division of lymphocytes into B and T cell types. However, it would seem appropriate to retain the present scheme, which has repeatedly proved of great practical value, until the conclusions obtained from these new techniques on pathologic material are duly tested and agreed upon.

Undifferentiated (stem cell) lymphoma

Undifferentiated lymphoma is a malignant proliferation of primitive cells having scanty cytoplasm and a round or oval nucleus with delicate chromatin, thin nuclear membrane, and a small, distinct nucleolus.[103] The large majority are diffuse. *Burkitt's lymphoma* is regarded as a specific variant of this type of lymphoma. It has a peculiar geographic distribution, the endemic areas being tropical Africa and New Guinea.[112] However, sporadic cases clinically, microscopically, and ultrastructurally identical to the African cases have been reported from all over the world[90, 91, 100] (Fig. 949).

Typically, Burkitt's lymphoma affects children and young adults. It has a great tendency for extranodal involvement, such as the jaws, ovaries, abdominal organs, retroperitoneum, and the central nervous system. Peripheral or mediastinal lymph node involvement, splenic enlargement, and a leukemic picture are exceptional. Untreated cases follow a rapid fatal course. On the other hand, chemotherapy often results in dramatic and durable remissions. Microscopically, the most striking feature is the "starry sky" pattern, resulting from a scattering of nonneoplastic histiocytes containing phagocytosed nuclear debris among a monomorphic infiltrate of highly primitive cells.[111, 113] It should be remarked

that this microscopic appearance *is not* pathognomonic of Burkitt's lymphoma. We have seen it in other lymphoreticular malignancies, in nonlymphoid sarcomas, in thymomas, and in carcinomas. A "starry sky" pattern was found in 10% of 602 cases of histiocytic lymphoma (reticulum cell sarcoma) by Diamandopoulos and Smith[89] and in 18% of eighty-five cases of poorly differentiated lymphocytic lymphoma by Oels et al.[101] The latter authors suggested that this feature is associated with a decrease in the survival rates.

Histiocytic lymphoma

Lymph nodes involved by histiocytic lymphoma (reticulum cell sarcoma) may be matted together and may contain large necrotic areas even leading to sinus formation. The nodal architecture is totally or partially obliterated by a proliferation of malignant histiocytes. Variations in cellular and nuclear shape are marked. The nuclei are large and vesicular, with a prominent nucleolus and thick nuclear membrane. Many are indented or lobulated (Fig. 950). Mitoses are common. Fibrosis with hyalinization of the stroma is sometimes prominent, separating the tumor cells in clusters or cords.[105]

It is possible that many, if not most, of the malignant lymphomas presently designated as histiocytic purely on the basis of morphologic criteria are actually composed of "large lymphoid cells"—i.e., transformed lymphocytes of either bone marrow or thymic origin.[86] The application of recently described immunohistochemical techniques for the identification of the latter should provide the evidence to substantiate this hypothesis.[92, 102a, 110]

Lymphocytic lymphoma

Grossly, the nodes of lymphocytic lymphoma may form large masses, but the individual nodes are not adherent. They appear highly cellular and occasionally contain areas of necrosis (Fig. 951). In the poorly differentiated variant, formerly called lymphoblastic, the cells are larger

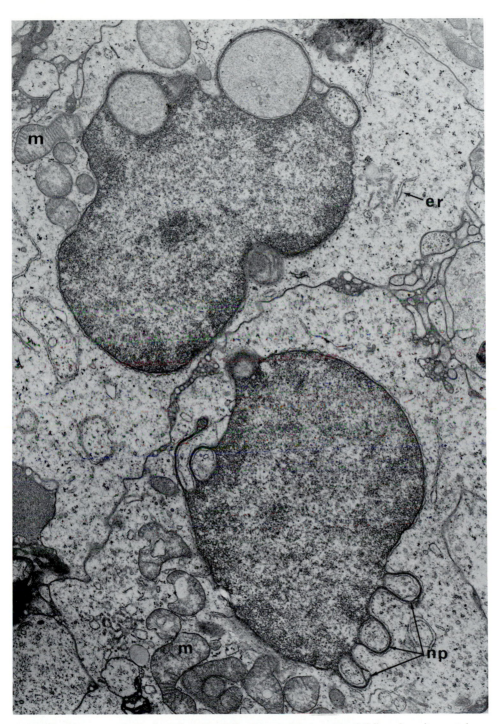

Fig. 949 These neoplastic lymphocytic cells, from patient with childhood malignant lymphoma of Burkitt variety in St. Louis, Mo., have numerous peculiar, although not unique, nuclear projections, **np,** polar aggregates of mitochondria, **m,** sparse endoplasmic reticulum, **er,** and scattered ribosomes. (Approximately ×13,000.)

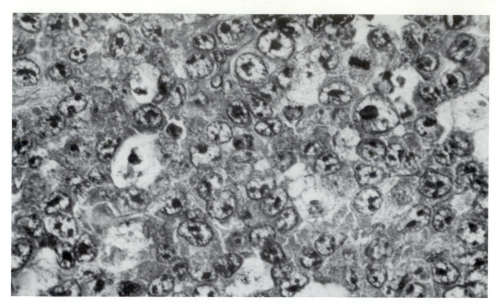

Fig. 950 High-power view of histocytic lymphoma involving inguinal lymph node. As may rarely occur, phagocytosis was present. Individual tumor cells have large vesicular nuclei, prominent nucleoli, and abundant cytoplasm. (×720; WU neg. 52-4080.)

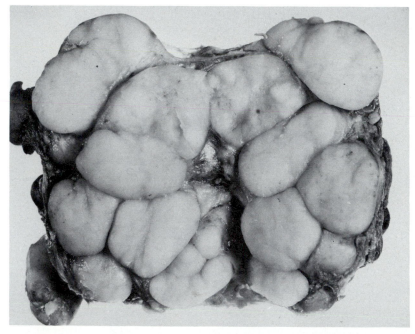

Fig. 951 Mass of nodes in lymphocytic malignant lymphoma. Note separation of lymph nodes and occasional areas of necrosis. (WU neg. 49-3387.)

than mature lymphocytes but smaller than histiocytes. The nuclei are round or oval and irregular, with focal chromatin clumping and a distinct nucleolus. Nuclear indentations are often present (Fig. 952).

In the well-differentiated lymphocytic lymphoma, the cells are remarkably similar to normal mature lymphocytes, by both light and electron microscopic criteria (Figs. 953 and 954). We have not found

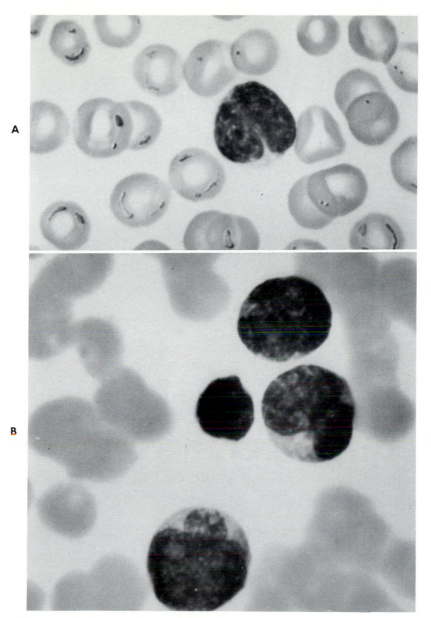

Fig. 952 A, Blood smear from patient with mixed type of nodular malignant lymphoma showing so-called "notched nucleus cell." **B,** Blood smear from same patient. Abnormal lymphocytes in smear are interpreted as neoplastic (poorly differentiated lymphocytes). (**A** and **B,** Wright; ×1,080; from Rappaport, H., Winter, W. J., and Hicks, E. B.: Follicular lymphoma; a reevaluation of its position in the scheme of malignant lymphoma, based on a survey of 253 cases, Cancer **9**:792-821, 1956.)

it possible to distinguish this type of lymphoma from chronic lymphocytic leukemia on the basis of histologic sections. The clinical history, the peripheral blood count, and the bone marrow findings are required to make such distinction, which is desirable in view of the different natural history of the two diseases.[114] Occasionally, nodes involved by lymphocytic lymphoma are composed of lymphoid nodules separated by abundant fibrous tissue. This pattern, which should be distinguished

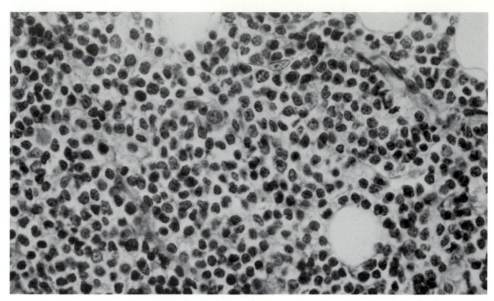

Fig. 953 Malignant lymphoma of lymphocytic type invading perinodal fat. We cannot differentiate this tumor from lymphocytic leukemia. (×600; WU neg. 49-6948.)

from the classical nodular lymphoma, is seen most commonly in inguinal and retroperitoneal lymph nodes of elderly individuals.[102] According to Bennett and Millett,[88] this feature is associated with a better prognosis.

Mixed (histiocytic-lymphocytic) lymphoma

The designation of mixed (histiocytic-lymphocytic) lymphoma should be restricted to tumors in which both histiocytes and lymphocytes are present in significant amounts. A nodular pattern of growth is common in the early stages of mixed lymphoma. The majority, however, eventually develop into a diffuse lymphoma of histiocytic type.

Whether the concept of a mixed lymphoma is a valid one needs to be substantiated. The alternative possibility that the lymphocytes are nonneoplastic but that they represent instead either a reaction to the tumor or residual normal lymph node cells seems to be at least as credible.

Clinicopathologic correlation

The pathologic features of malignant lymphoma bearing a direct relation to prognosis are extension of the disease, cell type, nodular or diffuse pattern of growth, and fibrosis. Stage I lesions have a good prognosis.[97] Unfortunately, they comprise only one-third of all cases. The routine use of lymphangiography has demonstrated that most patients with non-Hodgkin's malignant lymphoma have widespread disease at the time of diagnosis. In a series of 405 cases of non-Hodgkin's lymphoma reviewed by Jones et al.,[94] 39% were stage IV at the time of diagnosis. In another series of forty patients with apparently localized disease, only three were found to have normal lymphangiograms and inferior venacavograms.[95] The high diagnostic accuracy of lymphangiography in the evaluation of malignant lymphoma has been amply demonstrated[108, 109] (Fig. 955). Malignant lymphoma involving a high cervical lymph node is the one most likely to be localized. Spread by involvement of contiguous lymph node groups was found by Jones et al.[94] in 86% of their cases of non-Hodgkin's lymphoma; it was more common in the diffuse than in the nodular type. Contiguous pattern of spread is even more common in Hodgkin's disease.[93, 106] A notable exception to this rule is lymphoma of the left side of the neck,

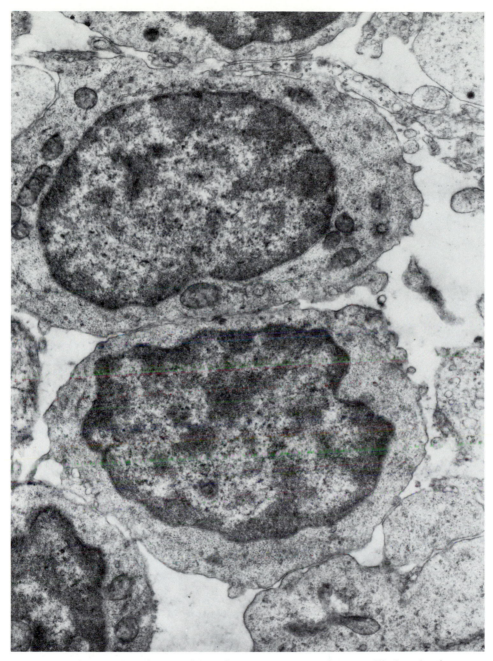

Fig. 954 Malignant lymphoma of lymphocytic type. Cytoplasm is filled with ribosomes. Few mitochondria are present. These cells are not structurally different from normal lymphocytes. (×14,000.)

which may spread to the retroperitoneal para-aortic nodes, sparing the mediastinum.

In regard to cell type, the average survival is longer for the well-differentiated lymphocytic type, shorter for the histiocytic variety, and intermediate for the poorly differentiated lymphocytic type.[98, 107] In all groups, the survival rates are better in patients with tumors with a nodular pattern

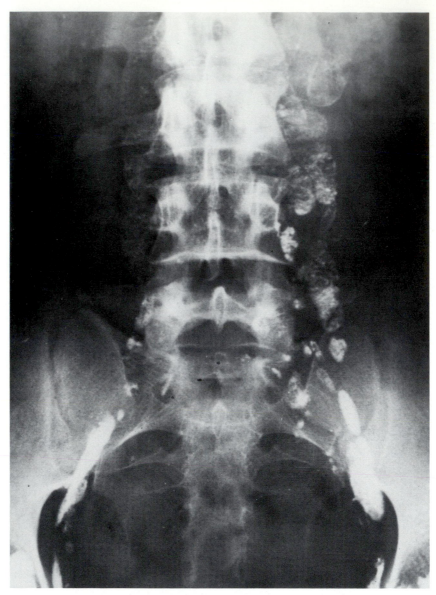

Fig. 955 Positive retroperitoneal lymphangiogram in patient with Hodgkin's disease. Lymph nodes are enlarged and have coarse reticulated appearance.

of growth and those associated with a significant degree of stromal fibrosis. Involvement of mesenteric lymph nodes is exceptional in Hodgkin's disease but quite common in the other types of lymphoma.[92a] Non-Hodgkin lymphomas have a much greater tendency to begin (or at least to present clinically) as extranodal tumors than Hodgkin's disease.[87] The bone marrow and the spleen are the most common sites of extranodal spread. Marrow involvement is

better demonstrated by histologic sections of the aspiration than by the conventional smear.[92a, 96]

Occasionally, patients with malignant lymphoma develop a leukemic blood picture, a condition designated by Sternberg as "leukosarcoma."[107a] The typical case is represented by a child or adolescent who comes to the emergency room in acute respiratory distress. Roentgenograms show a large anterior mediastinal mass. If the

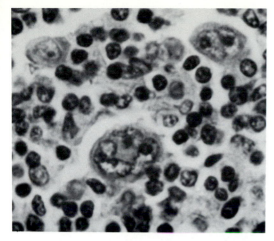

Fig. 956 Classic Sternberg-Reed cells with multilobated nuclei and prominent nucleoli. (High power; WU neg. 48-4608.)

patient survives the acute episode, leukemia inevitably develops.[88a] The microscopic appearance is that of a lymphocytic lymphoma, sometimes with a "starry sky" pattern. Smith et al.[107b] suggest a thymic origin for this neoplasm in view of the fact that the neoplastic cells in their case formed rosettes with normal sheep red blood cells, as normal T lymphocytes do.

Hodgkin's disease

Hodgkin's disease lacks the monomorphic appearance of the other malignant lymphomas. Lymphocytes, eosinophils, plasma cells, and histiocytes may all be present, in greater or lesser amount depending on the microscopic type. The initial diagnosis depends on the presence of the Sternberg-Reed cell. This cell is of relatively large size, its cytoplasm is abundant, either basophilic or amphophilic, and two or more vesicular nuclei are present, each having a thick nuclear membrane and a single, prominent, acidophilic or amphophilic nucleolus, surrounded by a clear halo (Fig. 956). Cells with only one nucleus should not be designated as Sternberg-Reed cells. On the other hand, we often see patients with morphologically documented Hodgkin's disease in whom a biopsy of bone marrow, liver, or some other organ done for staging purposes shows a

polymorphic infiltrate *with atypical mononuclear histiocytes* but without identifiable Sternberg-Reed cells. Our policy in these cases has been to regard these organs to be involved by Hodgkin's disease.

The Sternberg-Reed cell, although necessary for the initial diagnosis of Hodgkin's disease, is not pathognomonic of this entity. Megakaryocytes can simulate it closely in hematoxylin-eosin sections, but they can be identified by the presence of a strongly PAS-positive substance in their cytoplasm.[118] Cells morphologically indistinguishable from Sternberg-Reed cells have been seen in infectious mononucleosis, mycosis fungoides, and several types of malignant neoplasms.[136, 137] In all of these, the architecture and cell composition of the remaining elements were indicative of their respective nature. These findings restrict even further the diagnostic requirements of Hodgkin's disease. These can be summarized by saying that for the initial diagnosis of this disease, Sternberg-Reed cells not only need to be present but must be situated in the proper architectural and cytologic background.

The mixed cell composition and the presence of necrosis and fibrosis result in a heterogeneous gross appearance, quite dissimilar in most cases from that of the other malignant lymphomas. In the early stages, only focal involvement of a lymph node may be encountered.[132] Noncaseating granulomas are sometimes present in nodes and other organs involved by Hodgkin's disease.[127] They may be quite numerous and obscure the diagnostic features of the disease. In other instances, these granulomas may be seen within otherwise uninvolved organs of patients with Hodgkin's disease.[122] Their significance is unknown. Perhaps they represent an expression of delayed hypersensitivity. Their presence does not indicate involvement of that organ by Hodgkin's disease and should therefore not influence the staging criteria.

Growing dissatisfaction with the time-honored Jackson-Parker division of Hodgkin's disease into a granuloma, paragranu-

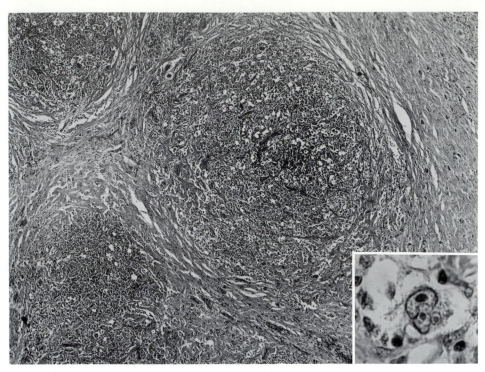

Fig. 957 Nodular sclerosis Hodgkin's disease. Bands of collagen separate nodules. **Inset** shows lacunar Sternberg-Reed cell. (×38; WU neg. 66-13059A; **inset**, ×800; WU neg. 66-13056.)

loma, and sarcoma variant[121] led to an improved classification by Lukes et al.[128] which was adopted with some modifications by the Nomenclature Committee at the Rye Conference on Hodgkin's disease. Four major categories are accepted. In *lymphocytic predominance Hodgkin's disease,* Sternberg-Reed cells are scanty, scattered among a large number of mature lymphocytes, and sometimes accompanied by proliferation of benign-appearing histiocytes. In Hodgkin's disease of *mixed cell type,* a significant number of eosinophils, neutrophils, plasma cells, and atypical histiocytes accompany the ubiquitous Sternberg-Reed cells and lymphocytes. *Lymphocytic depletion* results in an infiltrate predominantly formed by malignant-appearing histiocytes, some of which fulfill the criteria of Sternberg-Reed cells. Areas of necrosis and fibrosis are common. This rare type of Hodgkin's disease should be differentiated from the pleomorphic variant of histiocytic lymphoma.[129] *Nodular sclero-*

sis, which in many recent series has been the most common variant of Hodgkin's disease, is characterized by broad collagen bands separating the lymphoid tissue in well-defined nodules (Fig. 957). The fibrosis often centers around blood vessels. The cytologic pattern within the nodules may be one of lymphocyte predominance, lymphocyte depletion, or mixed cell type. Clumps of foamy macrophages are sometimes present.[138] In addition to the typical Sternberg-Reed cell, a variant designated as "cytoplasmic" or "lacunar" is seen. It is quite large (40μ to 50μ in diameter), with an abundant clear cytoplasm and several nuclei having complicated infoldings and inconspicuous nucleolus. Characteristically, formalin fixation results in shrinking of the cytoplasm, leaving the cell in an artifactually created "lacuna." Some observers regard this peculiar variant of the Sternberg-Reed cell as more typical of this type of Hodgkin's disease than the fibrosis itself and make the diagnosis of

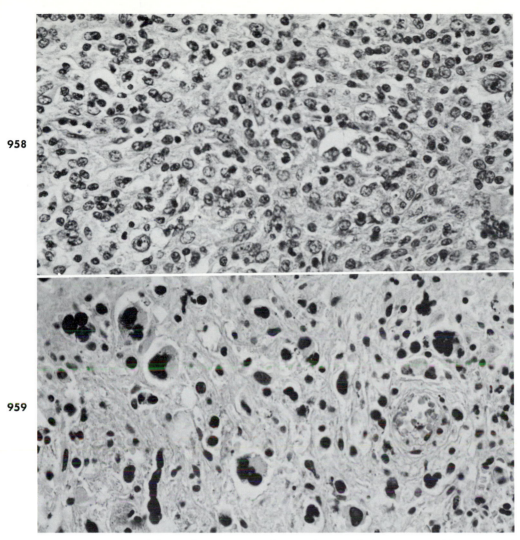

Fig. 958 Typical Hodgkin's disease. Note pleomorphism with histiocytic proliferation and numerous Sternberg-Reed cells. (×480; WU neg. 50-5996.)

Fig. 959 Lymph node from patient who had transient response to nitrogen mustard and died. This node shows fibrosis and prominent nuclear abnormalities. Patient had not received irradiation therapy. (×480; WU neg. 50-5994.)

nodular sclerosis Hodgkin's disease in their presence even if fibrosis is totally lacking.[133] Nodular sclerosis often presents in the neck and mediastinum of young females.[116] The long controversy over the nature of "granulomatous thymoma" has now been settled. It represents Hodgkin's disease of the nodular sclerosis type involving the thymus and adjacent lymph nodes and accompanied by a peculiar proliferation of the thymic epithelium.[117, 125] It should be re-membered that practically all types of Hodgkin's disease can exhibit some degree of fibrosis, particularly after therapy. If the pathologist is too liberal in his criteria for the diagnosis of nodular sclerosis, the clinical and prognostic connotations associated with this microscopic type will lose most of their meaning. Strum and Rappaport[133] showed that the histologic types of Hodgkin's disease remain constant over long follow-up periods in the large majority of

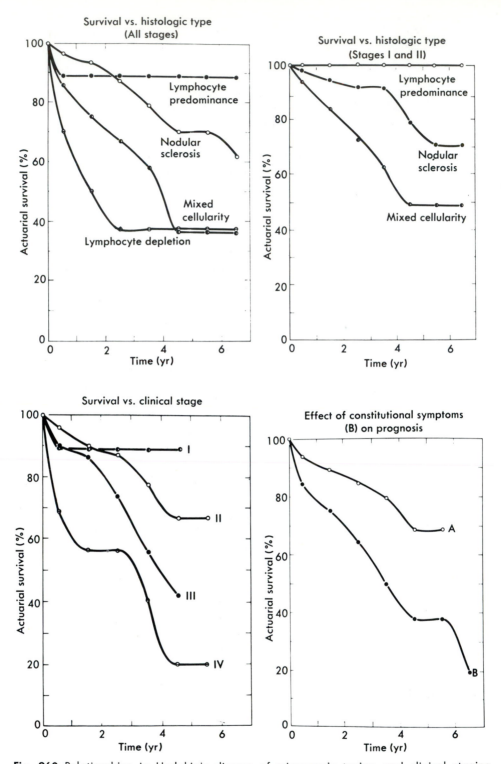

Fig. 960 Relationships in Hodgkin's disease of microscopic typing and clinical staging with prognosis and age of onset. (From Keller, A. R., Kaplan, H. S., Lukes, R. J., and Rappaport, H.: Correlation of histopathology with other prognostic indicators in Hodgkin's disease, Cancer **22:**487-499, 1968.)

the cases. They found this to be especially the case in the nodular sclerosis variety. When change occurred, it was usually toward a histologically more malignant form.

The microscopic typing of Hodgkin's disease should always be made on examination of a biopsy obtained prior to the institution of treatment. Radiation therapy and chemotherapy result in focal necrosis, fibrosis, and profound nuclear aberrations (Figs. 958 and 959). features that render impossible a proper pathologic evaluation.

Clinicopathologic correlation

The two main factors influencing the prognosis of Hodgkin's disease are the clinical staging and microscopic typing. There is a definite correlation between types and stages. Most lymphocyte predominance and nodular sclerosis cases are in Stages I and II, whereas most lymphocyte depletion cases are in Stages III and IV. However, the differences in survival rates among the different types are maintained even within clinical staging groups[126] (Fig. 960). Lymphocytic predominance and nodular sclerosis are most

favorable, mixed cellularity is intermediate, and the lymphocytic depletion type has an ominous prognosis.

Mediastinal involvement is the rule in nodular sclerosis, inconstant in mixed cellularity, and exceptional in lymphocyte predominance. On the other hand, the risk of abdominal involvement is highest in mixed cellularity and lymphocyte predominance, as compared with nodular sclerosis. We have seen several cases of Hodgkin's disease in elderly persons presenting as a febrile illness with pancytopenia or lymphocytopenia, hepatomegaly, abnormal liver function tests, and absence of peripheral lymphadenopathy. Most of these were of the lymphocytic depletion type.[129]

Most cases of Hodgkin's disease spread by involvement of adjacent lymph node groups.[124] This contiguous manner of spread is particularly common in the nodular sclerosis and lymphocytic predominance types.[126] The most common sites of extranodal involvement by Hodgkin's disease are the spleen, liver, bone marrow, lung, and skin. New important information has been acquired in regard to the frequency and significance of extranodal involvement as a result of a more aggressive diagnostic approach, particularly with the use of laparotomy as a routine staging procedure.[119, 120, 123] Of the nodes biopsied at

Fig. 960 cont'd For legend, see opposite page.

laparotomy, the most likely to be involved are those located in the splenic hilum and retroperitoneum. Mesenteric nodes are almost always spared. A spleen weighing 400 gm or more is practically always histologically positive. The converse is not true: spleens below this weight are involved in a high proportion of cases. The focal nature of the disease calls for a careful gross examination of this organ.

Spleens should be sectioned throughout in thin slices, and every suspicious area should be examined microscopically. If no nodules are detected on gross inspection, the chances of finding Hodgkin's disease in random microscopic sections are negligible. Hepatic disease is almost invariably associated with splenic involvement. Clinical assessment of liver involvement is quite unreliable. Lymphangiography is effective in detecting involvement below the level of the second lumbar vertebra but inconsistent for nodes situated higher in the periaortic area. About 30% of patients with negative lymphangiograms in whom the para-aortic nodes are left untreated will later demonstrate lymphoma below the diaphragm.[115] Involvement of lung or chest wall by the nodular sclerosis type often represents direct extension from mediastinal nodes and does not result in an ap-

preciable decrease in survival.[126] Bone marrow involvement is better detected with a surgical biopsy than by the conventional smear. Elevation of serum alkaline phosphatase level is the most reliable sign of marrow disease.[131]

Vascular invasion has been detected microscopically in 6% to 14% of the cases of Hodgkin's disease by the use of elastic tissue stains.[135] This finding is apparently associated with an increased incidence of extranodal organ involvement.[130]

Aggressive radiation therapy and chemotherapy are often successful in controlling Hodgkin's disease, but total eradication is rarely achieved. Of nineteen autopsied patients who died after having survived Hodgkin's disease for ten years or more, Strum and Rappaport[134] found residual disease in sixteen.

The main clinical differences between Hodgkin's disease and the other malignant lymphomas are summarized in Table 43.

Lymphoma and dysproteinemia

There is evidence suggesting that many malignant lymphomas arise from B lymphocytes (bone marrow–derived)—i.e., cells normally engaged in humoral immune responses.[139, 154] This being the case, it is not surprising that in some lymphomas the

Table 43 Clinical differences between Hodgkin's disease and other malignant lymphomas*

	Non-Hodgkin's malignant lymphoma	Hodgkin's disease
Age	Common at extremes of life	Peak between 18 and 38 yr of age; rare at puberty
General condition of patient in early stages	Often affected	Usually excellent
Pruritus	Usually not present	May precede and fairly frequently accompanies
Fever	Very rarely observed in early cases	May be found in early cases
Lesions in upper air passages or gastrointestinal tract	Common	Rare
Lymph node involvement	Often symmetrical	Often unilateral
Cervical lymph nodes	Often bilateral, upper cervical, spinal, and jugular chains	Often unilateral, lower cervical, jugular chain
Physical character	Often voluminous, ovoid mass	Often polylobated
Sternal lymph nodes	Practically never involved	Sometimes involved
Epitrochlear lymph nodes	May be involved	Practically never involved
Basal metabolic rate (afebrile cases)	May be elevated	Invariably normal
Contiguous spread	Rare	Common
Response to radiations	Immediate	Delayed

*Modified from Ackerman, L. V., and del Regato, J. A.: Cancer, ed. 4, St. Louis, 1970, The C. V. Mosby Co.

tumor cells express their potentialities by producing immunoglobulins of one sort or another.[150] Ranging in between the typical malignant lymphoma without globulin abnormalities and the typical plasma cell myeloma with monoclonal peak and Bence Jones proteinuria, all types of morphologic and biochemical hybrids have been encountered. Tumors have been described that secrete completely assembled immunoglobulins of the IgG, IgA, IgM, IgD, or IgE type, with or without concomitant production of isolated light chains; isolated light chains to the almost total exclusion of complete immunoglobulin molecules, and "heavy chains" (or, more accurately, Fc fragments) of IgG, IgM, or IgA specificity. This remarkably diverse expression of function has led to the introduction of such names as Waldenstrom's macroglobulinemia, light chain disease, Franklin's heavy chain disease, etc., and even to the proposal of grouping all immunoglobulin-secreting lymphoid and plasmocytic tumors under the term *immunocytoma*.[143, 144, 147, 148]

This practice has led to considerable confusion, as happens whenever morphologic and functional parameters are mixed in a common terminology. We believe that these neoplasms should be classified according to conventional morphologic criteria rather than by the biochemical findings in the patient's serum—i.e., a well-differentiated lymphocytic lymphoma should be designated as such whether it produces macroglobulins, heavy chains, light chains or no detectable globulins. Three main cytologic patterns are observed:

1 Malignant lymphomas of conventional type, indistinguishable from those not associated with immunoglobulin abnormalities.

2 Plasma cell myelomas, in which most of the tumor cells have the characteristic light and electron microscopic features of plasma cells.

3 Tumors having the overall appearance of a malignant lymphoma but in which a certain proportion of the tumor cells

has undergone a plasmocytic differentiation, as evidenced light microscopically by lateralization of the nucleus, coarse chromatin clumping, appearance of a perinuclear clear halo, and/or increased basophilic cytoplasm and ultrastructurally by prominence of the Golgi apparatus and abundance of granular endoplasmic reticulum (Fig. 961). We designate these lesions as malignant lymphoma with plasmocytic differentiation and suggest that the clinician investigate for the possibility of immunoglobulin abnormalities.[141]

Attempts to correlate the microscopic appearance with the secretory activity of these tumors have been made by several authors. The results have been largely discouraging, although a few more or less distinctive patterns have emerged.[147a, 149] In general, tumors producing IgM globulin or "heavy chains" have the anatomic distribution and cytologic appearance of malignant lymphoma, whereas most of those secreting IgG globulin or a light chain are clinically and microscopically classifiable as plasma cell myeloma. There is no reliable light microscopic or fine structural criteria which allow one to predict the type of immunoglobulin secreted by a plasma cell myeloma. Not even the rare "nonsecretory" plasma cell myelomas can be separated from the others by morphology alone.[142] Presence of Russell bodies, a rare occurrence in plasma cell myeloma, correlates with lack of Bence Jones protein in the urine.[146] Intranuclear and cytoplasmic inclusions are not specific for any type of immunoglobulin. However, those composed of IgM or IgA are often PAS positive due to their high carbohydrate content, whereas those composed of IgG are not.[145] Tumors which have been reported as secreting IgA "heavy chains" have always involved the gastrointestinal tract.[153] Of all the anatomic varieties of malignant lymphoma, Hodgkin's disease and lymphomas with nodular pattern of growth are the least likely to be associated with immunoglobulin production. The

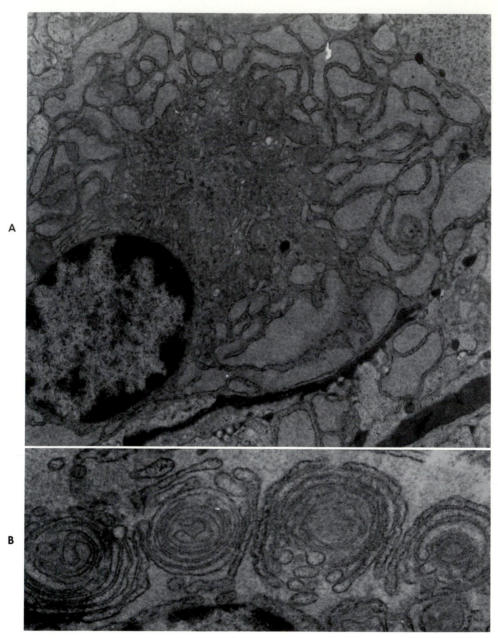

Fig. 961 Electron micrograph of lymph node involved by malignant lymphoma associated with production of heavy chains. **A,** Most cells show plasmocytic differentiation, as evidenced by chromatin clumping and margination, prominent perinuclear Golgi apparatus, and numerous dilated cisternae of granular endoplasmic reticulum. **B,** Peculiar ''fingerprint'' arrangement of endoplasmic reticulum is present in some of tumor cells.

more obvious the plasmocytic differentiation, the higher the chances if immunoglobulin alterations. However, it should be remembered that even fully differentiated plasma cell myelomas may sometimes be associated with complete lack of detectable immunoglobulin production. These "nonsecretory" plasma cell myelomas, as well as those that produce only light chains, seem to run an accelerated clinical course.[148]

The term *benign monoclonal gammopathy* has been applied to the presence on serum electrophoresis of a discrete, homogeneous protein ("M-protein") in the absence of clinical manifestations of plasma cell myeloma or lymphoma.[155] The incidence of this condition in the adult population is close to 1%, many times higher than that of overt myeloma.[140] Migliore and Alexanian[152] believe that its association with carcinomas of various organs is coincidental. It is possible that some of the cases of "benign monoclonal gammopathy" represent an early phase of plasma cell myeloma.[151] Bone marrow examination shows an increased number of mature plasma cells. In order to make a diagnosis of plasma cell myeloma, there should be cytologic abnormalities of the plasma cells, not just a numerical increase of them. Production of immunoglobulin fragments, suppression of normal immunoglobulin production, serum paraprotein levels higher than 1 gm/100 ml, and progressive rise in paraprotein levels all strongly suggest the malignant nature of a lymphocytic or plasmocytic proliferation.[148]

Malignant histiocytosis

A rare condition, malignant histiocytosis is differentiated from histiocytic malignant lymphoma mainly by virtue of the systemic involvement present even in the early stages of the disease.[158] Later in its evolution, this distinction may become impossible. Most of the cases we have seen have been in children. Microscopically, the affected lymph nodes often show a sinusal pattern of involvement, in contrast to the diffuse or nodular configuration of malignant lymphoma.

Two more or less distinct varieties of malignant histiocytosis have been described. The first, known as **histiocytic medullary reticulosis,** is characterized clinically by hepatosplenomegaly, jaundice, and rapidly fatal outcome.[156] Pathologically, prominent erythrophagocytosis is seen among the tumoral histiocytes. The second, also systemic and uniformly fatal, is accompanied by generalized skin rash and marked peripheral eosinophilia. Microscopically, the malignant histiocytes are accompanied by a mixed cellular infiltrate rich in eosinophils and lymphocytes, which may cause a mistaken diagnosis of Hodgkin's disease. Sternberg-Reed cells, however, are not present.[157]

Malignant histiocytosis, including its variants, should be clearly differentiated from the group of diseases sometimes designated as histiocytosis X. In the latter, the histiocytes are well differentiated and lack the malignant cytologic features of the former (Fig. 962).

Metastatic tumors

Lymph nodes frequently contain unexpected malignant processes. We are often asked to decide whether the malignant cells are epithelial or mesenchymal in character and their probable site of origin. In some instances, the microscopic changes are sufficiently diagnostic to give this information, but in others the changes warrant only a shrewd guess or a listing of possibilities in order of likelihood, based on the morphologic pattern and the exact location of the lymph node.[159, 160]

A small, firm supraclavicular lymph node may contain well-differentiated papillary tumor. Tumors with this pattern, forming acini and having psammoma bodies, do not originate within the oral cavity. Such tumors could arise from the thyroid gland. However, if the specific stain for mucin is positive, the tumor could not be primary in the thyroid gland. Such a papillary tumor would be unusual from the breast or lung, although the location of the metastases would be compatible with such origin. The most likely source of the primary tumor might well be the ovary (Fig. 963). There are many cases, however, in which all the pathologist can say is that the lymph node is replaced by a highly undifferentiated malignant tumor, source unknown.

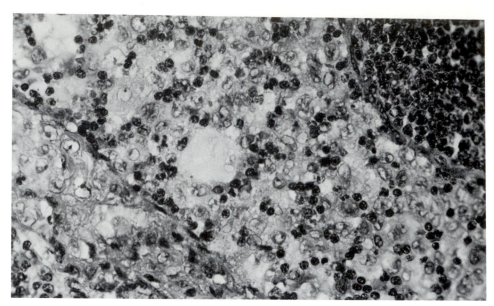

Fig. 962 Lymph node involved by differentiated histiocytosis of Letterer-Siwe type. Well-differentiated histiocytes, with large vesicular nuclei and abundant acidophilic cytoplasm, distend peripheral sinuses. Eosinophils also are present. (×460; WU neg. 50-475; slide contributed by Dr. A. R. Crane, Philadelphia, Pa.)

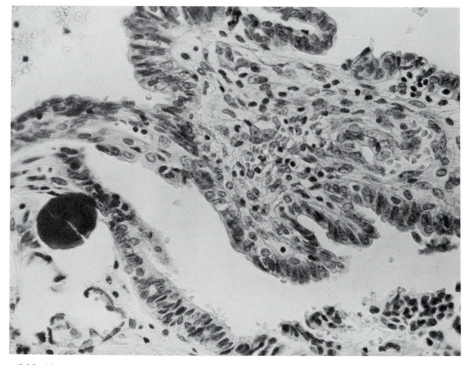

Fig. 963 Metastatic carcinoma in cervical lymph node. Tumor is epithelial with papillary arrangement. Primary neoplasm arose from ovary. (×300; WU neg. 52-4089.)

Biopsy of a peripheral lymph node may obviate a major operation. A small supraclavicular node may be biopsied and found to contain carcinoma metastatic from the breast. In such cases, breast surgery is fruitless. When well-differentiated squamous carcinoma replaces a lymph node, central necrosis may make the node cystic (Fig. 964). We have seen such lesions diagnosed clinically and pathologically as branchial cleft cysts (Fig. 965). Carcinoma may be so undifferentiated that it cannot be distinguished from malignant lymphoma. Under these circumstances, the reticulin stain and the cytologic details are not helpful. By light microscopy, the pattern of tumor cells growing in small nests separated by stroma is often the *only* feature suggesting carcinoma (Fig. 966). Electron microscopic examination of some of these nodes may be diagnostic of metastatic carcinoma by demonstrating complex desmosomes and tonofibrils.[161]

Other lesions

Disseminated lupus erythematosus rarely may be diagnosed by lymph node biopsy

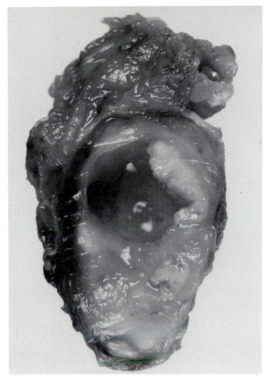

Fig. 964 Metastatic squamous cell carcinoma in lymph node. Cavitation incident to necrosis is evident. (WU neg. 66-8430.)

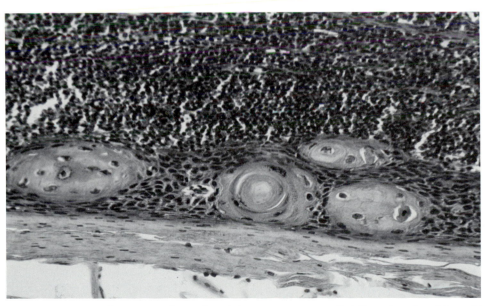

Fig. 965 Margin of cystic node replaced by metastatic, weil-differentiated epidermoid carcinoma. This pattern can easily be mistaken for branchial cleft cyst, for inner layer consists of keratin and squamous cells and next layer is composed of lymphoid tissue (×300; WU neg. 62-8260.)

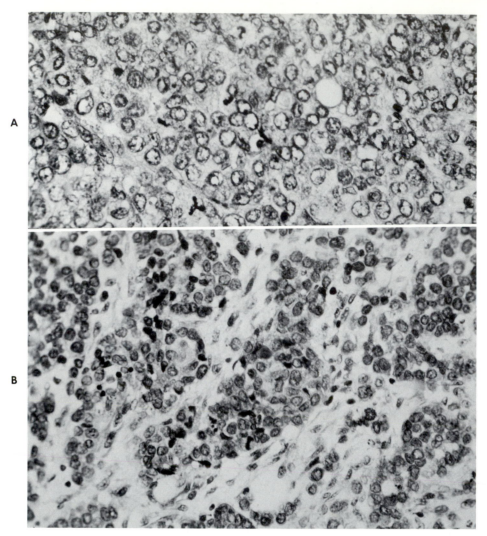

Fig. 966 **A,** Area in lymph node of replacement by carcinoma which is impossible to differentiate from malignant lymphoma. **B,** Another lymph node from same patient from whom node shown in **A** was taken. Diagnosis of carcinoma can be made from this node because of carcinoma cells growing in small nests. (**A,** ×420; WU neg. 51-4668; **B,** ×300; WU neg. 51-4669.)

(Fig. 967). In such nodes, there is a peculiar form of necrosis associated with hematoxylin bodies that have been found histochemically to be aggregates of smudged lymphocytes.[166] Moore et al.[169] described PAS-positive cytoplasmic bodies in plasma cells within the lymph nodes in disseminated lupus erythematosus.

Kaposi's sarcoma involving lymph nodes may be associated with the classic cutaneous involvement or be present without skin lesions. The latter occurrence is seen almost exclusively in African children.[163] Microscopically, the involved nodes show the typical proliferation of spindle cells separated by slitlike spaces containing red blood cells and accompanied by marked follicular hyperplasia and plasmocytic infiltration.[170]

It is not uncommon for lymph nodes, especially those situated in the aortoiliac region, to contain wide bands of *hyaline material* among the lymphoid elements.[167] Its presence has no pathologic significance.

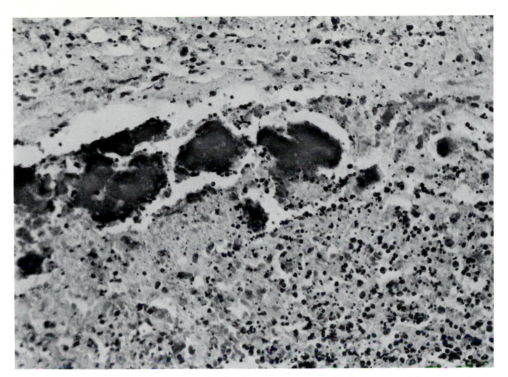

Fig. 967 Lymph node with hematoxylin bodies in patient with disseminated lupus erythematosus. Diagnosis of this disease was made on basis of pathologic alterations in lymph node. This finding is rare in our experience. (×260; WU neg. 55-3684.)

We have seen it confused with amyloidosis and radiation effect.

Inclusions of different types of benign tissue can occur within lymph nodes. Lack of awareness of this phenomenon can lead to the mistaken diagnosis of metastatic carcinoma. Salivary gland tissue is commonly seen in high cervical nodes.[162] Thyroid follicles may be found within the marginal sinus of a midcervical node in the absence of any pathologic change of the thyroid gland.[168] Inclusions of müllerian or coelomic epithelium, regarded by some as endometriosis, are not rare in pelvic lymph nodes of females.[165] Johnson and Helwig[164] reported six cases in which the capsule of a lymph node contained clusters of nevus cells, without involvement of the nodal parenchyma. Five of the six nodes were located in the axilla. Exceptionally, ectopic breast tissue is found in axillary lymph nodes.[163a] We have seen a "benign metastasis" from a mammary intraductal papilloma to the peripheral sinus of an axillary node, probably as a result of a too energetic manipulation of the primary tumor.

Another lesion worth mentioning in this regard is the *ectopic thymus* occasionally seen in supraclavicular lymph node biopsies. The pathologist unaware of this occurrence might easily interpret the Hassall's corpuscles as islands of metastatic epidermoid carcinoma.

REFERENCES
Biopsy

1 Butler, J. J.: Non-neoplastic lesions of lymph nodes of man to be differentiated from lymphomas, Nat. Cancer. Inst. Monogr. **32:**233-255, 1969.

2 Dawson, P. J., Cooper, R. A., and Rambo, O. M.: Diagnosis of malignant lymphoma, Cancer **17:**1405-1413, 1964.

3 Moore, R. D., Weisberger, A. S., and Bowerfind, E. S., Jr.: An evaluation of lymphadenopathy in systemic disease, Arch. Intern. Med. **99:**751-759, 1957.

4 Slaughter, D. P., Economeu, S. G., and Southwick, H. W.: Surgical management of

Hodgkin's disease, Ann. Surg. **148**:705-710, 1958.

5 Symmers, W. St. C.: Survey of the eventual diagnosis in 600 cases referred for a second histological opinion after an initial biopsy diagnosis of Hodgkin's disease, J. Clin. Pathol. **21**:650-653, 1968.

6 Symmers, W. St. C.: Survey of the eventual diagnosis in 226 cases referred for a second histological opinion after an initial biopsy diagnosis of reticulum cell sarcoma, J. Clin. Pathol. **21**:654-655, 1968.

7 Velez-Garcia, E., Fradera, J., Grillo, A. J., Velazquez, J., and Maldonado, N.: A study of lymph node and tumor imprints and aspirations, Bol. Asoc. Med. P. R. **63**:188-203, 1971.

8 Weed, L. A., and Dahlin, D. C.: Bacteriologic examination of tissues removed for biopsy, Am. J. Clin. Pathol. **20**:116-132, 1950.

Microscopic examination

8a Cottier, H., Turk, J., and Sobin, L.: A proposal for a standardized system of reporting human lymph node morphology in relation to immunological function, Bull. WHO **47**:375-408, 1972.

Immunodeficiencies

9 Baehner, R. L., and Nathan, D. G.: Quantitative nitroblue tetrazolium test in chronic granulomatous disease, N. Engl. J. Med. **278**:971-976, 1968.

10 Carson, M. J., Chadwick, D. L., Brubaker, C. A., et al.: Thirteen boys with progressive septic granulomatosis, Pediatrics **35**:405-412, 1965.

11 Fudenberg, H.: Primary immunodeficiencies; report of a World Health Organization Committee, Pediatrics **47**: 927-946, 1971.

12 Gitlin, D., Janeway, C. A., Apt. L., and Craig, J. M.: Agammaglobulinemia. In Lawrence, H., editor: Cellular and humoral aspects of hypersensitivity states, New York, 1959, Paul B. Hoeber, Inc., pp. 375-441.

13 Holmes, B., Park, B. H., Malawista, S. E., Quie, P. G., Nelson, D. L., and Good, R. A.: Chronic granulomatous disease in females; a deficiency of leukocyte glutathione peroxidase, N. Engl. J. Med. **283**:217-221, 1970.

14 Johnston, R. B., and McMurry, J. S.: Chronic familial granulomatosis, Am. J. Dis. Child. **114**:370-378, 1967.

15 Landing, B. H., and Shirkey, N. S.: A syndrome of recurrent infection and infiltration of viscera by pigmented lipid histiocytes, Pediatrics **20**:431-438, 1957.

15a Stiehm, E. R., and Fulginiti, V. A.: Immunologic disorders in infants and children, Philadelphia, 1973, W. B. Saunders Co.

Hyperplasia

16 Carter, R. L.: Review of some recent observations on "glandular fever cells," J. Clin. Pathol. **19**:448-455, 1966.

17 Cooper, R. A., Dawson, P. J., and Rambo, O. N.: Dermatopathic lymphadenopathy; a clinicopathologic analysis of lymph node biopsy over a fifteen-year period, Calif. Med. **106**:170-175, 1967.

18 Custer, R. P., and Smith, E. B.: The pathology of infectious mononucleosis, Blood **3**:830-857, 1948.

19 Dawson, P. J., Cooper, R. A., and Rambo, O. M.: Diagnosis of malignant lymphoma, Cancer **17**:1405-1413, 1964.

20 Dorfman, R. F., and Herweg, J. C.: Live, attenuated measles virus vaccine; inguinal lymphadenopathy complicating administration, J.A.M.A. **198**:320-321, 1966.

21 Evans, N.: Lymphadenitis of secondary syphilis (its resemblance to giant follicular lymphadenopathy), Arch. Pathol. **37**:175-179, 1944.

22 Gall, E. A., and Rappaport, H.: Seminar on diseases of lymph nodes and spleen. In Proceedings of the 23rd Seminar of the American Society of Clinical Pathologists, Chicago, 1958, American Society of Clinical Pathologists, pp. 7-9.

23 Goldenberg, G. J., Paraskevas, F., and Israels, L. G.: The association of rheumatoid arthritis with plasma cell and lymphocytic neoplasms, Arthritis Rheum. **12**:569-579, 1969.

24 Hartsock, R. J.: Postvaccinial lymphadenitis; hyperplasia of lymphoid tissue that simulates malignant lymphomas, Cancer **21**:632-649, 1968.

25 Hartsock, R. J., Halling, W., and King, F. M.: Luetic lymphadenitis: a clinical and histologic study of 20 cases, Am. J. Clin. Pathol. **53**:304-314, 1970.

26 Hyman, G. A., and Sommers, S. C.: The development of Hodgkin's disease and lymphoma during anticonvulsant therapy, Blood **28**:416-427, 1966.

27 Keller, A. R., Hochholzer, L., and Castleman, B.: Hyaline-vascular and plasma-cell types of giant lymph node hyperplasia of mediastinum and other locations, Cancer **29**:670-683, 1972.

28 Kreyberg, L., and Iversen, O. H.: Early diagnosis of malignant conditions in lymph nodes, Br. J. Cancer **13**:26-32, 1959.

29 Laipply, T. C.: Lipomelanotic reticular hyperplasia of lymph nodes, Arch. Intern. Med. **81**:19-36, 1948.

30 Levine, P. H., Stevens, D. A., Coccia, P. F., Dabich, L., and Roland, A.: Infectious mononucleosis prior to acute leukemia: a possible role for the Epstein-Barr virus, Cancer **30**:1-6, 1972.

31 McMahon, N. J., Gordon, H. W., and Rosen,

R. B.: Reed-Sternberg cells in infectious mononucleosis, Am. J. Dis. Child. **120**:148-150, 1970.

32 Metcalf, D.: Reticular tumours in mice subjected to prolonged antigenic stimulation, Br. J. Cancer **15**:769-779, 1961.

33 Motulsky, O. G., Weinberg, S., Saphir, O., and Rosenberg, E.: Lymph nodes in rheumatoid arthritis, Arch. Intern. Med. **90**:660-676, 1952.

34 Nosanchuk, J. S., and Schnitzer, B.: Follicular hyperplasia in lymph nodes from patients with rheumatoid arthritis; a clinicopathologic study, Cancer **24**:343-354, 1969.

35 Rappaport, H., Winter, W. J., and Hicks, E. B.: Follicular lymphoma; a re-evaluation of its position in the scheme of malignant lymphoma, based on a survey of 253 cases, Cancer **9**:792-821, 1956.

36 Robertson, M. D. J., Hart, F. D., White, W. F., Nuki, G., and Boardman, P. L.: Rheumatoid lymphadenopathy, Ann. Rheum. Dis. **27**:253-260, 1968.

37 Rosai, J., and Dorfman, R. F.: Sinus histiocytosis with massive lymphadenopathy: a pseudolymphomatous benign disorder; analysis of 34 cases, Cancer **30**:1174-1188, 1972.

38 Saltzstein, S. L.: The fate of patients with nondiagnostic lymph node biopsies, Surgery **58**:659-662, 1965.

39 Saltzstein, S. L., and Ackerman, L. V.: Lymphadenopathy induced by anticonvulsant drugs clinically and pathologically mimicking malignant lymphomas, Cancer **12**:164-182, 1959.

40 Salvador, A. H., Harrison, E. G., and Kyle, R. A.: Lymphadenopathy due to infectious mononucleosis: its confusion with malignant lymphoma, Cancer **27**:1029-1040, 1971.

41 Schwartz, R., André-Schwartz, J., Armstrong, M. Y. K., and Beldotti, L.: Neoplastic sequelae of allogenic disease. I. Theoretical considerations and experimental design, Ann. N.Y. Acad. Sci. **129**:804-821, 1966.

42 Sieracki, J. C., and Fisher, E. R.: Diagnostic problems involving nodal lymphomas. In Sommers, S. C., editor: Pathology Annual, vol. 5, New York, 1970, Appleton-Century-Crofts, pp. 91-124.

43 Stevens, D. A.: Infectious mononucleosis and malignant lymphoproliferative diseases, J.A.M.A. **219**:897-898, 1972.

44 Tung, K. S. K., and McCormack, L. J.: Angiomatous lymphoid hamartoma, Cancer **20**:525-536, 1967.

Granulomatous inflammation

45 Anderson, R., James, D. G., Peters, P. M., and Thomson, A. D.: Local sarcoid-tissue reactions, Lancet **1**:1211-1213, 1962.

46 Azar, H. A., and Lunardelli, C.: Collagen nature of asteroid bodies of giant cells in sarcoidosis, Am. J. Pathol. **57**:81-92, 1969.

47 Boitnott, J. K., and Margolis, S.: Mineral oil in human tissues. II. Oil droplets in lymph nodes of the porta hepatis, Bull. Hopkins Hosp. **118**:414-422, 1966.

48 Carithers, H. A., Carithers, C. M., and Edwards, R. O., Jr.: Cat-scratch disease; its natural history, J.A.M.A. **207**:312-316, 1969.

49 Carter, C. J., Gross, M. A., and Johnson, F. B.: The selective staining of curious bodies in lymph nodes of patients as a means for diagnosis of sarcoid, Stain Technol. **44**:1-4, 1969.

50 Chears, W. C., Jr., Smith, A. G., and Ruffin, J. M.: Diagnosis of Whipple's disease by peripheral lymph node biopsy; report of a case, Am. J. Med. **27**:351-353, 1959.

51 Cunningham, J. A.: Sarcoidosis. In Sommers, S. C., editor: Pathology Annual, vol. 2, New York, 1967, Appleton-Century-Crofts, pp. 31-46.

52 Cushard, W. G., Jr., Simon, A. B., Caterbury, J. M., and Reiss, E.: Parathyroid function in sarcoidosis, N. Engl. J. Med. **286**:395-398, 1972.

53 Daniels, W. B., and MacMurray, F. G.: Cat scratch disease, J.A.M.A. **154**:1247-2151, 1954.

54 Fisher, E. R.: Whipple's disease: pathogenetic considerations; electron microscopic and histochemical observations, J.A.M.A. **181**:396-403, 1962.

55 Gall, E. A., and Rappaport, H.: Seminar on diseases of lymph nodes and spleen. In Proceedings of the 23rd Seminar of the American Society of Clinical Pathologists, Chicago, 1958, American Society of Clinical Pathologists, pp. 7-9.

56 Gorton, G., and Linell, F.: Malignant tumours and sarcoid reactions in regional lymph nodes, Acta Radiol. (Stockh.) **47**:381-392, 1957.

57 Jansson, E., Wallgren, G. R., and Ahvenen, P.: Y. enterocolitica as a cause of acute mesenteric lymphadenitis, Acta Paediatr. Scand. **57**:448-450, 1968.

58 Johnson, W. T., and Helwig, E. B.: Cat-scratch disease; histopathologic changes in the skin, Arch. Dermatol. **100**:148-154, 1969.

59 Kadin, M. E., Donaldson, S. S., and Dorfman, R. F.: Isolated granulomas in Hodgkin's disease, N. Engl. J. Med. **283**:859-861, 1970.

60 Kelsall, G. R., and Blackwell, J. B.: The occurrence and significance of lipophage clusters in lymph nodes and spleen, Pathology **1**:211-220, 1969.

61 Knapp, W.: Mesenteric adenitis due to Pasteurella pseudotuberculosis in young people, N. Engl. J. Med. **259**:776-778, 1958.

62 Llewelyn, D. M., and Dorman, D.: Mycobacterial lymphadenitis, Aust. Paediatr. J. 7:97-102, 1971.

63 Määtta, K. T.: Histological study of mediastinal lymph nodes in clinical sarcoidosis; a report of 86 cases, Ann. Acad. Sci. Fenn. [Med.] 138:1-106, 1968.

64 Mackellar, A., Hilton, H. B., and Masters, P. L.: Mycobacterial lymphadenitis in childhood, Arch. Dis. Child. 42:70-74, 1967.

65 Mitchell, D. N.: The Kveim test. In Dyke, S. C., editor: Recent advances in clinical pathology, series 5, Boston, 1968, Little, Brown and Co., chap. 4.

66 Nadel, E., and Ackerman, L. V.: Lesions resembling Boeck's sarcoid, Am. J. Clin. Pathol. 20:952-957, 1952.

67 Naji, A. F., Carbonell, F., and Barker, H. J.: Cat scratch disease; a report of three new cases, review of the literature, and classification of the pathologic changes in the lymph nodes during various stages of the disease, Am. J. Clin. Pathol. 38:513-521, 1962.

68 Nethercott, S. E., and Strawbridge, W. G.: Identification of bacterial residues in sarcoid lesions, Lancet 2:1132, 1956.

69 Nilthn, B.: Studies on Yersinia enterocolitica with special reference to bacterial diagnosis and occurrence in human enteric disease, Acta Pathol. Microbiol. Scand. [suppl.] 206:1-48, 1969.

70 Piringer-Kuchinka, A., Martin, I., and Thalhammer, O.: Ueber die vorzuglich cerviconuchale Lymphadenitis mit kleinherdiger Epitheloid-zellwucherung, Virchows Arch. Pathol. Anat. 331:522-535, 1958.

71 Ravel, R.: Histopathology of lymph nodes after lymphangiography, Am. J. Clin. Pathol. 46:335-355, 1966.

72 Reid, J. D., and Wolinsky, E.: Histopathology of lymphadenitis caused by atypical mycobacteria, Am. Rev. Respir. Dis. 99:8-12, 1969.

73 Saxen, L., Saxen, E., and Tenhunen, A.: The significance of histological diagnosis in glandular toxoplasmosis, Acta Pathol. Microbiol. Scand. 56:284-294, 1962.

74 Sieracki, J. C., and Fisher, E. R.: The ceroid nature of the so-called "Hamazaki-Wesenberg bodies," Am. J. Clin. Pathol. 59:248-253, 1973.

75 Siltzbach, L. E.: Results of Kveim testing; an international Kvein test study (Proceedings of the Third International Conference on Sarcoidosis), Acta Med. Scand. 176(suppl. 425): 178-190, 1964.

76 Siltzbach, L. E.: Geographic aspects of sarcoidosis, Trans. N.Y. Acad. Sci. 29(Ser. II): 364-374, 1967.

77 Smith, E. B., and Custer, R. P.: The histopathology of lymphogranuloma venereum, J. Urol. 63:546-563, 1950.

78 Stansfeld, A. G.: The histological diagnosis of toxoplasmic lymphadenitis, J. Clin. Pathol. 14:565-573, 1961.

79 Vaněk, J., and Schwarz, J.: Demonstration of acid-fast rods in sarcoidosis, Am. Rev. Respir. Dis. 101:395-400, 1970.

80 Watson, J. H., and Haubrich, W. S.: Bacilli bodies in the lumen and epithelium of the jejunum in Whipple's disease, Lab. Invest. 21: 347-357, 1969.

81 Weed, L. A., and Dahlin, D. C.: Bacteriologic examination of tissues removed for biopsy, Am. J. Clin. Pathol. 20:116-132, 1950.

82 Wesenberg, W.: Saurefeste, Spindelkorper Hamazaki bei Sarkoidose, Arch. Klin. Exp. Med. 227:101-112, 1966.

83 White, J. D., and McGavran, M. H.: Identification of Pasteurella tularensis, J.A.M.A. 194: 180-182, 1965.

84 Winnacker, J. L., Becker, K. L., Friedlander, M., Higgins, G. A., and Moore, C. F.: Sarcoidosis and hyperparathyroidism, Am. J. Med. 46:305-312, 1969.

85 Winship, T.: Pathologic changes in so-called cat-scratch fever; review of findings in lymph nodes of 29 patients and cutaneous lesions of 2 patients, Am. J. Clin. Pathol. 23:1012-1018, 1953.

Malignant lymphoma
Undifferentiated (stem cell) lymphoma/Histiocytic lymphoma/Lymphocytic lymphoma

86 Aisenberg, A. C.: Malignant lymphoma, N. Engl. J. Med. 288:883-890 and 935-941, 1973.

87 Banfi, A., Bonadonna, G., Carnevali, G., Oldini, G., and Salvini, E.: Preferential sites of involvement and spread in malignant lymphomas, Eur. J. Cancer 4:319-324, 1968.

88 Bennett, M. H., and Millett, Y. L.: Nodular sclerotic lymphosarcoma; a possible new clinico-pathological entity, Clin. Radiol. 20:339-343, 1969.

88a Cooke, J. V.: Mediastinal tumor in acute leukemia, Am. J. Dis. Child. 44:1153-1177, 1932.

89 Diamandopoulos, G. T., and Smith, E. B.: Phagocytosis in reticulum cell sarcoma, Cancer 17:329-337, 1964.

90 Dorfman, R. F.: Diagnosis of Burkitt's tumor in the United States, Cancer 21:563-574, 1968.

91 Fagundes, L. A., de Oliveira, R. M., and Amaral, R.: Childhood lymphosarcoma in the state of Rio Grande do Sul, Brazil, Cancer 22:1283-1291, 1968.

92 Fröland, S., Natvig, J. B., and Bordal, P.: Surface-bound immunoglobulin as a marker of β lymphocytes in man, Nature (New Biol.) 234:251, 1971.

92a Goffinet, D. R., Castellino, R. A., Kim, H.,

Dorfman, R. F., Fuks, Z., Rosenberg, S. A., Nelson, T., and Kaplan, H. S.: Staging laparotomies in unselected previously untreated patients with non-Hodgkin's lymphomas, Cancer 32:672-681, 1973.

93 Han, T., and Stutzman, L.: Mode of spread in patients with localized malignant lymphoma, Arch. Intern. Med. 120:1-7, 1967.

94 Jones, S. E., Fuks, Z., Bull, M., Kadin, M. E., Dorfman, R. F., Kaplan, H. S., Rosenberg, S. A., and Kim, H.: Non-Hodgkin's lymphomas. IV. Clinicopathologic correlation in 405 cases, Cancer 31:806-823, 1973.

95 Lee, B. J., Nelson, J. H., and Schwarz, G.: Evaluation of lymphangiography, inferior venacavography and intravenous pyelography in the clinical staging and management of Hodgkin's disease and lymphosarcoma, N. Engl. J. Med. 271:327-337, 1964.

95a Levine, G. D., and Dorfman, R. F.: Nodular lymphoma: an ultrastructural study of its relationship to germinal centers and a correlation of light and electron microscopic findings, Cancer (in press).

96 Liao, K. T.: The superiority of histologic sections of aspirated bone marrow in malignant lymphomas; a review of 1,124 examinations, Cancer 27:618-628, 1971.

97 Lipton, A., and Lee, B. J.: Prognosis of Stage I lymphosarcoma and reticulum-cell sarcoma, N. Engl. J. Med. 284:230-233, 1971.

98 Lumb, G., and Newton, K. A.: Prognosis in tumors of lymphoid tissue; an analysis of 602 cases, Cancer 10:976-993, 1957.

99 Lukes, R. J., Butler, J. J., and Hicks, E. B.: Natural history of Hodgkin's disease as related to its pathologic picture, Cancer 19:317-344, 1966.

100 O'Conor, G. T., Rappaport, H., and Smith, E. B.: Childhood lymphoma resembling Burkitt's tumor in the United States, Cancer 18:411-417, 1965.

101 Oels, H. C., Harrison, E. G., Jr., and Kiely, J. M.: Lymphoblastic lymphoma with histiocytic phagocytosis ("starry sky" appearance) in adults; guide to prognosis, Cancer 21:368-375, 1968.

102 Millett, Y. L., Bennett, M. H., Jelliffe, A. M., and Farrer-Brown, G.: Nodular sclerotic lymphosarcoma; a further review, Br. J. Cancer 23:683-692, 1969.

102a Papamichail, M., Holborow, E. J., Keith, H. I., and Currey, H. L. F.: Subpopulations of human peripheral blood lymphocytes distinguished by combined rosette formation and membrane immunofluorescence, Lancet 2:64-66, 1972.

103 Rappaport, H.: Tumors of the hematopoietic system. In Atlas of tumor pathology, Sect. III, Fasc. 8, Washington, D. C., 1966, Armed Forces Institute of Pathology, pp. 91-206.

104 Rappaport, H., Winter, W. J., and Hicks, E. B.: Follicular lymphoma; a re-evaluation of its position in the scheme of malignant lymphoma, based on a survey of 253 cases, Cancer 9:792-821, 1956.

105 Rosas-Uribe, A., and Rappaport, H.: Malignant lymphoma, histiocytic type with sclerosis (sclerosing reticulum cell sarcoma), Cancer 29:946-953, 1972.

106 Rosenberg, S. A., and Kaplan, H. S.: Evidence for an orderly progression in the spread of Hodgkin's disease, Cancer Res. 26(Part I): 1225-1231, 1966.

107 Rosenberg, S. A., Diamond, H. D., and Craver, L. F.: Lymphosarcoma; survival and the effects of therapy, Am. J. Roentgenol. Radium Ther. Nucl. Med. 85:521-532, 1961.

107a Sternberg, C.: III. Leukosarkomatose und Myeloblastenleukämie, Z. Pathol. Anat. Pathol. 61:75-100, 1916.

107b Smith, J. L., Barker, C. R., Clein, G. P., and Collins, R. D.: Characterisation of malignant mediastinal lymphoid neoplasm (Sternberg sarcoma) as thymic in origin, Lancet 1:74-77, 1973.

108 Takahashi, M., and Abrams, H. L.: The accuracy of lymphangiographic diagnosis in malignant lymphoma, Radiology 89:448-460, 1967.

109 Wallace, S., and Jackson, L.: Diagnostic criteria for lymphangiographic interpretation of malignant neoplasia, Cancer Chemother. Rep. 52:125-145, 1968.

110 Wilson, J. D., and Nossal, G. J. V.: Identification of human T and B lymphocytes in normal peripheral blood and in chronic lymphocytic leukemia, Lancet 2:788-791, 1971.

111 World Health Organization: Histopathological definition of Burkitt's tumour, Bull. WHO 40:601-607, 1969.

112 Wright, D. H.: The epidemiology of Burkitt's tumor, Cancer Res. 27:2424-2438, 1967.

113 Wright, D. H.: Burkitt's lymphoma: a review of the pathology, immunology and possible etiologic factors, Path. Annu. 6:337-363, 1971.

114 Zacharski, L. R., and Linman, J. W.: Chronic lymphocytic leukemia versus chronic lymphosarcoma cell leukemia; analysis of 496 cases, Am. J. Med. 47:75-81, 1969.

Hodgkin's disease

115 Aisenberg, A. C.: Malignant lymphoma, N. Engl. J. Med. 288:883-890, 935-941, 1973.

116 Cross, R. M.: A clinicopathological study of nodular sclerosing Hodgkin's disease, J. Clin. Pathol. 21:303-310, 1968.

117 Fechner, R. E.: Hodgkin's disease of the thymus, Cancer 23:16-23, 1969.

118 Fisher, E. R., and Hazard, J. B.: Differen-

tiation of megakaryocyte and Reed-Sternberg cell, Lab. Invest. **3**:261-269, 1954.

119 Glatstein, E., Guernsey, J. M., Rosenberg, S. A., and Kaplan, H. S.: The value of laparotomy and splenectomy in the staging of Hodgkin's disease, Cancer **24**:470-718, 1969.

120 Glatstein, E., Trueblood, H. W., Enright, L. P., Rosenberg, S. A., and Kaplan, H. S.: Surgical staging of abdominal involvement in unselected patients with Hodgkin's disease, Radiology **97**:425-432, 1970.

121 Goldman, L. B., and Victor, A. W.: Hodgkin's disease, New York J. Med. **45**:1313-1318, 1945.

122 Kadin, M. E., Donaldson, S. S., and Dorfman, R. F.: Isolated granulomas in Hodgkin's disease, N. Engl. J. Med. **283**:859-861, 1970.

123 Kadin, M. E., Glatstein, E., and Dorfman, R. F.: Clinicopathologic studies of 117 untreated patients subjected to laparotomy for the staging of Hodgkin's disease, Cancer **27**:1277-1294, 1971.

124 Kaplan, H. S.: Contiguity and progression in Hodgkin's disease, Cancer Res. **31**:1811-1813, 1971.

125 Katz, A., and Lattes, R.: Granulomatous thymoma or Hodgkin's disease of thymus? A clinical and histologic study and a re-evaluation, Cancer **23**:1-15, 1969.

126 Keller, A. R., Kaplan, H. S., Lukes, R. J., and Rappaport, H.: Correlation of histopathology with other prognostic indicators in Hodgkin's disease, Cancer **22**:487-499, 1968.

127 Lennert, K., and Mestdagh, J.: Lymphogranulomatosen mit konstant hohem Epitheloidzellgehalt, Virchows Arch. [Pathol. Anat.]**344**:1-20, 1968.

128 Lukes, R. J., Butler, J. J., and Hicks, E. B.: Natural history of Hodgkin's disease as related to its pathologic picture, Cancer **19**:317-344, 1966.

129 Neiman, R. S., Rosen, P. J., and Lukes, R. J.: Lymphocyte-depletion Hodgkin's disease; a clinicopathologic entity, N. Engl. J. Med. **288**:751-755, 1973.

130 Rappaport, H., Strum, S. B., Hutchison, G., and Allen, L. W.: Clinical and biological significance of vascular invasion in Hodgkin's disease, Cancer Res. **31**:1794-1798, 1971.

131 Rosenberg, S. A.: Hodgkin's disease of the bone marrow, Cancer Res. **31**:1733-1736, 1971.

132 Strum, S. B., and Rappaport, H.: Significance of focal involvement of lymph nodes for the diagnosis and staging of Hodgkin's disease, Cancer **25**:1314-1319, 1970.

133 Strum, S. B., and Rappaport, H.: Interrelations of the histologic types of Hodgkin's disease, Arch. Pathol. **91**:127-134, 1971.

134 Strum, S. B., and Rappaport, H.: The persistence of Hodgkin's disease in long-term survivors, Am. J. Med. **51**:222-240, 1971.

135 Strum, S. B., Hutchison, G. B., Park, J. K., and Rappaport, H.: Further observations on the biologic significance of vascular invasion in Hodgkin's disease, Cancer **27**:1-6, 1971.

136 Strum, S., Park, J. K., and Rappaport, H.: Observation of cells resembling Sternberg-Reed cells in conditions other than Hodgkin's disease, Cancer **26**:176-190, 1970.

137 Tindle, B. H., Parker, J. W., and Lukes, R. J.: "Reed-Sternberg cells" in infectious mononucleosis? Am. J. Clin. Pathol. **58**:607-617, 1972.

138 Variakojis, D., Strum, S. B., and Rappaport, H.: The foamy macrophages in Hodgkin's disease, Arch. Pathol. **93**:453-456, 1971.

Lymphoma and dysproteinemia

139 Aisenberg, A. C., and Bloch, K. J.: Immunoglobulins on the surface of neoplastic lymphocytes, N. Engl. J. Med. **287**:271-276, 1972.

140 Axelsson, V., Bachmann, R., and Hallen, J.: Frequency of pathological proteins (M-components) in 6995 sera from an adult population, Acta Med. Scand. **179**:234-247, 1966.

141 Azar, H. A., Hill, W. T., and Osserman, E. F.: Malignant lymphoma and lymphatic leukemia associated with myeloma-type serum proteins, Am. J. Med. **23**:239-249, 1957.

142 Azar, H. A., Zaino, E. C., Pham, T. D., and Yannopoulos, K.: "Non-secretory" plasma cell myeloma; observations on seven cases with electron microscopic studies, Am. J. Clin. Pathol. **58**:618-629, 1972.

143 Ballard, H. S., Hamilton, L. M., Marcus, A. J., and Illes, C. H.: A new variant of heavy-chain disease (μ-chain disease), N. Engl. J. Med. **282**:1060-1062, 1970.

144 Cohen, R. J., Bohannon, R. A., and Wallterstein, R. O.: Waldenstrom's macroglobulinemia; a study of ten cases, Am. J. Med. **41**:274, 1966.

145 Dutcher, T. F., and Fahey, J. L.: The histopathology of the macroglobulinemia of Waldenstrom, J. Natl. Cancer Inst. **22**:887-917, 1959.

146 Fisher, E. R., and Zawadski, Z. A.: Ultrastructural features of plasma cells in patients with paraproteinemias, Am. J. Clin. Pathol. **54**:779-789, 1970.

147 Franklin, E. C., Lowenstein, J., Bigelow, B., et al.: Heavy chain disease—a new disorder of serum gamma-globulins: report of the first case, Am. J. Med. **37**:332-350, 1964.

147a Harrison, C. V.: The morphology of the lymph node in the macroglobulinaemia of Waldenstrom, J. Clin. Pathol. **25**:12-16, 1972.

148 Hobbs, J. R.: Immunocytoma o' mice an' men, Br. Med. J. **2**:67-72, 1971.

149 Kim, H., Heller, P., and Rappaport, H.: Monoclonal gammopathies associated with lymphoproliferative disorders; a morphologic study, Am. J. Clin. Pathol. **59**:282-294, 1973.

150 Krauss, S., and Sokal, J. E.: Paraproteinemia in the lymphomas, Am. J. Med. **40**:400-413, 1966.

151 Kyle, R. A., and Bayrd, E. D.: Benign monoclonal gammopathy—a potentially malignant condition? Am. J. Med. **40**:426-430, 1966.

152 Migliore, P. J., and Alexanian, R.: Monoclonal gammopathy in human neoplasia, Cancer **21**:1127-1131, 1968.

153 Seligmann, M., Danon, F., Hurez, D., Mihaesco, E., and Preud'homme, J.-L.: Alpha-chain disease: a new immunoglobulin abnormality, Science **162**:1396-1397, 1968.

154 Stein, H., Lennert, K., and Parwaresch, M. R.: Malignant lymphomas of B-cell type, Lancet **2**:855-857, 1972.

155 Zawadski, Z. A., and Edwards, G. A.: Dysimmunoglobulinemia in the absence of clinical features of multiple myeloma and macroglobulinemia, Am. J. Med. **42**:67-88, 1967.

Malignant histiocytosis

156 Friedman, R. M., and Stiegbigel, N. H.: Histiocytic medullary reticulosis, Am. J. Med. **28**:130-133, 1965.

157 Liao, K. T., Rosai, J., and Daneshbod, K.: Malignant histiocytosis with cutaneous involvement and eosinophilia, Am. J. Clin. Pathol. **57**:438-448, 1972.

158 Rappaport, H.: Tumors of the hematopoietic system. In Atlas of tumor pathology, Sect. III, Fasc. 8, Washington, D. C., 1966, Armed Forces Institute of Pathology, pp. 91-206.

Metastatic tumors

159 Kinsey, D. L., James, A. G., and Bonta, J. A.: A study of metastatic carcinoma of the neck, Ann. Surg. **147**:366-374, 1958.

160 Lindbergh, R.: Distribution of cervical lymph node metastases from squamous cell carcinoma of the upper respiratory and digestive tracts, Cancer **29**:1446-1449, 1972.

161 Rosai, J., and Rodriquez, H. A.: Application of electron microscopy to the differential diagnosis of tumors, Am. J. Clin. Pathol. **50**: 555-562, 1968.

Other lesions

162 Brown, R. B., Gaillard, R. A., and Turner, J. A.: The significance of aberrant or heterotopic parotid gland tissue in lymph nodes, Ann. Surg. **138**:850-856, 1953.

163 Davies, J. N. P., and Lothe, F.: Kaposi's sarcoma in African children. In Ackerman, L. V., and Murray, J. F., editors: Symposium on Kaposi's sarcoma, Basel, Switzerland, 1963, S. Karger, AG, pp. 81-86.

163a Edlow, D. W., and Carter, D.: Heterotopic epithelium in axillary lymph nodes, Am. J. Clin. Pathol. **59**:666-673, 1973.

164 Johnson, W. T., and Helwig, E. B.: Benign nevus cells in the capsule of lymph nodes, Cancer **23**:747-753, 1969.

165 Karp, L. A., and Dcernobilsky, B.: Glandular inclusions in pelvic and abdominal para-aortic lymph nodes, Am. J. Clin. Pathol. **52**: 212-218, 1969.

166 Klemperer, P., Boris, G., Lee, S. L., Leuchtenberger, C., and Pollister, A. W.: Cytochemical changes of acute lupus erythematosus, Arch. Pathol. **49**:503-516, 1950.

167 Lasersohn, J. T., Thomas, L. B., Smith, R. R., Ketcham, A. S., and Dillon, J. S.: Carcinoma of the uterine cervix; a study of surgical pathological and autopsy findings, Cancer **17**: 338-351, 1964.

168 Meyer, J. S., and Steinberg, L. S.: Microscopically benign thyroid follicles in cervical lymph nodes; serial section study of lymph node inclusions and entire thyroid gland in 5 cases, Cancer **24**:302-311, 1969.

169 Moore, R. D., Weisberger, A. S., and Bowerfind, E. S., Jr.: An evaluation of lymphadenopathy in systemic disease, Arch. Intern. Med. **99**:751-759, 1957.

170 Rywlin, A. M., Recher, L., and Hoffman, E.: Lymphoma-like presentation of Kaposi's sarcoma, Arch. Dermatol. **93**:554-561, 1966.

21 Spleen

Introduction

The functions of the spleen and their relation to morphology are poorly understood. The surgical pathologist often is frustrated by the lack of pathologic alterations of diagnostic value. The spleen is removed from patients with diverse clinical syndromes. If the pathologist does not know the clinical and laboratory data, particularly the hematologic findings, he may be unable to make a specific diagnosis.

Tabulation of positive pathologic changes from numerous articles and textbooks aids very little. We have tried unsuccessfully to chart the significant pathologic changes seen in each clinical syndrome. Only the changes that appear to be most significant are mentioned. Even these frequently are not diagnostic.

Biopsy and pathologic examination

In the United States, biopsy of the spleen is not done as a rule because of the technical difficulty at operation and the fear of hemorrhage after needle biopsy. When a large liver and spleen are encountered, the liver is usually biopsied, but the spleen is sacrosanct because of the danger of hemorrhage. However, biopsying both organs can produce a diagnosis that may not be made by liver biopsy alone. Cer-

tainly, splenic puncture should not be performed upon patients with bleeding tendency. However, the risk of this diagnostic procedure has been grossly exaggerated. For instance, Moeschlin[5] punctured the spleen in 300 patients and Soderström[6] in over 800 without mortality and essentially without morbidity.

The method of Block and Jacobson[1] (splenic puncture using the Vim-Silverman needle) would seem the most effective. Tissue so obtained may be fixed, cut, and stained as a conventional section. Block and Jacobson[1] and Ferris and Hargraves[3] reported a large number of splenic punctures resulting in a definitive diagnosis which was not possible by bone marrow biopsy, lymph node biopsy, or clinical data.

Surgically excised spleens obtained for diagnostic purposes should be cut in the fresh state into 2 cm to 3 cm slices, fixed overnight in formalin, and then sliced as thinly as possible (2 mm to 3 mm). We have used for this purpose an electrically driven meat-cutting machine with excellent results. The cut slices are then carefully examined, and all suspicious areas are submitted for microscopic examination. Ferrer-Brown et al.[2] mentioned three cases of Hodgkin's disease in which the areas of involvement appeared grossly as foci of slight prominence of the malpighian corpuscles. A careful search also should be made for hilar lymph nodes.

For the evaluation of the red pulp in states associated with hypersplenism, we have found it very helpful to inject the specimen with formalin through the splenic artery. A sharp distinction between sinuses and cords is thus obtained.[4] A lesser sub-

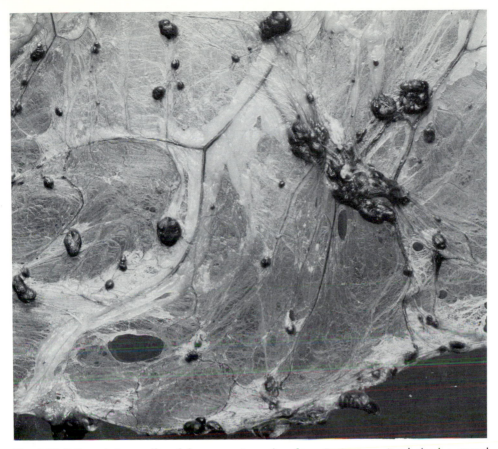

Fig. 968 Splenosis in small nodules on peritoneal surface. Patient previously had ruptured spleen. (WU neg. 55-3599.)

stitute for those unwilling to perform this time-consuming procedure is the examination of special stains that delineate the sinusal wall, such as periodic acid–Schiff or silver impregnation.

Rupture; splenectomy

Blunt trauma to the abdomen and surgical intervention within the abdominal cavity are the two most common factors responsible for rupture of the normal spleen.[14] In most instances, hemoperitoneum is an immediate consequence, leading to an emergency splenectomy. In about 15% of the cases, the rupture is "delayed" anywhere from forty-eight hours to several months.[10] Examination of the excised spleen will reveal the ruptured area which, in many cases, is limited to a deceivingly small capsular tear. Microscopically, leu-

kocytic infiltration is often seen along the edges of the tear.

Following traumatic rupture, splenic tissue in small nodules may grow as implants on the peritoneal surface, and even within the pleural cavity[8] (Fig. 968). The process is known as *splenosis*. These nodules are surrounded by a capsule, but malpighian follicles with a central arteriole do not form.[7]

The diseases most commonly associated with *spontaneous rupture* of the spleen are infectious mononucleosis, malaria, pregnancy, typhoid fever, subacute bacterial endocarditis, splenic tumors, and leukemias.[16] In every case of ruptured spleen without history of trauma or in which the trauma seems insignificant, a careful microscopic study should be performed in order to rule out all these possibilities. Rupture of the spleen with the resulting hemoperitoneum is the most frequent cause of death in infectious mononucleosis. This complication usually occurs from ten to twenty-one days after the onset of the disease.[15] Exceptionally, "spontaneous" rupture may occur in a perfectly normal spleen.[12]

Splenectomy performed in adults for traumatic rupture of the spleen does not seem to result in any sequelae of significance.[13] On the other hand, an increased incidence and severity of infections has been reported following splenectomy in young children.[11] Ellis and Smith[9] have shown that this is the result of a decrease in immunoglobulin production and phagocytic activity during transient bacteremia.

Hypersplenism (dyssplenism)

The splenic red pulp acts primarily as a biologic filter for the removal of abnormal or aged blood cells and their pathologic inclusions. This mechanism operates during the transit of the cells through the splenic cords from the *penicilli* arteries to the splenic sinuses and results from a combination of mechanical, rheologic, metabolic, and immunologic factors.[46] When this normal function increases to a significant degree, the resulting condition is designated as *hypersplenism* or *dyssplenism.*[22] Any of the cellular elements of the blood may be affected, singly or in combination. Thus, neutropenia, thrombocytopenia, hemolytic anemia, or pancytopenia may all be present. In some conditions, such as spherocytic hemolytic anemia or idiopathic thrombocytopenic purpura, the basic abnormality resides in the blood elements themselves. In others, the hypersplenism results from widening of the splenic cords with an increase in macrophages and/or connective tissue fibers and premature destruction of the normal elements of the blood. The latter phenomenon has been reproduced experimentally by the intraperitoneal injection of methyl cellulose.[34] Hypersplenism resulting from this mechanism can be seen with splenomegaly, Gaucher's disease (Fig.

969), malignant lymphoma, leukemia, differentiated histiocytosis, hemangioma, hamartoma, angiosarcoma, and practically any condition involving more or less diffusely the splenic parenchyma.[35]

Harrington et al.[27] demonstrated that if small amounts of blood from a patient with *idiopathic thrombocytopenic purpura* are given to a normal person, a humoral factor will cause a precipitous fall in platelets, thus establishing an immunologic basis for the disease. Subsequent studies showed that this antiplatelet factor has the physico-chemical characteristics of an immunoglobulin.[42, 43] Karpatkin and Siskind[29] demonstrated antiplatelet activity in the serum of 73% of patients with idiopathic thrombocytopenic purpura. The antibody-coated platelets have a short life span because they are rapidly removed by the reticuloendothelial system of the spleen and liver.[25, 26] There is some evidence that the number of antibody molecules bound to the platelets may determine the main site of removal. Heavily coated platelets are removed by the liver phagocytes, whereas lightly coated platelets pass through the liver but are sequestered in the spleen.[42]

The changes found in the spleen in idiopathic thrombocytopenic purpura have been summarized well by Bowman et al.[19] The spleen is slightly to moderately enlarged with moderately dilated sinusoids and a prominent increase in the number of germinal centers. The latter change, as well as the increased immunoglobulin production by the spleen in this condition,[32] is evidence of an immunologic humoral response. The normal marginal zone of large lymphocytes around many follicles persists, and there is a nonspecific moderate increase in megakaryocytes. The red pulp contains a "normal" number of eosinophilic and neutrophilic leukocytes.

Phospholipid deposits in the histiocytes of the splenic pulp were observed by Saltzstein[40] in seven spleens removed for thrombocytopenic purpura (Fig. 970). This microscopic finding was not seen in over 700 other spleens removed for other rea-

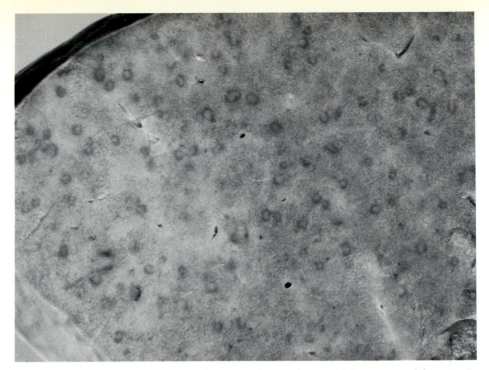

Fig. 969 Huge spleen in Gaucher's disease. White pulp is widely separated by massive red pulp replaced by cells of Gaucher's disease. (WU neg. 72-6653.)

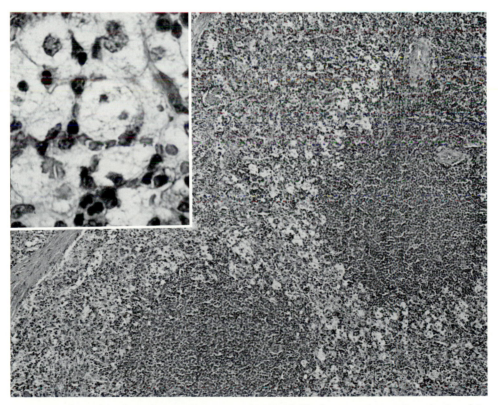

Fig. 970 Idiopathic thrombocytopenic purpura. Lipid-filled macrophages in splenic white pulp immediately around malpighian corpuscles. **Inset,** high power, demonstrates foamy nature of cytoplasm. Patient had no platelets before splenectomy. (×85; WU neg. 60-4376; **inset,** WU neg. 60-4379.)

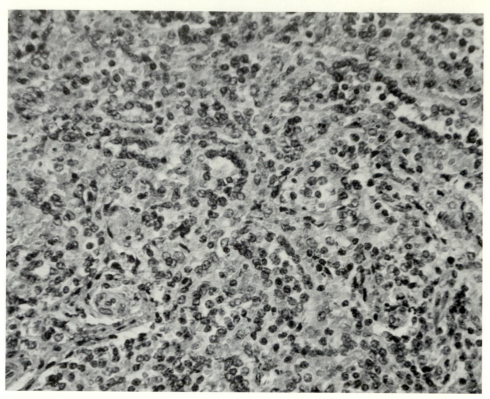

Fig. 971 Spleen of 4-year-old girl with hereditary spherocytosis. Splenic cords are congested, but sinusoids as seen on light microscopy are practically empty. (×350; WU neg. 67-1570.)

sons, although foamy cells with a similar appearance in routinely stained sections can be found in Gaucher's disease, Niemann-Pick disease, thalassemia,[24] hyperlipemic states,[39] the sea-blue histiocyte syndrome,[44] and follicular lipoidosis. Biochemical studies in the latter condition have demonstrated the presence of saturated hydrocarbons, thus implying ingestion of exogenous mineral oil.[30] Histochemical techniques usually allow for a distinction among these different conditions.[37]

Splenectomy in idiopathic thrombocytopenic purpura is reserved for the patients unresponsive to steroid or immunosuppressive therapy. It achieves sustained remission in 50% to 80% of the cases. Unfortunately, at present there is no method that can accurately predict the effect of splenectomy.[18] Occasionally, thrombocytopenic purpura is seen as a manifestation of lupus erythematosus, viral infection, drug hypersensitivity,[18] chronic lymphocytic leukemia,[23] or Hodgkin's disease.[38]

Hereditary spherocytosis is a hemolytic disease in which the red blood cells are abnormal (spherocytes). The abnormality lies in the cell membrane of the red blood cell, but the basic biochemical disorder has not yet been elucidated.[28] The erythrocytes lack the plasticity of normal red blood cells and become trapped in the interstices of the spleen.[45] If washed normal red blood cells are given to a patient with congenital hemolytic anemia, the cells survive normally. Conversely, if spherocytes are given to a normal individual, the survival of the cells remains short, supporting the concept that the erythrocyte is defective. Furthermore, this defect persists after removal of the spleen, but hemolysis is decreased.

About one-half of the cases of *acquired (autoimmune) hemolytic anemia* are unassociated with other significant pathologic abnormalities. We have seen acquired hemolytic anemia in various forms of leukemia, Hodgkin's disease, sarcoidosis, lupus erythematosus, tuberculosis, and brucellosis. The Coombs test is used to distinguish between the acquired and congenital types of hemolytic anemia. The patient's washed red cells are mixed with antihuman globulin rabbit serum. If the test is positive, agglutination occurs. Young et al.[48] called this type of anemia chronic hemolytic disease with erythrocyte-bound antibody.

The pathologic changes in the congenital and acquired types are somewhat different. In both, the spleen is enlarged (100 gm to 1000 gm), fairly firm and deep red, has a thin capsule, and has no grossly discernible malpighian follicles. In hereditary spherocytosis, the splenic cords are congested whereas the sinusoids are relatively empty[47] (Fig. 971). The lining cells of the sinuses are prominent, sometimes resulting in an adenoid appearance. Hemosiderin deposition and erythrophagocytosis are present in both conditions but are usually more pronounced in the acquired variety. Ultrastructural studies have shown that the splenic cords are not empty but rather contain red blood cells that have lost their electron density, thus corresponding to the red cell ghosts of light microscopy.[33]

In acquired hemolytic anemia, the congestion may predominate in the cords or sinuses or be equally prominent in both. Rappaport and Crosby[36] found a high correlation between spherocytosis and increased osmotic fragility on one hand and the degree of cord congestion on the other. Foci of extramedullary hematopoiesis may be present. Splenic infarcts are found in 24% of the cases.[36]

Hereditary spherocytosis is the hematologic disease that most benefits from splenectomy. The clinical cure rate is practically 100%, although the intrinsic red cell abnormality persists.[21] In acquired hemolytic anemia, splenectomy is usually reserved for cases which cannot be controlled by steroid or immunosuppressive

Table 44 Splenectomies performed at Barnes Hospital, 1947-1961*

Condition	Number of patients	Sustained remission†
Idiopathic thrombocytopenic purpura	111	60
Acquired (autoimmune) hemolytic anemia	24	16
Hereditary spherocytosis	38	36
Chronic lymphocytic leukemia	29	16
Malignant lymphoma	19	6
Aplastic anemia (hypoplastic anemia)	13	4
Agnogenic myeloid metaplasia	7	0
Hypersplenism	41	20
Disseminated lupus erythematosus	4	2
Total	286	158

*Statistics from James T. Adams, M.D., Barnes Hospital, St. Louis, Mo.
†Over two years.

therapy.[31] A sustained remission rate is obtained in about 50% of the cases and an objective improvement in an additional 25%. Studies of splenic sequestration using Cr^{51}-tagged red cells give a rough estimation of the benefit to be expected from splenectomy.[17]

The conditions for which splenectomy is done and the results obtained in our institution are indicated in Table 44.[20, 21, 41]

Agnogenic myeloid metaplasia (myelofibrosis)

In myeloid metaplasia, a rare, poorly understood condition, there is a great variation in the degree of myelofibrosis and myelosclerosis of the bone marrow.[49] The extramedullary hematopoiesis present in the spleen, liver, lymph nodes, and other organs was considered by some to be a compensatory mechanism and an expression of a systemic myeloproliferative disorder by others. At the present time, the latter view is almost universally accepted.[57] The spleens are extremely large (430 gm to 4,100 gm, averaging 2,013 gm).[55]

Microscopically, there are congestion, small and diluted follicles, and hemosiderosis. Most important, all bone marrow elements are present. Large numbers of

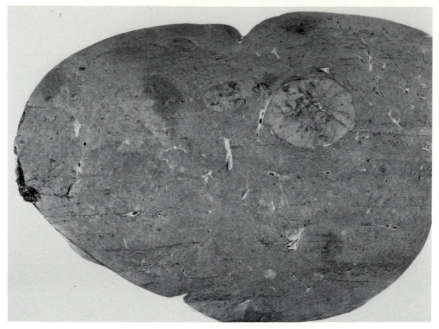

Fig. 972 Huge spleen (3,200 gm) from patient with extreme myelosclerosis and myelo-fibrosis, with subsequent anemia and failure to respond to all therapeutic measures. Nodule represents area of extreme extamedullary hematopoiesis. (WU neg. 52-3980.)

megakaryocytes and erythroid precursors are prominent (Figs. 972 and 973). The megakaryocytes often have atypical nuclear features and can simulate closely Stern-berg-Reed cells.[51] Biopsy of the liver shows extensive hematopoiesis among and within the sinusoids. Exceptionally large nodular masses of extramedullary hematopoiesis develop in the mediastinum and simulate a primary malignant tumor of this location.[53] This phenomenon also has been described in congenital spherocytosis and other types of anemia.[50, 56]

The relation of agnogenic myeloid metaplasia to chronic granulocytic leukemia is still debated. Some believe there is no relation, whereas others maintain that it is merely a leukemia with secondary fibrotic changes.[52]

Factors that serve to distinguish myelofibrosis from chronic myelocytic leukemia include a lower total white cell count, normal numbers of eosinophils and basophils, nucleated red cells in the peripheral blood, organ infiltrates consisting of several cell lines, greater marrow fibrosis

with less cellular immaturity, higher values of leukocyte alkaline phosphatase, and difficulty in performing a successful marrow aspiration. Usually, the evaluation of all such factors will enable one successfully to classify a given case as either myelofibrosis or leukemia, but transitional or intermediate cases are frequent.[55]

A test of greater significance in the differential diagnosis between these two conditions is chromosome analysis. It has been shown that approximately 90% of patients with chronic myelocytic leukemia have an abnormality in the twenty-second chromosome, known as the Philadelphia chromosome and characterized by a deletion of part of its longer arm.[49a] This abnormality, which apparently is acquired, is also present in cells of the erythroid series and megakaryocytes of patients with this disease, suggesting a common stem origin for these cell lines. On the other hand, it is practically never found in agnogenic myeloid metaplasia or in other myeloproliferative diseases.[54]

Splenectomy is sometimes carried out for

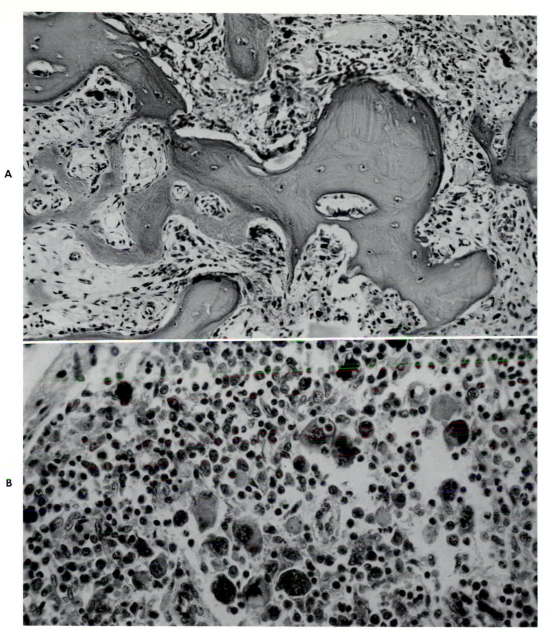

Fig. 973 A, Extreme myelofibrosis and myelosclerosis. Note fibrosis and thickened bone trabeculae. **B,** Extensive extramedullary hematopoiesis found at postmortem examination of patient referred to in **A.** It involved practically every organ in body, including such tissues as epididymis, retroperitoneal soft tissues, and adrenal gland. This section shows large clusters of atypical megakaryocytes within lymph node. (**A,** ×200; WU neg. 52-4493; **B,** ×400; WU neg. 52-4492.)

agnogenic myeloid metaplasia, especially when hemolytic phenomena or thrombocytopenia is severe. The results are not spectacular, but in some cases a moderate improvement has been noted.

Congestive and idiopathic splenomegaly

In *congestive splenomegaly,* there are enlargement of the spleen, signs of hypersplenism (anemia, leukopenia and/or thrombocytopenia), and often alarming gastric hemorrhages secondary to a collateral circulation that develops between the portal and peripheral venous systems. This condition develops in the presence of increased pressure in the portal circulation as reflected through the splenic vein. The etiology can be extrahepatic or intrahepatic. If intrahepatic, it is usually some form of cirrhosis. In the extrahepatic type, there may be stenosis, thrombosis, sclerosis, or cavernous transformation of the portal vein or a major tributary. The thrombosis may be the result of inflammation, trauma, or extrinsic pressure by inflammatory or neoplastic tissue.[67] Stenotic or sclerotic changes may be the result of extension into the main portal vein of the physiologic obliterative process that takes place at birth in the umbilical vein and the ductus venosum as they empty into the left portal vein.

The portal circulation, which has no valves, carries about three-fourths of the circulation of the liver. The hepatic artery carrying oxygen supplies the other one-fourth. Both vessels have a common exit channel, the hepatic veins, which empty into the inferior vena cava. According to Herrick,[61] in a normal liver the portal pressure rises 1 mm for every 40 mm of arterial pressure, whereas in the cirrhotic liver, it rises 1 mm for every 6 mm of arterial pressure. McIndoe[62] could not confirm these findings. He demonstrated the important fact that in advanced cirrhosis, if fluid was perfused through the portal circulation, all but 13% escaped through the collateral circulation. Because of this, the hepatic artery carries an increased blood flow, and when the arterial pressure falls, hepatic insufficiency occurs. The prominent increase of portal pressure leads to long-continued congestion of the spleen. The spleen enlarges, anemia develops, and collateral circulation becomes prominent. With still further time, the spleen becomes firmer and darker. Microscopically, there is marked dilatation of veins and sinuses, fibrosis of the red pulp, and accumulation of hemosiderin-containing macrophages. Lymphoid follicles are inconspicuous. Iron incrusta-

tion of the connective tissue and sclerosiderotic nodules ("Gamna-Gandy bodies") develop as a result of focal hemorrhages.

Splenectomy without shunt is successful when the coronary vein joins the portal system central to the point of obstruction. Otherwise, shunt is indicated.[64] Various types have been done, including anastomosis of the splenic vein to the renal vein and anastomosis of the portal vein to the vena cava.[59] The results from these operations have been encouraging as a means of controlling repetitive hemorrhage from esophageal varices. However, such procedures do not seem to prolong life.[66]

When a similar set of functional and pathologic changes occur in the absence of an anatomic explanation for increased portal pressure, the condition is designated as *idiopathic splenomegaly*.[60] Bagshawe[58] compared the relative features of hypersplenism among forty-six patients with congestive splenomegaly and twenty-nine with reactive splenomegaly and found no significant differences among them. Massive splenomegaly is commonly seen in several tropical countries, such as Zaire, Malagasy Republic, Nigeria, and New Guinea.[63] Spleens removed for this "tropical splenomegaly syndrome" are often extremely heavy (mean, 3,270 gm) and exhibit a uniform dark red cut surface. Microscopically, there are marked dilatation of sinuses and foci of extramedullary hematopoiesis but no significant fibrosis or hemosiderin deposition.[63] Signs of hypersplenism are the rule. Epidemiologic and therapeutic studies suggest a causal relationship with malaria.[63, 65] In this regard, it is interesting that the cases of idiopathic splenomegaly reported by Banti in 1883 were from an area which at the time was endemic for malaria.

Cysts

Approximately 75% of the nonparasitic *cysts* of the spleen are of the *false (secondary) type*.[69] Their wall is composed of dense fibrous tissue, often calcified, with no epithelial lining. The content is a mix-

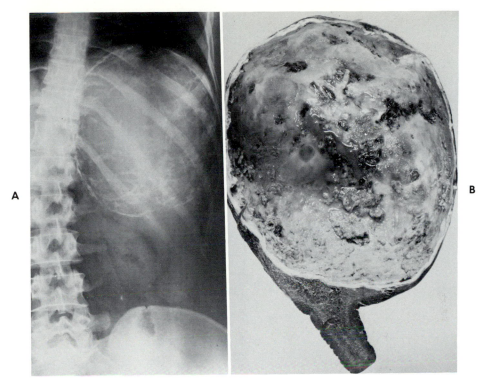

Fig. 974 A, Large cyst of spleen. **B,** Gross specimen of lesion illustrated in **A** showing calcified cyst partially lined by stratified squamous epithelium. (**A,** WU neg. 50-3794; **B,** WU neg. 50-3542.)

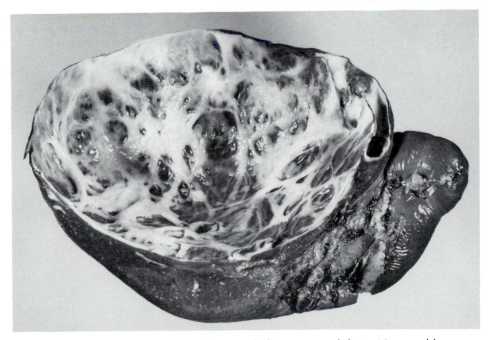

Fig. 975 Splenic cyst lined by squamous epithelium removed from 19-year-old woman. Note prominent trabeculation. (WU neg. 70-3125.)

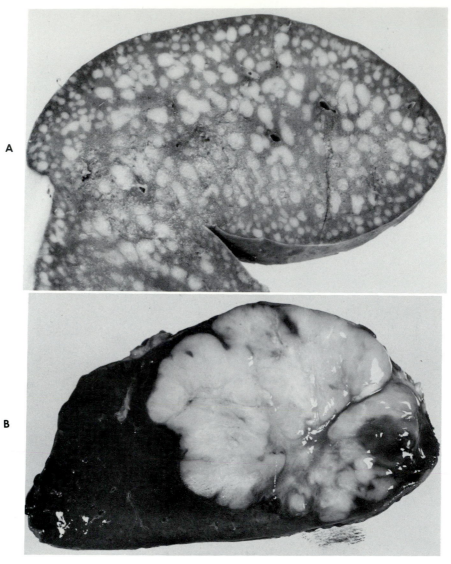

Fig. 976 Two distinct types of splenic gross involvement by malignant lymphoma. **A,** "Miliary" type of involvement. Any type of lymphoma can produce this pattern. Patient was 63-year-old woman in whom only findings were splenomegaly and neutropenia. Microscopically, it was nodular lymphocytic lymphoma. Two years after splenectomy, disseminated disease developed. **B,** Malignant lymphoma producing solitary mass. This pattern is seen only in Hodgkin's disease and histiocytic lymphoma. In this case, it was the latter. Patient, 66-year-old woman, later developed disseminated disease. (**A,** WU neg. 64-5358; **B,** WU neg. 54-3654.)

ture of blood and necrotic debris. If the cyst ruptures, massive hemoperitoneum may result. The majority of these cysts are solitary and asymptomatic. Trauma is the most likely etiologic factor, although it is possible that some represent epithelial cysts in which part or all of the lining has been destroyed (Fig. 974). There have been more than 400 reported cases of *epithelial cysts* of the spleen.[70] Most cases have occurred in children and young adults. Grossly, a glistening inner surface with marked trabeculation is often seen (Fig. 975). Microscopically, the wall is

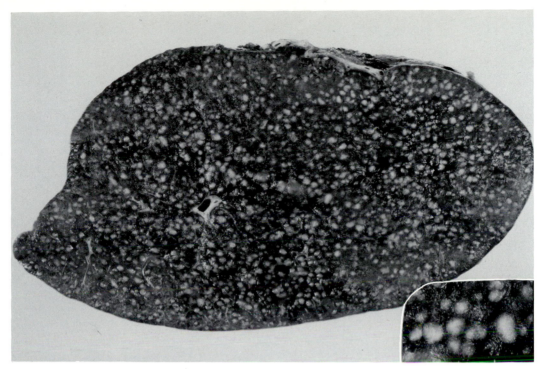

Fig. 977 Splenic involvement by Hodgkin's disease. Innumerable white nodules are scattered throughout parenchyma. (WU neg. 72-2001.)

lined by mature squamous epithelium, without skin adnexa.[68]

Tumors

Of the primary benign tumors, *hemangioma* is the most common.[78] It is often of the cavernous variety. Rupture is the commonest complication. Rappaport[79] described a *hamartoma (splenadenoma)* composed of red pulp only, resulting in marked sequestration of red cells. A case of intrasplenic *lipoma* was reported by Easler and Dowlin.[75]

Malignant lymphoma is by far the most common malignant tumor involving the spleen.[73, 74] Although usually affected as part of a generalized process, in some cases the spleen represents the only detectable site of disease. Spleen involvement by malignant lymphoma may present as an asymptomatic splenomegaly or result in a picture of hypersplenism.[80] Ahmann et al.[71] described four gross patterns of involvement: homogeneous, miliary, multiple masses, and solitary mass (Figs. 976 and 977). The first two were seen with all microscopic types of lymphoma. Conversely, the presence of masses, either solitary or diffuse, was encountered only in histiocytic lymphoma and Hodgkin's disease. Of their forty-eight cases, twenty-six (54%) had a nodular pattern of growth on microscopic examination. The prognosis was better for tumors composed of well-differentiated lymphocytes, for those growing in a nodular fashion, and for the Stage I (limited to the spleen) and Stage II (limited to the spleen and splenic lymph node) neoplasms. The overall five-year survival rate was 31%.

The microscopic diagnosis is obvious in most cases, but it may be extremely difficult with some well-differentiated lymphocytic lymphomas. The lymph nodes of the splenic hilum should be carefully dissected and examined microscopically, since they may show obvious lymphoma when the changes in the spleen are only equivocal. We have found the presence of nodular

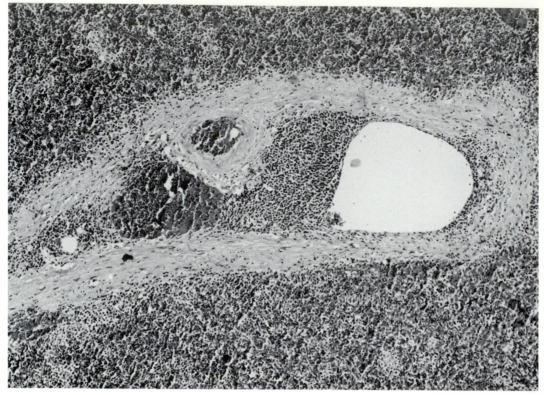

Fig. 978 Involvement of subendothelial space of large splenic vein in well-differentiated lymphocytic lymphoma. This is important diagnostic sign. (×90; WU neg. 73-7012.)

collections of lymphocytes beneath the endothelium of trabecular veins (presumably lodged in subendothelial lymphatic vessels) a helpful feature for the diagnosis of lymphocytic lymphoma or lymphocytic leukemia in the spleen[76] (Fig. 978). The only other condition in which we have seen it in a significant degree in an adult has been infectious mononucleosis. The features of Hodgkin's disease involving the spleen are discussed in Chapter 20. *Angiosarcoma* may present as a well-defined hemorrhagic nodule or involve the spleen diffusely. Metastases may be widespread. The clinical course is rapid and almost invariably fatal.[81]

Metastatic carcinoma of the spleen is uncommon, although widely disseminated neoplasms such as *melanoma* and *mammary carcinoma* may involve this organ.[72] Herbut and Gabriel[77] reported twenty-three patients with splenic metastases.

Other lesions

Congenital absence of the spleen *(asplenia)* is associated in more than 80% of the cases with malformations of the heart, nearly always involving the atrioventricular endocardial cushion and the ventricular outflow tracts.[85] Anomalies of the blood vessels, lung, and abdominal viscera also are frequent.[82] A hereditary form of splenic *hypoplasia* has recently been reported.[83]

Splenic-gonadal fusion occurs in two forms: "Continuous, in which the main spleen is connected by a cord of splenic and fibrous tissue to the gonadal mesonephric structures, and discontinuous, in which discrete masses of splenic tissue are found fused to these same structures."* Of the fifty-two cases reviewed by Watson,[87] only four were in females. Eleven

---

*From Putschar, W. G. J., and Manion, W. C.: Splenic-gonadal fusion, Cancer **32:**15-34, 1956.

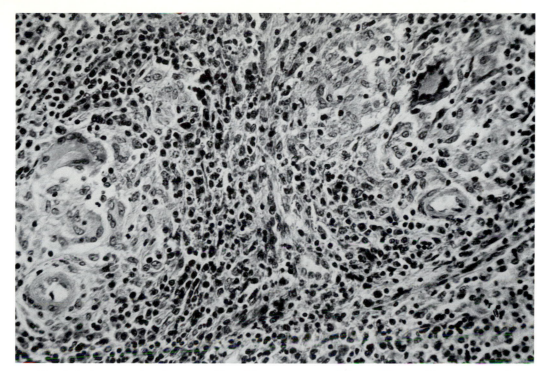

Fig. 979 Section of spleen weighing 750 gm removed from 31-year-old woman with fever and hepatosplenomegaly. These granulomatous lesions with giant cells were proved to be reaction to *Histoplasma capsulatum.* (×350; WU neg. 66-11901A.)

were associated with other congenital defects, such as peromelus and micrognathia. Various degrees of testicular ectopia and inguinal hernias are common. All of the reported cases have been on the left side.[86]

Thrombosis of the splenic vein of unknown etiology may cause *infarction.* If the artery is tied, usually infarction does not occur.

We have examined twenty enlarged spleens that contained *disseminated granulomas.*[84] In most instances, the etiology was not established, but in a few a definite diagnosis was made (Fig. 979). The splenic involvement was always the expression of generalized granulomatous disease. None of the patients developed malignant lymphomas. Discrete small foci of *calcification,* either solitary or scattered throughout the spleen, are usually the end results of focal granulomatous lesions. In the United States, they are particularly common in areas of endemic histoplasmosis.[88]

REFERENCES

Biopsy and pathologic examination

1 Block, M., and Jacobson, L. O.: Splenic puncture, J.A.M.A. **142:**641-647, 1950 (extensive bibliography).
2 Ferrer-Brown, G., Bennett, M. H., Harrison, C. V., Millett, Y., and Jelliffee, A. M.: The diagnosis of Hodgkin's disease in surgically excised spleens, J. Clin. Pathol. **37:**294-300, 1972.
3 Ferris, D. O., and Hargraves, M. M.: Splenic puncture, Arch. Surg. **67:**402-407, 1953.
4 Ham, A. W.: The structure of the spleen. In Blaustein, A., editor: The spleen, New York, 1963, McGraw-Hill Book Co.
5 Moeschlin, S.: Spleen puncture (translated from German by A. Piney), London, 1951, William Heinemann, Ltd.
6 Soderström, N.: Cytologie der Milz in Punktaten. In Lennert, K., and Harms, D., editors: Die Milz, Berlin, 1970, Springer-Verlag.

Rupture; splenectomy

7 Cohen, E. A.: Splenosis; review and report of subcutaneous splenic implant, Arch. Surg. **69:**777-784, 1954.
8 Dalton, M. L., Jr., Strange, W. H., and Downs, E. A.: Intrathoracic splenosis; case report and

review of the literature, Am. Rev. Respir. Dis. **103:**827-830, 1971.

9 Ellis, E. F., and Smith, R. T.: The role of the spleen in immunity, Pediatrics **37:**111-119, 1966.

10 Foster, R. P.: Delayed haemorrhage from the ruptured spleen, Br. J. Surg. **57:**189-192, 1970.

11 Nordøy, A.: The spleenless state in man. In Lennert, K., and Harms, D., editors: Die Milz, Berlin, 1970, Springer-Verlag.

12 Orloff, M. J., and Peskin, G. W.: Spontaneous rupture of the normal spleen; a surgical enigma, Int. Abstr. Surg. **106:**1-11, 1958.

13 Pedersen, B., and Videbaek, A.: On the late effects of removal of the normal spleen; a follow-up study of 40 persons, Acta Chir. Scand. **131:**89-98, 1966.

14 Pratt, D. B., Andersen, R. C., and Hitchcock, C. R.: Splenic rupture; a review of 114 cases, Minn. Med. **54:**177-184, 1971.

15 Rawsthorne, G. B., Cole, T. P., and Kyle, J.: Spontaneous rupture of the spleen in infectious mononucleosis, Br. J. Surg. **57:**396-398, 1970.

16 Stites, T. B., and Ultmann, J. E.: Spontaneous rupture of the spleen in chronic lymphocytic leukemia, Cancer **19:**1587-1590, 1966.

Hypersplenism (dyssplenism)

17 Amorosi, E. L.: Hypersplenism, Semin. Hematol. **2:**249-285, 1965 (excellent bibliography).

18 Baldini, M.: Idiopathic thrombocytopenic purpura, N. Engl. J. Med. **274:**1245-1251; 1301-1306; and 1360-1367, 1966.

19 Bowman, H. E., Pettit, V. D., Caldwell, F. T., and Smith, E. B.: Morphology of the spleen in idiopathic thrombocytopenic purpura, Lab. Invest. **4:**206-216, 1955.

20 Coller, F. A., and Orebaugh, J. E.: Indications for splenectomy, Surgery **37:**858-872, 1955.

21 Crosby, W. H.: Splenectomy in hematologic disorders, N. Engl. J. Med. **286:**1252-1254, 1972.

22 Doan, C. A.: Hypersplenism, Bull. N. Y. Acad. Med. **25:**625-650, 1949.

23 Ebbe, S., Wittels, B., and Dameshek, W.: Autoimmune thrombocytopenic purpura ("ITP" type) with chronic lymphocytic leukemia, Blood **19:**23-27, 1962.

24 Gupta, P. C. Sen, Chatterjea, J. B., Mukherjee, A. M., and Chatterji, A.: Observations on the foam cell in thalassemia, Blood **16:**1039-1044, 1960.

25 Harrington, W. J., and Arimura, G.: Platelet autoimmunization and thrombocytopenia, International Society of Hematology, Proceedings of Sixth Congress, 1956, New York, 1958, Grune & Stratton, Inc., p. 836.

26 Harrington, W. J., and Arimura, G.: Immune reactions of platelets. In Johnson, S. A., Monto, R. W., Rebuck, J. W., and Horn, R. C., Jr., editors: Blood platelets (Henry Ford Hospital International Symposium), New York, 1961, Little, Brown and Co., pp. 659-670.

27 Harrington, W. J., Minnich, V., and Hollingsworth, J. W.: Demonstration of a thrombocytopenic factor in the blood of patients with thrombocytopenic purpura, J. Lab. Clin. Med. **38:**1-10, 1951.

28 Jacob, H. S.: The defective red blood cell in hereditary spherocytosis, Annu. Rev. Med. **20:**41-46, 1969.

29 Karpatkin, S., and Siskind, G. W.: In vitro detection of platelet antibody in patients with idiopathic thrombocytopenic purpura and systemic lupus erythematosus, Blood **33:**795-812, 1969.

30 Liber, A., and Rose, H. G.: Saturated hydrocarbons in follicular lipidosis of the spleen, Arch. Pathol. **83:**116-122, 1967.

31 Loeb, V., Jr., Moore, C. V., and Dubach, R.: The physiologic evaluation and management of chronic bone marrow failure, Am. J. Med. **15:**499-517, 1953.

32 McMillan, R., Longmire, R. L., Yelenosky, B. S., Smith, R. S., and Craddock, C. G.: Immunoglobulin synthesis in vitro by splenic tissue in idiopathic thrombocytopenic purpura, N. Engl. J. Med. **286:**681-684, 1972.

33 Molnar, Z., and Rappaport, H.: Fine structure of the red pulp of the spleen in hereditary spherocytosis, Blood **39:**81-98, 1972.

34 Palmer, J. G., Eichwald, E. J., Cartwright, G. E., and Wintrobe, M. M.: The experimental production of splenomegaly, anemia and leukopenia in Albino rats, Blood **8:**72-80, 1953.

35 Rappaport, H.: The pathologic anatomy of the splenic red pulp. In Lennert, K., and Harms, D., editors: Die Milz, Berlin, 1970, Springer-Verlag.

36 Rappaport, H., and Crosby, W. H.: Autoimmune hemolytic anemia. II. Morphologic observations and clinicopathologic correlation, Am. J. Pathol. **33:**429-458, 1957.

37 Reidbord, H. R., Branimir, L. H., and Fisher, E. R.: Splenic lipidoses: histochemical and ultrastructural differentiation with special reference to the syndrome of the sea-blue histiocyte, Arch. Pathol. **93:**518-524, 1972.

38 Rudders, R. A., Aisenberg, A. C., and Schiller, A. L.: Hodgkin's disease presenting as "idiopathic" thrombocytopenic purpura, Cancer **30:**220-230, 1972.

39 Rywlin, A. M., Lopez-Gomez, A., Tachimes, P., and Pardo, V.: Ceroid histiocytosis of the spleen in hyperlipemia: relationship to the syndrome of the sea-blue histiocyte, Am. J. Clin. Pathol. **56:**572-579, 1971.

40 Saltzstein, S. L.: Phospholipid accumulation in histiocytes of splenic pulp associated with

thrombocytopenic purpura, Blood **18**:73-88, 1961.

41 Sandusky, W. R., Leavell, B. S., and Burton, I. B.: Splenectomy: indications and results in hematologic disorders, Ann. Surg. **159**:695-710, 1964.

42 Shulman, N. R., Marder, V. J., Hiller, M. C., and Collier, E. M.: Platelet and leukocyte isoantigens and their antibodies: serologic, physiologic and clinical studies, Prog. Hematol. **4**:222-304, 1964.

43 Shulman, N. R., Marder, V., and Weinrach, R. A.: Similarities between known antiplatelet antibodies and factor responsible for thrombocytopenia in idiopathic purpura, Ann. N. Y. Acad. Sci. **124**:499-542, 1965.

44 Silverstein, M. N., Ellefson, R. D., and Ahern, E. J.: The syndrome of the sea-blue histiocyte, N. Engl. J. Med. **282**:1-4, 1970.

45 Weed, R. I.: The importance of erythrocyte deformability, Am. J. Med. **49**:147-150, 1970.

46 Weiss, L., and Tavassoli, M.: Anatomical hazards to the passage of erythrocytes through the spleen, Semin. Hematol. **7**:372-380, 1970.

47 Wiland, O. K., and Smith, E. B.: The morphology of the spleen in congenital hemolytic anemia (hereditary spherocytosis), Am. J. Clin. Pathol. **26**:619-629, 1956.

48 Young, L. E., Platzer, R. F., Ervin, D. M., and Izzo, M. J.: Hereditary spherocytosis. II. Observations on the role of the spleen, Blood **6**:1099-1113, 1951.

Agnogenic myeloid metaplasia (myelofibrosis)

49 Bouroncle, B. A., and Doan, C. A.: Myelofibrosis; clinical, hematologic and pathologic study of 110 patients, Am. J. Med. Sci. **243**:697-715, 1962.

49a Caspersson, T., Gahrton, G., Lindsten, J., and Zech, L.: Identification of the Philadelphia chromosome as a number 22 by quinacrine mustard fluorescence analysis, Exp. Cell Res. **63**:238-240, 1970.

50 Condon, W. B., Safarik, L. R., and Elzi, E. P.: Extramedullary hematopoiesis simulating intrathoracic tumor, Arch. Surg. **90**:643-648, 1965.

51 Fisher, E. R., and Hazard, J. B.: Differentiation of megakaryocyte and Reed-Sternberg cell, Lab. Invest. **3**:261-269, 1954.

52 Heller, E. L., Lewisohn, M. G., and Palin, W. E.: Aleukemic myelosis; chronic nonleukemic myelosis, agnogenic myeloid metaplasia, osteosclerosis, leuko-erythroblastic anemia, and synonymous designations, Am. J. Pathol. **23**:327-365, 1947.

53 Lowman, R. M., Bloor, C. M., and Newcomb, A. W.: Roentgen manifestations of thoracic extramedullary hematopoiesis, Dis. Chest **44**:154-162, 1963.

54 Nowell, P. C., and Hungerford, D. A.: Chromosome changes in human leukemia and a tentative assessment of their significance, Ann. N. Y. Acad. Sci. **113**:654-662, 1964.

55 Pitcock, J. A., Reinhard, E. H., Justus, B. W., and Mendelsohn, R. A.: A clinical and pathological study of seventy cases of myelofibrosis, Ann. Intern. Med. **57**:73-84, 1962.

56 Seidler, R. C., and Becker, J. A.: Intrathoracic extramedullary hematopoiesis, Radiology **83**:1057-1059, 1964.

57 Silverstein, M. N., Gomes, M. R., Re Mine, W. H., and Elveback, L. R.: Agnogenic myeloid metaplasia, Arch. Intern. Med. **120**:546-550, 1967.

Congestive and idiopathic splenomegaly

58 Bagshawe, A.: A comparative study of hypersplenism in reactive and congestive splenomegaly, Br. J. Haematol. **19**:729-737, 1970.

59 Blakemore, A. H., and Lord, J. W.: The technic of using Vitallium tubes in establishing portacaval shunts for portal hypertension, Ann. Surg. **122**:476-489, 1945.

60 Dacie, J. V., Brain, M. C., Harrison, C. V., Lewis, S. M., and Worlledge, S. M.: Nontropical idiopathic splenomegaly (primary hypersplenism): a review of ten cases and their relationship to malignant lymphomas, Br. J. Haematol. **17**:317-333, 1969.

61 Herrick, F. C.: An experimental study into the cause of the increased portal pressure in portal cirrhosis, J. Exp. Med. **9**:93-104, 1907.

62 McIndoe, A. H.: Vascular lesions of portal cirrhosis, Arch. Pathol. **5**:23-42, 1928.

63 Pitney, W. R.: The tropical splenomegaly syndrome, Trans. R. Soc. Trop. Med. Hyg. **62**:717-728, 1968.

64 Rousselot, L. M.: The late phase of congestive splenomegaly (Banti's syndrome) with hematemesis but without cirrhosis of the liver, Surgery **8**:34-42, 1940.

65 Sagoe, A. S.: Tropical splenomegaly syndrome: long-term proguanil therapy correlated with spleen size, serum IgM, and lymphocyte transformation, Br. Med. J. **3**:378-382, 1970.

66 Satterfield, J. V., Mulligan, L. V., and Butcher, H. R., Jr.: Bleeding esophageal varices, Arch. Surg. **90**:667-672, 1965.

67 Whipple, A. O.: The problem of portal hypertension in relation to the hepatosplenopathies, Ann. Surg. **122**:449-475, 1945 (extensive bibliography).

Cysts

68 Fowler, R. H.: Nonparasitic benign cystic tumors of the spleen, Surg. Gynecol. Obstet. **96**(suppl.):209-227, 1953.

69 Park, J. Y., and Song, K. T.: Splenic cyst:

a case report and review of literature, Am. Surg. 37:544-547, 1971.

70 Talerman, A., and Hart, S.: Epithelial cysts of the spleen, Br. J. Surg. 57:201-204, 1970.

Tumors

71 Ahmann, D. L., Kiely, J. M., Harrison, E. G., Jr., and Payne, S.: Malignant lymphoma of the spleen, Cancer 19:461-469, 1966.

72 Berge, T.: The metastasis of carcinoma with special reference to the spleen, Acta Pathol. Microbiol. Scand. [suppl.] 188:5-128, 1967.

73 Bostick, W. L.: Primary splenic neoplasms, Am. J. Pathol. 21:1143-1165, 1945.

74 Das Gupta, T., Coombes, B., and Brasfield, R. D.: Primary malignant neoplasms of the spleen, Surg. Gynecol. Obstet. 120:947-960, 1965.

75 Easler, R. E., and Dowlin, W. M.: Primary lipoma of the spleen; report of a case, Arch. Pathol. 88:557-559, 1969.

76 Goldberg, G. M.: A study of malignant lymphomas and leukemias. VII. Lymphogenous leukemia and lymphosarcoma involvement of the lymphatic and hemic bed, with reference to differentiating criteria, Cancer 17:277-287, 1964.

77 Herbut, P. A., and Gabriel, F. R.: Secondary cancer of the spleen, Arch. Pathol. 33:917-921, 1942.

78 Husni, E. A.: The clinical course of splenic hemangioma with emphasis on spontaneous rupture, Arch. Surg. 83:681-688, 1961.

79 Rappaport, H.: The pathologic anatomy of the splenic red pulp. In Lennert, K., and Harms, D., editors: Die Milz, Berlin, 1970, Springer-Verlag.

80 Skarin, A. T., Davey, F. R., and Moloney, W. C.: Lymphosarcoma of the spleen, Arch. Intern. Med. 127:259-265, 1971.

81 Wilkinson, H. A., III, Lucas, J. C., and Foote, F. W., Jr.: Primary splenic angiosarcoma; a case report, Arch. Pathol. 85:213-218, 1968.

Other lesions

82 Esterly, J. R., and Oppenheimer, E. H.: Lymphangiectasis and other pulmonary lesions in the asplenia syndrome, Arch. Pathol. 90:553-560, 1970.

83 Kevy, S. V., Tefft, M., Vawter, G. F., and Rosen, F. S.: Hereditary splenic hypoplasia, Pediatrics 42:752-757, 1968.

84 Kuo, T., and Rosai, J.: Granulomatous inflammation in splenectomy specimens; clinicopathologic analysis of twenty cases (in preparation).

85 Putschar, W. G. J., and Manion, W. C.: Congenital absence of the spleen and associated anomalies, Am. J. Pathol. 26:429-470, 1956.

86 Putschar, W. G. J., and Manion, W. C.: Splenic-gonadal fusion, Cancer 32:15-34, 1956.

87 Watson, R. J.: Splenogonadal fusion, Surgery 63:853-858, 1968.

88 Young, J. M., Bills, R. J., and Ulrich, E.: Discrete splenic calcification in necropsy material, Am. J. Pathol. 33:189-197, 1957.

22 Bone and joint

Introduction

The European pathologists have studied bone thoroughly, their knowledge for the most part having come from thorough postmortem study of osseous lesions. The student need only examine German books of pathology such as Henke-Lubarsch's work to realize how extensive has been their study. The usual autopsy in the United States is considered thorough if small segments of femur, vertebra, and sternum are removed. In most instances, only a fragment of vertebra is examined. Even this specimen may not be studied microscopically.

American pathologists should study bone more thoroughly. The routine removal at autopsy of rib, the anterior half of the vertebral column, femur, and even humerus would prove worthwhile. The correlation of roentgenographic and microscopic findings in large sections of bone would add to the understanding of osseous pathologic processes. Excellent books on osseous pathology are available.[1, 4-7, 9]

Primary neoplasms of bone are rare.[13] Their rarity plus the technical difficulty of section preparation have made the diagnosis and proper treatment of bone tumors

1011

fraught with error. There are only a few centers in this country where much orthopedic pathology is seen. Consequently, many pathologists and radiologists have little real knowledge of these tumors. Before making a diagnosis, it is imperative that the clinical history be complete, that x-ray examination be adequate, and that the pathologic material be well prepared and representative of the lesion.[11]

In most instances, the clinical story is not diagnostic. The radiologic pattern may be diagnostic in some, but there are many exceptions. Radiologic examination must be thorough.[3] Often roentgenograms of other bones are necessary. The biopsy material must be representative, adequate, and well prepared. Pathologists should not attempt to interpret poorly prepared slides, nor should the radiologist attempt to interpret poor radiographs.

Too often, poorly prepared and incorrectly diagnosed slides are referred for diagnosis by experienced pathologists. The reasons are obvious. Most technicians do not know how to prepare and stain bone sections properly, many surgeons submit inadequate biopsies, and the pathologist, until recently, has found little to help him in the literature. Complicated classifications of bone tumors and bewildering discussions of embryology are confusing. Most important, it must be realized that osseous reactions to injury, tumors, and metabolic conditions are limited. They vary merely in degree.

The pathologist must acquire a thorough knowledge of the histology and development of bones.[2] He must know how to tell living bone from dead bone (Fig. 980) and bone production from bone destruction (Fig. 981). Once he has established these fundamental properties of bone clearly in his mind, he can help the orthopedic surgeon select representative material for biopsy, decalcify the specimen with care, stain the sections properly, and correlate the microscopic findings with the clinical history and roentgenograms.[10] Needle biopsy can be diagnostic at times and as out-

lined by Schajowicz and Derqui,[12] should be used more often. It is particularly valuable in vertebral lesions.

The surgical pathologist must have all data before attempting a diagnosis. If he does not, he may incorrectly diagnose an exuberant callus as an osteogenic sarcoma. We have observed an instance in which a large piece of bone was submitted and good sections were made but no significant pathology was seen. A review of the x-ray examination demonstrated that the surgeon had biopsied bone adjacent to the pathologic lesion. In our laboratory, we refuse to make a diagnosis on poorly prepared outside slides and in the absence of roentgenograms. These two items are essential. The clinical history is also of importance.

Brief descriptions of some of the fundamental processes of bone are given in the following paragraphs.

Dead bone can be recognized by its staining reaction. It stains a deeper blue than does normal bone. Lacunar cells are absent, and the margins of the bone are ragged (Fig. 980).

New bone can be recognized by the presence of well-stained small spicules of bone with cells in their lacunae and osteoblasts along their margins (Fig. 981). New bone formation can be studied in a variety of pathologic processes such as fibrous dysplasia, in a healing fracture, and in osteitis fibrosa cystica. The presence of fiber bone indicates a pathologic process as in fibrous dysplasia. In a callus, fiber bone eventually becomes lamellar bone.

Bone destruction can be recognized by the presence of large multinucleated cells called osteoclasts which are present on the ragged margins of bone that is being destroyed. Some of this bone will already be partially dead bone. The osteoclast and osteoblast may be differentiated by electron microscopy (Figs. 982 and 983).

The diaphysis of the bone is its shaft. The epiphysis represents the growing ends of a bone. When a bone has reached its adult length, the epiphyses close. Enchon-

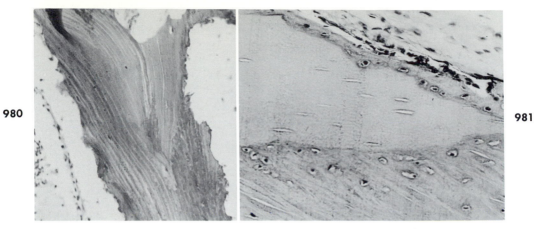

Fig. 980 Dead bone with empty lacunae and ragged bone margins. (×270; WU neg. 49-5373.)

Fig. 981 Appositional bone growth proceeding on surface of spicule of dead bone. Living bone is sharply demarcated, and its lacunae contain nuclei. (×300; WU neg. 49-5640.)

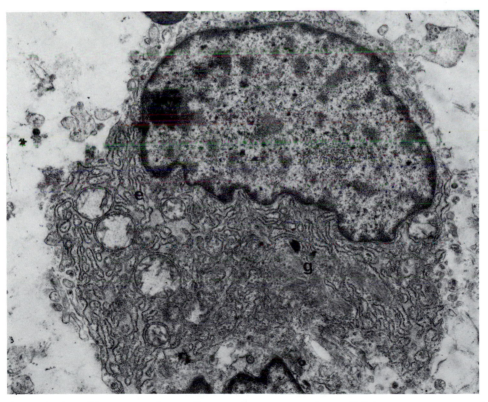

Fig. 982 Osteoblast in ossifying fibroma showing prominent Golgi apparatus, **g,** and much ergastoplasm, **e.** These are features that correlate with osteoid (collagen) synthesis. (Approximately ×9,000.)

dral ossification occurs at the epiphysis in a growing bone. Longitudinal, regularly spaced columns of vascularized cartilage are replaced by bone. When this process finally ends, the epiphysis becomes calcified and ossified.

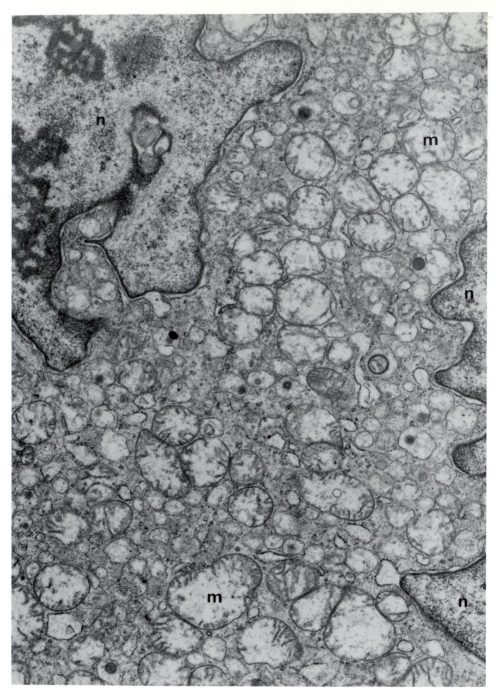

Fig. 983 Portion of giant cell, osteoclast, from giant cell tumor of bone. Portions of multiple nuceli, **n,** with irregular nuclear outlines are shown. Cytoplasm of normal and neoplastic osteoclasts is filled with mitochondria, **m.** Occasional dense bodies and vesicular profiles of endoplasmic reticulum are interspersed. (Approximately ×8,000.)

The time of closure of the epiphysis differs in various bones and in the sexes. Whether the epiphysis is closed or open influences the extension of pathologic processes. For instance, cartilage is often a barrier to spreading osteosarcoma. If the

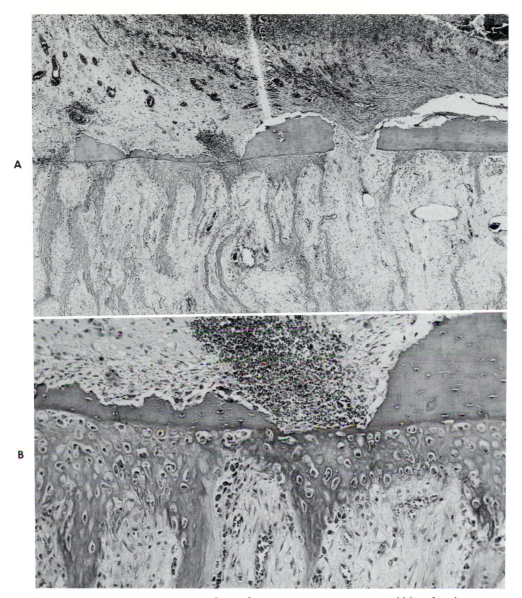

Fig. 984 Extreme periosteal new bone formation occurring in mandible after hematoma had almost completely destroyed bone through interference with blood supply. Only fragments of dead mandible remain, but exuberant periosteal bone proliferation is extending from periosteum in long columns. (**A,** Low power; WU neg. 52-3874; **B,** ×150; WU neg. 52-3873.)

epiphysis is closed and cartilage is no longer present, this area is more easily invaded.

An understanding of the blood supply of bone helps to explain spread and limitation of infection, the healing of fractures, and the involvement of bone by primary or secondary neoplasms. The metaphysis is supplied by nutrient end arteries entering from the diaphysis. These vessels terminate at the epiphyseal plate. Vessels also enter from the periphery. The epiphyses receive their blood supply from widely anastomosing vessels. Diaphyseal cortex is supplied by vessels that enter through Volkmann's canals and communicate with the haversian system. A nutrient artery enters the medullary canal at about the center of the shaft, divides, and extends both distally and proximally. The metabolic exchange of calcium and phosphorus occurs primarily in the metaphysis.

The localization of various pathologic processes occurs in different areas of the same bone and in different bones at different ages. The biologic reasons for such localizations are often unknown, but it is important for the pathologist to be able to answer certain questions about a given lesion of bone. What bone or bones are involved? In what part of the bone is the lesion located? Is it a localized or a diffuse process? What is the age and sex of the patient?

As an example of how to apply this knowledge, let us consider a lesion in a 13-year-old boy located in the diaphyseal area of the tibia. It is an eccentric, sharply delineated lesion. There are no other lesions in other bones. The eccentric localization of this lesion rules out the simple bone cyst which has a different configuration. The patient is too young to have giant cell tumor. In fact, there is only one lesion that will fit in this case, the metaphyseal fibrous defect of Hatcher (Fig. 1054). This diagnostic approach should be used for all bone lesions. In many instances, it will resolve the problem without difficulty.

The *periosteum* is closely applied to bone. It is a specialized connective tissue. It may become detached and elevated from the bone in such pathologic processes as trauma, infection, and primary or secondary malignant tumors. Under certain conditions, its elevation causes periosteal bone proliferation.

New bone formation between the elevated periosteum and the bone may be seen by radiographic examination as fine spicules placed perpendicular to the long axis of the bone. This finding, to the inexperienced radiologist and surgeon, is often considered a manifestation of a malignant neoplasm. We have seen conspicuous periosteal bone proliferation in syphilis, tuberculosis, metastatic carcinoma, osteosarcoma, Ewing's tumor, and even after trauma (Fig. 984). In some lesions, such as plasma cell myeloma, the periosteum may be destroyed or encroached upon so that no radiographic changes occur.

If a section of periosteum is transplanted beneath the capsule of a kidney of an experimental animal, its independent property of forming bone can be demonstrated.[8] Nerve filaments are present in the periosteum and carry proprioceptive and sensory impulses. Small nerve filaments may also pass with the nutrient vessels into the medullary canal.

Osteoporosis and osteomalacia

Metabolic bone disease is outside the scope of this chapter. Some metabolic bone diseases will be mentioned briefly, but there are entire books and monographs written on the problem.[18, 21] If one considers only osteoporosis and osteomalacia, it becomes apparent that these two processes are not well understood.

Osteoporosis develops when an individual is unable to repair and maintain the mass of bone tissue that has been acquired throughout growth and maturation.[22] Jowsey et al.[19] have demonstrated by quantitative microradiographic studies that the main difference between the bone in most forms of osteoporosis and normal bone is an increase in the amount of resorption, bone formation levels being generally normal. Osteoporosis occurs frequently after the menopause, perhaps related to estrogen deficiency.[17] The causes for osteoporosis are multiple. Fluoride consumption is probably important in its prevention.[15]

A good biopsy from the iliac crest corresponds well with changes in the spine.[14] However, radiographic examination of the spine is not reliable, for the changes have to be advanced before they can be seen. Studies made at autopsy by Caldwell[16] help to clarify the pathology. For instance, he showed that vertebral biconcavity is not a reliable index of osteoporosis.

Osteomalacia (comparable to rickets in

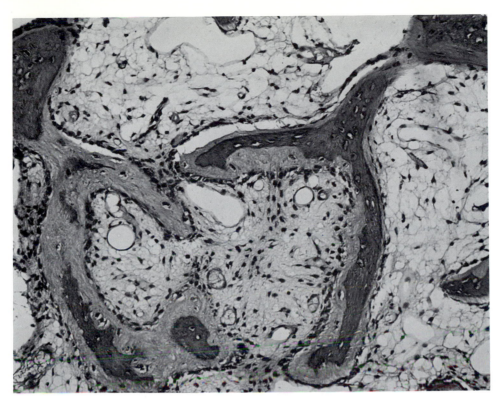

Fig. 985 Osteomalacia. Note wide noncalcified matrix around bone trabeculae. Patient had hyperparathyroidism of long duration with profound renal insufficiency. (×140; WU neg. 61-7452.)

a young person in whom the epiphyses are not yet closed) can be recognized pathologically. In this condition, the bone matrix is formed, but its calcification is incomplete, and this gives rise to a noncalcified matrix around the bone trabeculae[23] (Fig. 985). We have had good success in demonstrating these changes in adequate biopsies from long bones and iliac crests with preparation of nondecalcified specimens. The changes are emphasized when looked at under the phase microscope.

Many methods of investigating these metabolic bone processes have been devised, and many of them are difficult to institute in the usual pathology laboratory.[20, 22]

Fractures

Fractures are breaks in the continuity of bone usually with severance of periosteum, blood vessels, and perhaps muscles. The return of bone to normal following fracture depends upon factors such as treatment, age of the patient, severity of the fracture, vascularity of the area, and nutrition of the patient (Fig. 986). Fractures fail to heal because of improper immobilization, complete devascularization of segments of the fractured bone, persistent infection, and the interposition of soft tissue between the ends of the bone (Fig. 987). A hematoma forms between the two severed ends of bone. Organization of this hematoma begins with the ingrowth of young capillaries. After about three days, the devitalized bone fragments begin to be reabsorbed. Intramembranous bone growth makes its appearance from the cambium layer of the periosteum, both proximal and distal to the fracture site (Figs. 988 and 989). The newly formed trabeculae begin to calcify as the cartilage is replaced by bone.[27, 29, 30] This process on each side of

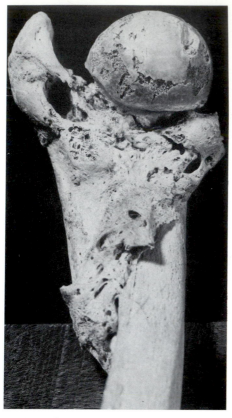

Fig. 986 Exuberant callus formation following fracture.

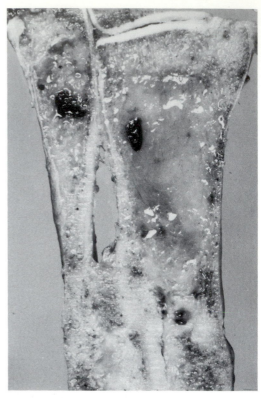

Fig. 987 Nonunion of old fracture of tibia and fibula in 53-year-old white man. Multiple fractures had occurred two years previously and necessitated bone grafting. (WU neg. 62-3316.)

the fracture meets at the fracture site to form the primary callus. The periosteum is composed of an outer fibrous layer and an inner osteogenic layer.[28] This inner osteogenic layer and the endosteum contribute to the formation of callus. "Lines of stress through the fracture site do not dictate the alignment of trabeculae in the primary callus."[*] The secondary callus is made up of mature lamellar bone. The primary callus is absorbed. The new bone is laid down predominantly along lines of stress (Figs. 990 and 991). The formation and persistence of cartilage is largely dependent upon mechanical factors.[31]

The early reduction of fractures promotes rapid healing.[32] With proper reduction of the fracture, adequate blood

supply, no infection, and normal metabolism, the fracture heals rapidly with little visible callus. Exuberant callus usually means slow fracture healing (Fig. 986). In children, even with prominent angulation or deformity, the bone remodels itself to an astonishing degree.[24, 33] For this reason, open reduction and internal fixation of fractures in children are seldom justified. Shortening of a long bone due to overriding of fragments will nearly always correct itself in children by overgrowth of bone.

The sequence of events in a rapidly forming primary callus such as the formation of exuberant cartilage and disorderly membranous bone may produce a bewildering microscopic pattern. Such callus formation may be excessive in osteogenesis imperfecta.[34] The microscopic picture may be difficult to differentiate from osteosarcoma.

---

[*]From Luck, J. V.: Bone and joint diseases, Springfield, Ill., 1950, Charles C Thomas, Publisher.

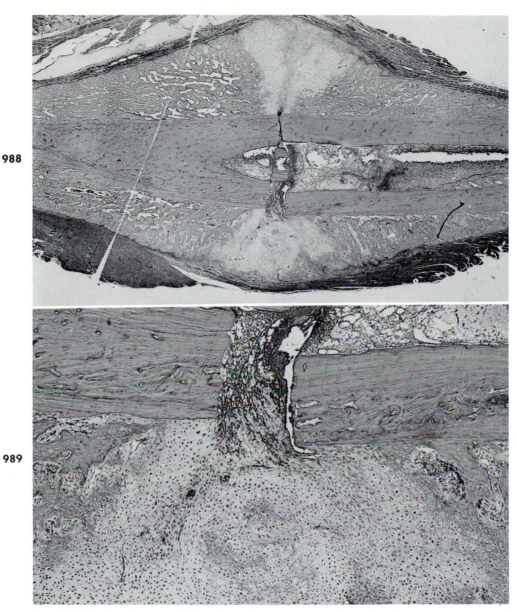

Fig. 988 Healing fracture of long bone in rat at seven days. Note intact periosteum and intramembranous bone formation. (Low power; WU neg. 52-4346.)

Fig. 989 Detailed view of point of fracture shown in Fig. 988. Granulation tissue has been replaced with cartilage, and new bone is gradually replacing this cartilage. Fragment of dead bone within marrow cavity is being reabsorbed. (Low power; WU neg. 52-4344.)

Changes in bone produced by nails, screws, and prostheses

When a noncorrosive nail, such as a Smith-Petersen nail, is driven into a bone to immobilize a fracture, it eventually becomes completely sequestered. The nail is separated from the medullary cavity by fibrous tissue which is continuous with the periosteum. Bone similar to cortical bone forms adjacent to the fibrous tissue (Fig. 992). This cortical bone, in turn, forms an uninterrupted continuity with the cortex of the bone. No foreign body giant cell reaction is observed.[25] The changes pro-

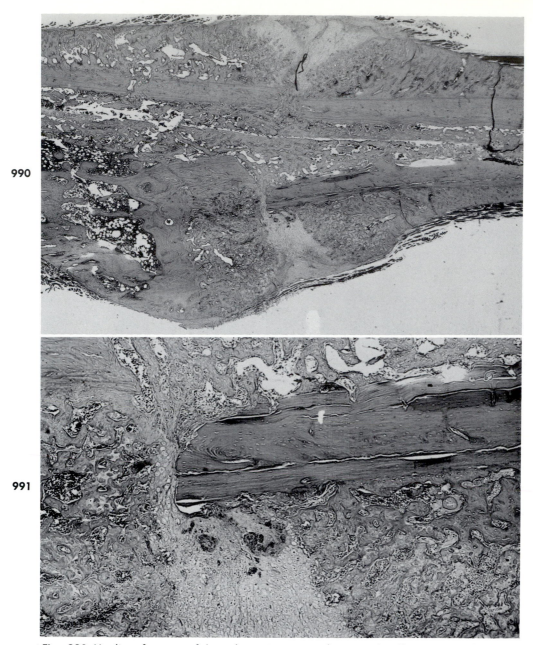

Fig. 990 Healing fracture of long bone in rat at three weeks. (Low power; WU neg. 52-4345.)

Fig. 991 Detailed view of fracture site shown in Fig. 990. Bone has almost completely bridged gap. Small amount of cartilage can still be seen near dead bone fragments. (Low power; WU neg. 52-4344.)

duced by other inert types of prostheses are similar to those produced by the Smith-Petersen nail.[26]

Osteomyelitis

Osteomyelitis may be caused by practically any bacteriologic agent. About 90% of the cases are caused by the coagulase-positive staphylococci. Other organisms such as the streptococcus, pneumococcus, gonococcus, and meningococcus and rare organisms such as *Brucella*, *Histoplasma capsulatum*, and *Actinomyces* also cause it. Patients with abnormal hemoglobin disease,

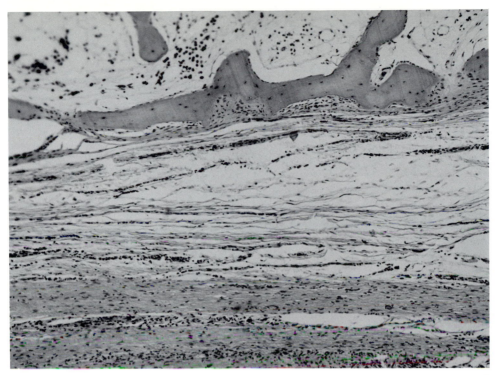

Fig. 992 Sequestration within nail tract. Lower margin shows fibrous tissue next to nail tract which is continuous with periosteum. Layer of bone above fibrous tissue is continuous with cortical bone. (Low power; WU neg. 58-4088.)

particularly sickle cell disease, are prone to develop osteomyelitis due to *Salmonella* infection.[41] Osteomyelitis may follow compound fractures. Hematogenous infections of bone occur most often in patients under 20 years of age. About 75% of cases occur in the lower extremity. The changes in the bone are conditioned by the bone involved, virulence of the organism, resistance of the host, and the age of the patient.

Trueta[42] has emphasized that the involvement of the bone varies with the age of the patient and the vascular supply of the bone. In the infant under 1 year of age, permanent epiphyseal damage and joint infection occur with little damage to the shaft and metaphysis. In children over 1 year of age, there is extensive cortical damage with involucrum formation. Permanent damage to cartilage and joints is rare. Usually with treatment, chronicity is absent.

Acute osteomyelitis of the long bones in the adult is infrequent (Fig. 993). When it occurs, joint infection develops, and the cortex is often absorbed without formation of a sequestrum. The entire bone is involved. Chronicity is more likely to occur.

The introduction of the strong antimicrobial drugs led initially to the treatment of acute hematogenous osteomyelitis without open drainage or saucerization. The mortality and morbidity dropped precipitously after the use of these drugs. However, more recently, saucerization and drainage have been instituted in combination with antibiotics in the treatment of acute osteomyelitis and have resulted in further improvement of results. The frequency of late recrudescence of osseous infection has been much less. Combined surgical and drug therapy has also proved much more effective in treating the staphylococcal infections that are partially or totally resistant to antibiotic therapy. Infections of the latter type appear to be increasing in frequency (Fig. 994). Hematogenous pyogenic vertebral osteomyelitis is frequently

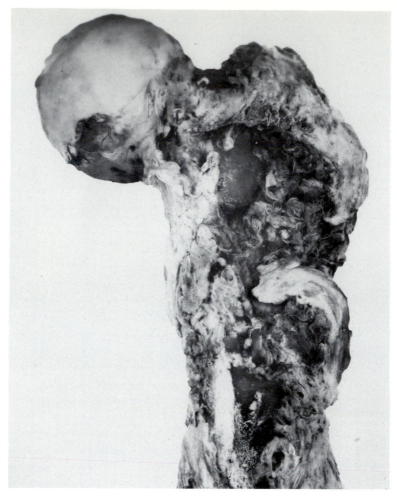

Fig. 993 Osteomyelitis of upper femur with massive bone destruction and reactive sclerosis. (Courtesy Dr. H. Rodriguez, Mexico City, Mexico.)

not diagnosed because of the subtle nature of the disease.[38]

If the infection is massive in the child, the inflammatory process in the metaphyseal area is complicated by an infected thrombus, leading to infarction and subsequent destruction of bone. The infectious material invades the cortex through the vessels of the Volkmann canals. The infection may spread along the medullary canal, through the cortex, or into the joint space. If pus develops beneath the periosteum, perforation through it usually takes place. With the process tending to localize, the cambium layer of the periosteum responds to the presence of dead bone (the sequestrum) by forming new bone (the involucrum). The involucrum eventually extends around the entire bone (Figs. 995 and 996). The sequestrum, if not too large, may be extruded through cutaneous sinuses. Chronic osteomyelitis may show prominent periosteal bone proliferation (Fig. 997). Osteomyelitic sinuses in the adult may become lined by squamous epithelium that may extend deeply into the bone.

Long-standing squamous-lined sinuses that extend into the bone may become discontinuous with the cutaneous surface. Despite apparent healing of the overlying skin, large epidermal inclusion cysts slowly

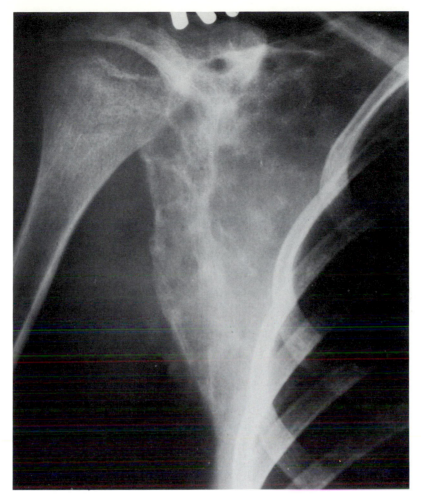

Fig. 994 Extensive involvement of scapula of osteomyelitis of staphylococcal origin in 8-year-old child. This was apparently the only bone involved. (WU neg. 62-8972; courtesy Dr. P. Flynn, Redding, Calif.)

develop in the underlying bone. These are filled with keratin-containing debris similar to that in epidermal inclusion cysts of the skin. Rarely, after a long period, squamous carcinoma develops within these sinuses. Pain and increasingly malodorous discharge heralds the development of carcinoma in such sinuses.[37, 39]

The chronic osteomyelitis persists as long as infected dead bone remains. The dead bone is surrounded by granulation tissue that attacks the sequestrum, making it pitted on the surface next to the marrow cavity. The cortical surface remains smooth. Operative removal of the sequestrum at the proper time usually allows the osteomyelitis to heal. The osteomyelitis may recur many years later if bacteria remain within the scar.

Tuberculous osteomyelitis as a hematogenous infection usually seen in young adults or children. Wherever pasteurization of milk is mandatory, the incidence of bone tuberculosis is low. The bones most often infected are the vertebrae and bones of the hip, knee, ankle, elbow, and wrist. Tuberculosis usually involves the metaphyseal area, the epiphysis, and the synovium.[35] There has been considerable controversy concerning the area primarily involved.

Metaphyseal infection is common in chil-

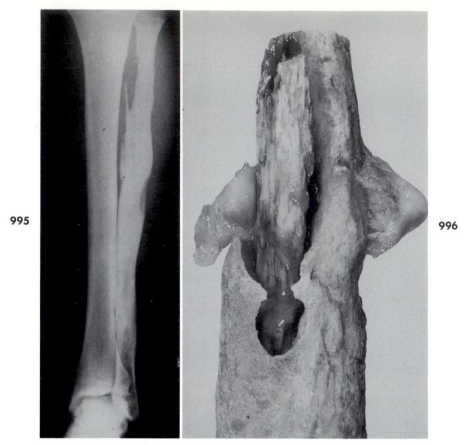

Fig. 995 Chronic osteomyelitis of fibula. Note dense, irregular bone. (WU neg. 50-1493.)
Fig. 996 Resected fibula showing dense outer involucrum surrounding loosened sequestrum with its pitted surface. (WU neg. 50-652.)

dren and epiphyseal infection common in adults. This does not have too much significance, for all zones eventually become involved (Fig. 998). Tuberculous granulation tissue forming in the synovia destroys the synovial attachments. The cartilage, no longer nourished from the synovia, undergoes progressive destruction, allowing tuberculous granulation tissue to extend into the epiphysis and finally into the metaphyseal area. If the process begins in the epiphysis, the tuberculous granulation tissue extends into the adjacent joint. When the process begins in the metaphyseal area, extension into the joint may be heralded by the development of fluid in it. Cutaneous sinuses may occur in advanced tuberculosis. These sinuses allow entry of secondary bacterial infection

which modifies the pathologic changes. When the tuberculous process begins to heal, fusion of the joint may be associated with complete or partial denudation of cartilage and "kissing sequestra." Sequestra are cortical in pyogenic processes, but in tuberculous disease they are cancellous. Tuberculosis of the diaphysis also occurs.[36]

The pathologic changes in tuberculosis of bone have been greatly modified by antimycobacterial drugs. Tuberculous tenosynovitis of the hand may form multiple soft tissue masses that are mistaken for neoplasm.[40]

Tertiary syphilis may involve the bone and cause both osseous destruction and production. It frequently is associated with conspicuous periosteal bone proliferation[43] (Fig. 999). The necrotic, well-defined de-

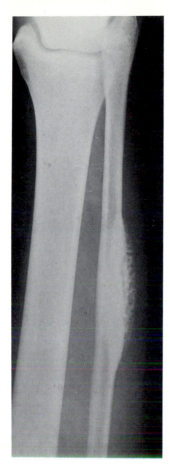

fects are mainly cortical and periosteal and are surrounded by sclerotic bone.

These lesions may be in the vertebrae, flat bones of the hands and feet, and the diaphysis of the long tubular bones. If a single x-ray film is taken, a diagnosis of osteosarcoma may be made. Biopsy will show a granulomatous process with bone destruction and production. The diagnosis usually will be apparent if multiple films of the bones are studied. In single or isolated lesions, the diagnosis may be difficult. The presence of a positive serology does not eliminate the possibility of osteosarcoma. In such instances, a biopsy is required to make an exact diagnosis.

Aseptic (avascular) bone necrosis

Osseous aseptic necrosis is an important orthopedic pathologic abnormality that has been reported as osteochondritis in practically every secondary epiphysis and in many primary epiphyses (Figs. 1000 and 1001). Unfortunately, each site has been

Fig. 997 Prominent periosteal bone proliferation in chronic osteomyelitis. (WU neg. 51-1883.)

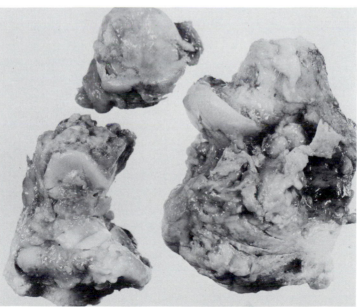

Fig. 998 Extensive involvement of synovium of elbow joint by tuberculous granulation tissue. (WU neg. 49-978.)

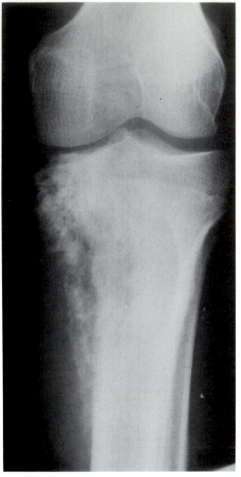

Fig. 999 Gummatous involvement of tibia in 45-year-old woman. (Courtesy Dr. R. J. Reed, New Orleans, La.)

described independently and often given individual names such as the following:

Tibial tubercle (Osgood-Schlatter disease) (Osgood, 1903)
Patella—primary epiphysis (Kohler, 1908)
Tarsal navicular (Kohler, 1908)
Capital epiphysis femur (osteochondritis deformans juvenilis; Legg-Perthes' disease) (Legg, 1909)
Head of humerus (Lewin, 1930)

The etiology of many cases is unknown and is thought possibly to be traumatic or related to endocrine imbalance. In some, etiology is related to obliteration of the epiphyseal blood supply because of fracture or dislocation.[44] Phemister[47] clarified the pathogenesis of femoral head avascular necrosis secondary to complete interrup-

tion of blood supply occurring in fractures of the femoral neck.

The sequence of events implies death of the epiphysis which, in time, becomes more clearly seen roentgenographically. This death of bone is followed by hyperemia of the neighboring tissues. The overlying cartilage of the epiphysis may or may not remain viable, for it receives nourishment from the overlying synovium. The dead bone gradually undergoes resorption. There may be osteoclasis on one side of necrotic trabeculae, with osteoblastic activity on the other.[46] This bone is gradually replaced by "creeping substitution." This replacement of the dead epiphysis by new bone is a slow process, taking months or even years. This is illustrated by the sclerosis that is seen after fractures of the neck of the femur. The dense appearance of the femoral head is often incident to new bone formation upon the dead trabecular bone.[44] The new soft bone may flatten because of pressure. If this change occurs, degenerative joint disease soon follows. Aseptic necrosis of the femoral head may occur in sickle cell disease.[45]

Osteochondritis dissecans

Osteochondritis dissecans is a small area of necrosis involving the articular cartilage and subchondral bone that totally or partially separates from adjacent structures. The etiology is uncertain but is probably related to trauma. It occurs most frequently on the lateral aspect of the medial femoral condyle, near the intercondylar notch[46] (Fig. 1002). If an osteochondromatous body remains attached to the joint surface or synovium, both components remain viable. If, however, such a body becomes completely detached, its osseous portion dies but the cartilage remains alive, apparently through nutrients obtained from the synovial fluid. Patients with bilateral symmetrical involvement and cases with familial incidence have been described.

Paget's disease

About 90% of the patients with Paget's disease are over 55 years of age. The dis-

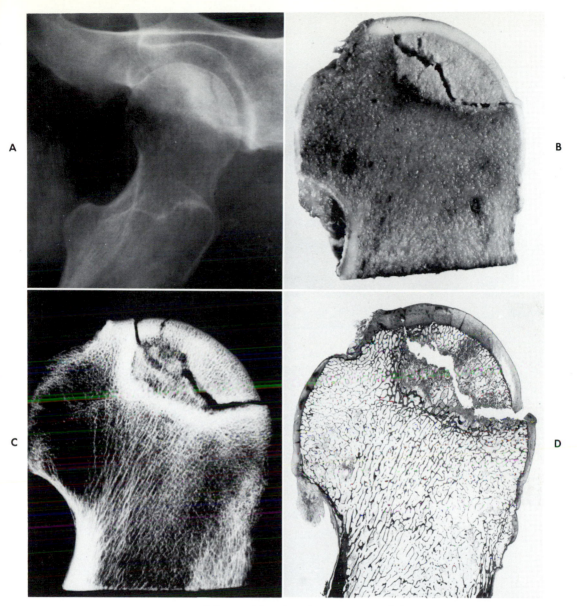

Fig. 1000 Aseptic necrosis of femoral head with superimposed fracture. **A,** Roentgenogram. **B,** Cross section of excised specimen. **C,** Roentgenogram of slice of same specimen, emphasizing peripheral eburnation. **D,** Whole-mount specimen showing well-delimited focus of necrosis. (**A,** WU neg. 73-4617; **B,** WU neg. 73-4420; **C,** WU neg. 73-5609; **D,** WU neg. 73-7722.)

ease is rare before the age of 40 years and uncommon between the ages of 40 and 55 years.[51] It affects men slightly more often than women (4:3). It has a very peculiar geographic distribution. The highest incidence is in England, Australia, and the Western European plain.[48] Collins[49] reported that at autopsy about one of every thirty patients over 40 years of age had Paget's disease in one of several locations. The most common sites are the lumbosacral spine, the pelvis, and the skull. It may occur in the femur, tibia, clavicle, and fibula but is extremely rare in the ribs (Fig. 1003). The process may involve only a portion of a single bone.

Initially, this lesion is osteoclastic.[50] Abnormal hyperplasia soon follows, as evi-

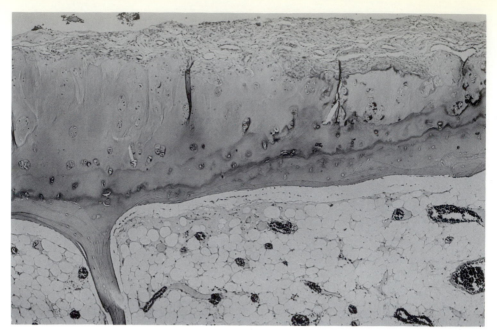

Fig. 1001 Aseptic bone necrosis in head of femur. Note fibrillation and almost complete absence of cartilage. Subchondral bone is dead with empty lacunae. (Low power; WU neg. 52-4090.)

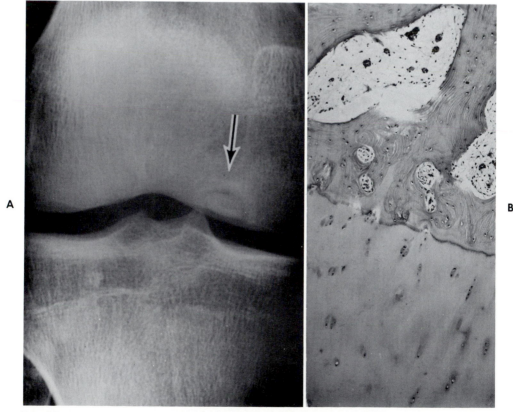

Fig. 1002 **A**, Sharply delimited area of osteochrondritis dissecans of medial condyle (arrow). This was easily enucleated. **B**, Same lesion shown in **A** demonstrating viability of bone removed from defect. Bone was alive because of its loose attachment to normal adjacent osseous tissue. (**A**, WU neg. 62-7783; **B**, WU neg. 62-8266.)

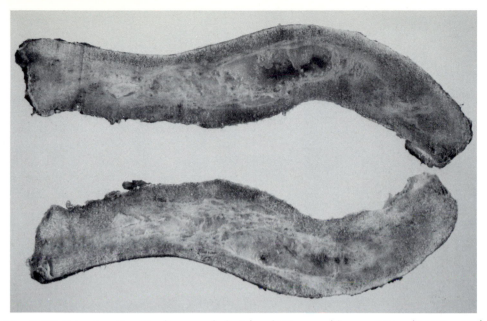

Fig. 1003 Extensive Paget's disease of clavicle of 60-year-old man. Note distortion and changes in cortex. (WU neg. 66-2557.)

denced by primitive coarse-fibered bone in discontinuous trabeculae. Later, massive, thick trabeculae with disjointed lamellar patterns occur. Reticulin stains are often very helpful in studying the pattern of growth. The use of polarized light is less instructive. When lamellar bone becomes disorganized, a mosaic of cement lines appears. This is caused by the abrupt interruptions and changes in direction of bone lamellae and fibers resulting from resorption and regeneration of masses of bone during the course of the disease. These lines are outlined clearly by Ehrlich's acid hematoxylin.

Collins[49] stressed the fact that the incidence of superimposed osteosarcoma is quite low if one considers the frequency of Paget's disease. The complications of fracture and sarcoma in Paget's disease, however, represent a significant number of clinical problems because of the frequency of the disease. Fractures in Paget's disease usually are transverse.[52] In addition to osteosarcoma, Paget's disease may rarely be complicated by the development of chondrosarcoma, fibrosarcoma, or giant cell tumor.[53] The most common location of sarcomas arising in Paget's disease are the

femur, humerus, innominate bone, tibia, and skull.

Rarely, Paget's disease is predominantly a monostotic process in a long bone.[56] We have seen it in an apparent monostotic phase in the maxilla, in the mandible, and in a collapsed vertebra. Under these conditions, the alkaline phosphatase level may be normal (Figs. 1004 and 1005).

The key to the microscopic pattern of the disease is the mosaic of numerous and scalloped cement lines.[55] There are many pathologic processes that undergo active reparative change accompanied by new bone formation with cement lines. If careful attention is given to the pattern of these normal cement lines which are orderly and structurally well oriented, these processes will not be confused with the microscopic appearance of Paget's disease. These lesions include irradiation effect, chronic osteomyelitis, reactive bone surrounding metastatic cancer, and polyostotic fibrous dysplasia. Uehlinger[57] pointed out that eccentric atrophy of the cortical bone is invariably present in polyostotic fibrous dysplasia but absent in Paget's disease. Rapid dissolution of bone substance may occur if a patient with Paget's disease of a

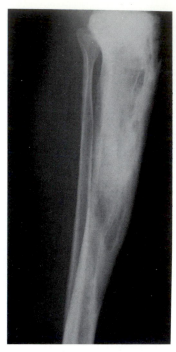

Fig. 1004 Monostotic Paget's disease of tibia with both bone destruction and bone formation. Nature of process was obscure until biopsy. (WU neg. 51-3657.)

long bone is immobilized because of fracture.[54]

Melorheostosis

Melorheostosis is a term derived from Greek words meaning flowing limb. The proliferation of ivorylike bone may be periosteal or endosteal. Osseous tissue also is deposited in soft tissues in the region of joints. In five biopsied lesions, the trabeculae were compact, the haversian canals were normally outlined, and the marrow was fibrotic.[58]

The excessive bone may cause locking of joints and bowing of long bones.[59] Associated soft tissue calcification is frequent.

Tumors
Classification and distribution

Many of the classifications of bone tumors are so complicated that they discourage the embryo pathologist. Much of this stems from the unjustified subdivision of a tumor in morphologic varieties which

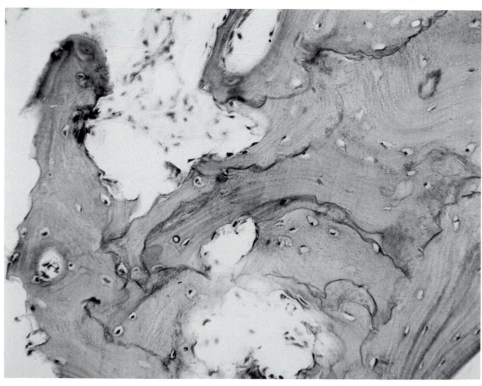

Fig. 1005 Paget's disease. Note numerous irregular but well-defined mosaic patterns of cement lines. (×275; WU neg. 66-9183.)

not only overlap but also lack any clinical or prognostic significance. This is the case, for instance, with osteosarcomas in the classification of the American College of Surgeons. The classification of bone tumors and tumorlike lesions and terminology we use are largely those recommended by the WHO International Reference Center for the Histological Definition and Classification of Bone Tumours[60]*:

Bone-forming tumors
  Benign
    Osteoma
    Osteoid osteoma and osteoblastoma
  Malignant
    Osteosarcoma
    Juxtacortical (parosteal) osteosarcoma
Cartilage-forming tumors
  Benign
    Chondroma
    Osteochondroma
    Chondroblastoma
    Chondromyxoid fibroma
  Malignant
    Chondrosarcoma
    Mesenchymal chondrosarcoma
Giant cell tumor
Marrow tumors
  Ewing's sarcoma
  Malignant lymphoma
  Plasma cell myeloma
Vascular tumors
  Benign
    Hemangioma
    Lymphangioma
    Glomus tumor
  Malignant
    Angiosarcoma, low grade
    Angiosarcoma, high grade
Other connective tissue tumors
  Benign
    Desmoplastic fibroma
    Lipoma
  Malignant
    Fibrosarcoma
    Liposarcoma
    Malignant mesenchymoma
    Undifferentiated sarcoma
Other primary tumors
  Chordoma
  "Adamantinoma" of long bones
  Neurilemoma

Metastatic tumors
Unclassified tumors
Tumorlike lesions
  Solitary bone cyst
  Aneurysmal bone cyst
  Ganglion cyst of bone
  Metaphyseal fibrous defect (nonossifying fibroma)
  Fibrous dysplasia
  Myositis ossificans
  Osteitis fibrosa cystica (discussed in Chapter 8)
  Differentiated histiocytosis (eosinophilic granuloma, Hand-Schüller-Christian disease, and Letterer-Siwe disease)

Tumors of the skeletal system, more than tumors arising anywhere else in the body, are relatively constant in their pattern of presentation. The five basic parameters in this regard are age of the patient, bone involved, specific area within the bone (epiphysis, metaphysis, or diaphysis; cortex, medulla, or periosteum), radiographic appearance, and microscopic appearance. The pathologist should be fully aware of the first four before trying to evaluate the fifth. Otherwise, serious mistakes will inevitably occur. Table 45 should help in providing a quick orientation to the pathologist confronted with a bone neoplasm.

At Washington University Medical Center, there is an extremely active orthopedic service. The distribution of 640 bone tumors seen in fourteen years is rather characteristic with the possible exception of a disproportionately large number of chondrosarcomas. The benign bone tumor seen most frequently is the osteochondroma, and the malignant bone tumor seen most frequently is the metastatic carcinoma (Table 46).

Bone-forming tumors
Osteoma

It is doubtful whether osteoma is a true neoplasm. It is seen almost exclusively in the bones of the skull and face and is always benign. It may protrude inside a paranasal sinus, particularly the frontal and ethmoid, and block the normal drainage from these sinuses.[62] Microscopically, it is composed of dense, mature, predomi-

---

*Adapted, with minor modifications, from Schajowicz, F., Ackerman, L. V., and Sissons, H. A.: Histological typing of bone tumours, International Histological Classification of Tumours, No. 6, Geneva, 1972, World Health Organization.

Table 45 Usual age and sex of patient and location and behavior of most common primary bone tumors and tumorlike lesions*

Tumor or tumorlike lesion	Age (yr)	Sex M:F	Bones more commonly affected (in order of frequency)	Usual location within long bone	Behavior
Osteoma	40-50	2:1	Skull and facial bones	—	Benign
Osteoid osteoma	10-30	2:1	Femur, tibia, humerus, hands and feet, vertebrae, fibula	Cortex of metaphysis	Benign
Osteoblastoma	10-30	2:1	Vertebrae, tibia, femur, humerus, pelvis, ribs	Medulla of metaphysis	Benign
Osteosarcoma	10-25	3:2	Femur, tibia, humerus, pelvis, jaw, fibula	Medulla of metaphysis	Malignant; 20% 5-yr survival rate
Juxtacortical (parosteal) osteosarcoma	30-60	1:1	Femur, tibia, humerus	Juxtacortical area of metaphysis	Malignant; 80% 5-yr survival rate
Chondroma	10-40	1:1	Hands and feet, ribs, femur, humerus	Medulla of diaphysis	Benign
Osteochondroma	10-30	1:1	Femur, tibia, humerus, pelvis	Cortex of metaphysis	Benign
Chondroblastoma	10-25	2:1	Femur, humerus, tibia, feet, pelvis, scapula	Epiphysis, adjacent to cartilage plate	Practically always benign
Chondromyxoid fibroma	10-25	1:1	Tibia, femur, feet, pelvis	Metaphysis	Benign
Chondrosarcoma	30-60	3:1	Pelvis, ribs, femur, humerus, vertebrae	Central—medulla of diaphysis Peripheral—cortex or periosteum of metaphysis	Malignant; 5-yr survival rate—low grade, 78%; moderate grade, 53%; high grade, 22%
Mesenchymal chondrosarcoma	20-60	1:1	Ribs, skull and jaw, vertebrae, pelvis, soft tissues	Medulla or cortex of diaphysis	Malignant; extremely poor prognosis
Giant cell tumor	20-40	4:5	Femur, tibia, radius	Epiphysis and metaphysis	Potentially malignant; 50% recur; 10% metastasize

	Age	Sex	Bones	Location	Character
Ewing's sarcoma	5-20	1:2	Femur, pelvis, tibia, humerus, ribs, fibula	Medulla of diaphysis or metaphysis	Highly malignant; 20%-30% 5-yr survival rate in recent series
Malignant lymphoma, histiocytic (reticulum cell sarcoma) and mixed cell types	30-60	1:1	Femur, pelvis, vertebrae, tibia, humerus, jaw, skull, ribs	Medulla of diaphysis or metaphysis	Malignant; 22%-50% 5-yr survival rate
Plasma cell myeloma	40-60	2:1	Vertebrae, pelvis, ribs, sternum, skull	Medulla of diaphysis, metaphysis, or epiphysis	Malignant; diffuse form uniformly fatal; localized form often controlled with radiation therapy
Hemangioma	20-50	1:1	Skull, vertebrae, jaw	Medulla	Benign
Desmoplastic fibroma	20-30	1:1	Humerus, tibia, pelvis, jaw, femur, scapula	Metaphysis	Benign
Fibrosarcoma	20-60	1:1	Femur, tibia, jaw, humerus	Medulla of metaphysis	Malignant; 28% 5-yr survival rate
Chordoma	40-60	2:1	Sacrococcygeal, spheno-occipital, cervical vertebrae	—	Malignant; slow course; locally invasive; 48% distant metastases
Solitary bone cyst	10-20	3:1	Humerus, femur	Medulla of metaphysis	Benign
Aneurysmal bone cyst	10-20	1:1	Vertebrae, flat bones, femur, tibia	Metaphysis	Benign; sometimes secondary to another bone lesion
Metaphyseal fibrous defect	10-20	1:1	Tibia, femur, fibula	Metaphysis	Benign
Fibrous dysplasia	10-30	3:2	Ribs, femur, tibia, jaw, skull	Medulla of diaphysis or metaphysis	Locally aggressive; rarely complicated by sarcoma
Eosinophilic granuloma	5-15	3:2	Skull, jaw, humerus, rib, femur	Metaphysis or diaphysis	Benign

*It should be emphasized that these data correspond to the typical case and that they should not be taken in an absolute sense. Isolated exceptions to practically every one of these statements have occurred.

Table 46 Frequency of bone tumors at Washington University Medical Center from 1948 to 1962

Tumor	Total*
Cartilage-forming tumors	
Chondroblastoma	18 (14)
Chondromyxoid fibroma	15 (11)
Osteochondroma	122 (8)
Osteochondromatosis	1
Chondroma	16 (5)
Ollier's disease	2
Chondrosarcoma	91 (33)
Bone-forming tumors	
Osteoid osteoma	25 (5)
Osteoblastoma	4 (1)
Osteosarcoma	108 (55)
Juxtacortical osteosarcoma	11 (1)
Osteosarcoma in Paget's disease	4
Postirradiation osteosarcoma	3 (3)
Giant cell tumor	51 (22)
Marrow tumors	
Ewing's sarcoma	26 (9)
Malignant lymphoma	40 (17)
Plasma cell myeloma	36 (5)
Vascular tumors	
Hemangioma	4 (2)
Hemangioma of joints	2
Maffucci's syndrome	1 (1)
Massive osteolysis	2 (1)
Glomus tumor	2 (2)
Lymphangioma	1 (1)
Angiosarcoma	5 (2)
Other tumors	
Lipoma	3 (1)
Liposarcoma	1 (1)
Desmoplastic fibroma	4 (2)
Fibrosarcoma	30 (11)
Neurilemoma	4 (2)
Neurofibroma	1
"Adamantinoma" of long bones	4 (3)

*Figures in parentheses represent cases seen in consultation.

nantly lamellar bone. Patients with Gardner's syndrome (intestinal polyposis and soft tissue tumors) may have multiple osteomas and other bone abnormalities.[61]

Osteoid osteoma and osteoblastoma

Osteoid osteoma is a benign neoplasm of bone occurring in men about twice as often as in women.[66] It is found most frequently in patients between 10 and 30 years of age. This lesion should not be confused with a local area of chronic osteo-myelitis,[63] as it has been in the past. It has been reported in practically every bone but occurs most frequently in the femur, tibia, humerus, bones of hands and feet, vertebrae, and fibula. Lesions of long bones are usually metaphyseal; vertebral lesions often occur in the pedicle or in the arch.[68] Osteoid osteoma usually begins in the cortex (85%), but it also may be located in the spongiosa (13%) or subperiosteal tissues (2%).[69]

The central nidus of this tumor seldom is larger than 1.5 cm and is surrounded by an area of dense bone (Fig. 1006). When the lesion appears in the cortex, the area of reaction may extend for several centimeters along the bone as well as around it. The nidus itself is radiolucent with or without a dense center (Fig. 1007).

Microscopically, the lesion is sharply delineated and made up of more or less calcified osteoid growing within highly vascular osteoblastic connective tissue and surrounded by dense bone (Figs. 1008 and 1009). There is no evidence of inflammation. We have seen one osteoid osteoma of a vertebra misdiagnosed as an osteosarcoma. If the lesion is removed piecemeal, it can still be diagnosed because of the characteristics of the nidus (Fig. 1009).

The most prominent symptom is increasing pain, often well localized. Clinical and laboratory evidence of infection is lacking. If the lesion is in the cortex of the bone, a diagnosis of Garré's osteomyelitis may be made because of the adjacent bone reaction. Removal of the lesion relieves symptoms.

Osteoblastoma (benign osteoblastoma; giant osteoid osteoma) is a tumor closely related to osteoid osteoma.[64] Microscopically, the two lesions are quite similar. Osteoblastoma is distinguished by the larger size of the nidus, the absence or inconspicuousness of a surrounding area of reactive bone formation, and the lack of intense pain.[65, 67] Most cases arise in the spongiosa of the bone, but cortical and subperiosteal forms also occur.[69]

We have seen several cases of well-

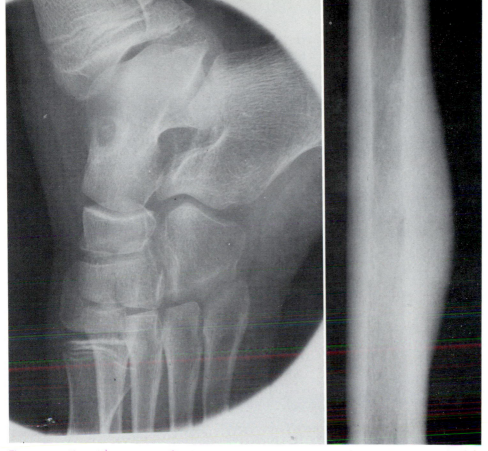

1006

1007

Fig. 1006 Osteoid osteoma of talus. Note small central osteolytic nidus surrounded by dense bone. (WU neg. 48-3921.)

Fig. 1007 Osteoid osteoma of femur obscured by area of reacting bone extending up, as well as around, bone. In past, such lesions were often diagnosed as Garré's osteomyelitis. (WU neg. 50-1910.)

differentiated osteosarcomas misinterpreted as osteoblastomas. The cytologic atypia present in the osteoblasts is the distinguishing feature of the latter.

Osteosarcoma

Osteosarcoma is the most frequent primary malignant bone tumor. It usually occurs in patients between 10 and 25 years of age, being slightly more frequent in male patients. Another peak age incidence occurs after 40, with most of the patients being men in whom osteosarcoma is superimposed on Paget's disease. The latter is not infrequently multicentric. Rarely, multiple foci of origin appear without antecedent Paget's disease, particularly in children.[70, 83]

Osteosarcoma may follow poorly planned irradiation therapy. Cahan et al.[73] reported eleven cases, and Hatcher[75] reported twenty-seven. Martland and Humphries[79] reported the development of osteosarcoma in factory workers who moistened brushes in their mouths when applying radium paint to luminous numerals on watches.

Trauma, as far as is known, does not cause bone tumors. If it did, one would expect to find bone tumors arising after fractures, the trauma of various orthopedic procedures, bullet wounds, or other severe injuries. Trauma usually only calls atten-

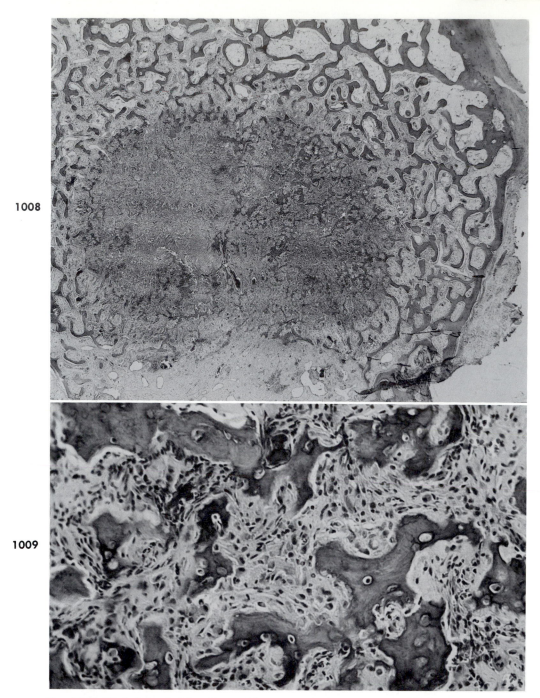

Fig. 1008 Well-defined nidus of osteoid osteoma. (×13; WU neg. 54-5990.)
Fig. 1009 Variably calcified osteoid growing within highly vascular osteoblastic connective tissue. These changes are typical of osteoid osteoma. (Moderate enlargement; WU neg. 52-4539.)

tion to an already present advanced bone tumor.

Recently, immunologic studies have strongly implicated the presence of an infectious agent, probably a virus, in association with human osteosarcoma.[80,81]

Osteosarcomas develop for the most part in the metaphyseal area of the long bones, particularly the lower end of the femur, the upper end of the tibia, and the upper end of the humerus.[74] When superimposed on Paget's disease, the most common sites are femur, humerus (Fig. 1010), innominate bone, tibia, and skull.

Grossly, these tumors vary in vascular, fibrous, catilaginous, and osseous content. As they grow, they extend along the marrow cavity (Fig. 1011) and elevate or perforate the periosteum. If they elevate the periosteum, they may produce the radiographic picture designated as Codman's triangle (a nonspecific finding). This angle is formed by the elevated periosteum and the underlying bone (Fig. 1012). If the epiphysis is closed, the tumor may extend through the entire epiphysis. Rarely following fractures or extension through the periosteum, the tumor may break into the joint. It practically never ulcerates through the skin or involves regional lymph nodes. In a rather wide experience, we have seen involvement of lymph nodes in only three instances. On the other hand, metastases through the bloodstream to distant sites, particularly the lung, are common.

Microscopically, the tumor may exhibit changes ranging from extremely well-differentiated tissue to highly anaplastic lesions (Figs. 1013 and 1014). Biopsy of an undifferentiated osteosarcoma may show a highly vascular lesion with tumor cells of greatly variable size and shape growing between and lining blood vessels without evidence of osteoid formation. These telangiectatic osteosarcomas may mimic aneurysmal bone cysts radiographically and pathologically, although their arteriographic patterns are usually diagnostic. The diagnosis can be made if the pathologist pays attention to the infrequent atypical osteoid in the septa of these sarcomas (Fig. 1015).

By contrast, a tumor may produce a disorderly arrangement of well-differentiated bone and large amounts of osteoid (Figs. 1013 and 1016). Wide areas of neoplastic

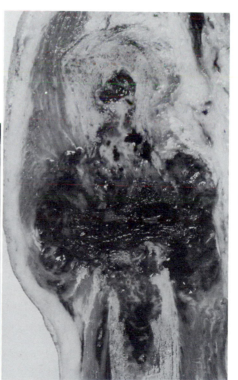

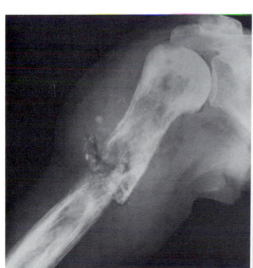

Fig. 1010 **A,** Osteosarcoma of upper end of humerus associated with fracture and Paget's disease. **B,** Point of fracture in humerus shown in **A** demonstrating extension of hemorrhagic neoplasm up shaft and out into soft tissues. Note porous, thickened cortical bone of Paget's disease. (**A,** WU neg. 48-6536; **B,** WU neg. 48-5008.)

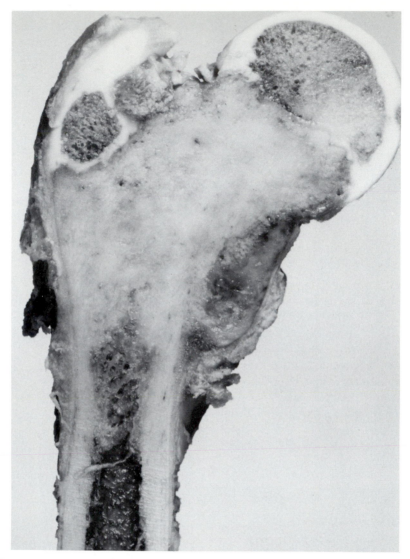

Fig. 1011 Osteosarcoma of proximal femur in 10-year-old boy. There are massive involvement of medullary cavity, invasion of cortex and soft tissues, and periosteal elevation. Note how tumor growth is restrained by epiphyseal cartilage. (WU neg. 68-6392.)

cartilage occur in some tumors, a feature that may prompt a mistaken diagnosis of chondrosarcoma. By definition, a malignant tumor in which osteoid and bone is being formed by the sarcomatous cells is an osteosarcoma, whether or not there is tumor cartilage production in other areas. Conversely, a cartilage-forming malignant tumor lacking the former feature should be designated as chondrosarcoma whether or not the malignant cartilage is being partial-ly replaced by nonneoplastic bone through a mechanism of endochondral ossification. The easily identified osteosarcoma contains sarcomatous stroma and immature osteoid recognized by its faint eosinophilic and glassy appearance. The demonstration of alkaline phosphatase activity may help in identifying as osteosarcoma an apparently undifferentiated neoplasm or in distinguishing tumor bone from hyaline fibrous tissue or cartilage.

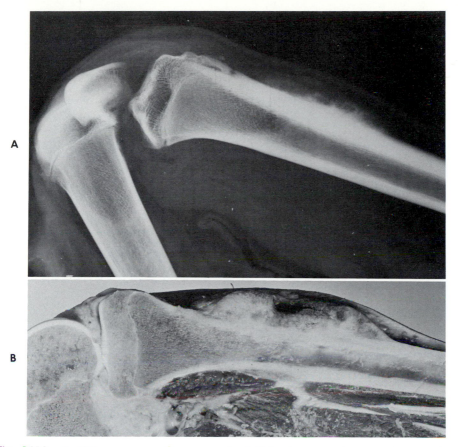

Fig. 1012 **A,** Osteosarcoma of upper end of tibia demonstrating prominent periosteal bone proliferation. **B,** Same tumor shown in **A** demonstrating elevation of periosteum in metaphyseal and diaphyseal areas. (**A,** WU neg. 48-6537; **B,** WU neg. 48-5884.)

The lesions mistaken for osteosarcoma include any in which there is rapid bone growth. We have seen slides of exuberant callus formation misdiagnosed because they were examined without knowledge of an antecedent fracture. The callus may be secondary to a pathologic fracture in a benign localized lesion (such as metaphyseal fibrous defect or aneurysmal bone cyst), in a metastatic carcinoma, or in osteogenesis imperfecta.[72, 76] On several occasions, the highly proliferative lesions of soft tissue designated as myositis ossificans have been diagnosed by competent authorities as osteosarcoma. Lichtenstein[77] cited an instance of gumma of the bone that was diagnosed incorrectly as osteosarcoma.

The prognosis for patients with osteosarcoma is not so dismal as many believe. Even if lesions such as chondrosarcoma, fibrosarcoma, juxtacortical osteosarcoma, and osteogenic sarcoma of the jaw (which have a better prognosis) are excluded, the five-year survival approaches 20%.[78] Sex, microscopic type (whether osteoblastic, chondroblastic, or fibroblastic), and grading bear no significant relationship with prognosis.[74, 82] Osteosarcomas arising on the basis of Paget's disease are usually highly malignant. Osteosarcomas located below elbows and knees have a slightly better prognosis than those situated more centrally.[74] In the series of twenty-eight radiation-induced osteosarcomas reported by Arlen et al.,[71] the prognosis was surprisingly good; an overall five-year survival rate of 28% was achieved.

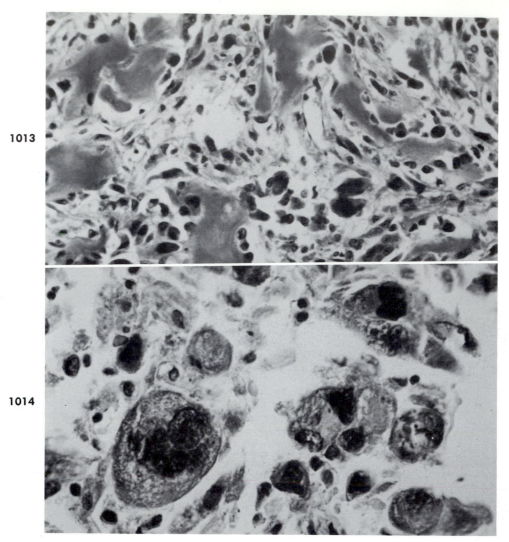

1013

1014

Fig. 1013 Osteosarcoma producing large amounts of neoplastic osteoid and sarcomatous stroma. (High power.)
Fig. 1014 Osteosarcoma with bizarre tumor giant cells. (×600; WU neg. 52-4081.)

Juxtacortical (parosteal) osteosarcoma

Juxtacortical (parosteal) osteosarcoma is an infrequent primary, slowly growing malignant tumor of bone. It arises in a juxtacortical position in the metaphyses of long bones and may have a life history of ten to fifteen years.[87] It forms a large, lobulated mass and has a tendency to encircle the bone (Fig. 1017). Later in the evolution, it may penetrate into the medullary cavity. The diagnosis is suggested by the roentgenographic picture[88] (Fig. 1018, A).

If a biopsy is taken of the soft tissue extension of the tumor, it will show a disorderly pattern of well-formed bone, osteoid, and an abnormal stromal pattern (Fig. 1018, B). The cytologic signs of malignancy in the fibrous stroma are often subtle, thus accounting for the great frequency of misdiagnoses made in this tumor type. Of ten cases of juxtacortical osteosarcoma we studied recently, in only two was the initial histologic diagnosis correct.[85] This lesion has to be differentiated from

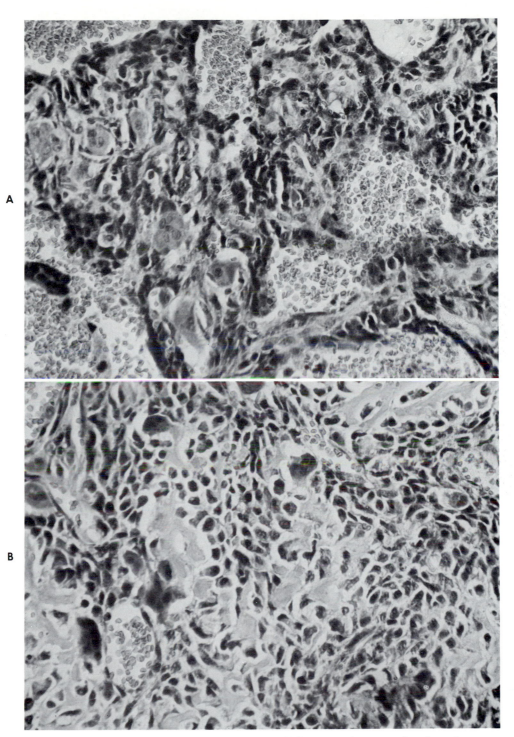

Fig. 1015 A, Pseudoaneurysmal bone cyst which, in reality, is telangiectatic osteo-sarcoma of tibia. This area would be almost impossible to distinguish from aneurysmal bone cyst. **B,** Same lesion shown in **A** demonstrating atypical osteoid growing in sarco-matous stroma. This finding makes the diagnosis of osteosarcoma. Patient died of dis-seminated disease. (**A,** ×300; WU neg. 67-1946; **B,** ×350; WU neg. 67-1945A.)

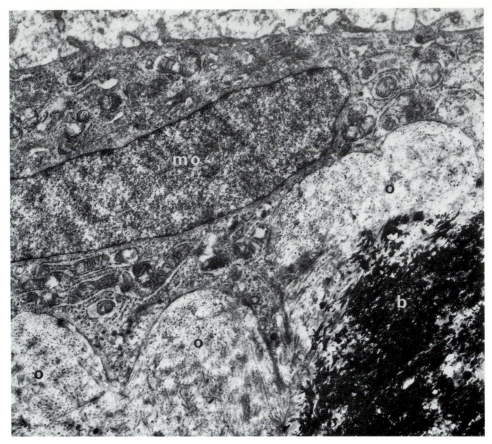

Fig. 1016 In this osteosarcoma, malignant osteoblast, **mo,** osteoid, **o,** and bone, **b,** have similar relationship as they normally do. (Approximately ×9,000.)

myositis ossificans, which has an orderly pattern of bone formation without a sarcomatous stroma. With adequate treatment, the prognosis in juxtacortical osteosarcoma is excellent.[84] Occasionally, local excision is possible. Some tumors having the radiologic and gross features of juxtacortical osteosarcoma have highly malignant cytologic features. Both the microscopic appearance and the clinical behavior of these neoplasms approach those of conventional osteosarcomas.[86]

Cartilage-forming tumors
Chondroma

Chondroma is a common benign cartilaginous tumor that occurs most frequently in the small bones of the hands and feet, particularly the proximal phalanges. Most cases begin in the central portion of the diaphysis (enchondromas), from which they expand and thin the cortex. Chondromas of the thumb and terminal phalanges are distinctly uncommon. In Takigawa's series[94] of 110 cases, thirty-five were multiple. Multiple enchondromas having a predominantly unilateral distribution are referred to as Ollier's disease. The association of multiple enchondromas with soft tissue hemangiomas is known as Maffucci's syndrome (Fig. 1019). In both conditions, there is a significant risk of malignant transformation in the form of chondrosarcoma.[89, 90] Enchondromas of the rib and long bones are distinctly unusual, although we have seen several examples. A variant of the latter, presenting in the metaphysis of long bones, is characterized by massive calcification within the neoplasm.[91] Rarely, chondromas arise in a juxtacortical (peri-

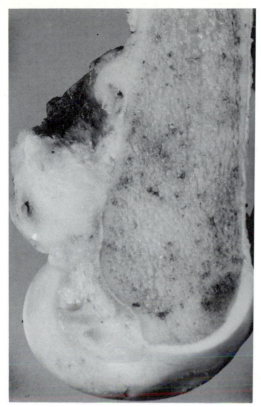

Fig. 1017 Classic juxtacortical osteosarcoma occurring in 57-year-old man. Patient remains well over ten years following amputation. (WU neg. 68-473.)

osteal) area of a long bone or a small bone of the hand and foot.[92] They characteristically erode and induce sclerosis of the contiguous cortex. Recurrence may follow incomplete excision.[93]

Chondromas are composed of lobules of hyaline cartilage which microscopically appear mature. Foci of necrosis, myxoid degeneration, calcification, and endochondral ossification are common. Juxtacortical chondroma tends to be more cellular than its medullary counterpart and may contain occasional plump or double nuclei.

Osteochondroma

The **osteochondroma** is the most frequent benign bone tumor. The most common locations are the lower femur, upper tibia, upper humerus, and pelvis. In forty cases studied at Washington Univer-

sity, the average age of the patient at onset was 10.9 years. In thirty-six cases, the tumor appeared before the patients were 20 years old. The average greatest dimension was 3.7 cm, and the largest tumor measured 8.5 cm. The smaller tumors were sessile and the larger ones pedunculated. All had a cap of cartilage covered by a fibrous membrane continuous with the periosteum of the adjacent bone. The average thickness of the cartilage cap was 0.6 cm (0.1 cm to 3 cm). In only seven cases was the cap thicker than 1 cm. The cartilaginous cap tended to be lobulated in large tumors (Fig. 1020). The gross and microscopic appearance of a single lesion of the familial condition known as osteochondromatosis or multiple cartilaginous exostoses (Ehrenfried's hereditary deforming chondrodysplasia, diaphyseal aclasis) cannot be distinguished from osteochondroma.[95]

Chondroblastoma

Chondroblastoma of bone is often confused with giant cell tumor and chondrosarcoma but is much rarer and bears no relation to these lesions.[100] It was classified in the past with other giant cell tumors as the chondromatous variant.[96]

This tumor occurs particularly in male individuals under 20 years of age. It arises in the epiphyseal end of long bones before epiphyseal cartilage has disappeared, particularly in the femur, humerus, and tibia (Figs. 1021 and 1022). We also have seen it involve small bones of the feet.

Radiographically, the tumor usually is fairly well delimited, contains areas of rarefaction, and may extend from the epiphysis into the metaphyseal areas. Transarticular spread occurred in two of the patients reported by Valls et al.[104] This lesion rarely may recur following curettage.[97]

Microscopically, this lesion often is confusing because of its extreme cellularity and variability. The occasional scattered collections of giant cells may lead to an erroneous diagnosis of giant cell tumor. The basic cell is an embryonic chondroblast without sufficient differentiation to

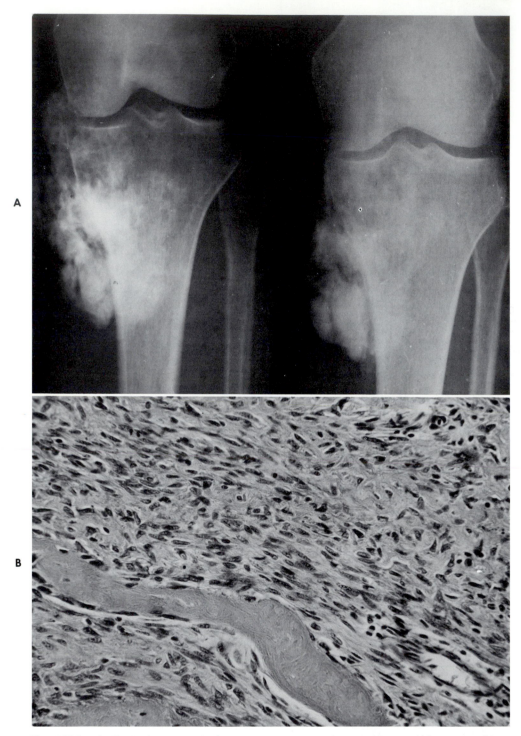

Fig. 1018 **A,** Typical juxtacortical osteosarcoma occurring in 40-year-old woman. Note large extracortical component. **B,** Same lesion shown in **A** demonstrating well-differentiated character of sarcomatous stroma. This lesion had been present for several years. (**A,** WU neg. 57-5271; **B,** WU neg. 58-3094.)

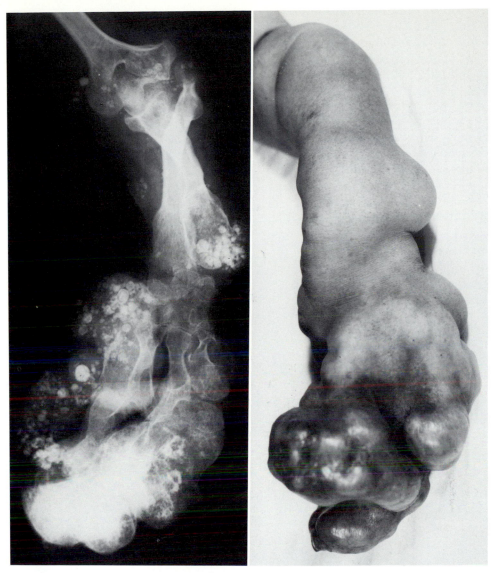

Fig. 1019 Arm of patient affected by Maffucci's syndrome. Innumerable chondromas are seen concentrated in distal aspect of extremity. Patient developed chondrosarcoma in innominate bone, with pulmonary metastases. (Courtesy Dr. O. Urteaga A., Lima, Peru.)

produce intercellular chondroid.[98] The shape is usually polyhedral, although spindle elements also can be present. The cell membrane is thick and sharply defined. The nuclei vary in shape from round to indented and lobulated, a feature emphasized by Levine and Bensch.[102] Mitoses are exceptional. Intracytoplasmic glycogen granules are present, sometimes in large numbers. Reticulin fibers surround each individual cell. Recurrent lesions may show some degree of atypia, a feature that needs not to be interpreted as a sign of malignant change.

The distinctive microscopic changes are small zones of focal calcification (Fig. 1023). These zones range from faintly discernible bluish areas to obvious deposits surrounded by giant cells. This lesion can be distinguished from giant cell tumor by these focal areas of calcification and the absence of the characteristic stroma of giant cell tumors. By electron microscopy, the cells of chondroblastoma closely resemble those of normal epiphyseal cartilage cells grown in tissue culture.[105] They often have a prominent "fibrous lamina" lying against the inner aspect of the nuclear membrane, this resulting in the membrane thickening seen by light microscopy.[99] A portion of a chondroblastoma cell from the humerus showing scattered glycogen particles and sparse cytoplasmic organelles is shown in Fig. 1024. In 24% of the cases reported by Huvos et al.,[99] areas resembling aneurysmal bone cyst were seen engrafted on the primary bone lesion. In patients with recurrent lesions, the incidence rose to 50%.

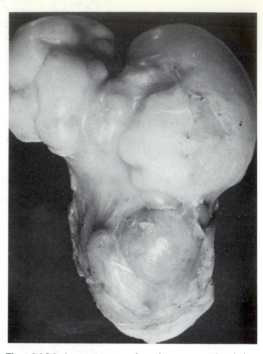

Fig. 1020 Large osteochondroma with lobulated cartilaginous cap. (WU neg. 51-3690.)

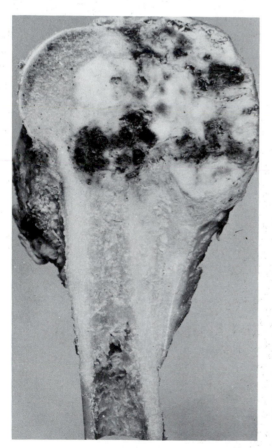

Fig. 1021 Well-outlined chondroblastoma involving epiphysis of humerus in young adult. (WU neg. 57-863; gross specimen contributed by Dr. A. J. Ramos, Manila, Philippines.)

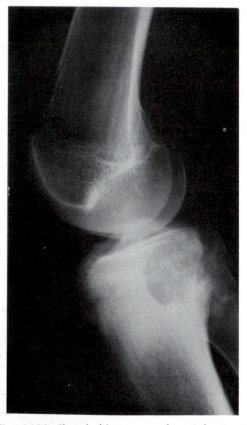

Fig. 1022 Chondroblastoma of epiphysis of tibia in young man. (WU neg. 59-3188.)

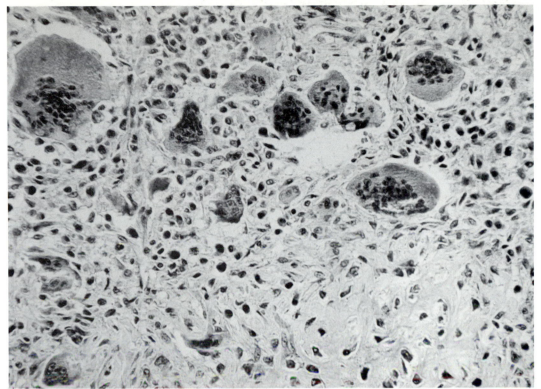

Fig. 1023 Chondroblastoma showing small cuboidal tumor cells, osteoclasts, and areas of chondroid differentiation. (WU neg. 66-9185.)

Levine and Bensch[102] have provided convincing histochemical and ultrastructural support for the truly cartilaginous nature of the basic tumor cells of chondroblastoma.

Clinically, patients with this lesion have pain that may become severe. Curettement is the indicated treatment. We have now seen several cases of chondroblastoma behaving locally in an aggressive fashion, invading the soft tissues and developing tumor thrombi in lymphatic channels. Most of them were located in the innominate bone. In addition, we have seen a chondroblastoma of the femur resulting in widespread visceral metastases.[101] Two instances of malignant change in chondroblastoma were recorded by Schajowicz and Gallardo.[103] Careful study of the primary lesion in our cases failed to show any characteristics that would permit them to be differentiated from other ordinary chondroblastomas.

Chondromyxoid fibroma

Chondromyxoid fibroma of bone is an unusual benign tumor of cartilaginous origin, often confused with chondrosarcoma.[107] The tumors usually occur in young adults, often in a long bone, but they also have been reported in the small bones of the hands and feet, pelvis, ribs, and vertebrae.

This lesion may become large and radiographically is sharply defined (Fig. 1025). It is solid, has a yellowish white or tan color, replaces bone, and thins the cortex. It is highly cellular, has a myxoid matrix, and contains areas suggesting cartilage and often giant cells (Fig. 1026). A lobular pattern can be discerned grossly and microscopically. It is formed by intersecting bands of fibrous tissue lined on the sides by an increased concentration of tumor cells. The occasional presence of large pleomorphic cells may result in an erroneous diagnosis of chondrosarcoma.[109]

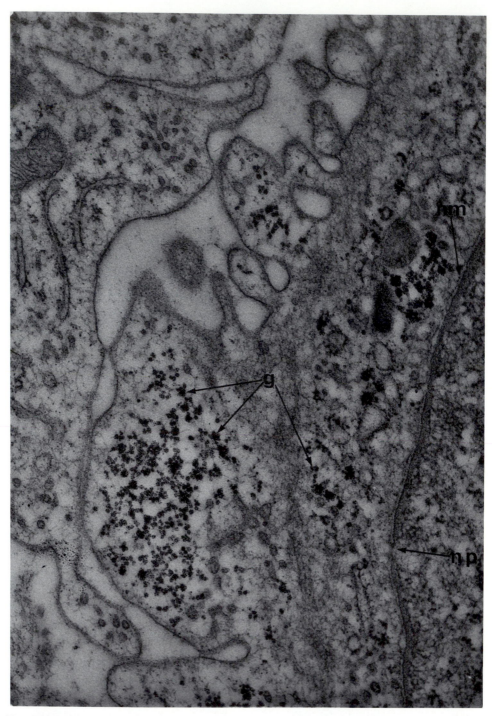

Fig. 1024 Portion of chondroblast from patient with chondroblastoma of humerus. Dense particulate material in cytoplasm is glycogen, **g.** Abnormal density is present beneath inner nuclear membrane, **nm,** and nuclear pore, **np,** can be readily seen at tip of arrow. (Lead stained; ×38,000; courtesy Dr. H. J. Spjut, Houston, Texas.)

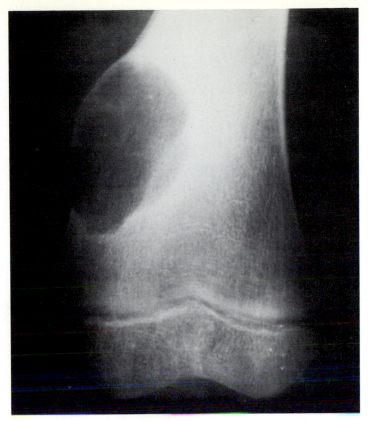

Fig. 1025 Sharply delimited chondromyxoid fibroma of lower femoral metaphysis in young boy. (WU neg. 65-779.)

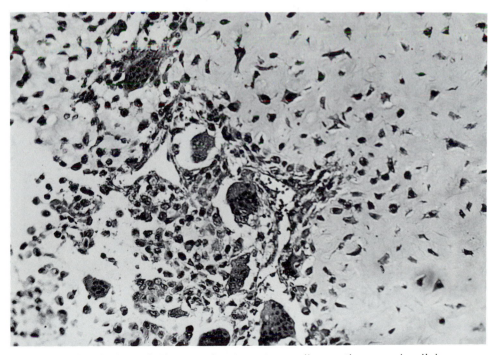

Fig. 1026 Chondromyxoid fibroma showing giant cells, cartilage, and cellular zones. (×200; WU neg. 54-1345.)

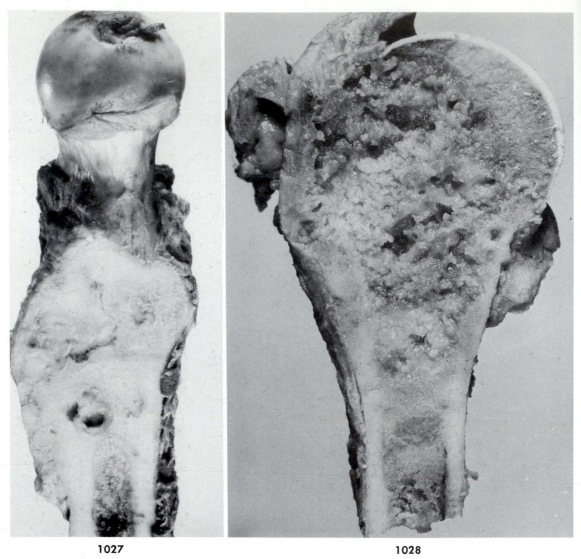

1027   1028

Fig. 1027 Chondromyxoid fibroma of proximal femur extending into soft tissue. This rare event should not be regarded as evidence of malignancy. (WU neg. 72-6210.)
Fig. 1028 Chondrosarcoma of head of humerus. (WU neg. 54-5003.)

However, mitotic figures are exceptional. We have seen several tumors showing a combination of the features of chondroblastoma and chondromyxoid fibroma.[106]

Local recurrence follows curettage in about 25% of the cases. Because of this, en bloc excision is regarded as the treatment of choice whenever possible. Soft tissue extension may occur, but we have never seen instances of distant metastases (Fig. 1027).

A tumor probably representing a variant of chondromyxoid fibroma occurring in older individuals was designated as *fibromyxoma* by Marcove et al.[108]

Chondrosarcoma

Chondrosarcoma is differentiated from osteosarcoma by the lack of osteoid or bone formation by the tumor cells. Bone can be present in a bona fide chondrosarcoma, but this is nonneoplastic and prob-

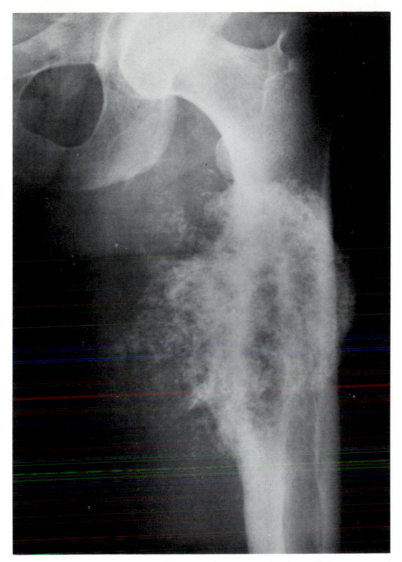

Fig. 1029 Typical chondrosarcoma of femur showing splotchy calcification and extensive cortical destruction. (WU neg. 61-6356.)

ably originates from reabsorption of the tumor cartilage by a mechanism of endochondral ossification. The distinction is important not only because of distinctive gross and microscopic differences, but also because of their better prognosis. The majority of the patients are between 30 and 60 years of age. Chondrosarcoma in childhood is distinctly uncommon. Most malignant bone tumors in this age group exhibiting cartilage formation are actually osteosarcomas with a predominant cartilaginous component. Most chon-

drosarcomas are located in the central portion of a bone (Fig. 1028). Radiographically, they present a rather characteristic picture of an osteolytic lesion with splotchy calcification (Fig. 1029). Ill-defined margins, fusiform thickening of the shaft, and perforation of the cortex are three important diagnostic signs.[110] In advanced stages, they may break through the cortex but only rarely grow beyond the periosteum. The pelvic bones, ribs (usually at the costochondral junction), and shoulder girdle are the commonest locations. The overwhelming majority of the central chondrosarcomas arise *de novo* rather than from a preexisting chondroma. Enchondromas of hands and feet, with the exception of the os calcis, practically never undergo malignant change.[110, 114] In our experience, the large majority of the central cartilaginous tumors of long bones and ribs behave in a malignant fashion.

Peripheral chondrosarcomas may arise de novo or from the cartilaginous cap of a preexisting osteochondroma. Multiple osteochondromatosis is particularly prone to this complication (three out of twenty-eight patients reported by Jaffe[113] and three out of seven patients seen by us). In the 212 cases of chondrosarcoma reported by Dahlin and Henderson,[112] nineteen apparently arose from osteochondroma. The risk of malignant transformation in a solitary osteochondroma is less than 5%. The signs of malignancy in an osteochondroma include increased growth during adolescence, a diameter over 8 cm, and a cartilaginous cap thicker than 3 cm. The average thickness of the caps of benign osteochondromas examined at Barnes Hospital was 0.6 cm, the thickest measuring 3 cm. Conversely, and with only one exception, the caps of chondrosarcomas were all thicker than 2 cm. The greatest diameter of the peripheral chondrosarcomas examined by us varied from 8 cm to 25 cm (Fig. 1030). Radiographically, peripheral chondrosarcomas present as large tumors, with a heavily calcified center surrounded by a lesser denser periphery with splotchy calcification (Fig. 1031).

The diagnosis of well-differentiated chondrosarcoma may not be made for such reasons as a long history of growth, lack of follow-up, and the failure of the pathologist to recognize the subtle microscopic changes that indicate a malignant cartilaginous tumor.

The microscopic diagnosis rests on the identification of abnormal nuclei in cartilage cells.[115] The nuclei are plump, atypical, and at times multinucleated (Fig. 1032). Areas near the growing edge are particu-

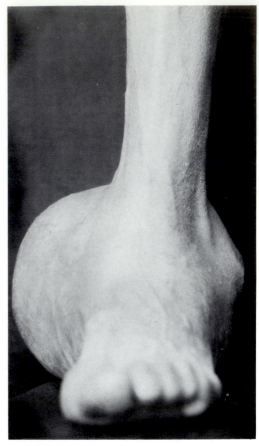

Fig. 1030 Large peripheral chondrosarcoma of os calcis in 36-year-old man. Tumor was of long duration. Patient finally came to clinic because he could no longer put on shoe.

larly diagnostic. Rarely, a poorly differentiated spindle cell component resembling fibrosarcoma or osteosarcoma is seen at the periphery of otherwise typical low-grade chondrosarcomas. This change can occur in the primary lesion or, more commonly, in the recurrent tissue. Dahlin and Beabout[111] found this phenomenon, which they call "dedifferentiation," in thirty-three of 370 well-differentiated chondrosarcomas that they examined. The prognosis was considerably worse than in the tumors lacking this component.

Frequently the statement is made that a benign central cartilaginous tumor became malignant or that it recurred. We have had the opportunity of examining tissue on two or more occasions over periods of five

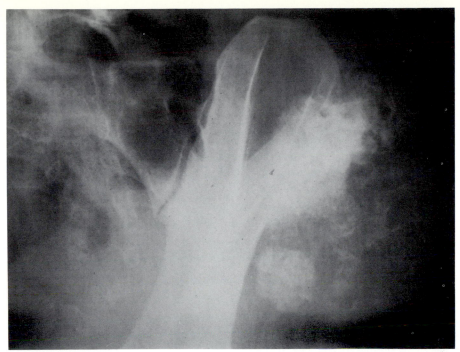

Fig. 1031 Typical radiographic appearance of peripheral chondrosarcoma of innominate bone. (WU neg. 66-766; courtesy Dr. W. T. Hill, Houston, Texas.)

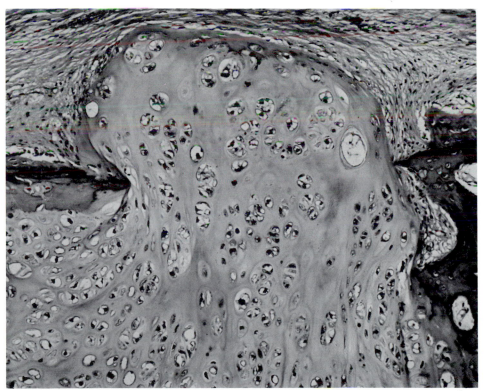

Fig. 1032 Bizarre and "plump" nuclei in rather well-differentiated chondrosarcoma from pelvis. This histologic section also shows tumor protruding through cortical bone into surrounding soft tissues. This pattern and lobular pattern seen grossly illustrate danger of enucleating these tumors. Persistent tumor is almost inevitable. (×125; WU neg. 58-3091; courtesy Dr. M. Ernest, Moose Jaw, Saskatchewan, Canada.)

months to twelve years from sixteen patients subjected to repeated operations for recurrences. *In none of these was the initial tumor clearly benign.* We believe, therefore, that in these instances the pathologist diagnosed the initial tumor incorrectly.

There is good correlation between poor differentiation, rapid growth rate, and metastases. The poorly differentiated tumors and those with elevated mitotic count metastasize early, usually to the lungs. Bloodstream invasion is particularly ominous. We have seen lymph node metastases (axillary) on only one occasion.

The correlation of the microscopic features with the clinical and radiographic findings is important in all bone tumors, but in the case of the cartilaginous neoplasms *it is essential.* Large tumors of long bones or ribs or those which begin to grow rapidly over adolescence and reach a size of 8 cm or more are almost invariably malignant.[117] Minor degrees of atypia in the cartilaginous cells under these circumstances justify a diagnosis of chondrosarcoma, whereas similar or even greater atypical changes in cartilaginous tumors of the hands and feet, osteochondromas, synovial osteochondromatosis, and soft tissue neoplasms are much less significant.[115] It also should be noted that the minor atypical changes on which the diagnosis of malignancy are based are often focal, a point to remember when examining a small sample of a cartilaginous neoplasm.

Soft tissue implantation following biopsy is a well known property of chondrosarcoma. Therefore, if a large cartilaginous tumor is so located that the biopsy site cannot be entirely excised, the initial surgery should be radical. If an extremely large tumor involves the pelvic bone, wide block excision or even hemipelvectomy is justified without prior histologic diagnosis. About 90% of the patients cured by hemipelvectomy had the operation for chondrosarcoma.[119] Chondrosarcomas of the rib should be excised radically, with removal of adjacent uninvolved ribs and the pleura en bloc with the lesion.[117, 118]

In contrast to what is seen in osteosarcoma, microscopic grading of chondrosarcomas is of value in predicting the final outcome. In the series reported by McKenna et al.,[116] the five-year survival rates were 78%, 53%, and 22% for low-grade, moderate-grade, and high-grade tumors, respectively.

We have seen a few examples of a malignant tumor of extravertebral bones and soft tissues with a microscopic appearance that closely resembles that of chordoma.[115a] It probably represents a variant of chondrosarcoma.

Mesenchymal chondrosarcoma

A specific variant of chondrosarcoma, mesenchymal chondrosarcoma is characterized microscopically by a dimorphic pattern, areas of well-differentiated cartilage alternating with undifferentiated stroma.[120, 123] The boundaries between the two components are usually abrupt. The undifferentiated element can be confused with malignant lymphoma and hemangiopericytoma. It should be noted that despite the apparently undifferentiated nature of this component, pleomorphism and mitotic activity are remarkably inconspicuous.[123] The flat bones are those most commonly affected. A significant number of these neoplasms involve extraosseous structures, such as the orbit, paraspinal region, meninges, or soft tissues of extremities.[121, 122] The prognosis is generally poor, although there is great variability in the clinical course.[123]

Giant cell tumor

Giant cell tumor is usually seen in patients over 20 years of age.[127] It is more common in women than in men. The classical location is the epiphysis of a long bone, from which it may spread into the metaphyseal area, break through the cortex, invade intermuscular septa, or even cross a joint space.[133] The sites most commonly affected, in order of frequency, are the lower end of the femur, the upper end of the tibia, and the lower end of the

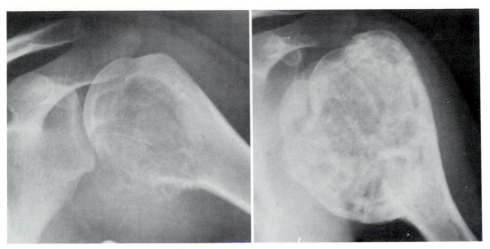

Fig. 1033 Giant cell tumor of upper end of humerus in 20-year-old girl who refused treatment. There was interval of nineteen months between x-ray films. (WU negs. 48-6970 and 48-6971.)

radius. Naturally, exceptions occur. For instance, we have seen giant cell tumors in the metaphysis of the radius in two children in the absence of epiphyseal involvement. We also have seen giant cell tumors in the patella, fibula, humerus, and sphenoid bone[125] (Fig. 1033). Involvement of the bones of the hands and feet, jaw, and vertebrae (other than sacrum) is distinctly unusual.

Giant cell tumors thin the cortex of the bone but only rarely produce periosteal bone formation. On section, they contain loculated spaces transversed by fibrous trabeculae (Fig. 1034). Areas of hemorrhage are frequent within them. They may be small or large. If they become large in long bones, fractures may follow.

X-ray examinations often show changes purported to be diagnostic. However, we have seen lesions diagnosed as giant cell tumors that proved to be plasma cell myeloma, fibrosarcoma, or chondrosarcoma. Whether a giant cell tumor is benign or malignant cannot be determined radiographically.

Microscopically, the giant cell tumor is mainly composed of two components, stromal cells and giant cells. Osteoid or bone, apparently of a reactive nature, is seen in one-third of the cases. The giant cells often are large and have many nuclei (twenty or

thirty are usual) that frequently occupy the center of the cell. The prominence of the giant cells gives the tumor its name. However, it is likely that the so-called stromal cells are the basic tumor elements. It is their relative number and appearance that correlate with the clinical evolution, not those of the giant cells. Therefore, the microscopic evaluation of a given giant cell tumor depends on careful study of the stromal cells. In the obvious malignant tumor, the stroma shows increased cellularity and mitotic activity.[132]

It is imperative that several sections of curettings be examined. We have had a giant cell tumor in which the original sections of the curettings showed no malignant tumor, but in time this tumor recurred, invaded the soft tissue, and metastasized to the lungs as a fibrosarcoma. Only two sections had been made of the initial curettings. Further sections of them showed malignant tumor in the primary lesion (Fig. 1035). Unfortunately, this lesion may appear to be entirely benign histologically, yet metastasize and kill.[124] The metastases in these instances may also appear to be cytologically benign. Except for the obviously sarcomatous (Grade III) lesions, microscopic grading of these neoplasms is of little practical value. Instead,

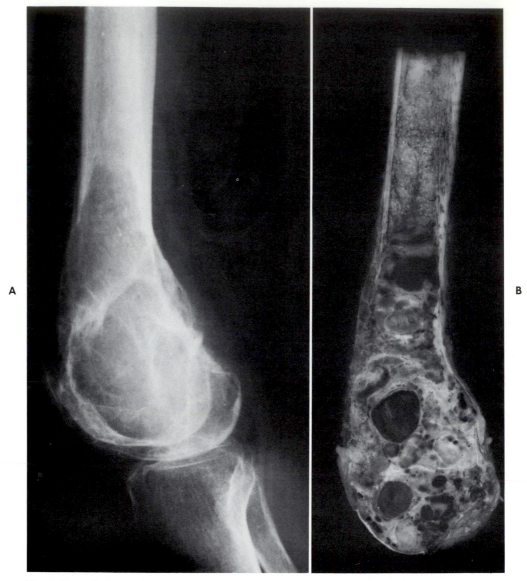

Fig. 1034 **A,** Typical roentgenogram of giant cell tumor of distal end of femur involving epiphysis and metaphyseal area. Lesion was resected surgically. **B,** Gross specimen that faithfully reproduces roentgenographic changes. (From Sissons, H. A.: Malignant tumours of bone and cartilage. In Raven, R. W., editor: Cancer, vol. 2, London, 1958, Butterworth & Co., Ltd.)

we regard all giant cell tumors as potentially malignant in view of the fact that as many as 50% of them recur after curettage and approximately 10% give rise to distant metastases.

Many benign pathologic lesions with giant cells have been called giant cell tumors. These lesions include such diverse entities as metaphyseal fibrous defect, chondromyxoid fibroma, chondroblastoma, eosinophilic granuloma, solitary bone cyst, osteitis fibrosa cystica of hyperparathyroidism, aneurysmal bone cyst, and osteoid osteoma. So-called giant cell tumors of tendon sheath are not related to giant cell tumors of bone. One of the main microscopic differences between true giant cell tumor and these so-called variants re-

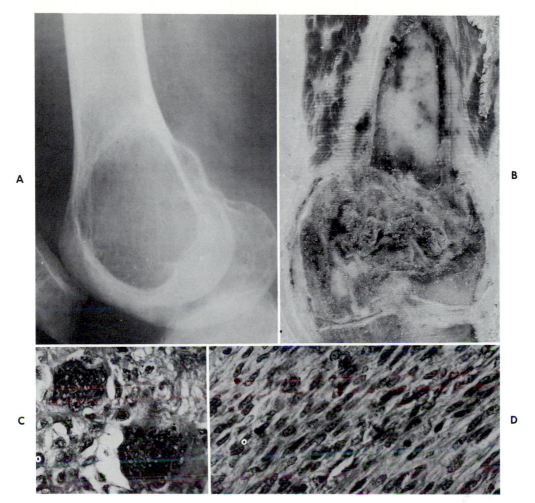

Fig. 1035   A, Giant cell tumor of distal end of femur. Lesion was curetted and replaced with bone chips. **B,** Giant cell tumor shown in **A** recurred, necessitating amputation.
Gross specimen demonstrates bone chips still in place with tumor replacing femur. Review
of original sections showed benign giant cell tumor, but recuts of curetted material
demonstrated malignant stroma. **C,** Original section of curettings referred to in **B** showing
areas of rather innocuous-appearing stroma with typical multinucleated giant cells.
These changes were called benign. **D,** Later tissue section of malignant giant cell tumor
referred in **B** and **C** that has appearance of fibrosarcoma. There was no evidence of
osteoid formation. Patient died of pulmonary metastases. (**A,** WU neg. 49-5963; **B,** WU
neg. 50-663; **C,** high power; WU neg. 51-1535; **D,** ×460; WU neg. 50-3550.)

sides in the spatial relationship between
giant and stromal cells. They tend to be
distributed regularly and uniformly in giant
cell tumor, whereas in the lesions that
simulate it, foci of numerous, clumped
giant cells alternate with large areas completely lacking this component. It also
should be remembered that nearly all multifocal giant cell lesions are other than

giant cell tumors. The inclusion of the
aforementioned entities has been responsible for the high cure rates reported in
the past. Histochemical studies unfortunately are of no aid in differentiating giant
cell tumor from its so-called variants.[130]

Willis[132a] and many of the English school
believe that the giant cells are osteoclasts
and that the tumors should be designated

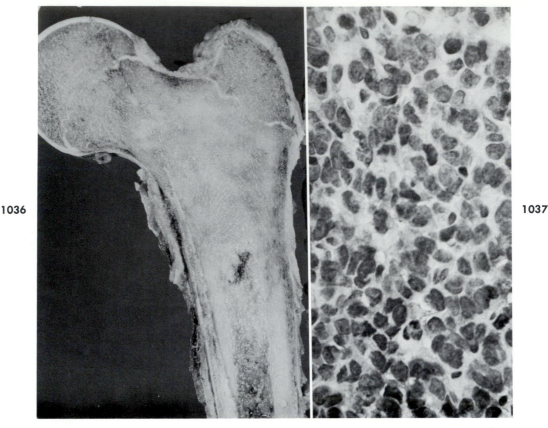

1036

1037

Fig. 1036 Resected end of femur involved by Ewing's sarcoma. Note complete replacement of marrow cavity and prominent cortical thickening. Microscopically, destruction and invasion of epiphysis were present. (WU neg. 50-1409.)

Fig. 1037 Ewing's sarcoma with uniform cells, inconspicuous cytoplasm, and no osteoid. (×600; WU neg. 51-294.)

as osteoclastomas. Electron microscopic and histochemical studies have confirmed the close similarity, if not identity, between the giant cell of this tumor and the osteoclast.[126, 131] On the other hand, the ultrastructural appearance of the stromal cells is suggestive of either a fibroblastic or osteoblastic derivation. If a giant cell lesion occurs in the maxilla or mandible or in some atypical location such as the small bones of the hand, a parathyroid adenoma must be suspected. We have seen three patients with functioning parathyroid adenomas seek medical care initially for giant cell lesions in the small bones of the fingers. In most reported series, the incidence of clinical malignancy in giant cell tumors is in the range of 10%.[124, 129] The

incidence of recurrence within the bone after curettage is much higher. Therefore, we recommend excision en bloc of the entire lesion, whenever possible, as the treatment of choice. Special care should be taken to prevent implantation of the tumor into the adjoining soft tissues.[128] Irradiation therapy is indicated for giant cell tumors located in areas not amenable to resection.

Marrow tumors
Ewing's sarcoma

Ewing's tumor of bone occurs in children and in adults under 30 years of age, most patients being between the ages of 5 and 20 years. This tumor occurs most often in the long bones (femur, tibia, humerus, and fibula) and in bones of the pelvis, rib, vertebra, mandible, and clavicle. It arises in the medullary canal of the shaft, from which it permeates the cortex and invades the soft tissues. We have now seen several cases of Ewing's sarcoma presenting clinically as soft tissue neoplasms with a normal roentgenographic appearance of the underlying bone. Microscopic examination of these cases revealed that the tumor originated in the medullary canal and had diffusely permeated the marrow spaces to extend outside the bone without destroying a significant amount of bone trabeculae and thus remaining undetectable by conventional radiographic examination. The first radiographic changes are cortical thickening and widening of the medullary canal. With progress of the lesion, reactive periosteal bone may be deposited in layers parallel to the cortex (onionskin appearance) or at right angles to it (sun-ray appearance)[141] (Fig. 1036). The radiographic appearance is not diagnostic.

Microscopically, Ewing's tumor consists of solid sheets of cells divided into irregular masses by fibrous strands. Individual cells are uniform with round nuclei, small nucleoli, and inconspicuous cytoplasmic outlines (Fig. 1037). The tumor is fairly well vascularized. It often contains cellular areas with necrosis, and the tumor cells may be grouped around blood vessels, producing a false rosette. This tumor does not form reticulin or osteoid. The glycogen stain is positive. This is not the case in neuroblastoma and histiocytic malignant lymphoma[140] (Fig. 1038).

The histogenesis of Ewing's sarcoma is still undecided. Recent tissue culture and ultrastructural studies favor the hypothesis of an origin from primitive marrow elements (the so-called reticular cells).[134, 135, 137]

Willis[141a] correctly pointed out that metastatic neuroblastoma may easily be confused with primary Ewing's tumor both roentgenographically and microscopically. Features that can be used for the differential diagnosis between these two neoplasms are indicated in Table 47.

Ewing's tumor can also be confused with undifferentiated carcinoma, malignant lymphoma, or even eosinophilic granuloma.

Clinically, Ewing's sarcoma in a young adult may simulate osteomyelitis because of the pain, disability, fever, and leukocytosis. The lesion is highly radiosensitive. The spread of this tumor is to the lungs and to other bones, particularly those of the skull.

Conventional treatment with surgery or radiation therapy resulted in the past in five-year survival rates of 5% to 8%. Recent series in which adjuvant therapy was employed have dramatically improved this gloomy outlook. Irradiation followed by chemotherapy is being presently used.[136, 138] A 24% five-year survival rate was obtained in fifty-four children reviewed by Phillips and Higinbotham.[139]

Malignant lymphoma

Malignant lymphoma of bone is a definite entity.[146] About 60% of the patients are over 30 years of age, although the tumors do occur in younger persons. The sex distribution is about equal.

Table 47 Differential features between Ewing's sarcoma and metastatic neuroblastoma

	Ewing's sarcoma	Metastatic neuroblastoma
Age	Most patients between 5 and 20 yr	Most patients under 3 yr
Number of lesions when first seen	Usually solitary	Usually multiple
Glycogen	Present; often abundant	Absent
Tissue culture	Grows as undifferentiated cells	Grows neurites in 24-48 hr
Electron microscopy[134, 135]	Undifferentiated cells; abundant glycogen	Neural processes; junctional complexes; neurosecretory granules
Urinary catecholamine derivatives	Normal	Almost always elevated

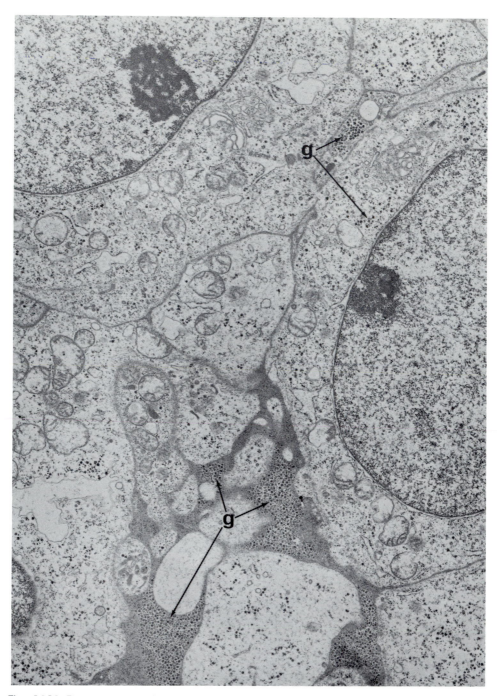

Fig. 1038 Fine structure of neoplastic cells in Ewing's sarcoma is distinct from that of malignant lymphoma of histiocytic and lymphocytic (Fig. 954) types. Accumulations of glycogen, **g**, are numerous. These are readily demonstrable in paraffin sections by use of PAS reaction with and without diastase digestion. (Lead citrate; approximately ×9,000.)

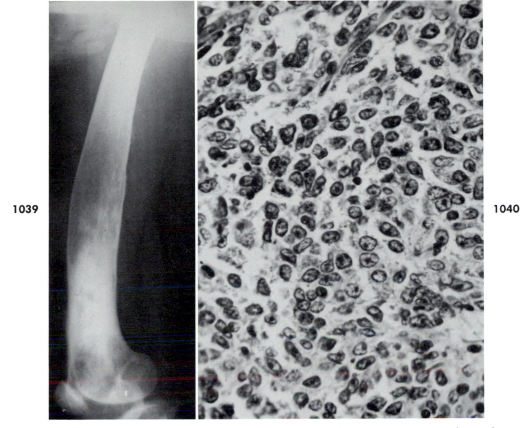

1039   1040

Fig. 1039 Malignant lymphoma involving lower end of femur demonstrating bone destruction and bone production. Such lesions are often erroneously diagnosed as chronic osteomyelitis. (WU neg. 49-4628.)
Fig. 1040 Malignant lymphoma of histiocytic type. Note large cells with prominent nucleoli. Reticulin was present. (×600; WU neg. 50-3840.)

Grossly, this tumor involves the shaft or metaphysis of the bone, producing cortical and medullary destruction. The destruction within the bone is patchy and associated with minimal to moderate periosteal reaction, usually of the lamellated type. The tumor is pinkish gray and granular, and it frequently extends into the soft tissues and invades the muscle. Lichtenstein[145] commented on a case invading the joint space.

Radiographically, a combination of bone production and bone destruction often involves a wide area of a long bone (Fig. 1039). This combination of changes is very suggestive of the diagnosis.[147] However, osteosarcoma and chronic osteomyelitis may result in a very similar appearance.

Microscopically, most malignant lymphomas presenting as primary bone tumors are of the histiocytic type (reticulum cell sarcoma) or mixed cell (histiocytic-lymphocytic) type. The main source of difficulty resides in their separation from Ewing's sarcoma. Malignant lymphoma has larger reticulum-like cells which may exhibit phagocytosis. The nuclei are somewhat pleomorphic; many are indented or horseshoe-shaped. They usually have prominent nucleoli, unlike the fine nucleoli of Ewing's sarcoma (Fig. 1040). Cytoplasmic outlines of histiocytic lymphoma are well defined, whereas those of Ewing's tumor are indistinct. The cytoplasm is more abundant and often eosinophilic. Reticulin is between individual cells and groups of cells, whereas in Ewing's sarcoma it is mainly restricted to the perivascular areas. Classically, malignant lymphoma of bone has been regarded as a tumor of better prognosis than Ewing's sarcoma, five-year survival rates varying from 22% to 50% in several series.[144, 148, 151] With recent improvements in the treatment of Ewing's sarcoma, this difference has narrowed considerably.

Hodgkin's disease produces radiographically detectable bone lesions in approximately 15% of the cases. In Horan's series,[143] the involvement was multifocal in 60%. The most frequent sites were the vertebrae, pelvis, ribs, sternum, and femur. Radiographically, the foci may be osteolytic, mixed, or purely osteoblastic. The latter appearance is particularly common in vertebrae.

Acute leukemia of childhood is associated with radiographic abnormalities in the skeletal system in 70% to 90% of the cases.[150] In the large majority of the instances, the changes are widespread and therefore unlikely to be confused with a primary bone neoplasm.[149] In contrast, destructive bone lesions are extremely rare in the chronic leukemias. Chabner et al.[142] reported six cases in a series of 205 patients with chronic granulocytic leukemia. In three of the patients, the bone lesion appeared at the time of blastic transformation.

Plasma cell myeloma

The pathologic expressions of plasma cell tumors are many.[152] Disseminated myeloma is the most frequent. It occurs slightly more often in men than in women. It usually occurs between 40 and 60 years of age, rarely before the age of 30 years. The tumor, when disseminated, produces osteolytic lesions in the vertebrae, pelvis, ribs, sternum, and skull. Under these circumstances, the life expectancy is usually less than two years. In advanced disease, extraskeletal spread may be seen. Most of the cases are confined to the soft tissues adjacent to bones involved by myeloma, but

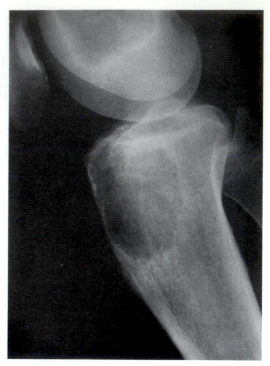

Fig. 1041 Osteolytic lesion of upper end of tibia due to localized lesion of plasma cell myeloma. Such lesion has osteolytic appearance of metastatic carcinoma. (WU neg. 50-417.)

distant metastases to the spleen, liver, lymph nodes, and kidney also can occur.[160]

Plasma cell tumors may first appear clinically in the soft tissue. The most frequent extraosseous locations are the nasopharynx, nose, and tonsil. We have seen these tumors in such areas as the mediastinum, skin, and lymph nodes. Rarely, plasma cell tumors occur with the clinical and hematologic manifestations of a leukemia.[159]

The majority of the lesions initially of soft tissue eventually become disseminated in bone. Christopherson and Miller[155] collected all the apparently localized cases of plasma cell tumors. Only five of the entire group still had localized disease after a ten-year follow-up. Of the ninety-two tumors reported by Carson et al.,[154] only one could be considered to be possibly localized. Kotner and Wang[157] analyzed twenty cases of plasmacytomas of the upper air and food passages, most of which had

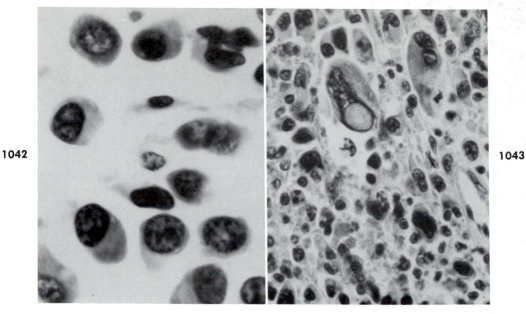

1042　　　　　　　　　　　　　　　　　　　　　　　　　　　　1043

Fig. 1042 Well-differentiated plasma cell tumor showing plasma cells with eccentric nuclei and characteristic arrangement of chromatin. (High power; WU neg. 50-228.)
Fig. 1043 Highly undifferentiated plasma cell tumor with tumor giant cells. (×600; WU neg. 50-3224.)

been treated aggressively by radiation therapy. They remarked that if systemic disease develops in a patient with soft tissue plasmacytoma, it may occur many years later and even then run a prolonged course.

Bones involved by plasma cell tumors often fracture. The tissue is hemorrhagic and cellular (Fig. 1041). The focal, slowly growing tumor may have a fairly well-defined border, is grayish yellow, homogeneous, and firm.

Microscopically, an obvious well-differentiated plasma cell tumor grows in sheets separated by fine trabeculae that are seen well by reticulin stain. We agree with Lichtenstein and Jaffe[158] that myeloma should not be divided into subvarieties and that the neoplasm arises from a single cell type, the plasma cell and its precursors.

Plasma cells are commonly found in chronic inflammatory conditions. They are particularly common within the oral cavity. The mere presence of large numbers of plasma cells should not be diagnosed as plasma cell tumor. The plasma cells of a granulomatous process are well differentiated and often contain Russell bodies (aggregates of eosinophilic material in the cytoplasm). Other chronic inflammatory cells will be interspersed between the abundant plasma cells. Such plasma cell granulomas may become large enough to be mistaken for a true neoplasm. Certainly, the lesions of the conjunctiva are granulomas, and we have seen other plasmacytic granulomas in the oral cavity, mediastinum, lung, stomach, kidney, testis, and bone. The importance of the differentiation of this granuloma from plasma cell myeloma is obvious.

Plasma cell tumors may be highly undifferentiated and difficult to identify. They may even have the pattern of histiocytic malignant lymphoma (Figs. 1042 and 1043). However, careful examination of many fields invariably reveals small zones of recognizable plasma cells. The well-differentiated plasma cell has an eccentric nucleus, a cartwheel arrangement of the chromatin, and often two nuclei. Electron microscopic study may provide the diagnosis in controversial cases.[161] Unfortunately, there seems to be no correlation between the ultrastructural appearance of the tumor cells and the type of immunoglobulin being secreted.[156]

Thorough study of a patient with an apparently single lesion of bone often demonstrates it to be only a localized manifestation of a disseminated process. Trephine biopsy of the sternal marrow is particularly important, for it may show increased plasma cells in the marrow. This finding often is present in the face of otherwise normal skeletal series, serum proteins, electrophoretic pattern of serum proteins, and absence of Bence Jones protein. Long-time follow-up, particularly of all localized lesions, is mandatory. In the patient referred to in Fig. 1041, the local lesion was treated and sterilized by irradiation and the defect replaced by bone chips. At that time, all laboratory and x-ray examinations were normal except for slight elevation of the plasma cells in the sternal marrow. The patient was still working eight years later but had disseminated disease evidenced by massive replacement of the sternal marrow by plasma cells. This patient illustrates the effectiveness of irradiation therapy in controlling localized lesions as well as the fact that patients with myeloma may live well over five years.

In a series of 112 patients studied by Carbone et al.,[153] 87% had a detectable protein abnormality. IgG proteins were found in 61%, IgA in 18%, and light chains only (Bence Jones protein) in 9%. Of the ninety patients with abnormal serum proteins, 69% had type kappa and 31% type lambda proteins. No association between the presence or type of immunoglobulin abnormality and the survival was encountered.

For a discussion on the clinicopathologic features of tumors associated with dysproteinemia, see p. 980.

Patients with disseminated multiple myeloma due to extensive involvement of the vertebrae and ribs develop a typical hunchback deformity. Rib fractures are frequent, anemia is prominent, and death occurs rather quickly. In one series, death occurred in fifty-seven of sixty patients with disseminated myeloma in the first two years. Thirty-one of these patients died within three months of initial diagnosis.[154] Irradiation therapy may sterilize or operation may eradicate localized lesions of bone. Chlorambucil occasionally gives striking palliation.

Vascular tumors

Hemangiomas of bone are often reported in the vertebra as a postmortem finding. In 2,154 autopsies studied by Töpfer,[170] hemangiomas occurred in 11.9%. They were multiple in 34%. These lesions should probably be regarded as vascular malformations rather than true neoplasms. The most common locations of clinically significant osseous hemangiomas are the skull, vertebrae, and jawbones.[171]

Hemangiomas in the long bones are extremely rare.[162] We have seen cavernous hemangioma of the clavicle and ribs and have observed a lesion of the fibula causing irregular bone destruction in the shaft, that was incorrectly diagnosed as Ewing's tumor. When a lesion involves the flat bones, (particularly the skull), sunburst trabeculation occurs because of elevation of the periosteum. On section, they often have a currant jelly appearance. They do not undergo malignant change. Microscopically, the appearance is classical, with a thick-walled latticelike pattern of endothelial-lined cavernous spaces filled with blood. Bone hemangiomas may be multiple. This rare condition, mainly seen in children, is associated in about half of the cases with cutaneous, soft tissue, or visceral hemangiomas.[168]

Massive osteolysis (Gorham's disease) is probably not a vascular neoplasm but is included in this discussion because of its microscopic similarities with skeletal angiomatosis. It has a destructive character that the latter lacks. It results in reabsorption of a whole bone or several bones and the filling of the residual spaces by a heavily vascularized fibrous tissue.[164, 165]

Glomus tumor of the subungual soft tissues may erode the underlying bone. Much rarer is the occurrence of a purely intraosseous glomus tumor involving the terminal phalanx.[166]

Malignant vascular tumors, which we prefer to designate as *angiosarcoma,* are best divided into two microscopic types that vary in their behavior. Both tend to be multicentric. Low-grade angiosarcoma (sometimes designated as hemangioendothelioma) is characterized by the formation of anastomosing cell cords, some with a central lumen. The tumor cells lining the spaces are prominent but without bizarre cytologic or nuclear features. Ultrastructurally, the large majority of the cells have the appearance of endothelial cells, with only an occasional admixture of pericytes.[169] The clinical course is prolonged, often characterized by repeated local recurrences but no distant metastases.[163, 167] High-grade angiosarcoma has a similar architectural pattern but differs from the low-grade tumor by the obvious atypia of the tumor cells, the formation of solid areas, and the presence of necrotic foci. Distant metastases are common, particularly to the lungs. Before making the diagnosis of high-grade angiosarcoma in a bone lesion, the more common possibilities of well-vascularized osteosarcoma and metastatic carcinoma (particularly of renal origin) should be ruled out.[171]

Lymphangiomas are exceptional. Most cases have multiple osseous involvement and are associated with soft tissue tumors of similar appearance.

Other connective tissue tumors
Desmoplastic fibroma

A rare neoplasm, desmoplastic fibroma is formed by mature fibroblasts separated by abundant collagen.[179] Pleomorphism, necrosis, and mitotic activity are lacking. This lesion probably represents the osseous counterpart of soft tissue fibromatosis. Local recurrences are common, but metastases do not occur.[177]

Fibrosarcoma

Fibrosarcomas of bone are specific neoplasms arising in the metaphyseal area of long bones.[172, 175] Approximately 50% of these occur in the distal segment of the femur or proximal portion of the tibia.[176] They destroy the cortex, are osteolytic, and often extend into the soft tissues. In our experience, fibrosarcomas only rarely arise from the periosteum. The diagnosis of this specific tumor is seldom made radiographically. Only a diagnosis of malignant bone neoplasm is suggested.

Microscopically, this tumor is a fibroblastic neoplasm similar to soft tissue fibrosarcomas (Figs. 1044 and 1045). This tumor is distinct from other bone tumors. We have seen examples in which innumerable sections of the primary tumor and its metastases showed no osteoid formation.

Fibrosarcomas must be treated radically. The rare tumors arising from periosteum have an excellent prognosis. Only one of thirteen reported by Stout[178] metastasized. Fibrosarcomas may arise in an area of bone infarct[174] (Fig. 1046). Extremely well-differentiated fibrosarcomas may be diagnosed as benign lesions of fibrous tissue, but invariably the radiographic appearance suggests its malignant nature. Microscopically, the presence of cellular areas, mitotic figures, hyperchromatism, and pleomorphism are all features that favor a diagnosis of fibrosarcoma over one of desmoplastic fibroma. Fibrosarcoma also should be differentiated from the variety of osteosarcoma mainly composed of fibroblastic elements.[173]

Other primary tumors
Chordoma

Chordoma, a malignant tumor, arises from the remnants of the fetal notochord, which is situated within the vertebral bodies and intervertebral discs and, rarely, in the presacral soft tissues.[181] Most chordomas arise from notochordal rem-

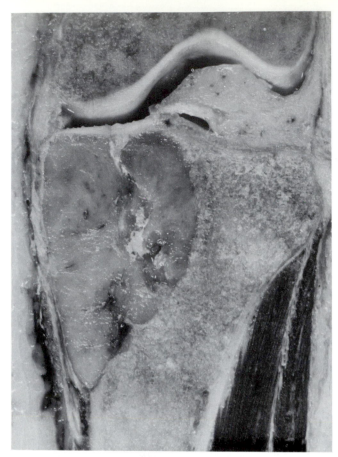

Fig. 1044 Fibrosarcoma of tibia. Lesion produced osteolytic defect and was confused radiographically with giant cell tumor. (WU neg. 57-789.)

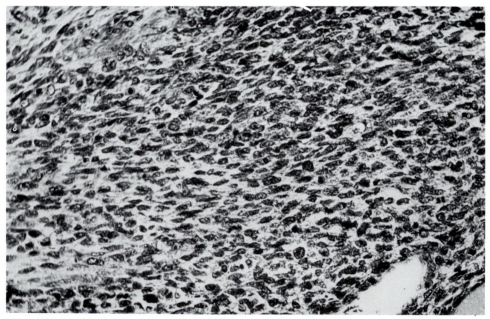

Fig. 1045 Histologic pattern of this cellular, poorly differentiated fibrosarcoma, primary in right femur, is similar to fibrosarcoma of soft tissues. (×275; WU neg. 53-623.)

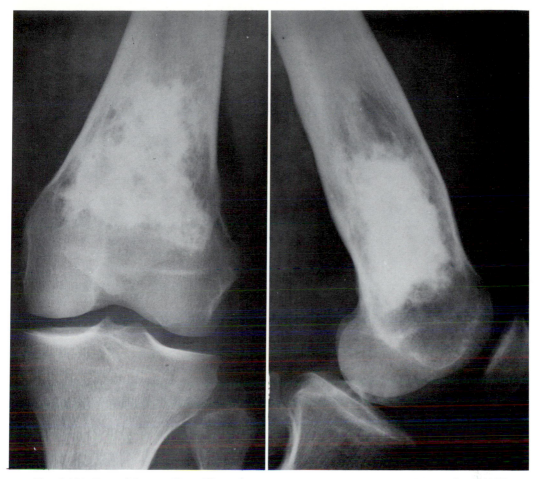

Fig. 1046 Typical bone infarct. These lesions are rare. (WU negs. 59-4049 and 59-4050; courtesy Dr. H. Danziger, Welland, Ontario.)

nants in bone rather than from those located inside the discs. They are more frequent in the fifth and sixth decades but occur at all ages and in both sexes.[184] They grow slowly, the duration of the symptoms before diagnosis usually being over five years. Fifty percent arise in the sacrococcygeal area, 35% in the spheno-occipital area, and the remaining along the cervicothoracolumbar spine.[184a] The sacrococcygeal tumors are more common in the fifth and sixth decades of life, whereas the spheno-occipital neoplasms occur predominantly in children. In the former, a portion of the sacrum is seen destroyed by an osteolytic or rarely an osteoblastic process (Fig. 1047). If the tumor encroaches upon the spine, symptoms of

spinal cord compression arise. The retroperitoneal space is often involved by direct extension. The tumor may grow large enough to narrow the lumen of the large bowel or impinge upon the bladder. It can be felt as a firm extrarectal mass.

Grossly, the chordoma is gelatinous and soft and contains areas of hemorrhage. Microscopically, it closely resembles normal notochord tissue in its different stages of development.[180] It grows in cell cords and lobules separated by a variable amount of mucoid intercellular tissue (Fig. 1048). Some of the tumor cells are extremely large with vacuolated cytoplasm and prominent vesicular nucleus. They are sometimes designated as physaliferous. Some of the vacuoles contain glycogen.[182, 188]

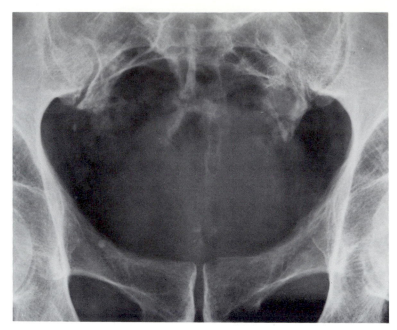

Fig. 1047 Osteolytic destruction of sacrum by chordoma. (WU neg. 52-2398.)

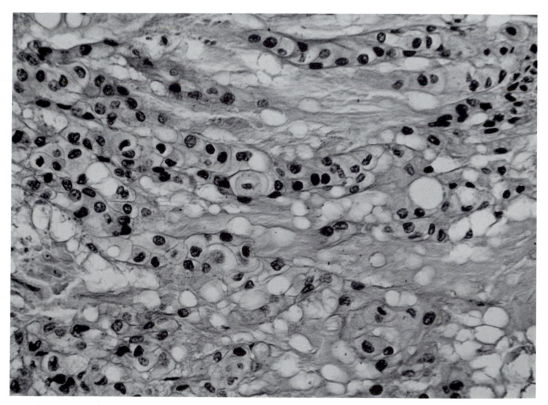

Fig. 1048 Chordoma of spheno-occipital region. Cuboidal and polyhedral cells of central nucleus form rows and nests among abundant myxoid matrix (×350; WU neg. 73-2685; courtesy Dr. J. E. Olvera-Rabiela, Mexico City, Mexico.)

Other tumor cells are small, with small nuclei and no visible nucleoli. Mitotic figures are scanty or absent. Areas of cartilage and bone may be present.[186] In some areas, the tumor may simulate carcinoma or spindle cell sarcoma. The microscopic differential diagnosis has to be made with chondrosarcoma, rectal signet-cell adenocarcinoma, and myxopapillary ependymoma. Erlandson et al.[183] examined three chordomas by electron microscopy and found in each case peculiar mitochondrial-endoplasmic reticulum complexes, an interesting even if nonspecific feature.

The natural history of chordoma is characterized by repeated episodes of local recurrence and an almost uniformly fatal outcome. Distant metastases are usually late in the evolution of the disease. They occurred in 43% of a series of patients reviewed by Higinbotham et al.[185] Total surgical excision is usually impossible. Thus radiation therapy remains as the only practical treatment.[187]

"Adamantinoma" of long bones

A locally aggressive neoplasm, "adamantinoma" occurs predominantly in the tibia but has been reported in other long bones, such as the femur, ulna, and fibula.[190, 192] It may arise in the shaft or in the metaphyseal area of the bone and be associated with a lesion of fibrous dysplasia.[191] Microscopically, several patterns of growth have been described. The most classical is one formed by solid nests of epithelial-appearing cells with palisading at the periphery and sometimes a stellate configuration in the center. Electron microscopic studies of this tumor type have confirmed the epithelial nature of the cells.[189, 193]

What epithelium is doing inside a long bone remains a mystery. A possible explanation is that these tumors originate in deep-seated (very deep seated!) sweat glands. Other tumors reported in the literature as adamantinomas have an altogether different appearance, some resembling vascular neoplasms and other synovial tissues.

It is likely, as Schajowicz and Gallardo[194] suggest, that the term adamantinoma is often applied too loosely to probably unrelated tumors of the tibia having a similar clinicoradiographic appearance.

Bona fide adamantinoma is best treated by amputation, for local recrudescence and even distant metastases may develop.

Neurilemoma

A few instances of intraosseous neurilemoma have been reported.[195] Although Recklinghausen's disease often results in several types of skeletal abnormalities (such as scoliosis, bowing, pseudoarthrosis, and other disorders of growth),[196] intraosseous neurofibromas are virtually nonexistent.

Metastatic tumors

The incidence of osseous metastases varies with the primary neoplasm and the thoroughness of postmortem examination. We are concerned chiefly with those metastatic lesions that may be confused clinically with primary benign or malignant osseous lesions. In most instances of bone metastases, the primary tumor is known. Excluding these, metastatic tumors are still the most frequent of all malignant neoplasms of bone. These lesions are usually osteolytic but may be osteoblastic or mixed. Tumors with a tendency to produce pure osteoblastic metastases are prostatic carcinoma and carcinoid tumor.[201] The bone or bones involved and the character of the changes seen radiographically are helpful in predicting the primary neoplasm. Certain occult primary carcinomas (carcinoma of the thyroid gland and kidney) may develop only a single bone metastasis. They also may manifest single bone metastases many years after removal of the primary neoplasm.

Thyroid carcinoma usually metastasizes to the bones of the shoulder girdle, skull, ribs, and sternum. Carcinoma of the kidney may involve the skull, sternum, flat bones of the pelvis, and upper end of the femur. Both thyroid carcinoma and carcinoma of the kidney produce osteolytic defects. If the tumor extends through the bone into soft tissue, pulsating masses may be present. Carcinomas of almost every organ may produce an apparently single metastasis to bone. The area involved in the long bones is usually the metaphyseal region.

It is often stated that metastases do not occur below the knees or elbows. However, numerous exceptions occur. We have seen metastatic epidermoid carcinoma of the lung in a terminal phalanx, carcinoma of the breast in the small bones of the feet, and carcinoma of the cervix appearing as a poorly defined cyst in the lower end of the tibia.

Periosteal bone proliferation may accompany a metastatic lesion.[199] This is likely to

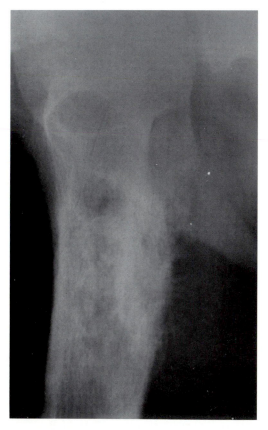

Fig. 1049 Metastatic carcinoma in femur, with extensive callus formation, which simulated osteosarcoma both radiographically and microscopically. Primary tumor was probably in lung. (WU neg. 67-9392.)

occur in certain sclerosing metastatic lesions such as those of the prostate. However, these metastases are usually multiple and often in ribs. We have seen a single metastasis in a long bone produce excessive periosteal proliferation simulating primary osteosarcoma.[198] Such changes are unusual but have occurred in metastatic rectal, pancreatic, and lung carcinoma (Fig. 1049).

It is imperative that such metastatic lesions be biopsied in order to avoid treatment designed for primary malignant bone tumors. Once a biopsy is available, the microscopic recognition usually is simple. The source of the bone metastasis may be suggested microscopically, particularly if carcinoma of the kidney, thyroid gland, or large bowel exists. If the tumor is squamous carcinoma in a thoracic vertebra and the patient is a man in the sixth decade, metastatic carcinoma of the lung is likely.

Sarcomas of soft tissue origin do not frequently involve bone except by direct invasion. The outstanding exception is embryonal rhabdomyosarcoma of childhood, which is complicated by blood-borne bone marrow metastases in a high percentage of cases.[197]

Most metastatic bone lesions cause pain. Treatment is for its relief. Irradiation therapy of localized lesions is the treatment of choice. When a pathologic fracture supervenes, internal fixation and radiation therapy provide the best results.[200] Palliative measures such as estrogen therapy and/or orchiectomy may afford relief in patients with disseminated metastases from carcinoma of the prostate. The pain of metastatic carcinoma from the breast is commonly relieved by testosterone. Occasionally, striking objective improvement in the condition of the bone is obtained. Other types of hormonal therapy than testosterone are thought less effective in the palliation of generalized bone metastases. In a few rare instances, a single metastatic focus, particularly from the thyroid gland and kidney, may be excised with benefit.

Laboratory findings

The only specific test of value in the diagnosis of bone tumors is the acid phosphatase test. Elevation of this enzyme in serum is usually evidence of metastatic carcinoma arising from the prostate (a rare exception is infarction of the prostate).

Elevation of the alkaline phosphatase level is merely an expression of bone production and is nonspecific. It can be elevated in bone-producing lesions such as osteosarcoma, hyperparathyroidism, Paget's disease, and metastatic carcinoma of the breast or prostate as well as incident to hepatic metastases. The alkaline phosphatase level is normal in many processes that predominantly destroy bone, such as osteolytic osteosarcoma, metastatic carcinoma from the kidney, and plasma cell myeloma.

Plasma cell myeloma is practically the only other tumor in which there are laboratory findings that lend weight to the diagnosis. However, these findings occur only when the process is disseminated. When a localized plasmacytoma of bone exists, all laboratory findings, including bone marrow, are usually normal. In disseminated multiple myeloma, the serum protein concentration frequently is elevated (as high as 20 gm%). This elevation involves mainly the globulin fraction. The electrophoretic pattern of the serum proteins may be diagnostic, but in certain instances of apparently localized plasma cell myeloma, it is normal.

Bence Jones protein is present in about half the cases. Serum calcium and phosphorus levels may be elevated because bone is being destroyed so fast that the kidneys do not have time to excrete it. The uric acid may be increased through catabolism of nucleoproteins derived from myeloma cells.[202] Elevation of the sedimentation rate may be the first evidence of recurrence of Ewing's tumor.

Biopsy and frozen section

The therapy of malignant tumors of bone often implies amputation in a young person. Before such a procedure, it is imperative that the pathologic diagnosis be correct.

The surgeon must obtain adequate material for pathologic diagnosis even though the lesion is confined entirely within the bone. If possible, he should excise a segment of bone that includes both involved and uninvolved areas. He should avoid excessive trauma to the tumor while securing a biopsy and should so place the biopsy incision that it may be entirely removed if subsequent radical operation is indicated. Theoretically, the use of a tourniquet proximal to bone lesions in the extremities while securing the biopsy may reduce the possibility of distant spread.

If there is any question of infection, the material obtained at biopsy must be properly studied bacteriologically.

Aspiration biopsy of bone tumors has been performed extensively at the Memorial Hospital for Cancer and Allied Diseases. Snyder and Coley[206] reported 385 cases, of which 67.5% were definitely and specifically diagnostic. In no case did a false aspiration diagnosis lead to amputation for a benign process. We believe that aspiration biopsy after preparation of paraffin sections is similar to a small biopsy and is particularly valuable in lesions that are deeply located.[205] Needle biopsy of bony lesions is usually diagnostic.[203, 204]

Frozen section diagnosis may be technically difficult. On the other hand, osseous lesions that extend into the soft tissue are easily diagnosed by frozen section. On some occasions, a frozen section may lead to an unexpected diagnosis. An osteolytic lesion of the pelvis was thought to be a primary malignant bone tumor, and hemipelvectomy was contemplated. Frozen section, however, demonstrated metastatic carcinoma. An osteolytic lesion of the femur with extension into the soft tissue was considered Ewing's tumor but proved to be eosinophilic granuloma.

At times, an exact diagnosis cannot be made, but the pathologist can usually say whether the lesion is benign or malignant.

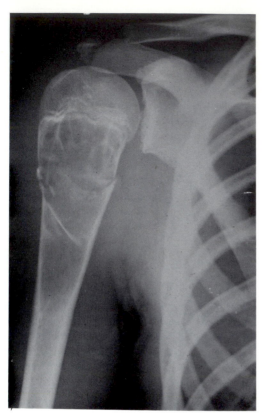

Fig. 1050 Typical solitary bone cyst of upper end of humerus abutting against epiphyseal plate in 13-year-old boy. (WU neg. 49-5897.)

Tumorlike lesions
Solitary bone cyst

Solitary (unicameral) bone cysts occur in long bones, most often in the upper portion of the shaft of the humerus and femur (Fig. 1050). Seventeen of the cases reported by James et al.[208] were in the humerus. These cysts occur predominantly in males (fourteen out of nineteen patients in Jaffe and Lichtenstein's series[207]), and almost all occur in patients under 20 years of age.

These lesions are usually advanced when first seen. They are usually metaphyseal in position and do not involve the epiphysis. In time, they tend to migrate away from the epiphysis.[211] The cortex is thinned, and periosteal bone proliferation does not take place except in areas of fracture. Bones affected by these lesions often frac-

ture, usually in the proximal portion of the cystic area.[207]

The cyst contains a clear or yellow fluid and is lined by a smooth connective tissue membrane that may be brown. The fluid may be hemorrhagic if a previous fracture has occurred. Microscopically, vascular connective tissue, hemosiderin (often within phagocytes), and cholesterol clefts are frequent. The diagnosis may be difficult in the presence of reparative changes following fracture, recurrence after bone grafting, and when articular cartilage is included in the curettings. The diagnosis becomes clear if the history and the x-ray films are available.

Pommer[210] believes that these cysts develop after mild trauma without fracture but with intramedullary hemorrhage. Conversely, von Mikulicz[209] believes that this lesion has its basis in a local disorder of development and bone growth. The latter theory is the more widely accepted.

The treatment of choice is curettement and replacement of the cyst with bone chips. Treatment of these cysts may be correlated with their activity. Good results are obtained when the cyst has migrated away from the epiphyseal line. Recurrences may appear if the cyst treated is lying close to the epiphyseal line.[211]

Aneurysmal bone cyst

Aneurysmal bone cyst is a rare lesion that may be mistaken for a peculiar giant cell tumor, a hemangioma, or even an osteosarcoma.[216] This large cystic lesion occurs usually in patients between 10 and 20 years of age. It occurs mainly in the vertebra and flat bones but can arise in the shaft of long bones.[214] Multiple involvement of the vertebrae was observed in seven of fifteen cases studied by Tillman et al.[217]

Radiographically, the lesion shows an eccentric expansion of the bone, erosion and destruction of the cortex, and a small border area of periosteal bone formation (Fig. 1051). Grossly, it forms a spongy hemorrhagic mass that may extend into

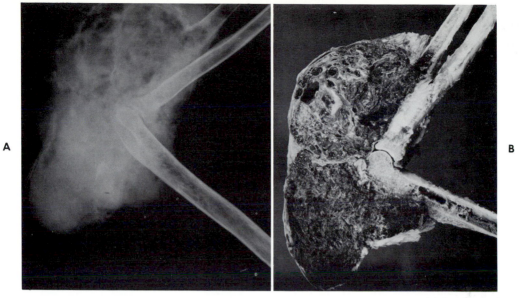

A

B

Fig. 1051 **A,** Aneurysmal bone cyst in region of elbow. Functional **disability** forced resection. **B,** Cyst shown in **A.** (Courtesy Dr. L. Litchtenstein, San Francisco, Calif.)

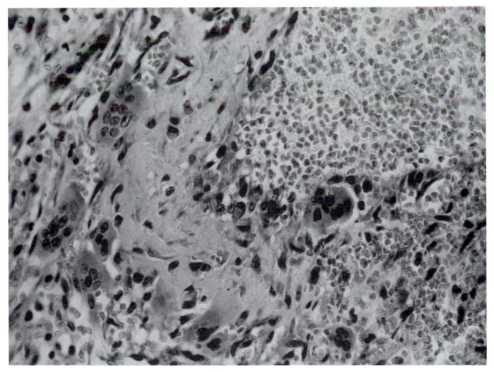

Fig. 1052 Aneurysmal bone cyst showing characteristic septum covered with giant cells and osteoid within its substance. (×400; WU neg. 54-5987.)

the soft tissues and be covered by a thin shell of reactive bone. Microscopically, large spaces filled with blood often are ac-companied by numerous giant cells. The septa contain osteoid[214] (Fig. 1052).

The differential diagnosis has to be made

with solitary bone cyst, giant cell tumor, "telangiectatic" osteosarcoma and, for the lesions located in the jaw, giant cell reparative granuloma.

The pathogenesis of aneurysmal bone cyst remains elusive. The findings in recent series suggest that this condition arises in some preexisting bone lesion as a result of changed hemodynamics.[212, 215] We have seen areas grossly and microscopically indistinguishable from aneurysmal bone cyst in chondroblastoma, giant cell tumor, fibrous dysplasia, osteoblastoma, and osteosarcoma. On the other hand, in most of the aneurysmal bone cysts that we have examined, we have been unable to demonstrate the existence of a previous lesion, an experience similar to that of Tillman et al.[217] Naturally, this might have been the result of sampling or the fact that the aneurysmal bone cyst destroyed all evidence of the preexisting lesion. Careful morphologic studies of future cases are needed to evaluate this interesting possibility.

Ganglion cyst of bone

On rare occasions, ganglion cysts, morphologically indistinguishable from those commonly seen in the periarticular soft tissue, are found in an intraosseous location, always close to a joint space (Fig. 1053).

The cyst is surrounded by a zone of condensed bone, often multiloculated, and has a gelatinous content and a wall of attenuated fibrous tissue. The bones of the ankle, particularly the tibia, are those most commonly affected.[218] Intraosseous ganglia need to be distinguished from solitary (unicameral) bone cysts and the periarticular cysts seen in association with degenerative joint diseases.

Metaphyseal fibrous defect (nonossifying fibroma)

Metaphyseal fibrous defects are distinctive lesions of bone that occur in adolescents, most often in long tubular bones, particularly the upper or lower tibia or the lower femur.[219, 221] They are eccentric,

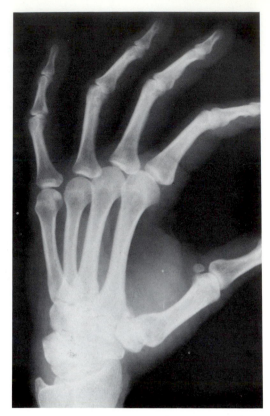

Fig. 1053 Intraosseous ganglion cyst involving base of first metacarpal. It was associated with larger ganglion of adjacent soft tissue, which is also apparent in roentgenogram. (WU neg. 71-6934; courtesy Dr. G. Davis, St. Louis, Mo.)

sharply delimited lesions not too distant from the epiphysis (Fig. 1054). They may involve the entire width of the bone (Fig. 1056). Fourteen of forty-five patients reported by Hatcher[220] had concomitant epiphyseal disorders. Because of this association, Hatcher[220] doubts that this lesion is a true neoplasm. Furthermore, several facts indicate that the lesion arises as the result of some developmental aberration at the epiphyseal plate:

1 It has been found only in the metaphysis of a bone.
2 It migrates (relatively) away from the epiphysis as the bone grows in length.
3 It tends to be elongated in the longitudinal axis of the bone, as though the abnormal development had occurred over a period of time.
4 Ponsetti and Friedman[222] illustrated three successive lesions arising from the same area of

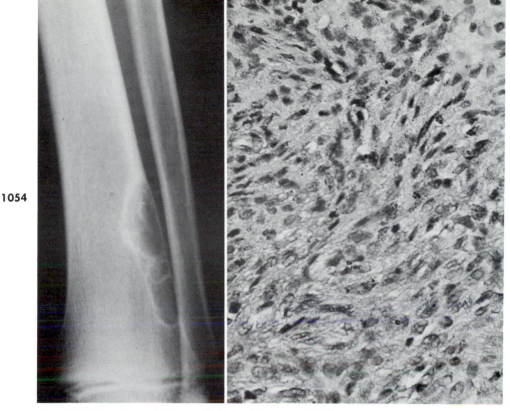

Fig. 1054 Metaphyseal fibrous defect of lower end of tibia. Note its sharp delineation and sclerotic margins. (WU neg. 52-3782.)

Fig. 1055 Area of metaphyseal fibrous defect demonstrating cellular whorllike masses of fibrous tissue. (×400; WU neg. 52-3453.)

the epiphyseal plate, indicating that the factors producing the defects may act intermittently.
5 No evidence of malignant transformation or unusual mitotic activity has been noted.*

Grossly, the lesion is granular and brown or dark red in color. Microscopically, it consists of cellular whorllike masses of fibrous tissue (Fig. 1055). Scattered giant cells and small collections of foam cells may be seen. It differs from fibrous dysplasia because it does not form bone. We have seen it diagnosed incorrectly as fibrosarcoma.

Clinically, there are few or no symptoms except pain. The lesion is usually found

incidentally on x-ray examination.[222] We have seen several fractures occurring through the thinned cortex.

Fibrous dysplasia

Fibrous dysplasia, a nonneoplastic condition, can be divided into two types: monostotic and polyostotic.[228] The monostotic variety occurs frequently in older children and young adults and most commonly affects the rib, femur, and tibia. The polyostotic type (an unusual variant) usually is associated with endocrine dysfunction, precocious puberty in female individuals, and areas of cutaneous hyperpigmentation.[223] There is frequently a unilateral distribution of these lesions. Schlumberger[230] believed that the two types of fibrous dysplasia are unrelated, although

---

*From Cunningham, J. B., and Ackerman, L. V.: Metaphyseal fibrous defects, J. Bone Joint Surg. [Am.] **38**:797-808, 1956.

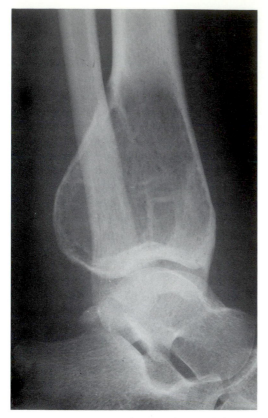

Fig. 1056 Large metaphyseal fibrous defect expanding lower tibial metaphysis. Lesions of this size are sometimes called nonossifying fibroma. (WU neg. 59-3916.)

they cannot be separated by examination of a single bone grossly or microscopically.

Roentgenograms of these lesions in the rib show a fusiform, expanded mass with thinning of the cortex. In the tibia, a lobulated, sharply delimited lesion of the shaft is formed (Fig. 1057). This lesion may produce a multilocular appearance because of endosteal cortical scalloping. Comparable lesions in membranous bone, particularly in the maxilla or the mandible, may show an overgrowth of dense bone.

The tissue cuts with a gritty consistency and is grayish yellow (Fig. 1058). The cortical bone often is thinned and expanded.

Microscopically, narrow, curved misshaped bone trabeculae usually are interspersed with fibrous tissue of variable cellularity (Fig. 1059). Harris et al.[224] and Reed[229] emphasized that fibrous dysplasia

represents a maturation defect. Coarse fiber bone never becomes tranformed to lamellar bone. Rows of cuboidal appositional osteoblasts do not appear on the surface of the trabeculae. Silver stains are helpful in showing failure of maturation. If a lesion of fibrous dysplasia is biopsied over a period of years, maturation is still absent. This fundamental histologic abnormality makes it possible to differentiate fibrous dysplasia from many lesions which, in the past, were confused with it.

Ossifying fibroma and desmoplastic fibroma must be differentiated from fibrous dysplasia.[231] The former is characterized by osteoblasts and osteoclasts rimming spicules of bone within a fibrous stroma. Ossifying fibroma has a tendency to recur and should be treated by resection of the involved area, stripping of the periosteum, and autogenous grafting.[226]

Highly cellular areas of fibrous dysplasia may be diagnosed incorrectly as sarcoma. The osseous metaplasia is close to preexisting bone. Focal areas of hyaline cartilage[227] and small cystic areas may be present. The transition of normal to abnormal bone is often abrupt. This is helpful in differentiating it radiographically from osteitis fibrosa cystica due to hyperparathyroidism. Huvos et al.[225] reported twelve cases of fibrous dysplasia associated with primary bone sarcoma. Eight of the tumors were osteosarcomas, two were chondrosarcomas, and two were labeled as spindle cell sarcomas. In half of the cases, the fibrous dysplasia was monostotic.

Resection cures fibrous dysplasia in bones such as the rib. Curettement is adequate in long bones such as the tibia. Indeed, in the maxilla, where some deformity may exist, partial removal of the lesion is all that is necessary.

Myositis ossificans

Myositis ossificans is a poor name for a group of conditions that are often mistaken microscopically for osteosarcoma.[234] It is a poor name because the lesion often does not involve muscle, show inflammation, or

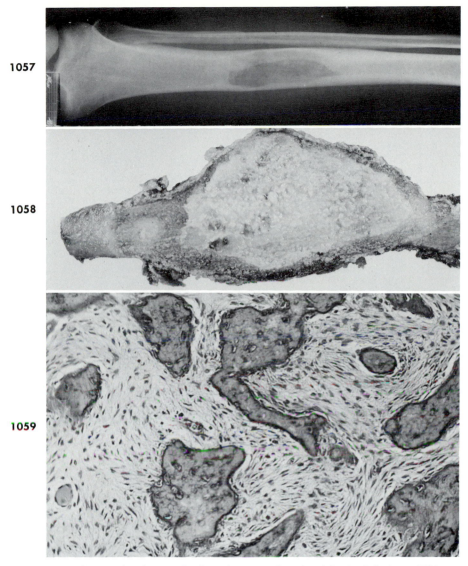

Fig. 1057 Fibrous dysplasia of tibia forming sharply delimited lesion. (WU neg. 49-5849.)

Fig. 1058 Fibrous dysplasia of rib forming fusiform, expanded mass which is grayish yellow. (WU neg. 49-4574.)

Fig. 1059 Typical fibrous dysplasia of rib demonstrating spicules of new bone formation with intervening cellular fibrous tissue. Trabeculae are not oriented along lines of stress. They form odd geometric patterns and have no osteoblasts on their surfaces. There is no maturation of this coarse fiber bone. (×140; WU neg. 52-333.)

form bone. About one-half of the patients have no history of trauma. It may arise in such atypical sites as the buttock. If found early in its evolution or in an atypical location, its biopsy diagnosis is difficult. Its distribution is indicated by the following statement:

Strauss' statistics[235] dealing with 127 cases of traumatic myositis ossificans show the following anatomic distribution: sixty-four of these occurred in the flexor muscles of the upper arm, the brachialis anticus being the one most frequently affected; forty-three occurred in the quadriceps femoris; thirteen in the adductor muscles of the thigh; two in the gluteal muscles; one in the

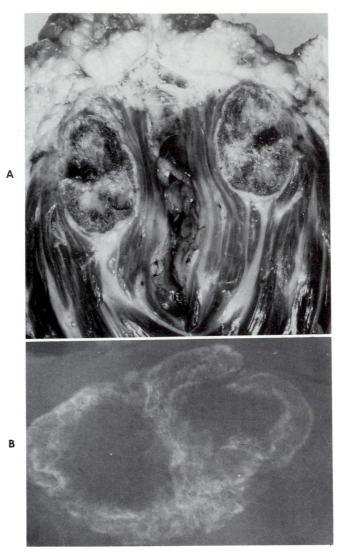

Fig. 1060 A, Well-defined myositis ossificans occurring in muscle. **B,** Same lesion shown in **A** illustrating bone formation in periphery. (**A,** WU neg. 56-6193; **B,** WU neg. 55-6190; **A** and **B,** from Ackerman, L. V.: Extraosseous localized nonneoplastic bone and cartilage formation (so-called myositis ossificans), J. Bone Joint Surg. [Am.] **40:**279-298, 1958.)

muscles of the ball of the thumb, and one in the temporal muscle.*

A typical history is as follows: A white 17-year-old youth complained of swelling of the thigh following a kick two weeks previously. X-ray examination showed calcification outside the femur. A segment of

---

*From Lewis, D.: Myositis ossificans, J.A.M.A. **80:**1281-1287, 1923; copyright 1923, American Medical Association.

fleshy white tissue was removed for biopsy. X-ray examination showed new bone formation in the periosteum and the soft tissues. Without a clinical history, an inexperienced radiologist could easily diagnose this lesion as osteosarcoma. The section of the lesion showed excessive new bone formation and a rather cellular stroma. An inexperienced pathologist also might easily diagnose this lesion incorrectly as osteosarcoma (Fig. 1062).

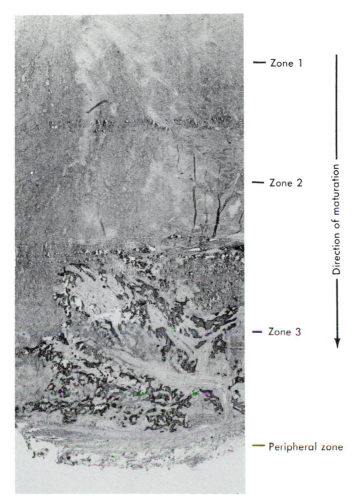

Fig. 1061 Schematic representation of zonal phenomena in myositis ossificans. (WU neg. 57-1317; from Ackerman, L. V.: Extraosseous localized nonneoplastic bone and cartilage formation (so-called myositis ossificans), J. Bone Joint Surg. [Am.] **40:**279-298, 1958.)

Zonal phenomenon is extremely helpful in the diagnosis.[232] During the evolution of the process, the newly formed bone matures peripherally. In a lesion approximately six weeks old, the centrally placed areas may be quite cellular and impossible to differentiate from osteosarcoma. Poorly defined osteoid, arranged in an orderly pattern, occurs in the intermediate zone. Excellent bone maturation with ossification occurs at the peripheral margins (Figs. 1060 to 1062).

This condition must be differentiated from extraosseous osteosarcoma. Undifferentiated tumor extends throughout the latter lesion without forming zones.[233] We have not seen myositis ossificans develop into osteosarcoma. We believe that previous cases reported represent juxtacortical osteosarcoma. The typical radiograph and the microscopic pattern of a sarcomatous stroma intermingled with adult bone are sufficient to make this differential diagnosis.

Differentiated histiocytosis (eosinophilic granuloma, Hand-Schüller-Christian disease, and Letterer-Siwe disease)

The unifying feature of the group of conditions designated as differentiated histiocytosis is an infiltration by differentiated

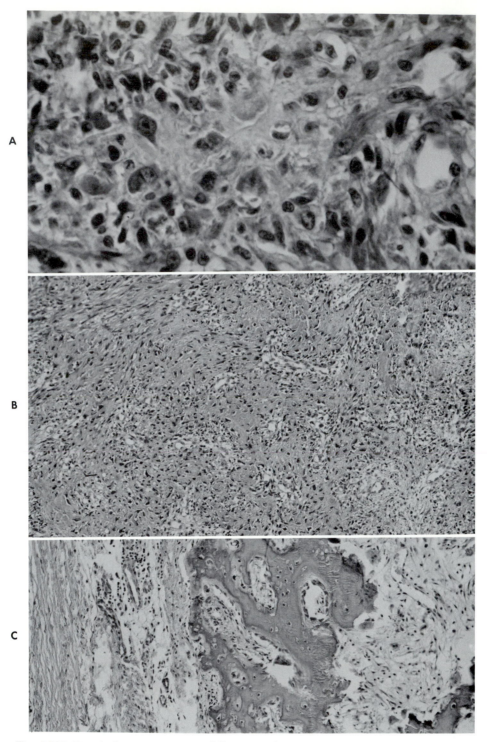

Fig. 1062 Zonal phenomena. **A,** Undifferentiated in pattern. **B,** Attempts at orientation of osteoid. **C,** Excellent bone formation at periphery. (**A** to **C,** ×450; **A,** WU neg. 55-6881; **B,** WU neg. 55-6880; **C,** WU neg. 55-6879; from Ackerman, L. V.: Extraosseous localized nonneoplastic bone and cartilage formation (so-called myositis ossificans), J. Bone Joint Surg. [Am.] **40:**279-298, 1958.)

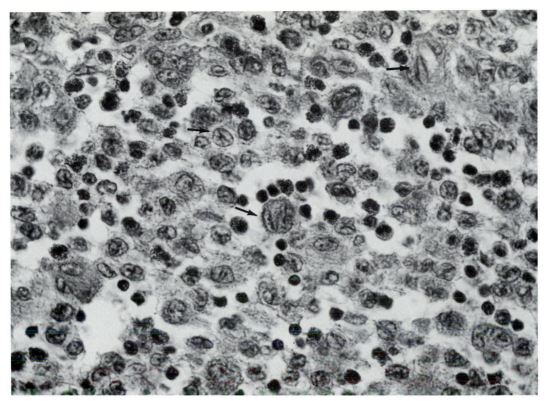

Fig. 1063 Eosinophilic granuloma of bone. Infiltrate is composed of histiocytes, lymphocytes, and eosinophils. Note lobulation and grooves in nuclei of many histiocytes (arrows). (×720; WU neg. 73-3404.)

histiocytes, accompanied by a variable admixture of eosinophils, giant cells, neutrophils, foamy cells, and areas of fibrosis. The histiocytes, which lack the cytologic stigmata of malignancy, have a characteristic appearance (Fig. 1063). Their nuclei are often lobulated or indented, sometimes with a longitudinal grove; their cytoplasm is, for the most part, distinctly acidophilic. Intracytoplasmic Langerhans' granules are regularly present on electron microscopic examination (Fig. 1064). Although not specific for this group of conditions, they occur in the cells of differentiated histiocytosis with striking regularity.[236] *Histiocytic proliferations with immature or undifferentiated cells should not be included in this category.* This is a mistake that has been made too frequently in the past.

The differentiated histiocytoses can be divided into three major categories on the basis of type and extent of the organ involvement:

1 Solitary bone involvement
2 Multiple bone involvement (with or without skin involvement)
3 Multiple organ involvement (bone, liver, spleen, etc.)

The cases with **solitary bone involvement,** which represent the most common variety, are usually referred to as *eosinophilic granuloma.*[237, 239, 242] Young adults are most commonly affected.[241] Any bone can be involved, with the possible exception of the hands and feet. The most common sites are the cranial vault, jaw, humerus, rib, and femur.[239] Radiographically, they present as an osteolytic lesion often in the metaphyseal area of long bones, sometimes associated with periosteal bone proliferation.[238] It can be confused radiographically with metastatic carcinoma (Fig. 1065) or Ewing's sarcoma (Fig. 1066). After fracture, this process may extend into adjacent soft tissues.[242] We have seen two recurrences in soft tissue after operation that disappeared with irradiation. These lesions may spontaneously regress but are radiosensitive and radiocurable with small

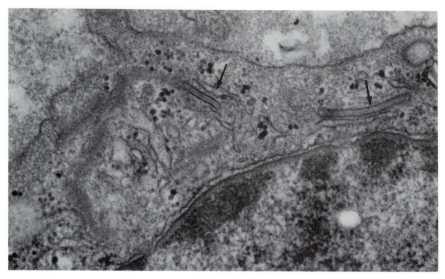

Fig. 1064 This histiocyte from eosinophilic granuloma of bone contains several Langerhans' granules (arrows). This is constant feature of histiocytes in this group of diseases. (Uranyl acetate–lead citrate; ×43,200.)

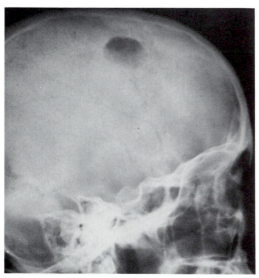

Fig. 1065 Osteolytic lesion of skull in 25-year-old woman. Radiographically, lesion was thought to be metastatic carcinoma but proved to be solitary lesion of eosinophilic granuloma. (WU neg. 48-4331.)

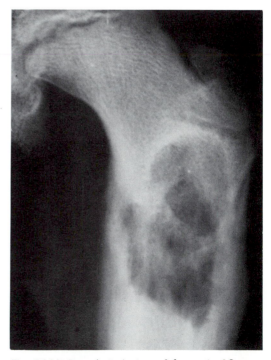

Fig. 1066 Osteolytic lesion of femur in 12-year-old boy. This was thought to be Ewing's tumor but proved microscopically to be eosinophilic granuloma. (WU neg. 48-6045.)

amounts of irradiation. All of our patients remained well. None of them developed other bone lesions or involvement of other organs.

Cases of *multiple bone involvement* are better designated as multiple eosinophilic granulomas.[240] When strategically located, the bony infiltration may result in proptosis, diabetes insipidus, or chronic otitis media or a combination of these conditions. The eponym of Hand-Schüller-Christian disease has been applied to this variety. Since the circumstances on which this designation is based are fortuitous and erratic, it would probably be better to drop the term entirely. Of the seven patients we reviewed (all of them children), all were alive but with persistent disease after a prolonged follow-up. The presence or absence of skin lesions (usually in the form of seborrheic dermatitis-like eruption of the scalp) did not influence the natural history of the disease.

Patients with *multiple organ involvement* are almost always under the age of 2 years. The disease, which is almost uniformly fatal, is known as Letterer-Siwe disease. The bone involvement is much more widespread than in the patients without extraskeletal involvement.

Articular and periarticular diseases
Ganglia

Ganglia occur about joints and rarely about tendon sheaths. They are annoying deformities that may cause some pain, weakness, partial disability of the joint, and bone changes.[244] Ganglia located in the popliteal space can produce pain or foot drop as result of compression of the common peroneal nerve.[247] Individuals using the wrist and fingers (pianists, typists) are prone to this condition. A history of injury preceding ganglion formation may exist.

Ganglia develop by myxoid degeneration and cystic softening of the connective tissue of the joint capsule or tendon sheath.[245, 246] The theory of a rent in the synovial membrane of a joint leading to the collection of synovial fluid and the formation of a false capsule[243] can seldom be substantiated.

The most common location is on the dorsal carpal area of the hand where the cystic lesion pushes its way toward the surface between the tendons of the extensor indices proprius and the extensor carpi radials (Fig. 1067). The second most frequent location is the volar surface of the wrist, superficial and medial to the radial artery. Ganglia also arise on the volar surfaces of the fingers just distal to the metacarpophalangeal joints in the dorsum of the foot, and around the ankle and knee. Ganglia are not lined by synovia and do not communicate with the joint cavity, two points distinguishing them from Baker's cysts (Fig. 1068).

Bursae; Baker's cyst

Bursae are found where muscles, tendons, and skin glide over bony prominences. They are subject to all the diseases that occur in large joint spaces. Inflammation may be associated with the formation of cysts, fluid, and loose bodies (Fig. 1069). The incomplete removal of loose bodies may be followed by the disappearance of the remaining ones from the bursa.

A related lesion is subdeltoid bursitis associated with calcareous tendonitis. This entity is primarily a degeneration of a tendon or muscle in the rotator cuff of the shoulder followed by deposition of calcium in necrotic collagenous tissue. This calcific material stimulates a secondary inflammatory reaction.[249]

A Baker's cyst occurs in the popliteal space from herniation of the synovial membrane through the posterior part of the capsule or from escape of joint fluid through normal anatomic connections of the knee joint with the semimembraneous bursa[248] (Fig. 1070). The cyst is lined by true synovium and may have cartilage in its wall. Any joint disease leading to increased intra-articular pressure, such as degenerative joint disease, neuropathic

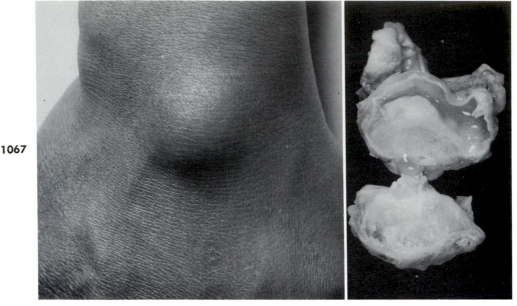

1067   1068

Fig. 1067 Typical location and appearance of ganglion. (WU neg. 49-1173.)
Fig. 1068 Ganglion illustrating mucoid appearance and poorly defined capsule. (WU neg. 50-3032.)

arthropathy, and rheumatoid arthritis, may result in the formation of a Baker's cyst.[250]

Fibrous histiocytoma of tendon sheath (nodular tenosynovitis)

Fibrous histiocytoma of the tendon sheath (also called giant cell tumor of the tendon sheath, xanthogranuloma, myeloplaxoma, and benign synovioma) is a common lesion that occurs more frequently in women than men, usually appearing in young and middle-aged persons. It is practically always distributed between the wrist and fingertips and between the ankle and toetips. It is more often proximal than distal on both the hands and feet and occurs most frequently on their flexor surfaces.

This tumor is a single lesion usually measuring between 1 cm and 3 cm in diameter. It has a fairly well-defined capsule, may be somewhat lobulated, and varies in color from whitish gray to yellowish brown. It arises from the inner layer of the tendon sheath.

Microscopically, this lesion contains closely packed polyhedral cells that have phagocytic properties. Giant cells containing fat and hemosiderin often are present (Fig. 1071). Cells in zones of active proliferation may show mitotic figures. Focal zones of hyalinization constitute the more quiescent areas.

The great cellularity of this tumor, its variable pattern, and the presence of mitotic figures may lead to an erroneous diagnosis of sarcoma. However, these tumors are not malignant. They may erode contiguous bone by pressure. If incompletely removed, they may recur locally. New lesions also possibly develop after excision.[251, 252]

The nature of this lesion is still controversial. Jaffe et al.[251] consider it a reactive process—hence the name of nodular tenosynovitis. We are impressed by the close similarities with other soft tissue lesions collectively called fibrous histiocytoma and believe that they may represent their tendon sheath counterpart (Chapter 23).

Pigmented villonodular synovitis and bursitis

Pigmented villonodular synovitis tends to occur in young adults.[256] Although the knee joint is the usual site,[253] the process

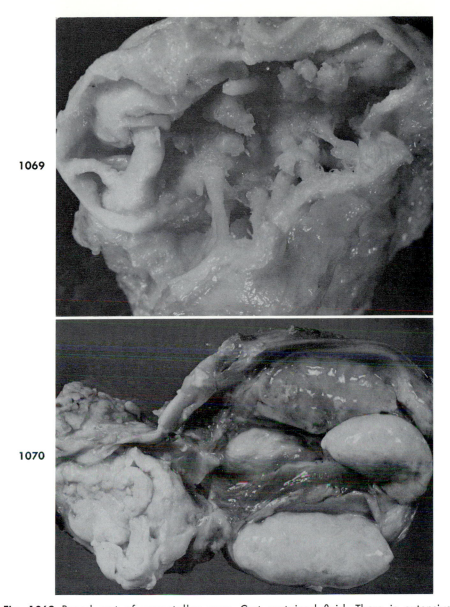

1069

1070

Fig. 1069 Bursal cyst of prepatellar area. Cyst contained fluid. There is extensive proliferation of synovia. (WU neg. 51-40.)
Fig. 1070 Large Baker's cyst. Synovial membrane is chronically inflamed, and loose bodies are present. (WU neg. 47-4094.)

may involve the ankle, hip, shoulder, or even the elbow joint. Usually only one articulation is affected, only one well-documented case of bilateral knee involvement having been reported.[255] Occasionally, the lesion may penetrate within the underlying bone.[257]

The synovitis may be focal or diffuse. When diffuse, it is made up of brownish yellow spongy tissue. Its appearance depends upon the content of hemosiderin pigment. Large amounts of tissue are often present, and complete removal may be impossible (Fig. 1072). Microscopically, the cellular component is similar to that of nodular tenosynovitis, but in addition there are papillary projections made up of foamy cells and hemosiderin-containing phagocytes (Fig. 1073).

This disease can be treated by excision.

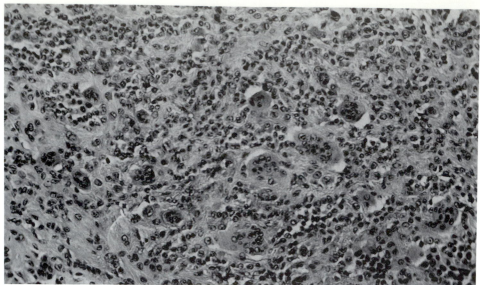

Fig. 1071 Rather cellular fibrous histiocytoma of tendon sheath origin. Giant cells are prominent, and mitotic figures are rare. (×200; WU neg. 50-1422.)

It may recur locally because complete removal is often impossible.[254] If it recurs locally, irradiation therapy may be helpful. In our experience, this lesion has not become malignant. Extensively recurrent lesions, however, have been misdiagnosed as fibrosarcoma and synovial sarcoma.

Synovial osteochondromatosis

Synovial osteochondromatosis is an infrequent disease of unknown etiology associated with the formation of osteocartilaginous bodies in the synovial membrane. This condition most often is monoarticular, affecting the knee or hip and communicating bursae. It is aggravated by infection and trauma.

Grossly, the osteocartilaginous bodies may remain confined to the synovium or be extruded within the joint cavity. They usually are partially calcified (Fig. 1074). Innumerable small bodies can be seen grossly in the resected lesion (Figs. 1075 and 1076). A single nodule beneath thinned synovium contains hyaline cartilage and at times bone (Fig. 1077).

In order to make a diagnosis of synovial osteochondromatosis, one should find cartilaginous or osteocartilaginous bodies attached to the synovial membrane in addition to those free in the joint spaces. The latter can also occur in degenerative joint disease, neuropathic arthropathy, and osteochondritis dissecans. Microscopically, the cartilage cells may show some degree of atypia and even binucleated forms, but this does not necessarily indicate malignancy.[260] Local recrudescence after treatment is rare.

Synovial osteochondromatosis needs to be differentiated from the exceptionally rare synovial chondrosarcoma, which it may closely resemble radiographically and grossly.[258] The distinction, which may be quite difficult, is made by the presence in the chondrosarcoma of obvious cytologic features of malignancy in the cartilaginous cells.[259]

Arthritis
Synovial biopsy

Needle biopsy of the synovium, particularly of the knee joint, is of aid in the assessment of synovial inflammatory conditions. For instance, it is possible to diagnose tuberculosis and other specific granulomatous lesions by this method.[261-265] By the use of a small-caliber synovial biopsy needle (Parker-Pearson technique), Schumacher and Kulka[263] were able to obtain sufficient synovial tissue for diagnosis in

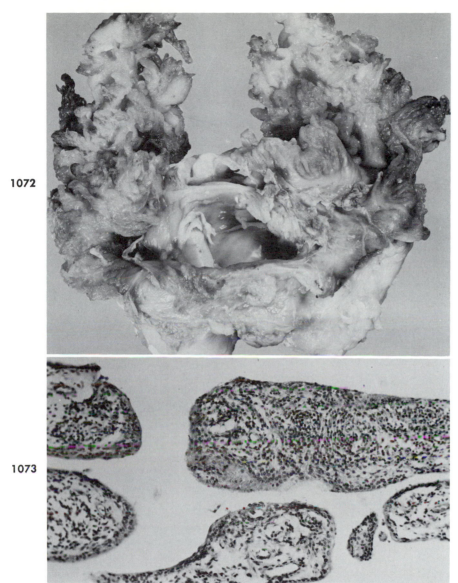

Fig. 1072 Large mass of papillary brown tissue removed from knee joint of patient with villonodular synovitis. (WU neg. 50-3300.)

Fig. 1073 Papillary projections in pigmented villonodular synovitis. (×120; WU neg. 50-3948.)

92% of the 109 joint biopsies they performed. Histologic examination proved to be of direct diagnostic value in thirty-eight cases.

Degenerative joint disease (osteoarthritis)

Surgical pathology specimens of legs amputated for traumatic reasons or because of gangrene secondary to vascular disease offer the unique opportunity for study of degenerative joint disease. The term osteoarthritis is inaccurate because this type of joint disease is degenerative and not inflammatory. The bone and joints affected are conditioned by use and occupation of the patient.[276]

Changes in the joints are related directly to age.[282] Both Bennett et al.[267] and Collins[268] described and illustrated these

1074

1075

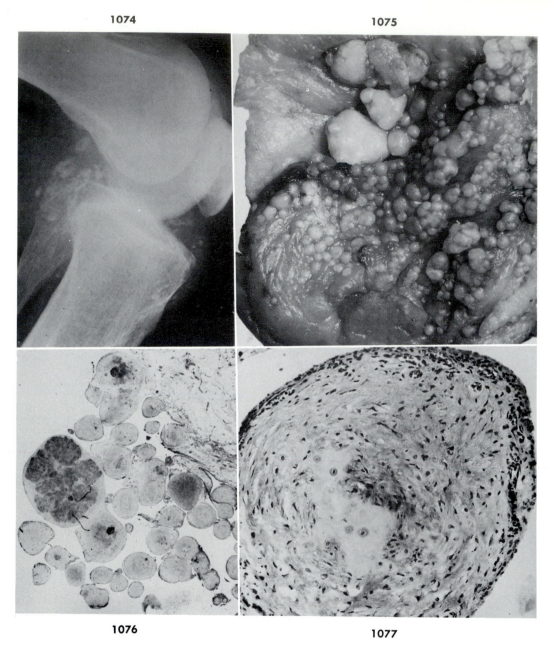

1076

1077

Fig. 1074 Synovial osteochondromatosis. Nodules can be seen clearly in joint space. (WU neg. 49-4113.)

Fig. 1075 Extensive involvement of synovium of knee joint by osteochondromatosis. (WU neg. 48-3983.)

Fig. 1076 Pattern and formation of synovial osteochondromatosis. (Low power; WU neg. 48-3981.)

Fig. 1077 Single nodule of osteochondromatosis forming beneath intact synovium. Note cartilage formation in center of this nodule. (High power; WU neg. 48-3972.)

changes in the knee joint beautifully. No less can be said of the work of Hirsch et al.[272] on similar changes in the cervical spine. The classic monograph by Nichols and Richardson[278] in 1909 described the pathologic alteration so well that we have

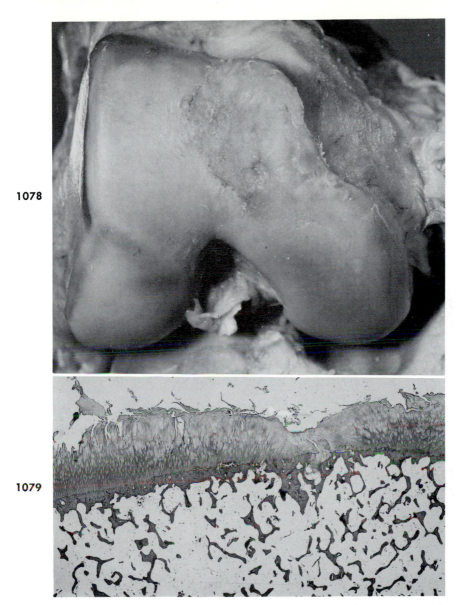

Fig. 1078 Pronounced degenerative joint disease in 55-year-old man. Note degeneration and destruction of cartilage over wide area. (WU neg. 52-3896.)
Fig. 1079 Section taken through zone shown in Fig. 1078 demonstrating fragmentation and fibrillation of thinned cartilage. (Low power; WU neg. 52-4490.)

little to add today. Bauer and Bennett[266] summarized their classic description as follows:

In degenerative arthritis, the earliest and primary change in the joints is a gradual and uneven degeneration of the hyaline cartilage of the articular surfaces. This is first detected as a fibrillation of the cartilaginous matrix which generally begins near the articular surface and is associated with a disappearance of the spindle-celled perichondrium. As a result of this fibrillation, which takes place usually at right angles to the articular surface, the neighboring cartilage cells are set free and finally disintegrate and disappear. Also, the original smooth articular surface takes on a papillary appearance. At times this fibrillation is responsible for the freeing of minute masses of cartilage and fibrillated matrix. The depth to which this fibrillation extends varies.

Sometimes it extends entirely through the cartilage down to the zone of provisional calcification so that masses of cartilage may be peeled away, exposing either the zone of provisional calcification or the underlying bone to the attrition of joint motion. [Fig. 1078.] Occasionally, only a portion of the articular cartilage undergoes degeneration, fibrillation, and destructon. [Fig. 1079.] This leads to thinning of the cartilage over a circumscribed area. To meet this erosion and depression, an overgrowth occurs on the opposite joint surface. This is brought about by increased activity of the perichondrium. As a result, an irregular or somewhat toothed joint line is formed, and finally, with ultimate disappearance of the

entire articular cartilage, the two bony surfaces are brought into contact. Since this change takes place gradually and is at first confined only to a portion of the joint, motion is continued with the result that the exposed bone undergoes marked thickening of the trabeculae and narrowing of the marrow spaces until an extremely dense bony structure has been produced. The friction of continued joint motion produces a high degree of polish on the exposed condensed bone which then acquires an appearance closely resembling ivory; hence the term "eburnation of bone."

While this process of fibrillation and destruction of cartilage with erosion is taking place in one portion of the joint and a corresponding over-

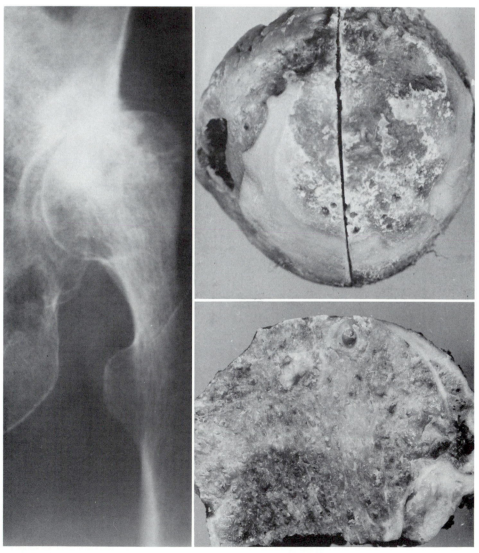

Fig. 1080 Head of femur demonstrating advanced osteoarthritic changes. There is loss of cartilage and cyst formation. (WU negs. 54-1439, 54-1273, and 54-1274.)

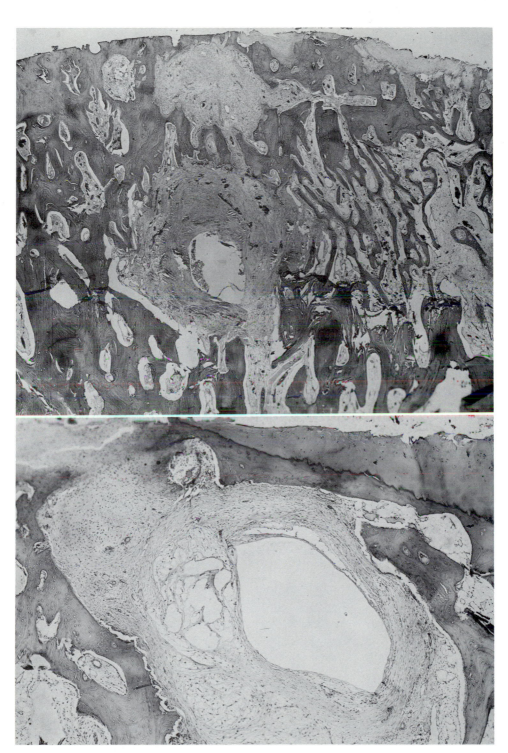

Fig. 1081 Loss of cartilage, eburnation, and cyst formation illustrated in Fig. 1080. (Low power; WU negs. 54-1493 and 55-34.)

growth is occurring on the opposite joint surface, secondary changes in the joint may be produced. Changes in the shape of the joint surface may gradually, over a period of months or years, lead to more or less extensive subluxations. As a result, the amount of joint motion may be diminished, or, in certain instances, the joint surfaces may become interlocked, producing "ankylosis by deformity." There is no true ankylosis in this type of joint disease. Common among these imperfectly understood secondary changes is an increased activity of the perichondrium at the periphery of the joint where the cartilage and capsule come together. This results in the new formation of cartilage which may be transformed into bone and thus causes an increase in the size of the bone end. As a rule this increase in circumference is not uniform, but is irregular and the contour is nodular, as exemplified by Heberden's node. Since this deposit of new bone is usually within the attachment of the joint capsule, it may in some cases lead to filling up of the original joint cavity, thus producing partial or complete dislocation.

As a rule, no great increase in the thickness of the joint capsules of these joints is observed, and, in many instances, the synovial membrane appears normal. However, in some cases, there is marked thickening of the synovial membrane with the production of papillary or pedunculated masses of connective tissue which may be converted by metaplasia into cartilage or bone or, in some cases, into fat tissue. Detachment of these pedunculated masses may give rise to loose bodies, the so-called joint mice. The breaking off of an osteophyte is another cause of loose-body formation. As a rule, in this type of joint disease there is very little tendency for the synovial membrane to extend over the articular surfaces and in no case does fibrous ankylosis occur.[*]

Nichols and Richardson[278] also called attention to the fact that there is no evidence of inflammatory exudation in early degenerative joint disease. On the other hand, some degree of synovial hyperplasia with hyperemia and lymphocytic infiltration can be seen in advanced stages, especially with osteoarthritis of the hip. This change should not be confused with rheumatoid arthritis.

The cartilage is the key to the changes in osteoarthrosis. Its capacity for repair

[*]From Bauer, W., and Bennett, G. A.: Experimental and pathological studies in the degenerative type of arthritis, J. Bone Joint Surg. 18: 1-18, 1936.

is feeble. Cartilaginous degeneration takes place in certain areas of the hip joint not exposed to pressure or friction,[271] although these changes occur most often on the joint surface exposed to friction, weight bearing, or movement.[269] There is loss of chondroitin sulfate matrix in the cartilage in advance of actual mechanical attrition.[277] With degeneration of cartilage, the stability of the chondro-osseous junction is lost. Narrowing of the joint space is, in fact, loss of cartilage thickness. If the osteoarthritic head of a femur is examined, cysts frequently are found close to the surface, where they may communicate with the joint and are surrounded by dense bone.[274, 281] The cyst may be replaced by fibrous tissue or may contain fluid[271] (Figs. 1080 and 1081).

Neuropathic arthropathy (Charcot's joint) is a particularly destructive variant of degenerative joint disease (Fig. 1082). The process is usually slowly progressive, although on rare occasions it may have an extremely rapid evolution.[279] Particles of dead bone and cartilage are often seen in large amounts embedded in the synovial membrane.[273] However, they are not specific for this condition.

Chondromalacia patella is the name given to a condition of obscure etiology characterized by softening, fibrillation, fissuring, and erosion of the articular cartilage of the patella.[280] Microscopically, the changes are indistinguishable from those of degenerative joint disease.[270, 275]

Rheumatoid arthritis

Rheumatoid arthritis is a chronic polyarticular arthritis of unknown etiology. It is most common in women during the second and third decades of life. The joints of the feet and hands are nearly always involved. Other joints frequently affected are the elbows, knees, wrists, ankles, hips, spine, and temporomandibular articulations.

Experimental studies carried out in recent years have indicated that lysosomes are one of the mediators of the inflamma-

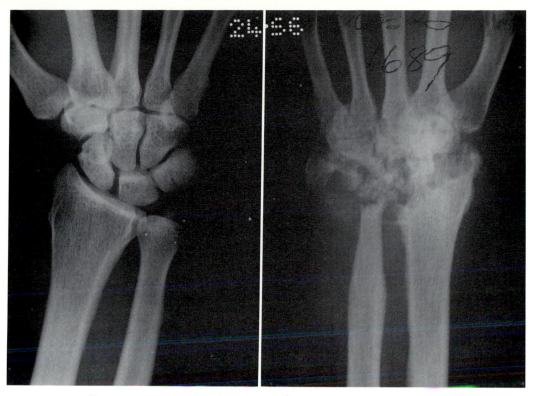

Fig. 1082 Neuropathic changes in wrist secondary to syringomyelia.

tory reaction seen in this disease and in other joint diseases.[312] The earliest morphologic changes occur in the synovial membrane. Hyperemia of the synovium is followed by proliferation of the synovial lining cells and infiltration by plasma cells and lymphocytes[283] (Fig. 1083). Lymphoid follicles are often present. The small synovial blood vessels are lined by plump endothelial cells, and fibrin deposits are often seen close to the synovial lining or within the stroma. Sokoloff[309] and Sherman[308] remarked that these changes, although certainly supporting a diagnosis of rheumatoid arthritis in a clinically compatible case, are not pathognomonic of this entity. Two additional microscopic features, which are also nonspecific, include the presence of synovial giant cells and of bone and cartilage fragments within the actual syovial membrane. Muirden[303] found synovial giant cells in one-third of the 100 biopsies he examined. They need to be distinguished from multinucleated plasma cells, foreign body cells, and Touton giant cells that can also occur in joints with rheumatoid arthritis. Grimley and Sokoloff[293] found them only in patients with active, seropositive disease, although they found no correlation with the serologic titer. On the other hand, Bhan and Roy[289] found them in seropositive and in seronegative cases, as well as in tuberculosis, traumatic arthritis, and villonodular synovitis. The cartilage and bone fragments tend to occur in joints with advanced disease. They appear to arise as a result of the erosive destructive process of the articular surface and can be distinguished by virtue of their position and clear demarcation from the metaplastic cartilage and bone that sometimes arises from synovial cells. They also have been seen in synovial membranes of osteoarthritis, osteochondritis dissecans, chondromalacia patella, and particularly in neuropathic joints[297, 303] (Fig. 1084).

In the second phase granulation tissue

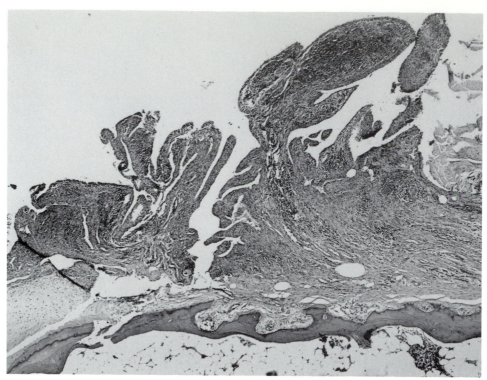

Fig. 1083 Exuberant papillary projections of inflamed synovium in rheumatoid arthritis involving wrist. (WU neg. 70-5932.)

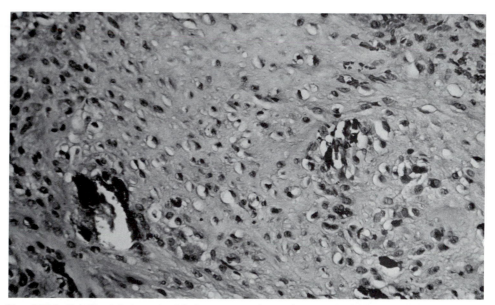

Fig. 1084 Calcific debris embedded in synovial membrane of Charcot's joint. (×250; WU neg. 62-9047.)

grows into the subchondral marrow of the bone. Osteoporosis occurs early and may result in spontaneous fractures of long bones (particularly the femoral neck) and the pelvis.[311] Prominent pannus is formed over the articular cartilage (Fig. 1085).

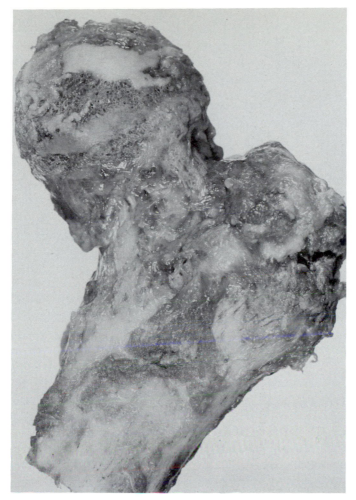

Fig. 1085 Advanced rheumatoid arthritis involving femur. There is prominent proliferation of synovium and almost complete destruction of overlying articular cartilage. (WU neg. 49-5578.)

Cartilage and even bone form in this pannus. The granulation tissue of the subchondral area and the pannus within the joint attack the cartilage.[290] Its destruction may be followed by fibrous ankylosis and eventually bony ankylosis. Mitchell and Shepard[301] have described the early changes seen by electron microscopy in the articular cartilage. Different pathologic stages of the process occur in different joints at the same time.[305] Increased articular pressure may lead to bursting of the joint capsule and acute joint rupture,[291] bone cysts ("rheumatoid geodes"),[304] or herniation of the capsule into the soft tissues.[298] The bone cysts are radiographically similar to those seen in association with degenerative joint disease, but in rheumatoid arthritis they contain granulation tissue instead of fluid or myxoid material.

Rheumatoid arthritis is now generally regarded as the expression of a systemic disease.[295, 296] Tenosynovitis and "rheumatoid nodules" are the two most common extra-articular manifestations. The latter, which are seen in approximately 20% of the patients, occur most often in tendons and tendon sheaths and periarticular subcutaneous tissue but also have been seen in the heart and large vessels, lung and pleura, kidney,

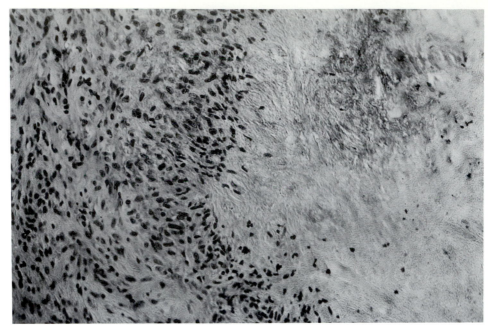

Fig. 1086 Typical rheumatoid nodule. There exist central necrosis, palisading of cells around margin of this area, and chronic inflammatory cells. (×200; WU neg. 49-4145.)

meninges, and in the synovial membrane itself.[284, 299, 306] In exceptional instances, they have occurred systemically and have been responsible for the patient's death.[288] Microscopically, they are composed of a necrotic center impregnated with fibrin, surrounded by a predominantly histiocytic inflammatory reaction often arranged in a palisading fashion (Fig. 1086). They are not specific of rheumatoid arthritis. Nodules morphologically indistinguishable can occur in rheumatic fever, systemic lupus erythematosus, and, in children, in the absence of any apparent disease.[285, 286, 294] Berardinelli et al.[287] followed ten cases of the latter and found rheumatoid factor two to sixteen years after the appearance of the nodules.

Sokoloff et al.[310] found nonnecrotizing arteritis in 10% of patients with rheumatoid arthritis. Necrotizing arteritis also has been described.[302, 307] Polyneuritis can be observed.[292]

The pulmonary manifestations of rheumatoid arthritis have been discussed in Chapter 6 and the lymph node changes in Chapter 20.

Amyloidosis is a significant complication of the disease. In the United States, rheumatoid arthritis has displaced tuberculosis as the most common underlying disorder associated with amyloid deposition.

Infectious arthritis

Bacterial, fungal, and parasitic infections can reach the joints either by hematogenous spread or by contiguous extension from a neighboring osteomyelitis (Fig. 1087).

Gout

About 2% to 5% of chronic joint disease is caused by gout. It may occur in families but is not restricted to man and has been reported in reptiles by Appleby.[313] The metatarsophalangeal joints are often the first to be involved, but other joints of the hands and feet are rather frequently involved, too. We also have seen gout involve the joints of the long bones.

Calcification and even ossification of tophi occur not infrequently.[315] The urate deposits progressively destroy the cartilage and may cause osteolytic, irregular destruc-

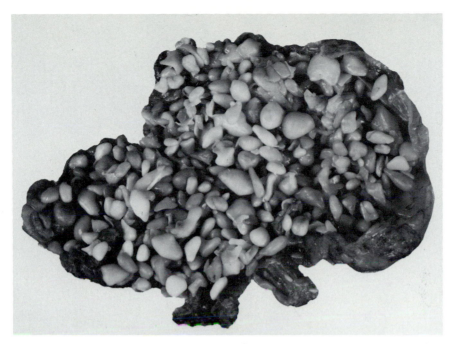

Fig. 1087 Tuberculous bursitis with innumerable "rice bodies." Latter are mainly composed of fibrin and have no diagnostic significance. (Courtesy Dr. E. F. Lascano, Buenos Aires, Argentina.)

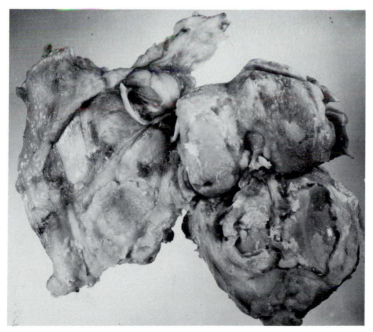

Fig. 1088 Extensive involvement of knee joint and synovium by gout. In some areas, cartilage of condyles is completely missing and there is involvement of semilunar cartilages as well. Grayish white plaques represent deposits of uric acid crystals. Patient, 83-year-old woman, had leg amputated because of arterial insufficiency, and finding of gout was unexpected. (WU neg. 59-5916.)

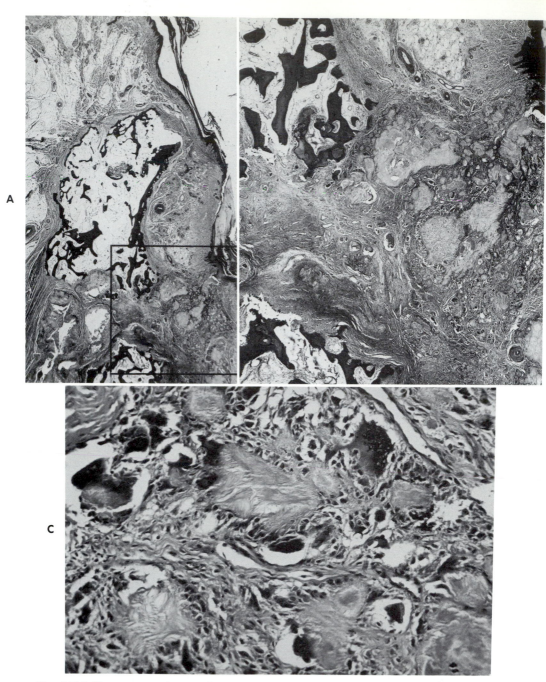

Fig. 1089 Characteristic lesion of gout. **A** and **B**, Tophaceous deposits that have destroyed joint, with complete destruction of cartilage and extension out into soft tissue and growth just beneath epidermis. **C**, Urate deposits surrounded by characteristic giant cells. Latter demonstrates characteristic picture of gout. Patient's trouble began in great toe. (**A**, ×10; WU neg. 63-73; **B**, ×40; WU neg. 63-72; **C**, ×275, WU neg. 63-74.)

tion of subchondral bone (Fig. 1088). These deposits may extend out from a joint into the soft tissue and cause destruction of the ligaments. This destruction eventually leads to subcutaneous deposits which may erode through the skin. The microscopic pattern of gout is unmistakable. Fixation in alcohol is important for the preservation of sodium urate monohydrate deposits which appear as needle-shaped, doubly refractile crystals. The deGalantha stain is particularly suited for their demonstration.[314] Even if alcoholic fixation is not done, the appearance of tophi is usually diagnostic because of the typical granulomatous response that they elicit (Fig. 1089). Histiocytes and foreign body giant cells predominate in the infiltrate. Palisading of the histiocytes sometimes occurs and may be a source of confusion with rheumatoid nodules.

Gout should be differentiated from chondrocalcinosis (pseudogout syndrome), a rare condition in which the symptoms result from diffuse calcification of the articular cartilage.[316]

REFERENCES
Introduction

1 Aegerter, E., and Kirkpatrick, J. A., Jr., Orthopedic diseases, ed. 3, Philadelphia, 1968, W. B. Saunders Co.
2 Bloom, W., and Fawcett, D. W.: Textbook of histology, ed. 9, Philadelphia, 1968, W. B. Saunders Co.
3 Brailsford, J. F.: The serious limitations and erroneous indications of biopsy in the diagnosis of tumours of bones, Proc. R. Soc. Med. 41:225-236, 1948.
4 Collins, D. H.: Pathology of bone, London, 1966, Butterworth & Co., Ltd.
5 Dahlin, D. C.: Bone tumors, ed. 2, Springfield, Ill., 1967, Charles C Thomas, Publisher.
6 Jaffe, H. L.: Tumors and tumorous conditions of the bones and joints, Philadelphia, 1958, Lea & Febiger.
7 Jaffe, H. L.: Metabolic, degenerative and inflammatory diseases of bones and joints, Philadelphia, 1972, Lea & Febiger.
8 La Croix, P.: The organization of bones, Philadelphia, 1951, The Blakiston Co.
9 Lichtenstein, L.: Bone tumors, ed. 4, St. Louis, 1972, The C. V. Mosby Co.
10 Luck, V. J.: Bone and joint diseases, Springfield, Ill., 1950, Charles C Thomas, Publisher.
11 Morse, A.: Formic acid-sodium citrate decalcification and butyl alcohol dehydration of teeth and bones for sectioning in paraffin, J. Dent. Res. 24:143-153, 1945.
12 Schajowicz, F., and Derqui, J. C.: Puncture biopsy in lesions of the locomotor system, J. Bone Joint Surg. 21:531-548, 1968.
13 Spjut, H. J., Dorfman, H. D., Fechner, R. E., and Ackerman, L. V.: Tumors of bone and cartilage. In Atlas of tumor pathology, Sect. II, Fasc. 5, Washington, D. C., 1971, Armed Forces Institute of Pathology.

Osteoporosis and osteomalacia

14 Beck, J. S., and Nordin, B. E. C.: Histological assessment of osteoporosis by iliac crest biopsy, J. Pathol. Bacteriol. 80:391-397, 1960.
15 Bernstein, D. S., Sadowsky, N., Hegsted, D. M., Guri, C. D., and Stare, F. J.: Prevalence of osteoporosis in high- and low-fluoride areas in North Dakota, J.A.M.A. 198:499-504, 1966.
16 Caldwell, R. A.: Observations on the incidence, aetiology and pathology of senile osteoporosis, J. Clin. Pathol. 15:421-431, 1962.
17 Davis, M. E., Strandjord, N. M., and Lanzl, L. H.: Estrogens and the aging process, J.A.M.A. 196:219-224, 1966.
18 Fourman, P.: Calcium metabolism and the bone, ed. 2, Philadelphia, 1968, F. A. Davis Co.
19 Jowsey, J., Kelly, P. J., Riggs, B. L., Bianco, A. J., Jr., Scholz, D. A., and Gershon-Cohen, J.: Quantitative microradiographic studies of normal and osteoporotic bone, J. Bone Joint Surg. [Am.] 47:785-806, 1965.
20 Mignani, G., Thurner, J., Marchetti, P. G., and Hussl, B.: Microradiographic investigations of various forms of bone disease (Paget's osteitis deformans, osteomalacia, Engel-Recklinghausen disease and Möller-Barlow disease), Frankfurt. Z. Pathol. 70:606-620, 1960.
21 Steendijk, R.: Metabolic bone disease in children, Clin. Orthop. 77:247-275, 1971.
22 Urist, M. R., Zaccalini, P. S., MacDonald, N. S., and Skoog, W. A.: New approaches to the problem of osteoporosis, J. Bone Joint Surg. [Br.] 44:464-484, 1962.
23 Van Buchem, F. S. P.: Osteomalacia—pathogenesis and treatment, Br. Med. J. 1:933-938, 1959.

Fractures

24 Blount, W. P., Schaefer, A. A., and Johnson, J. H.: Fractures of the forearm in children, J.A.M.A. 120:111-116, 1942.
25 Collins, D. H.: Structural changes around nails and screws in human bones, J. Pathol. Bacteriol. 65:109-121, 1953.
26 Collins, D. H.: Tissue changes in human femurs containing plastic appliances, J. Bone Joint Surg. [Br.] 36:458-563, 1954.
27 Ham, A. W.: A histological study of the early phases of bone repair, J. Bone Joint Surg. 12:827-844, 1930.

28 Ham, A. W.: Histology, ed. 6, Philadelphia, 1969, J. B. Lippincott Co.

29 Ham, A. W., and Gordon, S.: The origin of bone that forms in association with cancellous chips transplanted into muscle, Br. J. Plast. Surg. 5:154-160, 1952.

30 Ham, A. W., and Harris, W. R.: Repair and transplantation of bone. In Bourne, G. H., editor: The biochemistry and physiology of bone, London, 1956, Academic Press, Inc., pp. 475-505.

31 Mindell, E. R., Rodbard, S., and Kwasman, B. G.: Chondrogenesis in bone repair; a study of the healing fracture callus in the rat, Clin. Orthop. 79:187-196, 1971.

32 Murray, C. R.: Healing of fractures; its influence on the choice of methods of treatment, Arch. Surg. 29:446-464, 1934.

33 Odell, R. T., and Leydig, S. M.: The conservative treatment of fractures in children, Surg. Gynecol. Obstet. 92:69-74, 1951.

34 Schwarz, E.: Hypercallosis in osteogenesis imperfecta, Am. J. Roentgenol. Radium Ther. Nucl. Med. 85:645-648, 1961.

Osteomyelitis

35 Berney, S., Goldstein, M., and Bishko, F.: Clinical and diagnostic features of tuberculous arthritis, Am. J. Med. 53:36-42, 1972.

36 Carrell, W. B., and Childress, H. M.: Tuberculosis of the large long bones of the extremities, J. Bone Joint Surg. 22:569-588, 1940.

37 Farrow, R., and Cureton, R. J. R.: Carcinomatous invasion of bone in osteomyelitis, Br. J. Surg. 50:107-109, 1962.

38 Garcia, A., Jr., and Grantham, S. A.: Hematogenous pyogenic vertebral osteomyelitis, J. Bone Joint Surg. [Am.] 42:429-436, 1960.

39 Johnson, L. L., and Kempson, R. L.: Epidermoid carcinoma in chronic osteomyelitis: diagnostic problems and management, J. Bone Joint Surg. [Am.] 47:133-145, 1965.

40 Mason, M. L.: Tuberculous tenosynovitis of the hand, Surg. Gynecol. Obstet. 59:363-396, 1934.

41 Silver, H. K., Simon, J. L., and Clement, D. H.: Salmonella osteomyelitis and abnormal hemoglobin disease, Pediatrics 20:439-447, 1957.

42 Trueta, J.: The three types of acute haematogenous osteomyelitis, J. Bone Joint Surg. [Br.] 41:671-680, 1959.

43 Westermark, N., and Hellerström, S.: Zwei Fälle von Osteitis luetica, osteogenes Sarkom vortäuschend, Acta Radiol. 18:422-427, 1937.

Aseptic (avascular) bone necrosis

44 Bohr, H., and Larsen, E. J.: On necrosis of the femoral head after fracture of the neck of the femur, J. Bone Joint Surg [Br.] 47: 330-338, 1965.

45 Golding, J. S. R., Maciver, J. F., and Went, L. N.: The bone changes in sickle-cell anaemia and its genetic variants, J. Bone Joint Surg. [Br.] 41:711-718, 1959.

46 Luck, V. J.: Bone and joint diseases, Springfield, Ill., 1950, Charles C Thomas, Publisher.

47 Phemister, D. B.: Repair of bone in the presence of aseptic necrosis resulting from fractures, transplantations, and vascular obstruction, J. Bone Joint Surg. 12:769-787, 1930.

Paget's disease

48 Barry, H. C.: Paget's disease of bone, Edinburgh, 1969, E. & S. Livingstone, Ltd.

49 Collins, D. H.: Paget's disease of bone; incidence and subclinical forms, Lancet 2:51-57, 1956.

50 Collins, D. H., and Winn, J. M.: Focal Paget's disease of the skull (osteoporosis circumscripta), J. Pathol. Bacteriol. 69:1-9, 1955.

51 Dickson, D. D., Camp, J. D., and Ghormley, R. K.: Osteitis deformans; Paget's disease of the bone, Radiology, 44:449-470, 1945.

52 Lake, M. E.: The pathology of fracture in Paget's disease, Aust. N. Z. J. Surg. 27:307-312, 1958.

53 Price, C. H. G., and Goldie, W.: Paget's sarcoma of bone; a study of 80 cases from the Bristol and the Leeds bone tumour Registries, J. Bone Joint Surg. [Br.] 51:205-224, 1969.

54 Reifenstein, E. C., Jr., and Albright, F.: Paget's disease: its pathologic physiology and the importance of this in the complications arising from fracture and immobilization, N. Engl. J. Med. 231:343-355, 1944.

55 Schmorl, G.: Ueber Ostitis deformans Paget, Virchows Arch. Pathol. Anat. 283:694-751, 1931.

56 Seaman, W. B.: The roentgen appearance of early Paget's disease, Am. J. Roentgenol. Radium Ther. Nucl. Med. 66:587-594, 1951.

57 Uehlinger, E.: Osteofibrosis deformans juvenilis (Polyostotische fibröse Dysplasia Jaffe-Lichtenstein), Virchows Arch. Pathol. Anat. 306:255-299, 1940.

Melorheostosis

58 Franklin, E. L., and Matheson, I.: Melorheostosis, Br. J. Radiol. 15:185-191, 1942.

59 Kirby, S. V.: Melorheostosis; with report of a case, Radiology 37:62-67, 1948.

Tumors
Classification and distribution

60 Schajowicz, F., Ackerman, L. V., and Sissons, H. A.: Histologic typing of bone tumours, International Histological Classification of Tumours, No. 6, Geneva, 1972, World Health Organization.

Bone-forming tumors
Osteoma

61 Chang, C. H. J., Piatt, E. D., Thomas, K. E., and Watne, A. L.: Bone abnormalities in Gardner's syndrome, Am. J. Roentgenol. Radium Ther. Nucl. Med. **103**:645-652, 1968.

62 Hallberg, O. E., and Begley, J. W., Jr.: Origin and treatment of osteomas of the paranasal sinuses, Arch. Otolaryngol. **51**:750-760, 1950.

Osteoid osteoma and osteoblastoma

63 Brown, R. C., and Ghormley, R. K.: Solitary eccentric (cortical) abscess in bone, Surgery **14**:541-553, 1943.

64 Byers, P. D.: Solitary benign osteoblastic lesions of bone—osteoid osteoma and benign osteoblastoma, Cancer **22**:43-57, 1968.

65 Dahlin, D. C., and Johnson, E. W.: Giant osteoid osteoma, J. Bone Joint Surg. [Am.] **36**:559-572, 1954.

66 Jaffe, H. L.: Osteoid-osteoma of bone, Radiology **45**:319-334, 1945.

67 Lichtenstein, L.: Benign osteoblastoma, J. Bone Joint Surg. [Am.] **46**:755-765, 1964.

68 MacLennan, D. I., and Wilson, F. C., Jr.: Osteoid osteoma of the spine; a review of the literature and report of six new cases, J. Bone Joint Surg. [Am.] **49**:111-121, 1967.

69 Schajowicz, F., and Lemos, C.: Osteoid osteoma and osteoblastoma, Acta Orthop. Scand. **41**:272-291, 1970.

Osteosarcoma

70 Amstutz, H. C.: Multiple osteogenic sarcomata—metastatic or multicentric? Report of two cases and review of literature, Cancer **24**:923-931, 1969.

71 Arlen, M., Higinbotham, N. L., Huvos, A. G., Marcove, R. C., Miller, T., and Shah, I. C.: Radiation-induced sarcoma of bone, Cancer **28**:1087-1099, 1971.

72 Banta, J V., Schreiber, R. R., and Kulik, W J.: Hyperplastic callus formation in osteogenesis imperfecta simulating osteosarcoma, J. Bone Joint Surg. [Am.] **53**:115-122, 1971.

73 Cahan, W. G., Woodard, H. Q., Higinbotham, N. L., Stewart, F. W., and Coley, B. L.: Sarcoma arising in irradiated bone, Cancer **1**:3-29, 1948.

74 Dahlin, D. C., and Coventry, M. B.: Osteogenic sarcoma; a study of 600 cases, J. Bone Joint Surg. [Am.] **49**:101-110, 1967.

75 Hatcher, C. H.: The development of sarcoma in bone subjected to roentgen or radium irradiation, J. Bone Joint Surg. **27**:179-195, 1945.

76 Kahn, L. B., Wood, F. W., and Ackerman, L. V.: Fracture callus associated with benign and malignant bone lesions and mimicking osteosarcoma, Am. J. Clin. Pathol. **52**:14-24, 1969.

77 Lichtenstein, L.: Bone tumors, ed. 4, St. Louis, 1972, The C. V. Mosby Co.

78 Lindbom, A., Soderberg, G., and Spjut, H. J.: Osteosarcoma; a review of 96 cases, Acta Radiol. **56**:1019, 1961.

79 Martland, H. S., and Humphries, R. E.: Osteogenic sarcoma in dial painters using luminous paint, Arch. Pathol. **7**:406-417, 1929.

80 Morton, D. L., and Malmgren, R. A.: Human osteosarcomas: immunologic evidence suggesting an associated infectious agent, Science **162**:1279-1281, 1968.

81 Pritchard, D. J., Reilly, C. A., Jr., and Finkel, M. P.: Evidence for a human osteosarcoma virus, Nature [New Biol.] **234**:126-127, 1971.

82 O'Hara, J. M., Hutter, R. V. P., Foote, F. W., Jr., Miller, T., and Woodard, H. Q.: An analysis of 30 patients surviving longer than ten years after treatment for osteogenic sarcoma, J. Bone Joint Surg. [Am.] **50**:335-354, 1968.

83 Silverman, G.: Multiple osteogenic sarcoma, Arch. Pathol. **21**:88-95, 1936.

Juxtacortical (parosteal) osteosarcoma

84 Dwinnell, L. A., Dahlin, D. C., and Ghormley, R. K.: Parosteal (juxtacortical) osteogenic sarcoma, J. Bone Joint Surg. [Am.] **36**:732-744, 1954.

85 Edeiken, J., Farrell, C., Ackerman, L. V., and Spjut, H.: Parosteal sarcoma, Am. J. Roentgenol. Radium Ther. Nucl. Med. **111**:579-583, 1971.

86 Farr, G. H., and Huvos, A. G.: Juxtacortical osteogenic sarcoma, J. Bone Joint Surg. [Am.] **51**:1205-1216, 1972.

87 Scaglietti, O., and Calandriello, B.: Ossifying parosteal sarcoma, J. Bone Joint Surg. [Am.] **44**:635-647, 1962.

88 Van der Heul, R. O., and Von Ronnen, J. R.: Juxtacortical osteosarcoma; diagnosis, differential diagnosis, treatment, and an analysis of eighty cases, J. Bone Joint Surg. [Am.] **49**:415-439, 1967.

Cartilage-forming tumors
Chondroma

89 Anderson, I. F.: Maffucci's syndrome; report of a case with a review of the literature, S. Afr. Med. J. **39**:1066-1070, 1965.

90 Cowan, W. K.: Malignant change and multiple metastases in Ollier's disease, J. Clin. Pathol. **18**:650-653, 1965.

91 Laurence, W., and Franklin, E. L.: Calcifying enchondroma of long bones, J. Bone Joint Surg. [Br.] **35**:224-228, 1953.

92 Lichtenstein, L., and Hall, J. E.: Periosteal chondroma; a distinctive benign cartilage tumor, J. Bone Joint Surg. **34**:691-697, 1952.

93 Nosanchuk, J. S., and Kaufer, H.: Recurrent periosteal chondroma; report of two cases and

a review of the literature, J. Bone Joint Surg. [Am.] **51**:375-380, 1969.

94 Takigawa, K.: Chondroma of the bones of the hand, J. Bone Joint Surg. [Am.] **53**:1591-1600, 1971.

Osteochondroma

95 Fairbank, H. A. T.: An atlas of general affections of the skeleton, Edinburgh, 1951, E. & S. Livingstone, Ltd.

Chondroblastoma

96 Codman, E. A.: Epiphyseal chondromatous giant cell tumors of the upper end of the humerus, Surg. Gynecol. Obstet. **52**:543-548, 1931.

97 Coleman, S. S.: Benign chondroblastoma with recurrent soft-tissue and intra-articular lesions, J. Bone Joint Surg. [Am.] **48**:1554-1560, 1966.

98 Hatcher, C. H., and Campbell, J. C.: Benign chondroblastoma of bone: its histologic variations and a report of late sarcoma in the site of one, Bull. Hosp. Joint Dis. **12**:411-430, 1951.

99 Huvos, A. G., Marcove, R. C., Erlandson, R. A., and Mike, V.: Chondroblastoma of bone; a clinico-pathologic and electron microscopic study, Cancer **29**:760-771, 1972.

100 Jaffe, H. L., and Lichtenstein, L.: Benign chondroblastoma of bone; a reinterpretation of the so-called calcifying or chondromatous giant cell tumor, Am. J. Pathol. **18**:969-991, 1942.

101 Kahn, L. B., Wood, F. M., and Ackerman, L. V.: Malignant chondroblastoma; report of two cases and review of the literature, Arch. Pathol. **88**:371-376, 1969.

102 Levine, G. D., and Bensch, K. G.: Chondroblastoma—the nature of the basic cell; a study by means of histochemistry, tissue culture, electron microscopy, and autoradiography, Cancer **29**:1546-1562, 1972.

103 Schajowicz, F., and Gallardo, H.: Epiphysial chondroblastoma of bone; a clinico-pathological study of sixty-nine cases, J. Bone Joint Surg. [Br.] **52**:205-226, 1970.

104 Valls, J., Ottolenghi, C. E., and Schajowicz, F.: Epiphyseal chondroblastoma of bone, J. Bone Joint Surg. [Am.] **33**:997-1009, 1951.

105 Welsh, R. A., and Meyer, A. T.: A histogenetic study of chondroblastoma, Cancer **17**:578-589, 1964.

Chondromyxoid fibroma

106 Dahlin, D. C.: Chondromyxoid fibroma of bone, with emphasis on its morphological relationship to benign chondroblastoma, Cancer **9**:195-203, 1956.

107 Jaffe, H. L., and Lichtenstein, L.: Chondromyxoid fibroma of bone; a distinctive benign tumor likely to be mistaken especially for chondrosarcoma, Arch. Pathol. **45**:541-551, 1948.

108 Marcove, R. C., Kambolis, C., Bullough, P. G., and Jaffe, H. L.: Fibromyxoma of bone, Cancer **17**:1209-1213, 1964.

109 Schajowicz, F., and Gallardo, H.: Chondromyxoid fibroma (fibromyxoid chondroma) of bone; a clinico-pathological study of thirty-two cases, J. Bone Joint Surg. [Br.] **53**:198-216, 1971.

Chondrosarcoma

110 Barnes, R., and Catto, M.: Chondrosarcoma of bone, J. Bone Joint Surg. [Br.] **48**:729-764, 1966.

111 Dahlin, D. C., and Beabout, J. W.: Dedifferentiation of low-grade chondrosarcomas, Cancer **28**:461-466, 1971.

112 Dahlin, D. C., and Henderson, E. D.: Chondrosarcoma, a surgical and pathological problem, J. Bone Joint Surg. [Am.] **38**:1025-1038, 1956.

113 Jaffe, H. L.: Hereditary multiple exostoses, Arch. Pathol. **36**:335-357, 1943.

114 Lansche, W. E., and Spjut, H. J.: Chondrosarcoma of the small bones of the hand, J. Bone Joint Surg. [Am.] **40**:1139-1149, 1958.

115 Lichtenstein, L., and Jaffe, H. L.: Chondrosarcoma of bone, Am. J. Pathol. **19**:553-589, 1943.

115a Martin, R. F., Melnick, P. J., Warner, N. E., Terry, R., Bullock, W. K., and Schwinn, C. P.: Chordoid sarcoma, Am. J. Clin. Pathol. **59**:623-635, 1972.

116 McKenna, R. J., Schwinn, C. P., Soong, K. Y., and Higinbotham, N. L.: Sarcomata of the osteogenic series (osteosarcoma, fibrosarcoma, chondrosarcoma, parosteal osteogenic sarcoma, and sarcomata arising in abnormal bone), J. Bone Joint Surg. [Am.] **48**:1-26, 1966.

117 Marcove, R. C., and Huvos, A. G.: Cartilaginous tumors of the ribs, Cancer **27**:794-801, 1971.

118 O'Neal, L. W., and Ackerman, L. V.: Cartilaginous tumors of ribs and sternum, J. Thorac. Surg. **21**: 71-108, 1951 (extensive bibliography).

119 O'Neal, L. W., and Ackerman, L. V.: Chondrosarcoma of bone, Cancer **5**:551-577, 1952 extensive bibliography).

Mesenchymal chondrosarcoma

120 Dowling, E. A.: Mesenchymal chondrosarcoma, J. Bone Joint Surg. [Am.] **46**:747-754, 1964.

121 Goldman, R. L.: "Mesenchymal" chondrosarcoma, a rare malignant chondroid tumor usually primary in bone; report of a case arising in extraskeletal soft tissue, Cancer **20**:1494-1498, 1967.

122 Guccion, J. G., Font, R. L., Enzinger, F. M., and Zimmerman, L. E.: Extraskeletal mesenchymal chondrosarcoma, Arch. Pathol. **95**:336-340, 1973.

123 Salvador, A. H., Beabout, J. W., and Dahlin, D. C.: Mesenchymal chondrosarcoma; observations on 30 new cases, Cancer **28**:605-615, 1971.

Giant cell tumor

124 Dahlin, D. C., Cupps, R. E., and Johnson, E. W., Jr.: Giant-cell tumor; a study of 195 cases, Cancer **25**:1061-1070, 1970.

125 Emley, W. E.: Giant cell tumor of the sphenoid bone; a case report and review of the literature, Arch. Otolaryngol. **94**:369-374, 1971.

126 Hanaoka, H., Friedman, B., and Mack, R. P.: Ultrastructure and histogenesis of giant-cell tumor of bone, Cancer **25**:1408-1423, 1970.

127 Jaffe, H. L., Lichtenstein, L., and Portis, R. B.: Giant cell tumor of bone, Arch. Pathol. **30**:993-1031, 1940.

128 Joynt, G. H. C., and Ortved, W. E.: The accidental operative transplantation of benign giant cell tumor, Ann. Surg. **127**:1232-1239, 1948.

129 Murphy, W. R., and Ackerman, L. V.: Benign and malignant giant-cell tumors of bone, Cancer **9**:317-339, 1956.

130 Schajowicz, F.: Giant-cell tumors of bone (osteoclastoma); a pathological and histochemical study, J. Bone Joint Surg. [Am.] **43**:1-29, 1961.

131 Steiner, G. C., Ghosh, L., and Dorfman, H. D.: Ultrastructure of giant cell tumors of bone, Hum. Pathol. **3**:569-586, 1972.

132 Stewart, F. W., Coley, B. L., and Farrow, J. H.: Malignant giant cell tumor of bone, Am. J. Pathol. **14**:515-535, 1938.

132a Willis, R. A.: Pathology of tumours, ed. 4, New York, 1967, Appleton-Century-Crofts.

133 Windeyer, B. W., and Woodyatt, P. B.: Osteoclastoma: a study of thirty-eight cases, J. Bone Joint Surg. [Br.] **31**:252-267, 1949.

Marrow tumors
  Ewing's sarcoma

134 Friedman, B., and Gold, H.: Ultrastructure of Ewing's sarcoma of bone, Cancer **22**:307-322, 1968.

135 Friedman, B., and Hanaoka, H.: Round-cell sarcomas of bone; a light and electron microscopic study, J. Bone Joint Surg. [Am.] **53**:1118-1136, 1971.

136 Hustu, H., O., Holton, C., James, D. Jr., and Pinkel, D.: Treatment of Ewing's sarcoma with concurrent radiotherapy and chemotherapy, J. Pediatr. **73**:249-251, 1968.

137 Kadin, M. E., and Bensch, K. G.: On the origin of Ewing's tumor, Cancer **27**:257-273, 1971.

138 Millburn, L. F., O'Grady, L., and Hendrickson, F. R.: Radical radiation therapy and total body irradiation in the treatment of Ewing's sarcoma, Cancer **22**:919-925, 1968.

139 Phillips, R. F., and Higinbotham, N. L.: The curability of Ewing's endothelioma of bone in children, J. Pediatr. **70**:391-397, 1967.

140 Schajowicz, F.: Ewing's sarcoma and reticulum-cell sarcoma of bone; with special reference to the histochemical demonstration of glycogen as an aid to differential diagnosis, J. Bone Joint Surg. [Am.] **41**:349-356, 1959.

141 Swenson, P. C.: The roentgenological aspects of Ewing's tumor of bone marrow, Am. J. Roentgenol. Radium Ther. Nucl. Med. **50**:343-353, 1943.

141a Willis, R. A.: Pathology of tumours, ed. 4, New York, 1967, Appleton-Century-Crofts.

Malignant lymphoma

142 Chabner, B. A., Haskell, C. M., and Canellos, G. P.: Destructive bone lesions in chronic granulocytic leukemia, Medicine (Baltimore) **48**:401-410, 1969.

143 Horan, F. T.: Bone involvement in Hodgkin's disease, Br. J. Surg. **56**:277-281, 1969.

144 Ivins, J. C.: Reticulum-cell sarcoma of bone, J. Bone Joint Surg. [Am.] **35**:835-842, 1953.

145 Lichtenstein, L.: Bone tumors, ed. 4, St. Louis, 1972, The C. V. Mosby Co.

146 Parker, F., Jr., and Jackson, H., Jr.: Primary reticulum cell sarcoma of bone, Surg. Gynecol. Obstet. **68**:45-53, 1939.

147 Sherman, R. S., and Snyder, R. E.: The roentgen appearance of primary reticulum cell sarcoma of bone, Am. J. Roentgenol. Radium Ther. Nucl. Med. **58**:291-306, 1947.

148 Shoji, H., and Miller, T. R.: Primary reticulum cell sarcoma of bone; significance of clinical features upon the prognosis, Cancer **28**:1234-1244, 1971.

149 Simmons, C. R., Harle, T. S., and Singleton, E. B.: The osseous manifestations of leukemia in children, Radiol. Clin. North Am. **6**:115-129, 1968.

150 Thomas, L. B., Forkner, C. E., Frei, E., Besse, B. E., and Stabenau, J. R.: The skeletal lesions of acute leukemia, Cancer **14**:608-621, 1961.

151 Wang, C. C., and Fleischli, D. J.: Primary reticulum cell sarcoma of bone, with emphasis on radiation therapy, Cancer **22**:994-998, 1968.

Plasma cell myeloma

152 Azar, H. A.: Plasma cell myelomatosis and other monoclonal gammapathies, Pathol. Annu. **7**:1-17, 1972.

153 Carbone, P. P., Kellerhouse, L. E., and

Gehan, E. A.: Plasmacytic myeloma; a study of the relationship of survival to various clinical manifestations and anomalous protein type in 112 patients, Am. J. Med. **42:**937-948, 1967.

154 Carson, C. P., Ackerman, L. V., and Maltby, J. D.: Plasma cell myeloma, Am. J. Clin. Pathol. **25:**849-888, 1955.

155 Christopherson, W. M., and Miller, A. J.: A reevaluation of solitary plasma cell myeloma of bone, Cancer **3:**240-252, 1950.

156 Fisher, E. R., and Zawadzki, A.: Ultrastructural features of plasma cells in patients with paraproteinemias, Am. J. Clin. Pathol. **54:**779-789, 1970.

157 Kotner, L. M., and Wang, C. C.: Plasmacytoma of the upper air and food passages, Cancer **30:**414-418, 1972.

158 Lichtenstein, L., and Jaffe, H. L.: Multiple myeloma, Arch. Pathol. **44:**207-246, 1947.

159 Moss, W., and Ackerman, L. V.: Plasma cell leukemia, Blood **1:**396-406, 1946.

160 Pasmantier, M. W., and Azar, H. A.: Extraskeletal spread in multiple plasma cell myeloma; a review of 57 autopsied cases, Cancer **23:**167-174, 1969.

161 Rosai, J., and Rodriguez, H. A.: Application of electron microscopy to the differential diagnosis of tumors, Am. J. Clin. Pathol. **50:**555-562, 1968.

Vascular tumors

162 Bucy, P. C., and Capp, C. S.: Primary hemangioma of bone; with special reference to roentgenologic diagnosis, Am. J. Roentgenol. Radium Ther. Nucl. Med. **23:**1-33, 1930.

163 Dorfman, H. D., Steiner, G. C., and Jaffe, H. L.: Vascular tumors of bone, Hum. Pathol. **2:**349-376, 1971.

164 Gorham, L. W., and Stout, A. P.: Massive osteolysis (acute spontaneous absorption of bone, phantom bone, disappearing bone); its relation to hemangiomatosis, J. Bone Joint Surg. [Am.] **37:**985-1004, 1955.

165 Halliday, D. R., Dahlin, D. C., Pugh, D. G., and Young, H. H.: Massive osteolysis and angiomatosis, Radiology **82:**627-644, 1964.

166 Mackenzie, D. H.: Intraosseous glomus tumors; report of two cases, J. Bone Joint Surg. [Br.] **44:**648-651, 1962.

167 Otis, J., Hutter, R. V. P., Foote, F. W., Jr., Marcove, R. C., and Stewart, F. W.: Hemangioendothelioma of the bone, Surg. Gynecol. Obstet. **127:**295-305, 1968.

168 Spjut, H. J., and Lindbom, Å.: Skeletal angiomatosis; report of two cases, Acta Pathol. Microbiol. Scand. **55:**49-58, 1962.

169 Steiner, G. C., and Dorfman, H. D.: Ultrastructure of hemangioendothelial sarcoma of bone, Cancer **29:**122-135, 1972.

170 Töpfer, D. I.: Ueber ein infiltrierend wachsendes Hämangiom der Haut und multiple Kapillarektasien der Haut und innergen Organe. II. Zur Kenntnis der Wirbelangiome, Frankfurt. Z. Pathol. **36:**337-345, 1928.

171 Unni, K. K., Ivins, J. C., Beabout, J. W., and Dahlin, D. C.: Hemangioma, hemangiopericytoma, and hemangioendothelioma (angiosarcoma) of bone, Cancer **27:**1403-1414, 1971.

Other connective tissue tumors

172 Cunningham, M. P., and Arlen, M.: Medullary fibrosarcoma of bone, Cancer **21:**31-37, 1968.

173 Dahlin, D. C., and Ivins, J. C.: Fibrosarcoma of bone; a study of 114 cases, Cancer **23:**35-41, 1969.

174 Furey, J. G., Ferrer-Torells, M., and Reagan, J. W.: Fibrosarcoma arising at the site of bone infarcts; a report of two cases, J. Bone Joint Surg. [Am.] **42:**802-810, 1960.

175 Gilmer, W. S., Jr., and MacEwen, G. D.: Central (medullary) fibrosarcoma of bone, J. Bone Joint Surg. **40:**121-141, 1958.

176 McLeod, J. J., Dahlin, D. C., and Ivins, J. C.: Fibrosarcoma of bone, Am. J. Surg. **94:**431-437, 1957.

177 Rabhan, W. N., and Rosai, J.: Desmoplastic fibroma; report of ten cases and review of the literature, J. Bone Joint Surg. [Am.] **50:**487-502, 1968.

178 Stout, A. P.: Fibrosarcoma; the malignant tumor of fibroblasts, Cancer **1:**30-63, 1948.

179 Whitesides, T. E., and Ackerman, L. V.: Desmoplastic fibroma; a report of three cases, J. Bone Joint Surg. [Am.] **42:**1143-1150, 1960.

Other primary tumors
Chordoma

180 Alezais, H., and Peyron, A.: Sur l'histogenèse et l'origine des chordomes, C. R. Acad. Sci. (Paris) **174:**419-421, 1922.

181 Berard, L., Dunet, C. L., and Peyron, A.: Les chordomes de la region sacrococcygienne et leur histogenese, Bull. Assoc. Franc. Cancer **11:**28-66, 1922.

182 Crawford, T.: The staining reactions of chordoma, J. Clin. Pathol. **11:**110-113, 1958.

183 Erlandson, R. A., Tandler, B., Lieberman, P. H., and Higinbotham, N. L.: Ultrastructure of human chordoma, Cancer Res. **28:**2115-2125, 1968.

184 Gentil, F., and Coley, B. L.: Sacrococcygeal chordoma, Ann. Surg. **127:**432-455, 1948.

184a Heffelfinger, M. J., Dahlin, D. C., MacCarty, C. S., and Beabout, J. W.: Chordomas and cartilaginous tumors at the skull base, Cancer **32:**410-420, 1973.

185 Higinbotham, N. L., Phillips, R. F., Farr, H. W., and Hustu, O.: Chordoma; thirty-five-year study at Memorial Hospital, Cancer 20:1841-1850, 1967.

186 Mabrey, R. E.: Chordoma, Am. J. Cancer 25:501-517, 1935.

187 Pearlman, A. W., and Friedman, M.: Radical radiation therapy of chordoma, Am. J. Roentgenol. Radium Ther. Nucl. Med. 108:333-341, 1970.

188 Stewart, M. J., and Morin, J. E.: Chordoma: a review with report of a new sacrococcygeal case, J. Pathol. Bacteriol. 29:41-60, 1926.

"Adamantinoma" of long bones

189 Albores-Saavedra, J., Diaz Gutierrez, D., and Altamirano Dimas, M.: Adamantinoma de la tibia; observaciones ultraestructurales, Rev. Med. Hosp. Gral. Mex. 31:241-252, 1968.

190 Baker, P. L., Dockerty, M. B., and Coventry, M. B.: Adamantinoma (so-called) of the long bones, J. Bone Joint Surg. [Am.] 36:704-720, 1954.

191 Cohen, D. M., Dahlin, D. C., and Pugh, D. G.: Fibrous dysplasia associated with adamantinoma of the long bones, Cancer 15:515-521, 1961.

192 Moon, N. F.: Adamantinoma of the appendicular skeleton; a statistical review of reported cases and inclusion of 10 new cases, Clin. Orthop. 43:189-213, 1965.

193 Rosai, J.: Adamantinoma of the tibia; electron microscopic evidence of its epithelial origin, Am. J. Clin. Pathol. 51:786-792, 1969.

194 Schajowicz, F., and Gallardo, H.: Adamantinoma de tibia; revisión bibliográfica y consideración de un nuevo caso, Rev. Ortoped. Traumatol. Lat.-Am. 12:105-118, 1967.

Neurilemoma

195 Fawcett, K. J., and Dahlin, D. C.: Neurilemoma of bone, Am. J. Clin. Pathol. 47:759-766, 1967.

196 Hunt, J. C., and Pugh, D. G.: Skeletal lesions in neurofibromatosis, Radiology 76:1-19, 1961.

Metastatic tumors

197 Caffey, J., and Andersen, D. H.: Metastatic embryonal rhabdomyosarcoma in the growing skeleton: clinical, radiographic, and microscopic features, Am. J. Dis. Child. 95:581-600, 1958.

198 Kahn, L. B., Wood, F. W., and Ackerman, L. V.: Fracture callus associated with benign and malignant bone lesions and mimicking osteosarcoma, Am. J. Clin. Pathol. 52:14-24, 1969.

199 Norman, A., and Ulin, R.: A comparative study of periosteal new-bone response in metastatic bone tumors (solitary) and primary bone sarcomas, Radiology 92:705-708, 1969.

200 Perez, C. A., Bradfield, J. S., and Morgan, H. C.: Management of pathologic fractures, Cancer 29:1027-1037, 1972.

201 Thomas, B. M.: Three unusual carcinoid tumours, with particular reference to osteoblastic bone metastases, Clin. Radiol. 19:221-225, 1968.

Laboratory findings

202 Stewart, A., and Weber, F. P.: Myelomatosis, Q. J. Med. 7:211-228, 1938.

Biopsy and frozen section

203 Ottolenghi, C. E.: Diagnosis of orthopaedic lesions by aspiration biopsy; results of 1,061 punctures, J. Bone Joint Surg. [Am.] 37:443-464, 1955.

204 Schajowicz, F., and Derqui, J. C.: Puncture biopsy in lesions of the locomotor system; review of results in 4,050 cases, including 941 vertebral punctures, Cancer 21:531-548, 1968.

205 Sirsat, M. V.: Interpretation and evaluation of aspiration biopsy in sixty-six cases of bone tumors, J. Postgrad. Med. 2:32-36, 1956.

206 Snyder, R. E., and Coley, B. L.: Further studies on the diagnosis of bone tumors by aspiration biopsy, Surg. Gynecol. Obstet. 80:517-522, 1945.

Tumorlike lesions
Solitary bone cyst

207 Jaffe, H. L., and Lichtenstein, L.: Solitary unicameral bone cyst, Arch. Surg. 44:1004-1025, 1942.

208 James, A. G., Coley, B. L., and Higinbotham, N. L.: Solitary (unicameral) bone cyst, Arch. Surg. 57:137-147, 1948.

209 von Mikulicz, J.: Ueber cystische Degeneration der Knochen, Verh. Ges. Deutsch. Naturf. Aerzte 76:107, 1906.

210 Pommer, G.: Zur Kenntnis der progressiven Hämatom- and Phlegmasieveränderungen der Röhrenknochen, Arch. Orthop. Unfallchir. 17:17, 1920.

211 Stewart, M. J., and Hamel, H. A.: Solitary bone cyst, South. Med. J. 43:926-936, 1950.

Aneurysmal bone cyst

212 Buraczewski, J., and Dabska, M.: Pathogenesis of aneurysmal bone cyst; relationship between the aneurysmal bone cyst and fibrous dysplasia of bone, Cancer 28:597-604, 1971.

213 Dabska, M., and Buraczewski, J.: Aneurysmal bone cyst; pathology, clinical course and radiologic appearances, Cancer 23:371-389, 1969.

214 Dahlin, D. C., Besse, B. E., Pugh, D. G., and Ghormley, R. K.: Aneurysmal bone cysts, Radiology **64:**56-65, 1955.

215 Edling, N. P. G.: Is the aneurysmal bone cyst a true entity? Cancer **18:**1127-1130, 1965.

216 Lichtenstein, L.: Aneurysmal bone cyst; observations on fifty cases, J. Bone Joint Surg. [Am.] **39:**873-882, 1957.

217 Tillman, B. P., Dahlin, D. C., Lipscomb, P. R., and Stewart, J. R.: Aneurysmal bone cyst: an analysis of 95 cases, Mayo Clin. Proc. **43:**478-495, 1968.

Ganglion cyst of bone

218 Sim, F. H., and Dahlin, D. C.: Ganglion cysts of bone, Mayo Clin. Proc. **46:**484-488, 1971.

Metaphyseal fibrous defect
(nonossifying fibroma)

219 Cunningham, J. B., and Ackerman, L. V.: Metaphyseal fibrous defects, J. Bone Joint Surg. [Am.] **38:**797-808, 1956.

220 Hatcher, C. H.: Pathogenesis of localized fibrous lesion in the metaphyses of long bones, Ann. Surg. **122:**1016-1030, 1945.

221 Jaffe, H. L., and Lichtenstein, L.: Nonosteogenic fibroma of bone, Am. J. Pathol. **18:**205-221, 1942.

222 Ponsetti, I. V., and Friedman, B.: Evolution of metaphyseal fibrous defects, J. Bone Joint Surg. [Am.] **31:**582-585, 1949.

Fibrous dysplasia

223 Albright, F., Butler, A. M., Hampton, A. O., and Smith, P.: Syndrome characterized by osteitis fibrosa disseminata, areas of pigmentation and endocrine dysfunction, with precocious puberty in females, N. Engl. J. Med. **216:**727-746, 1937.

224 Harris, W. H., Dudley, H. R., and Barry, R. J.: The natural history of fibrous dysplasia, J. Bone Joint Surg. [Am.] **44:**207-233, 1962.

225 Huvos, A. G., Higinbotham, N. L., and Miller, T. R.: Bone sarcomas arising in fibrous dysplasia, J. Bone Joint Surg. [Am.] **54:**1047-1056, 1972.

226 Kempson, R. L.: Ossifying fibroma of the long bones, Arch. Pathol. **82:**218-233, 1966.

227 Lichtenstein, L.: Polyostotic fibrous dysplasia, Arch. Surg. **36:**874-898, 1938.

228 Lichtenstein, L., and Jaffe, H. L.: Fibrous dysplasia of bone, Arch. Pathol. **33:**777-816, 1942 (extensive bibliography).

229 Reed, R. J.: Fibrous dysplasia of bone; a review of 25 cases, Arch. Pathol. **75:**480-495, 1963.

230 Schlumberger, H. G.: Fibrous dysplasia of single bones (monostotic fibrous dysplasia), Milit. Surg. **99:**504-527, 1946.

231 Whitesides, T. E., Jr., and Ackerman, L. V.: Desmoplastic fibroma; a report of three cases, J. Bone Joint Surg. [Am.] **42:**1143-1150, 1960.

Myositis ossificans

232 Ackerman, L. V.: Extraosseous localized nonneoplastic bone and cartilage formation (socalled myostitis ossificans), J. Bone Joint Surg. [Am.] **40:**279-298, 1958.

233 Fine, G., and Stout, A. P.: Osteogenic sarcoma of the extraskeletal soft tissues, Cancer **9:**1027-1043, 1956.

234 Lewis, D.: Myositis ossificans, J.A.M.A. **80:**1281-1287, 1923.

235 Strauss: Cited by Lewis, D.: Myositis ossificans, J.A.M.A. **80:**1281-1287, 1923.

Differentiated histiocytosis (eosinophilic
granuloma, Hand-Schüller-Christian disease,
and Letterer-Siwe disease)

236 Basset, F., Escaig, J., and LeCrom, M.: A cytoplasmic membranous complex in histiocytosis X, Cancer **29:**1380-1386, 1972.

237 Green, W. T., and Farber, S.: "Eosinophilic or solitary granuloma" of bone, J. Bone Joint Surg. **24:**499-526, 1942.

238 Hatcher, C. H.: Eosinophilic granuloma of bone, Arch. Pathol. **30:**828-829, 1940.

239 Jaffe, H. L., and Lichtenstein, L.: Eosinophilic granuloma of bone, Arch. Pathol. **37:**99-118, 1944 (extensive bibliography).

240 Lieberman, P. H., Jones, C. R., Dargeon, H. W. K., and Begg, C. F.: A reappraisal of eosinophilic granuloma of bone, Hand-Schuller-Christian syndrome and Letterer-Siwe syndrome, Medicine (Baltimore) **48:**375-400, 1969.

241 McGavran, M. H., and Spady, H. A.: Eosinophilic granuloma of bone; a study of 28 cases, J. Bone Joint Surg. [Am.] **42:**979-992, 1960.

242 Otani, S., and Ehrlich, J. C.: Solitary granuloma of bone simulating primary neoplasm, Am. J. Pathol. **16:**479-490, 1940.

Articular and periarticular diseases
Ganglia

243 Doyle, R. W.: Ganglia and superficial tumours, Practitioner **156:**267-277, 1946.

244 Fisk, G. R.: Bone concavity caused by a ganglion, J. Bone Joint Surg. [Br.] **31:**220-221, 1949.

245 Lichtenstein, L.: Tumors of synovial joints, bursae, and tendon sheaths, Cancer **8:**816-830, 1955.

246 McEvedy, B. V.: Simple ganglia, Br. J. Surg. **49:**585-594, 1962.

247 Stack, R. E., Bianco, A. H., Jr., and MacCarthy, C. S.: Compression of the common peroneal nerve by ganglion cyst; report of

nine cases, J. Bone Joint Surg. [Am.] **47:** 773-778, 1965.

Bursae; Baker's cyst

248 Meyerding, H. W., and Van Denmark, R. E.: Posterior hernia of the knee, J.A.M.A. **122:**858-861, 1943.
249 Pederson, H. E., and Key, J. A.: Pathology of calcareous tendinitis and subdeltoid bursitis, Arch. Surg. **62:**50-63, 1951.
250 Wagner, T., and Abgarowicz, T.: Microscopic appearance of Baker's cyst in cases of rheumatoid arthritis, Reumatologia **8:**21-26, 1970.

Fibrous histiocytoma of tendon sheath (nodular tenosynovitis)

251 Jaffe, H. L., Lichtenstein, L., and Sutro, C. J.: Pigmented villonodular synovitis, bursitis, and tenosynovitis, Arch. Pathol. **31:**731-765, 1941.
252 Wright, C. J. E.: Benign giant cell synovioma; an investigation of 85 cases, Br. J. Surg. **38:**257-271, 1951.

Pigmented villonodular synovitis and bursitis

253 Atmore, W. G., Dahlin, D. C., and Ghormley, R. K.: Pigmented villonodular synovitis; a clinical and pathologic study, Minn. Med. **39:**196-202, 1956.
254 Byers, P. D., Cotton, R. E., Deacon, O. W., Lowy, M., Newman, P. H., Sissons, H. A., and Thomson, A. D.: The diagnosis and treatment of pigmented villonodular synovitis, J. Bone Joint Surg. [Br.] **50:**290-305, 1968.
255 Greenfield, M. M., and Wallace, K. M.: Pigmented villonodular synovitis, Radiology **54:**350-356, 1950.
256 Nilsonne, U., and Moberger, G.: Pigmented villonodular synovitis of joints; histological and clinical problems in diagnosis, Acta Orthop. Scand. **40:**448-460, 1969.
257 Scott, F. M.: Bone lesions in pigmented villonodular synovitis, J. Bone Joint Surg. **50:**306-311, 1968.

Synovial osteochondromatosis

258 Goldman, R. L., and Lichtenstein, L.: Synovial chondrosarcoma, Cancer **12:**1233-1240, 1964.
259 King, J. W., Spjut, H. J., Fechner, R. E., and Vanderpool, D. W.: Synovial chondrosarcoma of the knee joint, J. Bone Joint Surg. **49:**1389-1396, 1967.
260 Murphy, F. P., Dahlin, D. C., and Sullivan, C. R.: Articular synovial chondromatosis, J. Bone Joint Surg. [Am.] **44:**77-86, 1962.

Arthritis
  Synovial biopsy

261 Polley, H. F., and Bickel, W. H.: Experiences with an instrument for punch biopsy of synovial membrane, Mayo Clin. Proc. **26:** 273-281, 1951.
262 Rodnan, G. P., Yunis, E. J., and Totten, R. S.: Experience with punch biopsy of synovium in the study of joint disease, Ann. Intern. Med. **53:**319-331, 1960.
263 Schumacher, H. R., and Kulka, J. P.: Needle biopsy of the synovial membrane; experience with the Parker-Pearson technic, N. Engl. J. Med. **286:**416-419, 1972.
264 Schwartz, S., and Cooper, N.: Synovial membrane punch biopsy, Arch. Intern. Med. **108:** 400-406, 1961.
265 Zevely, H. A., French, A. J., Mikkelsen, W. M., and Duff, I. F.: Synovial specimens obtained by knee joint punch biopsy; histologic study in joint diseases, Am. J. Med. **20:**510-519, 1956.

Degenerative joint disease (osteoarthritis)

266 Bauer, W., and Bennet, G. A.: Experimental and pathological studies in the degenerative type of arthritis, J. Bone Joint Surg. **18:**1-18, 1936.
267 Bennett, G. A., Waine, H., and Bauer, W.: Changes in the knee joint at various ages, New York, 1942, Commonwealth Fund.
268 Collins, D. H.: The pathology of articular and spinal diseases, London, 1949, Edward Arnold & Co. (an excellent reference book).
269 Collins, D. H.: Recent advances in the pathology of chronic arthritis and rheumatic disorders, Postgrad. Med. J. **31:**602-608, 1955.
270 Haliburton, R. A., and Sullivan, C. R.: The patella in degenerative joint diseases; a clinicopathologic study, Arch. Surg. **77:**677-683, 1958.
271 Harrison, M. H. M., Schajowicz, F., and Trueta, J.: Osteoarthritis of the hip: a study of the nature and evolution of the disease, J. Bone Joint Surg. [Br.] **35:**598-626, 1953.
272 Hirsch, C., Schajowicz, F., and Galante, J.: Structural changes in the cervical spine; a study on autopsy specimens in different age groups, Acta Orthop. Scand. [Suppl.] **109:** 7-77, 1967.
273 Horwitz, T.: Bone and cartilage debris in the synovial membrane; its significance in the early diagnosis of neuro-arthropathy, J. Bone Joint Surg. [Am.] **30:**579-588, 1948.
274 Jayson, M. I., Rubenstein, D., and Dixon, A. S.: Intra-articular pressure and rheumatoid geodes (bone 'cysts'), Ann. Rheum. Dis. **29:**496-502, 1970.
275 Karlson, S.: Chondromalacia patellae, Acta Chir. Scand. **83:**347-381, 1940.
276 Keefer, C.: The etiology of chronic arthritis, N. Engl. J. Med. **213:**644-653, 1935.
277 Matthews, B. F.: Composition of articular cartilage in osteoarthritis; changes in colla-

gen/chondroitin-sulphate ratio, Br. Med. J. **2:**660-661, 1953.

278 Nichols, E. H., and Richardson, F. L.: Arthritis deformans, J. Med. Res. **16:**149-221, 1909.

279 Norman, A., Robbins, H., and Milgram, J. E.: The acute neuropathic arthropathy; a rapid, severely disorganizing form of arthritis, Radiology **90:**1159-1164, 1968.

280 Outerbridge, R. E.: The etiology of chondromalacia patellae, J. Bone Joint Surg. [Br.] **43:**752-757, 1961.

281 Rhaney, K., and Lamb, D. W.: The cysts of osteoarthritis of the hip; a radiological and pathological study, J. Bone Joint Surg. [Br.] **37:**663-675, 1955.

282 Silverberg, M., Frank, E. L., Jarrett, S. R., and Silberberg, R.: Aging and osteoarthritis of the human sternoclavicular joint, Am. J. Pathol. **35:**851-865, 1959.

Rheumatoid arthritis

283 Allison, N., and Ghormley, R. K.: Diagnosis in joint disease; a clinical and pathological study of arthritis, New York, 1931, William Wood & Co.

284 Baggenstoss, A. H., and Rosenberg, E. F.: Cardiac lesions in chronic infections (rheumatoid) arthritis, Am. J. Pathol. **16:**693-695, 1940.

285 Beatty, E. C., Jr.: Rheumatic-like nodules occurring in nonrheumatic children, Arch. Pathol. **68:**154-159, 1959.

286 Bennett, G. A., Zeller, J. W., and Bauer, W.: Subcutaneous nodules of rheumatoid arthritis and rheumatic fever, Arch. Pathol. **30:**70-89, 1940.

287 Berardinelli, J. L., Hyman, C. J., Campbell, E. E., and Fireman, P.: Presence of rheumatoid factor in ten children with isolated rheumatoid-like nodules, J. Pediatr. **81:**751-757, 1972.

288 Bevans, M., Nadell, J., Demartius, F., and Ragan, C.: The systemic lesions of malignant arthritis, Am. J. Med. **16:**197-211, 1954.

289 Bhan, A. K., and Roy, S.: Synovial giant cells in rheumatoid arthritis and other joint diseases, Ann. Rheum. Dis. **30:**294-298, 1971.

290 Cooper, N. S.: Pathology of rheumatoid arthritis, Med. Clin. North Am. **52:**607-621, 1968.

291 Dixon, A. St. J., and Grant, C.: Acute synovial rupture in rheumatoid arthritis; clinical and experimental observations, Lancet **1:**742-745, 1964.

292 Freund, H. A., Steiner, G., Leichtentritt, B., and Price, A. E.: Peripheral nerves in chronic atrophic arthritis, Am. J. Pathol. **18:**865-893, 1942.

293 Grimley, P. M., and Sokoloff, L.: Synovial giant cells in rheumatoid arthritis, Am. J. Pathol. **49:**931-954, 1966.

294 Hahn, B. H., Yardley, J. H., and Stevens, M. B.: "Rheumatoid" nodules in systemic lupus erythematosus, Ann. Intern. Med. **72:**49-58, 1970.

295 Hart, F. D.: Rheumatoid arthritis: extra-articular manifestations, Br. Med. J. **3:**131-136, 1969.

296 Hart, F. D.: Rheumatoid arthritis: extra-articular manifestations. Part II, Br. Med. J. **2:**747-752, 1970.

297 Horwitz, T.: Bone and cartilage debris in the synovial membrane; its significance in the early diagnosis of neuro-arthropathy, J. Bone Joint Surg. [Am.] **30:**579-588, 1948.

298 Jayson, M. I., Dixon, A. S., Kates, A., Pinder, I., and Coomes, E. N.: Popliteal and calf cysts in rheumatoid arthritis; treatment by anterior synovectomy, Ann. Rheum. Dis. **31:**9-15, 1972.

299 Kellgren, J. H.: Some concepts of rheumatic disease, Br. Med. J. **1:**1152-1157, 1952.

300 Luck, V. J.: Bone and joint diseases, Springfield, Ill., 1950, Charles C Thomas, Publisher.

301 Mitchell, N., and Shepard, N.: The ultrastructure of articular cartilage in rheumatoid arthritis; a preliminary report, J. Bone Joint Surg. [Am.] **52:**1405-1423, 1970.

302 Mongan, E. S., Cass, R. M., Jacox, R. F., and Vaughan, J. H.: A study of the relation of seronegative and seropositive rheumatoid arthritis to each other and to necrotizing vasculitis, Am. J. Med. **47:**23-25, 1969.

303 Muirden, K. D.: Giant cells, cartilage and bone fragments within rheumatoid synovial membrane: clinico-pathological correlations, Aust. Ann. Med. **2:**105-110, 1970.

304 Palmer, D. G.: Synovial cysts in rheumatoid disease, Ann. Intern. Med. **70:**61-68, 1969.

305 Pirani, C. R., and Bennett, G. A.: Rheumatoid arthritis: a report of three cases progressing from childhood and emphasizing certain systemic manifestations, Bull. Hosp. Joint Dis. **12:**335-367, 1951.

306 Roberts, W. C., Kehol, J. A., Carpenter, D. F., and Golden, A.: Cardiac valvular lesions in rheumatoid arthritis, Arch. Intern. Med. **122:**141-146, 1968.

307 Schmid, F. R., Cooper, N. S., Ziff, M., and McEwen, C.: Arteritis in rheumatoid arthritis, Am. J. Med. **30:**56-83, 1961.

308 Sherman, M. S.: The non-specificity of synovial reactions, Bull. Hosp. Joint Dis. **12:**335-367, 1951.

309 Sokoloff, L.: Biopsy in rheumatic diseases, Med. Clin. North Am. **45:**1171-1180, 1961.

310 Sokoloff, L., Wilens, S. L., and Bunim, J. J.: Arthritis of striated muscle in rheumatoid arthritis, Am. J. Pathol. **27:**157-173, 1951.

311 Taylor, R. T., Huskisson, E. C., Whitehouse, G. H., and Hart, F. D.: Spontaneous fractures of pelvis in rheumatoid arthritis, Br. Med. J. 4:663-664, 1971.

312 Weissmann, G.: Lysosomal mechanisms of tissue injury in arthritis, N. Engl. J. Med. 286:141-146, 1972.

Gout

313 Appleby, E. C.: Some cases of gout in reptiles, J. Pathol. Bacteriol. 80:427-430, 1960.

314 deGalantha, E.: Technic for preservation and microscopic demonstration of nodules in gout, Am. J. Clin. Pathol. 5:165-166, 1935.

315 Lichtenstein, L., Scott, H. W., and Levin, M. H.: Pathologic changes in gout—survey of eleven necropsied cases, Am. J. Pathol. 32:871-895, 1956.

316 Moskowitz, R. W., and Katz, D.: Chondrocalcinosis and chondrocalsynovitis (pseudogout syndrome); analysis of 24 cases, Am. J. Med. 43:322-334, 1967.

23 Soft tissues

Infections

Infections of subcutaneous tissues occur secondary to cutaneous, visceral, or osseous infections and trauma or as a complication of operations. Rarely, such infections may be hematogenous.

The severity of the inflammatory reaction and the type of tissue response observed pathologically depend upon the type, dose, and virulence of the infecting organism, the resistance of the host tissues, the presence or absence of necrotic tissue, hematoma, foreign body, and the anatomy of the infected area.

Clinical types of infectious processes such as hemolytic streptococcal gangrene, necrotizing fasciitis, and Meleney's synergistic gangrene must be diagnosed by clinical appearance and bacteriologic study. All advanced pyogenic and necrotizing infections produce acute inflammatory tissue reactions indistinguishable microscopically. However, in some instances the diagnosis of granulomatous infections may be made by proper staining and careful

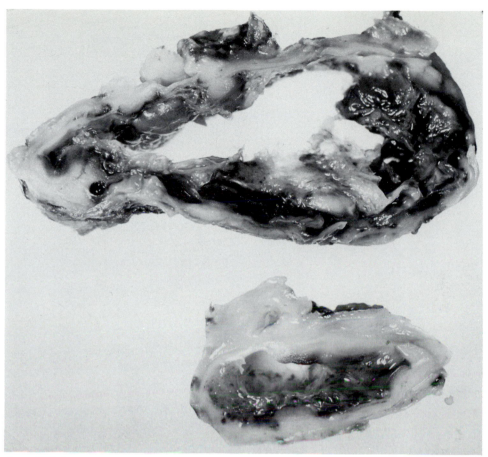

Fig. 1090 Cystic hematoma of left scapular region excised from 45-year-old black woman two weeks following injury. (WU neg. 55-4576.)

search of tissue sections for characteristic organisms (actinomycosis, blastomycosis, coccidioidomycosis, and sporotrichosis).

Tuberculosis also may be suspected histologically, but proof of the significance of the occasional acid-fast bacillus seen in tissue sections rests with culture and guinea pig inoculation. Certain granulomatous and chronic pyogenic infections, as well as encysted hematomas, mimic soft tissue tumors[1, 2] (Fig. 1090).

Pilonidal disease

Pilonidal sinuses appear as small openings in the intergluteal fold about 3.5 cm to 5 cm posterior to the anal orifice. Hairs are sometimes seen protruding from them. The opening is continued by a sinus tract, which is directed upward in 93% of the cases.[5] The disease is most often seen in young white males with dark, straight hair. Although congenital anomalies related to the closure of the neural canal can certainly occur in this area, it is now believed that the large majority of pilonidal sinuses have an acquired pathogenesis.[4] Hairs penetrate areas of inflammation from without, lodge in the dermis, and elicit a foreign body type of reaction (Fig. 1091). The sinus is lined by granulation tissue. In approximately 25% of the cases, hairs are not found within the lesion.

Pilonidal sinuses also have been described in other areas where skin folds are prominent, such as the axilla, umbilicus, clitoris, and axilla.[3] A further observation favoring the theory of the acquired origin is the fact that barbers and hairdressers occa-

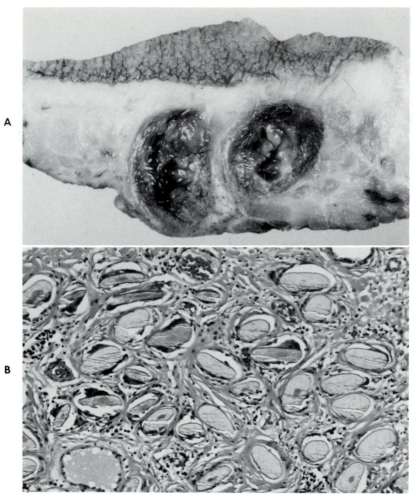

Fig. 1091   A, Pilonidal sinus removed from sacrococcygeal area of 19-year-old youth. Hair-containing cystic structures in dermis are characteristic. They communicated with each other in another plane of section. **B,** Microscopic appearance of pilonidal disease. Numerous hair shafts penetrate into dermis and elicit foreign body giant cell reaction. (**A,** WU neg. 73-1477; **B,** ×100; WU neg. 73-2073.)

sionally develop a disease equivalent to pilonidal sinus between their fingers, the sinuses containing somebody else's hairs!

Tumors
Introduction

The tumors of the soft tissue are a large heterogeneous group.[8] A marked difference in age distribution is seen among the different microscopic types. As a whole, a large proportion of soft tissue sarcomas affects children[7] and may even be present at birth. Kauffman and Stout[6] remarked that

congenital soft tissue tumors rarely behave malignantly, even when this behavior was to be expected from their microscopic appearance. In our institution, by far the most common soft tissue sarcomas are liposarcoma in adults and rhabdomyosarcoma in children. These tumors often are badly treated. Such poor treatment is related to ignorance of the pathology.

The soft tissue lesions discussed herewith exclude those of the mediastinum, retroperitoneum, and soft tissues of the visceral organs and those primarily involving the

Table 48 Clinical evaluation of preliminary biopsy of soft tissue masses*

	Cases	Local recurrences
Without biopsy	27	21 (78.8%)
With biopsy	12	2 (16.6%)
Total	39	23 (59.9%)

*From Lieberman, Z., and Ackerman, L. V: Principles in management of soft tissue sarcomas, Surgery 35:350-365, 1954.

dermis, such as Kaposi's sarcoma and mycosis fungoides.

Biopsy

The relatively untrained surgeon confronted by a soft tissue mass boldly excises or enucleates it, invariably inadequately. He is surprised to find it malignant. Because of poor primary treatment, the extent of the corrective operation may result in deformity or sacrifice of an extremity. The proper initial procedure is careful incisional biopsy. After accurate classification of the tumor, it can then be treated intelligently.

Biopsy is not dangerous and does not cause metastases. Indeed, incisional biopsy followed by adequate treatment is associated with a lower incidence of local recurrence than is primary excision of the malignant soft tissue tumor when the latter is performed without prior biopsy[9] (Table 48). At the definitive operation, the area of the biopsy should be excised in continuity with the tumor. Occasionally, aspiration or needle biopsy of a soft tissue neoplasm may be diagnostic. We have not hesitated to use frozen section. If a definite diagnosis can be made, the lesion may be treated immediately.

Of course, diagnosis by aspiration biopsy and/or frozen section may not be definitive. In these instances, treatment must be delayed until diagnosis from the permanent tissue sections can be made. The importance of this concept is evident in the following three cases.

A young ballet dancer noted a soft tissue tumor of the popliteal space. It was fairly firm and ap-

peared to be deeply attached. The tumor was not biopsied before its attempted removal. The surgeon found the tumor apparently infiltrating the deeper tissues and amputated the leg. Microscopic examination showed a fibrous tissue tumor of the desmoid type that could have been cured without amputation.

A young male patient with a soft tissue tumor in the region of the upper arm had careful incisional biopsy which showed desmoid tumor. The tumor was excised locally without sacrificing the arm. The patient is alive and well ten years later.

A young male patient had an apparently encapsulated soft tissue tumor on the upper, inner thigh enucleated without biopsy. The lesion was liposarcoma. It quickly recurred locally and required hemipelvectomy to encompass the recurrence. A primary diagnosis by incisional biopsy and a radical local excision might well have saved the lower extremity.

Many malignant soft tissue sarcomas appear grossly to be encapsulated. This encapsulation is false (Fig. 1092). Therefore, attempts to enucleate fail. This pseudoencapsulation occurs often with fibrosarcoma, liposarcoma, leiomyosarcoma, and synovial sarcoma.

The pathologist who studies these lesions should make every attempt to classify them accurately, for this classification has proved extremely useful from the standpoint of treatment and prognosis. He must know the orientation of the specimen and the tissue sections so that he can state with certainty whether or not the lesion was adequately excised.

Special stains may help in the classification of these tumors. Some examples are reticulin stain for vascular tumors and synovial sarcomas, periodic acid–Schiff for alveolar soft part sarcomas (for the demonstration of intracytoplasmic crystals), phosphotungstic acid–hematoxylin or Masson's trichrome for tumors of striated muscle, and mucin stains for synovial sarcomas and myxoid tumors in general. Electron microscopy also can be extremely helpful. Fibroblasts, smooth and striated muscle cells, Schwann cells, endothelial cells, pericytes, and the cells of granular cell tumor and alveolar soft part sarcoma have distinctive ultrastruc-

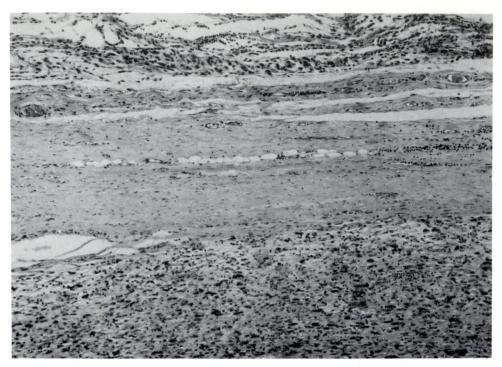

Fig. 1092 Liposarcoma. In center is broad band of connective tissue capsule. Tumor is present on both sides of capsule. Surgeon believed that he had excised neoplasm adequately. However, plane of dissection was close to capsule and through tumor. Therefore, lesion recurred locally. (×90; WU neg. 57-198.)

tural features that often provide a specific diagnosis.

Tumors and tumorlike conditions of fibrous tissue
Juvenile aponeurotic fibroma

A distinctive microscopic lesion, juvenile aponeurotic fibroma was described by Keasbey[12] in 1953. The classical presentation is that of a soft tissue mass in the hand or wrist of a child or an adolescent. At surgery, it may appear as a nodule or as an ill-defined infiltrating mass in the subcutaneous tissue or attached to a tendon. Sometimes, foci of calcification may be detected on gross inspection.

Microscopically, the lesion is characterized by a diffuse fibroblastic growth in which spotty calcification occurs (Fig. 1093). Infiltration of fat and striated muscle is often seen at the periphery. Mitoses are scarce, and atypical cytologic features are absent. Scattered osteoclast-like giant

cells are frequently seen. The cells inside and surrounding the calcified foci have a strong resemblance to chondrocytes. It is this feature that led Lichtenstein and Goldman[13] to postulate that this lesion is basically of cartilaginous origin and that it represents the cartilaginous analogue of fibromatosis. We basically agree with this view.[11]

Juvenile aponeurotic fibroma can be confused with rheumatoid nodule, neurilemoma, and fibromatosis. Local recurrence is common, especially in young children. However, distant metastases do not occur.[10]

Nodular fasciitis

The term **nodular fasciitis** is currently accepted for the condition originally designated as subcutaneous pseudosarcomatous fibromatosis.[17] It is a distinctive lesion and a very important one because of its ability to simulate a malignant process.[14] In the

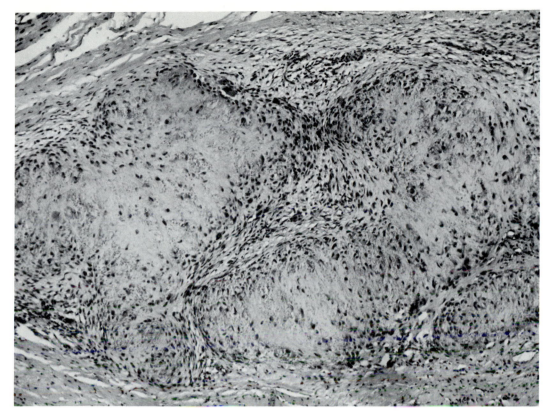

Fig. 1093 Localized nodular type of "juvenile aponeurotic fibroma" in 44-year-old man. It appeared as nodule on dorsal surface of wrist. Proliferating cells are cartilaginous in origin. (×90; WU neg. 67-1167; slide contributed by Dr. C. P. Schwinn, Los Angeles, Cailf.)

past, it was usually mislabeled as fibrosarcoma, liposarcoma, or rhabdomyosarcoma. Individuals in their fourth decade of life are most commonly affected. The most common locations are the upper extremities (particularly the flexor aspect of the forearms), trunk, and neck. Two important clinical features are the history of rapid growth (usually a few weeks) and the small size. It is usually located above the fascia, but it may be beneath it or in the fascia itself. Like most soft tissue growths of fibrous tissue origin, it has infiltrative margins.

Microscopically, the lesion is characterized by a cellular fibroblastic growth set in a loosely textured mucoid matrix (Fig. 1094). Vascular proliferation and chronic inflammatory cells also are present. The high cellularity of the lesion and the presence of mitotic figures and of occasional cells with bizarre nuclei are responsible for the frequent confusion of this lesion with sarcoma. However, follow-up studies have conclusively shown that it is perfectly benign.[15, 16, 18]

Elastofibroma

Elastofibroma is a benign, poorly circumscribed tumorlike condition involving almost exclusively the subscapular region of elderly individuals. There is often a history of hard manual labor. At surgery, the lesions are usually found at the apex of the scapula, beneath the rhomboid and latissimus dorsi muscles. The right side is affected more commonly than the left. Bilaterality is not infrequent.

Microscopically, collagen bundles alternate with homogeneous acidophilic material with the histochemical and ultrastructural appearance of degenerated elas-

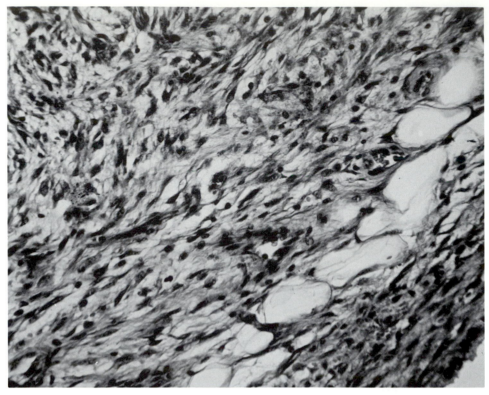

Fig. 1094 Typical nodular fasciitis in 47-year-old woman who had soft tissue mass just beneath skin in deltopectoral group which measured 3 cm × 2 cm × 1 cm and had been present for only two weeks. It is highly cellular and vascular and can easily be confused with fibrosarcoma. It infiltrates on its periphery and may show evidence of maturation. (×250; WU neg. 62-7387.)

tic tissue.[19, 21] Elastase digestion fully removes this material.[19] We agree with Järvi et al.[20] that this lesion is not a true neoplasm but rather a degenerative process probably produced by friction of the scapula against the rib cage. Surgery is curative.

Fibromatosis

The generic term *fibromatosis* was proposed by Stout[46] for a group of related conditions having in common the following features:

1 Proliferation of well-differentiated fibroblasts
2 Infiltrative pattern of growth
3 Presence of a variable (but usually abundant) amount of collagen between the proliferating cells
4 Lack of cytologic features of malignancy and scanty or absent mitotic activity
5 Aggressive clinical behavior, characterized by repeated local recurrences, but without the capacity to produce distant metastases

Grossly, these lesions are often large, firm, and whitish, with ill-defined outlines and an irregularly whorled cut surface (Figs. 1095 and 1096). They often arise in a muscular fascia. Microscopically, the fibroblastic nature of the cells is usually quite obvious. However, in some actively proliferating types, the plump nuclei with blunted ends can closely resemble those of smooth muscle cells. In these instances, the use of trichrome stains or electron microscopy can be decisive in the differential diagnosis. In an ultrastructural study of fibromatosis, Welsh[47] de-

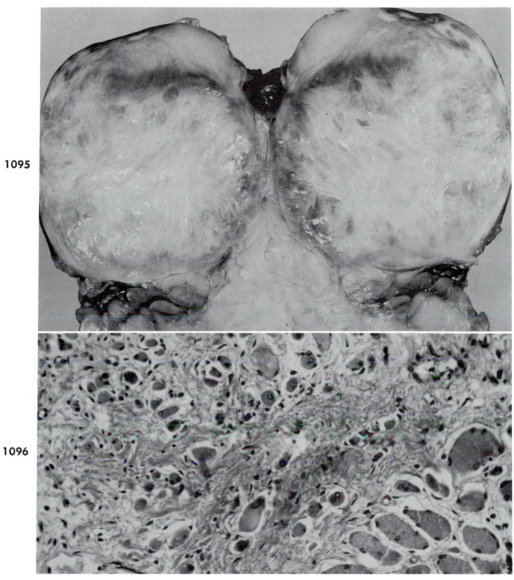

Fig. 1095 Large fibromatosis of abdominal wall. Note lack of circumscription and almost complete replacement of muscle. (WU neg. 50-5320.)
Fig. 1096 Fibromatosis with adult fibrous tissue growing between muscle bundles. (Low power.)

scribed intracytoplasmic collagen formation, probably representing a pathologic process in the course of collagen synthesis.

Some pathologists add the adjective *aggressive* to some forms of fibromatosis to emphasize the biologic behavior. We do not use the term, since we regard it as redundant; all fibromatoses are at least potentially aggressive. Besides, there is very little correlation between the cellularity or other microscopic features of these lesions and their biologic behavior. Other authors have gone even further and have used *differentiated fibrosarcoma* as a synonym for the histologically more cellular or clinically more aggressive types of fibromatosis.[46] We are opposed to this terminology, because the designation of sarcoma endowes this lesion in the mind of many surgeons with a truly malignant potential that it does not possess. Although we recognize the difficulties involved, we always attempt to make a distinction between fibromatosis and well-differentiated fibrosarcoma, reserving the latter term for tumors showing atypical cytologic features and/or a significant number of mitotic figures (more than one per high power field). As Enzinger[32] remarked, it is usually not possible on the basis of the histologic examination to predict whether or not a fibromatosis will recur, but it is possible to predict whether a fibrous tumor is or is not capable of metastases.

Most soft tissue fibromatoses are in intimate contact with skeletal muscles—hence their designation as *musculoaponeurotic fibromatosis*.[33] This is certainly preferable to the obsolete *desmoid tumor*, traditionally regarded as a neoplasm of the abdominal wall appearing in women during or following pregnancy, although in our experience it is almost as common in men and in other locations, such as the shoulder girdle, head and neck area, and thigh.[28, 36, 40] Enzinger and Shiraki[33] analyzed thirty cases located in the shoulder girdle that had been followed for a minimum of ten years. In 57% of the patients, the tumor recurred one or more times. However, at the end of the follow-up period, *all patients* were living without any evidence of continuing tumor growth. A higher incidence of recurrence was seen in young individuals and in those patients with tumors of large size.

The treatment of choice is a prompt radical excision, including a wide margin of involved tissue.[28] However, it should not sacrifice major blood vessels, nerves, or an extremity, even if recurrence is thought likely. Recurrences may still be treated by local excision with chance of control. In our experience, the incidence of local recurrence is lower in fibromatoses of the abdominal wall than in those located elsewhere.[36] Some of the latter have recurred as many as five or six times. Only rarely, however, has local aggressiveness forced amputation. Actually, cessation of

Table 49 Anatomic sites of fibrous tissue proliferations*

Site	Cases
Hands and feet	20
Neck	15
Shoulder and adjacent areas	14
Buttocks—thigh and leg	12
Scalp	3
Abdominal muscles	2
Ear	1
Eyelid	1
Suprapubic and perineal areas	1
Lung	1
Mesentery	1
Generalized	3

*From Stout, A. P.: Juvenile fibromatoses, Cancer 7:953-978, 1954.

attempts to excise persistent tissue locally may be followed by failure of the lesion to enlarge further.

The name *juvenile fibromatosis* has often been applied to examples of fibromatosis occurring in children and adolescents[35] (Table 49). In most cases, this is hardly justified. Except for their greater frequency in this age group and, in some specific instances, their greater propensity for local recurrence, there is very little either on clinical or microscopic grounds that differentiates fibromatosis in children from that occurring in other age groups.[31] We know of only two exceptions to this statement—i.e., two variants of fibromatosis apparently restricted to childhood and presenting a distinctive clinicopathologic picture: fibromatosis colli (congenital torticollis) and infantile digital fibromatosis.

Fibromatosis colli (congenital torticollis) is a type of fibromatosis affecting the lower third of the sternomastoid muscle and appearing at birth or shortly thereafter. Bilateral forms have been observed. Fibromatosis colli is frequently associated with various congenital anomalies. Thus, Iwahara and Iheda[37] found congenital (usually ipsilateral) dislocations of the hip in 14% of their patients. An association between complicated deliveries (particularly breech deliveries) and fibromatosis colli has been established.[29] Although some instances of spontaneous disappearance have been recorded, this condition usually necessitates resection of the muscle. Microscopically, the cellularity of the fibrous tissue depends upon the age of the process. This condition has been considered due to birth injury, but we have never seen evidence of previous hemorrhage.[26]

The so-called *infantile digital fibromatosis* is also a form of fibromatosis restricted to childhood.[42] The typical location is the exterior surface of the end phalanges of the fingers and toes. The lesions are either present at birth or appear during the first two years of life and are often multiple. A distinctive microscopic feature, not observed in the other forms of fibromatosis, is the presence of peculiar eosinophilic cytoplasmic inclusions. These have been examined ultrastructurally and found to be composed of compact masses of granules and filaments without a limiting membrane.[23, 27] Their significance is obscure, although their similarity with the "virus factories" seen in cells with certain viruses has been remarked. This disease has a high tendency for local recurrence.

Generalized fibromatosis may be present as multiple nodules limited to the superficial soft tissue or be associated with internal organ involvement.[24, 43] The latter form, which is usually congenital, can be fatal. Familial cases have been described.[30]

Fibromatosis hyalinica multiplex is a morphologically distinctive type of familial multiple fibromatosis. It affects children but is not present at birth.[36a, 48]

Some forms of fibromatosis derive their names from their particular location—i.e., *palmar fibromatosis* (Dupuytren's contracture), *plantar fibromatosis* (Ledderhose's disease), and *penile fibromatosis* (Peyronie's disease).[39, 44] The latter condition is discussed in Chapter 17. Both palmar and plantar fibromatosis can be extremely cellular.[41, 44] We have seen them confused with fibrosarcoma (Fig. 1097). It is well to remember that fibrosarcoma of the palmar and plantar areas is exceptional.[22] The differential diagnosis of a cellular spindle cell tumor of the sole is usually

between fibromatosis, synovial sarcoma, malignant melanoma, and Kaposi's sarcoma. Palmar and plantar fibromatosis occur predominantly in adults. Contracture of the fingers or toes is the leading clinical manifestation. In an excellent electron microscopic study, Gabbiani and Majno[34] found nuclear deformations such as are found in contracted cells (retrospectively identified by light microscopy as cross-banded nuclei) and a cytoplasmic fibrillary system similar to that found in smooth muscle cells. They suggested that the proliferating fibroblasts had modulated toward a contractile cell and that this was responsible for the contracture evident clinically. Multiple lesions involving the palmar as well as the plantar areas are frequenty observed. Bilaterality is also common. The plantar form of the disease tends to be more localized than its palmar counterpart.

Fibromatoses also have been named according to the presumed inciting cause, such as *cicatricial fibromatosis* and *post-irradiation fibromatosis*. The cicatricial form may follow accidental trauma or arise in the scar of surgical procedures. Post-irradiation fibromatosis differs from the other forms by virtue of the common occurence of bizarre cells with large hyperchromatic nuclei. This feature, which in the absence of radiation exposure would be strong evidence of malignancy, should be interpreted much more conservatively under these circumstances.

The association of soft tissue tumors, usually of the fibromatosis type, with multiple colonic polyposis and occasionally multiple osteomas is known as *Gardner's syndrome*.[25, 45] In this condition, the fibromatosis has a particular tendency to involve intra-abdominal structures, such as omentum and mesentery.[38]

Fibrosarcoma

Fibrosarcomas are commonly tumors of adults, although they can occur in any age group and even present as congenital neoplasms[50] (Fig. 1098). They arise from such superficial and deep connective tissues

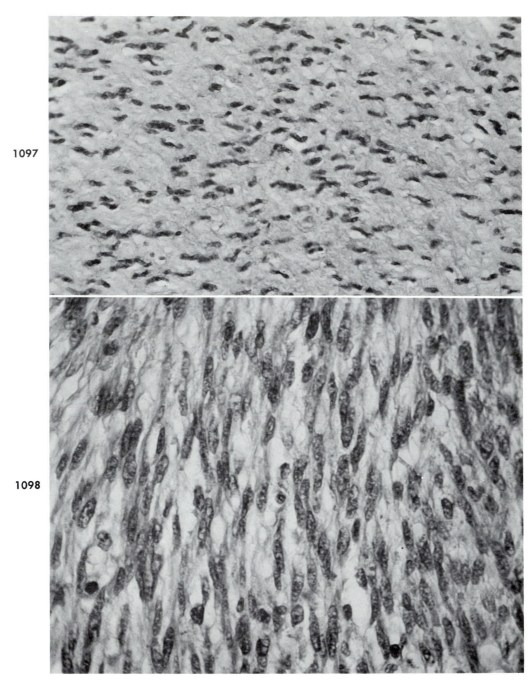

Fig. 1097 Cellular area in plantar fibromatosis, often incorrectly diagnosed as fibrosarcoma. Note uniformity of nuclei. Mitotic figures are exceptional. (×400; WU neg. 52-
3448.)
Fig. 1098 Fairly well-differentiated congenital fibrosarcoma of thigh. Lesion, which was
pseudoencapsulated mass, was locally excised and patient is living five years after operation. Patients with such tumor may have an unexpectedly good prognosis. (×600; WU neg.
62-7379.)

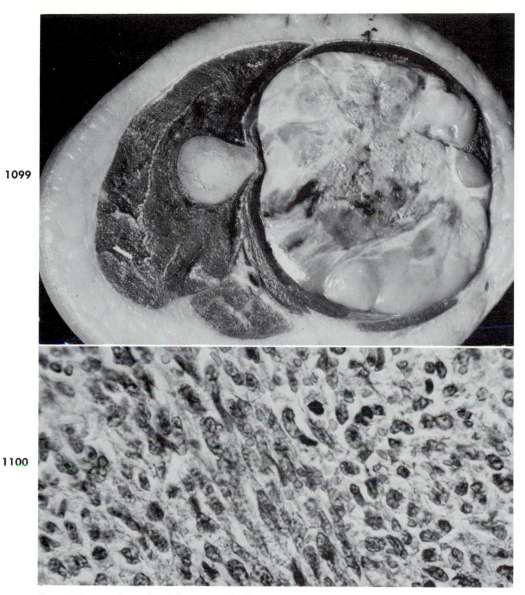

Fig. 1099 Moderately differentiated fibrosarcoma of thigh. Apparent encapsulation is in contrast to lack of circumscription in fibromatosis. (WU neg. 46-2006.)

Fig. 1100 Well-differentiated fibrosarcoma showing fibroblasts with occasional mitotic figures. (×600; WU neg. 52-3454.)

such as fascia, tendon, periosteum, and scar, grow slowly or rapidly, and often appear well circumscribed (Fig. 1099). They are usually soft and cellular and may contain areas of necrosis and hemorrhage.

Microscopically, the well-differentiated tumors are easily recognized as fibroblastic (Fig. 1100). The individual cells resemble fibroblasts, and a Wilder stain demonstrates abundant reticulin *wrapped around each cell.*[49] Phosphotungstic acid–hematoxylin demonstrates abundant fibroglia fibrils. The fibroblastic nature is more difficult to recognize in the undifferentiated tumors. It should be remembered that many other soft tissue tumors, particularly synovial sarcoma, liposarcoma, pleomorphic fibrous histiocytoma, and malignant schwannoma often contain areas closely resembling fibrosarcoma. Only careful examination of different blocks of the tumor will provide the correct diagnosis in these instances. The presence of tumor giant cells in a malignant soft tissue sarcoma usually means that it is not fibrosarcoma but more probably rhabdomyosarcoma, liposarcoma, or pleomorphic fibrous histiocytoma.

In contrast to the fibromatoses, fibrosarcomas are capable of distant metastases. Generally, the more superficial and differentiated the tumor, the better the prognosis. Increased mitotic activity is associated with an increased incidence of metastases.[51] The treatment of choice is radical excision.

Tumors of probable histiocytic origin

There has been in recent years a drastic reappraisal in the interpretation of soft tissue tumors of presumed histiocytic origin, largely initiated by the work of Stout and his colleagues at Columbia-Presbyterian Hospital.[54, 60, 61, 68, 72]

Lesions belonging to this category have been regarded by some authors as of reactive nature. We agree with Fisher and Hellstrom[55] that "the recognition that in some instances they may exhibit more aggressive growth, local recurrence and rarely metastasize would appear as ample evidence attesting to their neoplastic nature."[*] They are composed, wholly or in part, of cells with light microscopic, ultrastructural, and tissue cultural characteristics of histiocytes.[56, 65, 68] In addition, many of these tumors exhibit a more or less prominent fibroblastic component. Three hypotheses have been advanced to explain this mixed composition:

1 The tumors originate from primitive mesenchymal cells with a capacity for dual differentiation toward histiocytes and fibroblasts.

2 These are tumors of fibroblastic origin, some of the fibroblasts having the capacity to "transform" into histiocytes.

3 These are purely histiocytic neoplasms, some of the histiocytes becoming "facultative fibroblasts," a property also ascribed to Schwann cells, smooth muscle cells, and other mesenchymal cells.

The first theory is difficult to accept in view of the different histogenetic derivation of fibroblasts and histiocytes. Similarly, there is no good evidence in support of the second hypothesis. We agree with Stout and Lattes[72] that the third possibility is the most logical, and we have accepted it as a basis for the evaluation of these neoplasms, although we fully realize that the interpretation of the morphologic and tissue cultural data given as supportive evidence is open to serious questions.[59, 69, 74]

We have slightly modified the nomenclature presently in use and have devised the classification shown in Table 50. Tumors in which most or all of the cells have the appearance of histiocytes and in which the fibroblastic-like component is meager or absent are designated as **histiocytomas.** Tumors having a conspicuous fibroblastic element in addition to the histiocytes are referred to as **fibrous histiocytomas (fibrous xanthomas).** The name of **pleomorphic fibrous histiocytoma (pleomorphic fibrous xanthomas)** is proposed for a variant of the latter in which mononucleated or multinucleated bizarre cells of malignant appearance are added to the histiocytic and fibroblastic background. Approximately twenty "entities" described in the literature can be made to fit into one or another of these three major categories. It should be noted that the only criteria used for this classification are the presence or absence of a fibroblastic-like component and the presence or absence of bizarre atypical cells. Foamy cells, multinucleated cells of innocuous cytologic appearance (Touton's giant cells, osteoclast-like cells, etc), fibrosis, or hemosiderin is not significant in this regard. We prefer the designation "histio-

---

[*]From Fisher, E. R., and Hellstrom, H. R.: Dermatofibrosarcoma with metastases simulating Hodgkin's disease and reticulum cell sarcoma, Cancer **19:**1165-1171, 1966.

Table 50 Classification of soft tissue tumors of probable histiocytic origin

Type	Biologic behavior	Lesions included in this category
Histiocytoma	Benign	Juvenile xanthogranuloma (nevoxanthoendo-thelioma; nevoid histiocytoma) Reticulohistiocytoma (reticulohistiocytic granu-loma; multicentric reticulohistiocytosis; lipoid dermatoarthritis) Generalized eruptive histiocytoma
	Malignant	
Fibrous histiocytoma (fibrous xanthoma)	Benign	Subepidermal nodular fibrosis (fibrous xanthoma of skin; sclerosing hemangioma; dermatofi-broma; histiocytoma) Giant cell tumor of tendon sheath (fibrous xanthoma of tendon sheath; nodular teno-synovitis) Pigmented villonodular synovitis Xanthogranuloma
	Malignant	Dermatofibrosarcoma protuberans (progressive and recurring dermatofibroma; storiform fibrous xanthoma)
Pleomorphic fibrous histiocytoma (pleomorphic fibrous xanthoma)	"Benign"	Atypical fibroxanthoma of skin (paradoxical fibrosarcoma; pseudosarcomatous dermato-fibroma; pseudosarcomatous reticulohistiocy-toma) Postirradiation pseudosarcoma
	Malignant	Fibroxanthosarcoma (mixed storiform and giant cell fibrous xanthoma) ? Malignant giant cell tumor of soft parts ? Epithelioid sarcoma

cytoma" over that of "xanthoma" because it indicates the nature of the cell type. Besides, the term "xanthoma" merely refers to the morphologic appearance resulting from accumulation of cytoplasmic fat, which is a secondary and inconstant feature. Whenever possible, a label of benign or malignant should be added to tumors belonging to each one of these three major groups. Pure xanthomas, with or without accompanying serum lipid abnormalities, are regarded as nonneoplastic conditions and are excluded from this discussion.

Histiocytoma

The typical histiocytoma is made up of closely packed polygonal cells with little or no intervening stroma.[60] The cytoplasm is eosinophilic and may contain lipid droplets. Inflammatory cells are frequent. Fibrosis may be present in the older lesions; this should be differentiated from the active fibroblastic proliferation of fi-

brous histiocytomas. The benign tumors greatly predominate over those exhibiting a malignant behavior. The differential diagnosis between them may be difficult. Histiocytomas with clinical and/or pathologic features that single them out from the rest are juvenile xanthogranuloma, reticulohistiocytoma and generalized eruptive histiocytoma, all of which are benign. Most of these varieties are discussed in Chapter 3.

Fibrous histiocytoma (fibrous xanthoma)

Well-defined examples of the benign variant of fibrous histiocytoma include subepidermal nodular fibrosis, the so-called giant cell tumor to tendon sheath, and pigmented villonodular synovitis. The microscopic diagnosis is usually simple. A variable admixture of histiocytes (some foamy, others multinucleated, still others containing hemosiderin) and fibroblast-like cells is always present.[52, 66] Some lesions can be extremely cellular, but there is no atypia nor high mitotic activity.

The malignant variant differs microscopically from the former by virtue of a more monomorphic appearance, nuclear hyperchromasia, higher mitotic activity, and most of all, the presence of what has been called a *storiform* pattern of growth. The latter can be succinctly described as a peculiar arrangement of the tumor cells about a central point, producing radiating "spokes" grouped at right angles to each other. Although it can rarely occur in benign fibrous histiocytomas, its presence should always be regarded as a probable sign of malignancy. The best example of malignant fibrous histiocytoma is the tumor traditionally known as dermatofibrosarcoma protuberans.[53] Its typical location is the dermis, but it also can occur in deeper soft tissues. The malignancy of this neoplasm is of low grade, mainly manifested by local recurrence. Distant metastases are exceptional, but they are well documented.[55, 73]

We believe that most of the retroperitoneal and mediastinal lesions called *xanthogranulomas*[67] are examples of fibrous histiocytomas, either benign or malignant, whereas others probably represent idiopathic mediastinal or retroperitoneal fibrosis. Therefore, we suggest that this term be dropped entirely.

Pleomorphic fibrous histiocytoma (pleomorphic fibrous xanthoma)

Bizarre tumor cells, mononucleated, or multinucleated, are the hallmark of this tumor type, which otherwise resembles the group just described (Fig. 1101). Although we regard all tumors in this category at least as potentially malignant, we still divide them, for prognostic and therapeutic purposes, into a "benign" and a malignant variety. The "benign" form, generally known as atypical fibroxanthoma, typically presents as a small nodule in sun-exposed skin of elderly individuals.[63, 64] Less commonly, it appears as a larger mass in the trunk and limbs of younger patients.[57] We have seen it in areas previously subjected to radiation therapy and adjacent to other skin tumors

such as epidermoid carcinoma and sweat gland neoplasms.[70] The storiform pattern is usually absent. The large majority of these lesions are cured by local excision.[57, 58]

The malignant type, which is also known as fibroxanthosarcoma, tends to occur in deeper structures.[62] We have seen it in the soft tissues of the extremities, mediastinum, retroperitoneum, and breast and within bones (Fig. 1102). It differs from the "benign" variety mainly by its different location and the presence of a storiform pattern of growth. This tumor is prone to local recurrence and has the capacity to metastasize to distant sites, especially the lungs and regional lymph nodes.[71] Its malignant potential is higher than that of the ordinary malignant fibrous histiocytoma but lower than that of other soft tissue sarcomas which it resembles microscopically,—i. e., pleomorphic liposarcoma and pleomorphic rhabdomyosarcoma.[72]

It is probable that epithelioid sarcomas and malignant giant cell tumors of soft parts also represent malignant tumors of histiocytes. However, and until more definite evidence for this is obtained, we prefer to discuss them under the category of tumors of uncertain origin.

Tumors and tumorlike conditions of peripheral nerves

There are four distinct lesions of the peripheral nerves: *neuroma,* a benign nonneoplastic overgrowth of nerve fibers and Schwann cells; *neurilemoma* and *neurofibroma,* two benign neoplasms; and *malignant schwannoma,* formerly designated as neurofibrosarcoma. Despite the fact that these lesions may coexist, it is important to make a distinction among them in view of their markedly different natural history. For a discussion of the features of neurilemoma and neurofibroma in the mediastinum or retroperitoneal area, see Chapters 7 and 24, respectively.

Neuroma

The large majority of neuromas follow trauma—hence their designation of *trau-*

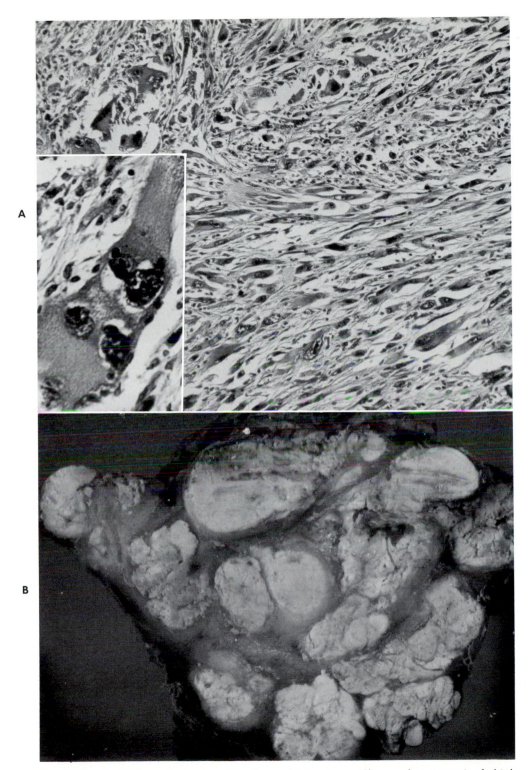

Fig. 1101   A, Malignant pleomorphic fibrous histiocytoma (fibroxanthosarcoma) of thigh (21 cm × 21 cm) excised from 38-year-old man. It recurred one year later. Note bizarre tumor giant cell, **inset,** and characteristic highly malignant spindle cell stroma. **B,** Tumoral calcinosis removed from buttock. Note nodularity with calcification. (**A,** ×150; WU neg. 68-6295; **inset,** WU neg. 68-6306; **B,** WU neg. 65-3865.)

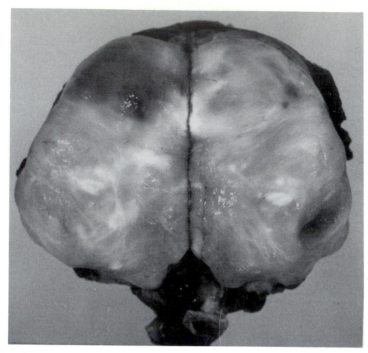

Fig. 1102 Malignant pleomorphic fibrous histiocytoma (fibroxanthosarcoma) excised from soft tissue of thigh in 27-year-old man. Lighter areas, which were yellow in color, are due to accumulation of foamy cells. (Courtesy Dr. M. R. Beck, San Francisco, Calif.)

matic neuromas. When a peripheral nerve is severed or crushed, the proximal end regenerates and, if it fails to meet the distal end, a tangled mass of nerve fibers results. Microscopically, all the elements of a nerve can be recognized: neurites, Schwann cells, and perineurial fibroblasts. In addition, scar tissue is often present. Not surprisingly, this lesion is often exquisitely painful. *Amputation neuroma,* a term made popular during World War I, is merely a type of traumatic neuroma in which the original trauma involved the loss of an extremity.

Morton's neuroma (Morton's metatarsalgia) can be regarded as a specific variant of traumatic neuroma. Its typical location is the interdigital plantar nerve between the third and fourth toes. The lesion is more common in female adults. Microscopically, the affected nerve is markedly distorted. There is extensive perineurial fibrosis often arranged in a concentric fashion. The arterioles are thickened and sometimes occluded by thrombi.[94, 96]

It is likely that the disease is secondary to repeated mild traumas to the region.

Neurilemoma

Neurilemoma is one of the few *truly encapsulated* neoplasms of the human body. It is almost always solitary and, for practical purposes, it never becomes malignant. The most common locations are the flexor surfaces of the extremities, neck, mediastinum, retroperitoneum, posterior spinal roots, and cerebellopontine angle.[91] The nerve of origin can often be demonstrated in the periphery, flattened along the capsule but not penetrating the substance of the tumor (Figs. 1103 and 1104). Since this is a benign neoplasm that only rarely recurs locally, every attempt should be made to preserve the nerve, if this is of any clinical significance (e. g., facial nerve or vagus nerve).

Grossly, the larger neurilemomas often contain cystic areas. The microscopic appearance is distinctive. Two different patterns can usually be recognized, designated

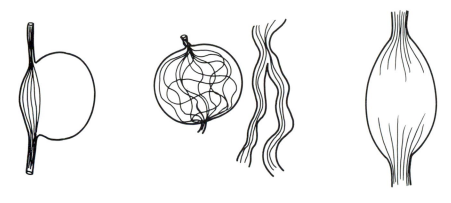

Neurilemoma   Neurofibroma   Malignant schwannoma

Fig. 1103 Schematic drawing emphasizing main differences between typical cases of three types of peripheral nerve tumors. Note diameter of nerve involved and behavior of neurites (thin black lines) in relation to neoplasm.

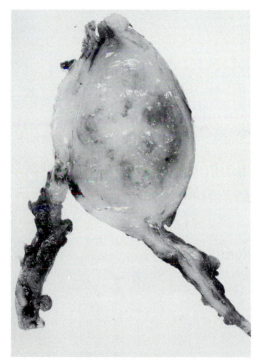

Fig. 1104 Encapsulated neurilemoma with small nerve entering its periphery. (WU neg. 52-1170.)

by Antoni as A and B. The type A areas, which in small tumors comprise almost their entirety, are quite cellular, composed of spindle cells often arranged in a palisading fashion or in an organoid arrangement (Verocay's bodies) (Figs. 1105 and 1106). In type B areas, the tumor cells are separated

by abundant edematous fluid that may form cystic spaces (Fig. 1105). Occasionally, isolated cells with bizarre hyperchromatic nuclei are observed. They are of no particular significance. Mitoses are absent or extremely scanty. The diagnosis of neurilemoma should be doubted if they are present more than occasionally. Blood vessels can be of such prominence as to simulate a vascular neoplasm. By electron microscopy, they have been found to be of the fenestrated type, a rather surprising feature.[87] Thrombosis and hyaline thickening of the adventitia are common. Palisading of nuclei is not unique for this neoplasm. We have seen it in leiomyoma, leiomyosarcoma, fibrous histiocytoma, juvenile aponeurotic fibroma, and even nonneoplastic smooth muscle of the appendiceal wall. Neurites are not present, except in the portion of the capsule where the nerve is attached. Collections of foamy macrophages are sometimes seen, especially in the larger neoplasms.

It is generally agreed that this neoplasm originates from Schwann cells. By electron microscopy, the cells of neurilemoma have a continuous basal lamina, numerous extremely thin cytoplasmic processes, and aggregates of intracytoplasmic microfibrils.[99] However, they lack what is probably the only pathognomonic feature of normal Schwann cells: mesoaxons. In this

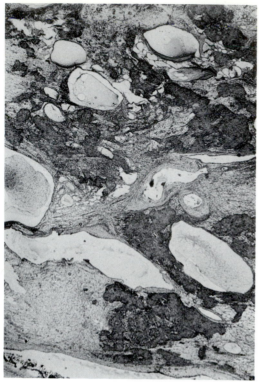

Fig. 1105 Antoni type A (cellular areas) and Antoni type B (cystic areas) tissue in neurilemoma. (Low power; WU neg. 50-438.)

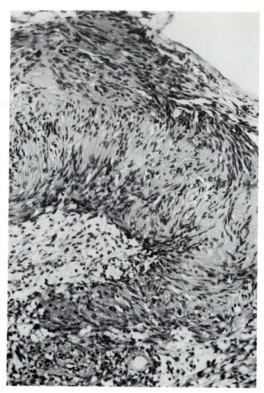

Fig. 1106 Area of Antoni type A tissue with palisading of cells. (×210; WU neg. 50-439.)

respect, they resemble the so-called *perineurial cell* of normal peripheral nerve, a cell whose possible participation in the development of these tumors deserves further investigations. "Long-spaced collagen" is frequently seen in the intercellular space, but its presence is not specific for this neoplasm.[82]

Neurofibroma

The gross, microscopic, and ultrastructural features of neurofibroma, as well as its natural history, are distinct from those of neurilemoma. Therefore, it is important to distinguish between these two types of benign neoplasms.[97] The fact that in some instances the differential diagnosis may be difficult or that in isolated cases features of both lesions may coexist does not justify lumping them together.

Neurofibromas can be solitary or multiple, the latter form being known as neuro-

fibromatosis or Recklinghausen's disease.[79] The gross appearance varies a great deal from lesion to lesion. As a rule, the tumors are not encapsulated and have a softer consistency than neurilemoma. The more superficial tumors appear as small, soft, pedunculated nodules protruding from the skin ("molluscum pendulum"). Deeper tumors grow larger. They may result in diffuse tortuous enlargement of peripheral nerves and are then designated as plexiform neurofibromas (Fig. 1107). The diffuse involvement of the nerves may make a complete resection impossible. This particular form of neurofibromatosis is more commonly seen in the orbit, neck, back, and inguinal region.

Microscopically, neurofibromas are formed by a combined proliferation of all the elements of a peripheral nerve: neurites, Schwann cells, fibroblasts, and probably perineurial cells. The former can be

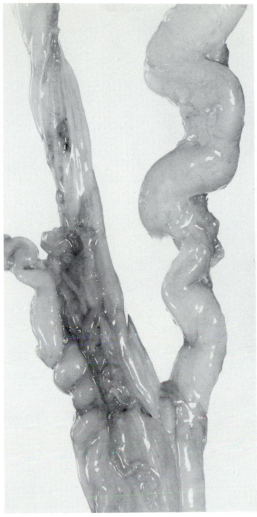

Fig. 1107 Plexiform neurofibroma involving nerves of lower extremity of young boy. Note enlargement and tortuosity of nerve bundles. (WU neg. 52-4785.)

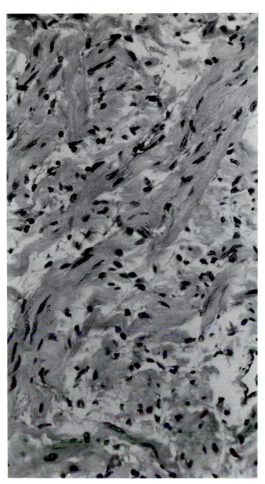

Fig. 1108 Typical neurofibroma. Note disorderly pattern of fibers. (×400; WU neg. 52-3602.)

demonstrated by silver stains. Schwann cells usually predominate. They usually have markedly elongated nuclei, with a wavy, serpentine configuration and pointed ends (Fig. 1108). Electron microscopically, they are seen to enclose axons in plasmalemmal invaginations (mesoaxons).[99] Mucinous changes in the stroma may be prominent and result in a mistaken diagnosis of myxoma or myxoid liposarcoma. Mitoses are exceptional. Their presence should arouse the suspicion of malignant degeneration. On the other hand, occasion-

al cellular pleomorphism is of no significance by itself (Fig. 1109). Numerous mast cells are present in the stroma.[92] Distorted organoid structures resembling Wagner-Meissner corpuscles are sometimes seen. Tumors in which these formations are particularly prominent have been sometimes designated as *tumors of tactile end-organs.*[86, 95] On the other hand, Verocay's bodies, palisading of nuclei, and hyaline thickening of the vessel wall are almost always absent. Exceptionally, otherwise typical neurofibromas are seen to contain melanin, a feature not unexpected in view of the embryologic relationship between Schwann cells and melanocytes.[75, 77] These

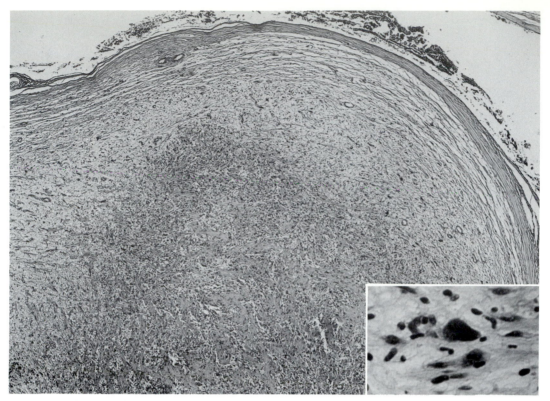

Fig. 1109 Neurofibroma excised from superficial soft tissues of arm in 38-year-old man. Focus of marked cellularity can be seen in center, surrounded by more typical areas. **Inset,** Cellular center contains scattered giant tumor cells with bizarre, hyperchromatic nuclei. This finding per se is not indication of malignant transformation. There were no mitoses. (×33; WU neg. 73-2072; **inset,** ×350; WU neg. 73-2076.)

tumors should be differentiated from blue nevi and malignant melanomas.

In Recklinghausen's disease, neurofibromas may occur in every conceivable site: axilla, thigh, buttocks, deep-lying soft tissue, orbit, mediastinum, retroperitoneum, tongue, gastrointestinal tract, etc.[93] Plexiform neurofibromas may result in massive enlargement of a limb or some other part of the body ("elephantiasis neuromatosa") (Fig. 1110). In addition to neurofibromas, patients with Recklinghausen's disease often have many other associated lesions, the most common being the *café au lait spot.* This consists microscopically of an increase in the amount of melanin in the epidermal basal layer and is sometimes seen overlying a neurofibroma. It can be distinguished from the pigmented spots associated with Albright's syndrome by virtue of its distribution and smooth, deli-

cate margins.[76] Solitary café au lait spots are common in normal individuals. Only when they are present in a number of five or more can a significant association with neurofibromatosis be detected.[101] Other lesions sometimes seen in patients with Recklinghausen's disease include congenital malformations of various types, neurilemoma (frequently multiple), meningioma and other intracranial neoplasms, lipoma, pheochromocytoma, medullary carcinoma of the thyroid gland, and ganglioneuroma.[78, 89]

A small proportion of patients with Recklinghausen's disease develop malignant schwannoma. The incidence usually given is in the range of 13%[88] but is probably much lower. The malignant tumors arise practically always in *large* nerve trunks of the neck or extremities. For practical purposes, peripheral superficial neu-

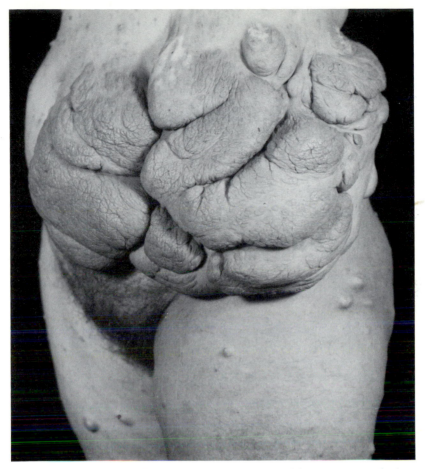

Fig. 1110 Florid case of Recklinghausen's disease. In addition to typical changes of elephantiasis in lower abdomen, multiple small neurofibromas of chest and extremities are evident. (WU neg. 64-5119.)

rofibromas never become malignant, and the only reasons for surgical removal are size and unsightliness (Fig. 1111).

A syndrome of multiple *mucosal neuromas,* pheochromocytoma, and medullary carcinoma of the thyroid gland has been recently described.[85, 102] The neuromas usually involve the tongue, lips, and conjunctiva. Despite their morphologic similarities with traumatic neuromas, they should probably be regarded as a morphologic variant of neurofibroma.

Malignant schwannoma

The term malignant schwannoma is the preferred name for a tumor also designated as neurogenic sarcoma and neurofibrosarcoma[83] (Figs. 1112 and 1113). It is the

malignant counterpart of neurofibroma and *not* of neurilemoma. Because of its difficult microscopic recognition, diagnostic errors are often made, more often than not by calling malignant schwannoma some other type of soft tissue sarcoma. We know of only two circumstances in which the diagnosis of malignant schwannoma should be the primary consideration in the presence of a malignant tumor of soft tissues composed of spindle cells: (1) when the tumor develops in a patient with Recklinghausen's disease and (2) when the tumor is obviously arising within the anatomic compartment of a major nerve or in continuity with an unquestionable neurofibroma.[80] In the absence of these circumstances, the microscopic diagnosis of malignant schwannoma

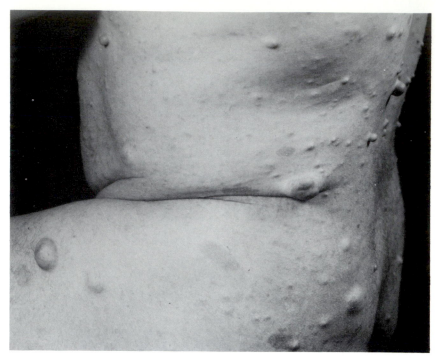

Fig. 1111 Recklinghausen's disease showing innumerable nodules and café au lait spots. (WU neg. 49-6545.)

can rarely be more than presumptive. It is true that in some tumors features suggestive of nerve sheath origin can be identified, such as serpentine cells, arrangement in palisades or whorls, or large gaping vascular spaces, but none of these features is pathognomonic. In most areas, the appearance is that of an extremely cellular spindle cell neoplasm. Mitoses are usually in abundance. Although most tumors are quite monomorphic, some can be extremely bizarre. Metaplastic cartilage, bone, and skeletal muscle have been described.[102a] Exceptionally, glandlike elements and primitive rosettes are present, suggesting an origin in more primitive neuroectodermal elements.[90]

The belief that these malignant neoplasms originate in Schwann cells is largely based on circumstantial evidence, the reasoning being that if these tumors represent the malignant counterpart of neurofibromas and the latter arise primarily from Schwann cells, then the former must also have that origin. Some of the microscopic

features just mentioned and tissue culture studies[98] support this hypothesis, which still necessitates more solid evidence.

A large majority of malignant schwannomas arise in adults. The most common locations are the neck, forearm, lower leg, and buttock. Grossly, the finding of a large mass producing fusiform enlargement of a major nerve is characteristic (Fig. 1103).

The clinical evolution is that of a highly malignant neoplasm, despite the relatively slow growth rate of some cases.[84] Local recurrence (often in the cut nerve ends) and distant metastases are frequent. In the series reported by D'Agostino et al.,[81] of thirteen patients with Recklinghausen's disease in whom malignant schwannoma occurred, nine died of tumor. This was also the case in nine of fifteen patients reported by White.[100]

Tumors of adipose tissue
Lipoma

Benign fatty tumors can arise in any location in which fat is normally present.

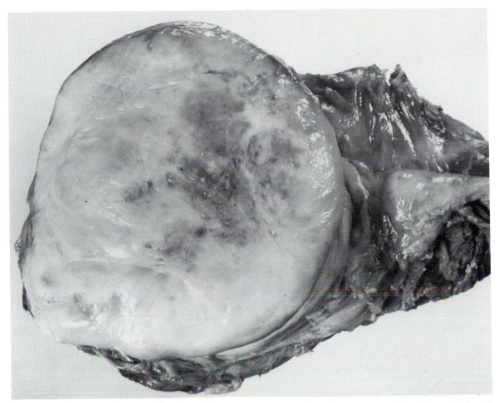

Fig. 1112 Malignant schwannoma removed from flank of 16-year-old girl with florid Recklinghausen's disease. (WU neg. 64-9254.)

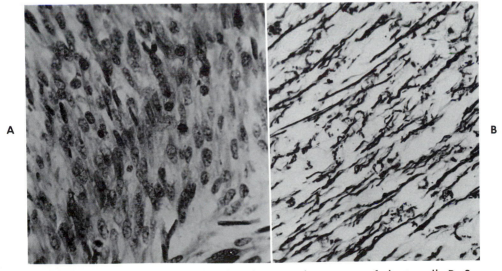

Fig. 1113   A, Fairly well-differentiated malignant schwannoma of chest wall. **B,** Same lesion shown in **A** stained for reticulin demonstrating thick, wiry fibers running in long parallel lines between tumor cells. (**A,** ×400; WU neg. 50-5445; **B,** ×400; WU neg. 50-5446.)

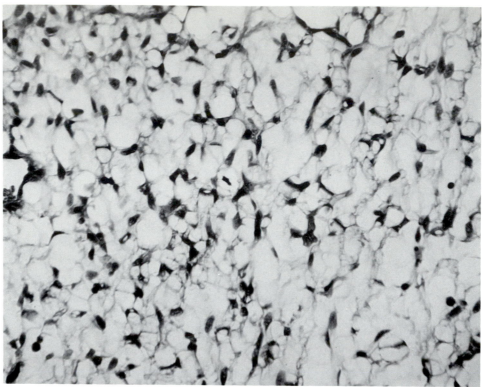

Fig. 1114 Lipoblastomatosis occurring in soft tissue of 8-year-old child. It was mistaken for liposarcoma. (×340; WU neg. 67-1169.)

The majority occur in the upper half of the body, particularly the trunk and neck. Paarlberg et al.[111] reviewed twenty-nine lipomas located in the hand. Although these tumors may be in the deep tissues, they are usually subcutaneous. In Pack and Pierson's series,[112] there were about 120 lipomas to 1 liposarcoma. Most patients are in the fifth or sixth decade of life. Children are only exceptionally affected.

Lipomas may be single or multiple. Patients with neurofibromatosis and multiple endocrine adenomatosis have an increased incidence of multiple lipomas. In *diffuse lipomatosis,* massive enlargement of a limb may be seen as a result of diffuse proliferation of mature adipose tissue. This rare condition is seen most exclusively in children. Lipomas grow to large size, are usually encapsulated when located in the superficial soft tissues but poorly curcumscribed when arising in deeper structures, and consist of bright yellow fat separated by fine fibrous trabeculae. Microscopically, they are composed of mature adipose tissue with no cellular atypia. Focal myxoid changes are sometimes present. Areas of infarction, necrosis, and calcification may occur. In contrast to subcutaneous lipomas, those located within skeletal muscle often have an infiltrative pattern of growth.[108]

Angiolipomas are small tumors occurring shortly after puberty. They are often painful and multiple. They are located in the subcutis, most commonly on the trunk or extremities. The vascularity often is limited to a band of tissue on the periphery of the neoplasm. Hyaline thrombi are common. The pain correlates well with the degree of vascularity.[109]

Lipoblastomatosis

Vellios et al.[115] described lipoblastomatosis, which is also known as embryonal or fetal lipoma. It predominates in children during the first year of life. Grossly, the

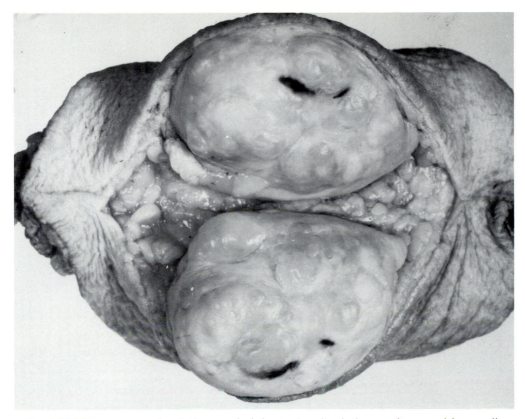

Fig. 1115 Liposarcoma of soft tissues of abdominal wall which was diagnosed by needle biopsy. Adequate excision was done. (WU neg. 66-1398.)

lesion is soft and lobulated. It can be well localized or diffusely infiltrate the soft tissues. Microscopically, it closely resembles fetal fat (Fig. 1114). It has often been confused with myxoid liposarcoma. It is differentiated from it by the young age of the patient, distinct lobulation, and absence of giant cells or pleomorphic nuclei.[104a]

Liposarcoma

Liposarcoma is the most frequent soft tissue sarcoma in adults. On the other hand, its occurrence in children is exceptional.[105] The tumors are usually large and occur most frequently in the lower extremities (popliteal fossa and medial thigh), retroperitoneal, perirenal, and mesenteric region, and shoulder area.[113] Grossly, they are well circumscribed, but this represents pseudoencapsulation[114] (Fig. 1115). The myxoid type has a mucoid, slimy surface

that is mistaken for a myxoma. The extremely well-differentiated type suggests a lipoma. Others may mimic brain tissue. The surfaces resemble cerebral convolutions.

Enzinger and Winslow[106] divided these tumors into four cellular types: myxoid, round cell, well differentiated, and pleomorphic. Mixed forms occur.

The myxoid type, which is by far the commonest, has no mitotic figures and suggests fetal fat. As in the latter, it contains proliferating lipoblasts in different stages of differentiation, a prominent anastomosing capillary network, and a mucoid matrix rich in hyaluronidase-sensitive acid mucopolysaccharides[116] (Fig. 1116). The presence of a prominent vascular component in myxoid liposarcoma is an important feature in the differential diagnosis with myxoma. The mucoid extracellular

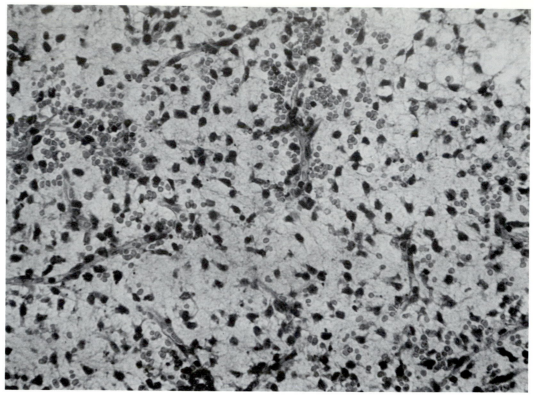

Fig. 1116 Myxoid type of liposarcoma, most common variant. Individual tumor cells have myxoidlike background with abundant proliferating vessels. (×350; WU neg. 72-10433.)

material may accumulate in large pools, thus simulating a tumor of lymphatic vessel origin.

In the round cell type, the tumor cells are small and have a distinctly acidophilic cytoplasm. The presence among them of scattered lipoblasts establishes the diagnosis. Mitoses are more common than in the myxoid form, but the vascular network is less prominent. Pseudoglandular arrangement of the tumor cells is frequent. We have seen several round cell liposarcomas misdiagnosed as hibernomas.

The well-differentiated type is often designated a lipoma, but careful examination always shows characteristic tumor cells with large, deep-staining nuclei (Fig. 1117). It is common for the malignant cells to be located within areas of dense fibrosis which are seen alternating with lipoma-like foci.

The pleomorphic type is highly undif-

ferentiated with many tumor giant cells and is often called a rhabdomyosarcoma (Fig. 1118). On the other hand, it is likely that many tumors formerly diagnosed as pleomorphic liposarcomas actually represent malignant pleomorphic fibrous histiocytomas, as evidenced by their storiform pattern of growth.

Fat stains are of little help in the diagnosis of liposarcoma. Fat may be totally lacking in some forms of this tumor and be present in a host of soft tissue neoplasms other than liposarcoma.

Both the myxoid and the well-differentiated types tend to recur locally rather than to metastasize. In contrast, the round cell and pleomorphic types often give rise to widespread metastases. In the series reported by Enzinger and Winslow,[106] the five-year survival rate of patients with myxoid and well-differentiated forms exceeded 70%, whereas in the round cell and pleo-

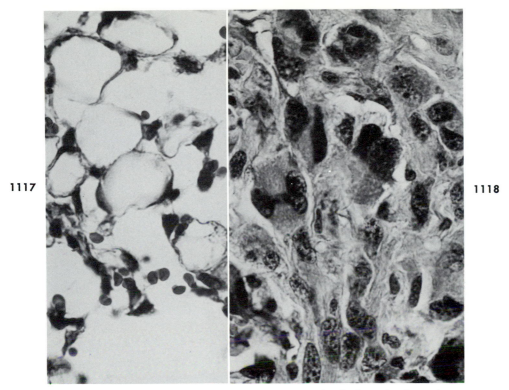

1117

1118

Fig. 1117 Well-differentiated liposarcoma in which individual nuclei have been compressed to crescentic shape. (×400; WU neg. 49-4502.)

Fig. 1118 Pleomorphic liposarcoma with innumerable tumor giant cells and great pleomorphism. Tumors with microscopic appearance are often incorrectly diagnosed as rhabdomyosarcomas. (×360; WU neg. 51-804.)

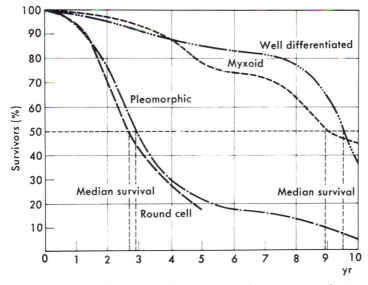

Fig. 1119 Survival rates according to histologic types in liposarcomas of retroperitoneum and lower extremity. (From Enzinger, F. M., and Winslow, D. J.: Liposarcoma; a study of 103 cases, Virchows Arch. Pathol. Anat. **355:**367-388, 1962; Berlin-Göttingen-Heidelberg: Springer.)

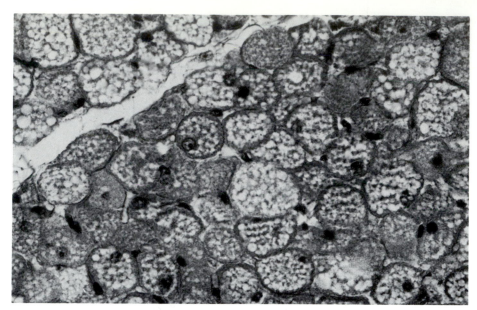

Fig. 1120 Hibernoma with large uniform cells. Vacuoles contain fat. (×40; WU neg. 49-6716.)

morphic varieties it amounted only to 18% (Fig. 1119). Rarely, liposarcomas have multiple foci of origin.[103, 107]

Hibernoma

The hibernoma is a rare benign neoplasm occurring usually in the intercapsular region and in the axilla. It forms a soft tissue mass, the cut surface of which is brown. The microscopic pattern is characteristic—an organoid arrangement of large cells that contain many vacuoles that stain with scarlet R (Fig. 1120).

This tumor received its name because it is thought to arise from brown fat similar to that seen in the hibernating glands of animals.[104] This similarity is maintained at an electron microscopic level.[110]

Tumors and tumorlike conditions of blood and lymph vesssels
Hemangioma

The classification of hemangiomas is unsatisfactory. In most cases, it is difficult to decide if these lesions are malformations (hamartomas) or true neoplasms. About three-fourths are present at birth. About 60% occur in the head and neck area.

The *port-wine type* (nevus flammeus) occurs frequently in the skin of the face, neck, and thorax and, at times, in the skin of the extremities. It is present at birth. This lesion grows very slowly, its increase in size being proportional to the growth of the patient. In time, it becomes nodular and soft. Microscopically, this vascular lesion is of the cavernous type. It contains scattered, thin-walled, superficial telangiectatic vessels.[125] It is resistant to radiotherapy and does not regress spontaneously. This lesion may become very large and unsightly. Its treatment is often difficult.

The *strawberry type* hemangioma is made up of cellular masses of closely packed endothelial cells with spaces containing relatively little blood. Only rarely does this type contain a significant cavernous component. It is present at birth or appears shortly afterward and grows rapidly during the first few months of life. At this time, it is highly cellular and contains many mitotic figures (Fig. 1121). This variety is also designated as benign hemangioendothelioma. The color is an intense crimson. When the infants cries, the surface of the nodule becomes smooth. The

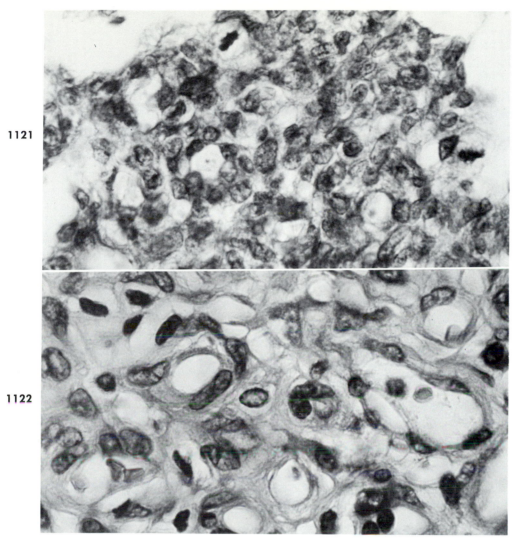

Fig. 1121 Highly cellular hemangioma (strawberry nevus) in 1-month-old infant. Note mitotic figures and solid masses of cells. (×480.)
Fig. 1122 Hemangioma (strawberry nevus) in 1-year-old child. Note vascular channels, decreased cellularity, and increased connective tissue. (×480.)

lesion stops growing and begins to fade when the baby is about 6 months old. It becomes flaccid, pale blue, and is covered with tiny wrinkles. Sections taken when the patient is 9 months of age or older show an absence of the intense cellularity and mitotic figures and the presence of increased connective tissue (Fig. 1122). Eventually it disappears completely (Fig. 1123).

In a group of ninety-three hemangiomas in seventy-seven patients studied by Lister[122] and followed from one to seven years, ninety-two out of the ninety-three lesions regressed. There is no exception to the rule that hemangiomas growing rapidly during the early months of life subsequently regress and disappear after about five years.[123] A rapid initial growth rate is not present in the port-wine type. The strawberry type must be sharply separated from the other varieties.

None of the hemangiomas become malignant. The so-called benign metastasizing hemangioma is a misnomer. It represents angiosarcoma. Large, deep cavernous hemangiomas may undergo thrombosis, ulceration, or infection and become lethal. Lelong et al.[120] collected fifty cases of large hemangiomas associated with thrombocytopenia. The hematologic abnormality is correctable by excision or irradiation of the hemangioma.[118, 124]

We have seen hemangiomas in the soft tissues of the thigh, back, and gluteal regions. They may form poorly circumscribed, hemorrhagic masses with areas of organization and calcification. Microscopically, they contain cavernous spaces lined by normal endothelial cells. Incomplete removal may cure or be followed by recurrence. The lack of circumscription should not be construed as evidence of malignancy.

Allen and Enzinger[117] reviewed eighty-nine hemangiomas of skeletal muscle. Some of their cases were extremely cellular, with plump nuclei, mitotic figures, intraluminal papillary projections, and even infiltration of perineurial spaces. They pointed out that bona fide metastasizing angiosarcomas of skeletal muscle are exceptionally rare.

All of the aforementioned types of angiomas are composed exclusively or predominantly by capillaries. Rarely, hemangiomas composed of veins (venous hemangiomas) or an admixture of arteries and veins (racemose or cirsoid hemangiomas) are encountered. Thrombosis and foci of calcification are common.

The association of varicose veins, soft tissue and bone hypertrophy, and cutaneous hemangioma is known as Klippel-Trenaunay syndrome.[121]

Koblenzer and Bukowski[119] reviewed the cases of multifocal angiomatosis of skin and soft tissues associated with involvement of internal organs.

Glomus tumor

Glomus tumor, also known as glomangioma, originates in the normal neuromyoarterial glomus, an arteriovenous shunt abundantly supplied with nerve fibers and fulfilling a temperature-regulating function.[129] The classical location of the glomus tumor is the subungual region, but it can occur elsewhere in the skin and soft tissues, particularly in the flexor surface of the arms and about the knee.[126, 131-133] It also has been reported in the stomach (Chapter 10), and we have seen one case in the nasal cavity. Subungual lesions are always supplied by numerous nerve fibers and are exquisitely painful, two features often absent in glomus tumors arising elsewhere. The tumor may erode the terminal phalanx or even present as an intraosseous lesion in this location.[128] Superficial lesions are well circumscribed. Glomus tumors in

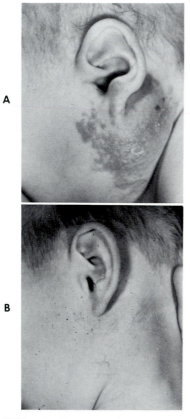

Fig. 1123 A, Extensive hemangioma (strawberry nevus) in 3-month-old infant. **B,** Same child four years later. Lesion completely disappeared without treatment.

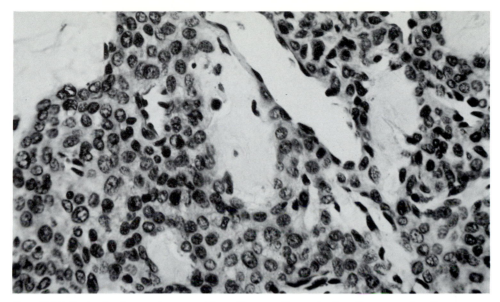

Fig. 1124 Typical glomus tumor with uniform cells and abundant vessels. It was exquisitely painful and located in subungual area. Cajal stain showed numerous neurites. (×500; WU neg. 52-3871.)

children tend to be multiple and of an infiltrative nature.[127]

Microscopically, glomus tumors consist of blood vessels lined by normal endothelial cells and surrounded by a solid proliferation of round or cuboidal "epithelioid" cells with perfectly round nucleus and acidophilic cytoplasm (Fig. 1124). By electron microscopy, the tumor cells have features of smooth muscle rather than of pericytes.[134] Three microscopic varieties were described by Masson: solid, angiomatous, and mucoid hyaline.[129, 130] The solid type can be confused with sweat gland tumor or metastatic carcinoma. Often the diagnostic relationship between tumor cells and blood vessels can be clearly seen only at the very periphery of the neoplasm. Rarely, glomus tumor recurs locally. However, cases with distant metastases have never been reported.

Hemangiopericytoma

Stout[140] regarded hemangiopericytoma as a less organoid type of glomus tumor, arising from Zimmerman's pericytes.[141] This theory was supported by the tissue culture studies of Murray and Stout.[137] The main differences with glomus tumor are summarized in Table 51. McCormack[136] has emphasized the characteristic brown color seen on gross inspection. Microscopically, the cells are spindle shaped, lack myofibrils, and have a close relationship with

Table 51 Clinical and anatomic features of glomus tumor and hemangiopericytoma*†

	Glomus tumor	Hemangio-pericytoma
Painful	Often	Rarely
Local invasion	Rare, usually in children	Frequent
Metastases	Never	Sometimes
Location	Skin, superficial soft tissues, stomach	Any tissue[138]
Multiple tumors	Sometimes	No
Histology	Organoid cells; round or oval vascular spaces, often dilated; axons are present	Diffuse elongated cells; vascular spaces often collapsed; axons are absent

*Based on the reported experience of Stout.[139, 140]
†From Kuhn, C., III, and Rosai, J.: Tumors arising from pericytes; ultrastructure and organ culture of a case, Arch. Pathol. 88:653-663, 1969; copyright 1969, American Medical Association.

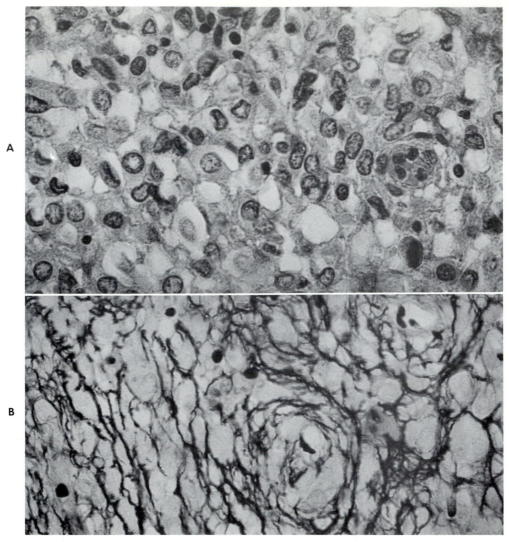

Fig. 1125 A, Hemangiopericytoma with uniform cells and abundant vascularization. **B,** Same lesion shown in **A.** Reticulin pattern shows tumor cells lying outside of reticulin sheaths. (**A** and **B,** High power.)

blood vessels, being separated from the normal-appearing endothelial cells by a layer of silver-staining material (which may be reticulin, basement membrane, or a mixture of both) (Fig. 1125). We studied a case by electron microscopy and found that most of the tumor cells had features comparable to those of normal pericytes, whereas others appeared as transitional forms with smooth muscle cells.[135] In Stout's series,[139] 11.7% of the cases resulted in distant metastases. He remarked that it is usually impossible to predict the

likelihood of malignant behavior on the basis of the microscopic appearance.

Angiosarcoma

The term angiosarcoma, if used without adjectives or prefixes, refers to a malignant neoplasm arising from the *endothelial cells of blood vessels*—i.e. a malignant hemangioendothelioma. Stout[144] could find only fourteen angiosarcomas in the soft tissues reported in the literature. The lesion is highly vascular, grows in skin, muscle, or deep tissues, and occurs at any age

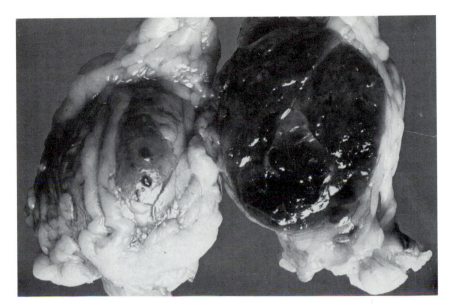

Fig. 1126 Angiosarcoma from omentum in 41-year-old woman. Tumor nodules also were present in retroperitoneum. On cross section, tumor is dark red, spongy, and of soft consistency. It proved rapidly fatal. (WU neg. 52-4780.)

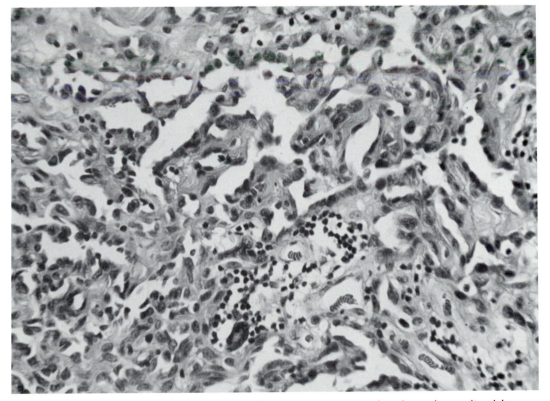

Fig. 1127 Soft tissue angiosarcoma. Freely anastomosing vascular channels are lined by atypical endothelial cells. (×350; WU neg. 73-3401.)

(Fig. 1126). The soft tissue of the female breast is one of the commonest sites (Chapter 19).

The microscopic pattern of angiosarcoma is accentuated by the silver reticulin stain. The tumor cells proliferate in the vascular lumina within a reticulin sheath. They form layers and communicating channels (Fig. 1127). The latter is an important diagnostic feature. It is also seen in organizing thrombi, but practically never in hemangiomas. Lymphoid foci and clumps of hemosiderin are common. In the more solid areas, the tumor cells acquire an epithelioid nature that we have seen confused with amelanotic melanoma and metastatic carcinoma. We have also seen the reciprocal error—i.e., misdiagnosing a well-vascularized liposarcoma or metastatic renal cell carcinoma as angiosarcoma.

We have reviewed nine angiosarcomas of skin. Characteristically, the tumors were multiple and involved the scalp or face of elderly individuals. The clinical course was that of repeated local recurrences over a long period of time, followed in four cases by lymph node and pulmonary metastases.[142, 144]

Lymphangioma

Most lymphangiomas represent malformations rather than true neoplasms. Three forms exist: capillary, cavernous, and cystic. The capillary form occurs in the skin, whereas the cavernous variety prefers deep soft tissues. Cystic lymphangioma is usually known as hygroma. It is a poorly defined soft tissue mass in the neck of children which consists of large lymphatic channels growing in loose connective tissue[149] (Fig. 1128). Large collections of lymphocytes may be present in the stroma and cause mistakes of interpretation. The lesion is usually posterior to the sternocleidomastoid muscle. It may extend into the mediastinum. It does not become malignant and is curable by excision.[147]

Lymphangiomyoma is the currently accepted term for a benign neoplasm originally described as lymphangiopericyto-

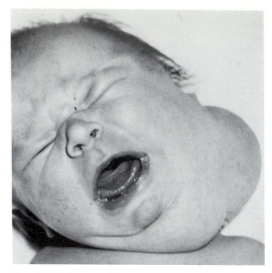

Fig. 1128 Large hygroma in infant. (From Maxwell, J. H.: Tumors of the face and neck in infancy and childhood, South. Med. J. **45:**292-299, 1952.)

ma.[146, 150] It is restricted to the mediastinum and retroperitoneum, in close association with the thoracic duct and its tributaries. It occurs exclusively in females. Chylothorax and pulmonary complications are almost always present.[145] Microscopically, a smooth muscle or pericytic component is seen in addition to the lymphatic proliferation. A relationship between lymphangioma and tuberous sclerosis was suggested by Jao et al.[148]

Lymphangiosarcoma

Lymphangiosarcomas arise rarely in patients who have had long-standing massive lymphedema after radical mastectomy.[151, 153] They may also develop secondary to chronic lymphedema of the lower leg.[152, 154] Clinically, they present as bluish or purple elevations in the edematous skin. They are frequently multiple, although in late stages they coalesce to form a large hemorrhagic mass.

Microscopically, the tumors are composed of areas resembling angiosarcoma and other zones with empty endothelium-lined spaces suggesting lymphatics. The malignant cells of this lesion lie within the vascular and lymphatic lumina in contrast to Kaposi's sarcoma, in which many of the cells lie outside the vessel wall. Lymphangiosarcoma occurs at an average age of 63.9 years and an average of ten years and three months after mastectomy. Of 129 patients reviewed by Woodward et al.,[155] only eleven had survived five years or more.

Tumors of smooth muscle
Leiomyoma

Three varieties of skin and soft tissue leiomyomas exist. *Multiple leiomyomas* of of the skin usually are superficial and small. They arise from the arrectores pilorum muscles. *Genital leiomyomas* are single tumors that arise from smooth muscle bundles in the superficial subcutaneous tissue of the nipple, axilla, anal region, scrotum, penis, and labia majora.[157]

Vascular leiomyomas (angioleiomyomas) arise from the wall of blood vessels. They occur most frequently in females and are usually located in the ankle or wrist regions. They constitute, together with traumatic neuroma, glomus tumor, eccrine spiradenoma, and angiolipoma, the classical five painful tumors of soft tissues.[156]

Grossly, these tumors are yellow or yellowish pink and fairly firm. Microscopically, those in soft tissues are made up of large numbers of vessels, usually without elastic fibers, which are mixed with smooth muscle bundles. Transitional forms with glomus tumor and hemangiopericytoma occur.

As is also the case with smooth muscle tumors of the gastrointestinal tract and uterus, soft tissue tumors may have a round cell or "epithelioid" configuration, in whole or in part. They are particularly common in the omentum and mesentery. The terms bizarre leiomyoma and leiomyoblastoma have been used for this variant. Benign and malignant forms occur. We prefer to designate these tumors as leiomyomas or leiomyosarcomas, round cell variant, classifying them as benign or malignant by using the same criteria we apply for smooth muscle tumors in general.

Leiomyosarcoma

Smooth muscle tumors of soft tissue origin are relatively rare.[158] They may occur at any site, including the wall of large veins, particularly the vena cava, the cubital vein, and the vena saphena.[159, 162] Despite their grossly well-circumscribed nature, the majority eventually give rise to distant metastases, sometimes fifteen or twenty years after the excision of the primary tumor. Both the benign and malignant variants are easily enucleated. If the tumor is malignant, such enucleation results in local recurrence.[160]

Microscopically, the individual cells have elongated, blunted nuclei. Occasionally, myofibrils are demonstrated. The phosphotungstic acid–hematoxylin stain of well-differentiated tumors infrequently shows terminal myofibrils with a hooklike appearance. The reticulin extends as wavy, undulating fibers between long lines of tumor cells. Palisading of nuclei should not be a reason for calling one of these tumors neurogenous.

The gross and microscopic differentiation between the benign and malignant variant usually is not too difficult. The benign variant invariably is small, less than 2 cm in diameter, and shows practically no mitotic activity. The malignant smooth muscle tumor, which rather closely resembles a leiomyoma, invariably shows a high degree of mitotic activity[161] (Fig. 1129). Leiomyosarcomas in children are exceedingly rare.[163]

Mitotic activity is the morphologic feature that best correlates with biologic behavior. However, we have seen cases with all the attributes of benignancy, including an extremely low mitotic count, which metastasized and killed the patient.

Tumors of striated muscle
Rhabdomyoma

So-called cardiac rhabdomyomas, seen in association with the tuberous sclerosis complex, are probably not true neoplasms. Bona fide benign tumors of skeletal muscle origin are exceedingly rare.[164, 166] They

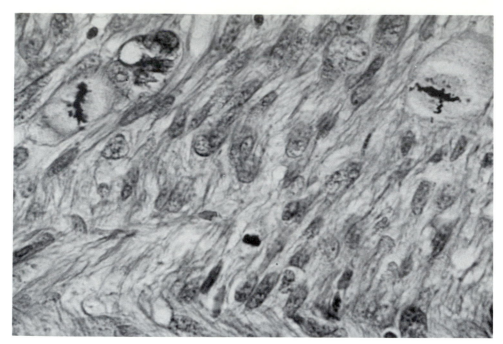

Fig. 1129 Fairly well-differentiated metastatic leiomyosarcoma. However, it showed numerous mitotic figures, both typical and atypical. (×600; WU neg. 62-8259.)

are found almost exclusively in the oral cavity and its vicinity. Adults are usually affected. Microscopically, the cells are well differentiated, and cross striations can usually be demonstrated. We have seen them confused with granular cell tumor and hibernoma. In contrast with the latter, the vacuolated cells of rhabdomyoma contain glycogen rather than fat.

Dehner and Enzinger[165] reported nine cases of a benign tumor they designated as *fetal rhabdomyoma.* Most patients were male children 3 years of age or under. The most common location was the head and neck region, particularly the posterior auricular area. Microscopically, the lesions were formed by immature skeletal muscle fibers (some containing cross striations) and undifferentiated mesenchymal cells. Nuclear aberrations were absent and mitoses exceedingly rare. Surgery was curative in every instance.

Rhabdomyosarcoma

One of the major changes in recent years in the field of soft tissue tumors has been

the realization that most childhood soft tissue sarcomas represent malignant tumors of skeletal muscle. Three major categories of rhabdomyosarcoma exist, which should be kept clearly separated: pleomorphic, embryonal, and alveolar.[170]

Pleomorphic rhabdomyosarcoma, which constituted practically all the cases in the older literature,[173] is actually the least common of the three categories. It arises from myotome-derived skeletal muscle and is therefore usually located in an extremity, especially the thigh.[176, 184] It occurs almost exclusively in adults. Grossly, it may be confined within fascial compartments and have the shape of the muscle from which it arises. The growth rate is often rapid. It may burst through the skin and form a fungating large mass (Fig. 1130). Microscopically, the differential diagnosis with liposarcoma and malignant pleomorphic fibrous xanthoma is often difficult. We make the unequivocal diagnosis of pleomorphic rhabdomyosarcoma *only* if we can detect cross striations in some of the tumor cells (Fig. 1131). This is a tumor

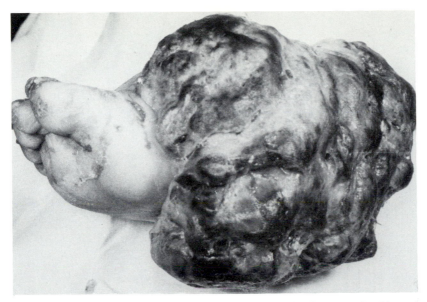

Fig. 1130 Large fungating rhabdomyosarcoma of soft tissue of ankle.

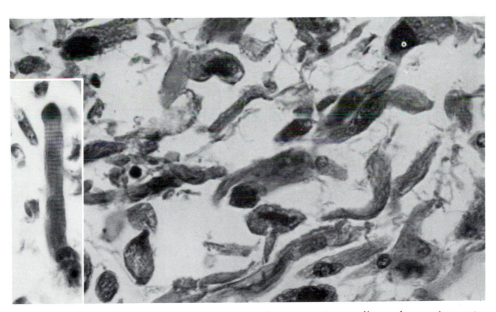

Fig. 1131 Pleomorphic rhabdomyosarcoma with tumor giant cells and tapering cytoplasmic processes. Cell in **inset** shows well-defined cross striations. (High power; WU neg. 46-1718.)

in which electron microscopy can have a definite diagnostic value.[171, 178] The five-year survival rate is in the range of 29%.[168, 174]

Embryonal rhabdomyosarcoma arises from unsegmented and undifferentiated mesoderm and is more common in the head and neck region (particularly the orbit, nasopharynx, and middle ear), retroperitoneum, bile ducts, and urogenital tract.[172, 175, 177] Less than 5% occur in the extremities. The large majority occur in children 5 years of age or younger. Grossly, it is poorly circumscribed, white, and

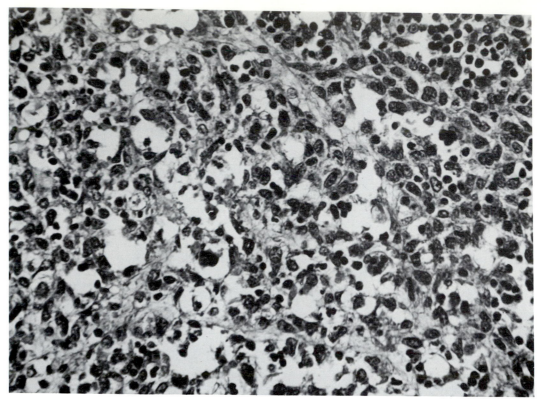

Fig. 1132 Embryonal rhabdomyosarcoma. It would be easy to confuse this tumor with malignant lymphoma. (×350; WU neg. 72-10435.)

soft. When growing beneath a mucosal membrane, such as vagina, urinary bladder, and nasal cavity, it frequently forms large polypoid masses resembling a bunch of grapes—hence the name sarcoma botryoides. The appearance is quite similar to that of an allergic nasal polyp. Microscopically, the tumor cells are small and spindle shaped. Some have a deeply acidophilic cytoplasm (Fig. 1132). A feature of diagnostic value is the presence of highly cellular areas usually centered by a blood vessel, alternating with parvicellular regions with abundant mucoid intercellular material.[183] A highly characteristic feature of the polypoid ("botryoid") tumors is the presence of a dense zone of undifferentiated tumor cells immediately beneath the epithelium, a formation known as Nicholson's *cambium layer*. The prognosis is exceedingly poor. In a series of sixty-five patients reviewed by Enzinger,[168] the five-

year survival rate was 8%. The most common sites of metastatic involvement are lung, bone marrow, and lymph nodes.

Alveolar rhabdomyosarcoma was well described by Riopelle and Thériault[181] and Enterline and Horn.[167] In the past, it was usually misinterpreted as primary reticulum cell sarcoma of soft tissues. Although clearly related to the embryonal form and occasionally coexisting with it, it should be regarded as a separate entity because of several clinical and pathologic differences with the latter. For instance, it predominates in a slightly older age group (10 to 25 years) and occurs more frequently in the extremities. In a series of 110 cases reported by Enzinger,[169] the most common locations were the forearms, arms, and the perirectal and perineal regions. Microscopically, the small, round or oval tumor cells are seen separated in nests by connective tissue septa. The tumor cells

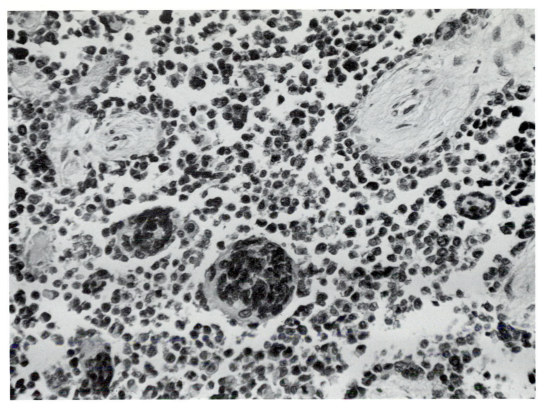

Fig. 1133 Alveolar rhabdomyosarcoma. Lack of cohesiveness of tumor cells and scattered multinucleated giant tumor cells are characteristic. (×300; WU neg. 73-2686.)

in contact with these fibrous strands remain firmly attached to them, but the others tend to detach due to lack of cohesiveness, thus resulting in a typical alveolar or pseudoglandular appearance. The deep acidophilia of the cytoplasm and the presence of occasional multinucleated giant cells are important diagnostic features (Fig. 1133). Cross striations are rarely found in alveolar and embryonal rhabdomyosarcomas. However, the appearance of these two types is sufficiently distinctive for a definite diagnosis to be made in their absence.[182] The prognosis of alveolar rhabdomyosarcoma is even worse than for the embryonal variety. In the series reported by Enzinger,[169] 92% of the patients had died from widespread metastasis within the first four years after diagnosis. Lung and regional lymph nodes were the most common metastatic sites.

Evidence has recently accumulated in-dicating that rhabdomyosarcoma can be locally controlled and even permanently cured by aggressive radiation therapy combined with appropriate chemotherapy.[179, 180, 185]

Tumors of synovial tissue
Synovial sarcoma

The synovial sarcoma is a highly malignant tumor arising in 80% of the cases about the knee and ankle joints in young adults[190] (Fig. 1134). It also occurs about the shoulder and elbow. We have also seen them in the region of hip, in the soft tissues of the neck (particularly the retropharyngeal area),[186] and in the anterior abdominal wall. This neoplasm grows very close to joints, tendon sheaths, and bursae, but it is rare for it to involve the synovial membrane. We have seen two exceptions. Grossly, this lesion forms circumscribed, firm, grayish pink tumors. Focal calcifica-

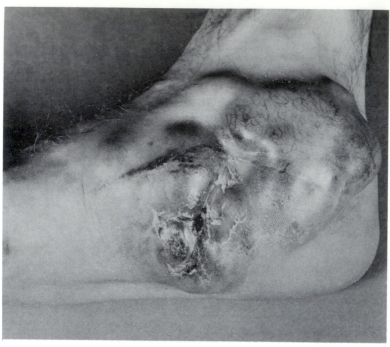

Fig. 1134 Recurrent synovial sarcoma of ankle in young man. It was inadequately excised, recurred, and distantly metastasized, causing death. (WU neg. 48-192.)

tion occasionally occurs (Fig. 1135). The circumscription is false.

Microscopically, the tumor has a sarcomatous stroma and pseudoglandular areas mimicking the arrangement of synovial membrane (Fig. 1136). Hyaluronidase-resistant mucin is often present within the glandular spaces and in the cytoplasm of the epithelial-like cells. Reticulin stains emphasize the differences between the two components. Hyalinization, calcification, and osseous or cartilaginous metaplasia can be present in the fibrosarcomatous component. According to Enzinger,[188] the former two features have favorable diagnostic connotations. If the fibrosarcomatous area predominates, the incorrect diagnosis may be fibrosarcoma. A careful search for an epithelial-like component should be carried out in any tumor with the appearance of fibrosarcoma located in a periarticular area. Enzinger[188] pointed out that the possibility of synovial sarcoma should be suspected in the presence of spindle cell tumors of monotonous appearance hav-

ing plump-appearing nuclei, scanty mitotic activity, a focally whorled pattern, a large number of mast cells, or occasional nests of large, pale cells. The pseudoglandular zones may be mistaken for metastatic adenocarcinoma. In all likelihood, most cases of synovial sarcoma do not arise from synovial cells but rather from mesenchymal elements with the capacity to differentiate into synovioblasts. Gabbiani et al.[189] have described the ultrastructural appearance of this neoplasm.

These tumors metastasize to regional lymph nodes (10% to 15%). The preferable treatment of such tumors is radical excision. Synovial sarcoma has been traditionally regarded as a tumor of ominous prognosis.[190] In recent series, however, the five-year survival rate has approached 50%.[187, 188, 191, 192]

Tumors of pluripotential mesenchyme
Mesenchymoma

Stout coined the term *mesenchymoma* for tumors consisting of two or more

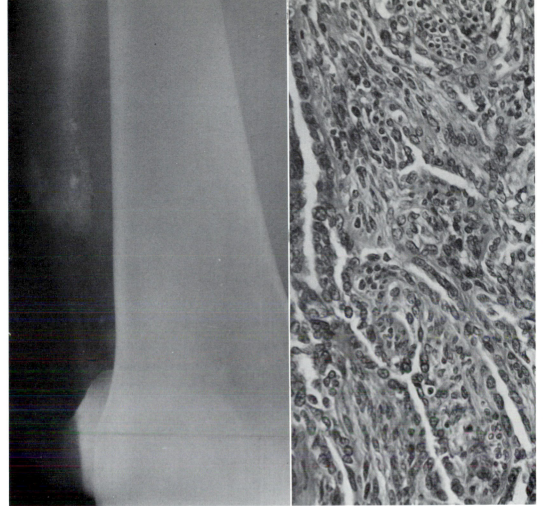

135

1136

Fig. 1135 Roentgenogram of synovial sarcoma of thigh in 28-year-old man. Tumor was partially calcified, a not uncommon finding in this type of neoplasm. (WU neg. 72-2175; courtesy Dr. R. Trinity, St. Louis, Mo.)

Fig. 1136 Typical synovial sarcoma with biphasic pattern composed of clefts and acinar structures lined by epithelial-like cells. These are separated by fibrosarcomatous stroma. (×350; WU neg. 72-10434.)

mesenchymal elements in addition to fibrous tissue. Benign and malignant forms exist. The most frequent benign variant is composed of smooth muscle, fat, and blood vessels. We are not sure that this is a true neoplasm. The malignant variants, well described by Stout,[194] contain multiple varieties of soft tissue sarcomas in the same neoplasm. In other words, chondrosarcoma, liposarcoma, and rhabdomyosarcoma may all be observed in a single tumor. Nash and Stout[193] reviewed forty-

two cases occurring in children, nine of them present at birth.

Tumors of metaplastic mesenchyme

Soft tissue chondromas are seen most frequently in the soft tissues of hands and feet.[199] Grossly, they are lobulated, have a typical hyaline appearance, and are often calcified (Fig. 1137). Some nuclear hyperchromasia may be present and should not be interpreted as evidence of malignancy. The occasional presence of a cellular fi-

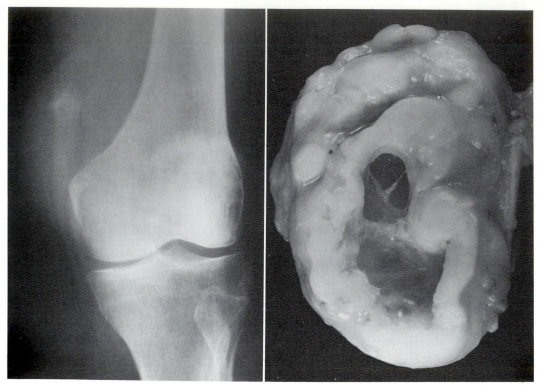

Fig. 1137 Soft tissue chondroma occurring in knee region of 71-year-old woman. As usual, tumor is partially calcified, lobulated, and focally cystic. (WU negs. 11139 and 11164.)

broblastic growth around the lobules suggests a possible histogenetic relationship with juvenile aponeurotic fibroma. Local recurrence is not infrequent.

Soft tissue chondrosarcomas are extremely rare.[198, 200] They occur in the extremities of adult patients and exhibit a less agressive behavior than their skeletal counterpart. Enzinger and Shiraki[196] studied thirty-four cases of a variant they designated as myxoid chondrosarcoma. Well-differentiated chondrocytes were absent, and this was responsible for the difficulties in diagnosis. Glycogen was demonstrated in many of the tumor cells. Acid mucopolysaccharides were abundant in the stroma. In contrast with those present in myxoma and myxoid liposarcoma, they were unaffected by testicular hyaluronidase treatment.

Soft tissue osteosarcoma is distinguished from chondrosarcoma by applying the same criteria used for the skeletal tumors. They usually occur in the extremities of adults.[197] The prognosis is much worse than for chondrosarcoma: of the twenty-six cases reviewed by Allan and Soule,[195] twenty-one of the patients died as a result of the tumor. Extraskeletal osteosarcoma should be differentiated from myositis ossificans. Nuclear atypia and lack of differentiation ("zone phenomena") are the most important distinguishing features. It also should be differentiated from other soft tissue tumors in which metaplastic bone is formed, such as fibrosarcoma and synovial sarcoma.

Tumors of probable extragonadal germ cell origin
Teratoma

Soft tissue teratomas are uncommon.[201] They are more frequent in females and are either present at birth or in early child-

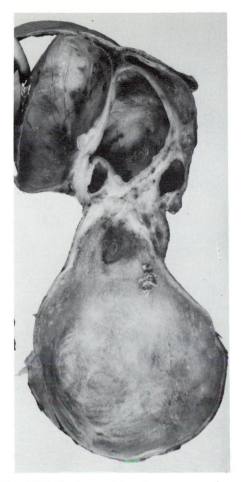

Fig. 1138 Benign multicystic teratoma of sacro-coccygeal region present at birth. It was mainly composed of adult skin and neural tissue. (WU neg. 68-5325.)

hood. In some cases, there is an association with twinning or malformations. The most common locations, in descending order of frequency, are retroperitoneum, mediastinum, sacrococcygeal area, base of skull, pineal region, and neck.[206] Taken as a whole, approximately three fourths are benign. However, there are important variations in the incidence of malignancy according to location, age, and sex.[203, 204] For instance, the large majority of sacrococcygeal teratomas present at birth are benign, whereas tumors in the same location discovered after the age of 2 months are often malignant.[203, 205] Presence of marked bowel or bladder dysfunction

indicates that the teratoma is probably malignant.

The terminology and diagnostic criteria used in the evaluation of these lesions is the same as for those of gonadal origin (Chapters 17 and 18). The benign form is often multicystic and contains a variety of well-differentiated tissues (Fig. 1138). The malignant types may have the appearance of teratocarcinoma, embryonal carcinoma, or yolk sac tumor. Chretien et al.[202] reviewed twenty-one cases of yolk sac tumor (which they refer to as embryonal adenocarcinoma) of the sacrococcygeal region. Seven of them had associated teratomatous elements. Local recurrence, often associated with distant metastases, resulted in the death of all twenty-one patients.

Tumors of neurogenic origin
Pigmented neuroectodermal tumor of infancy

The neurogenic origin of pigmented neuroectodermal tumor of infancy, also known as melanotic progonoma and retinal anlage tumor, is now established.[209, 212] The classical location is the maxilla, but it also has been reported in the skull and mediastinum.[210, 211] We also have seen it in the thigh, forearm, and epididymis. In most areas, the tumor cells are small and round, with the appearance of neuroblasts. As a matter of fact, we have seen this tumor misdiagnosed as neuroblastoma on several occasions. The diagnostic feature is the presence of pseudoglandular or alveolar formations lined by a wall of larger cells containing abundant melanin in their cytoplasm (Fig. 1139). The clinical course is invariably benign. Supposedly malignant varieties probably represent malignant teratomas with a pigmented neuroectodermal component.

Other neurogenic tumors

Exceptionally, *meningiomas* can present as a soft tissue mass at the base of the nose or scalp.[208] Anderson[207] reviewed seven benign *myxopapillary ependymomas* lo-

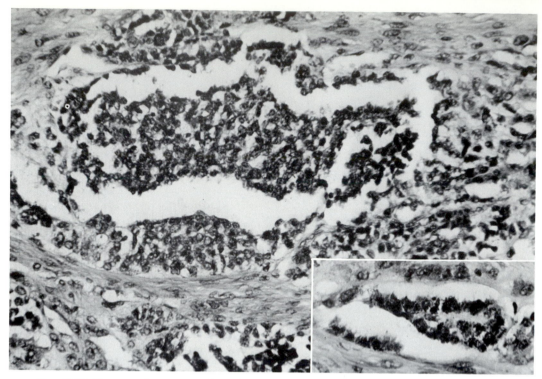

Fig. 1139 Pigmented neuroectodermal tumor of infancy. Clump of undifferentiated neu-roectodermal cells has detached from peripheral portion, resulting in alveolar pattern. **Inset,** Another area of same tumor illustrating melanin-containing elements. (×300; WU neg. 73-3402; **inset,** ×350; WU neg. 73-3403.)

cated in the soft tissues over the sacro-coccygeal area.

Tumors of hematopoietic origin

Rarely, *malignant lymphomas* first mani-fest themselves by the presence of a soft tissue tumor. This occurrence is more com-mon with histiocytic and lymphocytic malignant lymphomas than with Hodg-kin's disease. Most cases of *plasma cell myeloma* of soft tissue represent direct extension from underlying osseous foci. However, independent soft tissue masses also can occur. They inevitably become disseminated.

Exceptionally, nodules of *extramedullary hematopoiesis* develop in the mediastinum or other soft tissue areas; they have been described in agnogenic myeloid metaplasia and congenital spherocytosis and in other types of anemia.[212a]

Tumors of uncertain origin
Fibrous hamartoma of infancy

Enzinger[220] applied the term fibrous hamartoma of infancy to a tumorlike con-dition seen almost exclusively during the first two years of life and sometimes present at birth. It predominates in boys and the most common locations are the region of the shoulder, axilla, and upper arm. It is almost always solitary. Grossly, it is poorly circumscribed and composed of whitish tissue of fibrous appearance intermixed with islands of fat.

Microscopically, the distinctive feature of this lesion is an organoid pattern, three distinct types of tissue being present: (1) well-differentiated fibrous tissue, (2) ma-ture adipose tissue, and (3) immature, cellular areas arranged in a whorl-like pat-tern and resembling primitive mesenchyme. Although local recurrence may occur, the

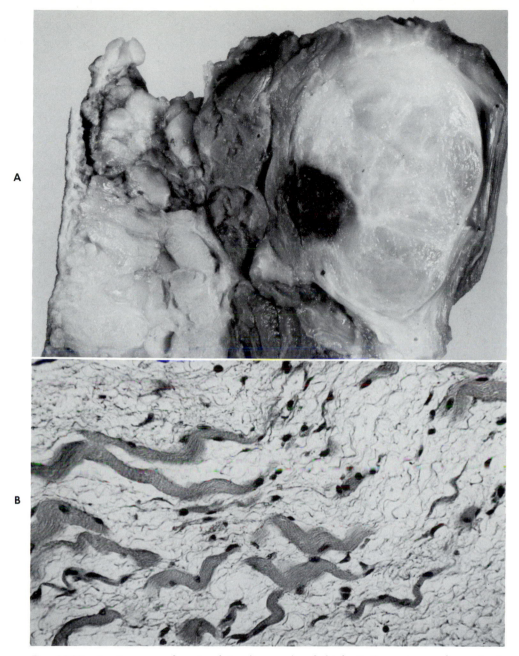

Fig. 1140   **A,** Myxoma of vastus lateralis muscle of thigh. **B,** Same tumor shown in **A.** Note myxomatous tissue infiltrating muscle bundles. (**A,** WU neg. 66-8361; **B,** ×300; WU neg. 67-1170.)

clinical course is basically that of a benign disease.[220]

Myxoma

Myxomas are rare neoplasms that have a mucoid, slimy gross appearance[237] (Fig. 1140, A). The majority are poorly circumscribed and may infiltrate neighboring structures. They occur almost always in adults. The diagnosis of myxoma in a child should be seriously questioned. Approximately 20% of all myxomas arise within

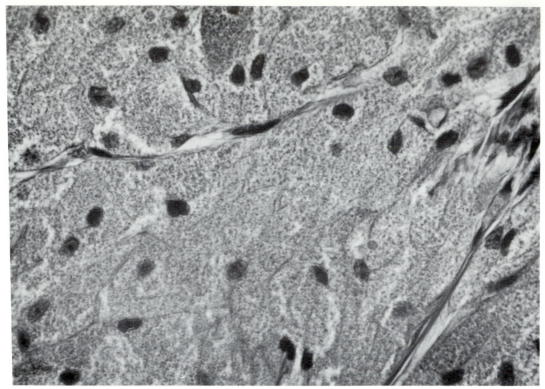

Fig. 1141 Granular cell tumor. Cells are large with finely granular cytoplasm and small dense nucleus. (×720; WU neg. 72-10437.)

skeletal muscle, especially those of the thigh. The prognosis is excellent. In a series of thirty-four cases reported by Enzinger,[218] there was not a single case of local recurrence. We have seen intramuscular myxomas in association with fibrous dysplasia of the bones of the same extremity.[240]

The differential diagnosis of myxoma should be made with two groups of diseases. The first is a group of neoplasms in which myxomatous change can be a prominent secondary feature, such as liposarcoma, chondrosarcoma, smooth muscle tumors, embryonal rhabdomyosarcoma, and neurofibroma. The second is a variety of conditions resulting in focal mucinous degeneration of the skin or soft tissues, such as localized myxedema, mucous (myxoid) cyst, ganglion, follicular mucinosis (alopecia mucinosa), papular mucinosis, and cutaneous focal mucinosis.[229] It should be remembered that in myxoma the cells have a bland *appearance* throughout, that mitot-

ic activity is practically absent, and that blood vessels are extremely scanty (Fig. 1140, *B*).

Granular cell tumor

The most common location of granular cell tumor, also known as granular cell myoblastoma, is the tongue. It has been seen, however, in many other locations such as the skin, vulva, breast, larynx, bronchus, esophagus, stomach, appendix, rectum, anus, bile ducts, urinary bladder, uterus, and soft tissue.[238, 239] Multiplicity of lesions can be observed, particularly in black patients.[231]

These tumors are usually small, although we have seen cases measuring up to 5 cm in diameter. They have a hard consistency and ill-defined margins. This, plus the ulceration sometimes complicating the larger cutaneous tumors, explains why they are often confused clinically and on

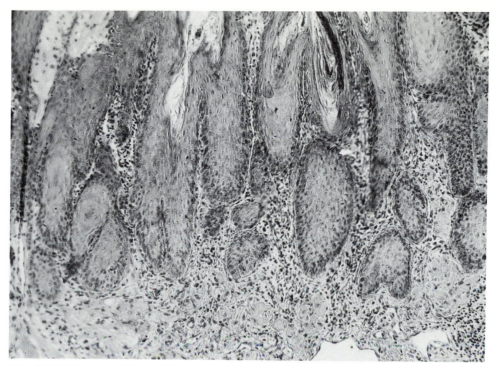

Fig. 1142 Bizarre epidermal changes overlying granular cell tumor. These changes often lead to incorrect diagnosis of cancer. (×125; WU neg. 52-3607.)

gross inspection with a malignant neoplasm. The individual cells are large and their cytoplasm highly granular (Fig. 1141). Most granules are small and regular. They alternate with larger round droplets having a homogeneous eosinophilic appearance. The histochemical reactions and ultrastructural appearance of these inclusions are those of lysosomes. If the tumor grows near an epithelial surface, such as the skin, vulva, or larynx, secondary epithelial hyperplasia occurs which is often incorrectly diagnosed as carcinoma (Fig. 1142).

The large majority of the granular cell tumors pursue a benign clinical course. Most cases reported in the literature as malignant granular cell myoblastomas are in reality examples of alveolar soft part sarcoma. On the other hand, we know of a few well-documented cases of tumors with a light microscopic appearance comparable to that of granular cell tumor which resulted in distant metastases.[213, 221]

The histogenesis of this lesion is still discussed, although recently most writers on the subject have favored a Schwann cell origin, based on histochemical and ultrastructural findings and on the occurrence of typical lesions within nerves.[216, 225, 227] On the other hand, changes histochemically and ultrastructurally indistinguishable from those above discussed have been documented in neoplastic and nonneoplastic smooth muscle cells and in tumoral ameloblasts.[217, 232, 235] We are therefore beginning to believe that granular cell tumor is not a specific entity but rather the expression of a degenerative change that can occur not only in schwann cells but also in a variety of other cell types, whether previously normal or forming part of a benign or a malignant neoplasm.

Alveolar soft part sarcoma

Alveolar soft part sarcoma, a malignant soft tissue tumor designated in the past as malignant organoid granular cell myoblastoma and malignant nonchromaffin para-

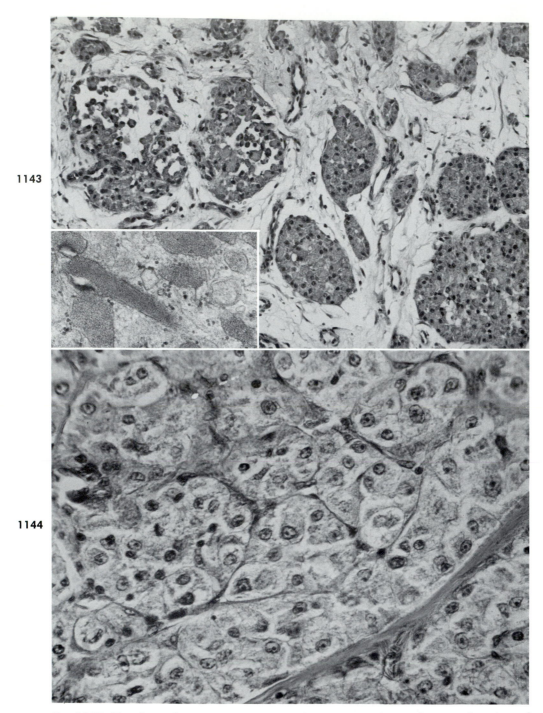

Fig. 1143 Alveolar soft part sarcoma persenting as mass in oropharyngeal region of young girl. Tumor forms well-defined lobules, some of which show central space simulating alveolus. **Inset,** Electron micrograph of same tumor. Crystalline inclusions characteristic of this lesion were found in some tumor cells. (×150; WU neg. 72-2016A; **inset,** uranyl acetate–lead citrate.)

Fig. 1144 Alveolar soft part sarcoma. Note arrangement of cells, prominent nuclei and nucleoli, and abundant granular cytoplasm. (×500; WU neg. 54-4754.)

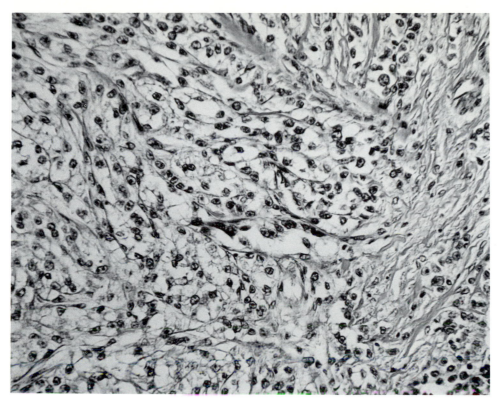

Fig. 1145 Clear cell sarcoma of soft tissue that occurred in 27-year-old woman and arose from left patellar tendon. (×300; WU neg. 66-9186; slide contributed by Dr. F. Enzinger, Washington, D. C.)

ganglioma, involves most often the deep soft tissues of the thigh and leg of young adults. Females are more commonly affected. We also have seen it in the oral cavity and mediastinum. Grossly, the tumors are well circumscribed, usually large, moderately firm, and gray or yellowish in color. Areas of necrosis or hemorrhage are common in the larger neoplasms.

Microscopically, the tumor cells are separated by fibrous tissue into well-defined nests. Detachment of the central cells results in a typical alveolar pattern (Fig. 1143). The individual cells are large and have vesicular nuclei, *prominent nucleoli*, and a granular cytoplasm (Fig. 1144). Mitoses are exceptional. PAS stain sometimes demonstrates the presence of diastase-resistant intracytoplasmic needle-like structures. These are seen by electron microscopy as membrane-bound crystals

with a periodicity of 58-100 Å, sometimes arranged in a cross-grid pattern. We have found this feature of diagnostic value in lesions of controversial nature[234] (Fig. 1143, *inset*).

The tumor is highly malignant, despite its deceivingly slow clinical course. Vein invasion is common. Blood-borne metastases appear in the lungs and other organs as long as fifteen years following excision of the primary tumor.[230]

The histogenesis of this strange neoplasm has not yet been definitely established. We believe there is no convincing evidence to support the theory that this tumor represents the malignant counterpart of granular cell tumor or that it arises from nonchromaffin paraganglia. We agree with Fisher et al.[224] that at the present time the bulk of evidence favors a myogenous derivation—i.e., that alveolar soft

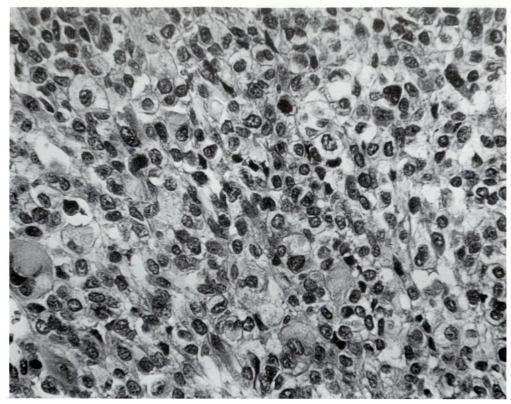

Fig. 1146 Epithelioid cell sarcoma. This rare tumor is highly cellular and at times has clear cytoplasm. (×350; WU neg. 72-10436.)

part sarcoma represents a distinct variant of rhabdomyosarcoma.

Clear cell sarcoma of tendons and aponeuroses

Enzinger[219] has described a malignant tumor arising chiefly from large tendons and aponeuroses of the extremities and having a distinctive microscopic appearance. The feet are the most common site. Grossly, the tumors are firm, well circumscribed, and gray or white and cut with a gritty sensation. Microscopically, solid nests and fascicles of pale fusiform or cuboidal cells are present (Fig. 1145). The nucleoli are large and deeply basophilic. Multinucleated giant cells are often seen. Abundant extracellular and intracellular iron was found in all twenty-one cases studied by Enzinger.[219]

The clinical course is characterized by slow but relentless progression with fre-

quent local recurrences and eventual distant metastases.[214, 219] The histogenesis is unknown.

Epithelioid sarcoma

Enzinger[222] reported sixty-two cases of a malignant soft tissue tumor having a characteristic multinodular growth. The necrosis invariably seen in the center of the nodules and the epithelioid appearance of the tumor cells often results in a mistaken diagnosis of granuloma.[233] Tumors of similar nature had been reported by Bliss and Reed[215] as "large cell sarcomas of tendon sheath." Enzinger[222] remarked on the striking acidophilia of the tumor tissue, due to the staining characteristics of the cytoplasm and the extensive desmoplasia (Fig. 1146). In his series, there was local recurrence in 85% of the patients and distant metastases in 30%. The histogenesis remains obscure. Histiocytes, fibroblasts,

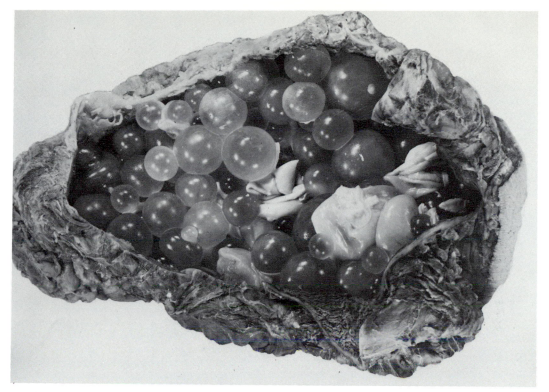

Fig. 1147 Hydatidosis presenting as soft tissue mass in gluteal region. (Courtesy Dr. E. F. Lascano, Buenos Aires, Argentina.)

and synovial cells have all been implicated.[223, 226, 236]

Malignant giant cell tumor of soft parts

Malignant giant cell tumor of soft parts is a rare neoplasm composed of a mixture of osteoclast-like giant cells, fibroblasts, and histiocytes. The appearance is similar to that of giant cell tumor of bone.[232a] Superficially located tumors are less aggressive than those situated in deeper structures. Guccion and Enzinger[228] favor a histiocytic derivation and a possible relationship with malignant fibrous histiocytoma.

Other tumorlike conditions

In **tumoral calcinosis,** large, painless calcified masses appear in the periarticular soft tissues, especially along extensor surfaces. The elbows and hips are the most common sites. Curiously, the knee is always spared. The serum calcium and phosphorus levels are normal. The disease may recur after excision.[243]

Kern[244] designated as **proliferative myositis** a reactive condition involving skeletal muscle and often confused microscopically with sarcoma of one type or another. The shoulder, thorax, and thigh are the regions most commonly affected. Most patients are over the age of 45 years. Grossly, the lesion is rather unimpressive. It appears as an ill-defined scarlike induration of muscle. Microscopically, a cellular proliferation is seen surrounding individual muscle fibers. Most of the cells are fibroblasts. They alternate with extremely large basophilic cells with vesicular nucleus and very prominent nucleolus, closely resembling ganglion cells or rhabdomyoblasts. Conservative surgery is curative.[241]

Bronchogenic cysts of skin and soft tissue were reported by Fraga et al.[242] The majority were discovered at or seen after birth in male infants. The most common location was the suprasternal notch and manubrium sterni.

In countries in which **hydatidosis** is

endemic, the disease may first present as a soft tissue mass (Fig. 1147).

REFERENCES
Infection

1 Michelson, E.: Syndrome of trauma to the psoas muscle, Arch. Surg. **50**:77-81, 1945.
2 Picket, W. J., and Friedell, M. T.: Large nonpulsating hematoma (false aneurysm), Surg. Clin. North Am. **27**:153-155, 1947.

Pilonidal disease

3 Culp, C. E.: Pilonidal disease and its treatment, Surg. Clin. North Am. **47**:1007-1014, 1967.
4 Davage, O. N.: The origin of sacrococcygeal pilonidal sinuses based on an analysis of four hundred sixty-three cases, Am. J. Pathol. **30**:1191-1205, 1954.
5 Notaras, M. J.: A review of three popular methods of treatment of postanal (pilonidal) sinus disease, Br. J. Surg. **57**:886-890, 1970.

Tumors
Introduction

6 Kauffman, S. L., and Stout, A. P.: Congenital mesenchymal tumors, Cancer **18**:460-476, 1965.
7 Soule, E. H., Mahour, G. H., Mills, S. D., and Lynn, H. B.: Soft-tissue sarcomas of infants and children; a clinicopathologic study of 135 cases, Mayo Clin. Proc. **43**:313-326, 1968.
8 Thompson, D. E., Frost, H. M., Hendrick, J. W., and Horn, R. C.: Soft tissue sarcomas involving the extremities and the limb girdles; a review, South. Med. J. **64**:33-44, 1971.

Biopsy

9 Lieberman, Z., and Ackerman, L. V.: Principles in management of soft tissue sarcomas, Surgery **35**:350-365, 1954.

Tumors and tumorlike conditions of fibrous tissue
Juvenile aponeurotic fibroma

10 Allen, P. M., and Enzinger, F. M.: Juvenile aponeurotic fibroma, Cancer **26**:857-867, 1970.
11 Goldman, R. L.: The cartilage analogue of fibromatosis (aponeurotic fibroma); further observations based on 7 new cases, Cancer **26**:1325-1331, 1970.
12 Keasbey, L. E.: Juvenile aponeurotic fibroma (calcifying fibroma), Cancer **6**:338-346, 1953.
13 Lichtenstein, L., and Goldman, R. L.: The cartilage analogue of fibromatosis, Cancer **17**:810-816, 1964.

Nodular fasciitis

14 Allen, P. W.: Nodular fasciitis, Pathology **4**:9-26, 1972.

15 Hutter, R. V. P., Stewart, F. W., and Foote, F. W., Jr.: Fasciitis; a report of 70 cases with follow-up proving the benignity of the lesion, Cancer **15**:992-1003, 1962.
16 Kleinstiver, B. J., and Rodriguez, H. A.: Nodular fasciitis; a study of 45 cases and review of the literature, J. Bone Joint Surg. [Am.] **50**:1204-1212, 1968.
17 Konwaler, B. E., Keasbey, L., and Kaplan, L.: Subcutaneous pseudosarcomatous fibromatosis (fasciitis); report of 8 cases, Am. J. Clin. Pathol. **25**:241-252, 1955.
18 Price, E. B., Jr., Silliphant, W. M., and Shuman, R.: Nodular fasciitis: a clinicopathologic analysis of 65 cases, Am. J. Clin. Pathol. **35**:122-136, 1961.

Elastofibroma

19 Banfield, W. G., and Lee, C. K.: Elastofibroma; an electron microscopic study, J. Natl. Cancer Inst. **40**:1067-1077, 1968.
20 Järvi, O. H., Saxén, A. E., Hopsu-Havu, V. K., Wartiovaara, J. J., and Vaissalo, V. T.: Elastofibroma; a degenerative pseudotumor, Cancer **23**:42-63, 1969.
21 Stemmermann, G. N., and Stout, A. P.: Elastofibroma dorsi, Am. J. Clin. Pathol. **37**:490-506, 1962.

Fibromatosis

22 Allen, R. A., Woolner, L. B., and Ghormley, R. K.: Soft-tissue tumors of the sole; with special reference to plantar fibromatosis, J. Bone Joint Surg. [Am.] **37**:14-26, 1955.
23 Battifora, H., and Hines, J. R.: Recurrent digital fibromas of childhood; an electron microscope study, Cancer **27**:1530-1536, 1971.
24 Beatty, E. C., Jr.: Congenital generalized fibromatosis in infancy, Am. J. Dis. Child. **103**:620-624, 1962.
25 Bochetto, J. F., Raycroft, J. E., and DeInnocentes, L. W.: Multiple polyposis, exostosis, and soft tissue tumors, Surg. Gynecol. Obstet. **117**:489-494, 1963.
26 Brown, J. B., and McDowell, F.: Wry-neck facial distortion prevented by resection of fibrosed sternomastoid muscle in infancy and childhood, Ann. Surg. **131**:721-733, 1950.
27 Burry, A. F., Kerr, J. F. R., and Pope, J. H.: Recurring digital fibrous tumour of childhood; an electron microscopic and virological study, Pathology **2**:287-291, 1970.
28 Conley, J., Healey, W. V., and Stout, A. P.: Fibromatosis of the head and neck, Am. J. Surg. **112**:609-614, 1966.
29 Coventry, M. B., Harris, L. E., Bianco, A. J., and Bulbulian, A. H.: Congenital muscular torticollis (wry neck), Postgrad. Med. **28**:383-392, 1960.
30 Drescher, E., Woyke, S., Markiewicz, C.,

and Tegi, S.: Juvenile fibromatosis in siblings (fibromatosis hyalinica multiplex juvenilis), J. Pediatr. Surg. 2:427-430, 1967.

31 Enzinger, F. M.: Fibrous tumors of infancy. In Tumors of bone and soft tissue, Houston, 1968, M. D. Anderson Hosp., pp. 375-396.

32 Enzinger, F. M.: Histological typing of soft tissue tumours, International histological classification of tumours, No. 3, Geneva, 1969, World Health Organization.

33 Enzinger, F. M., and Shiraki, M.: Musculoaponeurotic fibromatosis of the shoulder girdle (extra-abdominal desmoid); analysis of 30 cases followed up for ten or more years, Cancer 20:1131-1140, 1967.

34 Gabbiani, G., and Majno, G.: Dupuytren's contracture; fibroblast contraction? An ultrastructural study, Am. J. Pathol. 66:131-138, 1972.

35 Goslee, L., Clermont, V., Bernstein, J., and Woolley, P. W., Jr.: Superficial connective tissue tumors in early infancy, J. Pediatr. 65:377-387, 1964.

36 Hunt, R. T., Morgan, H. C., and Ackerman, L. V.: Principles in the management of extraabdominal desmoids, Cancer 13:825-836, 1960.

36a Ishikawa, H., and Mori, S.: Systemic hyalinosis or fibromatosis hyalinica multiplex juvenilis as a congenital syndrome; a new entity based on the inborn error of the acid mucopolysaccharide metabolism in connective tissue cells? Acta Dermatovenerol. 53:185-191, 1973.

37 Iwahara, T., and Ikeda, A.: On the ipsilateral involvement of congenital muscular torticollis and congenital dislocation of the hip, J. Jap. Orthop. Assoc. 35:1221-1226, 1962.

38 Kim, D.-H., Goldsmith, H. S., Quan, S. H., and Huvos, A. G.: Intra-abdominal desmoid tumor, Cancer 27:1041-1043, 1971.

39 Larsen, R. D., and Posch, J. L.: Dupuytren's contracture: with special reference to pathology, J. Bone Joint Surg. [Am.] 40:773-792, 1958.

40 Masson, J. K., and Soule, E. H.: Desmoid tumors of head and neck, Am. J. Surg. 112:615-622, 1966.

41 Pickren, J. W., Smith, A. G., Stevenson, T. W., Jr., and Stout, A. P.: Fibromatosis of the plantar fascia, Cancer 4:846-856, 1951.

42 Reye, R. D. K.: Recurring digital fibrous tumors of childhood, Arch. Pathol. 80:228-231, 1965.

43 Shnitka, T. K., Douglas, M. A., and Horner, R. H.: Congenital generalized fibromatosis, Cancer 11:627-639, 1958.

44 Skoog, T.: Dupuytren's contracture; pathogenesis and surgical treatment, Surg. Clin. North Am. 47:433-444, 1967.

45 Staley, C. J.: Gardner's syndrome; simultaneous occurrence of polyposis coli, osteomatosis and soft tissue tumors, Arch. Surg. 82:420-422, 1961.

46 Stout, A. P.: Juvenile fibromatoses, Cancer 7:953-978, 1954.

47 Welsh, R. A.: Intracytoplasmic collagen formations in desmoid fibromatosis, Am. J. Pathol. 49:515-535, 1966.

48 Woyke, S., Domagala, W., and Olszewski, W.: Ultrastructure of a fibromatosis hyalinica multiplex juvenilis, Cancer 26:1157-1168, 1970.

Fibrosarcoma

49 Stout, A. P.: Fibrosarcoma; the malignant tumor of fibroblasts, Cancer 1:30-63, 1948, (extensive bibliography).

50 Stout, A. P.: Fibrosarcoma in infants and children, Cancer 15:1028-1040, 1962.

51 van der Werf-Messing, B., and van Unnik, J. A. M.: Fibrosarcoma of the soft tissue; a clinicopathologic study, Cancer 18:1113-1123, 1965.

Tumors of probable histiocytic origin

52 Black, W. C., McGavran, M. H., and Graham, P.: Nodular subepidermal fibrosis; a clinical pathologic study emphasizing the frequency of clinical misdiagnoses, Arch. Surg. 98:296-300, 1969.

53 Burkhardt, B. R., Soule, E. H., Winkelman, R. K., and Ivins, J. C.: Dermatofibrosarcoma protuberans; study of 56 cases, Am. J. Surg. 111:638-644, 1966.

54 Feldman, F., and Norman, D.: Intra- and extraosseous malignant histiocytoma (malignant fibrous xanthoma), Radiology 104:497-508, 1972.

55 Fisher, E. R., and Hellstrom, H. R.: Dermatofibrosarcoma with metastases simulating Hodgkin's disease and reticulum cell sarcoma, Cancer 19:1165-1171, 1966.

56 Fisher, E. R., and Vuzevski, V. D.: Cytogenesis of schwannoma (neurilemoma), neurofibroma, dermatofibroma, and dermatofibrosarcoma as revealed by electron microscopy, Am. J. Clin. Pathol. 49:141-154, 1968.

57 Fretzin, D. F., and Helwig, E. B.: Atypical fibroxanthoma of the skin; a clinicopathologic study of 140 cases, Cancer 31:1541-1552, 1973.

58 Hudson, A. W., and Winkelmann, R. K.: Atypical fibroxanthoma of the skin; a reappraisal of 19 cases in which the original diagnosis was spindle-cell squamous carcinoma, Cancer 29:413-422, 1972.

59 Jacoby, F.: Macrophages (XIV. The problem of transformation). In Willmer, E. N., editor: Cells and tissues in culture; methods, biology

and physiology, vol. 2, London and New York, 1965, Academic Press, Inc., pp. 63-75.

60 Kauffman, S. L., and Stout, A. P.: Histiocytic tumors (fibrous xanthoma and histiocytoma) in children, Cancer 14:469-482, 1961.

61 Kaufman, S. L., and Stout, A. P.: Congenital mesenchymal tumors, Cancer 18:460-476, 1965.

62 Kempson, R. L. ,and Kyriakos, M.: Fibroxanthosarcoma of the soft tissues; a type of malignant fibrous histiocytoma, Cancer 29: 961-976, 1972.

63 Kempson, R. L., and McGavran, M. H.: Atypical fibroxanthoma of the skin, Cancer 17:1463-1471, 1964,

64 Kroe, D. J., and Pitcock, J. A.: Atypical fibroxanthoma of the skin; report of ten cases, Am. J. Clin. Pathol. 51:487-492, 1969.

65 Merkow L. P., Frich, J. C., Jr., Slifkin, M., Kyreages, C. G., and Pardo, M.: Ultrastructure of a fibroxanthosarcoma (malignant fibroxanthoma), Cancer 28:372-383, 1971.

66 Niemi, K. M.: The benign fibrohistiocytic tumours of the skin, Acta Derm. Venereol. (Stockh.) 50(suppl. 63):1-66, 1970.

67 Oberling, C.: Retroperitoneal xanthogranuloma, Am. J. Cancer 23:477-489, 1935.

68 O'Brien, J. E., and Stout, A. P.: Malignant fibrous xanthomas, Cancer 17:1445-1455, 1964.

69 Ozzello, L., Stout, A. P., and Murray, M. R.: Cultural characteristics of malignant histiocytomas and fibrous xanthomas, Cancer 16: 331-344, 1963.

70 Rachmaninoff, N., McDonald, J. R., and Cook, J. C.: Sarcoma-like tumors of the skin following irradiation, Am. J. Clin. Pathol. 36: 427-437, 1961.

71 Soule, E. H., and Enriquez, P.: Atypical fibrous histiocytoma, malignant fibrous histiocytoma, malignant histiocytoma and epithelioid sarcoma; a comparative study of 65 tumors, Cancer 30:128-143, 1972.

72 Stout, A. P., and Lattes, R.: Tumors of the soft tissues. In Atlas of tumor pathology, 2nd series, Fasc. I, Washington, D. C., 1967, Armed Forces Institute of Pathology.

73 Taylor, H. B., and Helwig, E. B.: Dermatofibrosarcoma protuberans; a study of 115 cases, Cancer 15:717-725, 1962.

74 Vernon-Roberts, B.: The macrophage, Cambridge, 1972, Cambridge University Press.

Tumors and tumorlike conditions of peripheral nerves

75 Bednář, B.: Storiform neurofibromas of skin, pigmented and nonpigmented, Cancer 10: 368-376, 1957.

76 Benedict, P. H., Szabó, G., Fitzpatrick, T. B., and Sinesi, S. J.: Melanotic macules in Albright's syndrome and in neurofibromatosis, J.A.M.A. 205:618-626, 1968.

77 Bird, C. C., and Willis, R. A.: The histogenesis of pigmented neurofibromas, J. Pathol. 97:631-637, 1969.

78 Bolande, R. P., and Towler, W. F.: A possible relationship of neuroblastoma to von Recklinghausen's disease, Cancer 26:162-172, 1970.

79 Crowe, F. W., Schull, W. J., and Neel, J. V.: Multiple neurofibromatosis, Springfield, Ill., 1956, Charles C Thomas, Publisher.

80 D'Agostino, A. N., Soule, E. H., and Miller, R. H.: Primary malignant neoplasms of nerves (malignant neurilemonas) in patients without manifestations of multiple neurofibromatosis (von Recklinghausen's disease), Cancer 16: 1003-1013, 1963.

81 D'Agostino, A. N., Soule, E. H., and Miller, R. H.: Sarcomas of the peripheral nerves and somatic soft tissues associated with multiple neurofibromatosis (von Recklinghausen's disease), Cancer 16:1015-1027, 1963.

82 Fisher, E. R., and Vuzevski, V. D.: Cytogenesis of schwannoma (neurilemoma), neurofibroma, dermatofibroma, and dermatofibrosarcoma as revealed by electron microscopy, Am. J. Clin. Pathol. 49:141-154, 1968.

83 Ghosh, B. C., Ghosh, L., Huvos, A. G., and Fortner, J. G.: Malignant schwannoma; a clinicopathologic study, Cancer 31:184-190, 1973.

84 Gore, I.: Primary malignant tumors of nerve; a report of eight cases, Cancer 5:278-296, 1952.

85 Gorlin, R. J., Sedano, H. O., Vickers, R. A., and Cervenka, J.: Multiple mucosal neuromas, pheochromocytoma and medullary carcinoma of the thyroid; a syndrome, Cancer 22:293-299, 1968.

86 Hill, R. P.: Neuroma of Wagner-Meissner tactile corpuscles, Cancer 4:879-882, 1951.

87 Hirano, A., Dembitzer, H. M., and Zimmerman, H. M.: Fenestrated blood vessels in neurilemoma, Lab. Invest. 27:305-309, 1972.

88 Hosoi, K.: Multiple neurofibromatosis (von Recklinghausen's disease), with special reference to malignant transformation, Arch. Surg. 22:258-281, 1931.

89 McCarroll, H. R.: Clinical manifestations of congenital neurofibromatosis, J. Bone Joint Surg. [Am.] 32:601-617, 1950.

90 Michel, S. L.: Epithelial elements in a malignant neurogenic tumor of the tibial nerve, Am. J. Surg. 113:404-413, 1967.

91 Oberman, H. A., and Sullenger, G.: Neurogenous tumors of the head and neck, Cancer 20:1992-2001, 1967.

92 Pineada, A.: Mast cells; their presence and ultrastructural characteristics in peripheral nerve tumors, Arch. Neurol. 13:372-382, 1965.

93 Raszkowski, H. J., and Hufner, R. F.: Neuro-fibromatosis of the colon; a unique manifestation of von Recklinghausen's disease, Cancer **27**:134-142, 1971.

94 Reed, R. J., and Bliss, B. O.: Morton's neuroma; regressive and productive intermetatarsal elastofibrositis, Arch. Pathol. **95**:123-129, 1973.

95 Saxen, E.: Tumours of tactile end-organs, Acta Pathol. Microbiol. Scand. **25**:66-79, 1948.

96 Scotti, T. M.: The lesion of Morton's metatarsalgia (Morton's toe), Arch. Path. **63**:91-102, 1957.

97 Stout, A. P.: Neurofibroma and neurilemoma, Clin. Proc. **5**:1-12, 1946.

98 Stout, A. P.: Discussion of case 5, Seventeenth Seminar of the American Society of Clinical Pathologists, October, 1951.

99 Waggener, J. D.: Ultrastructure of benign peripheral nerve sheath tumors, Cancer **19**:699-709, 1966.

100 White, H. R., Jr.: Survival in malignant schwannoma; an 18-year study, Cancer **27**:720-729, 1971.

101 Whitehouse, D.: Diagnostic value of the cafe-au-lait spot in children, Arch. Dis. Child. **41**:316-319, 1966.

102 Williams, E. D., and Pollock, D. J.: Multiple mucosal neuromata with endocrine tumors; a syndrome allied to von Recklinghausen's disease, J. Pathol. Bacteriol. **91**:71-80, 1966.

102a Woodruff, J. M., Chernik, N. L., Smith, M. C., Millett, W. B., and Foote, F. W.: Peripheral nerve tumors with rhabdomyosarcomatous differentiation (malignant "triton" tumors), Cancer **32**:426-439, 1973.

Tumors of adipose tissue

103 Ackerman, L. V.: Multiple primary liposarcomas, Am. J. Pathol. **20**:789-798, 1944.

104 Brines, O. A., and Johnson, M. H.: Hibernoma, a special fatty tumor; report of a case, Am. J. Pathol. **25**:467-479, 1949.

104a Chung, E. B., and Enzinger, F. M.: Benign lipoblastomatosis; an analysis of 35 cases, Cancer **32**:482-492, 1973.

105 Enterline, H. T., Culberson, J. D., Rochlin, D. B., and Brady, L. W.: Liposarcoma—a clinical and pathological study of 53 cases, Cancer **13**:932-950, 1960.

106 Enzinger, F. M., and Winslow, D. J.: Liposarcoma; a study of 103 cases, Virchows Arch. Pathol. Anat. **335**:367-388, 1962.

107 Georgiades, D. E., Alcalais, C. B., and Karabela, V. G.: Multicentric well-differentiated liposarcomas; a case report and a brief review of the literature, Cancer **24**:1091-1097, 1969.

108 Greenberg, S. D., Isensee, C., Gonzalez-Angulo, A., and Wallace, S. A.: Infiltrating lipomas of the thigh, Am. J. Clin. Pathol. **39**:66-72, 1963.

109 Howard, W. R., and Helwig, E. B.: Angiolipoma, Arch. Dermatol. **82**:924-931, 1960.

110 Levine, G. D.: Hibernoma; an electron microscopic study, Hum. Pathol. **3**:351-359, 1972.

111 Paarlberg, D., Linscheid, R. L., and Soule, E. H.: Lipomas of the hand; including a case of lipoblastomatosis in a child, Mayo Clin. Proc. **47**:121-124, 1972.

112 Pack, G. T., and Pierson, J. C.: Liposarcoma, Surgery **36**:687-712, 1954.

113 Reszel, P. A., Soule, E. H., and Coventry, M. B.: Liposarcoma of extremities and limb girdles: study of 222 cases, J. Bone Joint Surg. [Am.] **48**:229-244, 1966.

114 Stout, A. P.: Liposarcoma, the malignant tumor of lipoblasts, Ann. Surg. **119**:86-107, 1944.

115 Vellios, F., Baez, M. J., and Schumacher, H. B.: Lipoblastomatosis: a tumor of fetal fat different from hibernoma, Am. J. Pathol. **34**:1149-1155, 1958.

116 Winslow, D. J., and Enzinger, F. M.: Hyaluronidase-sensitive acid mucopolysaccharides in liposarcomas, Am. J. Pathol. **37**:497-505, 1960.

Tumors and tumorlike conditions of blood and lymph vessels
Hemangioma

117 Allen, P. W., and Enzinger, F. M.: Hemangioma of skeletal muscle; an analysis of 89 cases, Cancer **29**:8-22, 1972.

118 Brizill, H. E., and Raceuglia, G.: Giant hemangioma with thrombocytopenia, Blood **26**:751-756, 1965.

119 Koblenzer, P. J., and Bukowski, M. J.: Angiomatosis (hamartomatous hem-lymphangiomatosis); report of a case with diffuse involvement, Pediatrics **28**:65-76, 1961.

120 Lelong, M., Alagille, D., Habib, E.-C., and Steiner, A.: Memoires Originaux; L'hemangiome geant du nourrisson avec thrombopenie, Arch. Franc. Pédiatr. **21**:769-784, 1964.

121 Lindenauer, S. M.: The Klippel-Trenaunay syndrome: varicosity, hypertrophy and hemangioma with no arteriovenous fistula, Ann. Surg. **162**:303-314, 1965.

122 Lister, W. A.: The natural history of strawberry nevi, Lancet **1**:1429-1434, 1938.

123 Modlin, J. J.: Capillary hemangiomas of the skin, Surgery **38**:169-180, 1955.

124 Shim, W. K. T.: Hemangiomas of infancy complicated by thrombocytopenia, Am. J. Surg. **116**:896-906, 1968.

125 Watson, W. L., and McCarthy, W. D.: Blood and lymph vessel tumors, Surg. Gynecol. Obstet. **71**:569-588, 1940.

Glomus tumor

126 Carroll, R. E., and Berman, A. T.: Glomus tumors of the hand; review of the literature and report of 28 cases, J. Bone Joint Surg. [Am.] **54**:691-703, 1972.

127 Kohout, E., and Stout, A. R.: The glomus tumor in children, Cancer **14**:555-556, 1961.

128 Lattes, R., and Bull, D. C.: A case of glomus tumor with primary involvement of bone, Ann. Surg. **127**:187-191, 1948.

129 Masson, P.: Le glomus neuromyo-artériel des régions tactiles et ses tumeurs, Lyon Chir. **21**:259-280, 1924.

130 Masson, P.: Les glomus cutanés de l'homme, Bull. Soc. Fr. Dermatol. Syphiligr. **42**:1174-1245, 1935.

131 Murray, M. R., and Stout, A. P.: The glomus tumor; investigations of its distribution and behavior, and the identity of its "epithelioid" cell, Am. J. Pathol. **18**:183-203, 1942.

132 Shugart, R. R., Soule, E. H., and Johnson, E. W.: Glomus tumor, Surg. Gynecol. Obstet. **117**:334-340, 1963.

133 Stout, A. P.: Tumors of the neuromyoarterial glomus, Am. J. Cancer **24**:255-272, 1935.

134 Venkatachalam, M. A., and Greally, J. G.: Fine structure of glomus tumor: similarity of glomus cells to smooth muscle, Cancer **23**:1176-1184, 1969.

Hemangiopericytoma

135 Kuhn, C., III, and Rosai, J.: Tumors arising from pericytes; ultrastructure and organ culture of a case, Arch. Pathol. **88**:653-663, 1969.

136 McCormack, L. J.: Hemangiopericytoma, Cancer **7**:595-601, 1954.

137 Murray, M. R., and Stout, A. P.: The glomus tumor; investigation of its distribution and behavior, and the identity of its "epithelioid" cell, Am. J. Pathol. **18**:183-203, 1942.

138 O'Brien, P., and Brasfield, R. D.: Hemangiopericytoma, Cancer **14**:249-252, 1965.

139 Stout, A. P.: Hemangiopericytoma (a study of 25 new cases), Cancer **2**:1027-1954, 1949.

140 Stout, A. P.: Tumors featuring pericytes; glomus tumor and hemangiopericytoma, Lab. Invest. **5**:217-223, 1965.

141 Zimmerman, K. W.: Der feinere Bau der Blutcapillaren, Z. Anat. Entwicklungsgesch. **68**:29-109, 1923.

Angiosarcoma

142 Girard, C., Johnson, W. C., and Graham, J. H.: Cutaneous angiosarcoma, Cancer **26**:868-883, 1970.

143 Rosai, J., Kostianovsky, M., Sumner, H., and Perez-Mesa, C.: Angiosarcoma of skin; clinicopathologic study of 9 cases, with electron microscopic observations (in preparation).

144 Stout, A. P.: Hemangio-endothelioma: a tumor of blood vessels featuring vascular endothelial cells, Ann. Surg. **118**:445-464, 1943.

Lymphangioma

145 Cornog, J. L., Jr., and Enterline, H. T.: Lymphangiomyoma, a benign lesion of chyliferous lymphatics synonymous with lymphangiopericytoma, Cancer **19**:1909-1930, 1966.

146 Enterline, H. T., and Roberts, D.: Lymphangiopericytoma; case report of a previously undescribed tumor type, Cancer **8**:582-587, 1955.

147 Gross, R. E., and Hurwitt, E. S.: Cervicomediastinal and mediastinal cystic hygromas, Surg. Gynecol. Obstet. **87**:599-610, 1948.

148 Jao, J., Gilbert, S., and Messer, R.: Lymphangiomyoma and tuberous sclerosis, Cancer **29**:1188-1192, 1972.

149 Maxwell, J. H.: Tumors of the face and neck in infancy and childhood, South. Med. J. **45**:292-299, 1952.

150 Wolff, M.: Lymphangiomyoma: clinicopathologic study and ultrastructural confirmation of its histogenesis, Cancer **31**:988-1007, 1973.

Lymphangiosarcoma

151 Eby, C. S., Brennan, M. J., and Fine G.: Lymphangiosarcoma: a lethal complication of chronic lymphedema, Arch. Surg. **94**:223-230, 1967.

152 Hermann, J. B.: Lymphangiosarcoma of the chronically edematous extremity, Surg. Gynecol. Obstet. **121**:1107-1115, 1965.

153 Stewart, F. W., and Treves, N.: Lymphangiosarcoma in postmastectomy lymphedema; a report of six cases in elephantiasis chirurgica, Cancer **1**:64-81, 1948.

154 Whittle, R. J. M.: An angiosarcoma associated with an oedematous limb, J. Fac. Radiologists **10**:111-112, 1951.

155 Woodward, A. H., Ivins, J. C., and Soule, E. H.: Lymphangiosarcoma arising in chronic lymphedematous extremities, Cancer **30**:562-572, 1972.

Tumors of smooth muscle
Leiomyoma

156 Lendrum, A. C.: Painful tumours of the skin, Ann. R. Coll. Surg. Engl. **1**:62-67, 1947.

157 Stout, A. P.: Solitary cutaneous and subcutaneous leiomyoma, Am. J. Cancer **29**:435-469, 1937 (extensive bibliography).

Leiomyosarcoma

158 Bulmer, J. H.: Smooth muscle tumors of limbs, J. Bone Joint Surg. [Br.] **49**:52-58, 1967.

159 Dorfman, H. D., and Fishel, E. R.: Leiomyosarcomas of the greater saphenous vein, Am. J. Clin. Pathol. **39**:73-78, 1963.

160 Phelan, J. T., Sherer, W., and Perez-Mesa, C.: Malignant smooth-muscle tumors (leiomyosarcomas) of soft-tissue origin, N. Engl. J. Med. **266:**1027-1030, 1962.

161 Stout, A. P., and Hill, W. T.: Leiomyosarcoma of the superficial soft tissues, Cancer **11:**844-854, 1958.

162 Thomas, M. A., and Fine, G.: Leiomyosarcoma of veins; report of 2 cases and review of the literature, Cancer **13:**96-101, 1960.

163 Yannopoulos, K., and Stout, A. P.: Smooth muscle tumors in children, Cancer **15:**958-971, 1962.

Tumors of striated muscles
Rhabdomyoma

164 Czernobilsky, B., Cornog, J. L., and Enterline, H. T.: Rhabdomyoma; report of case with ultrastructural and histochemical studies, Am. J. Clin. Pathol. **49:**782-789, 1968.

165 Dehner, L. P., and Enzinger, F. M.: Fetal rhabdomyoma; an analysis of nine cases, Cancer **30:**160-166, 1972.

166 Morgan, J. J., and Enterline, H. T.: Benign rhabdomyoma of the pharynx; a case report, review of the literature, and comparison with cardiac rhabdomyoma, Am. J. Clin. Pathol. **42:**174-181, 1964.

Rhabdomyosarcoma

167 Enterline, H. T., and Horn, R. C.: Alveolar rhabdomyosarcoma; a distinctive tumor type, Am. J. Clin. Pathol. **20:**356-366, 1958.

168 Enzinger, F. M.: Recent trends in soft tissue pathology. In Tumors of bone and soft tissue, Houston, 1963, M. D. Anderson Hosp., pp. 315-332.

169 Enzinger, F. M.: Alveolar rhabdomyosarcoma; an analysis of 110 cases, Cancer **24:**18-31, 1969.

170 Horn, R. C., Jr., and Enterline, H. T.: Rhabdomyosarcoma; a clinicopathological study and classification of 39 cases, Cancer **11:**181-199, 1958.

171 Horvat, B. I., Caines, M., and Fisher, E. R.: The ultrastructure of rhabdomyosarcoma, Am. J. Clin. Pathol. **53:**555-564, 1970.

172 Jaffe, B. F., Fox, J. E., and Batsakis, J. G.: Rhabdomyosarcoma of the middle ear and mastoid, Cancer **27:**29-37, 1971.

173 Jönsson, G.: Malignant tumors of the skeletal muscles, fasciae, joint capsules, tendon sheaths and serous bursae, Acta Radiol. (suppl. 36), pp. 1-304, 1938.

174 Keyhani, A., and Booher, R. J.: Pleomorphic rhabdomyosarcoma, Cancer **22:**956-967, 1968.

175 Koop, E., and Tewarson, I. P.: Rhabdomyosarcoma of head and neck in children, Ann. Surg. **160:**95-103, 1964.

176 Linscheid, R. L., Soule, E. H., and Henderson, E. D.: Pleomorphic rhabdomyosarcomata of the extremities and limb girdles, J. Bone Joint Surg. [Am.] **47:**715-726, 1965.

177 Masson, J. K., and Soule, E. H.: Embryonal rhabdomyosarcoma of head and neck: report of 88 cases, Am. J. Surg. **110:**585-591, 1965.

178 Morales, A. R., Fine, G., and Horn, R. C., Jr.: Rhabdomyosarcoma: an ultrastructural appraisal, Pathol. Annu. **7:**81-106, 1972.

179 Nelson, A. J., III: Embryonal rhabdomyosarcoma; report of 24 cases and study of the effectiveness of radiation therapy upon the primary tumor, Cancer **22:**64-68, 1968.

180 Pratt, C. B., Hustu, H. O., Fleming, I. D., and Pinkel, D.: Coordinated treatment of childhood rhabdomyosarcoma with surgery, radiotherapy, and combination chemotherapy, Cancer Res. **32:**606-610, 1972.

181 Riopelle, J. L., and Thériault, J. P.: Sur une forme méconnue de sarcome des parties molles; le rhabdomyosarcome alvéolaire, Ann. Anat. Pathol. (Paris) **1:**88-111, 1956.

182 Soule, E. H., Geitz, M., and Henderson, E. D.: Embryonal rhabdomyosarcoma of the limbs and limb-girdles; a clinicopathologic study of 61 cases, Cancer **23:**1336-1346, 1969.

183 Stobbe, G. D., and Dargeon, H. W.: Embryonal rhabdomyosarcoma of head and neck in children and adolescents, Cancer **3:**826-836, 1950.

184 Stout, A. P.: Rhabdomyosarcoma of the skeletal muscles, Ann. Surg. **123:**447-472, 1946 (extensive bibliography).

185 Suit, H. D., Russell, W. O., and Martin, R. G.: Management of patients with sarcoma of soft tissue in an extremity, Cancer **31:**1247-1255, 1973.

Tumors of synovial tissue
Synovial sarcoma

186 Batsakis, J. G., Nishiyama, R. H., and Sullinger, G. D.: Synovial sarcomas of the neck, Arch. Otolaryngol. **85:**327-331, 1967.

187 Crocker, E. W., and Stout, A. P.: Synovial sarcoma in children, Cancer **12:**1123-1133, 1959.

188 Enzinger, F. M.: Recent trends in soft tissue pathology. In Tumors of bone and soft tissue, Houston, 1963, M. D. Anderson Hosp., pp. 315-332.

189 Gabbiani, G., Kaye, G. I., Lattes, R., and Majno, G.: Synovial sarcoma; electron microscopic study of a typical case, Cancer **28:**1031-1039, 1971.

190 Haagensen, C. D., and Stout, A. P.: Synovial sarcoma, Ann. Surg. **120:**826-842, 1944.

191 Mackenzie, D. H.: Synovial sarcoma; a review of 58 cases, Cancer **19:**169-180, 1966.

192 van Andel, J. G.: Synovial sarcoma; a re-

view and analysis of treated cases, Radiol. Clin. Biol. **41**:145-159, 1972.

Tumors of pluripotential mesenchyme
Mesenchymoma

193 Nash, A., and Stout, A. P.: Malignant mesenchymomas in children, Cancer **14**:524-533, 1961.
194 Stout, A. P.: Mesenchymoma, the mixed tumor of mesenchymal derivatives, Ann. Surg. **127**:278-290, 1948.

Tumors of metaplastic mesenchyme

195 Allan, C. J., and Soule, E. H.: Osteogenic sarcoma of the somatic soft tissues; clinicopathologic study of 26 cases and review of literature, Cancer **27**:1121-1133, 1971.
196 Enzinger, F. M., and Shiraki, M.: Extraskeletal myxoid chondrosarcoma; an analysis of 34 cases, Hum. Pathol. **3**:421-435, 1972.
197 Fine, G., and Stout, A. P.: Osteogenic sarcoma of the extraskeletal soft tissues, Cancer **9**:1027-1043, 1956.
198 Goldenberg, R. R., Cohen, P., and Steinlauf, P.: Chondrosarcoma of extraskeletal soft tissues: report of 7 cases and review of literature, J. Bone Joint Surg. [Am.] **49**:1487-1507, 1967.
199 Lichtenstein, L., and Goldman, R. L.: Cartilage tumors in soft tissues, particularly in the hand and foot, Cancer **17**:1203-1208, 1964.
200 Stout, A. P., and Verner, E. W.: Chondrosarcoma of the extraskeletal soft tissues, Cancer **6**:581-590, 1953.

Tumors of probable extragonadal germ cell origin

201 Berry, C. L., Keeling, J., and Hilton, C.: Teratomata in infancy and childhood: a review of 91 cases, J. Pathol. **98**:241-252, 1969.
202 Chretien, P. B., Milam, J. D., Foote, F. W., and Miller, T. R.: Embryonal adenocarcinomas (a type of malignant teratoma) of the sacrococcygeal region; clinical and pathologic aspects of 21 cases, Cancer **26**:522-535, 1970.
203 Conklin, J., and Abell, M. R.: Germ cell neoplasms of sacrococcygeal region, Cancer **20**:2105-2117, 1967.
204 Dehner, L. P.: Intrarenal teratoma occurring in infancy; report of a case with discussion of extragonadal germ cell tumors in infancy, J. Pediatr. Surg. **8**:369-378, 1973.
205 Donnellan, W. A., and Swenson, O.: Benign and malignant sacrococcygeal teratomas, Surgery **64**:834-846, 1968.
206 Willis, R. A.: Pathology of tumors, ed. 4, London, 1968, Butterworth & Co., Ltd.

Tumors of neurogenic origin

207 Anderson, M. S.: Myxopapillary ependymomas presenting in the soft tissue over the sacrococcygeal region, Cancer **19**:585-590, 1966.
208 Bain, G. O., and Shnitka, T. K.: Cutaneous meningioma (psammoma), Arch. Dermatol. **74**:590-594, 1956.
209 Borello, E. D., and Gorlin, R. J.: Melanotic neuroectodermal tumor of infancy—a neoplasm of neural crest origin; report of a case associated with high urinary excretion of vanilmandelic acid, Cancer **19**:196-206, 1966.
210 Clarke, B. E., and Parsons, H.: An embryological tumor of retinal anlage involving the skull, Cancer **4**:78-85, 1951.
211 Koudstaal, J., Oldhoff, J., Panders, A. K., and Hardonk, M. J.: Melanotic neuroectodermal tumor of infancy, Cancer **22**:151-161, 1968.
212 Neustein, H. B.: Fine structure of a melanotic progonoma or retinal anlage tumor of the anterior fontanel, Exp. Mol. Pathol. **6**:131-142, 1967.
212a Condon, W. B., Safarik, L. R., and Elzi, E. P.: Extramedullary hematopoiesis simulating intrathoracic tumor, Arch. Surg. **90**:643-648, 1965.

Tumors of uncertain origin

213 Al-Sarraf, M., Loud, A. V., and Vaitkevicius, V. K.: Malignant granular cell tumor; histochemical and electron microscopic study, Arch. Pathol. **91**:550-558, 1971.
214 Angervall, L., and Stener, B.: Clear-cell sarcoma of tendons; a study of 4 cases, Acta Pathol. Microbiol. Scand. **77**:589-597, 1969.
215 Bliss, B. O., and Reed, R. J.: Large cell sarcomas of tendon sheath; malignant giant cell tumors of tendon sheath, Am. J. Clin. Pathol. **49**:776-781, 1968.
216 Budzilovich, G. N.: Granular cell "myoblastoma" of vagus nerve, Acta Neuropathol. **10**:162-169, 1968.
217 Christ, M. L., and Ozzello, L.: Myogenous origin of a granular cell tumor of the urinary bladder, Am. J. Clin. Pathol. **56**:736-749, 1971.
218 Enzinger, F. M.: Intramuscular myxoma, Am. J. Clin. Pathol. **43**:104-113, 1965.
219 Enzinger, F. M.: Clear-cell sarcoma of tendons and aponeuroses; an analysis of 21 cases, Cancer **18**:1163-1174, 1965.
220 Enzinger, F. M.: Fibrous hamartoma of infancy, Cancer **18**:241-248, 1965.
221 Enzinger, F. M.: Histologic typing of soft tissue tumours, International histologic classification of tumours, No. 3, Geneva, 1969, World Health Organization.
222 Enzinger, F. M.: Epithelioid sarcoma; a sar-

coma simulating a granuloma or a carcinoma, Cancer 26:1029, 1041, 1970.

223 Fisher, E. R., and Horvat, B.: The fibrocytic derivation of the so-called epithelioid sarcoma, Cancer 30:1074-1081, 1970.

224 Fisher, E. R., and Reidbord, H.: Electron microscopic evidence suggesting the myogenous derivation of the so-called alveolar soft part sarcoma, Cancer 27:150-159, 1971.

225 Fisher, E. R., and Wechsler, H.: Granular cell myoblastoma—a misnomer; electron microscopic and histochemical evidence concerning its schwann cell derivation and nature (granular cell schwannoma), Cancer 15:936-957, 1962.

226 Gabbiani, G., Fu, Y.-S., Kaye, G. I., Lattes, R., and Majno, G.: Epithelioid sarcoma; a light and electron microscopic study suggesting a synovial origin, Cancer 30:486-499, 1972.

227 Garancis, J. C., Komorowski, R. A., and Kuzma, J. F.: Granular cell myoblastoma, Cancer 25:542-550, 1970.

228 Guccion, J. G., and Enzinger, F. M.: Malignant giant cell tumor of soft parts; an analysis of 32 cases, Cancer 29:1518-1529, 1972.

229 Johnson, W. C., and Helwig, E. B.: Cutaneous focal mucinosis; a clinicopathological and histochemical study, Arch. Dermatol. 93: 13-20, 1966.

230 Lieberman, P. H., Foote, F. W., Stewart, F. W., and Berg, J. W.: Alveolar soft-part sarcoma, J.A.M.A. 198:1047-1051, 1966.

231 Moscovic, E. A., and Azar, H. A.: Multiple granular cell tumors ("myoblastomas"); case report with electron microscopic observations and review of the literature, Cancer 20:2032-2047, 1967.

232 Navarrete, A. R., and Smith, M.: Ultrastructure of granular cell ameloblastoma, Cancer 27:948-955, 1971.

232a Salm, R., and Sissons, H. A.: Giant-cell tumours of soft tissues, J. Pathol. 107:27-39, 1972.

233 Santiago, H., Feinerman, L. K., and Lattes, R.: Epithelioid sarcoma; a clinical and pathologic study of nine cases, Hum. Pathol. 3: 133-147, 1972.

234 Shipkey, I. H., Lieberman, P. H., Foote, F. W., Jr., and Stewart, F. W.: Ultrastructure of alveolar soft part sarcoma, Cancer 17: 821-830, 1964.

235 Sobel, H. J., Marquet, E., and Schwarz, R.: Granular degeneration of appendiceal smooth muscle, Arch. Pathol. 92:427-432, 1971.

236 Soule, E. H., and Enriquez, P.: Atypical fibrous histiocytoma, malignant fibrous histiocytoma, malignant histiocytoma and epithelioid sarcoma; a comparative study of 65 tumors, Cancer 30:128-143, 1972.

237 Stout, A. P.: Myxoma, the tumor of primitive mesenchyme, Ann. Surg. 127:706-719, 1948.

238 Strong, E. W., McDivitt, R. W., and Brasfield, R. D.: Granular cell myoblastoma, Cancer 25:415-422, 1970.

239 Vance, S. F., III, and Hudson, R. P.: Granular cell myoblastoma; clinicopathologic study of 42 patients, Am. J. Clin. Pathol. 52:208-211, 1969.

240 Wirth, W. A., Leavitt, D., and Enzinger, F. M.: Multiple intramuscular myxomas; another extraskeletal manifestation of fibrous dysplasia, Cancer 27:1167-1173, 1971.

Other tumorlike conditions

241 Enzinger, F. M., and Dulcey, F.: Proliferative myositis; report of 33 cases, Cancer 20: 2213-2223, 1967.

242 Fraga, S., Helwig, E. B., and Rosen, S. M.: Bronchogenic cysts in the skin and subcutaneous tissue, Am. J. Clin. Pathol. 56: 230-238, 1971.

243 Harkess, J. W., and Peters, H. J.: Tumoral calcinosis, a report of six cases, J. Bone Joint Surg. [Am.] 49:721-731, 1967.

244 Kern, W. H.: Proliferative myositis; a pseudosarcomatous reaction to injury, Arch. Pathol. 69:209-216, 1960.

24 Peritoneum, omentum, mesentery, and retroperitoneum

PERITONEUM

Inflammation

Chemical peritonitis can be caused by bile, pancreatic juice, gastric juice, and barium sulfate.[23] The peritonitis associated with the intraperitoneal extravasation of barium primarily is the result of the bacteria accompanying it. Barium peritonitis practically always follows perforation of the colon during examination of the obstructed bowel.[38]

Extravasation following injury or disease of the gallbladder, bile ducts, or duodenum causes acute or subacute peritonitis initially in the upper quadrant of the abdomen.[8] Gastric juice produces a severe peritoneal reaction because of its hydrochloric acid content, although it may be bacteriologically sterile. The release of pancreatic juice causes fat necrosis. The formation of calcium salts in large areas of fat necrosis may cause hypocalcemia.

Bacterial peritonitis may be either primary or secondary. The primary form usually is caused by streptococci or pneumococci. Aspiration of intra-abdominal fluid discloses an inflammatory exudate containing only a single type of organism. Large amounts of extracellular fluid are lost into the exudate and edema associated with generalized peritonitis. The losses may be equivalent to those of a burn covering one-half to three-fourths of the cutaneous surface.[10]

Perforation of a viscus such as a colon produces secondary peritonitis. If the fluid is aspirated, a mixture of bacterial flora rather than a single organism is found. Tuberculous and actinomycotic peritonitis may occur with few constitutional symptoms, despite extensive involvement of the peritoneum.[15, 19, 41] In a review of forty-seven patients with tuberculous peritonitis, Singh et al.[39] found roentgenographic evidence of pulmonary parenchymal lesions in only 6% of the cases. Search for acid-fast organisms on a direct smear of ascitic fluid is often unrewarding. The best diagnostic methods are culture of the fluid and percutaneous biopsy of the peritoneum.[26, 27] Singh et al.[39] found the latter useful in 64% of their cases. These specific infections are in contrast to primary streptococcal peritonitis, which produces maximal constitutional symptoms with minimal gross findings.

Pseudocysts of the peritoneal cavity may be associated with some inflammatory process such as ulcerative colitis or may follow appendectomy complicated by abscess. The large multilocular cysts have a fibrous tissue wall and are lined by meso-thelium.

Adhesions

Adhesions, with the possibility of sub-sequent intestinal obstruction, complicate all intra-abdominal operations. They can be minimized by careful handling of tis-sues, reperitonealization where feasible, and removal of intraperitoneal blood clots. Ryan et al.[35] showed in an experimental model that drying of the serosa plus bleed-ing consistently resulted in the formation of adhesions.

Innumerable agents of every description (sodium citrate, heparin, olive oil, liquid paraffin, ACTH, cortisone, pepsin, fibri-nolysin, and amniotic fluid) have been used to prevent adhesions, but none has accom-plished this goal. Adhesions become col-lagenous and strong as the cellularity of their fibrous tissue decreases with matura-tion. Postoperative adhesions are the most frequent cause of intestinal obstruction today.

Reaction to talc and other foreign substances

The peritoneum reacts to all foreign substances. A great deal has been written about "talcum powder granuloma" of the peritoneum. This foreign body lesion fol-lows the spillage of talc into the peri-toneal cavity at operation. The use of talc on surgical gloves is presently recognized as a hazard and has been abandoned.[11] Talc (hydrated magnesium silicate) causes nodules to form on the peritoneum. These nodules are firm and may be mistaken for tuberculosis or metastatic cancer. Micro-scopic examination shows crystals in the tissue which are often better visualized by lowering the condenser of the microscope. They are best seen by polarized light[14] (Fig. 1148).

Intraperitoneal granulomas incident to the modified starch now used on surgical gloves occur less frequently than do talc granulomas.[18, 37] These can be identified by the presence of granules that are PAS

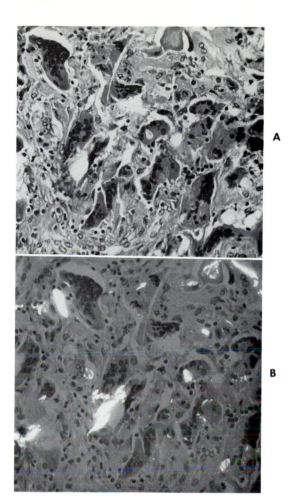

Fig. 1148 Histologic appearance of talc gran-uloma without, **A,** and with, **B,** polarized light. With latter, talc crystals can be seen vividly. (Moderate enlargement; **A,** WU neg. 47-1049; **B,** WU neg. 47-1050.)

positive and birefringent (with a Maltese cross pattern) within the cytoplasm of histiocytes and foreign body giant cells.[7, 9]

Mineral oil or paraffin placed in the peritoneal cavity to prevent adhesions may cause nodules that may be mistaken for metastatic carcinoma.[30] Frozen section of these nodules is sufficient to make the diag-nosis. It will show foreign body giant cells, chronic inflammation, and macrophages. Similar changes follow rupture of a cystic teratoma of the ovary, in which large amounts of oily material cause a profound nodular peritoneal reaction.[2]

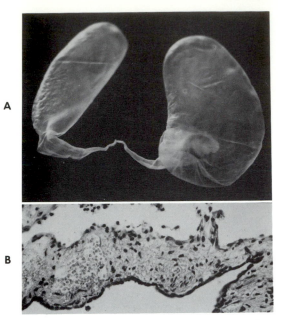

Fig. 1149 A, Thin-walled cyst containing clear fluid found free within abdominal cavity. **B,** Microscopically, it has fibrous wall and lining of flat mesothelial cells. (**A** and **B,** Courtesy Dr. E. F. Lascano, Buenos Aires, Argentina.)

Cysts

Lascano et al.[25] described five cases of cysts lying loose within the abdominal cavity. They varied in diameter from 1.5 cm to 6 cm and were lined by one or several layers of mesothelial cells (Fig. 1149).

Tumors
Primary tumors

The peritoneum has a great capacity to undergo metaplasia and form papillary projections, pseudoacini, squamous nests,[9] and even cartilaginous nodules (Fig. 1150). Cirrhosis with ascites is often associated with marked mesothelial proliferation (Fig. 1151).

In females, there is a layer of tissue sensitive to sex hormones situated underneath the peritoneal mesothelium which seems to be related to endometrial stroma.[33] It is more prominent in the pelvic parietal peritoneum and on the bladder dome. Although rather inconspicuous under normal conditions, it is probably responsible for the occurrence of ectopic decidual reaction and the exceptional cases of endometrial stromal sarcoma and mixed mesodermal tumor that have been found outside the genital system. In conjunction with the neighboring mesothelium, it may give rise to endometriosis and endosalpingiosis.[4]

Peritoneal mesotheliomas are very rare. Their very existence has been denied with the claim that they represent metastases from other neoplasms. Although we agree that sometimes metastatic tumors in the peritoneum, particularly those arising in the ovary, may be a source of confusion, we are convinced that true mesotheliomas exists. Most examples occur in patients more than 35 years of age, although they may appear at any age, including in childhood.[22] The frequency of mesothelioma has been on the increase, presumably as a result of asbestos exposure.[32, 40]

The types of mesothelioma seen in the peritoneum are similar to those of the pleura (Chapter 6), but the relative proportions vary a great deal. For example, the pure fibrous type, which is relatively common in the pleural space, constitutes only a minority of the peritoneal neoplasms.[17, 42] The large majority of the peritoneal mesotheliomas are of the papillary (tubular) or mixed type, and most of them are either *solitary and benign* or *diffuse and malignant*. A diffuse benign form and a solitary malignant form have been described, but these are curiosities. In a series of 114 peritoneal mesotheliomas reviewed by Stout,[43] there were twenty-five of the fibrous type, thirty-eight of the papillary benign solitary type, and thirty-six of the papillary diffuse malignant variety.

The fibrous type of mesothelioma presents the same bewildering microscopic picture as it does in the pleural cavity[42] (Chapter 6). The evidence of mesothelial origin is based on tissue culture studies rather than on the microscopic pattern.[36]

The solitary benign form of papillary mesothelioma presents as a small papillary structure resembling grossly and microscopically the appearance of choroid

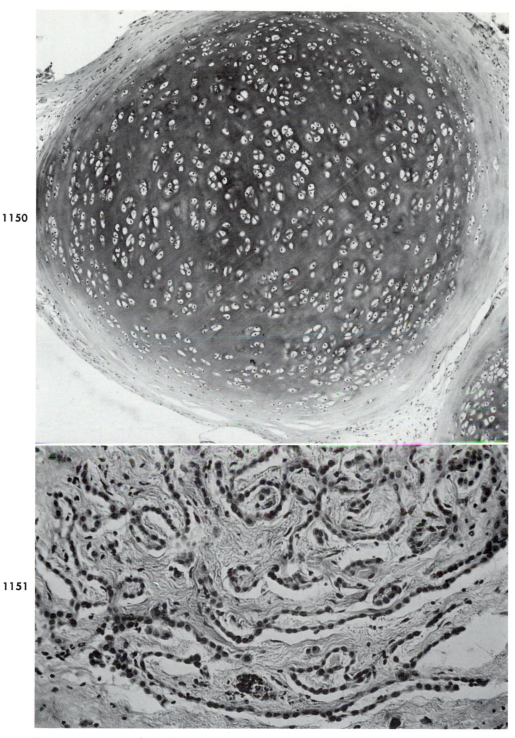

Fig. 1150 Peritoneal cartilaginous metaplasia. (Low power; WU neg. 62-90; slide contributed by Dr. J. Bauer, St. Louis, Mo.)

Fig. 1151 Localized area of proliferation of peritoneal mesothelium. These changes were associated with chronic inflammation. Note overproduction of fibrous tissue and pseudo-acini. (×240; WU neg. 52-4549.)

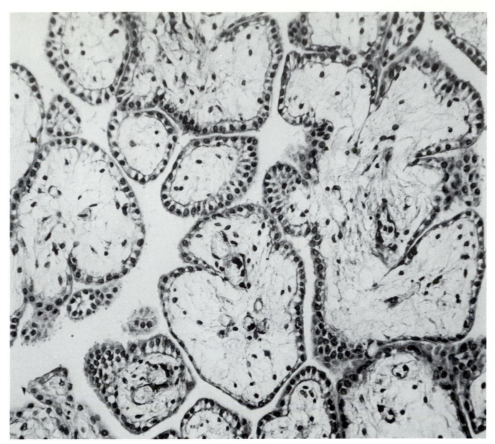

Fig. 1152 Benign papillary mesothelioma occurring in 41-year-old man. Lesion had been present for at least three years. (Low power; WU neg. 62-88; slide contributed by Dr. M. J. Zbar, Miami, Fla.)

plexus[45] (Fig. 1152). The diffuse malignant variety appears as multiple plaques or nodules scattered over the visceral and parietal peritoneum. It may be accompanied by dense intraperitoneal adhesions with shortening of the mesentery (Fig. 1153, A). Complete obliteration of the peritoneal cavity may actually develop. In advanced stages, the tumor may locally invade the intestinal wall, the hilum of the spleen and liver, and the gastric wall. However, distant metastases are unusual.[1, 46]

The microscopic pattern is highly variable. The most typical arrangement is that of papillae or tubules lined by atypical mesothelial cells, the former having vascularized fibrous cores (Fig. 1153, B). In other instances, the mesothelial-like cells alternate with a cellular spindle cell stroma in the manner of a synovial sarcoma. The individual cells are, in general, fairly uniform, with acidophilic or vacuolated cytoplasm and large vesicular nucleus.[3] Mitoses are often difficult to find. Intracellular and extracellular "mucin" can be present. This seems to represent acid mucopolysaccharides, since it stains with colloidal iron and Alcian blue, is removed at least partially by hyaluronidase digestion, and tends to be PAS negative.[12]

Pleural and peritoneal mesotheliomas may coexist. Hypoglycemia is occasionally encountered in association with extensive mesotheliomas and is often relieved by the removal of the tumor.[29]

Metastatic tumors

All types of metastatic tumors involve the peritoneal cavity. Their gross patterns vary from single, well-defined nodules to

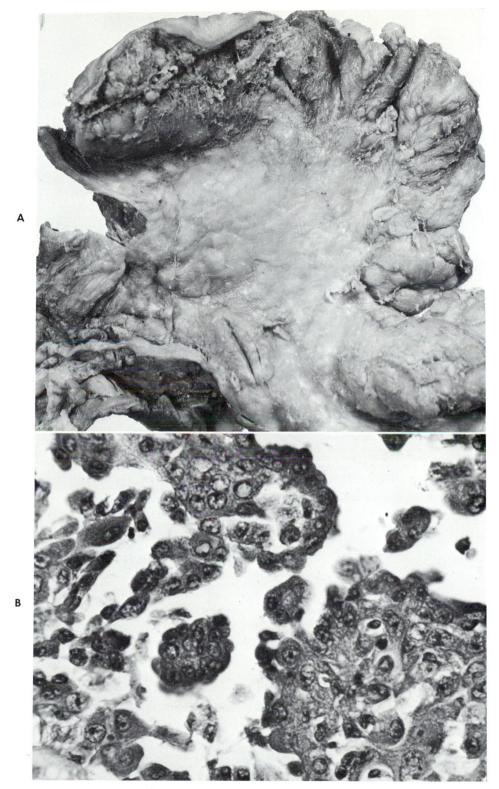

Fig. 1153 A, Malignant mesothelioma that diffusely involved peritoneal cavity. Fibrosis and shortening of mesentery are prominent. **B,** Same lesion shown in **A.** Papillary projections are prominent. (**A,** WU neg. 49-1666; **B,** ×600; WU neg. 49-1793.)

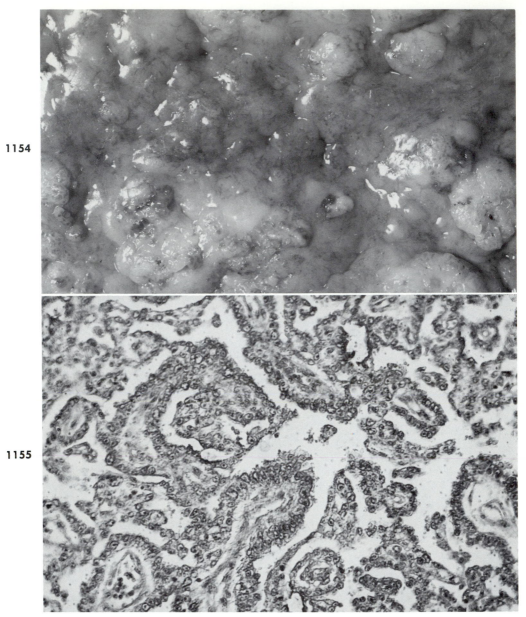

Fig. 1154 Diffuse involvement of peritoneum by metastatic squamous carcinoma simulating primary malignant peritoneal tumor. (WU neg. 52-383.)
Fig. 1155 Metastatic ovarian cancer of papillary serous type closely resembling primary malignant peritoneal tumor. (×240; AFIP 314863.)

diffuse lymphatic permeation. Variations in consistency depend upon their cellularity, amount of fibrous tissue, and mucin content. Metastatic carcinoma may simulate very closely primary malignant mesothelioma. We have observed this grossly with metastatic squamous carcinoma (Fig. 1154) and microscopically with papillary tumors of the ovary (Fig. 1155).

Pseudomyxoma peritonei is a form of peritoneal carcinomatosis in which the peritoneal cavity contains large amounts of mucinous material.[28] The primary tumor is usually a mucinous cystadenocarcinoma of

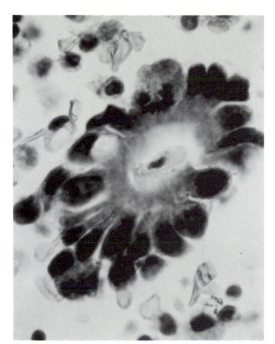

Fig. 1156 Easily identified metastatic malignant tumor. Note large, dense nuclei and atypical mitotic figure in acinus. (×900; WU neg. 52-1617.)

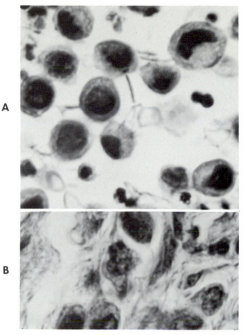

Fig. 1157 **A,** Ascitic fluid sediment with numerous tumor cells identified by their dense, large, atypical appearance. **B,** Same tumor shown in **A,** which was primary in stomach. (**A,** ×900; WU neg. 52-1621; **B,** ×900; WU neg. 52-1622.)

the ovary, rarely of the appendix. Microscopically, large pools of mucus are seen accompanied by hyperemic vessels and chronic inflammatory cells. *Viable epithelial glandular cells must be identified within the mucus in order to diagnose this condition.* Mucinous cystadenomas of the ovary and appendix can rupture and pour their content into the peritoneal cavity. The resulting condition, which is self-limited and microscopically lacks tumor cells, should not be designated as pseudomyxoma peritonei.[6, 16]

Cytology
Michael Kyriakos, M.D.

The report of a positive cytology in an effusion has great prognostic and therapeutic significance. A false positive diagnosis may delay therapy for a potentially remedial situation. For this reason, we are conservative in our interpretation of effusions, requiring the presence of cell clusters or fragments before rendering a diagnosis of carcinoma (Figs. 1156 and 1157). Only in cases of lymphoma do we base our positive diagnoses on the findings of isolated malignant-appearing cells. When sufficient material is available, we routinely use smears from the centrifuged specimen, in addition to membrane filter preparations and cell blocks. Clinicians somehow feel insecure unless the results are based on a cell block preparation. This insecurity is unfounded. We have seen cases in which the smear preparation was positive and the cell block negative or equivocal. A smear preparation contains fewer artifacts and usually gives better nuclear detail. The finding of tumor cells in the smear preparation means the patient has a malignancy regardless of what the cell block shows. We have, of course, had cases in which the smear was negative and the cell block positive. Although this is unusual, we still do the cell block, but only if enough material is available.

A negative cytology report does not exclude the presence of cancer in an effusion. In 207 patients with malignant effusion, the cytology was positive in 153 (74%), whereas in 162 patients with nonmalignant effusions, there was one false positive report (0.7%).[34] Cardozo[5] was able to diagnose 67% of malignant pleural effusions and 75% of malignant ascitic effusions, with a false positive rate of 0.1%.

Patients with effusions due to lymphomas and leukemias yield positive cytology in about 55% to 60% of the cases, with histiocytic lymphomas most likely to yield positive results (75%) and Hodgkin's disease least likely (25%).[31, 34] At Barnes Hospital, patients with positive effusion due to carcinoma had an average survival of 3.3 months, whereas the average for those with positive effusion due to lymphoma was 2 months. No patient with carcinoma of the lung and positive pleural cytology survived for more than one year. All patients who survived for longer than one year had either breast or ovarian carcinoma. These patients also had the longest average survival.[24]

The most common metastatic tumors to cause pleural effusions are lung and breast carcinomas and malignant lymphomas. In ascitic fluids, carcinomas of the ovary are the most commonly encountered.[5, 20, 24]

False positive diagnoses have been most commonly caused by hepatic cirrhosis, congestive heart failure, tuberculosis, and pulmonary infarction.[13] Such false positive diagnoses may be made because the mesothelial cells may form pseudoacini that closely resemble adenocarcinoma[44] (Fig. 1158). Furthermore, normal mitotic figures are frequent. Mesothelial cells also may have multiple nuclei and may assume a signet ring appearance.[21]

OMENTUM

Hemorrhagic infarct of the omentum may be due to torsion or strangulation in a hernia sac. Epstein and Lempke[47] reviewed the eighty-eight reported cases of primary idiopathic segmental infarction of the greater omentum, an acute abdominal lesion usually mistaken clinically for acute appendicitis or cholecystitis. Characteristically, the infarcted segment of omentum is on the right side adherent to the cecum, ascending colon, and anterior parietal peritoneum.

Stout et al.[48] examined twenty-four solid *tumors* of the great omentum. *Leiomyomas* predominated among the benign neoplasms and *leiomyosarcoma* was the most common malignant tumor.

MESENTERY

Mesenteric panniculitis, also called isolated lipodystrophy of the mesentery, is a rare condition grossly appearing as a multinodular thickening of the mesentery of the small bowel. Microscopically, there is an infiltration by inflammatory cells and foamy macrophages, the latter representing a reaction to fat necrosis.[50, 51] The differential diagnosis should include Weber-Christian disease and Whipple's disease.

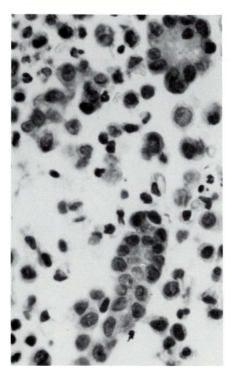

Fig. 1158 Pseudoacini in peritoneal fluid that easily can be mistaken for metastatic carcinoma. (×600; WU neg. 48-4070.)

A probably related condition is *retractile mesenteritis,* in which the inflammation and fibrosis lead to retraction, formation of adhesions, and distortion of the intestinal loops. Mesentery from both small and large bowel can be involved.[52]

Mesenteric cysts are usually incidental findings, but they may be large enough to produce symptoms. They are round and smooth, with a thin wall lined by a layer of flattened or low cuboidal cells of probably mesothelial origin.[49]

Yannopoulos and Stout[53] studied forty-four primary solid *tumors* of the mesentery. The majority were benign. There were twelve cases of fibromatosis, seven tumors of smooth muscle origin, six tumors of adipose tissue origin, six "xanthogranulomas," five vascular neoplasms, three neurofibromas, and five miscellaneous tumors.

RETROPERITONEUM

The retroperitoneal space is that indefinite area in the lumbar and iliac region which lies between the peritoneum and the posterior wall of the abdominal cavity. It extends from the twelfth rib and vertebra to the base of the sacrum and the iliac crest. The lateral margins correspond to the lateral borders of the quadratus lumbora muscles. The space contains the loose areolar tissue through which pass the inferior vena cava, aorta, ureters, renal vessels, and gonadal vessels. It contains numerous lymph nodes.

This potentially large space allows both primary and metastatic tumors to grow silently before clinical signs and symptoms appear. Symptoms are related to displacement of organs and obstructive phenomena. Objective evidence of retroperitoneal masses can best be demonstrated by retrograde pyelograms, angiography, and radiographic study of the gastrointestinal tract[84] (Fig. 1159).

Nonneoplastic conditions

Inflammatory processes from the kidney or the pancreas may form a retroperitoneal mass. We have seen perforation of the

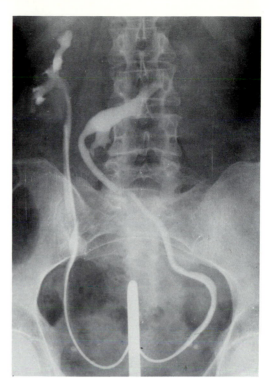

Fig. 1159 Extreme displacement of kidney and ureter in patient with large retroperitoneal tumor. (WU neg. 49-2913.)

biliary system with formation of a bile-containing cystic mass.[59] *Infection* from a tuberculosis vertebra may form a retroperitoneal cold abscess. Massive retroperitoneal *hemorrhage* in the adult is most often the result of a ruptured aortic aneurysm.[73] Less commonly, it is of adrenal origin. Lawson et al.[72] reviewed ten cases of the latter phenomenon. In five instances the adrenal gland was the site of a pheochromocytoma, but in the other five there was no demonstrable abnormality.

We have seen a few instances of benign retroperitoneal *cysts* not connected with the adrenal gland. Their inner lining was compatible with either a mesothelial or mesonephric origin.

Idiopathic retroperitoneal fibrosis (Ormond's disease) is a rare disease of obscure etiology that results in progressive renal failure by producing constriction and final obliteration of the ureters. Grossly, an ill-defined fibrous mass occupies the retroperitoneal midline, encircles the lower abdominal aorta, and displaces the ureters *medially.* The latter feature is of value to the radiologist in the differential diagnosis, since most retroperitoneal neoplasms displace the ureter laterally. Microscopically, a prominent inflammatory infiltrate composed of lymphocytes, plasma cells, and eosinophils, often containing germinal centers, is seen accompanied by foci of fat necrosis, fibroblastic proliferation, and collagen deposition.[77] The wall of veins is often involved by the inflammation.[67] Mitchinson[77] also found aortic involvement in three of his cases.

Idiopathic retroperitoneal fibrosis may be associated with a similar process in the mediastinum, sclerosing cholangitis, Riedel's thyroiditis, pseudotumor of the orbit, or generalized vasculitis.[58, 66] Several cases have been reported secondary to the administration of methysergide and other drugs.[64] The available evidence strongly suggests that Ormond's disease represents an immunologic hypersensitivity disorder. Occasionally, the clinical and pathologic features of idiopathic retroperitoneal fibrosis can be simulated by malignant neoplasms accompanied by chronic inflammation and fibrosis, notably malignant lymphoma and signet ring cell carcinoma of the stomach.[68, 71]

Tumors
Primary tumors

Primary tumors of the retroperitoneal area are relatively rare. They are of many types.[62, 74, 76, 80] Strickly speaking, neoplasms arising in the kidney, adrenal gland, and periaortic lymph nodes qualify in the category and are actually the commonest. However, the designation of retroperitoneal tumors has been traditionally reserved for tumors of this area arising outside these structures. Most of them have been already discussed elsewhere, particularly in Chapter 23. Here, only the peculiarities of these neoplasms when they occur in this region

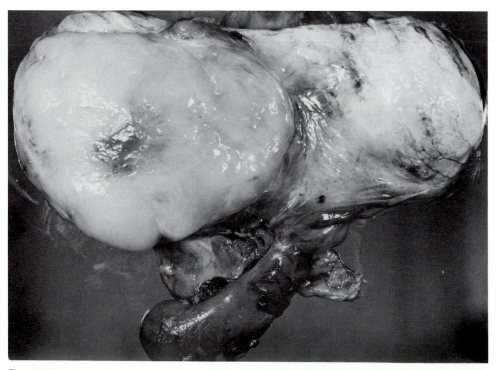

Fig. 1160 Large slimy retroperitoneal liposarcoma growing in region of kidney. (WU neg. 50-5055.)

will be described. Symptoms secondary to retroperitoneal neoplasms are vague and appear late in the course of the disease. The radiologic methods of evaluation include barium studies, intravenous pyelography, inferior vena cavography, and arteriography.[57]

Liposarcoma is the most frequent retroperitoneal sarcoma. It is particularly prone to grow in the perirenal region (Fig. 1160).

At the time of excision, it is usually extremely large.

Lipoma is less common than its malignant counterpart. As the latter, it is usually very large at the time of diagnosis. It can be multiple. We have seen one such case, in which the first symptom was a mass below the inguinal ligament. Many cases reported in the literature as retroperitoneal lipomas are actually liposarcomas, particu-

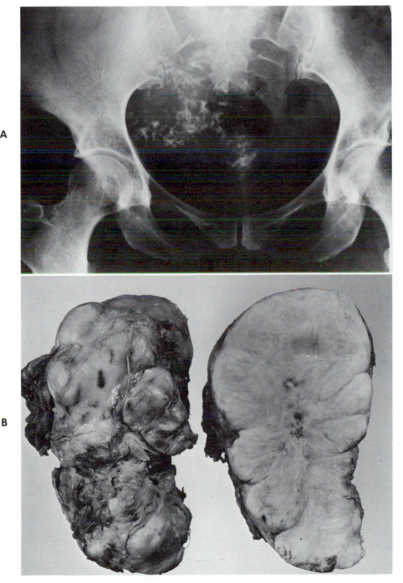

Fig. 1161   A, Partially calcified retroperitoneal malignant schwannoma. **B,** Same lesion shown in **A.** It was firm and grayish white and directly invaded vertebra, metastasized distantly, and caused death. (**A,** WU neg. 49-4366; **B,** WU neg. 49-4223.)

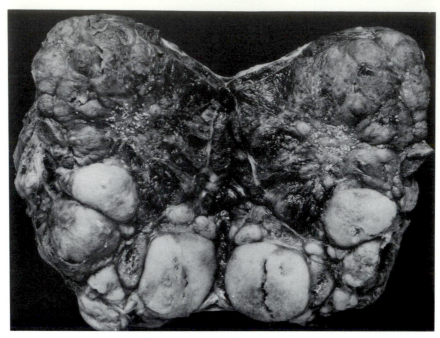

Fig. 1162 Hemorrhagic nodular ganglioneuroblastoma. (Courtesy Dr. M. Dockerty, Rochester, Minn.)

larly those in which a malignant transformation is said to have occurred.[82]

Leiomyosarcoma is the second most common sarcoma in this area.[63] This tumor has a particular tendency to undergo massive cystic degeneration when occurring in this region.[75] Of the thirteen cases reviewed by Kay and McNeill,[70] there was only one long-term survivor.

Leiomyoma is exceptionally rare as a primary neoplasm, although on occasion a uterine tumor may extend into the retroperitoneal space.

Rhabdomyosarcoma is practically always of the embryonal type and limited to infants and children. The prognosis is extremely poor.

Fibromatosis may occur, sometimes in association with mediastinal involvement. In contrast to idiopathic retroperitoneal fibrosis, it lacks a prominent inflammatory component.

Fibrosarcoma is one of the rarest retroperitoneal tumors in our experience. We believe that most cases so designated in the literature are actually liposarcomas, leiomyosarcomas, or fibrous histiocytomas.[55, 83]

Fibrous histiocytoma, on the other hand, is relatively frequent. The benign variant has often been designated as xanthogranuloma.[78] The malignant type has almost always a pleomorphic appearance on microscopic examination (fibroxanthosarcoma).[69]

Vascular tumors of several types have been described, including hemangioma, hemangiopericytoma, lymphangioma, lymphangiomyoma, and angiosarcoma.[61]

Neurogenic tumors are not nearly so common as in the mediastinum. We have seen neurilemomas, neurofibromas, and a single case of malignant schwannoma that invaded the bone and metastasized distantly (Fig. 1161).

Tumors of sympathetic nervous tissue of the type more commonly seen in the adrenal gland also can be present in the retroperitoneum outside this gland. This includes neuroblastoma, ganglioneuroblastoma, and ganglioneuroma. These lesions often are hemorrhagic, soft, and nodular (Fig. 1162).

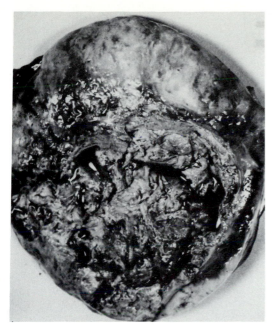

Fig. 1163 Paraganglioma arising from body of Zuckerkandl. (AFIP 270229.)

Paragangliomas arise outside the adrenal gland in approximately 10% of the cases. They may occur anywhere along the midline of the retroperitoneum, the best known location being Zuckerkandl's body[79] (Fig. 1163).

Tumors arising in *heterotopic adrenal cortex* and in *remnants of renal anlage* have been reported.[65]

Germ cell tumors are mainly represented by the *benign teratoma.*[60] This may grow large, is often cystic, and tends to occur in young children. It frequently involves the sacrococcygeal area[56] (Fig. 1164). It is often considered malignant by the surgeon because of its stubborn adherence to other structures. This fixation is of inflammatory nature, caused by reaction to extravasated material. *Malignant teratomas,* which comprise approximately one-fourth of the cases, may have the appearance of teratocarcinoma, embryonal carcinoma, or yolk sac tumor. *Seminomas* also can occur in this location. Here, even more than in the mediastinum, the possibility of a primary testicular neoplasm should be seriously investigated. However, its occurrence as a primary neoplasm in this area has been convincingly demonstrated.[54, 81]

Metastatic tumors

Secondary neoplasms may appear in the retroperitoneal space as a result of local extension or because of lymph node involvement. The former is mainly represented by pancreatic carcinoma and primary bone neoplasms, notably sacrococcygeal chordoma.

The carcinomas most commonly giving rise to retroperitoneal lymph node metastases are those originating in testis, pan-

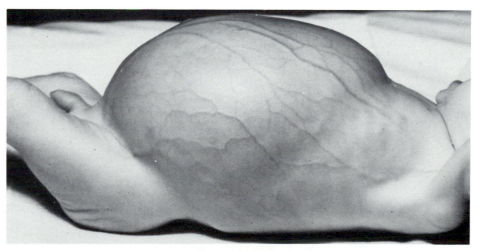

Fig. 1164 Huge benign cystic retroperitoneal teratoma in infant. Teratoma was removed successfully, and child is well. (WU neg. 52-760.)

creas, uterine cervix, endometrium, and kidney.

REFERENCES

PERITONEUM

1 Ackerman, L. V.: Tumors of the peritoneum and retroperitoneum. In Atlas of tumor pathology, Fasc. 23 and 24, Washington, D. C., 1953, Armed Forces Institute of Pathology.

2 Auer, E. A., Dockerty, M. B., and Mayo, C. W.: Ruptured dermoid cyst of the ovary simulating abdominal carcinomatosis, Mayo Clin. Proc. 26:489-497, 1951.

3 Bolio-Cicero, A., Aguirre, J., and Perez-Tamayo, R.: Malignant peritoneal mesothelioma, Am. J. Clin. Pathol. 36:417-426, 1961.

4 Burmeister, R. E., Fechner, R. E., and Franklin, R. R.: Endosalpingiosis of the peritoneum, Obst. Gynecol. 34:310-318, 1969.

5 Cardozo, P. L.: A critical evaluation of 3,000 cytologic analyses of pleural fluid, ascitic fluid and pericardial fluid, Acta Cytol. (Baltimore) 10:455-460, 1966.

6 Cariker, M., and Dockerty, M.: Mucinous cystadenomas and mucinous cystadenocarcinomas of the ovary; a clinical and pathological study of 355 cases, Cancer 7:302-310, 1954.

7 Coder, D. M., and Olander, G. A.: Granulomatous peritonitis caused by starch glove powder, Arch. Surg. 105:83-86, 1972.

8 Cope, V. Z.: Extravasation of bile, Br. J. Surg. 13:120-129, 1925.

9 Crome, L.: Squamous metaplasia of the peritoneum, J. Pathol. Bacteriol .62:61-68, 1950.

9a Davies, J. D., and Neely, J.: The histopathology of peritoneal starch granulomas, J. Pathol. 107:265-278, 1972.

10 Davis, J. H.: Current concepts of peritonitis, Am. Surg. 33:673-681, 1967.

11 Eiseman, B., Seelig, M. G., and Womack, N. A.: Talcum powder granuloma; frequent and serious postoperative complication, Ann. Surg. 126:820-832, 1947.

12 Enzinger, F. M.: Histologic typing of soft tissue tumours (Syllabus of tumors of synovial and mesothelial tissues), Geneva, 1969, World Health Organization.

13 Foot, N. C.: The identification of neoplastic cells in serous effusions, Am. J. Path. 32:961-977, 1956.

14 German, W. M.: Dusting powder granulomas following surgery, Surg. Gynecol. Obstet. 76:501-507, 1943.

15 Gonnella, J. S., and Hudson, E. K.: Clinical patterns of tuberculous peritonitis, Arch. Intern. Med. 117:164-169, 1966.

16 Higa, E., Rosai, J., Pizzimbono, C. A., and Wise, L.: Mucosal hyperplasia, mucinous cystadenoma and mucinous cystadenocarcino-

ma of appendix; a reevaluation of appendiceal "mucocele," Cancer (in press).

17 Hill, R. P.: Malignant fibrous mesothelioma of the peritoneum, Cancer 6:1182-1185, 1953.

18 Holmes, E. C., and Eggleston, J. C.: Starch granulomatous peritonitis, Surgery 71:85-90, 1972.

19 Hughes, H. J., Carr, D. T., and Geraci, J. E.: Tuberculous peritonitis: a review of 34 cases with emphasis on diagnostic aspects, Dis. Chest 38:42-50, 1960.

20 Jarvi, O. H., Kunnas, R. J., Laitio, M. T., and Tyrkko, J. E. S.: The accuracy and significance of cytologic cancer diagnosis of pleural effusions, Acta Cytol. (Baltimore) 16:152-158, 1972.

21 Johnson, W. D.: The cytological diagnosis of cancer in serous effusion, Acta Cytol. (Baltimore) 10:161-172, 1966.

22 Kauffman, S. L., and Stout, A. P.: Mesothelioma in children, Cancer 17:539-544, 1964.

23 Kay, S.: Tissue reaction to barium sulfate contrast medium: histopathologic study, Arch. Pathol. 57:279-284, 1954.

24 Konikov, N., Bleisch, V., and Piskie, V.: Prognostic significance of cytologic diagnoses of effusions, Acta Cytol. (Baltimore) 10:335-339, 1966.

25 Lascano, E. F., Villamayor, R. D., and Llauró, J. L.: Loose cysts of the peritoneal cavity, Ann. Surg. 152:836-844, 1960.

26 Levine, H.: Needle biopsy of peritoneum in exudative ascites, Arch. Int. Med. 120:542-545, 1967.

27 Levine, H.: Needle biopsy diagnosis of tuberculous peritonitis, Am. Rev. Resp. Dis. 97:889-894, 1968.

28 Long, R. T. L., Spratt, J. S., and Dowling, E.: Pseudomyxoma peritonei; new concepts in management with a report of 17 patients, Am. J. Surg. 117:162-168, 1969.

29 McPeak, C. J., and Papaioannou, A. N.: Nonpancreatic tumors associated with hypoglycemia, Arch. Surg. 93:1019-1024, 1966.

30 Marshall, S. F., and Forse, R. A.: Peritoneal adhesions: report of a case of paraffinoma, Surg. Clin. North Am. 32:903-908, 1952.

31 Melamed, M. R.: The cytological presentation of malignant lymphomas and related diseases in effusions, Cancer 16:413-431, 1963.

32 Newhouse, M. L., and Thompson, H.: Epidemiology of mesothelial tumors in the London area, Ann. N. Y. Acad. Sci. 132:579-588, 1965.

33 Ober, W. B., and Black, M. B.: Neoplasms of the subcoelomic mesenchyme, Arch. Pathol. 59:698-705, 1955.

34 Reagan, J. W.: Exfoliative cytology of pleural, peritoneal and pericardial fluids, CA 10:153-159, 1960.

35 Ryan, G. B., Grobety, J., and Majno, G.: Post-

operative peritoneal adhesions; a study of the mechanisms, Am. J. Pathol. **65**:117-140, 1971.

36 Sano, M. E., Weiss, E., and Gault, E. S.: Pleural mesothelioma, J. Thorac. Surg. **19**:783-788, 1950.

37 Saxen, L., and Saxen, E.: Starch granulomas as a problem in surgical pathology, Acta Pathol. Microbiol. Scand. **64**:55-70, 1965.

38 Seaman, W. B., and Wells, J.: Complications of the barium enema, Gastroenteology **48**:728-737, 1965.

39 Singh, M. M., Bhargava, A. N., and Jain, K. P.: Tuberculous peritonitis; an evaluation of pathogenetic mechanisms, diagnostic procedures and therapeutic measures, N. Engl. J. Med. **281**:1091-1094, 1969.

40 Smither, W. J.: Asbestos and mesothelioma of the pleura, Proc. Roy. Soc. Med. **59**:57-61, 1966.

41 Sochocky, S.: Tuberculous peritonitis; a review of 100 cases, Am. Rev. Respir. Dis. **95**:398-401, 1967.

42 Stout, A. P.: Solitary fibrous mesothelioma of the peritoneum, Cancer **3**:820-825, 1950.

43 Stout, A. P.: Discussion of case 2. Tumors of the soft tissues, Cancer Seminar of the Penrose Cancer Hospital **2**:173-177, 1960.

44 Takagi, F.: Studies on tumor cells in serous effusion, Am. J. Clin. Pathol. **24**:663-675, 1954.

45 Wells, A. H.: Papillomatous peritonei, Am. J. Pathol. **11**:1011-1014, 1935.

46 Winslow, D. J., and Taylor, H. B.: Malignant peritoneal mesotheliomas, Cancer **13**:127-136, 1960.

OMENTUM

47 Epstein, L. I., and Lempke, R. E.: Primary idiopathic segmental infarction of the greater omentum: case report and collective review of the literature, Ann. Surg. **167**:437-443, 1968.

48 Stout, A. P., Hendry, J., and Purdie, F. J.: Primary solid tumors of the great omentum, Cancer **16**:231-243, 1963.

MESENTERY

49 Barr, W. B., and Yamashita, T.: Mesenteric cysts; review of the literature and report of a case, Am. J. Gastroenterol. **41**:53-57, 1964.

50 Crane, J. T., Aguilar, M. J., and Grimes, O. R.: Isolated lipodystrophy, a form of mesenteric tumor, Am. J. Surg. **90**:169-179, 1955.

51 Ogden, W. M., Bradburn, D. M., and Rives, J. D.: Mesenteric panniculitis: review of 27 cases, Ann. Surg. **161**:864-875, 1965.

52 Tedeschi, C. G., and Botta, G. C.: Retractile mesenteritis, N. Engl. J. Med. **266**:1035-1040, 1962.

53 Yannopoulos, K., and Stout, A. P.: Primary solid tumors of the mesentery, Cancer **16**:914-927, 1963.

RETROPERITONEUM

54 Abell, M. R., Fayos, J. V., and Lampe, I.: Retroperitoneal germinomas (seminomas) without evidence of testicular involvement, Cancer **18**:273-290, 1965.

55 Ackerman, L. V.: Tumors of the peritoneum and retroperitoneum. In Atlas of tumor pathology, Fasc. 23 and 24, Washington, D. C., 1953, Armed Forces Institute of Pathology.

56 Arnheim, E. E.: Retroperitoneal teratomas in infancy and childhood, Pediatrics **8**:309-327, 1951 (excellent bibliography).

57 Bron, K. M., and Sherman, L.: Arteriography in evaluating retroperitoneal mass lesions, N. Y. State J. Med. **67**:1875-1888, 1967.

58 Comings, D. E., Skubi, K. B., van Eyes, J., and Motulsky, A. G.: Familial multifocal fibrosclerosis; findings suggesting that retroperitoneal fibrosis, mediastinal fibrosis, sclerosing cholangitis, Riedel's thyroiditis, and pseudo-tumor of the orbit may be different manifestations of a single disease, Ann. Intern. Med. **66**:884-892, 1967.

59 Cope, V. Z.: Extravasation of bile, Br. J. Surg. **13**:120-129, 1925.

60 Engel, R. M., Elkins, R. C., and Fletcher, B. D.: Retroperitoneal teratoma; review of the literature and presentation of an unusual case, case, Cancer **2**:1068-1973, 1968.

61 Gerster, J. C. A.: Retroperitoneal chyle cysts with special reference to the lymphangiomata, Ann. Surg. **110**:389-410, 1939 (extensive bibliography).

62 Gill, W., Carter, D. C., and Durie, B.: Retroperitoneal tumors; a review of 134 cases, J. R. Coll. Surg. Edinb. **15**:213-221, 1970.

63 Golden, T., and Stout, A. P.: Smooth muscle tumors of the gastrointestinal tract and retroperitoneal tissues, Surg. Gynecol. Obstet. **73**:784-810, 1941.

64 Graham, J. R., Suby, H. I., LeCompte, P. R., and Sadowsky, N. L.: Fibrotic disorders associated with methysergide therapy for headache, N. Engl. J. Med. **274**:359-368, 1966.

65 Hansmann, G. H., and Budd, J. W.: Massive unattached retroperitoneal tumors: an explanation of unattached retroperitoneal tumors based on remnants of the embryonic urogenital apparatus, J.A.M.A. **98**:6-10, 1932.

66 Hellstrom, H. R., and Perez-Stable, E. D.: Retroperitoneal fibrosis with disseminated vasculitis and intrahepatic sclerosing cholangitis, Am. J. Med. **40**:184-187, 1966.

67 Jones, J. H., Ross, E. J., Matz, L. R., Edwards, D., and Davies, D. R.: Retroperitoneal fibrosis, Am. J. Med. **48**:203-208, 1970.

68 Jonsson, G., Lindstedt, E., and Rubin, S.-O.: Two cases of metastasizing scirrhous gastric carcinoma simulating idiopathic retroperitoneal fibrosis, Scand. J. Urol. Nephrol. **1**:299-302, 1967.

69 Kahn, L. B.: Retroperitoneal xanthogranuloma and xanthosarcoma (malignant fibrous xanthoma), Cancer 31:411-422, 1973.

70 Kay, S., and McNeill, D. D.: Leiomyosarcoma of retroperitoneum, Surg. Gynecol. Obstet. 129: 285-288, 1969.

71 Kendall, A. R., and Lakey, W. H.: Sclerosing Hodgkin's disease vs. idiopathic retroperitoneal fibrosis, J. Urol. 35:284-291, 1961.

72 Lawson, D. W., Corry, R. J., Patton, A. S., and Austen, W. G.: Massive retroperitoneal adrenal hemorrhage, Surg. Gynecol. Obstet. 129:989-994, 1969.

73 Leake, R., and Wayman, T. B.: Retroperitoneal encysted hematomas, J. Urol. 68:69-73, 1952.

74 Lofgren, L.: Primary retroperitoneal tumors; a histopathological, clinical and follow-up study supplemented by follow-up study of a series from the Finnish Cancer Register, Ann. Acad. Sci. Fenn. [Med.] 129:5-86, 1967.

75 Lumb, G.: Smooth-muscle tumours of the gastrointestinal tract and retroperitoneal tissues presenting as large cystic masses, J. Pathol. Bacteriol. 63:139-147, 1951.

76 Melicow, M. M.: Primary tumors of the retroperitoneum; a clinico-pathologic analysis of 162 cases; review of the literature and tables of classification, J. Int. Coll. Surg. 19:401-449, 1953.

77 Mitchinson, M. J.: The pathology of idiopathic retroperitoneal fibrosis, J. Clin. Pathol. 23:681-689, 1970.

78 Oberling, C.: Retroperitoneal xanthogranuloma, Am. J. Cancer 23:477-489, 1935.

79 Olson, J. R., and Abell, M. R.: Nonfunctional nonchromaffin paragangliomas of the retroperitoneum, Cancer 23:1358-1367, 1969.

80 Pack, G. T., and Tabah, E. J.: Primary retroperitoneal tumors; a study of 120 cases, Surg. Gynecol. Obstet. 99(suppl.):209-231, 313-341, 1954.

81 Veraguth, P., Maillard, G.-F., and MacGee, W.: Retroperitoneal seminomas without evidence of primary growth, Oncology 24:193-209, 1970.

82 von Wahlendorf, A. R. L.: Ueber retroperitoneale Lipome, Arch. Klin. Chir. 115:751-768, 1921.

83 Warren, S., and Sommer, G. N. J., Jr.: Fibrosarcoma of the soft parts with special reference to recurrence and metastasis, Arch. Surg. 33:425-450, 1936.

84 Windholz, F.: Roentgen diagnosis of retroperitoneal lipoma, Am. J. Roentgenol. Radium Ther. Nucl. Med. 56:594-600, 1946.

25 Vessels

Arteries
Veins
Lymphatics

Arteries

Arteriosclerosis

Arteriosclerosis is a generalized progressive arterial disease associated with localized arterial occlusions and aneurysms. Its pathology has gained greater surgical significance in recent years with the development of direct operative therapy for lesions of major arteries.

The pathology of arteriosclerosis primarily consists of the following:

1 Formation of intimal *plaques*, composed of lipid deposits and prolifer-ated spindle cells; latter seem to be of heterogenous nature, fibroblasts and smooth muscle cells predominating[34]

2 Reduplication and fragmentation of the internal elastic lamina

3 Degeneration of the media indicated by fragmentation of elastic tissue network, by hyaline, mucinoid, and collagenous degeneration of the smooth muscle, and by medial calcification

4 Adventitial fibrosis and chronic inflammatory cellular infiltration

Arteriosclerosis in an artery may present as an occlusive process when the disease attacks the intima more rapidly than the media and adventitia but may present as an aneurysm when the reverse is true. Both occlusive disease and aneurysm may exist in the same arterial system.[41]

The cause of arteriosclerosis is unknown. Factors thought important in its pathogenesis include changes in lipid metabolism, increased endothelial permeability to serum lipoprotein complexes, the susceptibility of the intima to mechanical injury from flow turbulence at major bifurcations and in the presence of hypertension, elastic tissue fragmentation, and thrombosis or disruption of vasa vasorum.[27, 30, 46, 55]

The areas of the arterial tree involved by arteriosclerosis that frequently are successfully treated surgically have increased rapidly so that only occlusions of the small-

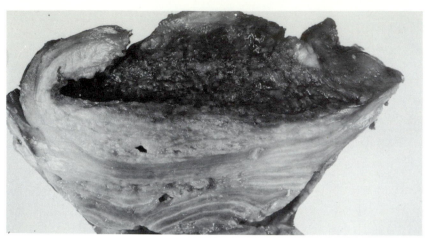

Fig. 1165 Resected abdominal aortic aneurysm that has been transected to show laminations of clot. (WU neg. 57-4850.)

er peripheral arteries of the extremities remain outside the realm of operative attack.

Surgical therapy for occlusive disease of the coronary, carotid, and mesenteric arteries is being undertaken more frequently. The principal manifestations of arteriosclerosis which at present are treated surgically with some success are fusiform and saccular aneurysms of the aorta or other major arteries, dissecting aneurysm, and occlusive disease of the abdominal aorta, the iliofemoral arterial system, and, less often, the popliteal, subclavian, brachial, renal, and carotid arterial systems.[15, 16, 18, 68]

Aneurysms
Aortic aneurysms

Aneurysms secondary to arteriosclerosis occur most frequently in the abdominal aorta. In the aorta and other arteries which become aneurysmal because of arteriosclerosis, the mechanism of development and the pathology of the arteriosclerotic aneurysms are similar.

Arterial dilatation is likely initiated by a loss of elasticity or weakening of the recoil strength in the arterial wall, which results in elongation and tortuosity as well as in dilatation. Initially, this dilatation is most often fusiform. At the same intraluminal pressure, tension developed in the arterial wall is greater the larger the diam-

eter of the artery. The tendency for dilatation thus increases rapidly after it has begun.[20] The progressive dilatation often results in a break in the arterial wall and in the development of sacculation of the aneurysm. In other words, most arteriosclerotic aneurysms probably begin as fusiform dilatations but, with the loss of structural integrity, become saccular. The sacculations nearly always are partially filled with laminated clot, which may be the source of emboli into the arteries peripheral to the aneurysm (Fig. 1165). Superimposed bacterial infection may complicate an aortic aneurysm of arteriosclerotic origin. *Salmonella* is the predominant organism, followed by *Staphylococcus*.[3]

The patient with an abdominal aneurysm may be asymptomatic and without clinical findings except for prominent abdominal aortic pulsations. The majority, however, seek treatment because of dull midabdominal or back pain associated with a pulsating, tender epigastric or retroumbilical mass that has enlarged rapidly or has been noted only recently. Painful and rapidly enlarging aneurysms will soon rupture if operative therapy is not undertaken. Retroperitoneal hemorrhages from small aneurysms may produce severe back pain with few abdominal symptoms or signs.

Patients with aneurysms of the thoracic aorta survive but a short time without surgical correction. Kampmeir[40] showed the average life expectancy after onset of symptoms to be six to eight months. The prognosis in abdominal aneurysm appears better than that in aneurysm of the thoracic aorta. Estes[25] found that one-third of patients with untreated abdominal aortic aneurysm die within one year, usually from rupture. He estimated that 90% of patients 65 years of age with untreated abdominal aortic aneurysm would be dead in eight years, whereas only 35% of persons of similar age without such an aneurysm could be expected to die.

Schatz et al.[60] reviewed 141 untreated cases of abdominal aortic aneurysms at the Mayo Clinic. The prognosis was poor when the aneurysms were accompanied by symptomatic heart disease, when they were symptomatic, and when they exceeded 7.5 cm in diameter. Only 20% of the patients with aneurysm associated with symptomatic heart disease survived five years. Of those in whom the cause of death was known, 44% died of ruptured aneurysm.

Klippel and Butcher[44] reported thirty patients with abdominal aortic aneurysms not treated operatively. Only two died of rupture. Szilagyi et al.[66] compared 223 untreated abdominal aortic aneurysms with a group of 480 treated surgically. They were able to show that modern operative mortality was significantly less than the likelihood of rupture without operation. Levy et al.[48] suggested that the presence of severe cerebral cardiovascular disease might be a contraindication to operation.

It may be concluded that once aneurysm of the aortic system is of significant size, its excision and aortic reconstitution are mandatory.[14, 17, 19]

Popliteal artery aneurysms

Arteriosclerotic aneurysms of arteries in the extremities are rare except for the popliteal artery, although Pappas et al.[56] reported eighty-nine aneurysms of the femoral artery. The pathologic changes and the progressive enlargement of these aneurysms are similar to those in larger arteries, although the rate of progressive dilatation usually is less. Their treatment is essential to avoid acute thrombosis, embolic phenomena, or rupture as causes of severe peripheral flow deficiency and gangrene. Most patients with popliteal aneurysms are first seen because of these complications. Occasionally, such patients seek medical aid because of anterior tibial muscular necrosis. The popliteal arterial elongation associated with aneurysm formation may kink and occlude the anterior tibial artery as it passes through the interosseous membrane.[38]

Patients with popliteal aneurysms frequently have multiple aneurysms. In sixty-nine patients having 100 popliteal aneurysms, hypertension and occlusive arterial disease were frequent.[28] Only three of these patients were women. Forty of the sixty-nine patients had multiple aneurysms. Thirty-one of them had bilateral popliteal aneurysms, and the remaining had aneurysms of arteries other than the popliteal artery. The most common sites of the second aneurysm in the latter group were the abdominal aorta and the femoral artery.

Ninety-two of the aneurysms were considered purely arteriosclerotic. Syphilis, mycotic infections, and trauma entered into the diagnosis of the remaining ones. In the absence of extensive gangrene, popliteal aneurysms with or without the presence of complications are best treated by excision of the aneurysm and the insertion of autologous vein grafts.

Dissecting aneurysms

Dissecting aneurysms of the aorta, if untreated, are associated with a rapidly fatal course in 75% to 90% of the patients. Their etiology is related to an underlying degeneration of the elements of the media. There is an increased risk of this complication during pregnancy, although the reason for this is unclear.[7, 52]

The process of dissection most commonly begins in a transverse intimal tear

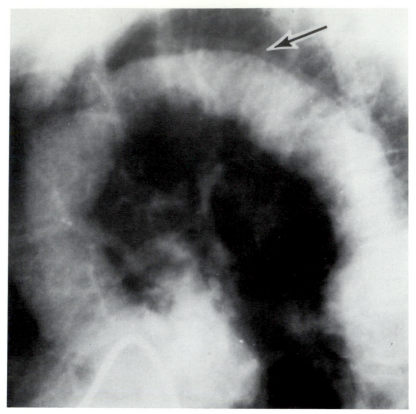

Fig. 1166 Dissecting aneurysm in 68-year-old man who died of rupture into pericardium on way to operating room. Double aortic shadow characteristic of dissecting aneurysm is indicated by arrow. (WU neg. 62-2999.)

associated with an intimal plaque located either in the ascending aorta or in the upper descending thoracic aorta near the origin of the left subclavian artery. Once this tear develops, the intramural layers of the aorta are rapidly separated by the force of the blood entering the wall. The dissection usually involves the entire circumference of the aorta as it progresses distally. Perforation often occurs through the adventitia, resulting in early death from hemorrhage into the pericardium or pleural cavity. Lower extremity symptoms and signs of acute occlusion of the abdominal aorta may be prominent because of distal aortic or iliac luminal occlusion by the leading point of the dissection.

A subacute clinical type characteristically begins abruptly and then progresses gradually for several days before rupture and death (Fig. 1166). Finally, a chronic

form occurs in a few patients who develop a reentry site from the dissected passage back into the lumen of the aorta. The occasional long-term survivor of dissecting aneurysm is encountered among these patients.

The pathologic and clinical features of dissecting aneurysms have been recognized for many years, but until recently definitive treatment has not existed. The surgical attack upon acute dissecting aneurysm of the aorta was introduced by DeBakey and Cooley,[13] who succeeded in salvaging some of these patients.

The fundamental principle in the surgical therapy initially introduced was the transection of the lower thoracic aorta and the establishment of a reentrance site through the intimal layer which had been dissected free by the aneurysmal process. This procedure is particularly applicable when the dissection begins in the ascending aorta. Aortic excision and graft, however, are thought to be superior if the site of beginning dissection is in the upper descending thoracic aorta. Excision is possible in most of the patients undergoing operation.[13, 50]

Wheat et al.[72, 73] reported the successful treatment of patients with acute dissecting aortic aneurysm by the use of antihypertensive agents. In a series of thirty-three patients so treated reported by McFarland et al.,[51] the survival rate was 52%, the mean follow-up period being more than three years. These authors emphasized the need for proper selection in deciding a surgical versus a medical therapy. Exceptionally, dissecting aneurysms can occur in arteries other than the aorta, such as the renal, coronary, pulmonary, and carotid vessels.[74]

Diffuse arterial tortuosity and dilatation

Occasionally, a more or less generalized arterial dilatation and extreme tortuosity are seen in patients suffering from generalized arteriosclerosis. Leriche[47] reported such instances as *dolicho et mega arteria*. The mechanism of the tortuosity and generalized dilatation is thought to relate to weakening of the arterial wall, but the cause for its generalized nature is not clearly understood.

We have encountered nine patients with this condition.[61] The arteriograms of one of these are illustrated in Fig. 1167. The patient presented with a nontender pulsatile abdominal mass diagnosed initially as an abdominal aortic aneurysm. However, because of the prominence of the femoral arterial pulsation, arteriography was performed. There was marked dilatation and tortuosity of the abdominal aorta with bilateral dilatation of the femoral and popliteal arteries. The posterior tibial and dorsalis pedis pulses were normal bilaterally.

One need know that such arterial dilatation and tortuosity may be mistaken for intra-abdominal aneurysm since surgical attack upon such generalized tortuosity is probably not warranted in the absence of complications.

Marked enlargement and tortuosity of the femoral arterial tree in one patient were associated with lamellar deposition of thrombotic material along the wall of the tortuous and enlarged artery, with maintenance of a lumen through the thrombosis. Embolization resulted in peripheral gangrene requiring amputation. Blood flow from the center of the laminated clot still was brisk at the time of amputation. The arterial wall showed marked loss of normal histologic structure, absence of elastic tissue, and marked fibrosis (Fig. 1168).

In another of our patients, marked tortuosity and enlargement of the brachial, axillary, and carotid arteries were present without localized aneurysmal formation.

Arterial substitution

Arteriosclerotic aneurysms of the abdominal aorta and the iliac arteries are best treated by excision and replacement of the involved arterial segment by synthetic cloth prostheses. Aneurysms of the popliteal arteries probably are best replaced by venous autografts. Arterial homografts are no longer used to replace diseased arterial segments because of the superiority of synthetic arterial prostheses. Degeneration of homografts resulted in an average yearly failure rate of 4.1% over ten years at the Massachusetts General Hospital.[53]

After implantation, homografts are partially replaced or encased by host collagenous tissue (Fig. 1169). In a few months they lose much of their elasticity, although fragmented elastic tissue is still demonstrable histologically over a year after implantation. The evolution of the intimal surface of both homografts and synthetic cloth prostheses after implantation consists of organization of the fibrin layer initially deposited and the development of a lining of flattened cells, which, by special staining techniques, appear

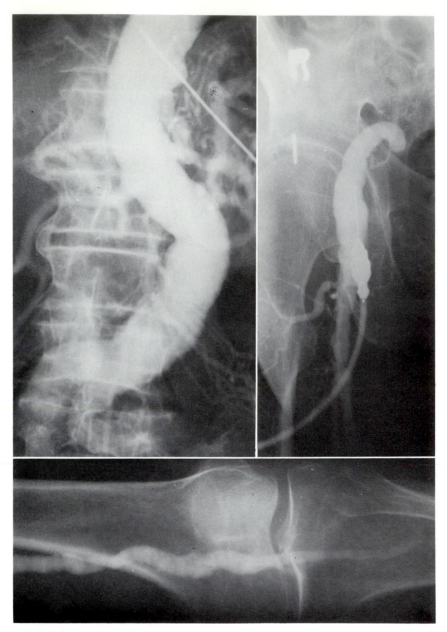

Fig. 1167 Arteriograms of abdominal aorta and femoral and popliteal arteries illustrating generalized arterial dilatation and tortuosity in patient who had pulsating intra-abdominal mass initially diagnosed as aneurysm. (WU neg. 57-4727.)

nearly like normal vascular endothelium.[63] True endothelial ingrowth from the host artery occurs across the suture line for a variable distance.

Szilagyi et al.[64] reported late aneurysm formation in two of fifty-five aortic homografts and tortuous dilatation in twelve of sixty-six femoral homografts within three years after insertion. Calcification may appear in the wall of homografts after long implantation. Implantation of synthetic cloth prostheses is followed by their encasement with collagen and a decline in tensile strength of some of them. Harrison[32] showed that nylon lost 60% to 90% of its strength two years after implantation

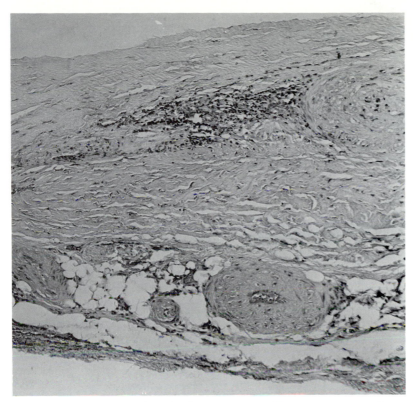

Fig. 1168 Appearance of arterial wall after amputation for gangrene secondary to embolization from mural thrombi in dilated and tortuous femoral artery. (WU neg. 57-5804.)

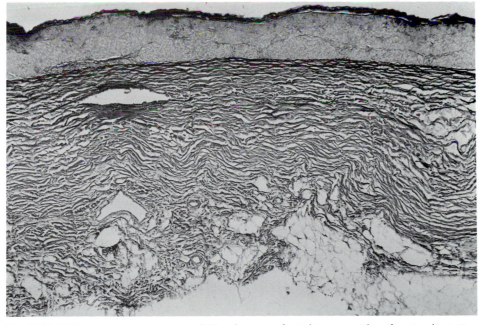

Fig. 1169 Collagenous encasement of iliac homograft eighteen months after implantation. (WU neg. 57-5807.)

in dogs. Dacron, Orlon, and Teflon proved much superior in this regard.

Controlled experimental hypercholesterolemia in the dog[10] and rabbit[26] produced atherosclerotic changes in lyophilized homografts that were greater than those in the host arteries. Synthetic arterial substitutes have been shown to develop intimal lipid deposits in hypercholesterolemic rabbits and, after months of implantation, in man.[67] Atheromas also developed in experimentally endarterectomized arteries.[29]

Although homografts have been used extensively to replace diseased larger arteries successfully, it appears that the synthetic prostheses are superior[8, 9, 11] if the cloth constituting them is of the proper porosity.[33, 71] Endoaneurysmorraphy and the intra-aneurysmal wiring are no longer indicated in the treatment of aneurysm.

Arterial occlusive disease

Thrombotic occlusions of the major arteries often are associated with arteriosclerotic changes such as calcification, atheromatosis, and ulceration of the intima. Jørgensen[37] made a thorough review of the different factors leading to thrombosis. The occlusive process is often insidious, although final thrombotic obliteration of the lumen is occasionally quite rapid and may be clinically indistinguishable from embolization. Indeed, the differentiation of the two pathologically and at operation is quite difficult in older individuals in whom arteriosclerosis of the abdominal aorta is nearly universal. The process of occlusion probably begins in the iliac arteries near the aortic bifurcation from which thrombus formation propagates cephalad in the aorta, occasionally to the level of the renal arteries. Thrombi and emboli can become secondarily infected by fungi, particularly *Aspergillus* and *Mucor* (Fig. 1170).

The syndrome of distal aortic thrombosis (Leriche syndrome) manifests itself with an insidious onset and gradual progression of symptoms of pain and easy fatigability in the legs, hips, and back, intermittent claudication, and sexual impotence (Fig. 1171). In this condition, arterial insufficiency in the lower extremities usually is manifested clinically by absence of pulses below the umbilicus. If the process is partial, weak pulsations may be felt or a characteristic systolic murmur heard over the abdominal aorta and the femoral arteries.

Despite the presence of intermittent claudication and the absence of pulses, many of the patients are found by arteriography to have near normal distal arteries. This patency of the peripheral arteries probably is responsible for the relative absence of muscular atrophy or of atrophy of skin appendages in the legs and feet of many of the patients despite their symptoms of peripheral blood flow insufficiency and lack of pulses.

Arteriosclerotic occlusive disease also frequently involves other major arterial bifurcations in the lower extremity such as those of the common iliac and common femoral arteries. In the latter instance, the intimal disease and thrombosis occur frequently in the external femoral artery just distal to the bifurcation. Other arterial segments in the lower extremity prone to early thrombotic occlusion are those associated with some degree of fascial fixation. Such areas exist (1) in the external iliac artery behind the inguinal ligament, (2) in the superficial femoral artery as it passes through the fascial ring beneath the adductor longus tendon, and (3) in the anterior tibial artery where it passes through the interosseous membrane.[23] Rodriguez-Martinez et al.[58] devised a practical, very useful dissecting technique for the pathologic evaluation of lower limbs with vascular occlusions. DeWolfe et al.[22] described in detail the correlation between clinical and arteriographic findings.

Although arteriosclerosis is a generalized arterial disease, the tendency for occlusive complications to develop early in its evolution at the sites just noted makes possible the successful treatment of patients

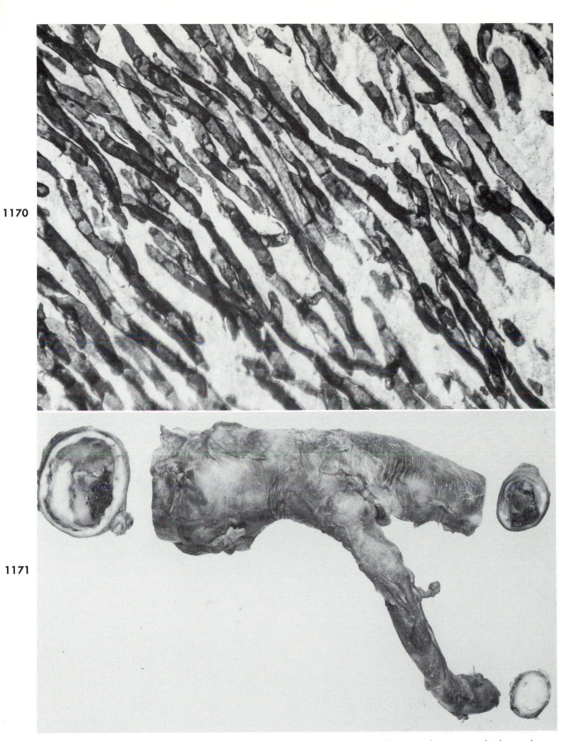

Fig. 1170 Infection of femoral artery embolus by *Aspergillus*. Hyphae are thick and septate and branch at acute angle. Patient, 59-year-old woman, had cold, pulseless lower extremity ten weeks following initial valve replacement. (Gomori's methenamine silver; ×600; WU neg. 73-55.)

Fig. 1171 Thrombotic occlusion of distal abdominal aorta and common iliac arteries (Leriche syndrome). (WU neg. 54-5749.)

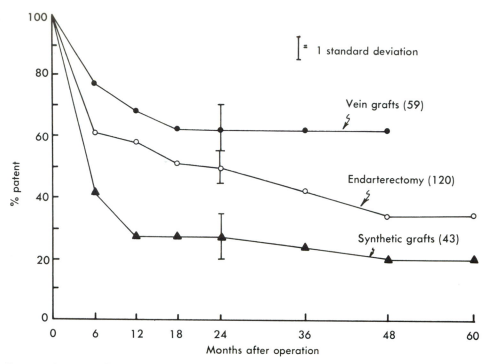

Fig. 1172 Accumulative patency rates after operations for femoral-popliteal occlusive disease. (WU neg. 66-7959.)

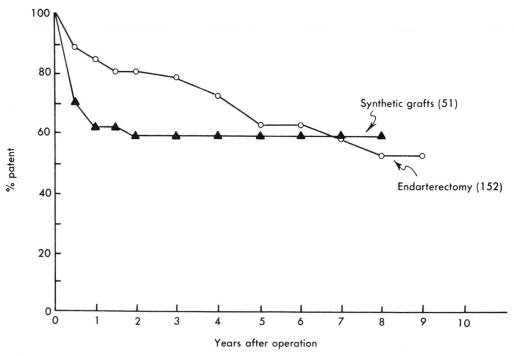

Fig. 1173 Accumulative patency rates after operations for aortic-iliac occlusive disease. (WU neg. 67-4325.)

with marked peripheral blood flow deficiency. Surgical correction of the obstructive disease, however, often only temporarily improves the peripheral blood flow because of the progressive nature of generalized arteriosclerosis.[69, 70] Successful operative therapy of arterial occlusive disease relieves symptoms of ischemia but actually prevents amputation of but a few extremities.[59] However, aggressive operative therapy in properly selected patients with limited gangrene of the extremities may permit healing after amputation of only the gangrenous part.[54]

The treatment of major arterial occlusive disease is being undertaken by surgeons today using two general methods: arterial substitutes and thromboendarterectomy (intimectomy).[65]

Data from Barnes Hospital show that thromboendarterectomy is superior to arterial replacement early after treatment of arterial occlusive disease of the aorta and iliac arteries[12] (Figs. 1172 and 1173). Autogenous venous bypass for femoral arterial occlusive disease appears to be associated with patency rates superior to those following endarterectomy and synthetic bypass grafts.[21, 45]

Successful results in 85% to 95% of patients with occlusions of the aortic and iliac arteries have been reported by both methods of treatment.[6, 39, 75] Postoperative aneurysm formation and vascular thrombosis have been reported following the use of both methods. Data which will allow one to analyze the relative frequency of these complications are not available. The correction of femoral occlusive disease by endarterectomy or by the bypass arterial substitution technique has proved less beneficial than grafts in larger arteries. Approximately 70% of the patients with femoral grafts develop late thrombosis.[69]

The incidence of late failure of both endarterectomy and arterial grafting procedures will likely always be higher in the smaller femoral artery than in the aorta and iliac arteries. Results after femoral endarterectomy reported by Cannon et al.[5]

indicate approximately 50% of the patients maintaining good results six months to two years after operation. Autogenous saphenous vein bypass is preferred by Linton and Darling.[49]

Thromboendarterectomy of major arteries is a technique in which the diseased intima and thrombotic material filling the lumen are dissected from the inner portion of the media in a smooth and uniform manner so that the remaining adventitia and media of the artery can continue to conduct blood (Figs. 1174 and 1175). The remaining arterial tube is lined rapidly by a fibrinoid layer which develops a pseudoendothelial surface similar to that lining an implanted arterial substitute. Likewise, early thrombosis does not occur in these segments if the transit time of the blood through them is rapid. Endarterectomized arterial segments, examined months after the operative procedure, show a fibrous type of intima with an endothelium-like covering and preservation of the remaining media and elastic tissue.[2]

Extensive medial calcification of the Mönckeberg type may occasionally be a contraindication to endarterectomy.

Studies of the elastic properties of normal human arteries and of arteriosclerotic arteries obtained at autopsy from patients of the same age have shown insignificant variations of elasticity coefficients between the two. The progressive encasement of synthetic prostheses with collagen and the similar encasement and invasion of fibrous tissue into the wall of homografts are associated with a reduction in the elastic properties of the implants. Their distensibility becomes much less after implantation[4] (Fig. 1176). Studies of both cloth prostheses and homografts at varying times after implantation indicate that the end result is a collagen-like tube through which the blood flows. The response of the wall of the graft to distention is no longer that of the adjacent host vessels.

In recent years, arterial embolism of atheromatous origin has become more often

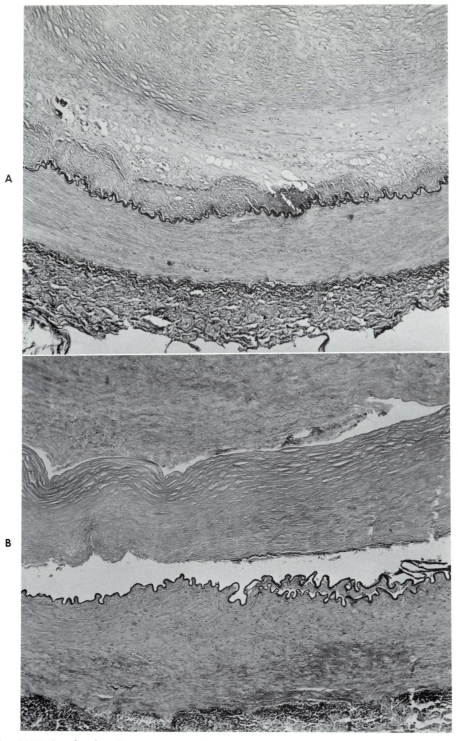

Fig. 1174 Result of endarterectomy performed upon occluded femoral artery removed at autopsy. **A,** Vessel was transected and section made from one of cut ends. **B,** Tissue section made from other cut end after simple wire loop endarterectomy. Freed intimal core was left in situ in order to demonstrate plane of cleavage developed. (**A,** WU neg. 57-5915A; **B,** WU neg. 57-5808.)

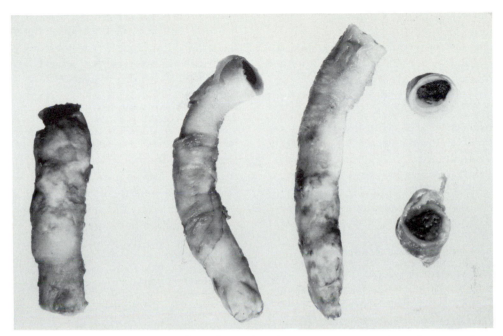

Fig. 1175 Operative specimen from femoral endarterectomy removed in cleavage plane similar to that shown in Fig. 1174. (WU neg. 61-6083.)

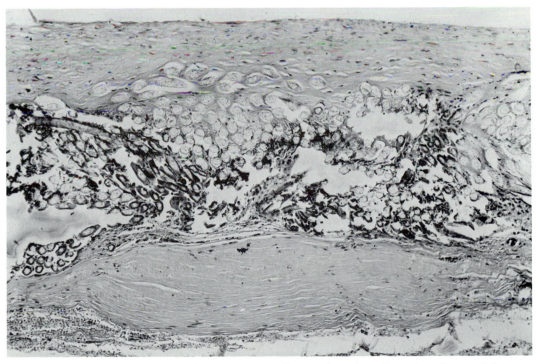

Fig. 1176 Nylon arterial prosthesis one year after implantation. Central graft material is encased in mature relatively acellular collagen, and endothelial-like lining is visible. (WU neg. 57-5805.)

recognized. It may occur spontaneously or following aortic surgery or angiographic procedures.[31, 62] The complications vary according to the vessels affected and include livedo reticularis and gangrene of the lower extremities, ocular symptoms, cerebral infarct, gastrointestinal bleeding, renal hypertention, and renal failure.[1, 24, 35, 36, 42, 43] The frequency of atheromatous embolism correlates with the severity of ulcerative atheromatous changes in the aorta. Simultaneous embolism to various organs may lead to a mistaken clinical diagnosis of polyarteritis nodosa.[57] Random biopsies of skeletal muscle may be diagnostic in these cases.[1]

Cystic adventitial degeneration

Cystic adventitial degeneration, a rare condition almost always affecting the popliteal artery, may cause luminal obstruction. A collection of jellylike material distends the wall and bulges into the lumen. Haid et al.[77] reported a case and reviewed forty previously described. Most cases occurred in young men without a history of trauma and without general arterial changes. The microscopic structure of the involved arterial segments suggested mucinous degeneration. The cysts were lined by flattened cells. The pathogenesis is probably related to that of soft tissue ganglion.[78] Other arteries may exceptionally be affected by this condition.[76]

Fibromuscular dysplasia

Although fibromuscular dysplasia was initially regarded as a renal disease, it is now recognized that this peculiar disorder may involve a wide variety of arteries, sometimes in a multicentric fashion.[79, 81, 82] It usually becomes manifest during the third or fourth decades of life, although it also can be seen in children.[84] It involves large and medium-sized muscular arteries, such as the renal, carotid, axillary, and mesenteric arteries. Morphologically, it is characterized by a disorderly arrangement and proliferation of the cellular and extracellular elements of the wall, particularly

the media, with the resulting distortion of the vessel lumen. The absence of necrosis, calcification, inflammation, and fibrinoid necrosis are important negative diagnostic features. Morphologic varieties with predominant intimal or adventitial involvement have been described.[80, 83]

Mesenteric vascular occlusion

Mesenteric vascular occlusion may originate in veins or arteries. Rarely, occlusion of both occurs simultaneously. Reports in recent years indicate arterial occlusion to be the more frequent (62% of cases).[98] After the initiation of arterial or venous thrombosis, hemorrhagic infarction of the intestine and its mesentery develops if the process is rapid in onset and extensive.

Johnson and Baggenstoss[89, 90] reported that venous mesenteric thrombosis often is associated with infection and cancer. This association was present in 25% of their ninety-nine patients. However, infection and cancer per se were not directly related to the mesenteric venous thrombosis. The true correlation in the 25% having infection and cancer was between portal venous and mesenteric venous obstruction.

The relative reduction in frequency of mesenteric venous occlusion has been attributed by Wilson and Block[98] to antibiotic control of many intra-abdominal infections. In the past, sepsis was thought to cause the majority of the mesenteric venous occlusions.

Occlusion of the mesenteric arterial system may be caused by emboli from thrombi in an arteriosclerotic aorta, from a fibrillating atrium, or from a mural thrombus secondary to myocardial infarction. Mesenteric arterial occlusion also may follow arteriosclerotic change in the superior mesenteric artery with local thrombosis and such rare conditions as polyarteritis or septic arteritis. Mesenteric arteries can be involved in rheumatoid disease and cause infarction.[87] Arterial and venous thrombosis, followed by ulceration and necrosis of the bowel, has been described following surgical repair of aortic coarctation.[88] The pathogenesis of this condition, which has been erroneously designated as "mesenteric arteritis," is probably related to the occurrence of hypertension during the first two postoperative days.

Infarction of the small intestine or colon, perforation, and peritonitis do not always follow mesenteric vascular occlusion, either arterial or venous. Johnson and Baggenstoss[89] reported the presence of infarction in only fifty-two of ninety-nine patients found to have mesenteric vascular occlusions post mortem. Conversely, mesenteric infarct can be seen in the absence of arterial or venous occlusion.[97] This was the case in sixty-seven of 136 patients studied by Ottinger and Austen.[95] In many of these cases, the infarction was secondary to diminished cardiac output or other hypotensive states.

Infarction of the bowel depends upon the location, the extent of the occlusion, the rapidity of its onset, and the state of the collateral circulation, as well as the general physical condition of the patient. Patients with cirrhosis of the liver and portal hypertension often have episodes of cramping abdominal pain associated with low-grade fever and moderate leukocytosis which gradually recede. Several such episodes may take place before a sufficient amount of the portal venous system is occluded to cause the clinical picture of intra-abdominal catastrophe.

The clinical diagnosis of mesenteric vascular thrombosis is difficult at times because the patient does not have the classical severe abdominal pain, distention, nausea, vomiting, leukocytosis, and shock. Such a picture depends upon a massive sudden occlusion of the superior mesenteric artery or vein.

Acute occlusion of mesenteric arteries produces bowel necrosis without the early marked hypovolemic disturbances seen with extensive venous thrombosis. Of the sixty-seven patients reported by Mavor,[93] only four were in a state of peripheral vascular collapse when first examined. Bloody

diarrhea is less common in arterial than in venous occlusions, although abdominal pain generally is more prominent in arterial occlusions. If the occlusion is sufficiently extensive to cause gangrene of the bowel, death from peritonitis follows if the bowel is not resected. A hypovolemic death in less than twenty-four hours, however, is often the outcome in the presence of massive venous occlusion.[85]

Of the two types of occlusion, arterial embolic occlusion is more likely to be amenable to successful treatment than is venous thrombosis. The treatment of both conditions consists primarily of early abdominal exploration and resection of nonviable bowel. The determination of viability at laparotomy may be quite difficult. The extent of small bowel resection compatible with subsequent life has been shown to be as much as three-fourths of the intestine in some patients.

To date, embolectomy has but rarely remedied occlusion of the superior mesenteric artery. However, because of the serious prognosis associated with extensive small intestinal and colonic resection, this procedure probably should be attempted more often.[91]

Postoperative anticoagulant therapy and prolonged extradural anesthesia have been recommended for acute vascular occlusion in the mesentery.[92]

We have encountered three patients in whom it appears that vascular impairment of a segment of small intestine was followed by pathologic changes and clinical findings that were quite similar to those seen in Crohn's disease. One patient developed cramping abdominal pain and tenderness in the right lower quadrant approximately one month after having had a coronary thrombosis. A diagnosis of appendicitis was made, and the abdomen was explored at another hospital. The terminal ileum was described as being edematous and blue in color. It was not removed. Following the operation, the patient entered Barnes Hospital with fever, leukocytosis, and guaiac-positive stools.

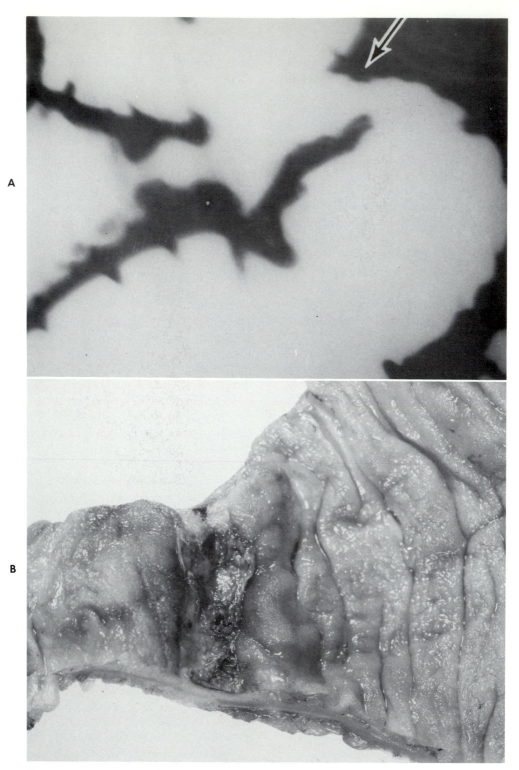

Fig. 1177 A, Segmental area of constriction (arrow) in small bowel interpreted as possible malignant neoplasm. **B,** Excised segment of lesion shown in **A** revealing well-delimited ulcer. Small segment of attached mesentery showed organized thrombi. Ulcer was on basis of vascular insufficiency. (**A,** WU neg. 64-7689; **B,** WU neg. 64-7576.)

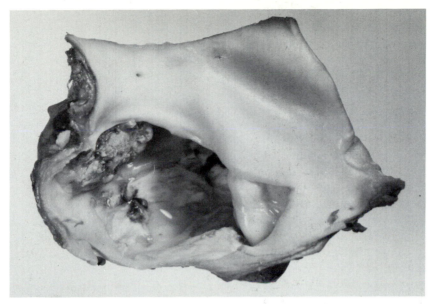

Fig. 1178 Classic traumatic aneurysm of thoracic aorta in 23-year-old man caused by automobile accident five years before operation. Note sharp line of demarcation between normal aorta and aneurysm. Aneurysm was excised and defect replaced with synthetic graft. (WU neg. 62-5338.)

Roentgenograms of the small intestine were interpreted as showing Crohn's disease. Symptoms persisted for approximately six weeks, at which time the patient died of pulmonary edema. Pathologic examination showed approximately 40 cm of the terminal ileum to have submucosal thickening, mucosal ulceration, and a few giant cells. A major branch of the superior mesenteric artery contained organized thrombus. The lymph nodes contained inflammatory cells but no granulomas.[96]

Chronic intestinal ischemia produces the syndrome of abdominal angina.[94] Segmental intestinal infarction may be incident to disease of small mesenteric arteries without involvement of the proximal superior mesenteric artery. So-called nonocclusive intestinal infarction probably is related to disease in these vessels in most instances[86] (Fig. 1177).

Renal artery disease and its relationship to hypertension is discussed in Chapter 16.

Traumatic injuries
Thrombosis

Nonpenetrating trauma may result in occlusive thrombosis of a major artery such as the carotid artery following blunt trauma to the paratonsillar area.[105, 108] In children, trauma and arteritis constitute the two most common causes of acquired occlusions of major arteries.[100, 109]

Pulsating hematoma

The pulsating hematoma or false aneurysm usually results from a small perforation in the artery produced usually by a sharp instrument or a small missile. However, traumatic aneurysms occasionally follow injury to an artery by blunt trauma[99] (Fig. 1178). The defect is only a few millimeters in diameter but is sufficiently large to allow the escape of blood into the immediately surrounding tissues.

Cohen[101] emphasized the role of the adventitial layer in the development of the aneurysmal sac because of its tendency to seal off the defect in the arterial wall. Of equal importance is the nature of the surrounding tissue and the strength of its fascial structures. When strong fascial surroundings are absent, the rate of aneurysmal enlargement is quite rapid. It is slower when the area of injury is within a circumscribed fascial channel such as

Hunter's canal. The blood collects about the defect in the artery until the pressure within the hematoma approaches the mean blood pressure. Enlargement of the hematoma then slows because blood returns to the arterial lumen during diastole. It is this situation that produces the characteristic to-and-fro murmur heard over the pulsating hematoma. This murmur has a rather harsh systolic component and a softer diastolic component. The murmur is not constant as is the murmur of arteriovenous fistula. The walls of the pulsating hematoma contain varying amounts of laminated clot, which in turn is surrounded by a rather dense fibrous tissue reaction.

The operative treatment of pulsating hematoma often is not difficult. Usually the arterial wall defect can be closed by simple suture after evacuation of the hematoma and excision of the fibrotic aneurysmal sac. Occasionally, however, arterial substitution is required.[111]

These lesions should be treated immediately upon diagnosis in order to prevent continued enlargement, pain upon compression of adjacent nerves and other structures, and ischemia of the tissues peripheral to them.[107] Since ligation of the afflicted artery, if it be a major one, is no longer the treatment of choice, waiting for collateral vessels to develop is not indicated.[106]

Acquired arteriovenous fistula

Acquired arteriovenous fistulas are seen most frequently during times of war and are produced in a manner quite similar to that of traumatic aneurysm. However, in this instance, the perforating injury involves both the artery and the adjacent vein. Such an injury usually results in a pulsating hematoma that communicates with both the arterial and the venous lumina.[103]

Following trauma, the fistula may be established almost immediately. However, the communication between the arterial and venous systems is frequently delayed until the wound is partially organized and the thrombus in the hematoma surrounding the artery and vein is partially absorbed. Most patients present with a pulsating mass in the region of injury which can be differentiated from simple pulsating hematoma in several ways. The murmur over the pulsating region is usually continuous because of a continuous flow of arterial blood into the vein. In other words, during diastole the pressure in the pulsating hematoma about the arteriovenous communication is never sufficient to produce reversal of blood flow. In some slowly developing long-standing arteriovenous communications in the absence of a pulsating hematoma, a massive sacculation of the adjacent vein may slowly develop. This is illustrated by the following case history.

A 68-year-old black woman suffered a shotgun wound of the right thigh at the age of 38 years. A mass was first noted on the medial side of the right knee twenty-one years later. It slowly enlarged over the intervening time until it reached sufficient size to interfere with walking (Fig. 1179, A). The large sacculation associated with the arteriovenous fistula in this patient did not contain any laminated clots but was covered by an endothelium-like surface. The popliteal vein entered the sacculation from below and the femoral vein left it above. There was a 6 mm communication between the femoral artery and the venous sac. The arteriogram showed marked femoral arterial dilatation, a characteristic finding in long-standing arteriovenous fistula. Branham's sign was positive. Occlusion of the femoral artery produced a sudden slowing of the pulse. The patient also exhibited significant cardiac enlargement but had not had difficulty with cardiac failure. Treatment consisted of ligation of the popliteal and the femoral veins near their communication with the aneurysmal sac and suture of the 6 mm arterial wall defect. There was rapid decrease in cardiac size following the operation (Fig. 1179, B and C). The diameter of the femoral artery and the prominence of its pulsation decreased in subsequent months.

Patients with an arteriovenous fistula usually show venous dilatation about and peripheral to the fistula, as well as increased skin temperature in the area of the fistula. Despite increased temperature near the lesion, the extremity peripheral

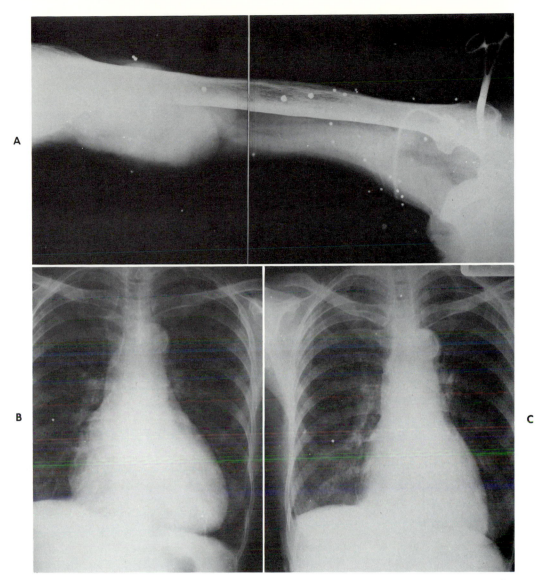

Fig. 1179 Arteriovenous fistula in 68-year-old woman. **A,** Arteriogram showing markedly enlarged femoral artery entering region of arteriovenous fistula. Pellets from original shotgun wound thirty years previously are visible. **B,** Roentgenogram before correction of arteriovenous fistula. **C,** Roentgenogram five days after operation. (**A,** WU neg. 57-980; **B** and **C,** WU neg. 57-9834.)

to it is usually cooler than normal since the actual peripheral blood flow is less.

When arteriovenous fistulas develop between smaller arteries and veins, the sac may be excised and the vessels ligated without difficulty. Those involving the larger arteries, such as the femoral, axillary, or popliteal artery, require the maintenance of arterial continuity. Some type

of arterial substitution may be necessary occasionally in larger arteriovenous aneurysms, although transvenous closure of the defect in the arterial wall usually can be accomplished satisfactorily.[110]

The dilatation of the major artery entering an arteriovenous fistula of long standing may be marked, and the degenerative changes in the arterial wall may be extensive.[104] These changes consist of atherosclerosis, calcification, disruption of the elastic tissue network, and fibrosis. If the degeneration is sufficiently advanced, it is irreversible. In such arteries, aneurysms may develop despite the cure of the arteriovenous fistula. The dilatation of the artery entering the arteriovenous fistula is thought to result from the increased flow of blood through it.

Arteriovenous fistulas are associated with increase in cardiac output, pulse rate, and blood volume, which may lead to congestive heart failure. Such systemic results rarely, if ever, develop from a single congenital arteriovenous fistula with the exception of those that appear in the pulmonary tree. Congenital arteriovenous fistulas usually present as tumefactions containing many relatively small arteries and veins surrounded by moderately large amounts of fibrous tissue. Their treatment is primarily excisional.[102]

Thromboangiitis obliterans

Thromboangiitis obliterans is a rare thrombotic and inflammatory disease of arteries and veins of unknown etiology which has no single diagnostic, clinical, or pathologic sign. Its inflammatory component may involve entire neurovascular bundles. Although it is a generalized vascular disease, the involvement of the arteries of the lower extremities is usually most advanced, and the resultant flow deficiency is the usual reason for the patient to seek therapy. The onset of the condition occurs most often in men between 20 and 35 years of age and may be heralded by superficial migratory acute thrombophlebitis that is precipitated by undue exertion or exposure to cold. Study of biopsies of such involved veins shows the histologic changes associated with acute intravascular thrombosis. Pathologic involvement in the arterial tree is segmental and usually is present primarily in the smaller arteries. There is a paucity of collateral flow.[113] This process has been reported with increased frequency in Korea and Japan.[116]

Microscopic examination of early arterial lesions shows panarteritis, periarteritis, and thrombosis. Endothelial proliferation and periarterial fibrosis soon become prominent. The inflammatory process attacks the entire thickness of the vessel wall and perivascular tissues. Where nerves are in close proximity to the vascular tree, it involves the perineural stroma. Extension of the inflammatory process about peripheral sensory nerves may be responsible in part for the severe pain so common in afflicted extremities. In other words, neuritis as well as vascular ischemia may contribute to peripheral pain in these patients. Calcification in the arterial wall is absent. Arterial calcification on x-ray examination indicates arteriosclerosis rather than Buerger's disease.

The arterial and venous thrombosis associated with the angiitic process becomes partially recanalized. Cellularity of the organizing fibrous tissue replacing the thrombus often is prominent. Recanalization of thrombi is incomplete and is characterized by numerous small vascular channels passing through the remaining fibrous tissue (Fig. 1180).

The pathologic process ascribed to Buerger's disease is difficult, if not impossible, to differentiate microscopically from inflammatory and fibrotic changes that may accompany arteriosclerotic thromboses.[115] There is no conclusive evidence of a primary angiitic etiology. The basic lesion seemed to be arterial thrombosis in the ten cases studied by Gore and Burrows.[112]

The vascular process tends generally to be progressive, but in some instances the acute manifestations seem to subside, particularly in patients who cease using tobacco. Little long-term improvement is attained with or without sympathectomy as long as patients use tobacco.[119] In many of those who stop smoking, the progressive vascular occlusion appears to cease. In nearly all who continue to smoke, however, the disease progresses eventually to gangrene.

Treatment is symptomatic and includes

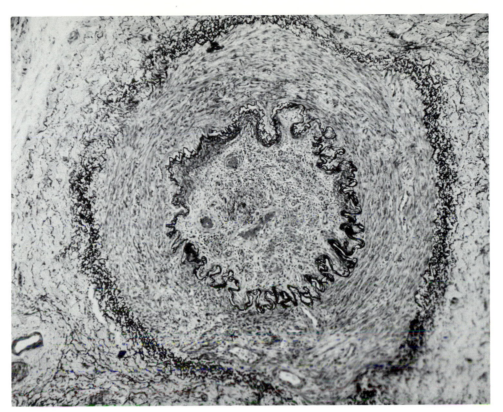

Fig. 1180 Cellular organization of occluding thrombus with small recanalizing channels thought to be compatible with Buerger's disease. Note absence of calcification. (WU neg. 58-643A.)

the control of pain, the avoidance of tobacco, and cleanliness of the extremity. Late in the disease, amputations may be necessary. Sympathectomy may benefit patients with cold, temperature-sensitive feet or hands and those with peripheral gangrenous ulcers.

The death of persons with Buerger's disease may follow complications attending gangrene of the extremities. However, many patients with this affliction die of myocardial infarction, renal insufficiency, occlusions of mesenteric vessels and strokes. Buerger's disease should be looked upon as a rare generalized vascular disease that attacks the smaller arteries more often than the aorta and its major branches.

During the past decade, with the use of arteriography and careful pathologic examination, a high proportion of cases of supposed Buerger's disease have been shown actually to be arteriosclerosis. This pathologic process can be mimicked with considerable exactitude by the development of embolism and thrombosis.[120, 121] This has led some investigators to postulate that Buerger's disease is not a distinct entity but rather a peculiar manifestation of arteriosclerosis. Although we agree that many cases originally diagnosed as Buerger's disease are indeed examples of arteriosclerosis, we believe that such an entity exists.[114, 118, 122]

Arteritis

Inflammatory disease of the arteries have been classified on the basis of the etiologic agent involved, the caliber and location of the vessel affected, and the type of microscopic change observed. The former is obviously the most desirable but, at present, impractical, since a specific etiologic

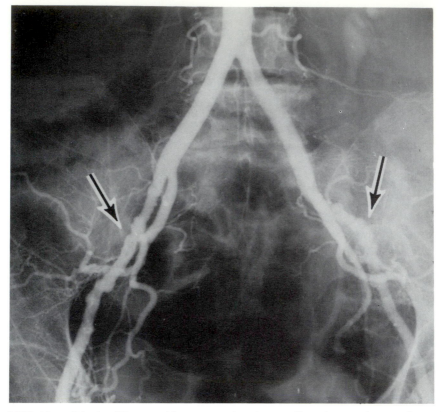

Fig. 1181 Vasculitis in 52-year-old woman showing scalloped irregularities limited to external iliac arteries. (WU neg. 62-3243.)

agent can be detected only for a minority of the cases, such as in syphilitic, mycotic, or tuberculous arteritis.[137] Gross as it seems, a division based on the vessel caliber is quite useful. Within each group, the arteritides can be further subdivided into more or less specific types on the basis of the associated condition and/or pathologic appearance.

Large vessel arteritis

There is a group of related nonsyphilitic diseases primarily affecting the aorta and its main branches and characterized by chronic inflammation and patchy destruction of the elements of the media.[124, 128, 131, 134] They may result in aortic insufficiency, diffuse aortic tortuosity and elongation, the aortic arch syndrome, aneurysm formation, and dissection of the vessel. They are more common in adults but also have been described in children.[125] In the variety known

as *Takayasu's disease,* there is chronic inflammation and fibrosis of the arterial wall, which predilects the aortic arch branches and results in absence of pulses in the upper extremities, ocular changes, and neurologic symptoms.[127, 130] Most patients are young, Asian, and female.

Aortic arteritis can be seen associated with rheumatoid arthritis, ankylosing spondylitis, and scleroderma.[132, 136]

We have encountered a single case of arteritis limited to the external iliac artery (Fig. 1181). This occurred in a 52-year-old woman whose only symptom was intermittent claudication. Arteriograms showed the aorta and peripheral arteries to be normal.

Medium-sized vessel arteritis

The classical example of medium-sized vessel arteritis is *polyarteritis nodosa,* formerly described at autopsy as visible nodu-

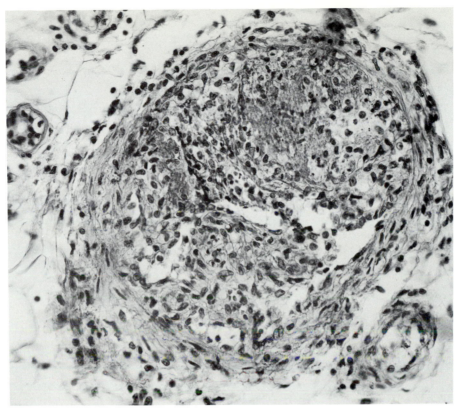

Fig. 1182 Vasculitis involving small vessel of subcutaneous tissue. Note thrombosis, inflammation, and eccentric involvement. (×340; WU neg. 51-6019.)

lar lesions at the points of arterial branchings. This condition should be suspected clinically if there is a history suggesting hypersensitivity, with fever, eosinophilia, and involvement of many organ systems. Infrequently, there are skin manifestations. A muscle or peripheral nerve biopsy may be diagnostic.[129] A biopsy is most rewarding in the presence of a nodule. Rarely, organs such as the gallbladder, appendix, or colon may show unsuspected lesions typical of polyarteritis. We also have seen isolated involvement of the stomach and pancreas.

In **Wegener's granulomatosis,** the arteritis is accompanied by necrosis and granulomatous reaction. Organs most commonly involved are the upper respiratory tract, lung, and kidney.

Giant cell arteritis was originally thought to be restricted to the temporal, cerebral, and retinal arteries. However, many cases with generalized arterial involvement have been described, indicating that this is a generalized disease.[123] This condition, which is most common in the older age group, is characterized by pain in the distribution of the temporal artery and localized tenderness. Sometimes, nodulations can be palpated along the course of the artery. Microscopically, partial destruction of the wall by an inflammatory infiltrate containing multinucleated giant cells is present. The syndrome of *polymyalgia rheumatica,* characterized by muscle pain and tenderness involving mainly the muscles of the neck, shoulder, and pelvic girdle and accompanied by elevated erythrosedimentation rate, is often a manifestation of generalized giant cell arteritis.[126, 133]

Degos' disease, a progressive subendothelial fibrous thickening of the wall of medium-sized arteries and arterioles, leads to vascular occlusions in many organs, particularly the skin and the digestive system, where ischemic infarcts result.[135]

Small vessel arteritis (arteriolitis)

Small vessel arteritis is the most common variety of arterial inflammation. Most examples are secondary to hypersensitivity to drugs or bacterial antigens or appear as a component of one of the "collagen" diseases. The two most important morphologic features to be determined are the nature of the inflammatory infiltrate (whether lymphocytic or neutrophilic) and the presence or absence of necrosis of the vessel wall. In the large majority of the cases, skin manifestations are prominent (Chapter 3) (Fig. 1182).

Tumors

Thirteen cases of primary malignant tumors of the aorta have been reported.[138] The majority have been labeled as fibrosarcomas or "fibromyxosarcomas."[138, 140] Cases with an appearance suggestive of endothelial origin also have been reported.[139] Distant metastases are common.

Tumors of smaller arteries and arterioles are discussed in Chapter 23.

REFERENCES
Arteriosclerosis

1 Anderson, W. R., Richards, A. M., and Weiss, L.: Hemorrhage and necrosis of stomach and small bowel due to atheroembolism, Am. J. Clin. Pathol. **48**:30-38, 1967.

2 Barker, W. J., Cannon, J. A., Zeldis, L. J., and Perry, A.: Anatomical results of endarterectomy, Surg. Forum **6**:266-269, 1955.

3 Bennett, D. E., and Cherry, J. K.: Bacterial infection of aortic aneurysms; a clinicopathological study, Am. J. Surg. **113**:321-326, 1967.

4 Butcher, H. R., and Newton, W. T.: Influence of age, arteriosclerosis and homotransplantation upon the elastic properties of major human arteries, Ann. Surg. **148**:1-20, 1958.

5 Cannon, J. A., Barker, W. F., and Kawakami, I. G.: Femoral popliteal endarterectomy in the treatment of obliterative atherosclerotic disease, Surgery **43**:76-93, 1958.

6 Cannon, J. A., Kawakami, I. G., and Barker, W. F.: The present status of aortoiliac endarterectomy for obliterative atherosclerosis, Arch. Surg. **82**:813-825, 1961.

7 Cavanzo, F. J., and Taylor, H. B.: Effect of pregnancy on the human aorta and its relationship to dissecting aneurysms, Am. J. Obstet. Gynecol. **105**:567-568, 1969.

8 Crawford, S., DeBakey, M. E., and Cooley, D. A.: Clinical use of synthetic arterial substitutes in three hundred seventeen patients, Arch. Surg. **76**:261-270, 1958.

9 Crawford, E. S., DeBakey, M. E., Morris, G. C., and Garrett, E.: Evaluation of late failures after reconstructive operations for occlusive lesions of the aorta and iliac femoral and popliteal arteries, Surgery **47**:79-104, 1960.

10 Creech, O., Jr., Jordan, G. L., Jr., DeBakey, M. E., Overton, R. C., and Halpert, B.: The effect of chronic hypercholesterolemia on canine aortic transplants, Surg. Gynecol. Obstet. **101**:607-614, 1955.

11 Creech, O., Jr., Deterling, R. A., Jr., Edwards, S., Julian, O. C., Linton, R. R., and Shumacker, H.: Vascular prostheses (report of Committee for Study of Vascular Prostheses of Society for Vascular Surgery), Surgery **41**: 62-80, 1957.

12 Darling, R. C., and Linton, R. R.: Aortoiliofemoral endarterectomy for atherosclerotic occlusive disease, Surgery **55**:184-194, 1964.

13 DeBakey, M. E., Cooley, D. A., and Creech, O., Jr.: Surgical considerations of dissecting aneurysm of the aorta, Ann. Surg. **142**:586-612, 1955.

14 DeBakey, M. E., Cooley, D. A., and Creech, O., Jr.: Resection of aneurysms of thoracic aorta, Surg. Clin. North Am. **36**:969-982, 1956.

15 DeBakey, M. E., Crawford, E. S., Cooley, D. E., and Morris, G. C., Jr.: Surgical considerations of occlusive disease of the abdominal aorta and iliac and femoral arteries: analysis of 803 cases, Ann. Surg. **148**:306-324, 1958.

16 DeBakey, M. E., Crawford, E. S., Cooley, D. A., Morris, G. C., Jr., Garrett, H. E., and Fields, W. S.: Cerebral arterial insufficiency; one to 11-year results following arterial reconstructive operation, Ann. Surg. **161**:921-945, 1965.

17 DeBakey, M. E., Crawford, E. S., Cooley, D. A., Morris, G. C., Jr., Royster, T. S., and Abbott, W. P.: Aneurysm of abdominal aorta —analysis of results of graft replacement therapy one to eleven years after operation, Ann. Surg. **160**:622-639, 1964.

18 DeBakey, M. E., Crawford, E. S., Morris, G. C., Jr., and Cooley, D. A.: Surgical considerations of occlusive disease of the innominate carotid, subclavian, and vertebral arteries, Ann. Surg. **154**:698-725, 1961.

19 DeBakey, M. E., Creech, O., Jr., and Morris, G. C., Jr.: Aneurysm of thoracoabdominal aorta involving the celiac, superior mesenteric, and renal arteries; report of 4 cases treated

by resection and homograft replacement, Ann. Surg. **144**:549-573, 1956.

20 de Takats, G., and Pirani, C. L.: Aneurysms: general considerations, Angiology **5**:173-208, 1954.

21 DeWeese, J. A., Barner, H. B., Mahoney, E. B., and Rob, C. G.: Autogenous venous bypass grafts and thromboendarterectomies for atherosclerotic lesions of the femoropopliteal arteries, Ann. Surg. **163**:205-214, 1966.

22 DeWolfe, V. G., and Beven, E. G.: Arteriosclerosis obliterans in the lower extremities: correlation of clinical and angiographic findings, Cardiovasc. Clin. **3**:65-92, 1971.

23 Dible, J. H.: The pathology of limb ischaemia, St. Louis, 1966, Warren H. Green, Inc.

24 Eliot, R. S., Kanjuk, V. J., and Edwards, J. E.: Atheromatous embolism, Circulation **30**:611-618, 1964.

25 Estes, J. E., Jr.: Abdominal aortic aneurysms; a study of 102 cases, Circulation **2**:258-264, 1950.

26 Fisher, E. R., and Fisher, B.: The effect of induced arteriosclerosis on fresh and lyophilized aortic homografts in the rabbit, Surgery **40**:530-542, 1956.

27 Getz, G. S., Vesselinovitch, D., and Wissler, R. W.: A dynamic pathology of atherosclerosis, Am. J. Med. **46**:657-673, 1969.

28 Gifford, R. W., Jr., Hines, E. A., Jr., and Janes, J. M.: An analysis and follow-up study of 100 popliteal aneurysms, Surgery **33**:284-293, 1953.

29 Gryska, P. F.: The development of atheroma in arteries subjected to experimental thromboendarterectomy, Surgery **45**:655-660, 1959.

30 Haimovici, H., editor: Atherosclerosis: recent advances, Ann. N. Y. Acad. Sci. **149**:585-1068, 1968.

31 Harrington, J. T., Sommers, S. C., and Kassirer, J. P.: Atheromatous emboli with progressive renal failure: renal arteriography as the probably inciting factor, Ann. Intern. Med. **68**:152-160, 1968.

32 Harrison, J. H.: Synthetic materials as vascular prostheses. II. A comparative study of nylon, Dacron, Orlon, Ivalon sponge, and Teflon in large blood vessels with tensile strength studies, Am. J. Surg. **95**:16-24, 1958.

33 Harrison, J. H., and Davalos, P. A.: Influence of porosity on synthetic grafts, Arch. Surg. **82**:8-13, 1961.

34 Haust, M. D., More, R. H., and Movat, H. Z.: The role of smooth muscle cells in the fibrogenesis of arteriosclerosis, Am. J. Pathol. **37**:377-389, 1960.

35 Hollenhorst, R. W.: Vascular status of patients who have cholesterol emboli in the retina, Am. J. Ophthalmol. **61**:1159-1165, 1966.

36 Hoye, S. J., Teitelbaum, S., Gore, I., and

Warren, R.: Atheromatous embolization: a factor in peripheral gangrene, N. Engl. J. Med. **261**:128-131, 1959.

37 Jørgensen, L.: Mechanisms of thrombosis, Pathobiology **2**:139-204, 1972.

38 Julian, O. C., Dye, W. S., and Javid, H.: The use of vessel grafts in the treatment of popliteal aneurysms, Surgery **38**:970-980, 1955.

39 Julian, O. C., Dye, W. S., Olwin, J. H., and Jordan, P. H.: Direct surgery of arteriosclerosis, Ann. Surg. **136**:459-474, 1952.

40 Kampmeir, R. H.: Saccular aneurysm of the thoracic aorta: a clinical study of 633 cases, Ann. Intern. Med. **12**:624-651, 1938.

41 Kannel, W. B., and Shurtleff, D.: The natural history of arteriosclerosis obliterans, Cardiovasc. Clin. **3**:37-52, 1971.

42 Kassirer, J. P.: Atheroembolic renal disease, N. Engl. J. Med. **280**:812-818, 1969.

43 Kazmier, F. J., Sheps, S. G., Bernatz, P. E., and Sayre, G. P.: Livedo reticularis and digital infarcts: a syndrome due to cholesterol emboli arising from atheromatous abdominal aneurysms, Vasc. Dis. **3**:12-24, 1966.

44 Klippel, A. P., and Butcher, H. R., Jr.: The unoperated abdominal aortic aneurysm, Am. J. Surg. **111**:629-631, 1966.

45 Kouchoukos, N. T., Levy, J. F., Balfour, J. F., and Butcher, H. R., Jr.: Operative therapy for femoral-popliteal arterial occlusive disease; a comparison of therapeutic methods, Circulation **35**(suppl. 1):174-182, 1967.

46 Lancet Editorial: Endothelium and arteriosclerosis, Lancet **2**:1239-1241, 1967.

47 Leriche, R.: Physiologie, pathologique et traitement chirurgical des maladies artérielles de la vasomotricité, Paris, 1945, Masson et Cie.

48 Levy, J. F., Kouchoukos, N. T., Walker, W. B., and Butcher, H. R., Jr.: Abdominal aortic aneurysmectomy, Arch. Surg. **92**:498-503, 1966.

49 Linton, R. R., and Darling, R. C.: Autogenous saphenous vein bypass grafts in femoropopliteal obliterative arterial disease, Surgery **51**:62-73, 1962.

50 Liotta, D., Hallman, G. L., Milam, J. D., and Cooley, M. D.: Surgical treatment of acute dissecting aneurysm of the ascending aorta, Ann. Thorac. Surg. **12**:582-592, 1971.

51 McFarland, J., Willerson, J. T., Dinsmore, R. E., Austen, W. G., Buckley, M. J., Sanders, C. A., and DeSanctis, R. W.: The medical treatment of dissecting aortic aneurysms, N. Engl. J. Med. **286**:115-155, 1972.

52 Mandell, W., Evans, E. W., and Walford, R. L.: Dissecting aortic aneurysm during pregnancy, N. Engl. J. Med. **251**:1059-1061, 1954.

53 Meade, J. W., Linton, R. R., Darling, R. C., and Menendez, C. V.: Arterial homografts—

a long-term clinical follow-up, Arch. Surg. 93: 392-399, 1966.

54 Morris, G. C., Jr., Wheeler, C. G., Crawford, E. S., Cooley, D. A., and DeBakey M. E.: Restorative vascular surgery in the presence of impending and overt gangrene of the extremities, Surgery 51:50-57, 1962.

55 National Research Council, Division of Medical Sciences: Symposium on atherosclerosis, Publication 338, Washington, D. C., 1954, National Research Council.

56 Pappas, G., Janes, J. M., Bernatz, P. E., and Schirger, A.: Femoral aneurysms—review of surgical management, J.A.M.A. 190:489-493, 1964.

57 Richards, A. M., Eliot, R. S., Kanjuh, V. I., Bloemendaal, R. D., and Edwards, J. E.: Cholesterol embolism; a multiple-system disease masquerading as polyarteritis nodosa, Am. J. Cardiol. 15:696-707, 1965.

58 Rodriguez-Martinez, H. A., Cruz-Ortiz, H., Alcantara-Vazquez, A., Alcorta-Anguizola, B., and Burgos-Mendivil, J.: Dissecting technique for gangrenous lower limbs with vascular occlusions, Patología (Mex.) 10:69-78, 1972.

59 Schadt, D. C., Hines, E. A., Jr., Juergens, J. L., and Barker, N. W.: Chronic atherosclerotic occlusion of the femoral artery, J.A.M.A. 175: 937-940, 1961.

60 Schatz, I. J., Fairbairn, J. F., II, and Juergens, J. L.: Abdominal aortic aneurysms; a reappraisal, Circulation 26:200-205, 1962.

61 Staple, T. W., Friedenberg, M. S. A., and Butcher, H. R., Jr.: Arteria magna et dolicho of Leriche, Acta Radiol. 4:293-305, 1966.

62 Stout, C., Hartsuck, J. M., Howe, J., and Richardson, J. L.: Atheromatous embolism after aortofemoral bypass and aortic ligation, Arch. Pathol. 93:271-275, 1972.

63 Stump, M. M., Jordan, G. L., Jr., DeBakey, M. E., and Halpert, B.: The endothelial lining of homografts and dacron prostheses in the canine aorta, Am. J. Pathol. 40:487-491, 1962.

64 Szilagyi, D. E., McDonald, R. T., Smith, R. F., and Whitcomb, J. G.: Biologic fate of human arterial homografts, Arch. Surg. 75:506-529, 1957.

65 Szilagyi, D. E., Smith, R. F., and Whitcomb, J. G.: The contribution of angioplastic surgery to the therapy of peripheral occlusive arteriopathy; a critical evaluation of eight years' experience, Ann. Surg. 152:660-677, 1960.

66 Szilagyi, D. E., Smith, R. F., DeRusso, F. J., Elliott, J. P., and Sherrin, F. W.: Contribution of abdominal aortic aneurysmectomy to prolongation of life, Ann. Surg. 164:678-699, 1966.

67 Tarizzo, R. A., Alexander, R. W., Beattie, E. J., Jr., and Economou, S. G.: Atherosclerosis

in synthetic vascular grafts, Arch. Surg. 82: 826-832, 1961.

68 Thompson, J. E., Kartchner, M. M., Austin, D. J., Wheeler, C. G., and Patman, R. D.: Carotid endarterectomy for cerebrovascular insufficiency (stroke); follow up of 359 cases, Ann. Surg. 163:751-763, 1966.

69 Warren, R., and Villavicencio, J. L.: Iliofemoropopliteal arterial reconstructions for arteriosclerosis obliterans, N. Engl. J. Med. 260:255-263, 1959.

70 Warren, R., Gomez, R. L., Marston, J. A. P., and Cox, J. S. T.: Femoropopliteal arteriosclerosis obliterans—arteriographic patterns and rates of progression, Surgery 55:135-143, 1964.

71 Wesolowski, S. A., Fries, C. C., Karlson, K. E., DeBakey, M., and Sawyer, P. N.: Porosity; primary determinant of ultimate fate of synthetic vascular grafts, Surgery 50:91-96, 105-106, 1961.

72 Wheat, M. W., Palmer, R. F., Bartley, T. D., and Seelman, R. C.: Treatment of dissecting aneurysms of the aorta without surgery, J. Thorac. Cardiovasc. Surg. 50:364-373, 1965.

73 Wheat, M. W., Jr., Harris, P. D., Malm, J. R., Kaiser, G., Bowman, F. O., Jr., and Palmer, R. F.: Acute dissecting aneurysms of the aorta: treatment and results in 64 patients, J. Thorac. Cardiovasc. Surg. 58:344-351, 1969.

74 Wychulis, A. R., Kincaid, O. W., and Wallace, R. B.: Primary dissecting aneurysms of peripheral arteries, Mayo Clin. Proc. 44:804-810, 1969.

75 Wylie, E. J.: Thromboendarterectomy for arteriosclerotic thrombosis of major arteries, Surgery 32:275-292, 1952.

Cystic adventitial degeneration

76 Backstrom, C. G., Linell, F., and Ostberg, G.: Cystic myxomatous adventitial degeneration of the radial artery with development of ganglion in the connective tissue, Acta Chir. Scand. 129:447-451, 1965.

77 Haid, S. P., Conn, J., Jr., and Bergan, J. J.: Cystic adventitial disease of the popliteal artery, Arch. Surg. 101:765-770, 1970.

78 Lewis, G. J. T., Douglas, D. M., Reid, W., and Watt, J. K.: Cystic adventitial disease of the popliteal artery, Br. Med. J. 3:411-415, 1967.

Fibromuscular dysplasia

79 Claiborne, T. S.: Fibromuscular hyperplasia: report of a case with involvement of multiple arteries, Am. J. Med. 49:103-105, 1970.

80 Crocker, D. W.: Fibromuscular dysplasias of renal artery, Arch. Pathol. 85:602-613, 1968.

81 Harrison, E. G., Hung, J. C., and Bernatz,

P. E.: Morphology of fibromuscular dysplasia of the renal artery in renovascular hypertension, Am. J. Med. 43:97-112, 1967.

82 Hill, L. D., and Anotononius, J. I.: Arterial dysplasia: an important surgical lesion, Arch. Surg. 90:585-595, 1965.

83 Hunt, J. C., Harrison, E. G., Jr., Kincaid, O. W., Bernatz, P. E., and Davis, G. P.: Idiopathic fibrous and fibromuscular stenoses of the renal arteries associated with hypertension, Mayo Clin. Proc. 37:181-216, 1962.

84 Price, R. A., and Vawter, G. F.: Arterial fibromuscular dysplasia in infancy and childhood, Arch. Pathol. 93:419-426, 1972.

Mesenteric

vascular occlusion

85 Allen, G. J.: Mesentery, splanchnic circulation and mesenteric thrombosis. In Rhoads, J. E., Allen, J. G., Harkins, H. N., and Moyer, C. A.: Surgery; principles and practice, ed. 4, Philadelphia, 1970, J. B. Lippincott Co.

86 Arosemena, E., and Edwards, J. E.: Lesions of the small mesenteric arteries underlying intestinal infarction, Geriatrics 22:122-138, 1967.

87 Bienenstock, H., Minick, R., and Rogoff, B.: Mesenteric arteritis and intestinal infarction in rheumatoid disease, Arch. Intern. Med. 119:359-364, 1967.

88 Ho, E. C. K., and Moss, A. J.: The syndrome of "mesenteric arteritis" following surgical repair of aortic coarctation; report of 9 cases and review of literature, Pediatrics 49:40-45, 1972.

89 Johnson, C. C., and Baggenstoss, A. H.: Mesenteric vascular occlusion. I. Study of 99 cases of occlusion of veins, Mayo Clin. Proc. 24:628-636, 1949.

90 Johnson, C. C., and Baggenstoss, A. H.: Mesenteric vascular occlusion. II. Study of 60 cases of occlusion of arteries and of 12 cases of occlusion of both arteries and veins, Mayo Clin. Proc. 24:649-565, 1949.

91 Kleitsch, W. P., Connors, E. K., and O'Neill, T. J.: Surgical operations on the superior mesenteric artery, Arch. Surg. 75:752-755, 1957.

92 Liang, H., Bernard, H. R., and Dodd, R. B.: The effect of epidural block upon experimental mesenteric occlusion, Arch. Surg. 83:409-413, 1961.

93 Mavor, G. E.: Superior mesenteric artery occlusion, Proc. R. Soc. Med. 54:356-359, 1961.

94 Morris, G. C., Jr., Crawford, E. S., Cooley, D. A., and DeBakey, M. E.: Revascularization of the celiac and superior mesenteric arteries, Arch. Surg. 84:95-107, 1962.

95 Ottinger, L. W., and Austen, W. G.: A study of 136 patients with mesenteric infarction,

Surg. Gynecol. Obstet. 124:251-261, 1967.

96 Pope, C. H., and O'Neal, R. M.: Incomplete infarction of ileum simulating regional enteritis, J.A.M.A. 161:963-964, 1956.

97 Williams, L. F., Anastasia, L. F., Hasiotis, C. A., Bosniak, M. A., and Byrne, J. J.: Non-occlusive mesenteric infarction, Am. J. Surg. 114:376-381, 1967.

98 Wilson, G. S. M., and Block, J.: Mesenteric vascular occlusion, Arch. Surg. 73:330-345, 1956.

Traumatic injuries

99 Bennett, D. E., and Cherry, J. K.: The natural history of traumatic aneurysms of the aorta, Surgery 61:516-523, 1967.

100 Bickerstaff, E. R.: Aetiology of acute hemiplegia in childhood, J. Neurosurg. 2:82-87, 1964.

101 Cohen, S. M.: Peripheral aneurysm and arteriovenous fistula, Ann. R. Coll. Surg. Engl. 11:1-30, 1952.

102 de Takats, G., and Pirani, C. L.: Aneurysms: general considerations, Angiology 5:173-208, 1954.

103 Gomes, M. M. R., and Bernatz, P. E.: Arteriovenous fistulas: a review of ten-year experience at the Mayo Clinic, Mayo Clin. Proc. 45:81-102, 1970.

104 Holman, E.: Fundamental principles governing the care of traumatic arteriovenous aneurysms, Angiology 5:145-166, 1954.

105 Houck, W. S., Jackson, J. R., Odom, G. L., and Young, W. G.: Occlusion of internal carotid artery in neck secondary to closed trauma to head and neck: report of two cases, Ann. Surg. 159:219-221, 1964.

106 Hughes, C. W., and Jahnke, E. J., Jr., The surgery of traumatic arteriovenous fistulas and aneurysms; a five-year follow up study of 215 lesions, Am. Surg. 148:790-797, 1958.

107 Julian, O. C., and Dye, W. S.: Peripheral vascular surgery. In Rhoads, J. E., Allen, J. G., Harkins, H. N., and Moyer, C. A.: Surgery; principles and practice, ed. 4, Philadelphia, 1970, J. B. Lippincott Co.

108 Pitner, S. E.: Carotid thrombosis due to intraoral trauma; an unusual complication of a common childhood accident, N. Engl. J. Med. 274:764-767, 1966.

109 Shillito, J., Jr.: Carotid arteritis: cause of hemiplegia in childhood, J. Neurosurg. 21:540-551, 1964.

110 Shumacker, H. B., Jr.: The problem of maintaining the continuity of the artery in the surgery of aneurysms and arteriovenous fistulae, Ann. Surg. 127:207-230, 1948.

111 Shumacker, H. B., Jr., and Carter, K. L.: Arteriovenous fistulas and arterial aneurysms in military personnel, Surgery 20:9-25, 1946.

Thromboangiitis obliterans

112 Gore, I., and Burrows, S.: A reconsideration of the pathogenesis of Buerger's disease, Am. J. Clin. Pathol. **29**:319-330, 1958.

113 Hershey, F. B., Pareira, M. D., and Ahlvin, R. C.: Quadrilateral peripheral vascular disease in the young adult, Circulation **26**:1261-1269, 1962.

114 Ishikawa, K., Kawase, S., and Mishima, Y.: Occlusive arterial disease in extremities, with special reference to Buerger's disease, Angiology **13**:398-411, 1962.

115 Kelly, P. J., Dahlin, D. J., and Janes, J. M.: Clinicopathological study of ninety-four limbs amputated for occlusive vascular disease, J. Bone Joint Surg. **40**:72-78, 1958.

116 McKusick, V. A., and Harris, W. S.: The Buerger syndrome in the Orient, Bull. Johns Hopkins Hosp. **109**:241-291, 1961.

117 McKusick, V. A., Harris, W. S., Ottesen, O. E., and Goodman, R. M.: The Buerger syndrome in the United States, Bull. Johns Hopkins Hosp. **110**:145-176, 1962.

118 McKusick, V. A., Harris, W. S., Ottesen, O. E., Shelley, W. M., and Bloodwell, D. B.: Buerger's disease: a distinct clinical and pathologic entity, J.A.M.A. **181**:93-100, 1962.

119 Selbert, S.: Etiology of thromboangiitis obliterans, J.A.M.A. **129**:5-9, 1954.

120 Theis, F. V.: Thromboangiitis obliterans: a 30-year study, J. Am. Geriatr. Soc. **6**:106-117, 1958.

121 Wessler, S., Ming, S.-C., Gurewich, V., and Greiman, D. G.: A critical evaluation of thromboangiitis obliterans; the case against Buerger's disease, N. Engl. J. Med. **262**:1149-1160, 1960.

122 Williams, G.: Recent views on Buerger's disease, J. Clin. Pathol. **22**:573-577, 1969.

Arteritis

123 Cardell, B. S., and Hanley, T.: A fatal case of giant cell or temporal arteritis, J. Pathol. Bacteriol. **63**:587-597, 1951.

124 Domingo, R. T., Maramba, M. D., Torres, L. F., and Wesolowski, S. A.: Acquired aortoarteritis; a worldwide vascular entity, Arch. Surg. **95**:780-790, 1967.

125 Gonzalez-Cerna, J. L., Villavicencio, L., Molina, B., and Bessudo, L.: Nonspecific obliterative aortitis in children, Ann. Thorac. Surg. **4**:193-204, 1967.

126 Hamilton, C. R., Jr., Shelley, W. M., and Tumulty, P. A.: Giant cell arteritis: including temporal arteritis and polymyalgia rheumatica, Medicine (Baltimore) **50**:1-27, 1971.

127 Judge, R. D., Currier, R. D., Gracie, W. A., and Figley, M. M.: Takayasu arteritis and the aortic arch syndrome, Am. J. Med. **32**:379-392, 1962.

128 Marquis, Y., Richardson, J. P., Ritchie, A. C., and Wigle, E. D.: Idiopathic medial aortopathy and arteriopathy, Am. J. Med. **44**:939-954, 1968.

129 Maxeiner, S. R., McDonald, J. R., and Kirklin, J. W.: Muscle biopsy in the diagnosis of periarteritis nodosa, Surg. Clin. North Am. **32**:1225-1233, 1952.

130 Nasu, T.: Pathology of pulseless disease: a systematic study and critical review of 21 autopsy cases reported in Japan, Angiology **14**:225-242, 1963.

131 Restrepo, C., Tejeda, C., and Correa, P.: Nonsyphilitic aortitis, Arch. Pathol. **87**:1-12, 1969.

132 Roth, L. M., and Kissane, J. M.: Panaortitis and aortic valvulitis in progressive systemic sclerosis (scleroderma); report of case with perforation of an aortic cusp, Am. J. Clin. Pathol. **41**:287-296, 1964.

133 Royster, T. S., and DiRe, J. J.: Polymyalgia rheumatica and giant cell arteritis with bilateral axillary artery occlusion, Am. Surg. **37**:421-426, 1971.

134 Schrire, V., and Asherson, R. A.: Arteritis of the aorta and its major branches, Q. J. Med. **33**:439-463, 1964.

135 Strole, W. E., Jr., Clark, W. H., and Isselbacher, K. J.: Progressive arterial occlusive disease (Kohlmeier-Degos); a frequently fatal cutaneosystemic disorder, N. Engl. J. Med. **276**:195-201, 1967.

136 Valaitis, J., Pilz, C. G., and Montgomery, M. M.: Aortitis with aortic valve insufficiency in rheumatoid arthritis, Arch. Pathol. **63**:207-212, 1957.

137 Whelan, T. J., Jr., and Baugh, J. H.: Nonatherosclerotic arterial lesions and their management (I. Trauma; II. Inflammatory lesions of arteries), Curr. Probl. Surg., pp. 3-76, Feb., 1967.

Tumors

138 Salm, R.: Primary fibrosarcoma of aorta, Cancer **29**:73-83, 1972.

139 Sladden, R. A.: Neoplasia of aortic intima, J. Clin. Pathol. **17**:602-607, 1964.

140 Stevenson, J. E., Burkhead, H., Trueheart, R. E., and McLaren, J.: Primary malignant tumor of the aorta, Am. J. Med. **51**:553-559, 1971.

Veins

Thrombophlebitis—thromboembolism
Stasis ulcers
Varicose veins

Thrombophlebitis—thromboembolism

Thrombophlebitis is a thrombotic disease of veins accompanied by varying degrees of inflammation. The venous wall is edematous, the intima irregularly ulcerated, and the media infiltrated with chronic inflammatory cells (Fig. 1183). As the acute inflammatory phase of the disease subsides, varying amounts of fibrous tissue and collagen are deposited in the adventitia and in the media. During the acute phase, the thrombus becomes attached more or less firmly to the denuded intima.

The process of thrombophlebitis is associated with edema of the part, which may be minimal or marked. When there is but little edema and few or no clinical signs of acute inflammation in the extremity, the venous thrombosis has been termed phlebothrombosis or bland noninflammatory venous thrombosis.[15] The noninflammatory type of thrombophlebitis probably is more frequently associated with pulmonary emboli than is thrombophlebitis with more marked signs of inflammation. However, the rigid separation of phlebothrombosis from thrombophlebitis is not possible pathologically or practical clinically. These conditions are merely different degrees of the same process.

Thrombophlebitis may involve only the superficial veins such as the saphenous vein. The vein is acutely inflamed and tender, and the overlying skin is usually red. When such thrombosis of the superficial veins occurs, there is usually little edema. However, thrombophlebitic edema may develop with marked rapidity and be of great volume if the process extends into the deep venous system. Rapid shifts of extracellular fluid into the leg may be sufficiently massive to cause shock.[12] In such instances, the extremity may become so swollen that cutaneous blebs develop, followed by cutaneous necrosis (phlegmasia cerulea dolens).[20] Thrombophlebitis of this severity, however, is rare. The usual postoperative or posttraumatic acute thrombophlebitis causes initially a painful, tender, swollen, cool, and mottled or grayish white extremity.

Purulent or septic thrombophlebitis occasionally is seen in association with abscess or other infection usually occurring in the peritoneal cavity or pelvis. Stein and Pruitt[21] found this complication in 4.6% of 521 burned patients who had been treated by venous catheterization. Purulent thrombophlebitis at any location is associated with marked chills and high temperature because of the bacteremia arising from the infected intravascular thrombus.

Pulmonary embolism is often thought to be primarily a complication of some surgical procedure or trauma such as fracture, particularly of the lower extremity, but the incidence of this complication is as high on medical as on surgical services.[10] Some of the factors thought to favor intravenous thrombosis and subsequent pulmonary embolism are neoplasms, cardiac disease, venous stasis from any cause, infection in the immediate area of veins, trauma, spasm of vessels, intimal injury, increased ability of the blood to coagulate, and immobilization of the limbs.[5] The use of oral contraceptives is causally related to the presence of thromboembolic phenomena[7, 19] Vessey and Doll[22] estimated that the risk of venous thromboembolism is approximately nine times greater in women taking contraceptives than in those who do not. Irey et al.[8] described distinctive vascular lesions in association with thrombosis

1215

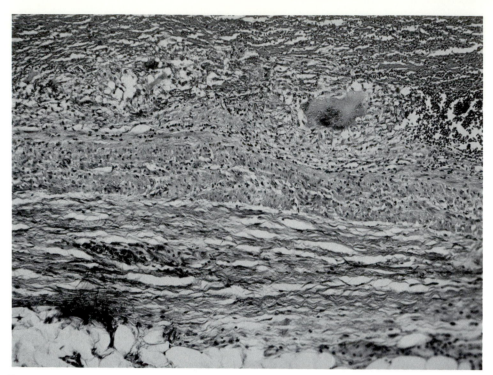

Fig. 1183 Acute venous thrombosis accompanied by inflammatory cellular infiltration containing giant cells. (WU neg. 58-6275.)

in arteries and veins of twenty young women receiving oral contraceptives. However, the basic etiology or initiating mechanisms of thrombosis are not known. The importance of endothelial surface injury and defects has been emphasized by Samuels and Webster,[18] using the technique devised by O'Neill.[16]

Pulmonary embolism is seen in all forms of thrombophlebitis. Sudden massive pulmonary emboli frequently occur in patients without antecedent symptoms or signs of peripheral thrombophlebitis.

The greatest percentage of thrombi resulting in pulmonary embolization are thought to originate in the veins of the lower extremity. Rössle[17] found that 27% of patients over 20 years of age harbored thrombi in the veins of the calf at autopsy. The study of Hunter et al.[6] confirmed these observations and indicated that the thrombosis occurred in over 50% of middle-aged or older persons confined to bed.

McLachlin and Paterson[11] stressed the finding of intravascular thromboses arising in relationship to the valve pockets. In 100 complete dissections of the veins of the pelvis and lower extremities, they showed gross venous thrombi in 34%, and in over one-half of these, there were pulmonary emboli (Fig. 1184). In their series, the thrombi found in thirty-four patients totaled seventy-six—six in the pelvic veins, forty-nine in the thigh veins, and twenty-one in the leg veins. In other words, they found that 75% of the venous thrombi arose in the veins of the thigh and pelvis and 25% in the smaller veins of the calf and feet, with 92% arising in the lower extremities. Similar findings were reported by Beckering and Titus.[2]

Crane[4] concluded that the evaluation of all data available concerning the origin of fatal pulmonary emboli indicates that approximately 85% of them arise in the legs. This figure may well be 90% in postsurgical patients and 80% in cardiac or medical patients.

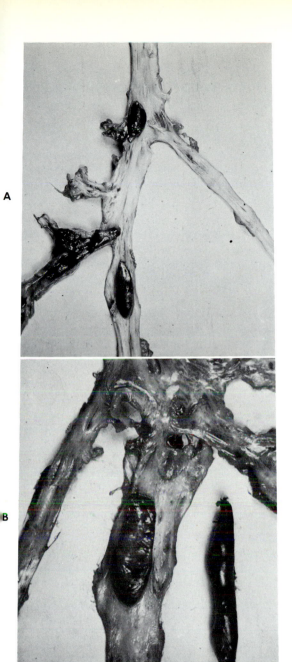

Fig. 1184 **A,** Multiple venous thrombi. Lower thrombus is lying in valve pocket at upper end of superficial femoral vein. Middle one on left is lying in proximal end of profunda femoris vein, while upper thrombus is lying in common femoral vein at junction of long saphenous vein. **B,** Thrombus arising in valve pocket at upper end of superficial femoral vein. Lines of Zahn can be clearly seen. Postmortem clot is shown for comparison. (**A** and **B,** From McLachlin, J., and Paterson, J. C.: Some basic observations on venous thrombosis and pulmonary embolism, Surg. Gynecol. Obstet. **93:**1-8, 1951; by permission of Surgery, Gynecology & Obstetrics.)

Stasis ulcers

The chief immediate complication of thrombophlebitis is pulmonary embolus, and the principal long-term complication is stasis ulceration.

The treatment of acute thrombophlebitis attempts to limit the extension of the process and to prevent pulmonary embolization. Elevation, rest with the maintenance of good hydration, elastic support, and possibly anticoagulant therapy are the initial measures. The effectiveness of anticoagulant therapy as usually administered for thromboembolic disease has been questioned.[3] Ligation of the venous system above the area of intravascular clotting is occasionally indicated when lesser measures fail to prevent pulmonary embolus.

As the acute phase of the disease subsides, measures must be taken to avoid later stasis disease in the lower extremity. The use of elastic supports to help control any dependent edema in the extremity is imperative and may be required for many months or years. With the passage of time, collateral venous channels may develop and communicate with the superficial venous systems, resulting in secondary superficial varicosities. Recanalization of the major deep veins usually is associated with this process. Any significant varicosities in the postphlebitic extremity should be removed.

For reasons not clearly understood, the prevention and control of stasis ulceration are quite difficult in the presence of subcutaneous varicosities. The preventive measures directed toward control of dependent edema often are not carried out by patients suffering from thrombophlebitis, so that after several years cutaneous pigmentation, brawny edema, dermal and subcutaneous fibrosis, extensive secondary varicosities, and ulceration of the skin in the lower one-third of the leg develop. Although stasis ulcers are seen in patients who have a history of past thrombophlebitis, such a history commonly is absent (only 50% of the patients seen in the Washington University Clinics have such a history). Even in patients having thrombophlebitis, the exact pathogenesis of the process leading to ulceration is unknown.

The diagnosis of stasis disease is usually not difficult. Only occasionally are ulceration, pigmentation, and surrounding fibrosis confused with other forms of ulceration. Before extensive treatment of a patient with advanced chronic leg ulcer, careful evaluation of the arterial blood supply should be made. Any significant arterial flow deficiency will likely result in failure of surgical therapy for ulceration. Correction of major arterial occlusion should be made when possible before treatment of the stasis ulcer in those patients in whom both are present. Obviously, the other rare causes of ulceration such as specific infections and neoplasms must be excluded. All ulcers should be cultured and any unusual-appearing ones biopsied before excisional therapy is undertaken.

If ulceration has not yet appeared or is not extensive or chronic in nature, the total removal of the varicose veins with ligation of perforating veins may control the process. If stasis ulceration is extensive, chronic, and long standing, it is best treated by excision and stripping of all superficial varicosities of the extremity after high ligation and division of the

saphena magna and its tributaries at the saphenal-femoral junction. The ulcer and its base should be excised down to normal tissue with removal of all the inelastic thickened skin and fascia about it. The cutaneous-fascial defect should then be covered with a partial thickness cutaneous autograft.[13] The results of this form of therapy at Barnes Hospital are shown in Table 52.

The extent of excision often required for advanced stasis ulceration is shown in Fig. 1185. In most instances, the depth of the excision should include the fascia overlying the muscle, for in the presence of long-standing stasis ulcers, the fascial fibrosis and thickening are quite extensive. This also facilitates ligation of the perforating veins which are invariably present beneath the area of stasis fibrosis.

Varicose veins

Varicose veins occur more frequently in women than in men. Their incidence is much higher in obese women, particularly those who have had several pregnancies. Varicosities developing in women after pregnancy may be secondary to deep venous thrombosis.

Larson and Smith[9] reported that 213 out of 491 patients (43%) had a definite family history of varicose veins, indicating some hereditary disposition. The superficial veins of the leg become dilated and tortuous and lose valvular function. Microscopically, there is fibrosis beneath the endothelium and in the wall, with secondary elastosis and loss of muscle. Calcification may occur.

Primary or simple varicosities often develop in the second and third decades of life and may be present for many years without causing symptoms or complications. The likelihood of thrombosis with propagation into the deep venous system and the likelihood of the development of the postphlebitic syndrome are sufficiently great to warrant the removal of varicose veins. The use of sclerosing agents is contraindicated because of the danger of deep

Table 52 Chronic stasis ulcer (time of recurrence of ulcer after operative therapy)*

Years after operation	At risk	Number of patients developing recurrent stasis ulcer in interval	Healed	Accumulative % of patients without ulcer
0-1	107	8	99	92
1-2	90	8	81	84
2-3	69	4	65	79
3-4	55	0	55	79
4-5	53	1	52	77
5-6	45	0	45	77
6-7	40	2	38	74
7-8	29	3	26	66
8+	16	0	16	66

*Three of five patients whose ulcer recurred after five postoperative years had had arterial occlusive disease develop.

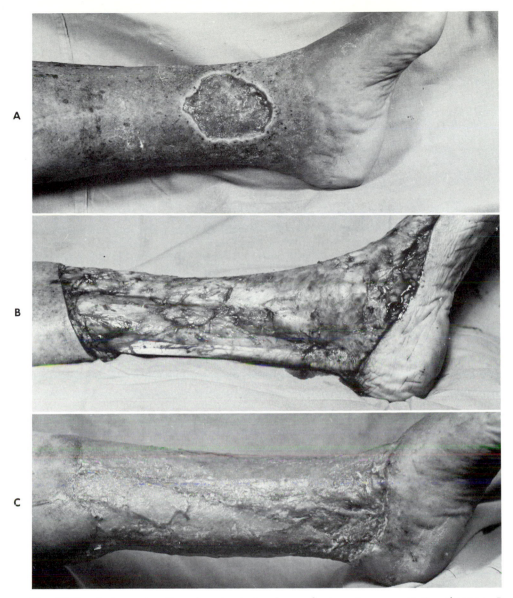

Fig. 1185   A, Long-standing chronic stasis ulcer refractory to nonoperative therapy. **B,** Fibrotic skin, subcutaneous tissue, and fascia have been widely excised. Periosteum and peritendineum were not removed. **C,** Extremity two years after operation. (**A,** WU neg. 57-5074; **B,** WU neg. 55-4561; **C,** WU neg. 57-5549.)

venous thrombosis as well as the temporary nature of the superficial venous occlusion obtained. The operative removal of varicosities is best performed by venous stripping techniques and excisions.[1, 14]

REFERENCES

1 Agrifoglio, G., and Edwards, E. A.: Results of surgical treatment of varicose veins, J.A.M.A. **178:**906-911, 1961.

2 Beckering, R. E., Jr., and Titus, J. L.: Femoral-popliteal venous thrombosis and pulmonary embolism, Am. J. Clin. Pathol. **52:**530-537, 1969.

3 Butcher, H. R., Jr.: Anticoagulant drug therapy for thrombophlebitis in the lower extremities—an evaluation, Arch. Surg. **80:**864-875, 1960.

4 Crane, C.: Deep venous thrombosis and pulmonary embolism, N. Engl. J. Med. **257:**147-157, 1957.

5 DeBakey, M. E.: Collective review: critical

evaluation of problem of thromboembolism, Int. Abstr. Surg. **98**:1-27, 1954.

6 Hunter, W. C., Krygier, J. J., Kennedy, J. C., and Sneedend, V. D.: Etiology and prevention of thrombosis of the deep leg veins, Surgery **17**:178-190, 1945.

7 Inman, W. H. W., and Vessey, M. P.: Investigation of deaths from pulmonary coronary and cerebral thrombosis and embolism in women in childbearing age, Br. Med. J. **2**:193-199, 1968.

8 Irey, N. S., Manion, W. C., and Taylor, H. B.: Vascular lesions in women taking oral contraceptives, Arch. Pathol. **89**:1-8, 1970.

9 Larson, R. A., and Smith, F. S.: Varicose veins: evaluation of observations in 491 cases, Mayo Clin. Proc. **18**:400-408, 1943.

10 McCartney, J. S.: Postoperative pulmonary embolism, N. Engl. J. Med. **257**:147-157, 1957.

11 McLachlin, J., and Paterson, J. C.: Some basic observations on venous thrombosis and pulmonary embolism, Surg. Gynecol. Obstet. **93**:1-8, 1951.

12 Moyer, C. A.: Nonoperative surgical care. In Rhoads, J. E., Allen, J. G., Harkins, H. N., and Moyer, C. A.: Surgery; principles and practice, ed. 4, Philadelphia, 1970, J. B. Lippincott Co.

13 Moyer, C. A., and Butcher, H. R.: Stasis ulcers: an evaluation of the effectiveness of three methods of therapy and the implication of obliterative cutaneous lymphangitis as a credible etiologic factor, Ann. Surg. **141**:577-587, 1955.

14 Myers, T. T.: Results of the stripping operation in the treatment of varicose veins, Mayo Clin. Proc. **29**:583-590, 1954.

15 Ochsner, A., DeBakey, M. E., and DeCamp, P. T.: Venous thrombosis, analysis of 580 cases, Surgery **29**:1-20, 1951.

16 O'Neill, J. F.: The effects on venous endothelium of alterations in blood flow through the vessels in vein walls and the possible relation to thrombosis, Ann. Surg. **126**:270-288, 1947.

17 Rössle, R.: Ueber die Bedeutung und die Entstehung der Wadenvenenthrombosen, Virchows Arch. Pathol. Anat. **300**:180-189, 1937.

18 Samuels, P. B., and Webster, D. R.: The role of venous endothelium in the inception of thrombosis, Ann. Surg. **136**:422-438, 1952.

19 Sartwell, P. E., Masi, A. T., Arthes, F. G., Greene, G. R., and Smith, H. E.: Thromboembolism and oral contraceptives: an epidemiological case-control study, Am. J. Epidemol. **90**:365-380, 1969.

20 Stallworth, J. M., Bradham, G. B., Kletke, R. R., and Price, R. G., Jr.: Phlegmasia cerulea dolens: a 10-year review, Ann. Surg. **161**:802-811, 1965.

21 Stein, J. M., and Pruitt, B. A., Jr.: Suppurative thrombophlebitis: a lethal iatrogenic disease, N. Engl. J. Med. **282**:1452-1455, 1970.

22 Vessey, M. P., and Doll, R.: Investigation of relation between use of oral contraceptives and thromboembolic disease; a further report, Br. Med. J. **2**:651-657, 1969.

Lymphatics

Introduction

With the exception of certain rare tumors related to lymph vessels, such as diffuse lymphangioma and lymphangiosarcoma (Chapter 23), the primary lymphatic disease encountered clinically is lymphedema. Of course, chylothorax and chyloascites occur, but in nearly all instances these processes are secondary to trauma, neoplastic disease, or some infectious process.

Lymphedema

Lymphedema may be classified as postinfectious, posttraumatic, obstructive, and idiopathic. Obstructive lymphedema is most often seen following the obstruction of regional lymph nodes by neoplastic invasion or following their removal, as in radical mastectomy or in radical groin dissection. The development of lymphedema of the arm after radical mastectomy is thought more likely to follow in those patients in whom postoperative infection has produced fibrosis in the axilla or in those patients having persistent cancer in the axilla. However, lymphedema is seen in patients who give a history of as little trauma as a severely sprained ankle or following such infections as a furuncle.

Many patients give no history of trauma or infection associated with the onset of their lymphedema. In such instances, the lymphedema usually is termed idiopathic or lymphedema praecox. Congenital lymphedema is usually considered in this category and is differentiated from lymphedema praecox only in that the patient has had some degree of swelling of the extremity since infancy. Idiopathic lymphedema may develop in persons up to the age of 40 years.[10]

Pathology

The obstructive nature of neoplastic involvement of regional lymph nodes is obvious. Improved injection techniques combined with magnification roentgenography may serve to delineate accurately normal fine lymphatic channels as well as tumor involvement[7, 8, 12] (Fig. 1186).

The swelling of lymphedema is usually slowly progressive. There is dilatation of the dermal lymphatics as well as the deeper fascial lymphatics[2] (Fig. 1187). When the degree of swelling is advanced, there is a depression of hair follicles and gross dermal edema. In such cases, the cutaneous lymphatics may be sufficiently dilated to be associated with lymphorrhea following minor cutaneous abrasions or needle punctures (Fig. 1188). Tissue sections of such skin usually show markedly dilated dermal lymphatics.

All forms of lymphedema probably are in some way associated with inadequate lymphatic drainage.[5] Drinker and Yaffey[3] postulated that the increased protein content of the lymph present in chronic lymphatic stasis stimulates the deposition of fibrous tissue in the skin, subcutaneous tissue, and fascia. Such fibrosis aggravates the degree of inadequate lymphatic drainage and makes the disease slowly progressive.

Whatever the mechanism is, the slowly progressive nature of lymphedema in many patients is associated with dermal thickening and collagenous deposition in the subcutaneous tissues and fascia. Bouts of superficial cellulitis and lymphangitis often become superimposed upon the lymphedema in an extremity. In some patients, recurrent bouts of such infections are com-

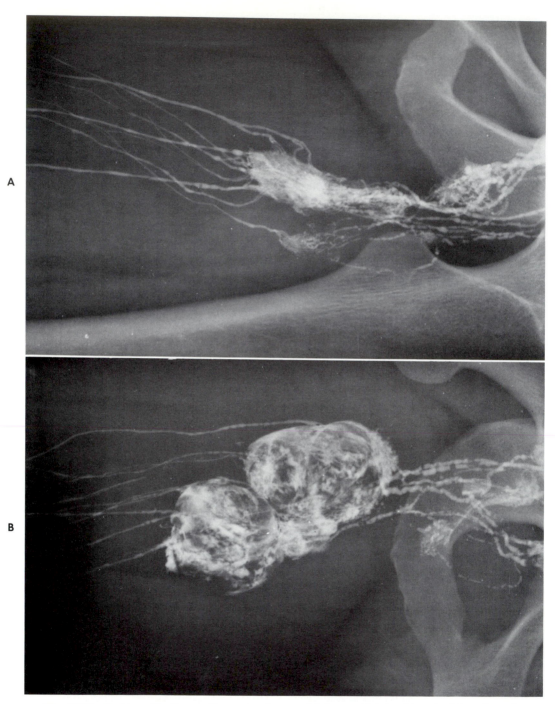

Fig. 1186 **A,** Magnification radiograph of normal left superficial subinguinal lymph node with afferent and efferent lymphatic channels in 40-year-old woman. **B,** Magnification radiograph of enlarged right superficial subinguinal lymph node with malignant infiltration secondary to primary melanoma of skin of heel. Same patient as shown in **A.** (**A** and **B,** From Isard, H. J., Ostrum, B. J., and Cullinan, J. E.: Magnification roentgenography; a "spot-film" technic, Med. Radiogr. Photogr. **38:**92-109, 1962.)

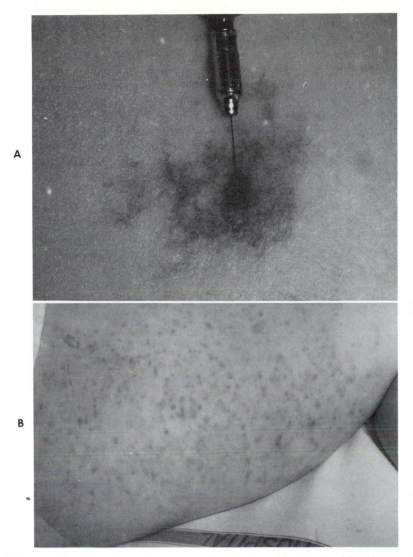

Fig. 1187 Injection of enlarged cutaneous lymphatics with 4% sky blue dye. Patient had obstructive lymphedema in inguinal region caused by Hodgkin's disease. **A,** Initial injection was made on lateral aspect of thigh. **B,** Four hours after injection, extensive retrograde filling of cutaneous lymphatics on skin of medial thigh had occurred. (**A** and **B,** From Butcher, H. R., Jr., and Hoover, A. L.: Abnormalities of human superficial cutaneous lymphatic cannulation, Ann. Surg. **142:**633-653, 1955.)

pletely incapacitating. The presence of recurrent infection in such an extremity appears to hasten the deposition of collagen and may result in such a large amount of fibrotic replacement of subcutaneous fat and normal dermal structures as to make demonstration of dermal lymphatics impossible.

Kinmonth et al.[6] reported the presence of dilated, valveless, deep lymphatic channels in idiopathic lymphedema. These were visualized at operation after the injection of patent blue dye and by roentgenologic lymphangiography. Although many varicose-like lymphatic trunks were found in their patients, in none was a definite proximal site of lymphatic channel obstruction discovered.

In a few patients with idiopathic lymphedema having no clinical evidence or

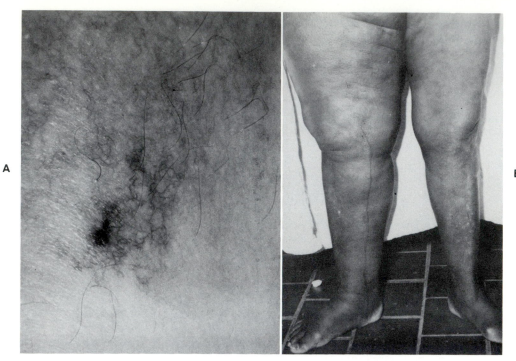

Fig. 1188   A, Dye-filled skin lymphatics in leg of patient with obstructive lymphedema.
B, Following cutaneous puncture for injection of lymphatics, dye-containing lymph flowed
from site. (**A** and **B,** From Butcher, H. R., Jr., and Hoover, A. L.: Abnormalities of human
superficial cutaneous lymphatic cannulation, Ann. Surg. **142:**633-653, 1955.)

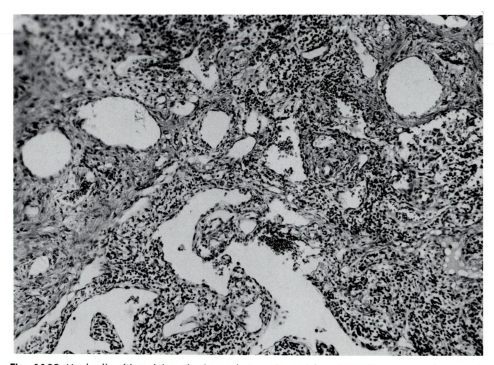

Fig. 1189 Markedly dilated lymph channels in enlarged lymph node removed from groin
of patient with idiopathic lymphedema of obstructive type.

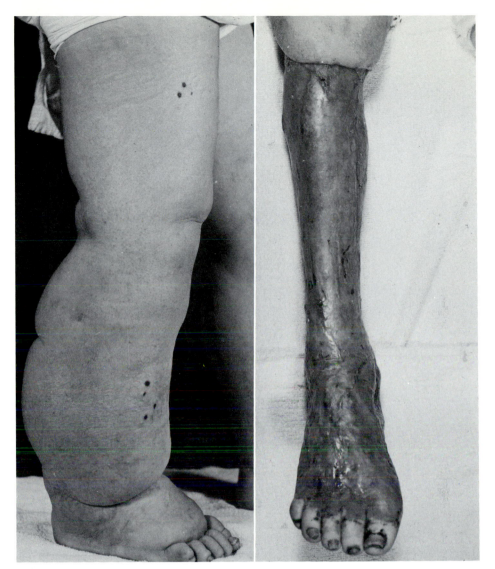

Fig. 1190 Preoperative and postoperative photographs of patient with long-standing infectious lymphedema. All fibrotic skin, subcutaneous tissue, and fascia were removed and defect was covered with split-thickness cutaneous autografts. (WU negs. 54-2266 and 54-2881; from Butcher, H. R., Jr., and Hoover, A. L.: Abnormalities of human superficial cutaneous lymphatic cannulation, Ann. Surg. **142:**633-653, 1955.)

history of lymphangitis or cellulitis in the extremity, enlarged regional lymph nodes have been removed. Microscopically, they contain a mild chronic inflammatory response, sinusoidal fibrosis, and markedly dilated lymphatic channels (Fig. 1189). Despite such findings, the pathogenesis responsible for the inadequate lymph drainage in most cases of lymphedema remains unknown.[1] Direct communication be-

tween lymph nodes and veins has been demonstrated by Pressman and Simon.[9]

Treatment

Treatment of lymphedema consists primarily of elevation of the extremity, compression, and massage, which must be maintained during many years of supervision. Recurrent bouts of streptococcal lymphangitis may be prevented by daily

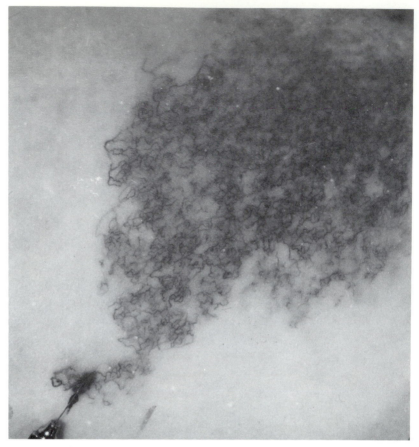

Fig. 1191 Unusually dilated superficial cutaneous lymphatics in skin of patient with idiopathic lymphedema. (From Butcher, H. R., Jr., and Hoover, A. L.: Abnormalities of human superficial cutaneous lymphatic cannulation, Ann. Surg. **142**:633-653, 1955.)

administration of penicillin orally. Such conservative measures will control the lymphedema sufficiently to avoid operation in many patients. Operative therapy is indicated only when the extent of subcutaneous fibrosis, infection, and massive swelling is sufficient to handicap the patient markedly.[10, 11]

The operation most useful is the excision of the thickened fibrotic skin, the edematous subcutaneous tissue, and the thickened fascia overlying the muscles, followed by the immediate application of split-thickness cutaneous autografts (Fig. 1190). The Sistrunk modification of the Kondoleon operation is no longer considered of value. The use of hyaluronidase and long, nonabsorbable subcutaneous sutures extending from the lymphedematous areas into the normal subcutaneous tissue have not proved of value.[4]

In patients with sufficiently severe lymphedema to require excision of the skin, subcutaneous tissue, and fascia of the extremity, gross examination of the excised portions shows dense fibrotic bands and sheets extending through the markedly swollen subcutaneous tissue. Pockets of fluid may be found in the intervening tissue spaces at operation. The skin over the fibrotic dermis may be atrophic in some areas and hyperplastic and keratotic in others. The collagenous thickening of the dermis is usually extreme. Lymphatic channels as such are often not seen histologically in such skin and subcutaneous tissue. This is particularly true if the process has been associated with multiple episodes of dermal infection. Dilated dermal lymphatics may be demonstrated histologically and by dye injection techniques in the skin of a lymphedematous extremity unassociated with long-standing episodes of infection (Fig. 1191).

The dermal and subcutaneous fibrosis similar to that seen in advanced forms of lymphedema also occurs about long-standing chronic stasis ulcers. The obliteration of dermal lymphatics, however, cannot be related primarily to the etiology of stasis ulcers since similar obliteration occurs in the fibrotic skin of long-standing lymphedema, a condition rarely associated with chronic ulceration of the lower extremity.

REFERENCES

1 Blocker, T. G., Jr., Smith, J. R., Dunton, E. F., Protas, J. M., Cooley, R. M., Lewis, S. R., and Kirby, E. J.: Studies of ulceration and edema of the lower extremity by lymphatic cannulation, Surgery **149**:884-896, 1959.

2 Butcher, H. R., Jr., and Hoover, A. L.: Abnormalities of human superficial cutaneous lymphatics associated with stasis ulcers, lymphedema, scars and cutaneous autographs, Ann. Surg. **142**:633-653, 1955.

3 Drinker, C. K., and Yaffey, J. M.: Lymphatics, lymph and lymphoid tissue; their physiological and clinical significance, Cambridge, Mass., 1941, Harvard University Press.

4 Foley, W. T.: The treatment of lymphedema, Surg. Gynecol. Obstet. **101**:25-34, 1955.

5 Kinmonth, J. B., and Taylor, G. W.: The lymphatic circulation in lymphedema, Ann. Surg. **139**:129-136, 1954.

6 Kinmonth, J. B., Taylor, G. W., Tracy, G. D., and Marsh, J. D.: Primary lymphoedema; clinical and lymphangiographic studies of a series of 107 patients in which the lower limbs were affected, Br. J. Surg. **95**:1-10, 1957.

7 McPeak, C. J., and Constantinides, S. G.: Lymphangiography in malignant melanoma; a comparison of clinicopathological and lymphangiographic findings in 21 cases, Cancer **17**:1586-1594, 1964.

8 Pomerantz, M., and Ketcham, A. S.: Lymphangiography and its surgical applications, Surgery **53**:589-597, 1963.

9 Pressman, J. J., and Simon, M. B.: Experimental evidence of direct communications between lymph nodes and veins, Surgery **113**:537-541, 1961.

10 Schirger, A., Harrison, E. G., Jr., and Janes, J. M.: Idiopathic lymphedema, J.A.M.A. **182**:124-132, 1962.

11 Thompson, N.: Surgical treatment of chronic lymphedema of extremities, Surg. Clin. North Am. **47**:445-503, 1967.

12 Wallace, S.: Dynamics of normal and abnormal lymphatic systems as studied with contrast media, Cancer Chemother. Rep. **52**:31-58, 1968.

26 Central nervous system

Congenital diseases

Most congenital malformations of the central nervous system that are amenable to surgical correction are associated with defects of the overlying bony structures. A less common group is represented by defects in the cerebrospinal fluid pathways.

Ectopia

Nodular collections of mature neural tissue, predominantly formed by astrocytic elements but occasionally also containing neurons and meningothelial cells, are sometimes found adjacent to the structures of the central nervous system. Nasal glioma, the most common variety, is discussed in Chapter 6. Goldring et al.[1] found ectopic neural tissue in the occipital bone of an adult. We have seen a well-circumscribed soft nodule in the soft tissues of the buttock composed of mature glial cells and ganglion cells, partially surrounded by a cleft lined by hyperplastic meningothelial cells, apparently not connected with the spinal canal. It is likely that all these lesions represent peculiar variants of the encephaloceles and meningomyeloceles described below.

Spina bifida

The group of malformations called spina bifida represent failures in the closure of

Despite such planning and the rather dire circumstances necessary to justify a biopsy, only about one-third yield a specific diagnosis, another third show abnormalities that are not diagnostic, and the remainder may yield normal tissue. Svennerholm[20] points out that most of the conditions specifically diagnosed can be easier diagnosed by other procedures and suggests that biopsy is really of more value for research than for diagnosis. As medical science is more successful in prolonging life, biopsy may be the only opportunity to learn more about the early phases of some diseases before late, nonspecific and secondary changes obliterate more essential features.[15]

Cellular inclusions in herpes, cytomegalic, and Dawson's encephalitis are examples of fairly specific morphologic landmarks, as are globoid cells in Krabbe's leukodystrophy and the brown granular bodies of metachromatic leukodystrophy.[16, 17] Fairly specific structural features in neurons in amaurotic familial idiocy, Alzheimer's disease, and Pick's disease may be demonstrated. Landing and Rubinstein[18] describe the features of many of these disorders in great detail and also point out other sites of biopsy that may yield helpful information, such as the liver in metachromatic leukodystrophy.[22]

Vascular diseases
Saccular aneurysms

Saccular aneurysms of the cerebral arteries comprise most of the acquired abnormalities of vessels that can be relieved by surgical treatment. They have been called congenital and berry aneurysms, but the fact that very few have ever been found in children and infants indicates that they are usually not present at birth, although certain important factors of formation may be congenital.

These lesions are the single most common cause of massive subarachnoid hemorrhage and occur most frequently in patients past the fourth decade and in those with hypertension. It has even been observed that patients with coarctation of the aorta and consequently hypertension in the carotid and brachial circulations have an apparently increased incidence of saccular aneurysms. About 80% of the lesions occur in that part of the circle of Willis derived from the carotid arteries, rostral to the posterior communicating arteries, with a great majority occurring within 3 cm of the terminations of the carotid arteries. The middle cerebral artery is most frequently involved, followed by the internal carotid and anterior cerebral arteries.

Multiple lesions may be found at postmortem examinations in perhaps one-fourth of the patients,[29] but it is unusual for more than one lesion to give symptoms. The problem of multiple lesions is important because the refinement of cerebral angiography has made the preoperative localization of these lesions much easier and has occasionally succeeded in demonstrating aneurysms that were not the site of the bleeding or symptoms. The coincidence of aneurysms and angiomas has been commented upon by Boyd-Wilson.[23]

The pathology of the saccular aneurysm is not of diagnostic importance, for the lesion is rarely examined before death. Nearly all occur in or very near the acute angles of bifurcations of the cerebral arteries, but when the sac is 1 cm or more in diameter, it is difficult, if not impossible, to define the site of its opening. This occurrence at the bifurcations has been explained by Forbus[26] as due to the maximum impact of the bloodstream at these points plus the presence of folds or defects in the muscle of the media in these sites.

Interpretation of the role of these medial defects has caused much controversy and misunderstanding.[24, 27] They occur in as many as one-third of the bifurcations of sizable cerebral arteries, even in newborn infants.[31, 33] It is therefore certain that they are not the sole factor in the formation of aneurysms, and probably they are more important in their localization than in their development. As Forbus[26] pointed out, the necessary prerequisite for initiation of the aneurysm is probably a defect or weaken-

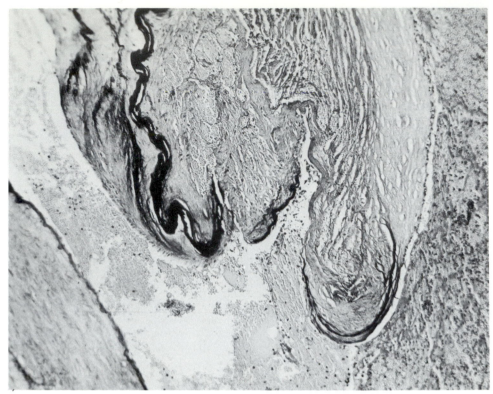

Fig. 1194 Saccular aneurysm of cerebral artery showing disruption of elastic lamella and muscularis at lip of mouth of aneurysm. Lumen of artery is to left and that of aneurysmal sac to right. (Verhoeff-van Gieson; ×125; WU neg. 52-4241.)

ing of the strongest layer of the wall—the elastic lamella (Fig. 1194). This would obviously be accelerated by increased intraluminal pressure and would most likely occur at the point of maximum impact, especially if that point overlies a discontinuity of the muscular media.

Other authors, particularly Dandy,[25] took exception to this view and maintained that most aneurysms occur on the straight parts of vessels at the sites of incomplete absorption of embryonic branches. They supported this contention with the observation that anomalies in the vessels of the circle of Willis in patients with aneurysms are more than usually frequent.

Regardless of the primeval nature of the origins of the aneurysms, the walls of the sacs are composed principally of fibrous connective tissue, and the elastic membrane and muscular media disappear at the edges of the mouth in ordinary microscopic sections. By electron microscopy,[28] smooth muscle cells, fine elastic fibers, and altered basement membranes can be observed and present appearances reminiscent of similar changes in the inner layers of arteries that are developing arteriosclerosis.

There are usually arteriosclerotic plaques in the wall of the sac or in the vessel about its mouth. Walker and Allegra[34] suggested that the fortuitous severity of such plaques may be the initiating factor that accomplishes the destruction of the elastic lamella and weakens the wall of the vessel. However, the correlation of aneurysms with general arteriosclerosis of the cerebral vessels is poor. Factors in the rupture of the lesions are not known other than the suggestion of overdistention of the fibrous sac.

After rupture, the effects on the surrounding brain vary with the site and direction of the rupture. The bleeding may occur simply into the subarachnoid space, or if the stream of blood under arterial pressure points toward cerebral substance, the effect may be much like that of a hose playing on sand with extensive dissection and destruction of tissue. Aneurysms of the anterior cerebral arteries sometimes dissect the opposite frontal lobe if the rupture is properly oriented, giving rise to evidence of hemorrhage and enlargement on the side of the normal artery. Rupture of the hemorrhage into the ventricles is not uncommon in fatal cases and usually occurs by dissection through the inferior and medial frontal lobe at the anterior extremity of the lateral ventricle.

Richardson and Hyland[30] reported that approximately 50% of patients with ruptured aneurysms recover with no therapy other than bed rest, and Slosberg[32] obtained successful results in twelve of fifteen patients treated only with induced hypotension. Repeated hemorrhages occur in one out of every seven patients.

Arteriovenous fistulas

Other than the communications between arteries and veins that arise in angiomas, intracranial arteriovenous fistulas develop principally between the internal carotid artery and the cavernous sinus because that is the only intracranial site where there is juxtaposition of a sizable artery and vein. Many are said to be of traumatic origin secondary to basilar skull fractures, but others develop from ruptured aneurysms of the internal carotid artery.

Symptoms include bruit, pulsating exophthalmos on the affected side, and evidence of disturbances of function of the third, fourth, and sixth nerves. Little can be said for the pathology of the lesions other than the gross observation of the communication between the artery and the vein, some surrounding fibrous reaction, and occasionally sclerotic plaques in the artery, fistula, or even the vein.

Cranial arteritis

Among the intrinsic diseases of the blood vessels of the head, cranial or granulomatous giant cell arteritis is most likely to come to the attention of the neurosurgeon. It is a febrile, self-limited disease of variable duration and unknown etiology. The greatest incidence is in women and in the seventh decade of life.

Prominent local signs are headache and pain in various structures of the head, but systemic symptoms such as malaise, anorexia, and weakness may be present. Involvement of the eye, with complete or partial loss of vision, may occur in as many as one-third of the patients. Cerebral symptoms may suggest focal ischemic damage or an encephalitis.[35]

A tender nodule is usually palpable along the course of the temporal artery. The disease may involve other cranial arteries and has been reported to occur concomitantly with similar lesions in arteries elsewhere, but there is some suggestion that it is related to a rather specific type of senile elastic degeneration and perielastic hyalinosis that occur in the normal temporal artery.

Histologically, cranial arteritis is a fibrosis of the intima with focal necrosis and granulomas of the media characterized by the presence of a few giant cells and an infiltrate of round cells but very few or no eosinophils. Kimmelstiel et al.[36] described the giant cells in association with the disrupted internal elastic membrane and considered the presence of fragments of that tissue in the cytoplasm of the giant cells as pathognomonic of this entity. Otherwise, the changes are similar to those of polyarteritis nodosa.

No specific therapy is known, but symptoms are often relieved by taking a biopsy, presumably due to the interruption of the periarterial plexus of nerves.

Another variety of giant cell granulomatous angiitis confined to the central nervous system has been distinguished from cranial arteritis.[37] This is a diffuse involvement of small arteries and veins. Necrosis within the granulomas is not a feature, and no elastic fragments are present in the giant cells, which may form the actual wall of small vessels. Therapy with steroids apparently has some beneficial effect. Earlier reports probably have not separated cases of this type from other examples of arteritis involving cranial arteries.

Effects of vascular insufficiency

The effects on the brain of vascular insufficiency are responsible for a great deal of morbidity but are usually common general pathologic processes of no special interest to the surgical pathologist. Two conditions, however, can give rise to a difficult symptomatology of acute intracranial pressure and may be recognized only on exploration and biopsy: acute encephalomalacia and pseudotumor cerebri.

Acute encephalomalacia

Acute encephalomalacia or ischemic infarction, in its early stages, may be accompanied by tremendous edema and swelling of the affected tissue and ventricular displacement suggestive of a tumor. The surgeon has no difficulty in recognizing the tissue as abnormal, and rarely is there an opportunity to demonstrate the actual causative lesion in the deeply buried blood vessel serving the involved region.

Although the arterial circulation of the brain is endarterial in pattern, there are innumerable communications at the capillary and precapillary levels between the distributions of the various major arteries. It is apparently by means of these connections that fluid enters the damaged tissue to cause the remarkable swelling. Pathologically, this tissue is usually seen only in the acute phase when its gross characteristics are principally its softness and moistness.

Microscopically, the elements of the tissue are irregularly separated, and perivascular and pericellular spaces are widened but empty. There may be small foci of diapedesis of erythrocytes. The most frequent definite histologic change is a leukostasis in the capillaries and small vessels with occasional small fibrin thrombi and migration of leukocytes through the vascular walls. Neurons may retain an essentially normal appearance for several days after the onset of symptoms. There is no evidence of proliferative glial reaction. The lack of lymphocytic cellular infiltrate about larger vessels and the lack of the evidence of damage or death of individual neurons distinguish this picture from that of an encephalitis. Not until three to five days after the onset do macrophages, peripheral vascular proliferation, and other better-recognized reactions to an infant appear.

Pseudotumor cerebri

Pseudotumor cerebri consists of the rather sudden appearance of the signs of increased intracranial pressure without other signs or symptoms suggestive of etiologic factors.[38, 39] Almost one-half the cases occur in persons in the third decade of life. The ventricular system is normal on ventriculography, and the cerebrospinal fluid is normal to examination and analysis. Zuidema and Cohen[40] determined by follow-up of a large series that there were three etiologic groups into which such cases could be eventually assigned:

1 Early and otherwise undetectable brain tumors
2 Dural sinus thrombosis that is usually a sequela of upper respiratory infection
3 A large idiopathic group in which the prognosis for recovery is very good

If the brain is biopsied, the tissue is usually remarkably normal, but occasionally it may present the histologic picture of acute encephalomalacia.

Traumatic diseases

Patients with acute traumatic lesions of the central nervous system comprise a high percentage of those treated by the neurosurgeon. Wounds create difficult and perplexing problems in diagnosis and therapy but supply very little material of pathologic interest. The physics of the distribution of forces about the skull and the physiology of acute cranial and spinal injuries are fields of study in themselves.[42]

Acute concussion leaves no recognizable morphologic equivalent. Contusion of the brain results only in physical disruption of its substance and acute hemorrhages. Material from more chronic lesions of traumatic origin, however, is more likely to come to the attention of the pathologist during the operative relief of posttraumatic epilepsy.[41]

Dural-cortical cicatrix

The dural-cortical cicatrix as the lesion responsible for much posttraumatic epilepsy has been ably investigated and explained by Penfield and Erickson.[43] A fibrous scar and adhesions develop between the dura mater and other extra-arachnoidal fibrous tissue and the brain substance.

Penetrating wounds of the brain and its coverings are most likely to be responsible for the development of this lesion, although it can follow skull fractures, hemorrhages, or abscesses.[44] It is less commonly a postoperative complication because its development is dependent upon the introduction of extraneous fibrous tissue into the brain wound rather than upon the amount of cerebral substance destroyed or removed. This connective tissue stimulates the proliferation of astrocytes that bind it to the surrounding viable brain. Capillaries grow out from the implant of fibrous tissue into the substance of the central nervous system and anastomose with the normal vascular bed in that site. This supplies a direct union of the external and internal carotid circulations.

Because the external carotid circulation is subject to much greater variation in flow due to greater vasomotor activity, the amount of blood in this newly formed abnormal bed is subject to considerable variation. This unstable vascular bed inevitably has at least an indirect effect on the blood supply of the surrounding cortex, and it is postulated that its variations are the trigger mechanism for the convulsions.

Surgical therapy of this condition consists of accurate delimitation of the electrically abnormal cortex by means of electrocorticograms and its excision along with the overlying fibrous adhesions. The pathologic specimen is an irregular mixture of fibrous and glial tissue that is usually characterized by distinct astrocytic gliosis. There may be macrophages, hemosiderin, or other evidences of the process of the acute injury depending upon its nature and the length of time since its occurrence.

Cortical excisions for jacksonian epilepsy are sometimes performed in the absence of cortical meningeal adhesions or scars. Such specimens are usually remarkably normal in appearance but deserve full examination since they occasionally contain evidence of an otherwise silent tumor.

Epidural hematoma

Hemorrhage in the epidural space is most often arterial and posttraumatic and is due to the rupture of an artery such as the middle meningeal incidental to a fracture involving the foramen by which the artery enters the skull.[45] These lesions are acute surgical emergencies. A much more rare epidural hemorrhage may be of venous origin following trauma and of chronic duration.[46]

Subdural hematoma

Subdural hematomas are of two varieties, occurring most commonly at the two extremes of life, infancy and old age.

The type seen in infants is the result of intracranial hemorrhage that usually has occurred at the time of birth. The infant's skull is deformed and distorted by the pressure and process of birth. This places a tension and shearing force on certain structures such as the tentorium, vein of Galen, and other bridging veins. If a major vessel ruptures, the infant dies during or soon after birth, but if bleeding is slow and slight, there may be only the symptoms of lethargy that later deepen into coma. Enlargement of the head may be one of the first noticeable signs. Because of the lack of full myelination in infancy, paralytic and motor phenomena that might be expected are often lacking.

The diagnosis and even the therapy can often be performed by aspiration through the fontanel. However, fluid tends to reaccumulate in the sacs. On exploration, a thin gray membrane is found forming a sac in the subdural space. It is filled with blood, bloody fluid, or sometimes yellow or clear fluid. The membrane itself may have yellow foci, especially on its inner surface. It is usually loosely adherent to the dura but not to the arachnoid.

Microscopically, these subdural hematomas are usually thin membranes composed of fibroblasts and relatively few blood vessels. The inner surface is often covered by a rather thick single layer of flattened cells that are probably fibroblasts. In the interstices of the tissue there are relatively few lymphocytes and histiocytes and, occasionally, foci of hemosiderin. The appearance is rarely as similar to granulation tissue as is often seen in subdural hematomas in adults. Once the blood has been removed, these membranes are apparently completely resorbed into the dura unless there is a bleeding point or a tear in the arachnoid that allows fluid to return. On rare occasions, the membranes may calcify.[48]

Essentially the same lesion sometimes develops in response to cerebrospinal fluid that has escaped into the subdural space, where it cannot be resorbed. Such lesions are called subdural hygromas. Their formation is apparently dependent upon the lack of absorptive abilities on the part of the subdural space. The fluid is supplied through the tear in the arachnoid that presumably has something of a valvular action. The membrane about the pocket of fluid is not essential to its formation or retention and may consist of little more than adhesions between the dura and the arachnoid.

Subdural hematomas in adults are considerably different lesions. Trauma to the head is almost always responsible for their formation, although there may be other factors such as a bleeding tendency or the widened subarachnoid spaces of arteriosclerotic cerebral atrophy that make it possible for this trauma to be so slight as to pass unnoticed.

The initial lesion must be a rupture of a small bridging vein in the subdural space, although some authors have suggested that bleeding from arteries or capillaries might also be responsible. This rupture often occurs in the contrecoup position because these veins are stretched by the displacement of the skull in the line of the blow and at the same time are subjected to the convergence of the transmitted forces that pass around the vault of the skull. The initial blow may cause a period of unconsciousness due to concussion or even contusion of the brain. In the latter instance, the patient's course is usually stormy from the very start, but it is also just as characteristic for the patient to recover consciousness and be essentially free of symptoms for a period of several weeks. There then appear, often rather suddenly, the signs and symptoms of increased intracranial pressure that may be accompanied by motor and paralytic phenomena, for these lesions are often near the motor cortex.

Pathologically, the well-developed lesion is a discoid sac filled with dark, partially laked blood (Fig. 1195). The gray membrane of the sac may be several millimeters thick. It is grossly similar on all sides of the hemorrhage but is attached to the dura on the outer side. It is smooth and unattached to the arachnoid on the inner side.

Microscopically, the membrane is composed of large fibroblasts, capillaries with thick endothelial walls, newly formed vessels and endothelial buds, and an infiltrate of histiocytes and lymphocytes (Fig. 1196). Many of the histiocytes contain hemosiderin, and hematoidin may be present to supply a grossly visible golden color. The histologic picture is quite similar to that of granulation tissue except for the

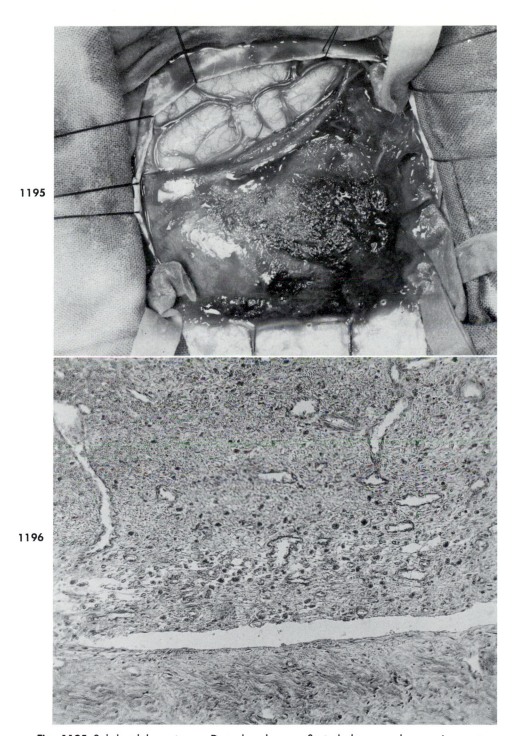

Fig. 1195 Subdural hematoma. Dura has been reflected downward, exposing neomembrane and hematoma in situ, and normal underlying pia-arachnoid and brain are exposed in upper part of field. (WU neg. 52-5356; courtesy Dr. H. G. Schwartz, St. Louis, Mo.)
Fig. 1196 Subdural hematoma. Cleft demarcates coarse collagenous tissue of dura from overlying organized membrane of hematoma. (Masson trichrome; ×125; WU neg. 52-4240.)

absence of prominent numbers of granular leukocytes.

The mechanisms of the development of the complete symptom-producing lesion have been well investigated. Leary[47] showed that there were four recognizable anatomic stages which could supply a basis for an estimate of the time from the onset of hemorrhage.

1 For the first eighteen hours, the subdural blood remained fluid or formed soft, nonadherent clots.

2 During the second and third days, the clots were recognizably firmer and adherent to the dura.

3 From the fourth day through the second week, the blood was very dark, clotted, and sometimes separated from a yellow fluid. Evidence of organization was visible on the dural surface, but there was no inner covering or neomembrane.

4 The last stage consisted of formation of the neomembrane, which was observed in one of his patients to be completely formed thirty-nine days after injury. After the complete double membrane is formed, it may persist for months or even years with no reliable anatomic changes to represent its age.

The mechanism of the production of symptoms of a space-occupying lesion by an old subdural hematoma is obscure because of contradictory results from the study of different cases. A most attractive thesis, although it has apparently never been demonstrated in experimental animals, is that the hematoma begins to behave as an osmometer. With completion of the enclosing membrane, the hemorrhage becomes a volume of fluid that contains cells, proteins, and salts. Zollinger and Gross[50] demonstrated that the surrounding sac had the properties of a semipermeable membrane when removed intact and connected to an osmometer. Furthermore, the protein content of the fluid in old subdural hematomas is one-third or less than that of whole blood due to disintegration of the proteins and imbibition

of fluid by means of osmotic forces. The source of this new fluid is probably the plasma of the capillaries in the surrounding membrane, and its method of accumulation accounts for the late onset of symptoms. The hemorrhage does not have a space-occupying effect until the sac is closed and its volume increased. However, there are also other phenomena that may help explain the clinical course.

Hemorrhages of various ages recognizable by the stage of preservation of erythrocytes are often seen within the membrane, so some of the increase of volume (particularly in hematomas that have been evacuated) may be due to fresh hemorrhages from the thin capillaries in the membrane. There is also a controversy as to the role of intradural hemorrhage in the formation of this lesion, but, to say the least, that theory has not gained general acceptance and would apparently apply more often to the lesions of vascular disease or hemorrhagic dyscrasias than to those of trauma.

Therapy consists of evacuation of the hemorrhage. The membranes often have been removed against the possibility of their refilling, but experience has shown this is not always necessary or advisable.[49] The success of treatment apparently depends more upon the condition of the underlying brain than upon the operative procedure itself. Since many persons with these lesions are elderly, their brains are atrophied by the effects of arteriosclerosis and arteriolosclerosis. With removal of the hematoma, the displaced and compressed cerebral tissue does not expand and return to its normal position, and functional improvement is equally unsatisfactory. Histologic examination of the underlying cortex will show principally thickening of the small vessels and loss of neurons with a slight hypertrophy and hyperplasia of astrocytes.

Chronic arachnoiditis and arachnoidal cyst

Chronic arachnoiditis may follow the introduction of foreign substances into the subarachnoid space. This is most likely to occur in the region of the lumbar sac and to be characterized by involvement of the spinal roots of the cauda equina, but occasionally a similar etiology is blamed for the formation of pockets of fluid in the subarachnoid space that are called arachnoidal cysts. The lesion may be a sequel of accidents during spinal anesthesia, and its crippling effects may be as severe as a paraplegia.[53]

The pathologic findings are usually more obvious in situ than they are in a histologic section. A distinct thickness, grayness, and opacity of the membrane can be observed at operation. Microscopically, the most that can usually be seen is a bland fibrous membrane that is several times thicker than the normal pia-arachnoid but that contains no evidence of inflammation beyond a few lymphocytes. Only very rarely are foreign substances, macrophages, and giant cells of a foreign body reaction identifiable.

Not all arachnoidal cysts are clearly of this origin. Some are undoubtedly congenital, but all are characterized by the nonspecific histologic character of their walls.

There are also other rare cystic lesions such as epidural cerebrospinal cysts that are due to herniation of a sac of pia-arachnoid through a congenital or acquired defect of the dura. These can occur in the spinal vertebral canal and give the signs and symptoms of cord compression like a tumor.[52] Miller and Elder[51] reported ten cases of paraspinal cysts occurring as a complication of laminectomy, probably the result of a tear in the dura-arachnoid layer. The cysts communicated with the arachnoid space and were lined by flattened connective tissue cells.

Cysts also occur at the intervertebral foramina, particularly of the sacrum, where they may compress the spinal nerves. These are often filled with a rather glairy fluid and are thought to be isolated diverticula of pia-arachnoid.

Ruptured intervertebral discs

Ruptured intervertebral discs are lesions of possibly traumatic origin and are of importance principally for the effects they produce on the central nervous system.[54] The great majority of these lesions occur between the lumbar vertebrae and produce signs of irritation and destruction of fibers in the roots of the cauda equina. They also occur at higher sites, where they cause pressure upon the spinal cord itself. In these instances, the root pain characteristic of the lower lesions is not prominent. Instead, there result confusing syndromes suggestive of such degenerative diseases as amyotrophic lateral sclerosis.

The material removed at operation is only fibroelastic cartilage which may show slight degenerative changes such as fibrillar stroma and focal calcification. The essential pathologic changes are probably in the outer layers of the intervertebral disc, which are weakened and destroyed and allow the central portions to herniate. As such, they are not observed or available for study.

Inflammatory diseases

Inflammatory diseases of the central nervous system that are subject to surgical treatment are of two types. In one, the process is focal and behaves as a space-occupying lesion (abscesses, granulomas). In the second, inflammatory changes in the meninges create the necessity of decompressing the underlying nerve tissue or of relieving the obstruction in the flow of cerebrospinal fluid (hydrocephalus following meningitis and an obscure condition that can be termed a chronic pachymeningitis).

Chronic pachymeningitis

Chronic pachymeningitis has been customarily ascribed to syphilis. The typical lesions is said to be a gummatous inflammation of the dura mater in the cervical region that forms a collar about the spinal cord and compresses it. There are, however, other cases in which there is great thickening of the dura mater in relatively wide expanses of the skull as well as in the vertebral canal. The membrane may reach a thickness of 1 cm and have the consistency of a tendon.

The symptomatology varies with the site of maximum involvement and is likely to include signs of pressure on various cranial nerves, the brainstem, or the spinal cord. Fever is sometimes present.[55]

Grossly, the tissue is a tough grayish yellow membrane several millimeters in thickness. Microscopically, it is composed of fibroblasts, collagenous fibers, and a light infiltrate of lymphocytes, plasma cells, and a few leukocytes and eosinophils. The cellular infiltrate is often concentrated in perivascular foci, and there may be small areas of necrosis. The blood vessels may be thickened and contain a few inflammatory cells in their walls.

The occurrence of fever in this disease and the localization of the lesion in the dura over the base of the skull have suggested that it may be related to chronic infection and inflammation of sinuses or retropharyngeal tissues. There is no evidence of syphilis in most patients. The course is apparently mildly progressive, and surgical removal of the thickened membrane can give worthwhile relief by decompression of involved structures.

Brain abscess

Experience with abscesses of the brain has changed greatly in the years since the introduction of modern chemotherapeutic agents.[57, 60] Although acute and chronic mastoiditis, which formerly anteceded a majority of brain abscesses, have declined markedly, the incidence of brain abscess appears to be about the same as it was previously.

This lesion occurs predominantly in the earlier decades of life. The symptoms are essentially those of an acute intracranial tumefaction. Headache, fever, and vomiting are the most common symptoms, and nausea, seizures, hemiplegia, and other neurologic symptoms may be observed. It is sometimes remarked that bradycardia is more common with abscesses than with tumors, presumably because of the more

acute development of elevated intracranial pressure.

Two-thirds or more of the abscesses formerly were associated with local suppurative disease in the adjacent ear or nasal sinuses and one-fourth with suppurative pulmonary disease or bacterial endocarditis. The remainder followed trauma or incidental conditions or were of idiopathic origin. In the series reported by Kerr et al.,[59] one-half arose from direct extension from the ear, sinuses, or skull, and one-third were of hematogenous origin. These groupings also indicate the principal methods by which the infection reaches the brain:

1 By contiguous spread, utilizing infected thrombi in veins

2 By emboli in the arterial bloodstream or possibly distant venous embolization by way of the vertebral veins

3 By direct inoculation or unknown methods

The abscesses of the first group are associated with infection of the middle ear or sinuses about equally, although formerly they arose from the mastoid from four to nine times as frequently as from the sinuses. Lesions arising by contiguous spread and localizing in the frontal lobe or anterior fossa are characteristically associated with frontal sinusitis and subsequent osteomyelitis. Those of the middle fossa follow chronic middle ear infection. The cerebellar abscesses are associated with infected thrombosis of the lateral sinus or chronic labyrinthitis which, in turn, follows infection of the middle ear or mastoid. The abscess is not always immediately adjacent to the focus of chronic infection, however, for the inoculum can apparently be carried as an infected embolus in cerebral or diploic veins for considerable distances. In general, the proportion of temporal lobe to cerebellar involvement in abscesses following ear disease is approximately two to one, but only one-eighth of all abscesses occur in the posterior fossa.

Lesions that arise by hematogenous

spread are distributed to the various parts of the brain according to their volumes. Many of the particularly unfavorable cases of multiple abscesses develop lesions by this mechanism.

The initial focus of involvement in an abscess is apparently immediately beneath the cortex which, with its high content of astrocytes, retains the developing lesion and prevents its outward rupture, although extension toward and into the ventricles is not so opposed.[56, 58] Judging by our knowledge of the development of abscesses elsewhere, there must be an early stage of diffuse pyogenic inflammation followed by liquefaction of tissue and then formation of a pyogenic membrane.

In the brain, this membrane is much like that of abscesses in other tissues. There is an inner zone of necrotic tissue and fibrin heavily infiltrated with leukocytes and a middle zone of proliferated capillaries and fibroblasts, which respond unusually extensively for lesions of the central nervous tissue. These zones are infiltrated with leukocytes and histiocytes which phagocytize the lipids of the destroyed brain. Beyond this, there is a zone of astrocytic glial proliferation that is naturally characteristic of abscesses in this tissue. A plane of cleavage often exists in this region so that well-encapsulated abscesses can be enucleated with removal of very little adherent surrounding brain. The pyogenic membrane about an abscess of the brain requires at least two weeks for complete development, but its first traces in wounds can be seen grossly in as few as four or five days.

The bacterial etiology of brain abscesses may be staphylococci, streptococci, pneumococci, or various other organisms, especially gram-negative rods. Pneumococci and beta hemolytic streptococci are much less frequent causative organisms than formerly, while anaerobic streptococci and enterococci are of increased importance. Many abscesses today are sterile by culture at the time of operation.

Many different methods of surgical treat-ment of abscesses have been used. The single most important contribution to their effective therapy has been the modern antibiotics. It has been long recognized that operation upon a well-encapsulated lesion may give the most favorable result, but many patients become desperately ill before complete encapsulation takes place. Mortality rates of greater than 40% were the rule before the spread of infection could be so well controlled by drugs, but a rate of less than 20% may now be expected if the abscesses are not multiple. Excision and treatment of early abscesses in the stages before encapsulation may be even more effective.[61] It is significant that in one series of cerebellar abscesses, only two of nine patients survived before the advent of penicillin, whereas eight of nine survived when penicillin was used. Chemotherapy is not the whole answer, however, and there remains the necessity of surgical drainage or removal of loculated suppuration.

Granulomatous diseases

Granulomas of the central nervous system are most frequently due to tuberculosis but may be caused by syphilis or various fungal diseases, such as cryptococcosis, actinomycosis, or mucormycosis. Because of their space-occupying properties, these lesions present a clinical picture essentially that of a tumor. They make up 2% to 3% of a group of lesions diagnosed at first as tumors. The infectious inoculum of these lesions is borne by the blood to the central nervous system, and its localization there is consequently dependent upon the relative size and vascularity of the various areas. Being a disease of adults, granulomas are, therefore, relatively more common in the posterior fossa than are primary glial tumors.

The histology of these lesions is comparable to that of the same diseases as they occur elsewhere with perhaps a relatively less prominent fibroblastic component in their composition. Fungal lesions vary from those that are more properly described as abscesses to others that are quite solid and like tuberculomas or gummas.[62, 63, 65] The specific diagnosis rests upon the recognition of the causative organisms either in tissues or by culture.

Parasitic infestation of the central nervous system by *Cysticercus, Amoeba,* or *Echinococcus* is rare in this country. Depending upon the number and size of the lesions, they can present the symptoms of either space-occupying masses or a more diffuse process suggestive of an encephalitis. Rayport et al.[64] have reported an interesting case in which hydatids of *Echinococcus* in the vertebra resulted in a compression myelopathy.

Tumors
Introduction

Neoplasms of the central nervous system have several unique features, some as the result of the very specialized tissue from which they originate and others from the anatomic peculiarities of this region. This should not detract from the fact that, by and large, their morphologic patterns and biologic behavior can be adequately studied by applying the same principles and techniques as those employed for tumors elsewhere in the body. Knowledge of the age of the patient, exact location of the tumor, and its gross appearance at operation are essential pieces of information that the pathologist should possess in order to properly evaluate a microscopic slide. Examination by frozen section at the time of operation is as accurate for neural neoplasms as it is for tumors in general.

Much has been argued about the value of silver and gold impregnation techniques (principally those of Golgi, Cajal, and del Rio Hortega) in the identification of central nervous system neoplasms. Some pathologists believe they are essential for the proper classification of these tumors and advocate their use as a routine procedure.[67] Others seriously doubt their diagnostic utility. It seems obvious that they have greatly contributed to our understanding of this family of neoplasms and that the researcher in the field might still profit from them, as he might profit from electron microscopic examination, tissue culture studies, or histochemical techniques. But we must agree with Willis,[69] Kernohan and Sayre,[66] Rubinstein,[68] and many others that, in the overwhelming majority of the cases, examination of sections from formalin-fixed, paraffin-embedded material stained with hematoxylin-eosin (sometimes supplemented by PTAH, reticulin, or other stains) is perfectly adequate for the classification and prognostic evaluation of tumors of the central nervous system.

Tumors of neuroglial cells
Astrocytoma

Tumors originated from adult astrocytes are the most common type of glioma and, for that matter, the most common primary neoplasms of the central nervous system. All ages are affected. It is very useful to divide astrocytomas into clinicopathologic varieties on the basis of their different age incidence, location, and biologic behavior.

Cerebral astrocytomas are generally tumors of adults. Their gross boundaries are very difficult to define. They are solid, whitish or gray, and may infiltrate the cortex, white matter, or basal ganglia. The microscopic diagnosis is often difficult, since the cells are mature and widely scattered between normal structures. The only clue to the diagnosis in a biopsy may be slight nuclear enlargement and hyperchromasia, with accumulation of cells beneath the pia, around neurons or surrounding the Virchow-Robin spaces.[85] The cytologic appearance seen in a small biopsy may not be representative of the whole neoplasm. We have seen many cases in which extremely well-differentiated astrocytes in the superficial portion of the tumor coexisted with highly atypical cells in deeper areas. Grading of these tumors is, therefore, of little prognostic value.

Cerebellar astrocytomas are predominantly tumors of children. They may oc-

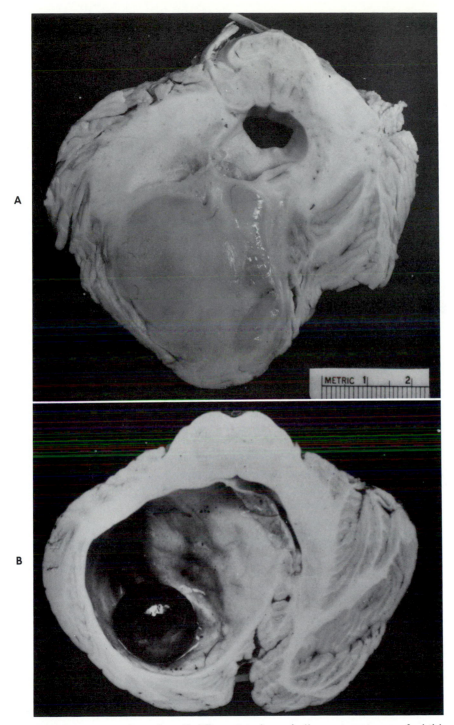

Fig. 1197 Two examples of well-differentiated cerebellar astrocytoma of children, illustrating two most common forms of gross presentation. **A,** Predominantly solid neoplasm of gray color and firm consistency. **B,** Cystic tumor with sharply circumscribed, hemorrhagic mural nodule. (**A,** UVa neg. 11,148; **B,** WU neg. 72-5924; from Rubinstein, L. J.: Seminario de Neuropatología, Mérida, Yucatán, Bol. Asoc. Mex. Patol., A. C., **7:**13-59, 1969; courtesy Dr. J. E. Olvera-Rabiela, Mexico City, Mexico.)

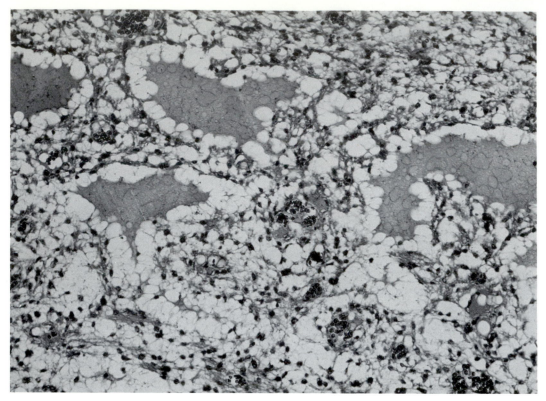

Fig. 1198 Well-differentiated astrocytoma of cerebellum in child. Multiple cystic spaces containing proteinaceous material are characteristic. (×175; WU neg. 73-2665.)

cupy the cerebellar hemispheres or the vermis or even extend within the cavity of the fourth ventricle. Grossly, they may appear solid, of a homogeneous gray color, firm consistency, and ill-defined borders, or as a cystic mass with a mural, frequently hemorrhagic nodule (Fig. 1197). Microscopically, cellular areas composed of mature fibrillary astrocytes are present, often surrounding microcystic formations containing an eosinophilic amorphous material (Fig. 1198). Multinucleated astrocytes may be seen, but mitoses are exceptional. Rosenthal fibers, representing amorphous aggregates of unknown composition in the glial cell processes, can often be identified.[75] Cerebellar astrocytomas are among the most benign tumors of the brain. Their successful removal will result in a complete and permanent cure.[71]

Astrocytomas of the third ventricle are sometimes called pilocytic (hairlike), be-

cause of the marked elongation of the tumor cells which has been responsible in the past for the erroneous designation of this tumor as polar spongioblastoma. Specific silver stains, growth in tissue culture, and electron microscopic studies have clearly demonstrated their astrocytic nature.[77, 84] Rosenthal fibers and microcystic areas are often encountered.

Astrocytomas of pons and medulla are generally tumors of children. Grossly, they are solid, gray or whitish, and result in a symmetrical enlargement of the pons and medulla (Fig. 1199). Microscopically, a whole spectrum of cytologic atypia can be found, even within the same neoplasm. A significant portion of the cells have a pilocytic configuration.

Astrocytomas of spinal cord are more common in the thoracic and cervical segments. They are solid, of firm consistency, and often elongated. Microscopically, they

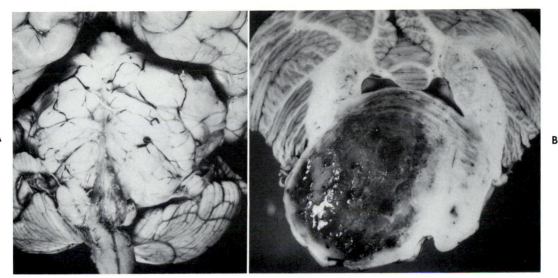

Fig. 1199   A, External appearance of astrocytoma of pons, illustrating symmetrical enlargement of structure often seen in this tumor. **B,** Cross section of astrocytoma of pons,
showing hemorrhagic tumor of ill-defined margins partially obliterating fourth ventricle.
(**A,** WU neg. 72-5923; **B,** WU neg. 72-5926; courtesy Dr. J. E. Olvera-Rabiela, Mexico
City, Mexico.)

display no specific characteristics. Like
those of the brainstem and third ventricle,
they may contain pilocytic elements.

Astrocytomas of the optic nerve constitute the majority of the tumors collectively
named "optic nerve glioma," the remaining
being oligodendrogliomas. The distinction
is difficult and often requires silver impregnation techniques. In children, optic nerve
astrocytomas are slow growing and usually behave as benign neoplasms. In adults,
this tumor is often highly aggressive and
fatal.[78]

In *diffuse astrocytoma (gliomatosis cerebri),* neoplastic astrocytes are seen occupying extensive areas of the cerebrum, cerebellum and brainstem without producing
a grossly evident tumor mass.[72] Most cells
are microscopically mature but, as in other
astrocytomas, anaplastic foci are occasionally detected.

It is obvious that age, location, and
gross features, in conjunction with the
microscopic appearance, play an important
role in the characterization of the varieties
of astrocytomas already mentioned. In addition, there are histologic features which

need to be recognized and evaluated independently of the above. The occurrence
of *pilocytic astrocytomas* has already been
alluded to. It probably represents a secondary feature dictated by the disposition of
the preexisting nerve fibers and has no
particular prognostic significance. Although
the pilocytic cells are almost always well
differentiated, this does not preclude the
existence of anaplastic elements in other
portions of the tumor. *Gemistocytic astrocytomas,* in which the tumor astrocytes are
characterized by an abundant, brightly
acidophilic cytoplasm, can be seen as a
pure form (particularly in the cerebellum
or, in patients with tuberous sclerosis, in
the wall of the lateral ventricles) or, most
commonly, intermingled with areas of ordinary astrocytoma. Their presence has no
prognostic significance but for the fact that
they appear most commonly in well-differentiated neoplasms. Astrocytic tumors
formed by compact small cells that arrange
themselves around blood vessels were
designated as *astroblastomas* by Bailey and
Bucy.[70] Only rarely are they present as a
pure form. In most instances, this pattern

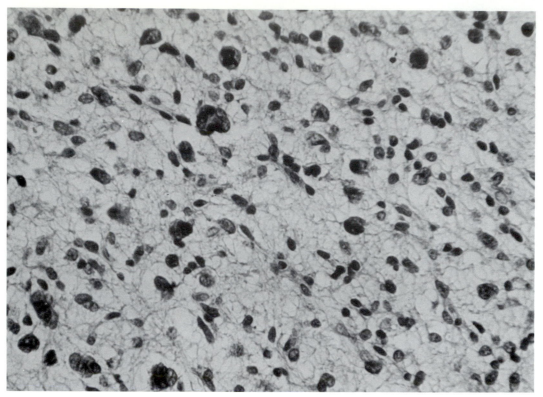

Fig. 1200 Malignant astrocytoma of cerebral hemisphere. Despite marked cytologic atypia, astrocytic nature of tumor is evident even in routinely stained sections. (×300; WU neg. 73-2689.)

of growth is seen focally as an otherwise typical astrocytoma or in an undifferentiated glioma.

The most important feature to evaluate in the microscopic examination of an astrocytoma is the presence of atypia of the tumor astrocytes, evidenced by nuclear enlargement, nucleolar prominence and mitotic activity, often accompanied by vascular proliferation and areas of necrosis. The occurrence of these alterations can be regarded as a reliable sign forecasting aggressive clinical behavior, which may be manifest by local invasion of the surrounding parenchyma and meninges, spread through the cerebrospinal fluid pathways, and, exceptionally, by metastatic involvement of distant organs. On the other hand, the absence of these atypical features in a biopsy specimen should not be used as conclusive evidence that the tumor lacks these properties. Astrocytomas are well

known for their marked variations in degrees of maturity from area to area. This variability, although rare in cerebellar tumors, is quite common in neoplasms of the cerebral hemispheres.

The astrocytic lineage of many cytologically malignant glial neoplasms is evident with the use of special stains or, in hematoxylin-eosin sections, by the common intermingling of well-differentiated elements. The term *malignant astrocytoma* is properly applied to this tumor type (Fig. 1200). In other cases, however, the dedifferentiation is so great that an astrocytic origin cannot be established. The designation of *glioblastoma multiforme* has traditionally been given to this variety. This term is unsatisfactory on several grounds. First, it implies an origin from (or at least a relationship with) the embryonal glioblast which probably does not exist. All the available evidence seems to

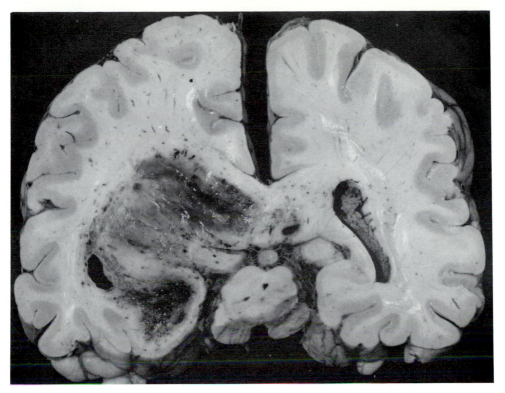

Fig. 1201 Undifferentiated glioma of left parietal and temporal lobes with extension into corpus callosum. Variegated surface and foci of hemorrhage are characteristic. (UVa neg. 11,026.)

indicate that this tumor is instead the result of progressive dedifferentiation in a neoplasm that originated in an adult cell. Second, it conveys the impression of a specific tumor type when it simply represents the undifferentiated form of all types of gliomas. Admittedly, the large majority of tumors called glioblastoma multiforme are of astrocytic origin, as demonstrated by special stains, tissue culture, and electron microscopy,[82] but oligodendrogliomas and ependymomas may result in an identical microscopic appearance. Therefore, it seems more logical to simply call these tumors *undifferentiated gliomas.* The majority occur in the cerebral hemispheres (particularly frontal lobes) of adults (Fig. 1201). Grossly, they often have a sharper border than their better differentiated counterparts. Areas of necrosis are almost always encountered. Cystic degeneration and hemorrhage may be present (Fig.

1202). Invasion of the meninges and ventricular cavities is a common event. Multiple foci are sometimes found.[88]

Microscopically, highly cellular areas, which are always present, alternate with large necrotic foci. In many cases, the tumor cells show a wide diversity of sizes and shapes—hence the designation of "multiforme." Round, polygonal, oval, and markedly elongated elements can all be present. Intranuclear "inclusion bodies" are frequent.[83] They represent cytoplasmic invaginations lying within nuclear folds.[81] It is not uncommon to find multinucleated tumor giant cells with abundant acidophilic cytoplasm (Fig. 1203). Tumors in which these cells represent the predominant type have been regarded in the past as sarcomas, but there is now convincing ultrastructural evidence for their glial derivation.[76, 80] It is characteristic for the tumor cells to concentrate around foci of the necrosis, resulting

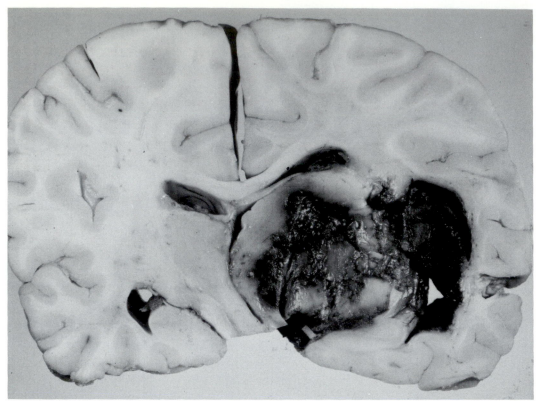

Fig. 1202 Massive hemorrhage within substance of undifferentiated glioma. This complication is often the first clinical manifestation of disease. Note marked displacement of
midline structures. (WU neg. 72-2479.)

in a palisading effect (Fig. 1204, A). This
is an important differential feature with
metastatic carcinoma, since in the latter
the necrosis tends to spare perivascular
collections of tumor cells, leading to the
so-called "perithelial" effect. Another constant microscopic feature of undifferentiated gliomas is represented by the vascular changes. The most common abnormality is a marked proliferation of the endothelium (and perhaps also the perithe-
lium) of the capillaries, resulting in the
formation of highly cellular nests with a
narrow central lumen (Fig. 1204, B). It
should be remarked that this change also
can be seen, although less commonly,
in oligodendrogliomas, well-differentiated
astrocytomas, and even metastatic carcinomas. Other vascular changes of undifferentiated gliomas include perivascular fibrosis,
marked dilatation of the lumen, and throm-

bosis. Cases have been described in which
glioblastoma multiforme seemed to coexist
with sarcoma, the latter presumably arising
from the proliferating endothelial cells or
fibroblasts of the stroma.[73, 74] An increased
incidence of extracranial metastases has
been observed in this particular variety.[87]
This exceptional occurrence should be differentiated from the more common spindle
cell metaplasia and desmoplastic reaction
which can occur in ordinary undifferentiated gliomas, especially in areas of meningeal invasion.

Of all primary tumors of the central
nervous system, undifferentiated gliomas
are the ones most commonly associated
with the production of extracranial metastases, these being preceded in most cases
by a surgical intervention.[86] The most common sites are the lungs and cervical lymph
nodes. Undifferentiated gliomas are among

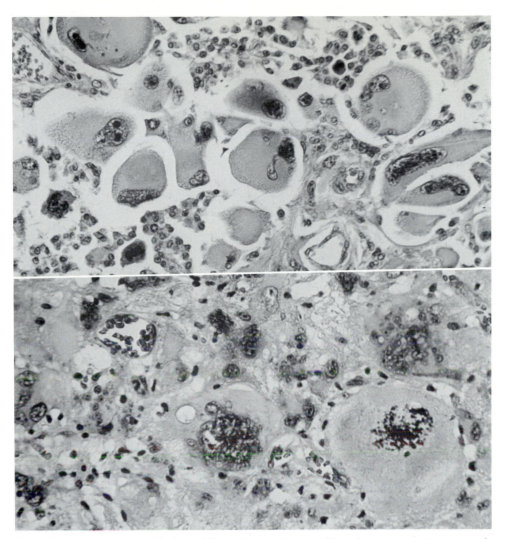

Fig. 1203 Bizarre tumor cells in undifferentiated glioma. Although tumors containing such elements have been interpreted by some as sarcomas, special staining techniques and electron microscopy have clearly evidenced their glial derivation. (×300; WU negs. 73-2683 and 73-2688.)

the most malignant tumors of the human body.[89] The two-year mortality following operation approaches 90%. Jelsma and Bucy[79] showed that two favorable prognostic signs, relatively speaking, are gross circumscription of the tumor and young age of the patient.

Oligodendroglioma

A rare form of glioma, oligodendroglioma presents most often as a slow-growing neoplasm in adults.[96] Grossly, it is well cir-

cumscribed, soft, and sometimes of a gelatinous appearance. Cystic changes are very common. Foci of calcification are present in 70% of the cases and are sufficiently numerous in 40% to be detectable radiographically. Microscopically, the most common and best known pattern is that of a uniformly cellular neoplasm composed of round cells with a small darkly staining nucleus, clear cytoplasm, and clearly defined cell membrane (Fig. 1205). This type is most commonly seen in the cerebral

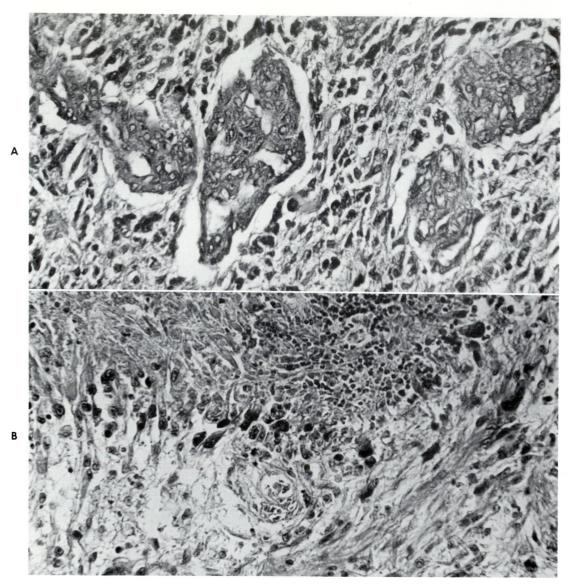

Fig. 1204 Two common microscopic features of undifferentiated glioma. Although not completely specific, they are of considerable diagnostic value. **A,** Marked proliferation of blood vessels within tumor mass. Both endothelial and perithelial cells participate. **B,** Palisading of tumor cells around foci of necrosis. Note fact that necrosis shows no particular relationship to blood vessels. (**A,** ×300; WU neg. 73-2687; **B,** ×300; WU neg. 73-2684.)

hemispheres, although the cerebellum and spinal cord also may be affected. In the second variety, most frequently seen in the optic nerve and chiasma and in the corpus callosum, the tumor cells are elongated. Transitions often occur. At the periphery of the neoplasm, it is not uncommon for the tumor cells to surround neu-rons in a fashion similar to that of reactive glial cells.[94] Morphologic variations which may result in diagnostic difficulties include separation into well-defined nests by connective tissue septa, accumulation of a PAS-positive cytoplasmic mucosubstance, and formation of signet ring cells.[93] In most cases, other glial elements (particularly

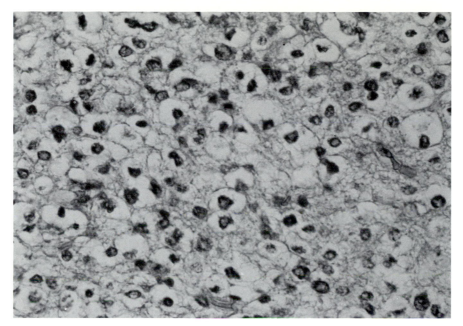

Fig. 1205 Oligodendroglioma with typical perinuclear clear zones of unstained cytoplasm. (×750; WU neg. 52-4237.)

astrocytes) are present in addition to the oligodendrocytes. Ultrastructurally, a striking concentric arrangement of cytoplasmic processes of the tumor cells was described by Robertson and Vogel.[92]

The behavior of this tumor is quite erratic. Presence of marked cytologic atypia can be correlated with a biologically aggressive tumor, but the reverse is not necessarily true. Local recurrence is to be expected in approximately 50% of the cases.[91] Clinical malignancy is manifested by dissemination through the cerebrospinal pathways and, exceptionally, by the appearance of distant metastases.[90, 95]

Ependymoma

Ependymoma constitutes only 5% of all intracranial gliomas in adults and 8% in children. On the other hand, it represents the most common intramedullary glioma. It may be seen in all ages. The most common locations are the ventricles (particularly the fourth), the lumbosacral portion of the spinal cord, and the filum terminale (Figs. 1206 and 1207). In a significant proportion of cases, anatomic con-

nection of the tumor with the ventricular cavity cannot be demonstrated.[100] We have seen extraneural ependymomas appearing in the soft tissues of the sacrococcygeal region.[97] The tumor is almost always solitary, except in the variant known as subependymoma and in patients with Recklinghausen's disease.

Grossly, the most common appearance of ependymoma is that of a well-circumscribed, granular, friable gray mass. When located in the filum terminale, it typically presents as a fusiform enlargement of this structure (Fig. 1208).

Microscopically, the most important distinguishing feature (although not always demonstrable in biopsy material) is the presence of ependymal rosettes. These are ductlike structures with a round or elongated central lumen around which columnar tumor cells are arranged concentrically. The nuclei lie in a basal position. Cilia and blepharoplasts can often be demonstrated. These rosettes, which in this location are diagnostis of ependymomas, should be clearly differentiated from Wright's rosettes of neuroblastomas and medullo-

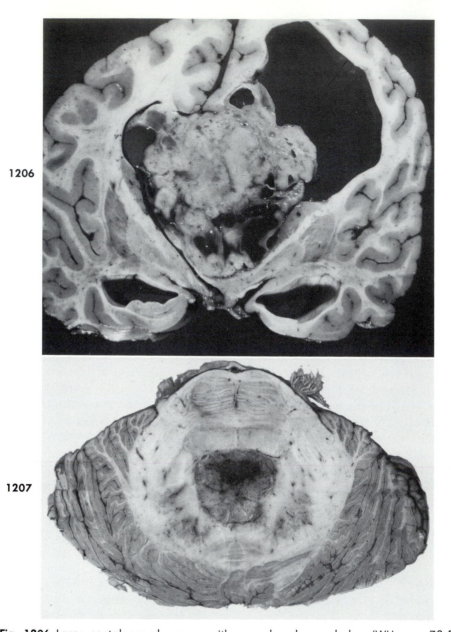

Fig. 1206 Large septal ependymoma, with secondary hyrocephalus. (WU neg. 72-5943; courtesy Dr. J. E. Olvera-Rabiela, Mexico City, Mexico.)
Fig. 1207 Ependymoma of fourth ventricle. This tumor should be distinguished from choroid plexus papilloma. (Courtesy Dr. E. Lascano, Buenos Aires, Argentina.)

blastomas. The latter are an expression of neuroblastic differentiation and are therefore never present in ependymomas. Formation of perivascular pseudorosettes is another feature of ependymoma and often the only clue to the diagnosis. In routinely stained sections, these structures appear quite similar to those of astroblastoma, although specific silver impregnations differentiate them easily.[103] Foci of calcification can be identified in 15% of the cases. Malignant histologic variants, which are rare, are recognized by the usual features of malignancy, such as invasive properties, cytologic atypia, and large foci of necrosis. These tumors can be properly called malignant ependymomas, and an aggressive clinical behavior can be predicted.[105] This implies seeding of the subarachnoid space and, exceptionally, extraneural metastases. On the other hand, a "benign" microscopic appearance does not guarantee a benign clinical evolution although this will be the case in the majority of the instances. Ultrastructurally, tumor ependymal cells retain many of the features of the normal parent cells, particularly their specialized connections, cilia, ciliary rootlets (blepharoplasts), and microvilli.[101]

There are two types of ependymomas that deserve to be treated separately because of their distinctive clinicopathologic features: myxopapillary ependymoma and subependymoma.

Myxopapillary ependymoma occurs exclusively in the region of the conus medullaris and filum terminale. It constitutes the majority of tumors of this region.[98, 102] Grossly, it presents as a fusiform enlargement of the filum terminale sometimes attached to the meninges. Microscopically, the distinctive feature is the presence of papillae centered by dilated blood vessels, surrounded by an abundant mucinous stroma and covered by one or more layers of regular cuboidal tumor cells (Fig. 1209). Fusion of adjacent papillae results in a complicated reticular pattern. A very common mistake is to confuse these tumors with chordomas. Rawlinson et al.[102a] have described the fine structural appearance of this neoplasm. The prognosis is generally good, although exceptional cases with distant metastases have been reported.[104]

Subependymomas are rarely a surgical problem. They most often represent an incidental necropsy finding in the cerebral ventricles, where they present as multiple small nodules protruding into the cavity. Microscopically, they seem to be composed of an admixture of ependymal cells and subependymal astrocytes.[99]

Tumors and tumorlike conditions of choroid plexus

Although tumors of the choroid plexus can be regarded as variants of ependymoma, their highly specialized nature and distinctive appearance justify a separation from the latter.

Choroid papilloma is by far the commonest variety. Young male children are most commonly affected. The cavity and lateral recesses of the fourth ventricle are the commonest sites of involvement. The appearance of a large tumor mass in the cerebellopontine angle is a frequent form of presentation. In younger children, the tumor prefers the lateral ventricles, where it may reach a large size. The internal hydrocephalus frequently encountered may be due to secretory activity by the tumor.[113] The primarily intraventricular growth is responsible for the paucity of symptoms in the early stages of the disease.

Grossly, choroid plexus papilloma appears as an intraventricular mass of obvious

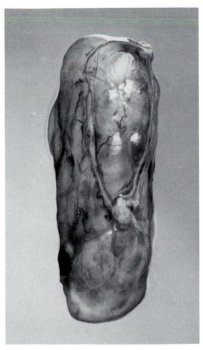

Fig. 1208 Ependymoma of spinal cord. Elongated shape and encapsulation are characteristic. (WU neg. 51-3014.)

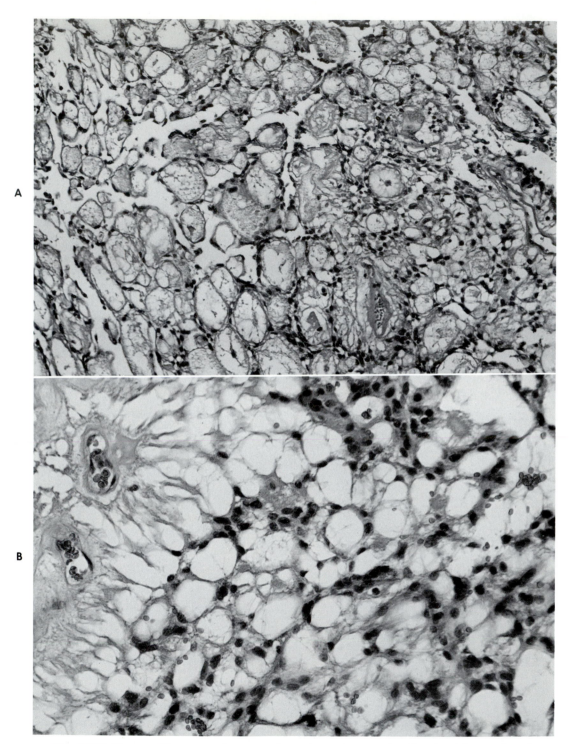

Fig. 1209 Myxopapillary ependymoma of cauda equina. **A,** Small cuboidal ependymal cells line papillae containing large amount of myxoid intercellular material. **B,** Reticulated appearance of tumor can result in mistaken diagnosis of chordoma. Note relationship with blood vessel wall. (**A,** ×150; WU neg. 73-2662; **B,** ×300; WU neg. 73-2953.)

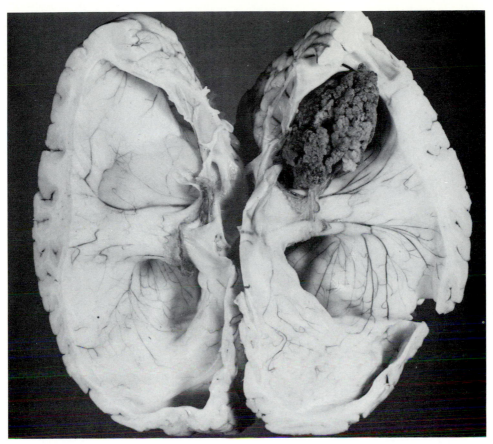

Fig. 1210 Choroid papilloma in right lateral ventricle of infant with accompanying advanced hydrocephalus. (WU neg. 50-3245.)

papillary configuration (Fig. 1210). Microscopically, the tumor duplicates the structure of the normal choroid plexus, with its formation of fibrovascular fronds lined by a single layer of uniform cuboidal or columnar cells of almost epithelial appearance (Fig. 1211). The similarities with benign[108] papillary mesothelioma are striking. Exceptionally, mucus-producing columnar cells are present. Excision is curative.

Choroid carcinomas are extremely rare.[112] Although they retain some of the papillary configuration of the papillomas, they differ from them because of invasion of the adjacent brain and the presence of malignant cytologic features (Fig. 1212). Most of the cases have occurred in children and have shown a marked propensity for spread throughout the ventricular and subarachnoid spaces. Great caution should

be exercised in the diagnosis of choroid carcinomas, especially in adults. *The large majority of papillary and/or glandular malignant tumors involving the ventricles represent metastatic carcinoma.*

Not infrequently, collections of foamy macrophages are found incidentally in the choroid plexus, resulting in the formation of a yellowish plaque or nodule. Although they have been sometimes dignified with the designation of *xanthogranuloma,* they do not represent true neoplasms and are of no clinical significance.[107]

Colloid (neuroepithelial) cysts occur most commonly in the anterior part of the third ventricle, but they can develop in any part of the cerebral ventricular system.[111] Whether they arise from the paraphysis, ependymal pouches from the diencephalon, or the choroid plexus epithelium

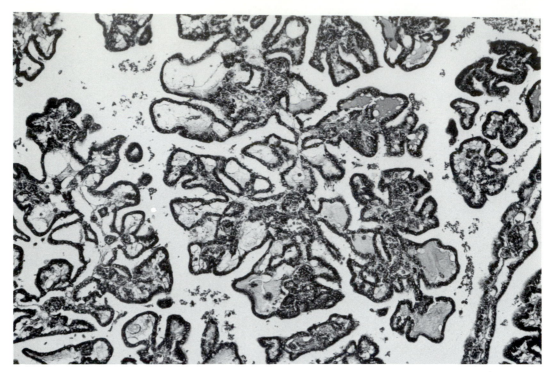

Fig. 1211 Choroid plexus papilloma removed from right lateral ventricle of 8-month-old male infant. Tumor is made of innumerable papillary fronds lined by cuboidal epithelium and supported by delicate fibrovascular cores. (×150; WU neg. 73-2661.)

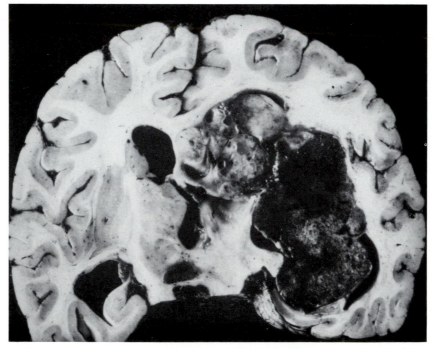

Fig. 1212 Carcinoma of choroid plexus filling lateral ventricle and invading brain substance. (Courtesy Dr. J. E. Olvera-Rabiela, Mexico City, Mexico.)

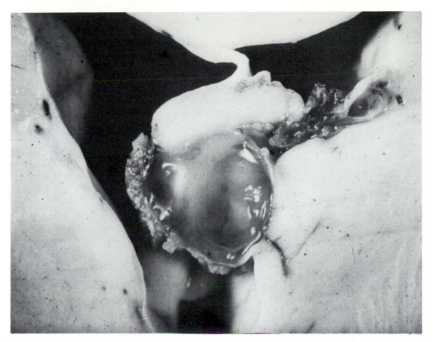

Fig. 1213 Typical gross appearance of colloid cyst of third ventricle. It is easy to imagine how this formation may result in acute hydrocephalus. (Courtesy Dr. J. E. Olvera-Rabiela, Mexico City, Mexico.)

is still unsettled.[106, 110] The cyst is usually unilocular and contains a fluid which may appear clear or milky (Fig. 1213). The wall is quite thin, made of fibrous tissue, and lined by one layer of low cuboidal epithelium, sometimes ciliated.[109] It may reach a diameter of 3 cm or 4 cm. Cysts measuring 1 cm or less are usually asymptomatic. The cases that become clinically manifest frequently do so during the third or fourth decade. Acute hydrocephalus, sometimes fatal, may develop as a result of blockage of the foramen of Monro. Operative removal of the cyst results in relief of almost all symptoms, except those due to permanent damage of neighboring structures.

Tumors of primitive neuroepithelial cells

Rubinstein[133] has lucidly discussed the cytogenesis, morphology, and possible relationships of embryonal tumors of the central nervous system—i.e., tumors which arise during embryonal, fetal, or early postnatal development from tissues that are still immature. Although in an individual case the distinction may not be easy, this group of neoplasms should be clearly separated from those previously discussed, which are presumed to arise from adult differentiated cells. As is usually the case with embryonal tumors in general, those originating in the central nervous system almost always affect infants or children. They may arise at any stage of the differentiation process and thereby acquire a wide spectrum of morphologic patterns. The best defined varieties are given specific names, as indicated in Table 53, but it should be realized that mixed and intermediate forms are not infrequently encountered.

Medulloepithelioma

Medulloepithelioma is the most undifferentiated member of the group, in the sense that it recapitulates the structure of the primitive medullary epithelium and shows minimal or no signs of neuroblastic, spongioblastic, or ependymal differentiation.[123] All of the few reported cases have occurred in infants or children.[137, 138] The

Table 53 Correlation between normal cytogenesis of central nervous system and embryonal neuroepithelial tumors

Stage of cytogenesis	Normal cell	Tumor
First	Neuroepithelial (matrix) cell	Medulloepithelioma
Second	Neuroblast	Medulloblastoma Neuroblastoma
Third	Spongioblast	Polar spongioblastoma
	Ependymoblast	Ependymoblastoma

cerebral hemispheres have been the preferred location, either in or near the ventricular system. Microscopically, the tumor is made up of tubules and papillae lined by columnar or cuboidal cells, often pseudostratified and with high mitotic activity. Since malignant teratomas may contain neural elements with an identical appearance, this possibility should always be eliminated by generous sampling of the tumor. The differential diagnosis should also include malignant ependymoma, choroid plexus carcinoma, and metastatic carcinoma. The former is identified by the presence of rosettes, blepharoplasts, and/or ependymal rosettes. The behavior of medulloepithelioma is that of a highly malignant tumor, prone to local recurrence, leptomeningeal spread, and distant metastases.

Medulloblastoma

Medulloblastoma is the commonest and most controversial of all the embryonal neuroectodermal tumors. Despite all the arguments and uncertainties regarding its cytogenesis and the justified criticisms that have been voiced to the term medulloblastoma, there is little doubt that it constitutes a definite clinicopathologic entity. More than one-half of the cases occur in the first decade of life.[119] Medulloblastoma accounts of over 25% of all intracranial tumors in children. *It occurs exclusively in the cerebellum.* The classical presentation is that of a midline tumor involving the vermis and often extending into

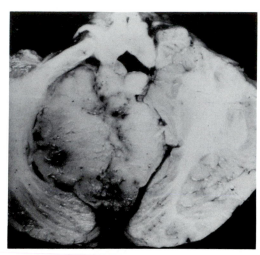

Fig. 1214 Cerebellar medulloblastoma in child. Tumor involves vermis and extends into fourth ventricle. (Courtesy Dr. J. E. Olvera-Rabiela, Mexico City, Mexico.)

the fourth ventricle. Rarely, it is found in one of the cerebellar hemispheres.

Grossly, it is soft, friable, and well circumscribed. Its color varies from gray to pinkish (Fig. 1214). Microscopically, it is a highly cellular neoplasm. The nuclei are closely packed, hyperchromatic, relatively uniform, and round, oval, or carrot-shaped. In the absence of previous radiation therapy, the presence of giant or bizarre cells makes the diagnosis of medulloblastoma very unlikely. The cytoplasm is scanty, and the cytoplasmic margins are indistinct.[118] Rosettes centered by neurofibrillary material are encountered in approximately one-third of the cases. These should not be confused with areas of perivascular ar-

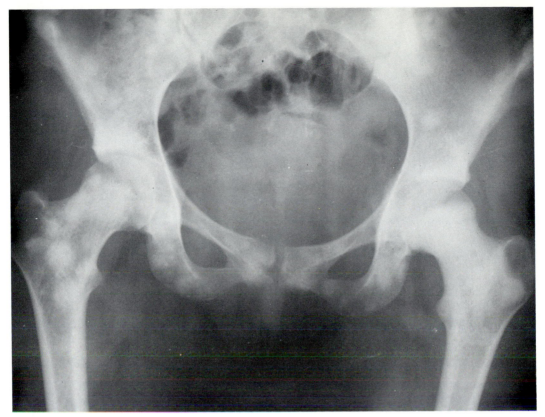

Fig. 1215 Widespread osteoblastic metastases of medulloblastoma in 12-year-old girl who also had local recurrence in posterior fossa of tumor treated by surgery and irradiation five years previously. (WU neg. 71-6738.)

rangement of the tumor cells, which may also occur. Matakas et al.[125] found no evidence of differentiation toward neuronal or glial structures in the nine cases they examined ultrastructurally.

Spread of medulloblastoma takes place through several routes. Subpial permeation is particularly common, as are also infiltration of the subarachnoid space and spread through the cerebrospinal fluid. Extraneural metastases also occur, particularly to bone and cervical lymph nodes.[120, 128] Osseous metastases may be osteoblastic, osteolytic, or mixed[115] (Fig. 1215). The treatment consists of surgical removal of as much tumor as possible, followed by radiation therapy to the entire cerebrospinal axis. In a series of eighty-two cases reviewed by Bloom et al.,[116] 40% of the patients completing treatment survived five years and 30% ten years. The major

cause of treatment failure is local recurrence in the posterior fossa.[124]

A well-defined variant of medulloblastoma (designated as "desmoplastic" by Rubinstein et al.[135]) has been described in an older age group, involving the cerebellar hemispheres, extending into the leptomeninges, and accompanied by abundant reticulin formation. Although originally regarded as a malignant mesenchymal tumor and designated "circumscribed arachnoidal cerebellar sarcoma," several authors have convincingly shown its link with the "classic" medulloblastoma.[135] Its prognosis is somewhat better than that of the latter.[118] Transitional and mixed forms have been described.[136] Another variant of medulloblastoma is characterized by the presence of embryonal skeletal muscle fibers in an otherwise typical neoplasm.[117, 127]

The cytogenesis of this tumor has been

a subject of heated discussions for decades. It is now more or less agreed that it arises from the primitive cells which originate in the neuroepithelial roof of the fourth ventricle to migrate upward and laterally to form the external granular layer of the cerebellar cortex.[121] Although cases with spongioblastic, astrocytic, and even oligodendroglial differentiation have been observed,[134] the differentiation, if present at all, is almost always in the direction of neuroblasts.[122] In this respect, medulloblastoma can be regarded in most instances as a peculiar clinicopathologic variant of neuroblastoma.[129, 130]

Other embryonal tumors

Rare embryonal tumors of controversial cytogenesis include cerebral neuroblastoma, polar spongioblastoma, and ependymoblastoma.

Cerebral neuroblastoma closely resembles adrenal neuroblastoma on the one hand and cerebellar medulloblastoma on the other. Like them, it probably represents a malignant tumor of neuroblastic derivation.[126, 135]

Polar spongioblastoma faithfully recapitulates the architectural patttern of normal migrating polar spongioblasts.[131] Microscopically, uniform elongated cells are seen growing in a parallel fashion with a striking palisading effect.

Rubinstein[132] suggested the designation of *ependymoblastoma* (in a quite different sense from that previously used by Bailey and Cushing[114]), for a highly malignant embryonal tumor in which differentiation toward ependymal cells can be demonstrated. Whether it is justified to regard this as a specific tumor type distinct from medulloepithelioma and malignant ependymoma remains to be determined.

Tumors of neuronal cells

Whereas tumors containing adult neurons are not uncommon in the autonomic nervous system, their occurrence in the central nervous system is exceptional. It is likely that, here too, they form as a result

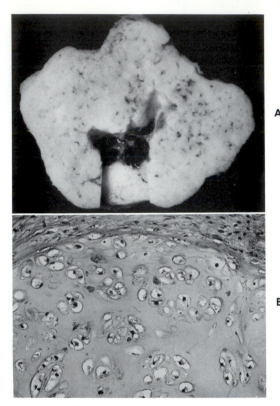

Fig. 1216 Chondroma of cerebral meninges. **A,** Gross appearance is that of well-circumscribed, lobulated mass of glistening white cut surface. **B,** Microscopic appearance of same tumor. Lobule of mature cartilage is partially surrounded by dense fibrous tissue. (**A,** WU neg. 66-7871; **B,** ×150; WU neg. 73-2682.)

of maturation of tumors originally composed of primitive neuroblastic cells. In a few reported examples, mature neurons make the bulk of the tumor, which is then designated as *ganglioneuroma.* In the majority of the cases, however, there is in addition a conspicuous astrocytic component (analogous to the schwannian element of peripheral tumors)—hence the term *ganglioglioma.*[139] Most cases have occurred in children and young adults, and the preferred locations have been the floor of the third ventricle, the hypothalamus, and the temporal lobe.[140] Occasionally, multiple foci are encountered.[141]

Microscopically, the abnormal neurons and astrocytes are characteristically surrounded by a prominent fibrovascular

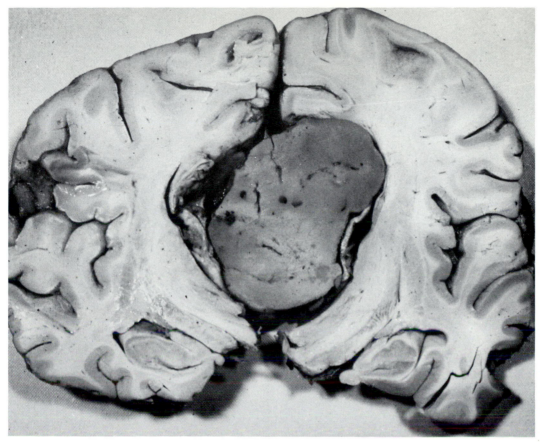

Fig. 1217 Meningioma of falx cerebri impinging upon corpus callosum and partially obliterating cerebral ventricles. There were no localizing symptoms, and clinical diagnosis was viral encephalitis. (WU neg. 73-2735.)

stroma, which we have seen confused with hemangioma. Ordinary astrocytomas can simulate gangliogliomas by entrapment of normal neurons. Also, some astrocytomas contain tumor glial cells with abundant acidophilic cytoplasm of polygonal shape and large vesicular necleus, thus simulating the appearance of a neuron.

If all the elements present in a ganglioneuroma or ganglioglioma appear microscopically mature, a benign clinical behavior will follow in the large majority of the cases.

Tumors of meningothelial cells

Tumors of several different origins may arise from, or be connected with, the anatomic structures composing the dura mater and leptomeninges.[144] It is unfortunate that the designation of meningioma has often been indiscriminately applied to such tumors regardless of their histogenesis. Following this nomenclature, a lipoma becomes a lipoblastic meningioma, a chondroma is designated a chondromatous meningioma, etc. (Fig. 1216). It is probably better to restrict the term meningioma to the specific neoplasm arising from, and composed of, meningothelial (arachnoid) cells.

Most examples occur in adults, and there is a definite predilection for females. These tumors may be encountered in many sites, including the parasagittal region, lateral cerebral convexity, falx cerebri (Fig. 1217), base of the brain (particularly the sphenoid ridge), olfactory grooves, pontocerebellar angles, petrous ridge of

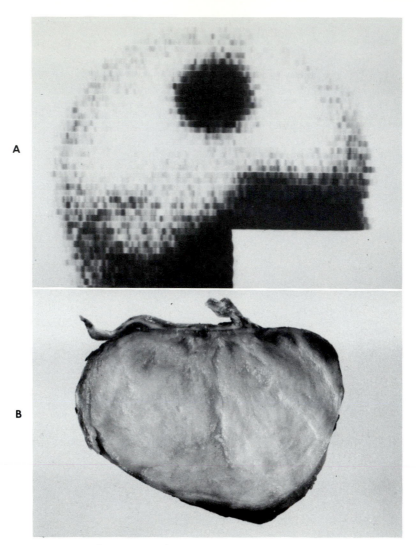

Fig. 1218 Parasagittal meningioma in 51-year-old man. **A,** Tc99ᵐ scan showing round hot area in frontoparietal region. **B,** Same tumor. It is well circumscribed, gray, homogeneous, and of firm consistency. Portion of dura attached to neoplasm may be seen at upper edge. (**A,** WU neg. 72-2786; **B,** WU neg. 72-2866.)

the temporal bone, spinal canal (especially the thoracic segments) and inside the cerebral ventricles (most often on the left side).[144, 147] We also have seen them in the orbit, nasal cavity, paranasal sinuses, bones of the skull, and soft tissues of the glabella.[146, 155]

The gross appearance of the meningioma is that of a well-circumscribed, often lobulated solid tumor of gray color and firm consistency (Fig. 1218). Calcification is common and can often be recognized radio-

graphically and on gross inspection. The cut section exhibits a whorling configuration not unlike that of uterine leiomyomas. Most meningiomas have a round or oval shape, but some (known as *meningiomas en plaque*) grow in a diffuse sheetlike manner over the convexity of the brain. Hyperostosis of the neighboring bone is a common finding and an important radiographic sign. Microscopically, the tumoral meningothelial cells may appear round, polygonal, oval, or spindle shaped (Fig.

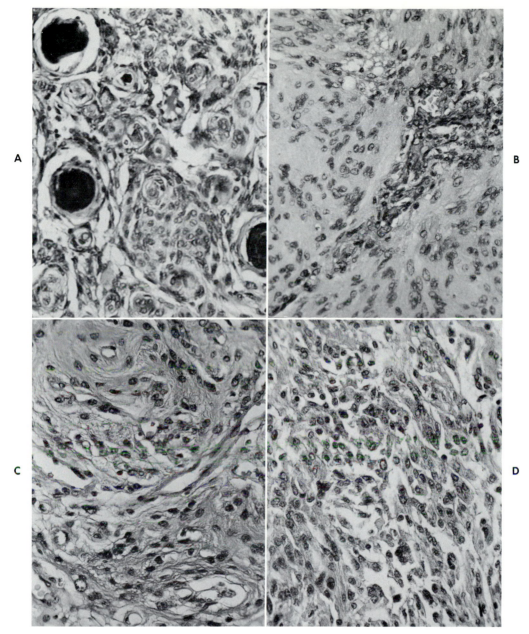

Fig. 1219 Four histologic appearances of meningioma. **A,** Small, well-defined whorls and psammoma bodies. **B,** Tumor cells with abundant fibrillary cytoplasm arranged in indistinct whorls. **C,** Tumor with marked vascularity and focal hyaline changes. **D,** Invasive meningioma, with atypical cytologic features. (**A** to **D,** ×280; **A,** WU neg. 49-3364; **B,** WU neg. 52-4262; **C,** WU neg. 52-4263; **D,** WU neg. 52-4264.)

1219). Their nuclei are regular, round or oval, and leptochromatic. The cytoplasm has a pale eosinophilic hue, and the cytoplasmic borders are indistinct. Mitoses are exceptional. Ultrastructurally, the most

distinctive features are the pronounced interdigitations of the plasma membrane, the abundance of cytoplasmic microfilaments, and the presence of desmosomes.[143, 149] The tumor cells are often arranged in nests

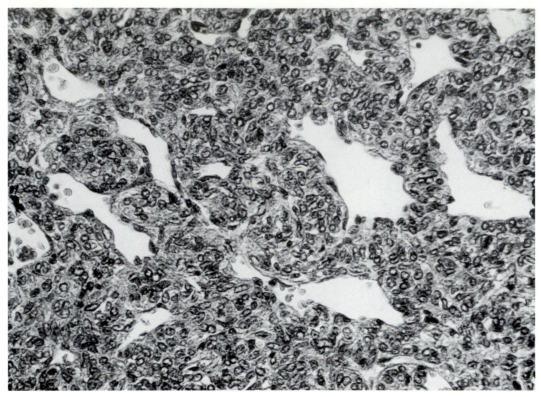

Fig. 1220 ''Angioblastic meningioma.'' Morphologic similarities with hemangiopericytoma of soft tissue are evident. (×350; WU neg. 73-2668.)

and concentric whorls, the latter sometimes containing psammoma bodies in their centers.[145] Blood vessels with thick hyaline walls are very prominent in some examples, to the point that a mistaken diagnosis of hemangioma can be made. Collections of foamy macrophages and foci of metaplastic bone are well recognized secondary features. The subdivision of meningiomas into microscopic types, such as syncytial, psammomatous, meningotheliomatous, etc. is probably unwarranted in view of their similar biologic behavior.

The large majority of meningiomas follow a benign clinical course and are permanently cured by surgical excision. Local recurrence supervenes in about 10% of the cases.[154] Extension into the dura mater, major sinuses, and skull is a feature inherent to this neoplasm and not a sign of malignancy. On the other hand, well-documented cases of bona fide *malignant menin-*

giomas exist. According to Rubinstein,[151] features in a meningioma which when present should raise the possibility of malignancy include invasion of the adjacent brain, papillary configuration, and presence of numerous mitotic figures. Distant metastases have been observed along the cerebrospinal fluid pathways as well as extracranially.[153]

The tumor that Bailey and Cushing[142] designated as **angioblastic meningioma** needs to be clearly separated from those just described. Microscopically, it is a highly vascular neoplasm, the blood vessels being separated by closely packed cells with ill-defined cytoplasm (sometimes containing neutral fat) and oval or fusiform nuclei. Some examples show a striking similarity to hemangiopericytoma of soft tissues (Fig. 1220). Others closely resemble cerebellar hemangioblastoma[152] (Fig. 1221). In one such case that we examined

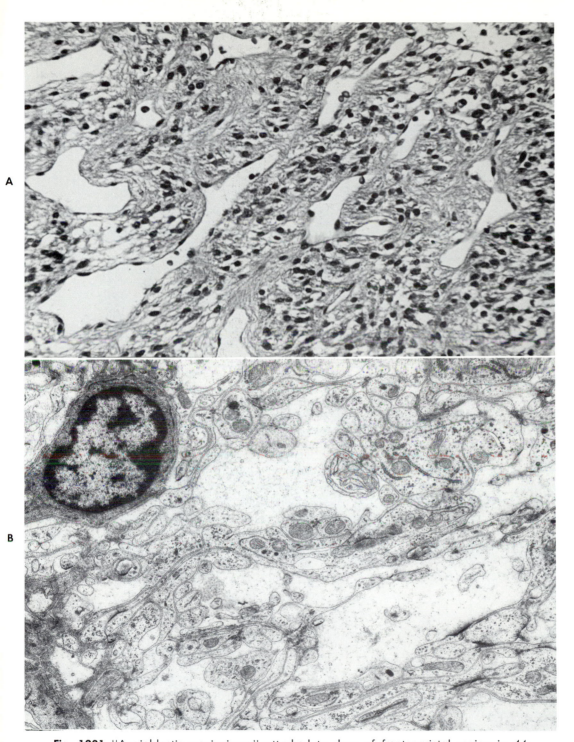

Fig. 1221 ''Angioblastic meningioma'' attached to dura of frontoparietal region in 44-year-old woman. **A,** Microscopic appearance of tumor. Resemblance to cerebellar hemangioblastoma is striking. **B,** Electron microscopic appearance of same tumor. There are complicated evaginations of plasmalemma, connected by desmosomes and partially surrounded by basal lamina. (**A,** ×300; WU neg. 73-2952; **B,** uranyl acetate—lead citrate; ×500; courtesy Dr. J. Bilbao, Toronto, Ontario, Canada.)

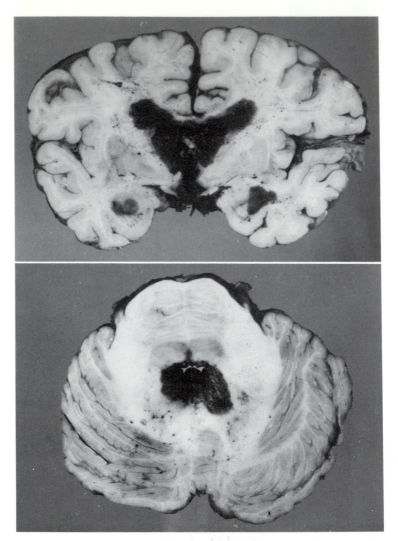

Fig. 1222 Leptomeningeal and ventricular spread of metastatic malignant melanoma. Primary tumor had been excised eighteen months previously from skin of back. (WU negs. 67-5089 and 67-5091.)

ultrastructurally, the tumor cells had unmistakable meningothelial features (Fig. 1221). The behavior of this neoplasm is, on the whole, more aggressive than that of the bona fide meningioma. Local recurrence is common, and extracranial metastases are not so rare as with the latter.[148, 150]

Tumors of melanocytes

The melanocytes normally present in the pia mater may give rise to a variety of disorders, most of which can be classified into one of two categories: neurocutaneous melanosis and primary meningeal melanoma.

In *neurocutaneous melanosis,* a disease of infants and children, diffuse pigmentation of the meninges resulting from proliferation of mature authoctonous melanocytes is associated with giant cutaneous nevi and occasionally with peripheral neurofibromas.[157] Internal hydrocephalus is the main complication of the central nervous system component of the disease.

Primary meningeal melanoma, which may occur as a complication of neurocutaneous melanosis, presents as a more or less circumscribed tumor mass or as a diffuse leptomeningeal process.[156] The latter form is differentiated from neurocutaneous melanosis by the atypia of the tumor cells, which is, however, less marked than that usually exhibited by cutaneous melanomas. Young adults are more commonly affected. The prognosis is poor. Metastasis from a cutaneous melanoma should be carefully ruled out before accepting any case as being of primary meningeal origin (Fig. 1222).

Tumors and malformations of blood vessels

Arteriovenous malformations are also known as arteriovenous angiomas, but the former designation is preferable since they are not true neoplasms.[160] Although congenital, they usually become manifest in late childhood and adolescence. A common complication is the production of repeated subarachnoid or intracerebral hemorrhages.[165] Most examples are found along the course of the middle cerebral artery. The cerebral choroid plexus, cerebellum, and spinal cord are less often affected. Usually, the lesion is quite superficial in character—i.e., restricted to the leptomeninges and the immediate cortical areas.

Grossly, large tortuous blood vessels are seen traversing thickened and hemorrhagic meninges and penetrating between atrophic cortical convolutions. Microscopically, some vessels can be identified as arteries and others as veins, but the majority represent hybrids difficult to classify. Secondary changes such as hyaline thickening, arteriosclerosis, calcification, and thrombosis are common.

Pure **venous malformations** are most commonly seen in the spinal cord and its meninges in adults.[168a] The thoracic and cervical portions are the sites of predilection.[159, 161, 173] A well-known variant of venous malformation is Sturge-Weber disease, in which extensive venocapillary malformations of a cerebral hemisphere are associated with a cutaneous "port-wine hemangioma" in the region of the trigemi-

nal nerve.[158, 172] Arteriovenous malformations of the spinal cord also can be associated with segmentally related cutaneous hemangiomas.[164]

Cavernous hemangiomas have a structure quite reminiscent of the similarly called cutaneous lesions. Markedly dilated capillaries are seen side by side with little intervening parenchyma. The subcortical region of the cerebral hemisphere is the preferred location. As with hemangiomas elsewhere, multiplicity and multicentric involvement of other organs are not infrequent.

Hemangioblastoma is the most enigmatic member of the group. Its classical location is the cerebellar hemispheres, but it also can occur in the vermis, spinal cord, medulla, and, exceptionally, the cerebral hemispheres.[166, 170] It usually becomes clinically manifest during the third or fourth decade of life. It may be the only abnormality present or represent a component of von Hippel–Lindau disease in association with angiomatosis of the retina, renal and pancreatic cysts, and, occasionally, renal cell carcinoma.[167] It also has been reported in association with syringomyelia,[169] pheochromocytoma,[168] and erythrocythemia,[163] the latter as the result of the secretion of an erythropoietin-like substance by the tumor.[171]

Grossly, hemangioblastoma is well circumscribed, soft, yellowish or brown, and often cystic (Fig. 1223). Microscopically, an anastomosing network of capillary vessels is invariably seen. This feature is responsible for the tumor name, its typical angiographic presentation, and the general belief that it represents a primary vascular neoplasm (Fig. 1224). We favor the alternative theory that the true tumor cells of this well-vascularized lesion are those located between the blood vessels and often designated as "stromal cells." They are large, round, or polygonal and have a pale cytoplasm that often contains abundant neutral fat (Fig. 1225). The nuclei are usually small and uniform. In some instances, however, bizarre hyperchromatic

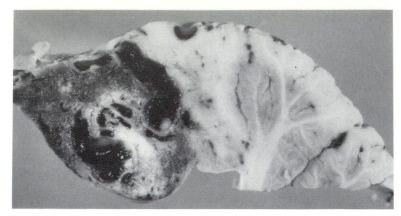

Fig. 1223 Hemangioblastoma of cerebellum. Tumor is well circumscribed, granular, and markedly vascular. (WU neg. 72-5929; courtesy Dr. J. E. Olvera-Rabiela, Mexico City, Mexico.)

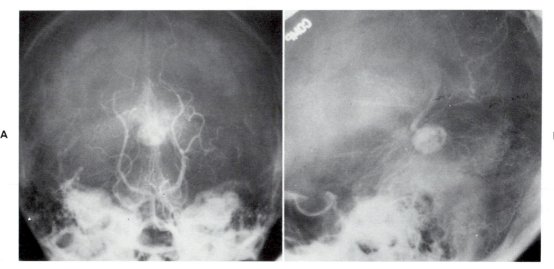

Fig. 1224 Arteriographic appearance of cerebellar hemangioblastoma. Vertebral arteriogram illustrated in **A** shows early in arterial phase a round dense homogeneous blush in midline of culmen of cerebellum. **B** corresponds to the venous phase. (**A,** WU neg. 73-3127; **B,** WU neg. 73-3128.)

forms are observed. They are of no particular prognostic significance. The nature of these cells is obscure. Ultrastructurally, their most prominent feature is a complex system of smooth membrane traversing the cytoplasm (Fig. 1226). The electron microscopic appearance does not resemble that of glial, meningothelial, endothelial, or perithelial cells or, for that matter, that of any normal cell known to occur in this area.[162] The treatment is surgical, and the prognosis is good. The main

hazard is local recurrence, either as a result of incomplete removal or because of multicentricity.

Tumors of lymphoreticular system

Secondary involvement of the central nervous system, particularly of the meninges, epidural space, and nerve roots, is a common event in malignant lymphoma and leukemia during the late stages of their evolution.[180, 183, 185] This includes Hodgkin's disease and the lymphomas associa-

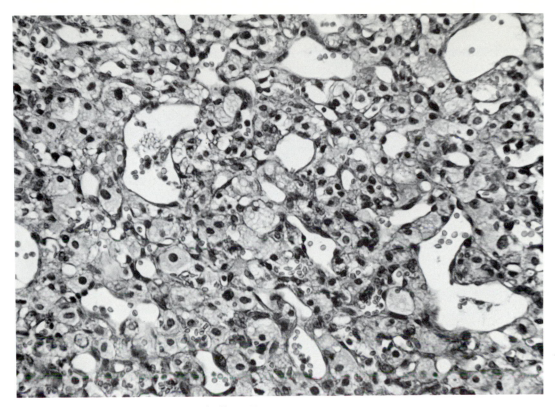

Fig. 1225 Hemangioblastoma of cerebellum. Tumor cells grow among intricate network of capillaries. They contain central normochromatic nuclei and abundant acidophilic (frequently foamy) cytoplasm. (×350; WU neg. 73-2667.)

ted with dysproteinemia.[179] It also can be seen, although exceptionally, in mycosis fungoides and plasma cell myeloma.[178, 187] In other instances, neurologic involvement represents the initial manifestation of a lymphoma or leukemia in which physical or radiographic examination shows to be in other organs as well. We are concerned here with the rarer instances in which a careful clinical study of the patient fails to uncover extraneural foci.

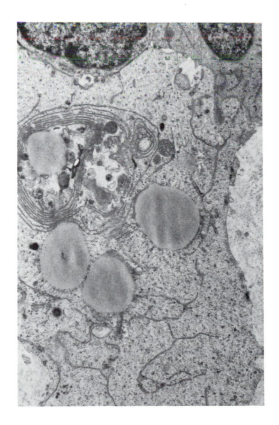

Fig. 1226 Ultrastructural appearance of "stromal cell" of cerebellar hemangioblastoma. Most conspicuous feature is presence of complex anastomosing membranous system in cytoplasm, sometimes arranged in concentric circles. Fat globules also are evident. (Uranyl acetate–lead citrate; ×8,400.)

Malignant lymphoma of histiocytic type (reticulum cell sarcoma) is sometimes referred to as microglioma or microgliomatosis.[184, 188] Since the microglial cell is but a histiocyte, we prefer the former term for the sake of consistency. This neoplasm is probably not so rare as the paucity of reported cases might suggest. Review of reference cases has convinced us that many cases go unrecognized because of the common tendency to label all poorly differentiated primary tumors of the central nervous system as malignant glioma or glioblastoma multiforme.[177] Some have been observed in patients with congenital immune deficiencies[175] or following immunosuppression.[190] Most patients are either young children or elderly adults.[174, 189] Any region of the central nervous system can be affected, although the cerebral hemispheres are the most common site. Multicentric foci are frequent.

Malignant lymphoma of the histiocytic type most commonly presents as an ill-defined gray, granular mass. Microscopically, the appearance is the same as that of histiocytic lymphoma elsewhere. This is also true electron microscopically.[181] The microglial nature of the cells can be well appreciated if the appropriate silver impregnation techniques are employed.[186] A striking perivascular distribution, accompanied by the deposition of concentric rings of reticulin fibers, is an important distinguishing feature. Leptomeningeal spread is frequent. Extraneural foci eventually develop in a minority of cases.[177] The clinical course is usually rapidly fatal,[189] although radiation therapy has resulted in prolonged survival in several instances.[182]

Malignant lymphoma of lymphocytic type primarily involving the central nervous system is almost always found in one of two sites: the meninges and the spinal epidural space, particularly in the thoracic portion.[176] We have seen a single case of *plasma cell tumor* apparently restricted to the meninges of the sphenoid ridge in a 58-year-old woman. We have never seen, and indeed doubt the existence of, primary Hodgkin's disease of the central nervous system.

Tumors of nerve roots

The morphologic appearance of tumors of the nerve roots, their biologic behavior, and the problems of histogenetic interpretation they present are those of the most common types occurring outside the cranial cavity and spinal canal, which are discussed in Chapter 23. *Neurilemomas* are by far the commonest. They have a strong predilection for two sites: the cerebellopontine angle and the spinal extramedullary space. The former arise practically always in the acoustic nerve, especially its vestibular branch (Fig. 1227). Enlargement of the internal auditory canal is an early finding and an important radiographic sign. Spinal neurilemomas have a predilection for the posterior (sensory) roots of the lumbar region.[197] Not infrequently, the tumor extends outside the spinal canal through an intervertebral foramen to form a large soft tissue mass ("dumbbell tumor").

Neurilemomas regularly present as solitary tumors in adults.[193] A few cases in children have been reported.[191] *The presence of bilateral acoustic neurilemomas should be regarded as a probable indication of Recklinghausen's disease.* Microscopically, the main source of difficulty lies in the differential diagnosis with meningioma. The presence of foci of microcystic degeneration (Antoni B areas), vascular changes, and collections of foamy macrophages should lead to the correct diagnosis. The electron microscopic appearance is distinctive.[192] The treatment is surgical. The outcome of the operation is directly related to the size of the neoplasm. The larger the tumor, the higher the operative mortality rate and the possibilities of permanent residual damage.[194] If the excision is only partial, recurrence of symptoms is common. Interruption of vital arterial supply to the tegmentum of the pons is the main hazard of the operation.[194]

Neurofibromas of the central nervous

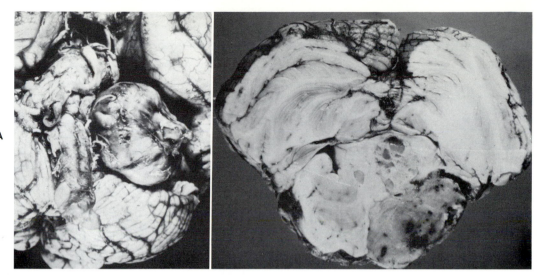

A   B

Fig. 1227 A, External appearance of neurilemoma of cerebellopontine angle. Tapered end of acoustic nerve on one side and compression of pons and medulla on other are well appreciated. **B,** Cross section of acoustic nerilemoma. Tumor compression has resulted in focal degenerative change of pons. (**A,** WU neg. 72-5942; **B,** WU neg. 72-5934; **A** and **B,** courtesy Dr. J. E. Olvera-Rabiela, Mexico City, Mexico.)

system are always multiple and an expression of Recklinghausen's disease. Both cranial and spinal nerve roots may be involved. In addition to neurofibromas, patients with Recklinghausen's disease may present with a bewildering variety of neural tumors and hamartomas. These include neurilemomas (particularly bilateral acoustic tumors), meningiomas, ependymomas, astrocytomas, and optic nerve gliomas.[196] Syringomyelia is another frequently associated abnormality.[195]

Tumors of germ cell origin

Tumors presumably arising from misplaced germ cell elements can occur within the cranial cavity. Like extragonadal germ cell tumors in general, they are located almost exclusively in midline structures, particularly within the pineal gland, in the parapineal area, and in a suprasellar or even intrasellar position.[201] Their common relationship with the pineal gland, plus a vague similarity with the embryonic structure of this organ, has resulted in many of these tumors being mistakenly regarded as pinealomas,[202] a misconception

still widely held in spite of convincing arguments to the contrary.[206-208]

All varieties of germ cell tumors have been described, including germinoma (a term proposed by Friedman[200] for neoplasms having the morphologic features of seminoma or dysgerminoma, regardless of site of origin), embryonal carcinoma, adult teratoma, choriocarcinoma, and yolk sac tumor.[198, 203] Combinations of these tumor types commonly occur. Their gross and microscopic features are identical to the homologous gonadal tumors. Grossly, germinomas are soft, grayish, friable, and granular. Two or more independent foci may be present. Microscopically, they consist of tumor cells with large, vesicular nuclei and pale, glycogen-containing cytoplasm that are irregularly divided in groups by thin fibrous strands infiltrated by inflammatory cells (Fig. 1228). The lymphocytic and sometimes granulomatous reaction accompanying these neoplasms is sometimes so intense that the true nature of the lesion may be missed in a small biopsy.[208] The ultrastructural appearance is identical to that of the corresponding gonadal neoplasm.[205]

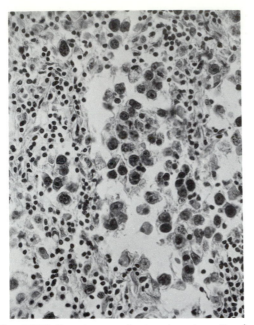

Fig. 1228 Germinoma of pineal region. Poorly cohesive nests of large tumor cells are surrounded by fibrous strands heavily infiltrated by lymphocytes. (×280; WU neg. 52-4267.)

The majority of the patients with germ cell neoplasms are young adult males.[199] Symptoms derive from pressure effects upon the regions of the rear of the third ventricle and over the mesencephalon. Oculomotor and visual disturbances are common. Diabetes insipidus, emaciation, and precocious puberty occur less frequently.[204] Local extension within the third ventricle is common. Occasionally, it spreads to other ventricles and even into the meningeal space.[199] The surgical approach is understandably difficult. Excision, whether partial or apparently complete, should be followed by radiation therapy. Germinomas are extremely radiosensitive neoplasms. Of seven patients with suprasellar germinoma who survived the operation and were treated with radiation therapy, five were alive and well from three to eighteen years later.[208] Adult teratomas, although radioresistant, can be cured by total removal. Conversely, embryonal carcinomas, choriocarcinomas, yolk sac tumors, and their combinations are almost invariably fatal.

Tumors of pineal gland

Once germ cell tumors are excluded from the category of tumors of the pineal gland, true neoplasms of the pineal gland become a curiosity. They supposedly arise from the pineal parenchymal cells and are classified into pineocytomas and pineoblastomas according to their degree of differentiation.

Pineocytomas present as solid, well-circumscribed tumors replacing the pineal body. Microscopically, the tumor cells are small and uniform, with round nucleus and eosinophilic cytoplasm, separated in nests by delicate connective tissue strands. The overall microscopic appearance and the argyrophilia that the tumor cells often exhibit have suggested to some a link with paraganglioma.[209, 211] Electron microscopic and biochemical studies should be instrumental in answering this intriguing possibility. The relationship of the tumor cells with blood vessels may cause confusion with ependymoma and astroblastoma. Actually, even a normal pineal gland may suggest ependymoma to the uninitiated. The majority of pineocytomas have behaved in a benign fashion, but the number of reported cases is too small to make any generalizations about their natural history.

The name *pineoblastoma* has been given to an extremely rare, highly malignant neoplasm histologically resembling medulloblastoma, mainly on the basis of its anatomic location.[210] Whether this tumor is indeed of pineal parenchymal origin remains to be determined.

Primary sarcomas

Primary sarcomas are extremely rare tumors, most frequently found in infants and children.[215] The majority arise from the dura, but leptomeningeal and parenchymal cases also have been observed. In some instances, the previous use of radiation therapy has been incrimated in their causation.[217, 219] A rare variant characterized by diffuse meningeal involvement has been designated *meningeal meningiomatosis.*[213] Sometimes a definite diag-

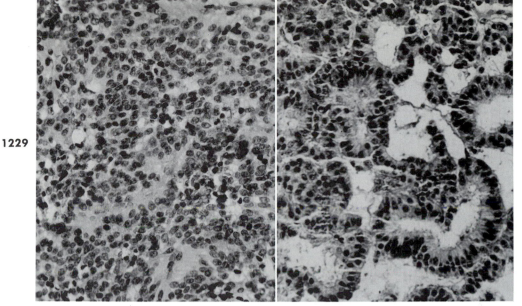

1229   1230

Fig. 1229 Pituitary adenoma of diffuse type. (×280; WU neg. 52-4265.)
Fig. 1230 Pituitary adenoma with glandular arrangement of tumor cells. This pattern is uncommon in our experience. (×280; WU neg. 49-3365.)

nosis of tumor type can be made, such as fibrosarcoma, malignant fibrous histiocytoma, rhabdomyosarcoma, chondrosarcoma, or mesenchymal chondrosarcoma.[212, 214-216, 218] In many cases, however, the specific cell type involved remains elusive despite the most exhaustive morphologic study.

Excluded from this group are the following "entities": circumscribed arachnoidal cerebellar sarcoma, monstruocellular sarcoma, giant cell fibrosarcoma, and gliosarcoma. The reasons why we do not regard them as authentic sarcomas have been given elsewhere in this chapter.

Tumors of pituitary gland

Pituitary neoplasms constitute approximately 10% of the intracranial tumors. The large majority arise from the endocrine cells of the adenohypophysis and are designated as *pituitary adenomas.* Naturally, most examples are found within the confines of the sella turcica. However, since aberrant adenohypophyseal cells are known to occur in the pituitary infundibulum, pituitary stalk, and floor of third ventricle and between the nasopharynx and the pituitary fossa, the appearance of pituitary adenomas in one of these locations is not unexpected, even if exceptional. Grossly, pituitary adenomas are usually solid and soft. Their color varies from gray to red according to the degree of vascularity. Cystic and hemorrhagic changes may occur in the larger tumors. A characteristic gross appearance is that of a tumor occupying both the intrasellar and suprasellar areas, with a central constriction produced by the diaphragm and the circle of Willis.

The microscopic pattern in hematoxylin-eosin sections varies from case to case, the differences being based on the relative degrees of cellularity and vascularity (Figs. 1229 and 1230). Kernohan and Sayre[241] classified their cases into a *diffuse* type, highly cellular, with scanty stroma and blood vessels; a *sinusoidal* type, having an architecture which recapitulates that of the normal gland; and a *papillary* type, in which pseudopapillae centered by a blood vessel and covered by tumor cells are noted. Transitional and mixed forms often

Table 54 Histochemical and ultrastructural features of normal pituitary cells and of the corresponding tumors

Hormone	Chemical composition and molecular weight	Normal cell				Tumor	
		Hematoxylin-eosin	Special stains	Granules (E.M.) in rat	Granules (E.M.) in human beings (tentative)	Hematoxylin-eosin	Granules (E.M.)
Growth hormone (STH or GH)	Protein ~21,000	Acidophil (alpha cell)	PAS, −; orange G, +; erythrosin, −	300-350 mμ; abundant; throughout cytoplasm	350-400 mμ	Acidophil or "chromophobe"	300-400 mμ
Adrenocorticotropic hormone (ACTH)	Protein ~4,500	? Basophil and chromophobe (beta, R, or zeta cell)	PAS, ±; orange G, −; erythrosin, −	200-300 mμ; more numerous in peripheral cytoplasm	200-300 mμ	Basophil or "chromophobe"	100-400 mμ
Thyrotropic hormone (TSH)	Glycoprotein ~28,000	Basophil (beta cell)	PAS, +; orange G, −; erythrosin, −	150-200 mμ; more numerous in peripheral cytoplasm	80-150 mμ	Basophil or "chromophobe"	?
Prolactin (LTH)	Protein ~25,000	Acidophil (eta cell)	PAS, −; orange G, ±; erythrosin, +	600-900 mμ; scanty of irregular shape	100-200 mμ in width; 600-900 mμ in length	Acidophil or "chromophobe"	500-600 mμ
Luteinizing hormone (LH or ICSH)	Glycoprotein ~26,000	Basophil (delta$_1$ cell)	PAS, +; orange G, −; erythrosin, −	200-250 mμ; throughout cytoplasm or concentrated in periphery	100-250 mμ	?	?
Follicle-stimulating hormone (FSH)	Glycoprotein ~50,000	Basophil (delta$_2$ cell)	PAS, +; orange G, −; erythrosin, −	200-250 mμ; throughout cytoplasm or concentrated in periphery	150-300 mμ	?	?

occur. There is apparently no relation between these microscopic types and prognosis. The tumor cells are similar in all three varieties. They are generally round or polygonal, and have a round or oval nucleus and a variable amount of cytoplasm, which may be basophilic, amphophilic, acidophilic, or clear. Mitoses are scanty or absent. Occasional bizarre hyperchromatic nuclei may occur. Rarely, the tumor cells have the morphologic features of oncocytes.[243] We have seen pituitary adenomas composed of uniform tumor cells of clear cytoplasm confused with oligodendrogliomas. We also have seen adenomas made up of oval cells with oval acidophilic cytoplasm and eccentric nucleus mistaken for plasma cell myeloma. The most common error, however, is the misinterpretation of a papillary type of pituitary adenoma as an ependymoma.

The time-honored classification of pituitary adenomas into chromophobe, acidophil, and basophil varieties is so grossly inadequate that there is little use in maintaining it.[226, 260] It has become evident that most normal "chromophobe" cells simply represent specific cells of one kind or another in which the number of granules is not large enough to be obvious at a light microscopic level.[234] The same seems to be true of the so-called chromophobe adenomas.[247]

There is now general agreement that each of the major hormones of the adenohypophysis is secreted by a single cell type. The identification of these cells and the correlation with a given hormone have been achieved in some animals (particularly the rat) by careful histochemical and electron microscopic studies under normal and abnormal conditions and, most of all, by immunocytochemical methods[221, 222, 235, 252, 253] (Table 54). Understandably, the corresponding information on the normal human pituitary gland is not nearly so complete. However, correlation with the animal models and studies in several disease processes has permitted at least a tentative classification of cell types[220, 224, 255, 257, 267]

(Fig. 1231). The same approach should be followed in the case of the neoplasms. Hematoxylin-eosin stains should be routinely supplemented by PAS–hematoxylin–light green–orange G,[247] and, if possible, by electron microscopic examination. Biochemical and immunochemical procedures in tumor extracts and in tumors grown in tissue culture should be even more informative.[242] The types of pituitary adenomas already identified include STH, ACTH, TSH, and LTH cell types.

Adenomas of the STH cell type may result in gigantism or acromegaly if functioning at a clinical level or, more commonly, be unaccompanied by signs of hyperfunction. If the series reported by McCormick and Halmi,[247] only 3% of the acidophilic adenomas produced typical acromegaly. The few tumors composed of highly granulated cells appear acidophilic in hematoxylin-eosin sections. The others, which constitute the majority, have the appearance of "chromophobe adenomas."[269] By electron microscopy, secretory granules measuring 300 mμ to 400 mμ can be identified in every case.[245] The endoplasmic reticulum is disposed in concentric arrays. Bundles of cytoplasmic microfilaments are sometimes encountered.[262]

The functioning examples of *adenomas of the ACTH cell type,* which constitute approximately 7% of the cases,[247] result in the production of Cushing's syndrome. Female patients predominate. Approximately 10% of all cases of Cushing's syndrome are secondary to a pituitary adenoma.[259, 261] Removal of the hyperplastic adrenal glands in these patients may result in rapid enlargement or even massive hemorrhagic infarct of the pituitary neoplasm. Nelson et al.[254] have estimated that about 10% of patients with Cushing's disease and adrenal cortical hyperplasia who undergo total adrenalectomy later develop clinical signs of a pituitary neoplasm. By light microscopy, the tumor cells are rarely basophilic, more often "chromophobe." Ultrastructurally, the secretory granules concentrate along the cell membrane and

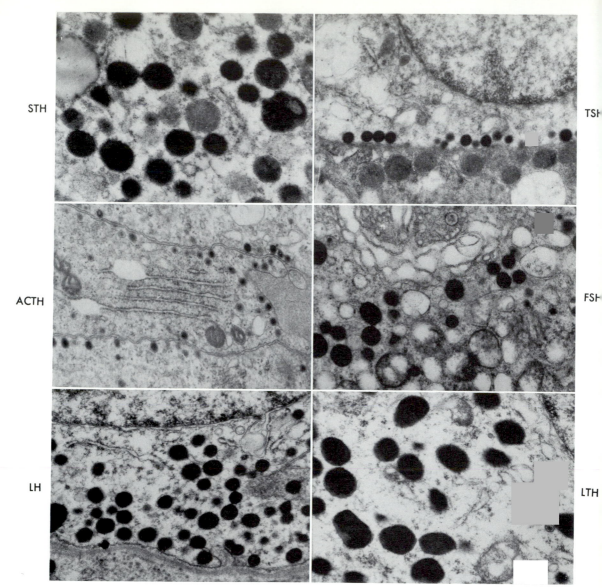

Fig. 1231 Electron microscopic appearance of secretory granules of six major cell types of human anterior pituitary gland. (Uranyl acetate–lead citrate; ×21,000; courtesy Dr. I. von Lawzewitsch, Buenos Aires, Argentina.)

measure from 100 mμ to 400 mμ (Fig. 1232).

The presence of *adenomas of THS cell type* had been suggested by the reports of pituitary adenomas associated with hyperthyroidism,[237] but only recently confirmed by Hamilton et al.[233] by the finding of elevated serum TSH levels on radioimmunoassay. The ultrastructural features of this tumor type remain to be determined.

The situation in regard to *adenomas of the LTH (prolactin) cell type* is somewhat similar. Their existence had been long suspected by the reported cases of pituitary adenomas associated with galactorrhea and amenorrhea (Forbes-Albright syndrome)[228, 229] and finally documented by the thoroughly investigated case of Peake et al.[256] The light microscopic appearance of this tumor is similar to that of *STH cell*

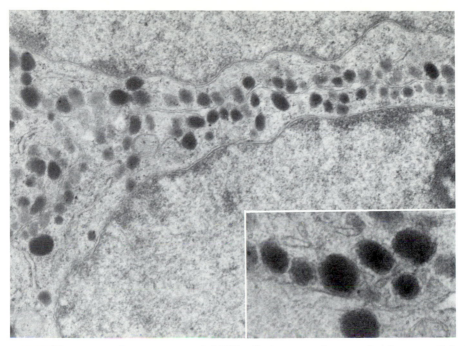

Fig. 1232 Ultrastructural appearance of ACTH cell pituitary adenoma that became clinically evident six years following bilateral adrenalectomy for Cushing's syndrome in 29-year-old woman. Secretory granules arrange themselves in parallel rows along cell membranes. **Inset,** Higher magnification of secretory granules. Their diameter ranges from 100 mμ to 300 mμ. (Uranyl acetate–lead citrate; ×21,900; **inset,** uranyl acetate–lead citrate; ×55,350.)

adenoma, but ultrastructurally it differs by the larger size of its secretory granules (500 mμ to 600 mμ).

As far as we know, the **FSH** and **LH** cells are the only ones for which no corresponding tumor in human beings has yet been conclusively demonstrated, although its occurrence in experimental animals is well known.[232] However, Kohler et al.[242] have found production of LH in several human pituitary adenomas grown in tissue culture. Tumors composed of more than one cell type, and therefore secreting two or more hormones, also occur.

Pituitary adenomas, as a group, are more frequent in adults and show a slight predilection for males. In a small percentage of patients, the pituitary tumor is one of the components of the multiple endocrine adenomatosis syndrome.[223] They may become clinically evident as a result of the increased secretion of a specific hormone by the tumor cell as previously outlined, by signs of hypopituitarism secondary to destruction of the normal gland, and/or by symptoms or signs resulting from the compression of adjacent structures. Enlargement and erosion of the floor of the sella turcica is a very common finding and an important radiologic sign. Suprasellar extension, present in 10% to 20% of the cases, results in visual symptoms as a result of compression of the optic chiasm. Extraocular tumor palsies occur in 5% to 10% of the patients. In 5% to 10% of all pituitary tumors, actual invasion of neighboring structures is encountered, such as the anterior, middle, or posterior fossa, cavernous sinus, optic nerves, chiasm, nasopharynx, or nasal cavity.[240, 250] We prefer to designate these tumors as "invasive adenomas" rather than as carcinomas. Exceptionally, pituitary neoplasms are found to implant along the subarachnoid space and

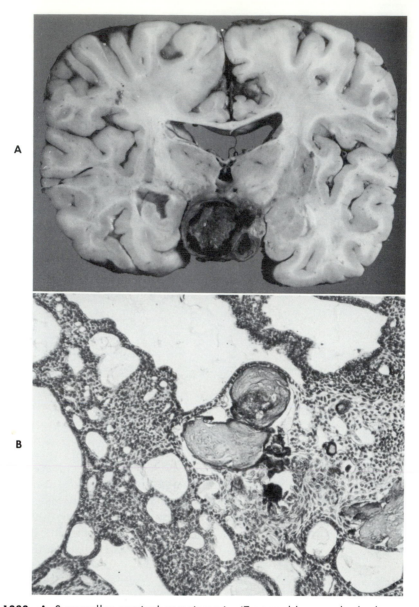

Fig. 1233 A, Suprasellar craniopharyngioma in 47-year-old man who had surgery fifteen years previously, but tumor could not be excised because of its size. Despite subsequent irradiation therapy, progressive tumor growth led to compression of optic chiasm, pituitary gland, and cerebral peduncles. Note good circumscription of tumor and its variegated appearance. **B,** Microscopic appearance of craniopharyngioma of suprasellar region. Solid epithelial nests with calcification, collections of "shadow cells," and peripheral palisading alternate with cystic areas. **(A,** WU neg. 62-5191; **B,** ×90; WU neg. 73-2681.)

even to metastasize distantly, particularly to the liver.[227, 248] This phenomenon has been reported with nonfunctioning tumors as well as with neoplasms associated with Cushing's syndrome.[259] As in most other endocrine tumors, the correlation between microscopic appearance and biologic behavior is poor. Some of the invasive or metastasizing neoplasms have an obviously malignant cytologic appearance, but the majority do not appreciably differ from the ordinary pituitary adenoma. "Pituitary apoplexy" is a rare complication of adenomas. It represents a massive hemorrhagic infarct within the tumor and is most often seen in adenomas associated with acromegaly or Cushing's syndrome.[259]

The therapeutic approach to pituitary adenomas varies in different clinics. Both surgical excision and radiation therapy can be employed, the results being largely comparable. The choice of therapy sometimes depends on the clinical circumstances but most often on local preference.[225, 244, 250, 264] A few cases of sarcoma developing as a possible late complication of radiation therapy for pituitary adenoma have been reported.[268] The average latent period is ten years, and the average tissue dose of irradiation is over 7,000 R.[231]

Craniopharyngioma is not a tumor of pituitary origin but is included in this discussion because of its invariable close correlation with the pituitary gland. Children and adults are equally affected. Its location is usually suprasellar, although it may occupy the sella as well (Fig. 1233, A). Cystic degeneration is an extremely common finding, the content of the cyst being a straw-colored or brown fluid rich in cholesterol crystals. Focal calcification is almost invariably present. In about 75% of the cases, it is prominent enough to be detectable radiographically. The microscopic appearance is very similar to that of ameloblastoma of the jaws. Anastomosing epithelial islands with a palisaded layer of cells and a center of stellate cells are characteristic (Fig. 1233, B). Foci of squamous metaplasia, microcystic degeneration, calcification, and reactive gliosis are often found. Small epithelial strands trapped in the peripheral reactive glial tissue may result in a mistaken diagnosis of carcinoma. Cystic adamantinomas also should be differentiated from epidermoid and other cysts occurring in this region. The electron microscopic appearance of craniopharyngioma has been well described by Ghatak et al.[230]

Although minor microscopic differences exist between craniopharyngioma and ameloblastoma of the jaws, comparative morphologic and histochemical studies and the finding in several cases of craniopharyngioma of undeniable tooth structures is conclusive evidence of a related embryologic origin, the intracranial tumor probably arising from a buccal equivalent of the embryonic enamel organ present in Rathke's pouch.[238, 263, 266]

Symptoms are dominated by those of hydrocephalus, especially in the younger patients, and of pressure upon the chiasm and optic tracts. Signs of hypothalamic involvement such as diabetes insipidus are common. Total surgical excision is the treatment of choice. In one series, most postoperative morbidity and all postoperative mortality occurred after second and third operations for recurrent tumor.[251]

Granular cell tumors arising from the stalk or posterior lobe of the pituitary gland usually represent an incidental autopsy finding,[246] but in a few cases they have attained enough size to produce symptoms and require surgical intervention.[265] Their morphologic appearance and histochemical reactions are similar to those of their more common peripheral counterpart. Granular cell tumors also can occur in the cerebral hemispheres.[249]

Metastatic carcinoma to the pituitary gland and sella turcica is a common finding in autopsy material, particularly in cases of breast carcinoma.[258] Microscopic examination of pituitary glands surgically removed as part of the treatment of breast carcinoma reveals a strikingly high incidence of unsuspected metastatic involvement.[239] This is always the expression of generalized disease and of little clinical significance, although on occasion it results in diabetes insipidus.[236]

Tumors of metastatic origin

Tumors of diverse origins can secondarily involve the central nervous system, either by direct extension or in the form of hematogenous metastases. They are important because they can mimic the features of primary neoplasms both clinically and pathologically. The excision of a solitary brain metastasis may precede the detection of a primary visceral neoplasm by several years. Furthermore, the neurologic manifestations may be so prominent that its removal permits an appreciably comfortable life.[272] Local extension is common in *pituitary adenomas,* as previously indicated. *Glomus jugulare tumors* often extend into the posterior fossa and present as pontocerebellar angle tumors (Chapter 15). *Carcinomas* of nasopharynx, paranasal sinuses, and ear may spread into the meninges and nerve roots of the base of the brain. This is also the case with *embryonal rhabdomyosarcomas* of the nasopharynx and ear. We have seen a *basal cell carcinoma* of the scalp penetrate into the skull and invade the cerebral meninges. *Sacrococcygeal chordomas* often produce symptoms of nerve root compression as a result of extension around the cauda equina. *Spheno-occipital chordomas* have a special propensity for penetrating the sella turcica, thus simulating a pituitary neoplasm.

Blood-borne metastatic tumors comprise approximately 4% of the intracranial tumors in surgical series and as many as 27% in some large autopsy series. Carcinomas predominate greatly over the sarcomas. The primary sites, in approximate order of frequency, are lung (65%), breast (30%), malignant melanoma (10%), kidney, colon, pancreas, prostate, stomach, and testis. The metastatic foci may appear as well-circumscribed nodules in the dura and neural parenchyma or as a diffuse meningeal and ventricular carcinomatosis (Fig. 1222). In general, metastatic nodules are better delimited than primary tumors and are surrounded by more pronounced edema (Fig. 1234). Vascular endothelial proliferation of the type most commonly seen with glial tumors is occasionally present. Any site of the brain can be affected, but the posterior portion of the sylvian fissure is a favorite location because of the

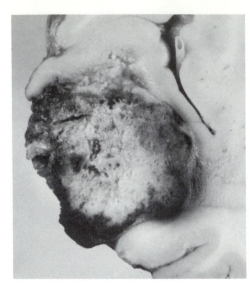

Fig. 1234 Metastatic carcinoma of temporal lobe. Primary tumor was in lung. Note sharp circumscription of tumor and surrounding edema. (WU neg. 72-1778.)

dominance of the middle cerebral artery as a continuation of the internal carotid artery. Metastatic tumors involving the spine have a strong preference for the thoracic segment of the epidural space, although intramedullary deposits also may occur.[270, 271]

Clinicopathologic correlation

Tumors of the central nervous system exhibit a rather close correlation between their microscopic types and certain clinical and anatomic parameters. Thus, knowledge of the age of the patient and exact location of the tumor frequently allows for a fairly accurate prediction of the tumor type to be expected, a piece of information that can prove quite useful to the pathologist when examining a small biopsy of a central nervous system neoplasm, particularly at the time of frozen section. The list on pages 1283 and 1284, compiled from the surgical cases seen at our institution and several published series,[273-281] summarizes this information. Each major anatomic heading contains the main tumor types to be expected, listed according to their relative frequency.

Cerebral meninges

Meningioma
Metastatic carcinoma
Direct extension from glial tumors
Direct extension from skull tumors
Malignant lymphoma
Primary sarcoma
Melanosis and malignant melanoma

Cerebral hemispheres—adults

Astrocytoma
Undifferentiated glioma
Metastatic carcinoma
Oligodendroglioma
Ependymoma
Arteriovenous malformation
Malignant lymphoma

Cerebral hemispheres—children

Astrocytoma
Ependymoma
Undifferentiated glioma
Sarcoma
Oligodendroglioma

Thalamus and basal ganglia

Undifferentiated glioma
Astrocytoma
Metastatic carcinoma

Corpus callosum and septum pellucidum

Undifferentiated glioma
Astrocytoma
Oligodendroglioma
Metastatic carcinoma

Third ventricle

Colloid cyst
Epidermoid cyst
Craniopharyngioma
Astrocytoma (pilocytic)
Ependymoma
Meningioma
Choroid plexus papilloma
Pituitary adenoma

Lateral ventricles

Ependymoma
Meningioma
Choroid plexus papilloma
Metastatic carcinoma

Pineal region

Germ cell tumors
Astrocytoma
Pinealoma

Region of sella turcica and chiasm—adults

Pituitary adenoma
Meningioma

Craniopharyngioma
Germ cell tumors
Malignant lymphoma
Chordoma

Region of sella turcica and chiasm—children

Craniopharyngioma
Germ cell tumors
Meningioma
Pituitary adenoma

Brainstem

Astrocytoma
Ependymoma
Undifferentiated glioma
Metastatic carcinoma

Fourth ventricle—adults

Ependymoma
Undifferentiated glioma
Astrocytoma
Choroid plexus papilloma
Metastatic carcinoma

Fourth ventricle—children

Ependymoma
Medulloblastoma
Choroid plexus papilloma
Astrocytoma

Cerebellar vermis—children

Medulloblastoma
Astrocytoma

Cerebellar hemispheres—adults

Astrocytoma
Metastatic carcinoma
Hemangioblastoma
Medulloblastoma

Cerebellar hemispheres—children

Astrocytoma
Medulloblastoma
Hemangioblastoma

Cerebellopontine angle

Neurilemoma
Meningioma
Astrocytoma
Choroid plexus papilloma
Paraganglioma

Spinal cord—intramedullary

Ependymoma
Astrocytoma

Spinal cord—extramedullary

Neurilemoma
Meningioma

Metastatic carcinoma
Malignant lymphoma

Cauda equina—adults

Myxopapillary ependymoma
Metastatic undifferentiated glioma
Metastatic carcinoma
Malignant lymphoma
Chordoma

Cauda equina—children

Metastatic medulloblastoma
Invasion by sacrococcygeal germ cell tumors
Myxopapillary ependymoma

Local and regional effects of intracranial tumors

The most common general signs of intracranial neoplasms are headache, papilledema, vomiting, giddiness, convulsions, abducens palsy, disturbances of mentation, and, less commonly, bradycardia and respiratory dysrhythmias. The plain roentgenogram supplies certain other signs of increased intracranial pressure or space-occupying lesions such as evidence of atrophy about the sella turcica and on the inner table of the skull and detectable shift in the position of a calcified pineal body, whereas special roentgenographic techniques such as ventriculography and arteriography can indicate specifically the location of a lesion. Echoencephalography with ultrasound may be helpful in detecting a shift of midline structures and even the position of parts of tumors or other lesions without subjecting the patient to an operative procedure.[282]

Examples of specific or focal signs are the uncinate fits that accompany involvement of the temporal lobe in the neighborhood of the hippocampus, field defects resulting from interruption of the optic tracts or projection fields, recognizable disturbance of cerebellar functions from involvement of the cerebellum, and, less frequently, recognizable deficit in extrapyramidal activity characteristic of the corpus striatum, or sensory disturbance of a nature that can be recognized as thalamic in origin. Lesions in the brainstem and spinal cord often can be almost pinpointed

by careful consideration of the disturbances of particular functions known to be associated with tracts or nuclei that are of constant location.

None of these signs, either general or focal, gives any but inferential evidence, however, of the nature of the underlying lesion.

In addition to the diagnostic import of the phenomenon underlying the signs and symptoms of increased intracranial pressure, certain pathologic conditions are created by this pressure and account for important complications that constantly lurk as unpleasant possibilities in the background of most neurosurgical cases. Principal among these are the herniations that occur at the foramen magnum and through the incisura tentorii. These are most likely to accompany supratentorial space-taking lesions. The compression of the medulla as a consequence of its being wedged between the cerebellar tonsils and the rim of the foramen magnum is rarely a lethal mechanism but has been blamed for death due to respiratory or cardiac arrest. This accounts for the general reluctance of neurosurgeons to consent to diagnostic lumbar punctures in patients suspected of having space-occupying cerebral lesions. Such events are fortunately rare, and careful examinations of the entire medical histories of a very high percentage of patients with brain tumors will reveal that a lumbar puncture was performed at some time after the onset of symptoms and before operation with no appreciable untoward effects.

Hemorrhages into the mesencephalon and pons are more commonly proved complications of increased intracranial pressure with herniations at the incisura and the foramen magnum (Fig. 1235). Poppen et al.[285] observed an incidence of 14% in 258 fatal cases of supratentorial lesions. The lesions are particularly prone to occur shortly after operations but may occur spontaneously. It is impossible to estimate how often they may develop without a fatal outcome, but their occurrence

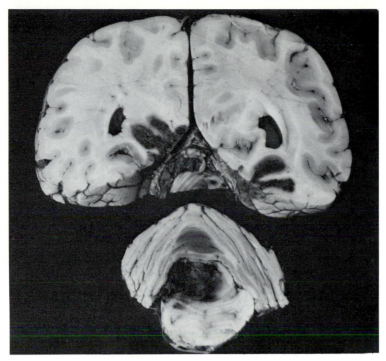

Fig. 1235 Bilateral hemorrhagic infarcts in distribution of posterior cerebral arteries and venous hemorrhages in tegmentum of pons that resulted from incisural and foramen magnum herniations in untreated astrocytoma of frontal lobe. (WU neg. 50-1272.)

in patients who survive is occasionally suggested by the signs of increased disturbance of oculomotor and pyramidal tract function with depression of consciousness or coma. The demonstration of old hemorrhages in these sites at autopsy, however, is very uncommon.

These hemorrhages appear to be of venous or capillary origin because of their infiltrative nature. Were they arterial, a lesion of more destructive and dissecting character would be expected. A satisfactory explanation of their pathogenesis is founded upon the fact that a large portion of the venous drainage of the brainstem flows upward to join the vein of Rosenthal and finally the vein of Galen. The herniation of tissue into the incisura tentorii compresses this path of venous outflow and is followed by congestion and rupture of vessels in the venous bed. On the other hand, there is interesting evidence that the hemorrhages are related rather specifically to the dynamics of the blood pressure and the in-

creased intracranial pressure[284] and might arise from focal arterial necrosis.[283]

Infarction of the medial and inferior temporal and occipital cortices also occurs as a complication of transtentorial herniation. In this event, the posterior cerebral arteries are compressed in their course around the mesencephalon, and the resulting lesions are usually symmetrical hemorrhagic infarcts. The lesions obviously involve the visual cortex, but the comatose condition of the patient generally prevents recognition of the resulting defects.

Cytology
Michael Kyriakos, M.D.

The use of spinal fluid cytology as a diagnostic method has, until recently, been impeded by the need for a simple and reliable concentration procedure for recovery of the limited number of cells found in spinal fluid specimens. The introduction of special membrane filters permits about 100% cellular recovery and a simplified approach to the problem. The method recommended by Rich[286] is used in our laboratory and is quite satisfactory.

Spinal fluid cytology is of value in patients in whom an intracranial tumor is suspected but other diagnostic procedures have been unrewarding. The recovery of tumor cells depends upon whether the tumor has made contact with the subarachnoid space and its ability to exfoliate cells. Meningiomas, although having access to the subarachnoid space, infrequently shed cells, whereas medulloblastomas do so quite readily. Metastatic tumors are more frequently identified than are primary intracranial neoplasms. Tumor cells have been diagnosed cytologically in 40% to 50% of patients with cranial metastases, whereas they are detected on an average of 30% to 40% in patients with primary lesions. Low-grade gliomas have yielded positive cytology in about 20% of cases studied; while the higher grade tumors have been positive in 40% of cases. Patients with acute lymphoblastic or myeloblastic leukemia have been shown to have immature leukocytes in the spinal fluid at some time during the course of their disease in over 60% of cases. Due to the scanty cellular material, the finding of even a few cells which are not consistent with cells normally found in a normal spinal fluid makes the diagnosis of tumor usually a simple task. False positives are rare.[286]

Diseases of skeletal muscle

Nonneoplastic diseases of the skeletal muscle system can be divided into six major categories:

1 *Neurogenic atrophy,* secondary to partial or total denervation of the muscle segment; the term *amyotrophy,* which simply means "muscle atrophy," sometimes used as synonym for neurogenic atrophy
2 *Muscular dystrophies,* thought to represent genetically determined primary degenerative diseases of the muscle fibers
3 *Myositis,* either infectious or immunologically induced

4 *Myopathies,* a term which in a generic sense embraces all muscle diseases but which is usually restricted to primary degenerative conditions that are noninflammatory, nondystrophic, and not caused by denervation
5 *Traumatic and circulatory disturbances*
6 *Disorders of function* not accompanied by significant structural changes by the usual microscopic examination; includes some disorders of neuromuscular transmission and of supraspinal tonal regulation

An internationally agreed comprehensive classification of the neuromuscular disorders has been published by the Research Group on Neuromuscular Diseases.[287]

Techniques of pathologic examination

The adequate study of muscle biopsies is a highly specialized endeavor, requiring a careful evaluation of the patient, a rigorous biopsy technique, and the performance of a battery of sophisticated techniques on the processed material.[298] When properly done, it often allows the disease to be classified into one of the five major categories previously noted and sometimes provides enough information for the diagnosis of a specific condition.[292] In selected cases, muscle biopsy should be combined with biopsy of the skin or of a peripheral nerve. The most common and successful application of muscle biopsy is in the differential diagnosis of progressive muscle wasting. When the morphologic abnormalities seen in the muscle biopsy are correlated with the results of other tests, such as enzyme determinations, electromyography, determination of motor and sensory nerve conduction times, and repetitive motor nerve stimulation, it is usually possible to determine whether the primary disease is in the spinal cord, peripheral nerves, neuromuscular function, or in the muscle fiber itself.[296, 297] To attempt to make a specific diagnosis with a single muscle biopsy without knowledge of the clinical and laboratory findings is simply to invite disaster. Many of the morphologic changes seen are nonspecific. There is often a marked dis-

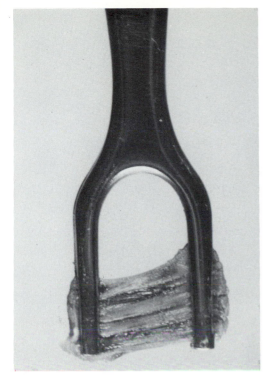

Fig. 1236 Clamp used for skeletal muscle biopsy. Specimen is maintained in this position throughout fixation step, thus minimizing retraction and distortion of muscle fibers. (WU neg. 71-10454.)

needed to obtain good fixation with a minimum of contraction of the muscle fragment. This is best accomplished by removing the sample of muscle in a special clamp that can hold the specimen throughout fixation (Fig. 1236). Ideally, at least two sections should be made to show muscle fibers in cross section as well as longitudinal section. Masson's trichrome and Mallory's phosphotungstic acid–hematoxylin are useful additions to the routine hematoxylin-eosin in the evaluation of formalin-fixed, paraffin-embedded material. Whenever possible, this should be supplemented by enzymatic histochemical techniques performed on fresh frozen sections. This allows a sharp separation of the muscle fibers into two distinct categories: *Type I fibers*, characterized by high mitochondrial oxidative enzyme activity, and *Type II fibers*, rich in myofibrillar enzymes[291] (Fig. 1237). We employ the DPNH dehydrogenase reaction for the identification of the first type and ATPase for the second. The distinction is important because these two fiber types show selective susceptibility to several diseases.[290] Finally, electron microscopic examination has proved of great value in the evaluation of the several types of myopathy.[289, 293]

crepancy between the severity of the symptoms and the degree of pathologic abnormalities. Furthermore, minor microscopic alterations in muscle are often seen in the absence of any specific muscle disease, as demonstrated by Pearson[295] and by Clawson et al.[288] in careful autopsy studies.

The muscle chosen for biopsy should be one *moderately* affected by the disease. Muscles with minimal changes or with total atrophy usually fail to provide diagnostic information. Pain to palpation and electromyographic changes may be of help in this selection. Care should be taken to avoid the muscle area needled at electromyography as the biopsy site, since marked degenerative and inflammatory changes always follow the procedure.[294] In some conditions, it is important to examine a piece of muscle that includes the terminal innervation, the latter having been located by surface electric stimulation. Care is

Neurogenic atrophy (amyotrophy)

The normal size of muscle fibers varies in different muscles as well as with the age and physical development of the individual. Most muscles of the extremities have fibers that average about 50μ in diameter, whereas external ocular muscles regularly contain uniformly small fibers of 20μ to 25μ in diameter.[301]

Skeletal muscle fibers hypertrophy with exercise and decrease in diameter and volume with disuse. Such atrophic changes are particularly pronounced if a fiber is denervated and loses its tonic stimuli.

The muscles in diseases characterized by neurogenic atrophy contain fibers that are reduced to 20μ or less in diameter, yet they retain normal structural features such as cross striations. The sarcolemmal nuclei may increase slightly in size, and their

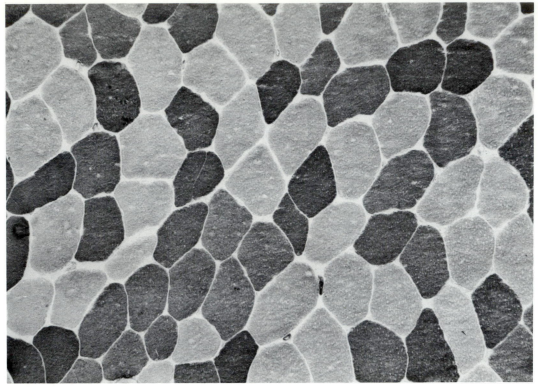

Fig. 1237 ATPase stain in normal skeletal muscle. Type I (light) and Type II fibers can be easily distinguished. (×150; WU neg. 73-3540.)

nucleoli become more prominent. Combined with the decreased fiber size, this results in a considerable apparent increase in the number of nuclei, although it is not certain whether an absolute increase actually takes place.

The most characteristic feature of biopsies from patients with neurogenic atrophy consists of large groups of small atrophic fibers with persisting islands of smaller groups of normal or hypertrophied fibers (Fig. 1238, A). This group is considered to be due to the atrophy of fibers by motor units as their anterior horn cells or major nerve fibers are destroyed. "Group lesions" often occur in neurogenic atrophy, but they are not pathognomonic of this condition. They also have been described in muscular dystrophy, malnutrition, and disuse atrophy.[305] In the early stages of neurogenic muscle disease, the atrophy may be represented only by scattered small angular fibers wedged between normal fibers. Histochemical staining often reveals "type grouping" instead of the normal mosaic pattern of type I and type II fibers.[300] "Target fibers" often appear. These are best demonstrated with the myofibrillary ATPase reaction and are regarded as characteristic of denervation atrophy.[304, 305] Intravital or supravital staining of motor nerve filaments and end-plates reveals a characteristic pattern of branching of subterminal intramuscular nerve fibers, with collateral reinnervation and degeneration of end-plates.[303]

Occasionally, focal degenerative changes simulating myopathy may appear during the late stages of neurogenic atrophy, perhaps due to reinnervation by neighboring motor neurons.[299, 302] It is not until late in these diseases that structural changes in the atrophied fibers and interstitial tissue occur. Sarcoplasm and myofibrils may disap-

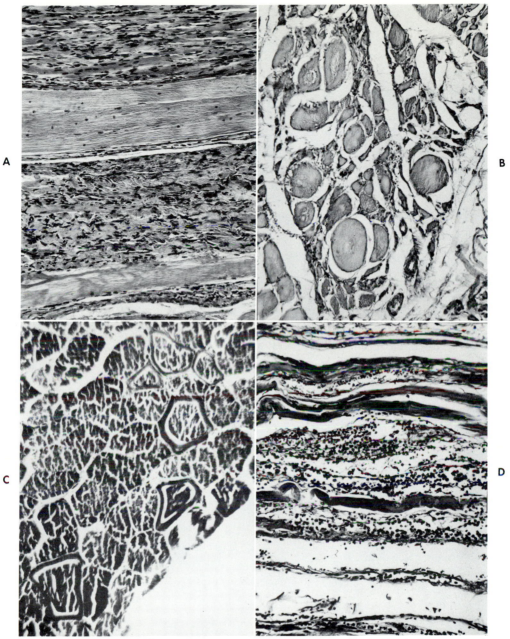

Fig. 1238 Four patterns of reaction in primary diseases of muscle. **A,** Fascicular atrophy in amyotrophic lateral sclerosis. **B,** Dystrophy with irregular, large, hyalinized fibers. **C,** Ringed fibers as occur in myotonic states, especially myotonic dystrophy. **D,** Polymyositis with disrupted fibers and heavy cellular infiltration. (**A,** ×125; UVa neg. 6308; **B,** ×125; UVa neg. 6308; **C,** Masson; ×260; UVa neg. 6308; courtesy Dr. A. G. Smith, Memphis, Tenn.; **D,** ×125; UVa neg. 6308; courtesy Dr. C. E. Wheeler, Chapel Hill, N. C.)

pear, sometimes with persistence of rows of sarcolemmal nuclei, and finally fibers are completely destroyed. Interstitial connective tissue increases slowly in amount, and there may be moderate infiltration of fat cells into the fascicles. It takes about eleven months for significant fibrosis to appear following denervation. Cellular infiltrations in the interstitial tissues and regenerative proliferation of fragments of muscle fibers form no part of the histologic pattern in these muscles.

Neurogenic atrophy can be secondary to diseases of the spinal cord, motor nerve roots, or peripheral nerves. Types of spinal muscular atrophies include the genetically determined infantile (Werdnig-Hoffmann) and juvenile spinal muscular atrophies, the amyotrophies due to congenital, infectious, and traumatic diseases of the spinal cord, and a large group of diseases of unknown etiology, such as motor neuron (Aran-Duchenne) disease.

Muscular dystrophies

The muscular dystrophies are an inherited group of conditions that has been classically regarded as a primary degenerative condition of the muscle, although the possibility of an aberration of the normal controlling influence of the nervous system on muscle also has been considered.[309] Muscular dystrophies are classified into different types on the basis of age of onset, regional distribution of the muscle involvement, and pattern of genetic transmission. The commonest varieties are *Duchenne's (pseudohypertrophic) type*, a severe generalized disease affecting children and inherited by either a sex-linked or a recessive gene, and the *facioscapulohumeral (Landouzy-Dejerine) type,* a disease of adults with a dominant pattern of inheritance and first involving the muscles of the face and shoulder girdle. Other recognized varieties of muscular dystrophy are the limb-girdle type, distal myopathy, ocular myopathy, and oculopharyngeal muscular type.[287] Also included in this category are the myotonic disorders, of which dystrophia myotonica is the commonest.

The microscopic appearance of the muscle is quite similar in all these clinical varieties of dystrophy and is mainly dependent on the stage of the disease at the time of biopsy. There is random variation in size of the muscle fibers (without the grouping of neurogenic atrophy), atrophy and disappearance of the muscle fibers with progressive replacement by fat and fibrous tissue and degenerative changes, characterized by increased eosinophilia, loss of cross striations, disorganization of myofibrils and granular, hyaline, or vacuolated appearance of the sarcoplasm (Fig. 1238, *B*). The sarcolemmal nuclei are enlarged, increased in number, and sometimes arranged in chains along the center of the muscle fiber.[307, 310] This latter change, as well as ringed fibers, is particularly prominent in dystrophia myotonica[314] (Fig. 1238, *C*). Inflammatory reaction, phagocytosis, and regeneration (as indicated by the presence of basophilic muscle fibers), although frequently present, rarely reach the severity seen in polymyositis.[312]

Histochemically, muscular dystrophies exhibit preservation of myofibrillary ATPase activity and focal loss of mitochondrial enzymatic activity.[308] Ultrastructurally, mitochondrial abnormalities and disruption and loss of myofilaments are constant findings.[306, 311] Muscular dystrophy carriers exhibit changes qualitatively similar but of lesser severity.[311] According to Schroder and Adams[313] the most characteristic fine structural feature of dystrophia myotonica is the presence of large sarcoplasmic aggregates of disordered myofilaments and other organelles.

Myositis

Inflammatory diseases of muscle can be divided into two groups: those of recognized infectious etiology (viral, bacterial, fungal, or parasitic) and those probably mediated by immunologic mechanisms. The better known forms of infectious myositis are due to trichinosis, superimposed bacterial infection in a muscle of an ischemic extremity, and gas gangrene. The infrequent granulomatous myositis due to tuberculosis, atypical mycobacteriosis, sarcoidosis, or syphilis also belongs to this category.[319] Immunologically mediated myositis is characterized by generalized involvement —hence the term polymyositis. The disease may be restricted to the skeletal muscle system or, more commonly, be a manifestation of a systemic "collagen disease," such as dermatomyositis, lupus erythematosus, rheumatic fever, rheumatoid arthritis, scleroderma, polyarteritis nodosa, or Sjogren's syndrome.[316] Polymyositis developing after the age of 40 years is associated with visceral carcinoma in a high percentage of patients.

Polymyositis primarily affects the girdle muscles. It can closely simulate various types of muscular dystrophy on clinical grounds,[318, 320] but the two diseases are easily distinguished by examination of a muscle biopsy. Microscopically, the acute form is expressed by a combination of inflammatory, degenerative, and regenerative changes, such as granular and floccular degeneration, fragmentation and phagocytosis of muscle fibers, and interstitial infiltrations of lymphocytes, plasma cells, macrophages and occasional neutrophils and eosinophils (Fig. 1238, *D*). Evidence of regeneration consists of buds or separate masses of basophilic sarcoplasm in which there are central large or multiple nuclei. This disease may be overwhelming and fatal, but many patients recover.

Chronic polymyositis, on the other hand, is a more relentlessly progressive disease. The histologic appearance of the muscles may be that of intense inflammation even late in the course of the disease in some patients, but in many the changes consist of a greater interstitial fibrosis with less inflammatory cellular infiltration and evidence of regenerative reaction by the muscle fibers. Adams et al.[315] emphasized the particular atrophy, vacuolation, and destruction of fibers at the periphery of muscle fascicles in this condition. It may progress to complete destruction of the muscle, fibrous contracture, and even metaplastic bone formation.

Histochemically, the affected muscle fibers show extensive loss of myosin ATPase as a result of destruction of myofibrils. On the other hand, mitochondrial oxidative enzymatic activity is usually preserved. Ultrastructurally, the most significant finding in polymyositis is the frequent occurrence of filamentous or tubular structures resembling paramyxovirus nucleocapsid.[317] Whether they indeed represent viral structures or a peculiar cytoplasmic reaction to injury, their almost constant occurrence in cases of dermatomyositis is of diagnostic significance. Other changes include disorganization and loss of myofilaments, mitochondial alterations, and dilation of endoplasmic reticulum.[321]

Myopathies

The nondystrophic, noninflammatory primary degenerative muscle diseases can be divided into two distinct categories. The first is comprised of a large group of acquired myopathies secondary to or at least associated with a variety of endocrine, metabolic, neoplastic, and immunologically mediated disorders or with the administration of drugs or toxins. We are referring to the myopathies seen in association with hyperthyroidism,[347] myxedema, hypopituitarism, acromegaly, Cushing's disease, Addison's disease, primary aldosteronism, hyperparathyroidism, osteomalacia, glycogen storage disease, nutritional deficiency, carcinomatosis,[322, 325, 326] and myasthenia gravis, as well as those appearing after the administration of chloroquine,[348] emetine,[327] plasmocid,[345] vincristine,[354] tri-ortho-cresylphosphate (TOCP),[346] steroid, ACTH, and alcohol.[338, 340, 344]

The microscopic appearance is nonspecific. In some cases, no morphologic alterations are present. In the majority, however, scattered degenerative changes of the muscle fibers are present, sometimes accompanied by an inflammatory infiltrate. The differential diagnosis with muscular dystrophy and polymyositis may be impossible on morphologic grounds. This is also the case at an electron microscopic level.[349]

Most types of glycogenosis involve skeletal muscle, their common morphologic denominator being the accumulation of glycogen in the sarcoplasm.[334] The tinctorial and ultrastructural appearance of the glycogen granules and their location within the sarcoplasm vary according to the types of glycogenosis.[336]

The second group of myopathies, sometimes referred to as "benign congenital myopathies," become symptomatic in infancy or childhood, the usual way of presentation being proximal or diffuse muscle weakness ("floppy infants"). They are unaccompanied by elevation of serum enzyme levels, run an essentially nonprogressive clinical course and have a definite familial incidence.[343] Among this group, an ever-increasing number of more or less distinct varieties have been singled out in recent years, principally on the basis of some supposedly specific fine structural feature.

In *nemaline myopathy,* threadlike or rodlike structures appear within an otherwise normal sarcoplasm.[353] These structures stain with Mallory's PTAH and Masson's trichrome. Ultrastructurally, the nemaline structures have a tetragonal filamentous structure with a perpendicular periodicity of 125Å to 200Å, thus closely resembling hypertrophic Z bands.[328, 331] *Central core disease* is characterized by the presence of "cores" in the central areas of the sarcoplasm which are PAS-positive and fail to rotate polarized light.[351] Ultrastructural study of the "core" shows focal decrease of mitochondria, myofibrillar degeneration, and decrease of glycogen and sarcotubular profiles.[332] *Multicore disease* shows qualitatively similar changes but differs from the former by virtue of the pleomorphism of the cores, their smaller size, and their greater number per unit area in the affected fibers.[330] In *centronuclear (myotubular) myopathy,* most of the myofibers contain central nuclei, the appearance thus resembling that of embryonal myotubules.[341, 355] *"Mitochondrial" myopathies* are so named because of the striking mitochondrial abnormalities seen on electron microscopic examination. These consist of enlargement, abnormal shapes, and presence of inclusions.[352] Other "entities" recently described are crystalline intranuclear inclusion myopathy,[337] reducing body myopathy,[323] and fingerprint body myopathy.[329]

It is becoming evident that many of these ultrastructural features are not specific for their respective entities. The sampling error inherent in any electron microscopic study and the limited present knowledge on the ultrastructural variations of normalcy or of physiologic reaction in human muscle call for caution in the interpretation of these findings. Rodlike structures and "cores" have been produced by tenotomy.[339] Mitochondrial abnormalities similar to those described by Shy et al.[352] have been found in hypothyroid myopathy,[335, 342] neuropathy,[333] myositis,[324] and muscular atrophy.[350]

Traumatic and circulatory disturbances

Several types of reaction may arise in muscle as the result of hemorrhage or ischemia. *Myositis ossificans* has been discussed in Chapter 23. *Volkmann's contracture* represents a complication of too tightly applied casts and bandages and is probably the result of ischemia due principally to interruption of the venous drainage. Microscopically, large amounts of cellular fibrous tissue are seen replacing a destroyed muscle, of which only a few fibers may eventually persist.

Violent contraction or hard exercise in the untrained individual may lead to rupture of muscle sheaths, with herniation or hemorrhages in the muscle. A particularly interesting form is the "anterior tibial compartment syndrome" in which initial edema or hemorrhage increases the volume of a rather rigidly confined muscle and results in progressive destruction of the remainder of the muscle apparently by ischemia.[356] The connective tissue in these muscles reacts rapidly with the formation of considerable fibrosis.

Diseases of peripheral nerves

Routinely processed biopsies of peripheral nerves can provide diagnostic information in a few selected diseases, such as periarteritis nodosa, amyloidosis, sarcoidosis, leprosy, and metachromatic leukodystrophy. On the other hand, they are of little use in the evaluation of the much more common primary degenerative conditions. Proper evaluation of a nerve biopsy in these cases includes a battery of special stains for neurites, myelin, and various enzymes, quantitative estimations, examination of teased fiber preparations, conduction velocity studies in vitro, and electron microscopic examination. The sural nerve is particularly suited for biopsy, because of its common involvement in peripheral nerve diseases, its superficiality, and its primarily sensorial nature. Dyck and Lofgren[362] have described a technique for fascicular biopsy of this nerve which results in only minimal sensory deficit.

Pathologically, degenerative peripheral neuropathies can be divided in two broad categories. In *axonal (wallerian) degeneration,* the central axon is the primary site of the disease, eventually leading to collapse of the myelin sheath. In *segmental demyelination,* the myelin sheath (and therefore the Schwann cell) is the site of degeneration. The disease begins near the nodes of Ranvier, eventually leading to disappearance of the myelin sheath of an entire internode.[364]

Many are the causes of peripheral neuropathy.[361, 366] Some are genetically determined, such as peroneal muscular atrophy (Charcot-Marie-Tooth disease) and hereditary hypertrophic interstitial neuropathy (Dejerine-Sottas disease). A large percentage arise on the basis of a metabolic derangement, such as nutritional deficiency, diabetes, chronic liver disease, uremia, or porphyria.[357, 363, 367] A form of neuropathy of special interest is that associated with malignant tumors. It is seen more commonly with carcinoma, particularly of the bronchogenic type,[359] but it also has been observed with malignant lymphoma and myeloma.[360, 368] It may present as a purely sensory neuropathy with paresthesias due to degeneration of dorsal root ganglion cells or as a symmetrical distal mixed neuropathy secondary to segmental demyelina-

tion.[359] The rare occurrence of direct metastatic involvement of the nerve by carcinoma and lymphoma has been reported by Barron et al.[358] In a large percentage of polyneuropathies, the cause remains undetermined.[365]

REFERENCES
Congenital diseases
Ectopia

1 Goldring, S., Hodges, F. H., Jr., and Luse, S. A.: Ectopic neural tissue of occipital bone, J. Neurosurg. **21**:479-484, 1964.

Spina bifida

2 Fisher, R. G., Uihlein, A., and Keith, H. M.: Spina bifida and cranium bifidum; study of 530 cases, Mayo Clin. Proc. **27**:33-38, 1952.
3 Mawdsley, T., Rickham, P. P., and Roberts, J. R.: Long term results of early operation of open myelomeningoceles and encephaloceles, Br. Med. J. **1**:663-666, 1967.
4 Russell, D. S.: Observations on the pathology of hydrocephalus, Medical Research Council Special Report Series, No. 265, London, 1949, His Majesty's Stationery Office.

Epidermoid, dermoid, and other congenital cysts

5 Leidler, F., Smith, D. E., and Woolsey, R. D.: Intracranial epidermoid cyst, Am. J. Clin. Pathol. **21**:852-857, 1951.
6 MacCarty, C. S., Leavens, M. E., Love, J. G., and Kernohan, J. W.: Dermoid and epidermoid tumors in the central nervous systems of adults, Surg. Gynecol. Obstet. **108**:191-198, 1959.
7 Manno, N. J., Uihlein, A., and Kernohan, J. W.: Intraspinal epidermoids, J. Neurosurg. **19**:754-765, 1962.
8 Mount, L. A.: Congenital dermal sinuses as a cause of meningitis, intraspinal abscess and intracranial abscess, J.A.M.A. **139**:1263-1268, 1949.
9 Scoville, W. B., Manlapaz, J. S., Otis, R. D., and Cabieses, F.: Intraspinal enterogenous cyst, J. Neurosurg. **20**:704-706, 1963.
10 Ulrich, J.: Intracranial epidermoids; a study of their distribution and spread, J. Neurosurg. **21**:1054-1058, 1964.

Hydrocephalus

11 Beckett, R. S., Netsky, M. G., and Zimmerman, H. M.: Developmental stenosis of the aqueduct of Sylvius, Am. J. Pathol. **26**:755-787, 1950.
12 Russell, D. S.: Observations on the pathology of hydrocephalus, Medical Research Council Special Report Series, No. 265, London, 1949, His Majesty's Stationery Office.

Arnold-Chiari deformity and platybasia

13 Fairman, D., and Horrax, G.: Classification of craniostenosis, J. Neurosurg. **6**:307-313, 388-395, 1949.

14 List, C. F.: Neurologic syndromes accompanying developmental anomalies of occipital bone, atlas and axis, Arch. Neurol. Psychiatry **45**:577-616, 1941.

Congenital cerebral diseases and brain biopsy

15 Borberg, A.: Clinical and genetic investigations into tuberous sclerosis and Recklinghausen's neurofibromatosis; contribution to elucidation of interrelationship and eugenics of syndromes, Acta Psychiatr. Neurol., Suppl. 71, pp. 3-239, 1951.

16 Davidson, C., and Jacobson, S. A.: Generalized lipoidosis in a case of amaurotic familial idiocy, Am. J. Dis. Child. **52**:345-360, 1936.

17 Hain, R. F., and LaVeck, G. D.: Metachromatic leuko-encephalopathy, Pediatrics **22**:1064-1073, 1958.

18 Landing, B. H., and Rubinstein, J. H.: Biopsy diagnosis of neurologic diseases in children, with emphasis on the lipidoses. In Aronson, S. M., and Volk, B. W., editors: Cerebral sphingolipidoses (A symposium on Tay-Sach's disease and allied disorders), New York, 1962, Academic Press, Inc. (this volume has other relative papers).

19 McMenemey, W. H.: Cerebral biopsy, and special methods for the study of cerebrospinal fluid. In Bailey, O. T., and Smith, D. E., editors: The central nervous system, Baltimore, 1968, The Williams & Wilkins Co.

20 Svennerholm, L.: Chemical examination of neural biopsy material; general aspects, Acta Neurol. Scand. **41**(suppl. 13):281-284, 1965.

21 Wagner, J. A., and Wisotzkey, H.: Cerebral cortical biopsy: a new vista for the pathologist, South. Med. J. **56**:415-418, 1963.

22 Wolfe, H. J., and Pietra, G. G.: The visceral lesions of metachromatic leukodystrophy, Am. J. Pathol. **44**:921-930, 1964.

Vascular diseases
Saccular aneurysms

23 Boyd-Wilson, J. S.: The association of cerebral angiomas with intracranial aneurysms, J. Neurol. Neurosurg. Psychiatr. **22**:218-223, 1959.

24 Crompton, M. R.: The pathogenesis of cerebral aneurysms, Brain **89**:797-814, 1966.

25 Dandy, W. E.: Intracranial arterial aneurysms, New York, 1969, Hafner Publishing Co.

26 Forbus, W. D.: On the origin of miliary aneurysms of the superficial cerebral arteries, Bull. Hopkins Hosp. **47**:239-284, 1930.

27 Glynn, L. E.: Medial defects in the circle of Willis and their relation to aneurysm formation, J. Pathol. Bacteriol. **51**:213-222, 1940.

28 Lang, E. R., and Kidd, M.: Electron microscopy of human cerebral aneurysms, J. Neurosurg. **22**:554-562, 1965.

29 McCormick, W. F., and Nofzinger, J. D.: Saccular intracranial aneurysms; an autopsy study, J. Neurosurg. **22**:155-159, 1965.

30 Richardson, J. C., and Hyland, H. H.: Intracranial aneurysms, Medicine (Baltimore) **20**:1-83, 1941.

31 Sahs, A. L.: Observations on the pathology of saccular aneurysms, J. Neurosurg. **24**:792-806, 1966.

32 Slosberg, P. S.: Medical treatment of intracranial aneurysm, Neurology **10**:1085-1089, 1960.

33 Smith, D. E., and Windsor, R. B.: Embryologic and pathogenic aspects of the development of cerebral saccular aneurysms. In Fields, W. S., editor: Pathogenesis and treatment of cerebro vascular disease, Springfield, Ill., 1961, Charles C Thomas, Publisher, pp. 367-386.

34 Walker, A. E., and Allegra, G. W.: The pathology and pathogenesis of cerebral aneurysms, J. Neuropathol. Exp. Neurol. **13**:248-259, 1954.

Cranial arteritis

35 Hollenhorst, R. W., Brown, J. R., Wagener, H. P., and Shick, R. M.: Neurologic aspects of temporal arteritis, Neurology **10**:490-498, 1960.

36 Kimmelstiel, P., Gilmour, M. T., and Hodges, H. H.: Degeneration of elastic fibers in granulomatous giant cell arteritis (temporal arteritis), Arch. Pathol. **54**:157-168, 1952.

37 Kolodny, E. H., Rebeiz, J. J., Caviness, V. S., Jr., and Richardson, E. P., Jr.: Granulomatous angiitis of the central nervous system, J. Neuropathol. Exp. Neurol. **27**:125-126, 1968.

Effects of vascular insufficiency Pseudotumor cerebri

38 Conn, H. O., Dunn, J. B., Newman, H. A., and Belkin, G. A.: Pulmonary emphysema simulating brain tumor, Am. J. Med. **22**:524-533, 1957.

39 Foley, J.: Benign forms of intracranial hypertension—"toxic" and "otitic" hydrocephalus, Brain **78**:1-41, 1955.

40 Zuidema, G. D., and Cohen, S. J.: Pseudotumor cerebri, J. Neurosurg. **11**:433-441, 1954.

Traumatic diseases

41 Penfield, W., and Flanigin, H.: Surgical therapy of temporal lobe seizures, Arch. Neurol. Psychiatry **64**:491-500, 1950.

42 Tedeschi, C. G.: Cerebral injury by blunt mechanical trauma; review of literature, Medicine (Baltimore) **24**:339-357, 1945.

Dural-cortical cicatrix

43 Penfield, W., and Jasper, H.: Epilepsy and the functional anatomy of the human brain, Boston, 1954, Little, Brown and Co.

44 Walker, A. E.: Posttraumatic epilepsy, Springfield, Ill., 1949, Charles C Thomas, Publisher.

Epidural hematoma

45 Gallagher, J. P., and Browder, E. J.: Extradural hematoma; experience with 167 patients, J. Neurosurg. **29**:1-12, 1968.

46 Stevenson, G. C., Brown, H. A., and Hoyt, W. F.: Chronic venous epidural hematoma at the vertex, J. Neurosurg. **21**:887-891, 1964.

Subdural hematoma

47 Leary, T.: Subdural hemorrhages, J.A.M.A. **103**:897-903, 1934.

48 McLaurin, R. L., and McLaurin, K. S.: Calcified subdural hematomas in childhood, J. Neurosurg. **24**:648-655, 1966.

49 Svien, H. J., and Gelety, J. E.: On the surgical management of encapsulated subdural hematomas; a comparison of the results of membranectomy and simple evacuation, J. Neurosurg. **21**:172-177, 1964.

50 Zollinger, R., and Gross, R. E.: Traumatic subdural hematoma; an explanation of the late onset of pressure symptoms, J.A.M.A. **103**:245-249, 1934.

Chronic arachnoiditis and arachnoidal cyst

51 Miller, P. R., and Elder, F. W., Jr.: Meningeal pseudocysts (meningocele spurius) following laminectomy; report of ten cases, J. Bone Joint Surg. [Am.] **50**:268-276, 1968.

52 Nugent, G. R., Odom, G. L., and Woodhall, B.: Spinal extradural cysts, Neurology **9**:397-405, 1959.

53 Rosenbaum, H. E., Long, F., Hinchey, T., and Trufant, S. A.: Paralysis following saddle-block anaesthesia, Arch. Neurol. Psychiatry **68**:783-790, 1952.

Ruptured intervertebral discs

54 Strully, K. J., Gross, S. W., Schwartzmann, J., and von Storch, T. J. C.: Progressive spinal cord disease; syndromes associated with herniation of cervical intervertebral discs, J.A.M.A. **146**:10-12, 1951.

Inflammatory diseases
Chronic pachymeningitis

55 Hassin, G. B.: Circumscribed suppurative (nontuberculous) peripachymeningitis, Arch. Neurol. Psychiatry **20**:110-129, 1928.

Brain abscess

56 Atkinson, E. M.: Abscess of the brain: its pathology, diagnosis and treatment, London, 1934, Medical Publications, Ltd.

57 Carey, M. E., Chow, S. N., and French, L. A.: Experience with brain abscesses, J. Neurosurg. **36**:1-9, 1972.

58 Carmichael, F. A., Kernohan, J. W., and Adson, A. W.: Histopathogenesis of cerebral abscess, Arch. Neurol. Psychiatry **42**:1001-1029, 1939.

59 Kerr, F. W. L., King, R. B., and Meagher, J. N.: Brain abscess—a study of forty-seven consecutive cases, J.A.M.A. **168**:868-872, 1958.

60 Samson, D. S., and Clark, R.: Current review of brain abscesses, Am. J. Med. **54**:201-210, 1973.

61 Wright, R. L., and Ballantine, H. T., Jr.: Management of brain abscesses in children and adolescents, Am. J. Dis. Child. **114**:113-122, 1967.

Granulomatous diseases

62 Canton, C. A., and Mount, L. A.: Neurosurgical aspect of cryptococcosis, J. Neurosurg. **8**:143-156, 1951.

63 Krueger, E. G., Norsa, L., Kenney, M., and Price, P. A.: Nocardiosis of the central nervous system, J. Neurosurg. **11**:226-233, 1954.

64 Rayport, M., Wisoff, H. S., and Zaiman, H.: Vertebral echinococcosis; report of case of surgical and biological therapy with review of the literature, J. Neurosurg. **21**:647-659, 1964.

65 Schneider, R. C., and Rand, R. W.: Actinomycotic brain abscess, J. Neurosurg. **6**:255-259, 1949.

Tumors
Introduction

66 Kernohan, J. W., and Sayre, G. P.: Tumors of the central nervous system, In Atlas of tumor pathology, Fasc. 35, Washington, D. C., 1952, Armed Forces Institute of Pathology.

67 Polak, M.: Blastomas del sistema nervioso central y periférico. Patología y ordenación histogenética, Buenos Aires, 1966, Lopez Libreros Ed.

68 Rubinstein, L. J.: Tumors of the central nervous system, In Atlas of tumor pathology, Second Series, Fasc. 6, Washington, D. C., 1972, Armed Forces Institute of Pathology.

69 Willis, R. A.: Pathology of tumours, ed. 4, London, 1967, Butterworth & Co.

Tumors of neuroglial cells
  Astrocytoma

70 Bailey, P., and Bucy, P. C.: Astroblastomas of the brain, Acta Psychiatr. Neurol. **5**:439-461, 1960.

71 Bucy, P. C., and Thieman, P. W.: Astrocytomas of the cerebellum; a study of a series of patients operated upon over 28 years ago, Arch. Neurol. **18**:14-19, 1968.

72 Dunn, J., Jr., and Kernohan, J. W.: Gliomatosis cerebri, Arch. Pathol. **64**:82-91, 1957.

73 Feigin, I. H., and Gross, S. W.: Sarcoma arising in glioblastoma of the brain, Am. J. Pathol. **31:**633-653, 1955.

74 Goldman, R. L.: Gliomyosarcoma of the cerebrum; report of a unique case, Am. J. Clin. Pathol. **52:**741-744, 1969.

75 Grcevic, N., and Yates, P. O.: Rosenthal fibres in tumours of the central nervous system, J. Pathol. Bacteriol. **73:**467-472, 1957.

76 Hadfield, M. G., and Silverberg, S. G.: Light and electron microscopy of giant-cell glioblastoma, Cancer **30:**989-996, 1972.

77 Hossman, K. A., and Wechsler, W.: Zur feinstruktur menschlicher spongioblastome, Dtsch. Z. Nervenheilk **197:**327-351, 1965.

78 Hoyt, W. F., Meshel, L. G., Lessell, S., Schatz, N. J., and Suckling, R. D.: Malignant optic glioma of adulthood, Brain **96:**121-132, 1973.

79 Jelsma, R., and Bucy, P. C.: The treatment of glioblastoma multiforme of the brain, J. Neurosurg. **27:**388-400, 1967.

80 Lynn, J. A., Panopio, I. T., Martin, J. H., Shaw, M. L., and Race, G. J.: Ultrastructural evidence for astroglial histogenesis of the monstruocellular astrocytoma (so-called monstruocellular sarcoma of brain), Cancer **22:** 356-366, 1968.

81 Robertson, D. M., and MacLean, J. D.: Nuclear inclusions in malignant gliomas, Arch. Neurol. **13:**287-296, 1965.

82 Rubinstein, L. J., Herman, M. M., and Foley, V. L.: *In vitro* characteristics of human glioblastomas maintained in organ culture systems; light microscopic observations, Am. J. Pathol. **71:**61-76, 1973.

83 Russell, D. S.: The occurrence and distribution of intranuclear "inclusion bodies" in gliomas, J. Pathol. Bacteriol. **35:**625-634, 1932.

84 Russell, D. S., and Bland, J. O. W.: Further notes on the tissue culture of gliomas with special reference to Bailey's spongioblastoma, J. Pathol. Bacteriol. **39:**375-380, 1934.

85 Scherer, H. J.: Structural development in gliomas, Am. J. Cancer **34:**333-351, 1938.

86 Smith, D. R., Hardman, J. M., and Earle, K. M.: Metastasizing neuroectodermal tumors of the central nervous system, J. Neurosurg. **31:** 50-58, 1969.

87 Smith, D. R., Hardman, J. M., and Earle, K. M.: Contiguous glioblastoma multiforme and fibrosarcoma with extracranial metastasis, Cancer **24:**270-276, 1969.

88 Solomon, A., Perret, G. E., and McCormick, W. F.: Multicentric gliomas of the cerebral and cerebellar hemispheres; case report, J. Neurosurg. **31:**87-93, 1969.

89 Weir, B.: The relative significance of factors affecting postoperative survival in astrocytomas, grade 3 and 4, J. Neurosurg. **38:**448-452, 1973.

Oligodendroglioma

90 Best, P. V.: Intracranial oligodendromatosis, J. Neurol. Neurosurg. Psychiatry **26:**249-256, 1963.

91 Roberts, M., and German, W. J.: A long term study of patients with oligodendrogliomas; follow-up of 50 cases, including Dr. Harvey Cushing's series, J. Neurosurg. **24:**697-700, 1966.

92 Robertson, D. M., and Vogel, F. S.: Concentric lamination of glial processes in oligodendrogliomas, J. Cell Biol. **15:**313-334, 1962.

93 Rubinstein, L. J.: Tumors of the central nervous system. In Atlas of tumor pathology, Second Series, Fasc. 6, Washington, D. C., 1972, Armed Forces Institute of Pathology.

94 Scharenberg, K.: Blastomatous oligodendroglia as satellites of nerve cells; a study with silver carbonate, Am. J. Pathol. **30:**957-967, 1954.

95 Spataro, J., and Sacks, O.: Oligodendroglioma with remote metastases; case report, J. Neurosurg. **28:**373-379, 1968.

96 Weir, B., and Elvidge, A. R.: Oligodendrogliomas; an analysis of 63 cases, J. Neurosurg. **29:**500-525, 1968.

Ependymoma

97 Anderson, M. S.: Myxopapillary ependymomas presenting in the soft tissue over the sacrococcygeal region, Cancer **19:**585-590, 1966.

98 Ayres, W. W.: Ependymoma of the cauda equina; a report of the clinicopathologic aspects and follow-up studies of eighteen cases, Milit. Med. **122:**10-35, 1958.

99 Chason, J. L.: Subependymal mixed gliomas, J. Neuropathol. Exp. Neurol. **15:**461-470, 1956.

100 Fokes, E. C., Jr., and Earle, K. M.: Ependymomas: clinical and pathological aspects, J. Neurosurg. **30:**585-594, 1969.

101 Goebel, H. H., and Cravioto, H.: Ultrastructure of human and experimental ependymomas; a comparative study, J. Neuropathol. Exp. Neurol. **31:**54-71, 1972.

102 Kernohan, J. W., and Fletcher-Kernohan, E.: Ependymomas; a study of 109 cases, Assoc. Res. Nerv. Ment. Dis., Proc. **16:**182-209, 1937.

102a Rawlinson, D. G., Herman, M. M., and Rubinstein, L. J.: The fine structure of a myxopapillary ependymoma of the filum terminale, Acta Neuropathol. **25:**1-13, 1973.

103 Rubinstein, L. J.: Tumors of the central nervous system. In Atlas of tumor pathology, Second Series, Fasc. 6, Washington, D. C., 1972, Armed Forces Institute of Pathology.

104 Rubinstein, L. J., and Logan, W. J.: Extraneural metastases in ependymoma of the cauda equina, J. Neurol. Neurosurg. Psychiatry **33:**763-770, 1970.

105 Wolff, M., Santiago, H., and Duby, M. M.:

Delayed distant metastasis from a subcutaneous sacrococcygeal ependymoma; case report with tissue culture, ultrastructural observations and review of the literature, Cancer **30**: 1046-1067, 1972.

Tumors and tumorlike conditions of choroid plexus

106 Ariëns-Kappers, J. A.: The development of the paraphysis cerebri in man with comments on its relationship to the intercolumnar tubercle and its significance for the origin of cystic tumors in the third ventricle, J. Comp. Neurol. **102**:425-509, 1955.

107 Ayres, W. W., and Haymaker, W.: Xanthoma and cholesterol granuloma of the choroid plexus; report of the pathologic aspects in 29 cases, J. Neuropathol. Exp. Neurol. **23**:431-445, 1964.

108 Carter, L. P., Beggs, J., and Waggener, J. D.: Ultrastructure of three choroid plexus papillomas, Cancer **30**:1130-1136, 1972.

109 Coxe, W. S., and Luse, S. A.: Colloid cyst of third ventricle; an electron microscopic study, J. Neuropathol. Exp. Neurol. **23**:431-445, 1964.

110 Shuangshoti, S., and Netsky, M. G.: Neuroepithelial (colloid) cysts of nervous system: further observations on pathogenesis, location, incidence and histochemistry, Neurology **16**: 887-903, 1966.

111 Shuangshoti, S., Roberts, M. P., and Netsky, M. G.: Neuroepithelial (colloid) cysts, Arch. Pathol. **80**:214-224, 1965.

112 Shuangshoti, S., Tangchai, P., and Netsky, M. G.: Primary adenocarcinoma of choroid plexus, Arch. Pathol. **91**:101-106, 1971.

113 Smith, J. F.: Hydrocephalus associated with choroid plexus papillomas, J. Neuropathol. Exp. Neurol. **14**:442-449, 1955.

Tumors of primitive neuroepithelial cells

114 Bailey, P., and Cushing, H.: A classification of the tumors of the glioma group on a histogenetic basis with a correlated study of prognosis, Philadelphia, 1926, J. B. Lippincott Co.

115 Banna, M., Lassman, L. P., and Pearce, G. W.: Radiological study of skeletal metastases from cerebellar medulloblastoma, Br. J. Radiol. **43**:173-179, 1970.

116 Bloom, H. J. G., Wallace, E. N. K., and Henz, J. M.: Treatment and prognosis of medulloblastoma in children: study of 82 verified cases, Am. J. Roentgenol. Radium Ther. Nucl. Med. **105**:43-62, 1969.

117 Bofin, P. J., and Ebels, E.: A case of medullomyoblastoma, Acta Neuropathol. (Berl.) **2**: 309-311, 1963.

118 Chatty, E. M., and Earle, K. M.: Medulloblastoma; a report of 201 cases with emphasis on the relationship of histologic variants to survival, Cancer **28**:977-983, 1971.

119 Crue, B. L., Jr.: Medulloblastoma, Springfield, Ill., 1958, Charles C Thomas, Publisher.

120 Drachman, D. A., Winter, T. S., III, and Karon, M.: Medulloblastoma with extracranial metastases, Arch. Neurol. **9**:518-530, 1963.

121 Kadin, M. E., Rubinstein, L. J., and Nelson, J. S.: Neonatal cerebellar medulloblastoma originating from the fetal external granular layer, J. Neuropathol. Exp. Neurol. **29**:583-600, 1970.

122 Kane, W., and Aronson, S. M.: Gangliogliomatous maturation in cerebellar medulloblastoma, Acta Neuropathol. (Berlin) **9**:273-279, 1967.

123 Karch, S. B., and Urich, H.: Medulloepithelioma: definition of an entity, J. Neuropathol. Exp. Neurol. **31**:27-53, 1972.

124 McFarland, D. R., Horwitz, H., Saenger, E. L., and Bahr, G. K.: Medulloblastoma; review of prognosis and survival, Br. J. Radiol. **42**: 198-214, 1969.

125 Matakas, F., Cervós-Navarro, J., and Gullotta, F.: The ultrastructure of medulloblastomas, Acta Neuropathol. (Berl.) **16**:271-284, 1970.

126 Miller, A. A., and Ramsden, F.: A cerebral neuroblastoma with unusual fibrous tissue reaction, J. Neuropathol. Exp. Neurol. **25**:328-340, 1966.

127 Misugi, K., and Liss, L.: Medulloblastoma with cross-striated muscle: a fine structural study, Cancer **25**:1279-1285, 1970.

128 Oberman, H. A., Hewitt, W. C., Jr., and Kalivoda, A. J.: Medulloblastomas with distant metastases, Am. J. Clin. Pathol. **39**:148-160, 1963.

129 Polak, M.: On the true nature of the so-called medulloblastoma, Acta Neuropathol. (Berl.) **8**:84-95, 1967.

130 Rio Hortega, P. del: Nomenclatura y clasificación de los tumores del sistema nervioso, Buenos Aires, 1945, Lopez & Etchegoyen.

131 Rubinstein, L. J.: Discussion on polar spongioblastomas, Acta Neurochir. (Wien) suppl. **10**:126-132, 1964.

132 Rubinstein, L. J.: The definition of the ependymoblastoma, Arch. Pathol. **90**:35-45, 1970.

133 Rubinstein, L. J.: Cytogenesis and differentiation of primitive central neuroepithelial tumors, J. Neuropathol. Exp. Neurol. **31**:7-26, 1972.

134 Rubinstein, L. J.: Tumors of the central nervous system, In Atlas of tumor pathology, Second Series, Fasc. 6, Washington, D. C., 1972, Armed Forces Institute of Pathology.

135 Rubinstein, L. J., and Northfield, D. W. C.: Medulloblastoma and so-called "arachnoidal cerebellar sarcoma": critical re-examination of a nosologic problem, Brain **87**:379-412, 1964.

136 Schenk, E. A.: Medulloblastoma; relationship to meningeal sarcoma, Arch. Pathol. **82**:363-368, 1966.

137 Treip, C. S.: A congenital medulloepithelioma of the midbrain, J. Pathol. Bacteriol. **74:**357-363, 1957.

138 von Epps, R. R., Samuelson, D. R., and McCormick, W. F.: Cerebral medulloepithelioma; case report, J. Neurosurg. **27:**568-573, 1967.

Tumors of neuronal cells

139 Courville, C. B.: Ganglioglioma, tumor of the central nervous system; review of the literature and report of two cases, Arch. Neurol. Psychiatry **24:**439-491, 1930.

140 Steegmann, A. T., and Winer, B.: Temporal lobe epilepsy resulting from ganglioglioma; report of an unusual case in an adolescent boy, Neurology **11:**406-412, 1961.

141 Wahl, R. W., and Dillard, S. H., Jr.: Multiple ganglioneuromas of the central nervous system, Arch. Pathol. **94:**158-164, 1972.

Tumors of meningothelial cells

142 Bailey, P., Cushing, H., and Eisenhardt, L.: Angioblastic meningiomas, Arch. Pathol. **6:**953-990, 1928.

143 Cervós-Navarro, J., and Vazquez, J. J.: An electron microscopic study of meningiomas, Acta Neuropathol. (Berl.), **13:**301-323, 1969.

144 Cushing, H. W., and Eisenhardt, L.: Meningiomas: their classification, regional behavior, life history and surgical end results, Springfield, Ill., 1938, Charles C Thomas, Publishers.

145 Kepes, J.: Observations of the formation of psammoma bodies in meningiomas, J. Neuropathol. Exp. Neurol. **20:**255-262, 1961.

146 Kjeldsberg, C. R., and Minckler, J.: Meningiomas presenting as nasal polyps, Cancer **29:**153-156, 1972.

147 Kobahashi, S., Okazaki, H., and MacCarthy, C. S.: Intraventricular meningiomas, Mayo Clin. Proc. **46:**735-741, 1971.

148 Kruse, F., Jr.: Hemangiopericytoma of the meninges (angioblastic meningioma of Cushing and Eisenhardt); clinicopathologic aspects and follow-up studies in 8 cases, Neurology **11:**771-777, 1961.

149 Napolitano, L., Kyle, R., and Fisher, E. R.: Ultrastructure of meningiomas and the derivation and nature of their cellular components, Cancer **17:**233-241, 1964.

150 Pitkethly, D. T., Hardman, J. M., Kempe, L. G., and Earle, K. M.: Angioblastic meningiomas; clinicopathologic study of 81 cases, J. Neurosurg. **32:**539-544, 1970.

151 Rubinstein, L. J.: Tumors of the central nervous system. In Atlas of tumor Pathology, Second Series, Fasc. 6, Washington, D. C., 1972, Armed Forces Institute of Pathology.

152 Russell, D. S., and Rubinstein, L. J.: Pathology of tumours of the nervous system, Baltimore, 1963, The Williams & Wilkins, Co.

153 Shuangshoti, S., Hongsaprabhas, C., and Netsky, M. G.: Metastasizing meningioma, Cancer **26:**832-841, 1970.

154 Simpson, D.: The recurrence of intracranial meningiomas after surgical treatment, J. Neurol. Neurosurg. Psychiatry **20:**22-39, 1957.

155 Suzuki, H., Gilbert, E. F., and Zimmerman, B.: Primary extracranial meningioma, Arch. Pathol. **84:**202-206, 1967.

Tumors of melanocytes

156 Pappenheim, E., and Bhattacharji, S. K.: Primary melanoma of the central nervous system, Arch. Neurol. **7:**101-113, 1962.

157 Slaughter, J. C., Hardman, J. M., Kempe, L. G., and Earle, K. M.: Neurocutaneous melanosis and leptomeningeal melanomatosis in children, Arch. Pathol. **88:**298-304, 1969.

Tumors and malformations of blood vessels

158 Alexander, G. L., and Norman, R. M.: The Sturge-Weber syndrome, Bristol, 1960, John Wright & Sons, Ltd.

159 Bailey, W. L., and Sperl, M. P.: Angiomas of the cervical spinal cord, J. Neurosurg. **30:**560-568, 1969.

160 Brihaye, J., and Blackwoord, W.: Arteriovenous aneurysm of the cerebral hemispheres, J. Pathol. Bacteriol. **73:**25-31, 1957.

161 Brion, S., Netsky, M. G., and Zimmerman, H. M.: Vascular malformations of the spinal cord, Arch. Neurol. Psychiatry **68:**339-361, 1952.

162 Castaigne, P., David, M., Pertviset, B., Escourolle, R., and Poirier, J.: L'ultrastructure des hémangioblastomes du système nerveux central, Rev. Neurol. **118:**5-26, 1968.

163 Cramer, F., and Kimsey, W.: Cerebellar hemangioblastomas; review of 53 cases, with special reference to cerebellar cysts and the association of polycythemia, Arch. Neurol. Psychiatry **67:**237-252, 1952.

164 Doppman, J. L., Wirth, F. P. Jr., Di Chiro, G., and Ommaya, A. K.: Value of cutaneous angiomas in the arteriographic localization of spinal-cord arteriovenous malformations, N. Engl. J. Med., **281:**1440-1444, 1969.

165 Henderson, W. R., and Gomez, R. de R. L.: Natural history of cerebral angiomas, Br. Med. J. **4:**571-574, 1967.

166 Hoff, J. T., and Ray, B. S.: Cerebral hemangioblastoma occurring in a patient with von Hippel-Lindau disease; case report, J. Neurosurg. **28:**365-368, 1968.

167 Melmon, K. L., and Rosen, S. W.: Lindau's disease; review of the literature and study of a large kindred, Am. J. Med. **36:**595-617, 1964.

168 Nibbelink, D. W., Peters, B. H., and McCormick, W. F.: On the association of pheochromocytoma and cerebellar hemangioblastoma, Neurology **19:**455-460, 1969.

168a Pia, H. W.: Diagnosis and treatment of spinal angiomas, Acta Neurochir. **28**:1-12, 1973.

169 Poser, C. M.: The relationship between syringomyelia and neoplasm, Springfield, Ill., 1956, Charles C Thomas, Publisher.

170 Silver, M. L., and Hennigar, G.: Cerebellar hemangioma (hemangioblastoma); a clinicopathological review of 40 cases, J. Neurosurg. **9**:484-494, 1952.

171 Waldmann, T. A., Levin, E. H., and Baldwin, M.: The association of polycythemia with a cerebellar hemangioblastoma; the production of an erythropoiesis stimulating factor by the tumor, Am. J. Med. **31**:318-324, 1961.

172 Wohlwill, F. J., and Yakovlev, P. I.: Histopathology of meningofacial angiomatosis (Sturge-Weber's disease); report of four cases, J. Neuropathol. Exp. Neurol. **16**:341-364, 1957.

173 Wyburn-Mason, R.: The vascular abnormalities and tumours of the spinal cord and its membrane, London, 1943, Henry Kimpton.

Tumors of lymphoreticular system

174 Adams, J. H., and Jackson, J. M.: Intracerebral tumours of reticular tissue: the problem of microgliomatosis and reticulo-endothelial sarcomas of the brain, J. Pathol. Bacteriol. **91**: 369-381, 1966.

175 Brand, M. M., and Marinkovich, V. A.: Primary malignant reticulosis of the brain in Wiskott-Aldrich syndrome, Arch. Dis. Child. **44**:536-542, 1969.

176 Bucy, P. C., and Jerva, M. J.: Primary epidural spinal lymphosarcoma, J. Neurosurg. **19**: 142-152, 1962.

177 Burstein, S. D., Kernohan, J. W., and Uihlein, A.: Neoplasms of the reticuloendothelial system of the brain, Cancer **16**:289-305, 1963.

178 Clarke, E.: Cranial and intracranial myelomas, Brain **77**:61-81, 1954.

179 Edgar, R., and Dutcher, T. F.: Histopathology of the Bing-Neel syndrome, Neurology **11**:239-245, 1961.

180 Griffin, J. W., Thompson, R. W., Mitchinson, M. J., de Kiewiet, J. C., and Wellard, F. H.: Lymphomatous meningitis, Am. J. Med. **51**: 200-208, 1971.

181 Horvat, B., Pena, C., and Fisher, E. R.: Primary reticulum cell sarcoma (microglioma) of brain, Arch. Pathol. **87**:609-616, 1969.

182 Kernohan, J. W., and Uihlein, A.: Sarcomas of the brain, Springfield, Ill., 1962, Charles C Thomas, Publisher.

183 Marshall, G., Roessmann, U., and van der Noort, S.: Invasive Hodgkin's disease of brain; Report of two new cases and review of American and European literature with clinical-pathologic correlations, Cancer **22**:621-630, 1968.

184 Miller, A. A., and Ramsden, F.: Primary reticulosis of the central nervous system; "microgliomatosis," Acta Neurochir. **11**:439-478, 1963.

185 Moore, E. W., Thomas, L. B., Shaw, R. K., and Freireich, E. J.: The central nervous system in acute leukemia; a postmortem study of 117 consecutive cases, with particular reference to hemorrhages, leukemia infiltrations, and the syndrome of meningeal leukemia, Arch. Intern. Med. **105**:451-468, 1960.

186 Polak, M.: Blastomas del sistema nervioso central y periférico. Patología y ordenación histogenética, Buenos Aires, 1966, Lopez Libreros Ed.

187 Rosai, J., and Spiro, J.: Central nervous system involvement by mycosis fungoides, Acta Derm. Venereol. (Stockh.) **48**:482-488, 1968.

188 Russell, D. S., Marshall, A. H. E., and Smith, F. B.: Microgliomatosis; a form of reticulosis affecting the brain, Brain **71**:1-15, 1948.

189 Samuelsson, S.-M., Werner, L., Poutén, J., Nathorst-Windahl, G., and Thorell, J.: Reticuloendothelial (perivascular) sarcoma of the brain, Acta Neurol. Scand. **42**:567-580, 1966.

190 Schneck, S. A., and Penn, I.: De-novo brain tumors in renal transplant recipients, Lancet **1**:983-986, 1971.

Tumors of nerve roots

191 Anderson, M. S., and Bentinck, B. R.: Intracranial schwannoma in a child, Cancer **29**: 231-234, 1972.

192 Cravioto, H.: The ultrastructure of acoustic nerve tumors, Acta Neuropathol. **12**:116-140, 1969.

193 Erickson, L. S., Sorenson, G. D., and McGavran, M. H.: A review of 140 acoustic neurinomas (neurilemmoma), Laryngoscope **75**: 601-627, 1965.

194 Olivecrona, H.: Acoustic tumors, J. Neurosurg. **26**:6-13, 1967.

195 Rodriguez, H. A., and Berthrong, M.: Multiple primary intracranial tumors in von Recklinghausen's neurofibromatosis, Arch. Neurol., **14**:467-475, 1966.

196 Rubinstein, L. J.: Tumors of the central nervous system. In Atlas of tumor pathology, Second Series, Fasc. 6, Washington, D. C., 1972, Armed Forces Institute of Pathology.

197 Sloof, J. L., Kernohan, J. W., and MacCarthy, C. S.: Primary intramedullary tumors of the spinal cord and filum terminale, Philadelphia, 1964, W. B. Saunders Co.

Tumors of germ cell origin

198 Bestle, J.: Extragonadal endodermal sinus tumours originating in the region of the pineal gland, Acta Pathol. Microbiol. Scand. **74**:214-222, 1968.

199 Dayan, A. D., Marshall, A. H. E., Miller, A.

A., Pick, F. J., and Rankin, N. E.: Atypical teratomas of the pineal and hypothalamus, J. Pathol. Bacteriol. **92**:1-28, 1966.

200 Friedman, N. B.: Germinoma of the pineal; its identity with germinoma ("seminoma") of the testis, Cancer Res. **7**:363-368, 1947.

201 Ghatak, N. R., Hirano, A., and Zimmerman, H. M.: Intrasellar germinomas: a form of ectopic pinealoma, J. Neurosurg. **31**:670-675, 1969.

202 Globus, J. H., and Silbert, S.: Pinealomas, Arch. Neurol. **25**:937-984, 1931.

203 Nishiyama, R. H., Batsakis, J. G., Weaver, D. K., and Simrall, J. H.: Germinal neoplasms of the central nervous system, Arch. Surg. **93**:342-347, 1966.

204 Puschett, J. B., and Goldberg, M.: Endocrinopathy associated with pineal tumor, Ann. Intern. Med. **69**:203-219, 1968.

205 Ramsey, H. J.: Ultrastructure of a pineal tumor, Cancer **18**:1014-1025, 1965.

206 Russell, D. S.: The pinealoma: its relationship to teratoma, J. Pathol. Bacteriol. **56**:145-150, 1944.

207 Russell, D. S.: "Ectopic pinealoma": its kinship to atypical teratoma of the pineal gland; report of a case, J. Pathol. Bacteriol. **68**:125-129, 1954.

208 Simson, L. R., Lampe, I., and Abell, M. R.: Suprasellar germinomas, Cancer **22**:533-544, 1968.

Tumors of pineal gland

209 Costero, I., and Earle, K. M.: Pinealoma: a variety of argentaffinoma? Nature (Lond.) **199**:190, 1963.

210 Rubinstein, L. J.: Tumors of the central nervous system. In Atlas of tumor pathology, Second Series, Fasc. 6, Washington, D. C., 1972, Armed Forces Institute of Pathology.

211 Smith, W. T., Hughes, B., and Ermocilla, R.: Chemodectoma of the pineal region, with observations on the pineal body and chemoreceptor tissue, J. Pathol. Bacteriol. **92**:69-76, 1966.

Primary sarcomas

212 Bailey, O. T., and Ingraham, F. D.: Intracranial fibrosarcomas of the dura mater in childhood: pathological characteristics and surgical management. J. Neurosurg. **2**:1-15, 1945.

213 Black, B. K., and Kernohan, J. W.: Primary diffuse tumors of the meninges (so-called meningeal meningiomatosis), Cancer **3**:805-819, 1950.

214 Kepes, J. J., Kepes, M., and Slovik, F.: Fibrous xanthomas and xanthosarcomas of the meninges and the brain, Acta Neuropathol. **23**:187-199, 1973.

215 Kernohan, J. W., and Vihlein, A.: Sarcomas of the brain, Springfield, Ill., 1962, Charles C Thomas, Publisher.

216 Raskind, R., and Grant, S.: Primary mesenchymal chondrosarcoma of the cerebrum; report of a case, J. Neurosurg. **24**:676-678, 1966.

217 Schrantz, J. L., and Araoz, C. A.: Radiation induced meningeal fibrosarcoma, Arch. Pathol. **93**:26-31, 1972.

218 Shuangshoti, S., Piyaratn, P., and Viriyapanich, P. L.: Primary rhabdomyosarcoma of cerebellum: necropsy report, Cancer **22**:367-371, 1968.

219 Waltz, T. A., and Brownell, B.: Sarcoma: a possible late result of effective radiation therapy for pituitary adenoma; report of two cases, J. Neurosurg. **24**:901-907, 1966.

Tumors of pituitary gland

220 Bain, J., and Ezrin, C.: Immunofluorescent localization of the LH cell of the human adenohypophysis, J. Clin. Endocrinol. Metab. **30**:181-184, 1970.

221 Baker, B. L.: Studies on hormone localization with emphasis on the hypophysis, J. Histochem. Cytochem. **18**:1-8, 1970.

222 Baker, B. L., and Yu, Y.-Y.: The thyrotropic cell of the rat hypophysis as studied with peroxidase-labelled antibody, Am. J. Anat. **131**:55-71, 1971.

223 Ballard, H. S., Frame, B., and Hartsock, R. J.: Familial multiple endocrine adenoma-peptic ulcer complex, Medicine (Baltimore) **43**:481-516, 1964.

224 Bergland, R. M., and Torack, R. M.: An ultrastructural study of follicular cells in the human anterior pituitary, Am. J. Pathol. **57**:273-297, 1969.

225 Chang, C. H., and Pool, L.: The radiotherapy of pituitary chromophobe adenomas: an evaluation of indication, technic and result, Radiology **89**:1005-1016, 1967.

226 Doniach, I.: Cytology of pituitary adenomas, J. R. Coll. Physicians Lond. **6**:299-307, 1972.

227 Epstein, J. A., Epstein, B. S., Molho, L., and Zimmerman, H. M.: Carcinoma of the pituitary gland with metastasis to the spinal cord and roots of the canda equina, J. Neurosurg. **21**:846-853, 1964.

228 Finn, J. W., and Mount, L. A.: Galactorrhea in males with tumors in the region of the pituitary gland, J. Neurosurg. **35**:723-727, 1971.

229 Forbes, A. P., Henneman, P. H., Griswold, G. C., and Albright, F.: Syndrome characterized by galactorrhea, amenorrhea and low urinary FSH: comparison with acromegaly and normal lactation, J. Clin. Endocrinol. Metab. **14**:265-271, 1954.

230 Ghatak, N. R., Hirano, A., and Zimmerman, H. M.: Ultrastructure of a craniopharyngioma, Cancer 27:1465-1475, 1971.

231 Greenhouse, A. H.: Pituitary sarcoma, J.A.M.A. 190:269-273, 1964.

232 Griesbach, W. E., and Purves, H. D.: Basophil adenomata in the rat; hypophysis after gonadectomy, Br. J. Cancer 14:49-59, 1960.

233 Hamilton, C. R., Jr., Adams, L. C., and Maloof, F.: Hyperthyroidism due to thyrotropin-producing pituitary chromophobe adenoma, N. Engl. J. Med. 283:1077-1080, 1970.

234 Harris, G. W., and Donovan, B. T., editors: The pituitary gland, Berkeley, 1966, University of California Press.

235 Herlant, M.: The cells of the adenohypophysis and their functional significance, Int. Rev. Cytol. 17:299-382, 1964.

236 Houck, W. A., Olson, K. B., and Horton, J.: Clinical features of tumor metastasis to the pituitary, Cancer 26:656-659, 1970.

237 Jackson, I. M. D.: Hyperthyroidism in a patient with a pituitary chromophobe adenoma, J. Clin. Endocrinol. Metab. 25:491-494, 1965.

238 Kalnins, V.: Calcification and amelogenesis in craniopharyngiomas, Oral Surg. Oral Med. Oral Pathol. 31:366-379, 1971.

239 Kaufman, B., Lapham, L. W., Shealy, C. N., and Pearson, O. H.: Transphenoidal yttrium 90 pituitary ablation, Acta Radiol. 5:17-25, 1966.

240 Kay, S., Lees, J. K., and Stout, A. P.: Pituitary chromophobe tumors of the nasal cavity, Cancer 3:695-704, 1950.

241 Kernohan, J. W., and Sayre, G. P.: Tumors of the pituitary gland and infundibulum, In Atlas of tumor pathology, Sect. X, Fasc. 36, Washington, D. C., 1956, Armed Forces Institute of Pathology.

242 Kohler, P. O., Bridson, W. E., Rayford, P. L., and Kohler, S. E.: Hormone production by human pituitary adenomas in culture, Metabolism 18:782-788, 1969.

243 Kovacs, K., and Horvath, H.: Pituitary "chromophobe" adenoma composed of oncocytes, Arch. Pathol. 95:235-239, 1973.

244 Levene, M. B.: Pituitary radiotherapy, Radiol. Clin. North Am. 5:333-348, 1967.

245 Lewis, P. D., and Van Noorden, S.: Pituitary abnormalities in acromegaly, Arch. Pathol. 94:119-126, 1972.

246 Luse, S. A., and Kernohan, J. W.: Granular cell tumors of the stalk and posterior lobe of the pituitary gland, Cancer 8:616-622, 1955.

247 McCormick, W. F., and Halmi, N. S.: Absence of chromophobe adenomas from a large series of pituitary tumors, Arch. Pathol. 92:231-238, 1971.

248 Madonick, M. J., Rubinstein, L. J., Dacso, M. R., and Ribner, H.: Chromophobe adenoma of pituitary gland with subarachnoid metastasis, Neurology 13:836-840, 1963.

249 Markesbery, W. R., Duffy, P. E., and Cowen, D.: Granular cell tumors of the central nervous system, J. Neuropathol. Exp. Neurol. 32:92-109, 1973.

250 Martins, A. N., Hayes, G. J., and Kempe, L. G.: Invasive pituitary adenomas, J. Neurosurg. 22:268-276, 1965.

251 Matson, D. D., and Crigler, J. F., Jr.: Management of craniopharyngioma in childhood, J. Neurosurg. 30:377-390, 1969.

252 Mikami, S.: Light and electron microscopic investigations of six types of glandular cells of the bovine adenohypophysis, Z. Zellforsch. Mikrosk. Anat. 105:457-482, 1970.

253 Nakane, P. K.: Classifications of anterior pituitary cell types with immunoenzyme histochemistry, J. Histochem. Cytochem. 18:9-20, 1970.

254 Nelson, D. H., Meakin, J. W., and Thorn, G. W.: ACTH-producing pituitary tumors following adrenalectomy for Cushing's syndrome, Ann. Intern. Med. 52:560-569, 1960.

255 Paiz, C., and Hennigar, G. R., Electron microscopy and histochemical correlation of human anterior pituitary cells, Am. J. Pathol. 59:43-73, 1970.

256 Peake, G. T., McKeel, D. W., Jarett, L., and Daughaday, W. H.: Ultrastructural, histologic and hormonal characterization of a prolactin-rich human pituitary tumor, J. Clin. Endocrinol. Metab. 29:1383-1393, 1969.

257 Phifer, R. F., Spicer, S. S., and Orth, D. N.: Specific demonstration of the human hypophyseal cells which produce adrenocorticotropic hormone, J. Clin. Endocrinol. Metab. 31:347-361, 1970.

258 Roessmann, U., Kaufman, B., and Friede, R. L.: Metastatic lesions in the sella turcica and pituitary gland, Cancer 25:478-480, 1970.

259 Rovit, R. L., and Duane, T. D.: Cushing's syndrome and pituitary tumors; pathophysiology and ocular manifestations of ACTH-secreting pituitary adenomas, Am. J. Med. 46:416-427, 1969.

260 Russfield, A. B.: Human pituitary tumors. In Sommers, S. C., editor: Pathology annual, vol. 2, New York, 1967, Appleton-Century-Crofts, pp. 332-350.

261 Salassa, R. M., Kearns, T. P., Kernohan, J. W., Sprague, R. G., and MacCarthy, C. S.: Pituitary tumors in patients with Cushing's syndrome, J. Clin. Endocrinol. Metab. 19:1523-1539, 1959.

262 Schochet, S. S., Jr., McCormick, W. F., and Halmi, N. S.: Acidophil adenomas with intracytoplasmic filamentous aggregates; a light and electron microscopic study, Arch. Pathol. 94:16-22, 1972.

263 Seemayer, T. A., Blundell, J. S., and Wigles-worth, F. W.: Pituitary craniopharyngioma with tooth formation, Cancer **29**:423-430, 1972.

264 Svien, H. J., Colby, M. Y., Jr., and Kearns, T. P.: Comparison of results after surgery and after irradiation in pituitary chromophobe ade-nomas, Acta Radiol. [Ther.] (Stockh.) **5**:53-66, 1966.

265 Symon, L., Ganz, J. C., and Burston, J.: Gran-ular cell myoblastoma of the neurohypophysis; report of two cases, J. Neurosurg. **35**:82-89, 1971.

266 Timperley, W. R.: Histochemistry of Rathke pouch tumours, J. Neurol. Neurosurg. Psychi-atry **31**:589-595, 1968.

267 von Lawzewitsch, I., Dickmann, G. H., Ame-zúa, L., and Pardal, C.: Cytological and ultra-structural characterization of the human pi-tuitary, Acta Anat. (Basel) **81**:286-316, 1972.

268 Waltz, T. A., and Brownell, B.: Sarcoma: possible late result of effective radiation ther-apy for pituitary adenoma; report of two cases, J. Neurosurg. **24**:901-907, 1966.

269 Young, D. G., Bahn, R. C., and Randall, R. V.: Pituitary tumors associated with acromeg-aly, J. Clin. Endocrinol. Metab. **25**:249-259, 1965.

Tumors of metastatic origin

270 Auld, A. W., and Buerman, A.: Metastatic spinal epidural tumors; an analysis of 50 cases, Arch. Neurol. **15**:100-108, 1966.

271 Edelson, R. N., Deck, M. D. F., and Posner, J. B.: Intramedullary spinal cord metastases; clinical and radiographic findings in nine cases, Neurology **22**:1222-1231, 1972.

272 Haar, F., and Patterson, R. H., Jr.: Surgery for metastatic intracranial neoplasm, Cancer **30**:1241-1245, 1972.

Clinicopathology correlation

273 Bodian, M., and Lawson, D.: The intracranial neoplastic diseases of childhood; a descrip-tion of their natural history based on a clinico-pathological study of 129 cases, Br. J. Surg. **40**:368-392, 1953.

274 Cheek, W. R., and Taveras, J. M.: Thalamic tumors, J. Neurosurg. **24**:503-513, 1966.

275 Dastur, D. K., and Lalitha, V. S.: Pathological analysis of intracranial space-occupying lesions in 1000 cases including children. Part 2. Inci-dence, types and unusual cases of glioma, J. Neurol. Sci. **8**:143-170, 1968.

276 Kernohan, J. W.: Tumors of the spinal cord; a review, Arch. Pathol. **32**:843-883, 1941.

277 Koos, W. T., and Miller, M. H.: Intracranial tumors of infants and children, St. Louis, 1971, The C. V. Mosby Co.

278 Low, N. L., Correll, J. W., and Hammill, J.

F.: Tumors of cerebral hemispheres in chil-dren, Arch. Neurol. **13**:547-554, 1965.

279 Marsden, H. B., and Steward, J. K.: Gliomas and other intracranial tumors. In Tumors in children, Recent Results in Cancer Research, vol. 13, New York, 1968, Springer-Verlag New York, pp. 86-130.

280 Pecker, J., Ferrand, B., and Javalet, A.: Tu-mors of 3rd ventricle, Neurochirurgie **12**:7-136, 1966.

281 Zülch, K. J.: Brain tumors; their biology and pathology, ed. 2, New York, 1965, Springer Publishing Co.

Local and regional effects of
intracranial tumors

282 Dreese, M. J., and Netsky, M. G.: Studies of lateral reflections in the echo-encephalogram, Neurology **14**:521-528, 1964.

283 Friede, R. L., and Roessmann, U.: The patho-genesis of secondary midbrain hemorrhages, Neurology **16**:1210-1216, 1966.

284 Klintworth, G. K.: The pathogenesis of second-ary brainstem hemorrhages as studied in a experimental model, Am. J. Pathol. **47**:525-536, 1965.

285 Poppen, J. L., Kendrick, J. F., and Hicks, S. F.: Brain stem hemorrhages secondary to su-pratentorial space-taking lesions, J. Neuro-pathol. Exp. Neurol. **11**:267-279, 1952.

Cytology

286 Rich, J. R.: A survey of cerebrospinal fluid cytology, Bull. Los Angeles Neurol. Soc. **34**:115-131, 1969.

Diseases of skeletal muscle

287 Classification of the neuromuscular disorders: Appendix A, minutes of the Meeting of the Research Group on Neuromuscular Diseases, Sept. 21, 1967, J. Neurol. Sci. **6**:165-177, 1968.

Techniques of pathologic examination

288 Clawson, B. J., Noble, J. F., and Lufkin, N. H.: Nodular inflammatory and degenerative lesions of muscles from 450 autopsies, Arch. Pathol. **43**:579-589, 1947.

289 Engel, A. G.: Ultrastructural reactions in mus-cle disease, Med. Clin. North Am. **52**:909-931, 1968.

290 Engel, W. K.: Selective and nonselective susceptibility of muscle fiber types, Arch. Neurol. **22**:97-117, 1970.

291 Engel, W. K.: The essentiality of histo- and cytochemical studies of skeletal muscle in the investigation of neuromuscular disease, Neu-rology **12**:778-794, 1962.

292 Engel, W. K., and Brooke, M. H.: Muscle biopsy as a clinical diagnostic aid. In Fields,

W. S., editor: Neurological diagnostic techniques, Springfield, Ill., 1966, Charles C
Thomas, Publisher, pp. 90-146.

293 Hudgson, P.: The value of electron microscopy in muscle biopsies, Proc. R. Soc. Med.
63:14-18, 1970.

294 Hughes, J. T., and Brownell, B.: Muscle biopsy in the diagnosis of neurological and
muscle disease. In Dyke, S. C., editor: Recent
advances in clinical pathology, ser. 5, London, 1968, J. & A. Churchill, Ltd., Chap. 20.

295 Pearson, C. M.: Incidence and type of pathologic alterations observed in muscle in a routine autopsy survey, Neurology **9:**757-766,
1959.

296 Samaha, F. J.: Electrodiagnostic studies in
neuromuscular disease, N. Engl. J. Med. **282:**
1244-1247, 1971.

297 Vassella, F., Richterich, R., and Rossi, E.:
The diagnostic value of serum creatine kinase
in neuromuscular and muscular disease, Pediatrics **35:**322-330, 1965.

298 Walton, J. N., editor: Disorders of voluntary
muscle, ed. 2, Boston, 1969, Little, Brown
and Co.

Neurogenic atrophy
(amyotrophy)

299 Emery, A. E. H.: The nosology of the spinal
muscular atrophies, J. Med. Genet. **8:**481-
495, 1971.

300 Engel, W. K., and Brooke, M. H.: Muscle
biopsy as a clinical diagnostic aid. In Fields,
W. S., editor: Neurological diagnostic techniques, Springfield, Ill., 1966, Charles C
Thomas, Publisher, pp. 90-146.

301 Greenfield, J. G., Shy, G. M., Alvord, E. C.,
and Berg, L.: An atlas of muscle pathology in
neuromuscular diseases, Edinburgh, 1957, E.
& S. Livingstone, Ltd.

302 Hasse, G. R., and Shy, G. M.: Pathological
changes in muscle biopsies from patients with
peroneal muscular atrophy, Brain **83:**631-637,
1960.

303 Pearce, J., and Harriman, D. G. F.: Chronic
spinal muscular atrophy, J. Neurol. Neurosurg. Psychiatry **29:**509-520, 1966.

304 Schotland, D. L.: An electron microscopic
study of target fibers, target-like fibers and related abnormalities in human muscle, J. Neuropathol. Exp. Neurol. **28:**214-228, 1969.

305 Zacks, S. I.: Recent contributions to the diagnosis of muscle disease, Hum. Pathol. **1:**465-
498, 1970.

Muscular dystrophies

306 Aleu, F. P., and Afifi, A. K.: Ultrastructure of
muscle in myotonic dystrophy, Am. J. Pathol. **45:**221-232, 1964.

307 Bell, C. D., and Conen, P. E.: Histopatho-

logical changes in Duchenne muscular dystrophy, J. Neurol. Sci. **7:**529-544, 1968.

308 Brooke, M. H., and Engel, W. K.: The histologic diagnoses of neuromuscular diseases: a
review of 79 biopsies, Arch. Phys. Med.
Rehabil. **47:**99-121, 1966.

309 Dubowitz, V.: Muscular dystrophy—where is
the lesion? Dev. Med. Child Neurol. **13:**238-
240, 1971.

310 Engel, W. K., and Brooke, M. H.: Muscle
biopsy as a clinical diagnostic aid. In Fields,
W. S., editor: Neurological diagnostic techniques, Springfield, Ill., 1966, Charles C
Thomas, Publisher, pp. 90-146.

311 Fisher, E. R., Cohn, R. E., and Denowski,
T. S.: Ultrastructural observations of skeletal
muscle in myopathy and neuropathy with
special reference to muscular dystrophy, Lab.
Invest. **15:**778-793, 1966.

312 Pearce, G. W., and Walton, J. N.: Progressive
muscular dystrophy; the histopathological
changes in skeletal muscle obtained by biopsy,
J. Pathol. Bacteriol. **83:**535-550, 1962.

313 Schroder, J. M., and Adams, R. D.: The
ultrastructural morphology of the muscle
fiber in myotonic dystrophy, Acta Neuropathol. **10:**218-241, 1968.

314 Wohlfart, G.: Dystrophia myotonica and
myotonia congenita. Histopathologic studies
with special reference to changes in the
muscle, J. Neuropathol. Exp. Neurol. **10:**
109-124, 1951.

Myositis

315 Adams, R. D., Denny-Brown, D., and Pearson, C. M.: Disease of muscle; a study in
pathology, ed. 2, New York, 1962, Harper
& Row, Publishers.

316 Brooke, M. H., and Engel, W. K.: The histologic diagnosis of neuromuscular diseases: a
review of 79 biopsies, Arch. Phys. Med. Rehabil. **47:**99-121, 1966.

317 Chou, S-M.: Myxovirus-like structures and
accompanying nuclear changes in chronic
polymyositis, Arch. Pathol. **86:**649-658, 1968.

318 Dowben, R. M., Vawter, G. F., Bradfon-
brenner, A., Sniderman, P., and Kaegy, R.
D.: Polymyositis and other diseases resembling muscular dystrophy, Arch. Intern. Med.
115:584-594, 1965.

319 Gardner-Thorpe, C.: Muscle weakness due to
sarcoid myopathy; six case reports and an
evaluation of steroid therapy, Neurology **22:**
917-928, 1972.

320 Munsat, T. L., Piper, D., Cancilla, P., and
Mednick, J.: Inflammatory myopathy with
facioscapulohumeral distribution, Neurology
22:335-347, 1972.

321 Rose, A. L., Walton, J. N., and Pearce, G.
W.: Polymyositis: an ultramicroscopic study

of muscle biopsy material, J. Neurol. Sci. 5:457-472, 1967.

Myopathies

322 Azzopardi, J. G.: Systemic effects of neoplasia: neuromyopathies. In Harrison, C. V., editor: Recent advances in pathology, ed. 8, Boston, 1966, Little, Brown and Co.

323 Brooke, M. H., and Neville, H. E.: Reducing body myopathy, a new disease, Neurology 21:412-413, 1971.

324 Cape, C. A., Johnson, W. W., and Pitner, S. E.: Nemaline structures in polymyositis; a nonspecific pathological reaction of skeletal muscles, Neurology 20:494-502, 1970.

325 Croft, P. B., and Wilkinson, M.: Carcinomatous neuromyopathy; its influence in patients with carcinoma of the lung and carcinoma of the breast, Lancet 1:184-188, 1963.

326 Croft, P. B., and Wilkinson, M.: The incidence of carcinomatous neuromyopathy in patients with various types of carcinoma, Brain 88:427-434, 1965.

327 Duane, D. D., and Engel, A. G.: Emetine myopathy, Neurology 18:274, 1968.

328 Engel, A. G., and Gomez, M. R.: Nemaline (Z disk) myopathy: observations on the origin, structure, and solubility properties of the nemaline structures, J. Neuropathol. Exp. Neurol. 26:601-619, 1967.

329 Engel, A. G., Angelini, C., and Gomez, M. R.: Fingerprint body myopathy; a newly recognized congenital muscle disease, Mayo Clin. Proc. 47:377-388, 1972.

330 Engel, A. G., Gomez, M. R., and Groover, R. V.: Multicore disease; a recently recognized congenital myopathy associated with multifocal degeneration of muscle fibers, Mayo Clin. Proc. 46:666-681, 1971.

331 Gonatas, N. K., Shy, G. M., and Godfrey, E. H.: Nemaline myopathy; the origin of nemaline structures, N. Engl. J. Med. 274:535-539, 1966.

332 Gonatas, N. K., Perez, M. C., Shy, G. M., and Evangelista, I.: Central core disease of skeletal muscle; ultrastructural and cytochemical observations in 2 cases, Am. J. Pathol. 47:503-524, 1965.

333 Gonatas, N., Evangelista, I., and Martin, J.: A generalized disorder of nervous system, skeletal muscle, and heart resembling Refsum's disease and Hurler's syndrome. II. Ultrastructure, Am. J. Med. 42:169-178, 1967.

334 Hers, H. G.: Glycogen storage disease, Adv. Metab. Disord. 1:1-44, 1964.

335 Hudgson, P., Brodley, W. G., and Jenkison, M.: Familial "mitochondrial" myopathy; a myopathy associated with disordered oxidative metabolism in muscle fibers, J. Neurol. Sci. 16:343-370, 1972.

336 Hug, G., Garancis, J. C., Schubert, W. K., and Kaplan, S.: Glycogen storage disease, Types II, III, VIII, and IX, Am. J. Dis. Child. 111:457-474, 1966.

337 Jenis, E. H., Lingquist, R. R., and Lister, R. C.: New congenital myopathy with crystalline intranuclear inclusions, Arch. Neurol. 20:281-287, 1969.

338 Kahn, L. B., and Meyer, J. S.: Acute myopathy in chronic alcoholism: a study of 22 autopsy cases, with ultrastructural observations, Am. J. Clin. Pathol. 53:516-530, 1970.

339 Karpati, G., Carpenter, S., and Eisen, A. A.: Experimental core-like lesions and membrane rods; a correlative morphological and physiological study, Arch. Neurol. 27:237-251, 1972.

340 Klinkerfuss, G., Bleisch, V., Dioso, M. M., and Perkoff, G. T.: A spectrum of myopathy associated with alcoholism. II. Light and electron microscopic observations, Ann. Intern. Med. 67:493-510, 1967.

341 Munsat, T. L., Thompson, L. R., and Coleman, R. S.: Centronuclear ("myotubular") myopathy, Arch. Neurol. 20:120-131, 1969.

342 Norris, F. H., and Panner, B. J.: Hypothyroid myopathy, Arch. Neurol. 14:574-589, 1966.

343 Pearson, C. M., Coleman, R. F., Fowlder, W. M., Jr., Mommaerts, W., Munsat, T. L., and Peter, J. B.: Skeletal muscle, Ann. Intern. Med. 67:614-650, 1967.

344 Perkoff, G. T., Dioso, M. M., Bleisch, V., and Klinkerfuss, G.: A spectrum of myopathy associated with alcoholism. I. Clinical and laboratory features, Ann. Intern. Med. 67:481-492, 1967.

345 Price, H. M., Pease, D. C., and Pearson, C. M.: Selective actin filament and Z-band degeneration induced by plasmocid; an electron microscopic study, Lab. Invest. 11:549-562, 1962.

346 Prineas, J.: Tri-ortho-cresyl-phosphate (TOCP) myopathy, Arch. Neurol. 21:150-156, 1969.

347 Ramsay, I. D.: Muscle dysfunction in hyperthyroidism, Lancet 2:931-934, 1966.

348 Rewcastle, N. B., and Humphrey, J. G.: Vacuolar myopathy; clinical, histochemical and microscopic study, Arch. Neurol. 12:570-582, 1965.

349 Santa, T.: Fine structure of the human skeletal muscle in myopathy, Arch. Neurol. 20:479-489, 1969.

350 Shafiq, S. A., Milhorat, A. T., and Gorycki, M. A.: Giant mitochondria in human muscle with inclusions, Arch. Neurol. 17:666-671, 1967.

351 Shy, G. M., and Magee, A. R.: A new congenital non-progressive myopathy, Brain 79:610-621, 1956.

352 Shy, G. M., Gonatas, N. K., and Perez, M.: Two childhood myopathies with abnormal mitochondria. I. Megaconial myopathy. II. Pleoconial myopathy, Brain **89**:133-158, 1966.
353 Shy, G. M., Engel, W. K., Somers, J. E., and Wanko, T.: Nemaline myopathy: a new congenital myopathy, Brain **86**:793-810, 1963.
354 Slotweiner, P., Song, S. K., and Anderson, P. J.: Spheromembranous degeneration of muscle induced by vincristine, Arch. Neurol. **15**:172-176, 1966.
355 Spiro, A. J., Shy, G. M., and Gonatas, N. K.: Myotubular myopathy: persistence of fetal muscle in an adolescent boy, Arch. Neurol. **14**:1-14, 1966.

Traumatic and circulatory disturbances

356 Leach, R. E., Hammond, G., and Stryker, W. S.: Anterior tibial compartment syndrome, J. Bone Joint Surg. [Am.] **49**:451-462, 1967.

Diseases of peripheral nerves

357 Appenzeller, O., Kornfeld, M., and MacGee, J.: Neuropathy in chronic renal disease; a microscopic, ultrastructural, and biochemical study of several nerve biopsies, Arch. Neurol. **24**:449-461, 1971.
358 Barron, K. D., Rowland, L. P., and Zimmerman, H. M.: Neuropathy with malignant tumor metastases, J. Nerv. Ment. Dis. **131**:10-31, 1960.
359 Brain, W. R., and Adams, R. D.: In Brain, W. R., and Norris, F. H., editors: The remote effects of cancer on the nervous system, New York, 1965, Grune & Stratton, Inc., p. 216.

360 Dayan, A. D., and Gardner-Thorpe, C.: Peripheral neuropathy and myeloma, J. Neurol. Sci. **14**:21-35, 1971.
361 Dyck, P. J.: Peripheral neuropathy; changing concepts, differential diagnosis and classification, Med. Clin. North Am. **52**:895-908, 1968.
362 Dyck, P. J., and Lofgren, E. P.: Nerve biopsy; choice of nerves, method, symptoms, and usefulness, Med. Clin. North Am. **52**:885-893, 1968.
363 Knill-Jones, R. P., Goodwill, C. J., Dayan, A. D., and Williams, R.: Peripheral neuropathy in chronic liver disease: clinical, electrodiagnostic, and nerve biopsy findings, J. Neurol. Neurosurg. Psychiatry **35**:22-30, 1972.
364 Locke, S.: Axons, Schwann cells and diabetic neuropathy, Bull. N. Y. Acad. Med. **43**:784-791, 1967.
365 Prineas, J.: Polyneuropathies of undetermined cause, Acta Neurol. Scand. [Suppl.] **44**:1-72, 1970.
366 Thomas, P. K.: Peripheral neuropathy, Br. Med. J. **1**:349-351, 1970.
367 Thomas, P. K., Hollinrake, K., Lascelles, R. G., O'Sullivan, D. J., Baillod, R. A., Moorhead, J. F., and Mackenzie, J. C.: The polyneuropathy of chronic renal failure, Brain **94**:761-780, 1971.
368 Walsh, J. C.: The neuropathy of multiple myeloma; an electrophysiological and histological study, Arch. Neurol. **25**:404-414, 1971.

27 Eyes and ocular adnexa*

Morton E. Smith, M.D.

Eyelids
  Developmental anomalies
  Inflammation
    Chalazion
  Metabolic disorders
  Cysts
  Tumors and tumorlike lesions
    Tumors of surface epithelium
    Nonneoplastic keratotic lesions
    Melanotic tumors
    Glandular and other adnexal tumors
    Stromal lesions
    Secondary tumors
Lacrimal passages
  Canaliculitis and dacryocystitis
  Mucocele
  Dacryolithiasis
  Tumors
Lacrimal gland
  Dacryoadenitis
  Atrophy; Sjögren's syndrome
  Tumors
Orbit
  Congenital and developmental conditions
    Angioma
    Neurofibroma
    Mucocele
  Systemic diseases
    Endocrine exophthalmos
    Histiocytoses and juvenile xanthogranuloma
  Inflammatory processes
  Primary tumors
    Connective tissue tumors
    Lymphoid tumors
    Glioma of optic nerve
    Meningioma
  Secondary tumors
Conjunctiva and cornea
  Congenital and developmental lesions
    Dermoid tumors
    Nevi
  Inflammation
  Degeneration

Tumors and related lesions
  Papilloma
  Carcinoma in situ
  Squamous cell carcinoma
  Malignant melanoma
    Nevus origin
    Acquired melanosis, benign and
      malignant
  Lymphoid tumors
Intraocular tissues
  Congenital and developmental malformations
    Congenital glaucoma
    Retrolental fibroplasia
    Phakoma
    Persistent hyperplastic primary vitreous
    Retinal dysplasia
    Other congenital entities
  Trauma
  Inflammation
    Acute inflammation
    Chronic nongranulomatous inflammation
    Granulomatous inflammation
      Toxoplasmosis
      Nematodiasis
    Posttraumatic uveitis
      Sympathetic uveitis
      Phacoanaphylaxis
  Degeneration
    Phthisis bulbi
    Glaucoma
      Primary glaucoma
      Secondary glaucoma
    Diabetes
  Tumors and pseudotumors
    Malignant melanoma
      Conditions confused with malignant
        melanoma of uvea
    Retinoblastoma
      Conditions confused with retinoblastoma
    Metastatic carcinoma
    Leukemia and malignant lymphoma
    Other tumors
Technique for examination and opening of
  enucleated eyes

---

*The author wishes to acknowledge the assistance of Dr. T. E. Sanders, Washington University School of Medicine, St. Louis, Mo. Dr. Lorenz E. Zimmerman, Armed Forces Institute of Pathology, Washington, D. C., wrote the original chapter, much of the text of which remains.

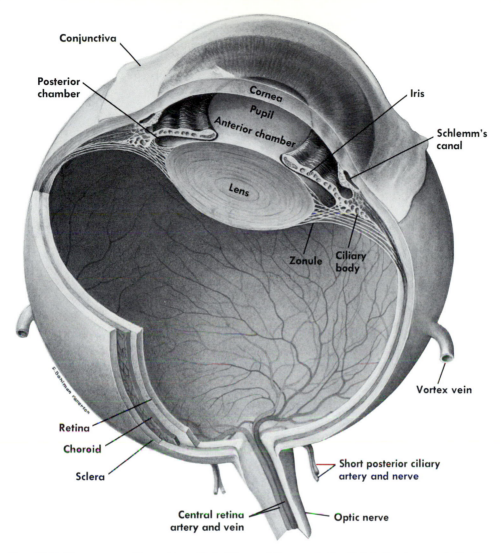

Fig. 1239 Human eye. (From Newell, F. W., and Ernest, J. T.: Ophthalmology, ed. 3, St. Louis, 1974, The C. V. Mosby Co.)

A myriad of diseases can affect the eyes and ocular adnexa,[1-4, 6, 7, 9, 11-13] but this chapter will concern itself only with those entities that would come to the attention of the surgical pathologist. For example, certain congenital anomalies will not be discussed since they would only be seen at postmortem examination.

It goes without saying that a knowledge of the normal topography of the eye and its adnexa is essential for the correct diagnosis of biopsy specimens from this region[5, 8, 10] (Fig. 1239). As with all surgical specimens, a complete description of the lesion is invaluable and good clinical photographs will often aid the pathologist.

Electron microscopy is playing an increasingly important role in diagnostic surgical pathology, and ophthalmic pathology is no exception. A variety of disease entities have become better understood via electron microscopy.[14]

EYELIDS

Most of the pathologic processes that involve the eyelids are those which involve the skin in general and are considered in detail in Chapter 3. Some consideration,

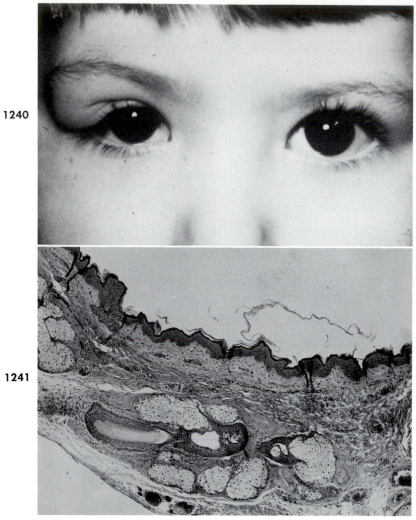

Fig. 1240 Dermoid cyst of right upper eyelid. (WU neg. 67-3508.)
Fig. 1241 Dermoid cyst of eyelid and brow. Cyst lumen is located in upper right corner. (×55; AFIP 722706.)

however, is given here to those lesions that are either peculiar to the lids or present particular problems in this location.

Developmental anomalies

Dermoid cysts typically involve the upper eyelid along the brow margin (Fig. 1240). Most of them represent forward extensions of masses that are primarily intraorbital. Some, however, are of palpebral origin.

Microscopically, the cysts are lined by well-differentiated epidermal and dermal tissues containing all of the usual skin appendages (Fig. 1241). The lumen is filled with keratinous debris, sebum, and hairs. In places where these contents have been extruded into the surrounding tissues, a severe foreign body inflammatory reaction may be observed.

Nevi dating from birth may be observed in either the cutaneous or the conjunctival surface of the eyelids. They tend to be of the junctional or compound type and, like those in other areas, may give rise to malignant melanoma.

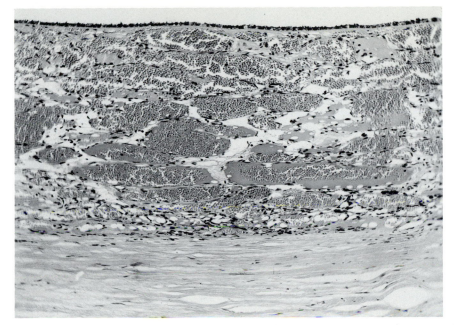

Fig. 1242 Hemangioma of choroid in eye enucleated from 42-year-old white woman who had had a port-wine facial hemangioma since birth and ipsilateral glaucoma since early childhood. (×115; AFIP 759801.)

A more diffuse and deeply situated melanotic lesion of the lids is the nevus of Ota (congenital oculodermal melanosis). This is a form of extrasacral mongolian spot involving the face in areas supplied by the first and second branches of the trigeminal nerve.[15, 16] Associated conjunctival, scleral, and orbital pigmentation is present in many of the cases. This type of nevus occurs more frequently in Orientals and blacks than in Caucasians. Caucasians with this condition seem to have a greater than normal predilection for ocular and orbital malignant melanomas.[17]

Angiomas may be small lesions confined to the eyelid or may extend deep into the orbit. Hemangiomas are more common than lymphangiomas. The histopathologic characteristics have been described elsewhere (Chapter 3).

The so-called port-wine stain (nevus flammeus) is of special interest not only because of its great cosmetic effect, but also because it may be associated with malformations in other tissues (Fig. 1242). In the Sturge-Weber syndrome, the facial hemangioma may be associated with a choroidal hemangioma, glaucoma, and a meningeal hemangioma, all on the ipsilateral side[18] (Fig. 1243).

Neurofibromas also may be isolated developmental lesions of the eyelid, or they may be merely a part of Recklinghausen's neurofibromatosis. Although believed to be present from birth, these tumors frequently show accelerated growth during childhood or later. When associated with Recklinghausen's disease, there may be marked asymmetry of the face due to diffuse hypertrophy and pendulousness of all of the facial tissues on one side (Fig. 1244).

Inflammation

Inflammation of the eyelids may be the result of viral, rickettsial, bacterial, mycotic, or parasitic infections, of chemical or physical irritants, of hypersensitivity states, or of systemic dermatologic disorders. These inflammatory processes are rarely biopsied and are of relatively little practical significance to pathologists.

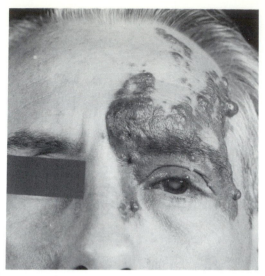

Fig. 1243 Sturge-Weber syndrome. Patient, 42-year-old white man, had had facial hemangioma all his life and was blind in ipsilateral eye because of retinal degeneration, glaucoma, and cataract. Choroidal hemangioma was found in enucleated eye, but clinical study failed to disclose evidence of intracranial lesion. (AFIP 761707; courtesy Veterans Administration Hospital, Hines, Ill.)

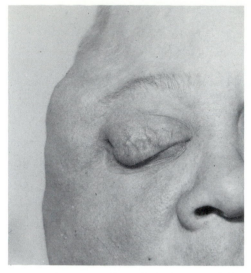

Fig. 1244 Severe unilateral deformity of face in patient with Recklinghausen's neurofibromatosis. (AFIP 55-17512; courtesy Dr. L. L. Calkins, Kansas City, Kan.)

Chalazion

A chalazion is a lipogranuloma that develops in and about a meibomian gland, presumably as a consequence of the combined effects of obstruction and nonspecific infection of the excretory passages of the gland. The sebaceous material, discharged into the tarsus as a result of the meibomitis, provokes an intense granulomatous inflammatory reaction.

Although it begins as a deep-seated process, the chalazion not infrequently erupts through the conjunctival surface of the eyelid. Ordinarily, this lesion is readily recognized and treated, but if, after curettage, one or more recurrences develop, the clinician should be alert to the possibility of a meibomian gland tumor that has previously escaped recognition. In such cases, excision and histopathologic study are indicated.

Microscopically, the typical chalazion reveals multiple foci of granulomatous inflammation (Fig. 1245). In the center of many of the focal granulomas there is a small globule of fat, which in paraffin sections presents simply as an empty round to ovoid space (Fig. 1246).

Metabolic disorders

Xanthelasmas are slightly elevated yellow plaques located on the medial aspect of the upper and lower eyelids (Fig. 1247). They are rarely indicative of any serious systemic disturbance and are usually removed for cosmetic reasons. Most of the patients are in the fifth or sixth decade of life. Patients with familial hypercholesterolemia may develop these lesions at a younger age.

Microscopically, these lesions show large pale-staining fat-laden histiocytes throughout the subepithelial tissues.

Localized **amyloidosis** can occur in the eyelids and conjunctiva. It presents as a chronic painless tumefaction usually not associated with any systemic disease.[19]

Cysts

Cysts of Moll's glands, referred to as sudoriferous cysts, form thin-walled transparent vesicles at the lid margin. Microscopically, they are simple cysts lined by atrophic cuboidal or flattened epithelial cells (Fig. 1248).

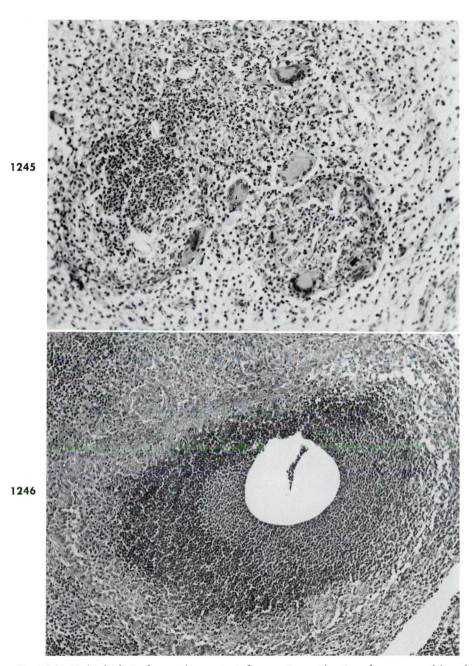

Fig. 1245 Multiple foci of granulomatous inflammation with microabscesses and Langhans' giant cells in chalazion. (×137; AFIP 91218.)

Fig. 1246 Presence of pools of fat in center of many of granulomas is characteristic of chalazia. (×115; AFIP 732397.)

Sebaceous cysts may arise from the ordinary pilosebaceous glands of the skin or from the more specialized Zeis and meibomian glands located along the lid margin and within the tarsus, respectively.

Tumors and tumorlike lesions
Tumors of surface epithelium

Basal cell carcinomas are by far the most frequent of all true neoplasms arising in any of the palpebral tissues.[20, 21] The over-

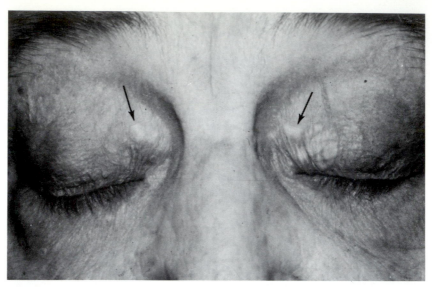

Fig. 1247 Xanthelasma of upper eyelids in patient who had no other systemic findings. (WU neg. 67-4281.)

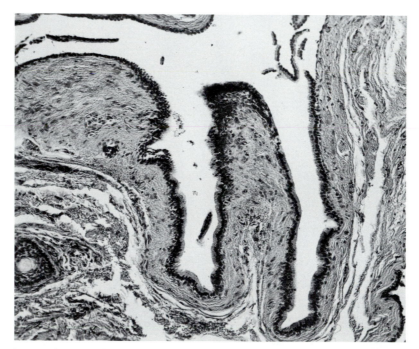

Fig. 1248 Simple cyst of lid margin believed to be secondary to obstruction of duct of Moll's gland (sudoriferous cyst). (×110; AFIP 750918.)

whelming majority are easily excised without sequelae. Larger lesions are best treated by radiation therapy. On rare occasion, they may invade the orbit or nose or both, and exenteration of the orbit may become necessary.

Basal cell carcinomas arise from the cu-

taneous surface of the lids and rarely, if ever, from the conjunctiva. This point is of some diagnostic significance, for papillomas of the palpebral conjunctiva may resemble basal cell carcinoma. When such a lesion is excised and sectioned in such a way that its topographic orientation in relation to

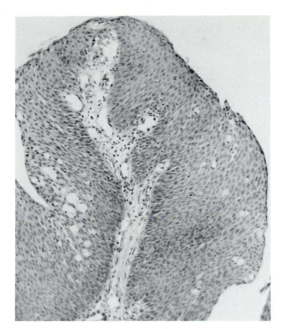

Fig. 1249 Conjunctival papilloma. Many mucous cells are scattered about in acanthotic nonkeratinized epithelium. (×125; AFIP 230075; from Friedenwald, J. S., et al: Ophthalmic pathology: an atlas and textbook, Philadelphia, 1952, W. B. Saunders Co.)

the conjunctival surface of the lid is not apparent and if the pathologist is not informed of the clinical appearance of the tumor, an erroneous diagnosis of basal cell carcinoma can be made (Fig. 1249).

Squamous cell carcinomas have often been cited as responsible for about 10% to 20% of all malignant epithelial tumors of the eyelid. Experience, however, indicates that squamous cell carcinoma is much less frequent than that, accounting for less than 3% of malignant tumors of the eyelids.[29]

Papillomatous lesions of the eyelids include true squamous papillomas and such other lesions as seborrheic keratosis, warts, and cutaneous horns.

Nonneoplastic keratotic lesions

Nonneoplastic keratotic lesions may resemble squamous cell carcinomas so closely that even experienced clinicians and pathologists have much difficulty in differential diagnosis.

The lesions include such entities as pseudoepitheliomatous hyperplasia, kera-

toacanthoma, inverted follicular keratosis, seborrheic keratosis, senile keratosis, and cutaneous horns.[23, 24] The histopathologic features of these lesions are described in Chapter 3.

Melanotic tumors

Nevi have already been mentioned (Chapter 3) since they are generally considered to be congenital or developmental tumors, even though their presence may not be recognized until growth or pigmentation takes place during adolescence or later.

Acquired melanosis is a condition that may involve either or both surfaces of the eyelid in association with the conjunctiva and is described under conjunctiva and cornea (p. 1332).

Malignant melanoma of the eyelid may originate from a nevus that has been present for many years, from an acquired melanosis of variable duration, or from what is believed to have been previously normal skin or conjunctiva.

In general, malignant melanomas of the lid carry a very grave prognosis, for they tend to metastasize early by lymphatics and the bloodstream. This is in decided contrast with malignant melanomas of the bulbar conjunctiva (p. 1330) and of the uvea (p. 1356), which have a much more favorable prognosis.

Glandular and other adnexal tumors

Sebaceous gland adenomas and adeno-carcinomas may arise from the cutaneous sebaceous glands, the glands of Zeis, or the meibomian gland.

Solitary adenomas of the meibomian and Zeis glands are rarely seen in the laboratory, although they may be more common than is generally believed. The meibomain gland tumors, for example, may simulate a chalazion and be removed by curetttage. Such curettings are rarely submitted for microscopic examination. Hence, one does not know how often such tumors are missed. In the case of malignant tumors, however, recurrence is likely. It is for this reason that recurrent chalazia are often excised and sent to the pathology labora-

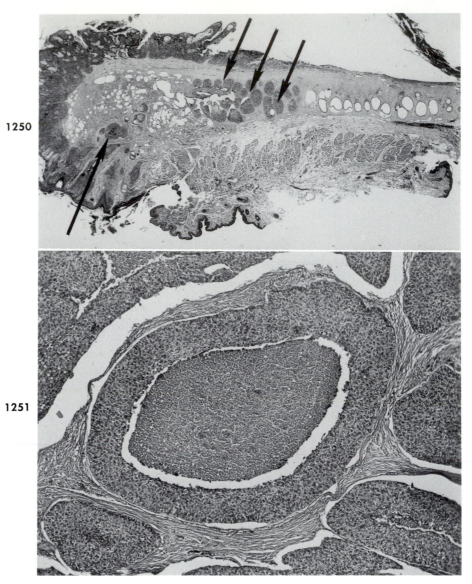

Fig. 1250 Full-thickness section of eyelid showing sebaceous gland carcinoma arising from meibomian glands (arrows) as well as pagetoid invasion of skin. (×5; WU neg. 72-6065.)

Fig. 1251 Adenocarcinoma of meibomian gland. Plugs of completely necrotic tumor fill central portions of ductlike tubular masses of neoplastic tissue. (×65; AFIP 541358.)

tory. In reviewing the histories of patients with meibomian gland carcinomas, it is impressive that the usual story is one of repeated currettages for chalazia before a neoplasm is suspected and a biopsy obtained.

In the series of seventy-eight sebaceous carcinomas of the eyelid recorded by Boniuk and Zimmerman,[25] thirty presented clinically as a chalazion. In twelve patients, the clinical picture was that of a chronic blepharoconjunctivitis, but seven tumors were mistaken for basal cell carcinoma. Following early complete excisional surgery, the prognosis is good. In Boniuk and Zimmerman's series,[25] however, orbital invasion occurred in 17%, lymph node metastasis developed in 28%, and the tumors

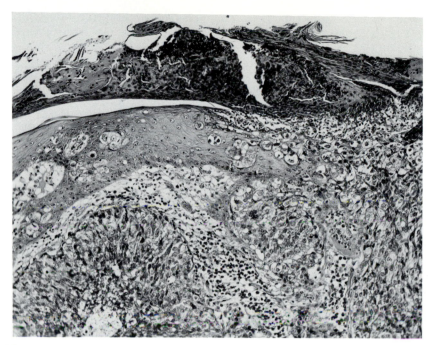

Fig. 1252 Pagetoid involvement of skin of eyelid in patient with carcinoma of meibomian gland. (×115; AFIP 804889.)

proved fatal in 14% of the patients.

Malignant meibomian gland tumors show considerable histologic and cytologic variation, merging with adenomas on the one hand and with very anaplastic epithelial tumors of uncertain histogenesis on the other. The former are easily recognized, first by their position within the tarsus and their obvious anatomic relation to the meibomian gland and second by their cytologic characteristics. In such tumors, the cells continue to exhibit sebaceous differentiation (Fig. 1250), which is very dramatically brought out by frozen sections stained for fat. More rapidly growing tumors may be characterized by extensive necrosis of the central areas of neoplastic lobules, giving rise to a comedocarcinoma pattern (Fig. 1251). Pagetoid involvement of the overlying skin can occur (Fig. 1252). The latter feature also can be seen with *carcinoma of Moll's glands,* a rare adenocarcinoma arising from the sweat glands of the eyelid.[30] *Pilomatrixoma* can occur in the eyelid and be confused with basal cell carcinoma.[22, 27]

Stromal lesions

Stromal lesions include *juvenile xanthogranuloma*[31] and *nodular fasciitis,*[26] which have been discussed in Chapters 3 and 23, respectively.

Secondary tumors

Malignant tumors of the nose and paranasal sinuses may first make their presence known as a result of their direct spread into the eyelids. Similarly, a tumor of the nasolacrimal sac may appear as a primary lesion of the conjunctiva about the punctum.

Leukemias, especially the acute leukemias of childhood, not uncommonly involve the eyelids. Tumefactions of the lids, with or without hemorrhage, may be the initial manifestation of the disease.

Metastases of malignant tumors of distant sites to the eyelids are encountered from time to time with or without other evidence of metastatic disease in the eye or orbit. Breast carcinoma metastatic to the eyelid can adopt a deceptive histiocytoid appearance.[28]

LACRIMAL PASSAGES

Diseases of the lacrimal passages that are of importance to the surgical pathologist are characterized by epiphora, the imperfect drainage of tears so that they flow over the lid margin onto the check, and by varying degrees of swelling, induration, and inflammation of the lower eyelid at its nasal end. While inflammatory obstructions of these passages are common, neoplastic lesions are rare.

Canaliculitis and dacryocystitis

Canaliculitis and dacryocystitis may be the result of direct spread of inflammatory processes in such neighboring structures as the conjunctiva or nose, but more often their pathogenesis is obscure. Acute and chronic types are recognized, and the inflammatory reaction may be suppurative, granulomatous, or necrotizing, with the formation of fistulous tracts to the skin surface below the eyelid near the base of the nose.

The lacrimal passages become filled with purulent exudate in the acute suppurative types, whereas in the chronic forms the passages are narrowed by the inflammatory thickening of the walls of the lacrimal canal or sac. Frequently, there are also hyperplasia of the lining epithelium and hypersecretion of mucus. At times, the degree of papillomatous or adenomatous hyperplasia of the sac may give rise to difficulties in differential diagnosis.

Mucocele

Lacrimal mucocele is another complication of chronic inflammation of the lacrimal sac. A low-grade obstructive lesion with a relatively intact and possibly hypersecreting mucosa may lead to great distention of the sac by accumulated secretions. A discrete swelling occurs just below the inner canthus, between the eyelid and the nose. If untreated, it may enlarge progressively to occupy much of the side of the face and hide the eye.

The contents of the cyst may be clear or milky, fluid or gelatinous, fibrinous or flocculent, sterile or infected. Microscopically, the cyst wall reveals varying degrees of atrophy, degeneration, hyperplasia, and hypersecretion of the mucosa and chronic inflammation of the subepithelial tissues.

Dacryolithiasis

Dacryolithiasis and concretions in the lacrimal canaliculus are of uncertain pathogenesis, but they are generally believed to be the result of a low-grade inflammatory process. Mycotic infections are believed by some authorities to account for most "tear stones." If such concretions are crushed and examined microscopically, they will be seen to contain myriad mycelial elements embedded in a relatively acellular matrix. Others, however, are laminated, mineralized stones without recognizable fungal or bacterial forms.

Tumors

Neoplasms of the lacrimal passages are rare. Papillomas similar to those arising in the conjunctival surface of the eyelid (p. 1328) may form in the punctum, within the canaliculus, or in the sac. Inflammatory pseudoepitheliomatous hyperplasia, however, is seen more often.

From the clinical point of view, it is usually not possible to differentiate malignant tumors of the lacrimal passages from benign neoplasms and pseudotumors. Dacryocystography has become an important part of the clinical evaluation of lacrimal sac tumors.

All malignant tumors of the lacrimal passages except carcinoma are exceedingly rare, and even carcinoma is distinctly uncommon. These tumors are usually moderately well-differentiated squamous carcinomas, similar in appearance to those arising from the mucosa of the nose or in the conjunctiva. They tend to form papillary projections into the lumen and spread along natural surfaces, but they also infiltrate directly into adjacent tissues.[32]

LACRIMAL GLAND

According to Reese,[37] the nature of an expanding mass in the lacrimal fossa cannot be determined without histopathologic examination. Biopsy or excision must be performed to exclude the possibility of a malignant tumor. In approximately one-half of the cases the lesion is nonepithelial, and in most of these it is a nonneoplastic process (inflammatory pseudotumor, lymphoid hyperplasia, etc.). Among those that prove to be epithelial tumors, about one-half are benign mixed tumors and the remainder carcinomatous.

Biopsies of the lacrimal gland are also made to assist in the differential diagnosis of Mikulicz's and Sjögren's syndromes.

Dacryoadenitis

When chronic dacryoadenitis is associated with enlargement of the parotid or other salivary glands, it has been referred to as *Mikulicz's syndrome*. This may be the result of a variety of specific diseases, including sarcoidosis, tuberculosis, syphilis, mumps, Graves' disease, malignant lymphoma, and leukemia.

The term *Mikulicz's disease* is being used less and less, for no one knows exactly what Mikulicz's patients had, and it is doubtful whether there is a specific disease of the lacrimal and salivary glands, other than that responsible for Sjögren's syndrome, that is sufficiently distinctive in its clinical and/or histopathologic picture to justify this eponymic designation.[35]

The benign lymphoepithelial lesion of the salivary glands described by Godwin[34] has been equated with Mikulicz's disease,[36] but the patients usually present clinical evidence of Sjögren's syndrome. The occurrence of the benign lymphoepithelial lesion in the lacrimal glands and its relationship to Sjögren's syndrome have been discussed by Font et al.[33] The typical lesion is shown in Fig. 529 (p. 498).

The lacrimal gland also may be involved in a unilateral chronic nongranulomatous inflammatory process with no associated involvement of salivary glands, no systemic manifestations, and no features of Sjögren's syndrome. As a matter of fact, this is the type of dacryoadenitis the surgical pathologist sees most frequently. Bilateral lacri-

mal gland enlargement with a histologic picture of chronic dacryoadenitis has been reported in a patient with diffuse elevation of IgG and IgA fractions.[38]

Atrophy; Sjögren's syndrome

Sjögren's syndrome is characterized by a failure of lacrimal and conjunctival secretions and consequent keratoconjunctivitis sicca, usually in postmenopausal women. Typically, there is evidence of a systemic disorder affecting mucous membranes and their associated glands. It is believed that degeneration of the secretory portions of the lacrimal and salivary glands is the essential feature of the pathologic anatomy in Sjögren's syndrome, although such secondary changes as lymphocytic infiltration, fibrosis, and hyalinization are commonly present.

The benign lymphoepithelial lesion (Fig. 529, p. 498), while not pathognomonic of Sjögren's syndrome, is so often associated with it that it carries more diagnostic significance than any other histopathologic finding.[33, 34, 36]

Tumors

Most neoplasms of the lacrimal gland arise in the orbital lobe where the gland is firmly attached to the orbital rim about the lacrimal fossa. The bone tends to restrict growth in its direction. Hence, the enlarging tumor characteristically displaces the eye downward and nasally (Fig. 1253).

The histopathologic characteristics of

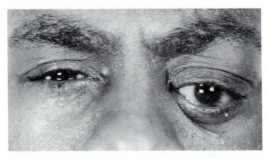

Fig. 1253 Pleomorphic adenoma of left lacrimal gland in 38-year-old black man. Proptosis was acompanied by severe visual loss. (AFIP 62-931; courtesy Veterans Administration Hospital, Jefferson Barracks, Mo.)

lacrimal gland tumors are similar to those of the salivary glands (Chapter 11). Whereas pleomorphic adenomas are by far the most common, they do not predominate to the degree that some writers have suggested (90%). Pleomorphic adenomas account for about 50% to 60%, carcinomas in pleomorphic adenomas for 5% to 10%, adenoid cystic carcinomas for 20% to 30%, and other carcinomas for 5% to 10%.

Because so many of these lacrimal gland tumors have not been completely and adequately removed at the initial operation, there has been an excessively high recurrence rate.[39] It is even more difficult to treat the recurrences, for these are often multiple. The carcinomas have a very poor prognosis.[40]

In addition to the epithelial tumors of the lacrimal gland, malignant lymphomas, lymphoid pseudotumors, and chronic inflammatory processes are important causes of enlargement of the gland. In a patient who is in good general health and who presents no evidence of a systemic disease, the discovery of a lymphomatous tumor in the lacrimal fossa rarely heralds the development of malignant lymphoma or leukemia. In fact, in the majority of cases there is a polymorphism suggestive of a reactive inflammatory process, although in other cases the rather pure proliferation of lymphocytes makes it quite impossible to rule out a lymphocytic lymphoma or leukemia. The lacrimal glands may, of course, become involved along with other tissues in a leukemia or malignant lymphoma.

ORBIT

The hallmark of disease of the orbit is exophthalmos.[42] This may not necessarily be caused by a true neoplasm, and therefore the surgical pathologist may never see any specimen from many patients who present with this finding. For example, the most common cause for exophthalmos is endocrine ophthalmopathy and rarely is a biopsy taken in these cases.

As for the relative frequency of lesions that cause exophthalmos, many of the statistics that have been reported merely reflect the bias of the specialist involved. For example, to the radiologist one of the most common orbital lesions producing displacement of the eye is a mucocele arising from a paranasal sinus. The ophthalmologist, however, would place mucocele far below such entities as endocrine exophthalmos, hemangioma, and malignant lymphoma.[41]

Congenital and developmental conditions
Angioma

Angiomas are generally considered to be the most common of all orbital tumors that require surgical treatment. These are generally of blood vessel origin, for lymphangiomas of the orbit are comparatively rare. Although encountered in any age group, angiomatous tumors typically make their presence known early in life.[43]

These tumors characteristically present as soft, compressible tumors with the eye itself usually unaffected. In the infant, these may be quite diffuse throughout the orbit and surgical removal may be difficult. Fortunately, most of the lesions spontaneously regress by the age of 3 years. In the young adult, the tumors may be encapsulated and can be surgically "shelled" out. X-ray examination frequently shows a characteristic symmetrical enlargement of the involved orbit.

These tumors rarely present difficulties in histopathologic diagnosis, for they are not significantly dissimilar from angiomas of other regions.

Neurofibroma

Neurofibromas are also basically hamartomatous lesions, but they are much less common in the orbit than are the vascular tumors. These orbital tumors may be merely one of a number of manifestations of Recklinghausen's disease, but on occasion they are also encountered as isolated lesions.

In the former situation, there may be gross deformity of the orbit and eyelids as well as diffuse involvement of the orbital

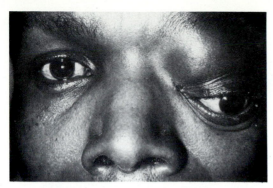

Fig. 1254 Mucocele producing downward and lateral displacement of left eye. (WU neg. 69-7637; from Ackerman, L. V., and del Regato, J. A.: Cancer, ed. 4, St. Louis, 1970, The C. V. Mosby Co.)

nerves. The bony defects are often easily recognized radiographically and may be responsible for a pulsating exophthalmos.

Mucocele

Chronic disease of the frontal or ethmoid sinuses may produce a mucocele that erodes through the wall of the sinus to produce an inferolateral displacement of the globe. The onset is usually insidious, and the enlargement is symptomless and slow (Fig. 1254).

Histopathologically, this cystic mass is lined by mucus-secreting sinus mucosa with variable degrees of inflammation and scarring.

Systemic diseases
Endocrine exophthalmos

The most common cause of unilateral exophthalmos is endocrine exophthalmos in which there is some dysfunction of the thyroid-pituitary axis. Although there is a certain amount of overlap, it has been customary to think of this entity in terms of two forms.

The thyrotoxic form is almost invariably associated with some degree of hyperthyroidism, whereas in the thyrotrophic form the patient may be euthyroid or hypothyroid.

Unilateral orbital involvement occurs with sufficient frequency in both forms of

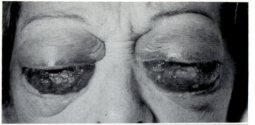

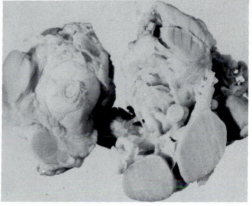

Fig. 1255   A, Malignant exophthalmos of about ten months' duration in 65-year-old white woman who finally died of congestive heart failure. **B,** At autopsy, extraocular muscles were found to be massively thickened. (**A** and **B,** AFIP 692463.)

endocrine exophthalmos to warrant these conditions always being considered in the differential diagnosis of orbital tumors (Fig. 1255).

Histopathologic changes observed in the severe cases which are most likely to come to the attention of surgical pathologists include widespread edema and chronic inflammation of all the orbital tissues. The most striking gross alterations are observed in the extraocular muscles, which may be massively enlarged. Muscle fibers degenerate and become hyalinized. A great increase in the interstitial connective tissue, including both cellular elements and ground substance, is observed particularly in the muscles but also in the other orbital tissues.

Histiocytoses and juvenile xanthogranuloma

Exophthalmos may rarely be caused by orbital involvement by Hand-Schüller-

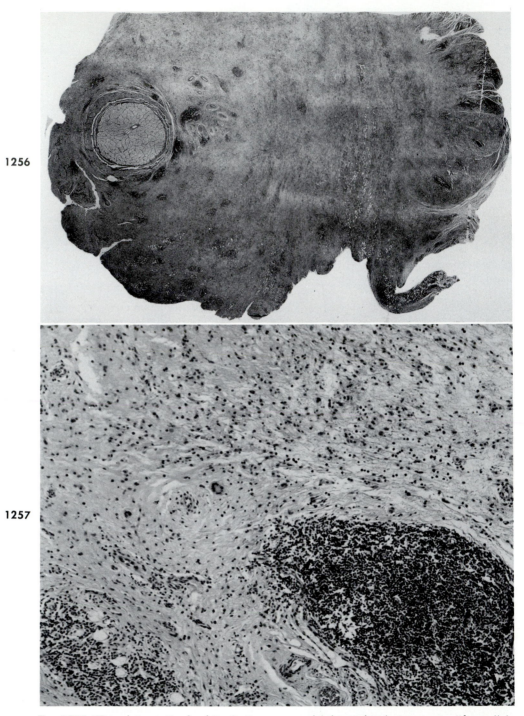

Fig. 1256 ''Pseudotumor'' of orbit. Optic nerve and other orbital tissues are ''frozen'' in dense mass of nonspecific chronic inflammatory tissue. (×5½; AFIP 35691.)
Fig. 1257 ''Pseudotumor'' of orbit showing infiltration by chronic inflammatory cells, giant cells, and generalized fibrosis. (×90; WU neg. 67-4223.)

Christian disease, Letterer-Siwe disease, eosinophilic granuloma, or juvenile xanthogranuloma.

Inflammatory processes

The orbit may become secondarily inflamed by lesions arising in the face, eyes, nose, sinuses, orbital bones, blood vessels, brain, and meninges. Generally, it is only when such inflammations simulate neoplasms that orbital exploration is undertaken and tissue is obtained for histopathologic diagnosis.

Specific granulomas, including those of tuberculosis and sarcoidosis, are rare.

Nonspecific chronic inflammations ("pseudotumors" of orbit) are very much more frequent than are the specific infectious granulomas.

Undoubtedly, these pseudotumors represent an etiologically and pathogenetically heterogeneous group. The pathologic features which they share include the following:

1 The formation of an indurated orbital mass often surrounding the optic nerve and incorporating one or more of the extraocular muscles (Fig. 1256)
2 A tissue reaction which includes exudation of fluid, excessive production of ground substance, the mobilization of chronic inflammatory cells, vascular proliferation, and hyperplasia of connective tissue (Fig. 1257)
3 The absence of demonstrable etiologic agents or of otherwise diagnostic histopathologic alterations indicative of such specific disease entities as Hodgkin's disease, cranial arteritis, etc.

This is not to say, however, that the microscopic features are uniform from case to case. In some instances, the proliferation of blood vessels and ground substance resembles that of exuberant granulation tissue. At times, the lymphoid hyperplasia with follicle formation is of such intensity that the picture resembles that which is characteristic of orbital malignant lymphomas (p. 1322). Other cases with prominent involvement of extraocular muscles suggest the possibility of thyrotropic exophthalmos.

A well-developed granulomatous reaction about small pools of fat is observed in certain cases. Such lesions may suggest traumatic fat necrosis. Others containing large numbers of cholesterol clefts and many foamy macrophages and giant cells suggest an area of old suppuration or hemorrhage. Periphlebitis is prominent in certain cases, and some of these may present a significant eosinophilia suggesting the possibility of a hypersensitivity angiitis. Rarely, the picture merges with that of sclerosing hemangioma or fasciitis.

Patients with pseudotumors are usually in their third to fifth decade and in good health. The exophthalmos is of relatively sudden onset and in at least one-half of the patients is associated with moderate to severe orbital pain. Diplopia is often present, secondary to limitation of ocular motility in one or more fields of gaze, but visual acuity is usually unimpaired.

The lesion often can be palpated as a firm, irreducible mass along the floor or roof of the orbit and firmly attached to the bone, so that the tumor edge and the orbital margin are indistinguishable. The amount of exophthalmos varies. It can be quite severe or not present at all. Usually, there is at least some degree of lid and conjunctival edema and injection. Radiographic changes are characteristically absent except for the occasional occurrence of hyperostosis.[45]

These tumors often regress spontaneously only to recur, sometimes in the contralateral orbit. Steroids often produce a marked improvement in the signs and symptoms. The patients usually remain in good general health,[44] but occasionally a necrotizing orbital granuloma is part of the picture of Wegener's granulomatosis.[46]

Primary tumors
Connective tissue tumors

Connective tissue tumors of the orbit, both benign and malignant, are extremely rare. Only the *rhabdomyosarcoma* is en-

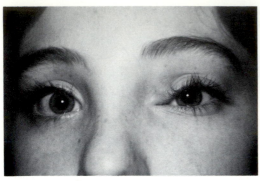

Fig. 1258 Rhabdomyosarcoma presenting as palpable mass in upper medial quadrant of left orbit with only minimal downward and lateral displacement of eye. (WU neg. 67-3507; from Smith, M. E.: The differential diagnosis of unilateral exophthalmos. In Gay, A. J., and Burde, R. M., editors: Clinical concepts in neuro-ophthalmology, International Ophthalmology Clinics, vol. 7, no. 4, Boston, 1967, Little, Brown and Co.)

countered with any degree of regularity, and this is the most frequently observed tumor in the orbit in children.[47, 50]

This neoplasm characteristically occurs between the ages of 5 and 15 years with a rather sudden onset and a rapidly progressive course. Although the tumor can occur anywhere in the orbit, there is a slightly higher incidence of an upper nasal location displacing the eye downward and outward (Fig. 1258). Microscopically, it resembles the undifferentiated rhabdomyosarcomas of childhood seen in other anatomic locations (Chapter 23).

Fibromas, lipomas, osteomas, and their malignant counterparts have all been reported, but they are of little importance. One possible exception to this statement concerns the occurrence of osteosarcomas and other sarcomas arising in the orbital tissues as a late complication of extensive radiation therapy. Several cases have already been reported.[49] In recent years, however, the amount of radiation used in the treatment of retinoblastoma in particular has been greatly reduced.

Reactive fibroblastic proliferations such as nodular fasciitis and fibrous histiocytomas may be mistaken for sarcomas.[48]

Lymphoid tumors

Lymphoid tumors of the orbit present great difficulties in histopathologic diagnoses. Such lesions may develop in the course of a previously recognized malignant lymphoma or leukemia, but much more often the lymphoid tumor of the orbit, lacrimal gland, or conjunctiva is not accompanied by any clinical or hematologic evidence of a systemic disease.

Microscopically, lymphoid tumors of the orbit fall into three main groups. The smallest but most important contains those lesions that are quite obviously malignant neoplasms. The two largest groups include the following:

1 Those lesions which are fairly obvious examples of severe reactive hyperplasia

2 Those lesions which are characterized by a rather uniform but widespread proliferation of lymphocytes

In the former, one frequently observes considerable polymorphism, a variety of cell types participating, vascular proliferation, and prominent follicles with reactive centers. It is the latter group, characterized by a monotonous lymphocytic proliferation, frequently with apparent infiltration of orbital fat, blood vessels, and nerves, that presents most of the exceedingly difficult problems in differential diagnosis. At present, we believe that such lymphocytomas are benign, for they generally respond to very small doses of radiation, are not associated with other evidence of systemic disease, and do not recur or metastasize following therapy. It is possible, however, that much longer periods of follow-up will be required to ascertain the behavior of these lesions properly. The orbit is a common site of involvement of Burkitt's lymphoma.[51-53]

Glioma of optic nerve

Gliomas of the optic nerve are relatively rare slow-growing tumors that usually arise within the orbital segment of the nerve.[55]

Considerable cytologic variation is observed among the gliomas, not only from

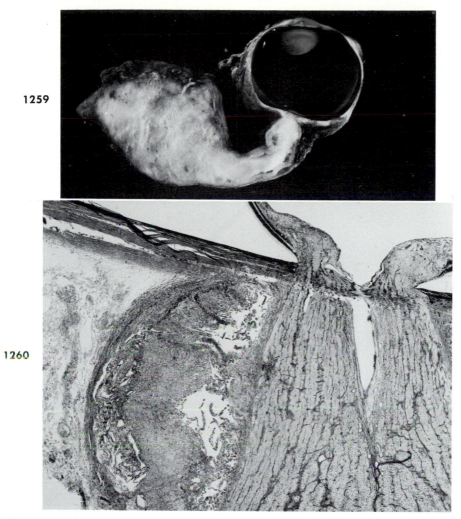

1259

1260

Fig. 1259 Glioma that has produced massive enlargement of orbital segment of optic nerve. Tumor has completely effaced characteristic architectural features of nerve and its meninges. (AFIP 842777.)

Fig. 1260 Section through optic nerve just anterior to main mass of this glioma reveals minimal alteration of parenchyma of nerve but greatly thickened meninges. Combination of infiltrating tumor and arachnoidal proliferation is responsible for this meningeal thickening. (×20; AFIP 65035.)

case to case but also in different portions of a given tumor. Varying degrees of cellularity are observed, but generally these neoplasms are characterized by a low order of anaplasia. This is especially true about the margins of the tumor, where it is often impossible to be certain where reactive gliosis ends and neoplasia begins. Typically, there are areas of intense mucinous degeneration within the tumor. Frequently in such areas the tumor cells appear to

be virtually lost in the abundant hyaluronidase-sensitive mucoid accumulations.

As these gliomas increase in size, they tend to form a bulbous enlargement of the nerve (Fig. 1259). They also extend along the nerve peripherally toward the eye and centrally toward the brain. In so doing, they often produce great enlargement of the optic canal, an important diagnostic sign for the radiologist. In such cases, the optic nerve fibers are likely to be com-

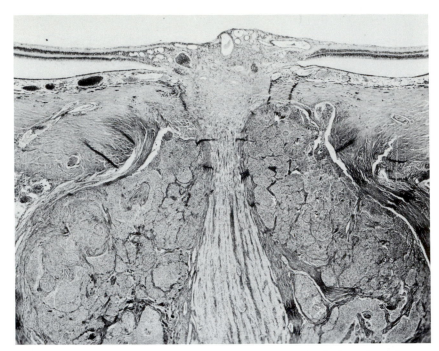

Fig. 1261 Meningioma of optic nerve. Meninges are greatly thickened, and optic nerve reveals severe compression atrophy. (×21; AFIP 55939.)

pletely destroyed, and the optic disc typically presents the ophthalmoscopic characteristics of primary optic atrophy.

Another growth pattern exhibited by a majority of optic nerve gliomas is for infiltration to take place through the pia. This leads to great thickening of the arachnoid (Fig. 1260). This is partly the result of more exuberant growth of the tumor cells once they have reached the arachnoid, but equally important is the reactive proliferation of arachnoidal cells. At times, this has created difficulties in differential diagnosis between glioma and meningioma.

Gliomas of the optic nerve typically make their presence known during the first decade of life. According to Davis,[54] there is a distinct association of these tumors and Recklinghausen's disease.

Meningioma

Meningiomas of the orbit may arise from the meninges of the optic nerve (Fig. 1261), but more often they represent orbital extension of sphenoidal ridge meningiomas. In many cases it is impossible to establish with certainty the site of origin of these slowly progressive neoplasms. In general, however, the site of origin and the position of the main tumor mass account for differences in the resultant clinical picture.[56]

Those tumors arising from the orbital meninges generally produce some visual loss, optic atrophy, and exophthalmos. Those arising from the inner portion of the sphenoidal ridge produce more severe compression of the optic nerve within the optic canal, resulting in papilledema or optic atrophy before proptosis. Those arising from the middle and outer thirds of the ridge tend to spare the optic nerve, although the associated hyperostosis frequently leads to proptosis or formation of a mass in the temporal area.

Secondary tumors

Direct spread from adjacent structures can occur with primary intraocular tumors such as retinoblastoma or uveal malignant melanomas. Carcinomas of the paranasal sinuses also may fail to produce diagnostic symptoms until orbital extension has occurred.

Hematogenous metastases to the orbit

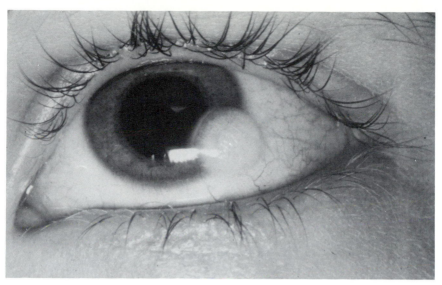

Fig. 1262 Limbal dermoid in child. (WU neg. 67-4282.)

may be seen, on occasion, with many different tumors, but rarely are these initial manifestations of a carcinoma. Even the neuroblastoma, which has a notorious reputation for its orbital metastases, rarely does so before other diagnostic signs appear.

Most important in this regard is the distinct possibility that a primary embryonal rhabdomyosarcoma might be misinterpreted as a metastatic tumor. Another important possibility to be considered when an undifferentiated "round cell sarcoma" is found in a child's orbital tissues is acute leukemia. Such orbital lesions may make their appearance before peripheral blood studies are diagnostic, but bone marrow aspirates will usually furnish a conclusive answer. In the case of adults, an orbital metastasis may, on rare occasions, be the initial manifestation of carcinoma of the breast, bronchus, or kidney.

CONJUNCTIVA AND CORNEA
Congenital and developmental lesions
Dermoid tumors

Dermoid tumors of the bulbar conjunctiva are firm, localized, elevated opaque masses which typically occur at the limbus, often encroaching upon the cornea (Fig. 1262). These are solid choristomatous masses, not to be confused with dermoid cysts of the orbit.[57]

Over the lesion, the surface epithelium and the subepithelial connective tissue present the histologic features characteristic of epidermis and dermis, respectively. Typically, a few hairs project from the tumor. The bulk of the mass is composed of thick bundles of collagen and masses of adult fat. In some lesions, skin appendages are few, and adipose tissue is abundant. These are known as dermolipomas, and they are usually situated in the upper outer fornix. Ocular dermoids may be part of Goldenhar's syndrome or merely associated with auricular appendages.[58]

Nevi

Nevi of the bulbar conjunctiva, like those of the skin, may be observed from birth, or they may become noticeable at any time during childhood, adolescence, or later. At times, a nevus known to have been present since infancy appears to become much larger and more pigmented at puberty.

Characteristically, conjunctival nevi are discrete, elevated lesions located on the globe in the interpalpebral zone near the limbus, but they vary greatly in size, shape, and position. They also exhibit much varia-

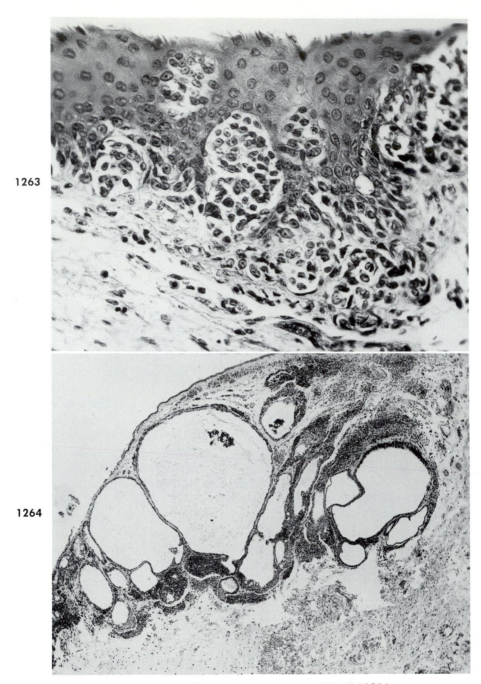

Fig. 1263 Junctional nevus of bulbar conjunctiva (×305; AFIP 819328.)
Fig. 1264 Conjunctival nevus with many associated cystic epithelial inclusions. Small round cells about large cysts are not inflammatory cells but nevus cells. This epibulbar lesion may be analogous to hairy dermal nevi of skin. (×48; AFIP 713602.)

tion in degree of pigmentation, about one-third being essentially amelanotic.

Microscopically, conjunctival nevi are al-

most always of the junctional (Fig. 1263) or compound varieties. Counterparts of the common dermal nevus of the skin are

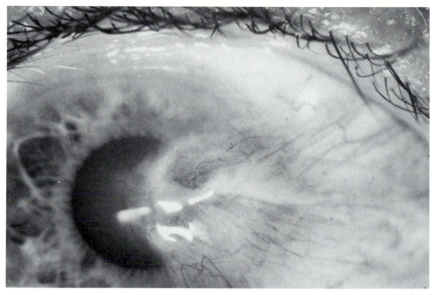

Fig. 1265 Pterygium that has grown over pupillary axis and has interfered with vision. (WU neg. 67-4284.)

rarely observed. Frequently, there are numerous solid and cystic inclusions of conjunctival epithelium intimately incorporated into the subepithelial component of these nevi. At times, the epithelial inclusions may so dominate the clinical and histopathologic picture (Fig. 1264) that the nevoid nature of the lesion is overlooked.

Inflammation

Inflammatory lesions of the conjunctiva do not often give rise to the type of diagnostic or therapeutic problem that requires excision and histopathologic study. Two lesions that deserve mention are the *chronic granulomas* characteristic of sarcoidosis and *ligneous conjunctivitis.*

In the former situation, a noncaseating granulomatous tubercle can be found in about one-fourth of patients with sarcoidosis.[59] Ligneous conjunctivitis is a peculiar form of chronic pseudomembranous conjunctivitis that presents as a woody induration of the eyelids plus the formation of a pseudomembrane on the tarsal conjunctiva. The cardinal feature histologically is the presence of large hyaline masses.[60]

Degeneration

Pinguecula is a very common degenerative process affecting primarily the subepithelial connective tissues of the bulbar conjunctiva in the interpalpebral region. This gives rise to an elevated yellowish lesion over which the eptihelium may become atrophic or thickened.

Histologically, the most characteristic feature is senile elastosis affecting a bandlike zone beneath the epithelium. Secondary hyalinization and calcareous degeneration also may be observed. Typically, the

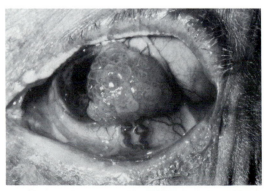

Fig. 1266 Extensive papilloma of bulbar conjunctiva. (WU neg. 72-6272.)

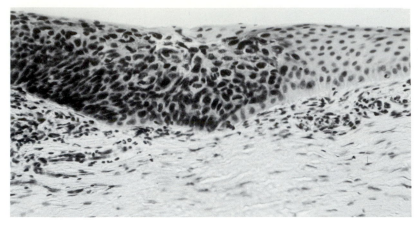

Fig. 1267 Carcinoma in situ in which there is abrupt transition from essentially normal conjunctival epithelium to intraepithelial neoplasm. (×160; WU neg. 67-5356.)

epithelium over pingueculae becomes atrophic, but at times it becomes so acanthotic and dyskeratotic that the erroneous diagnosis of carcinoma may be made.

Pterygium extends into the cornea and is therefore a more important lesion than the pinguecula (Fig. 1265).

Microscopically, there is usually some senile elastosis but also a variable amount of acute and chronic inflammation and congestion of blood vessels.

Tumors and related lesions
Papilloma

Papillomas may be sessile or fungating. Often a rather broad area of involvement is observed, and the lesion extends onto the cornea. Variable pigmentation occurs, and the lesion may be confused with a pedunculated malignant melanoma (Fig. 1266).

Microscopically, the typical papilloma reveals pronounced acanthosis and varying degrees of keratinization, dyskeratosis, and nonspecific inflammation (Fig. 1249).

Carcinoma in situ

Carcinoma in situ of the bulbar conjunctiva varies considerably in its clinical appearance. It may present as an area of leukoplakia, as a papilloma, or as a complication of pterygium or pinguecula.

The histopathologic characteristics of carcinoma in situ of the conjunctiva and

cornea are similar to those observed elsewhere in the mucous membranes (Fig. 1267), or the lesion may mimic Bowen's disease of the skin.[61]

Squamous cell carcinoma

Squamous cell carcinoma is encountered on the bulbar conjunctiva and cornea, but basal cell carcinoma arising in these tissues is of questionable occurrence.

Clinically, significant infiltrative carcinoma (Figs. 1268 and 1269) is seldom ob-

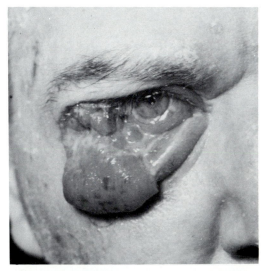

Fig. 1268 Epidermal carcinoma of conjunctiva. Tumor grew rapidly over four-month period. (WU neg. 64-3837.)

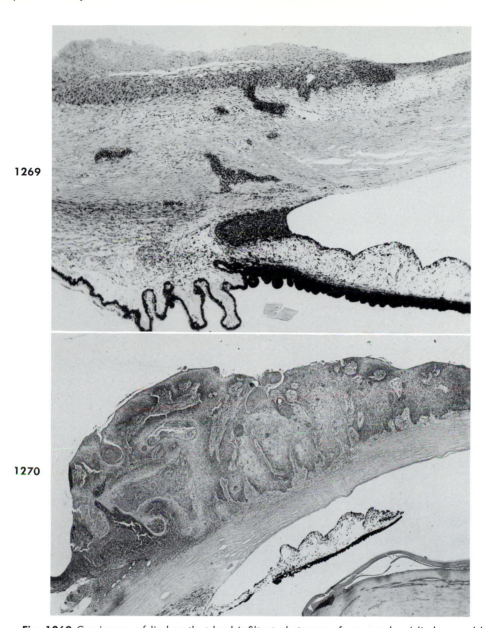

Fig. 1269 Carcinoma of limbus that had infiltrated stroma of corneoscleral limbus and had extended along aqueous outflow pathways into angle of anterior chamber, a very unusual complication of limbal tumors. (×50; AFIP 690246.)

Fig. 1270 Carcinoma of limbus that presented more characteristic picture than that shown in Fig. 1269. Exophytic growth pattern with formation of papillomatous mass is typical of more advanced limbal carcinomas. Even in such large tumors, corneoscleral stroma tends to prevent neoplasm from invading intraocular tissues. (×18; AFIP 785865.)

served in the United States, probably because it is a common practice to excise early "precancerous" or "in situ cancerous" lesions long before they become infiltrative. Such lesions, as well as the majority of early invasive carcinomas of the limbal area, can be adequately controlled by excisional therapy. Rarely in this country is it necessary to resort to radical surgery for these tumors[62] (Fig. 1270).

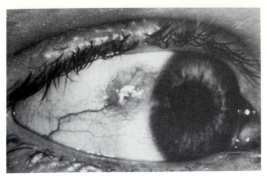

Fig. 1271 Pigmented lesion at limbus that proved to be benign nevus. (WU neg. 69-2209; from Ackerman, L. V., and del Regato, J. A.: Cancer, ed. 4, St. Louis, 1970, The C. V. Mosby Co.; courtesy Registry of Ophthalmic Pathology, Armed Forces Institute of Pathology.)

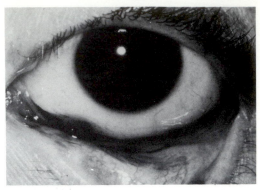

Fig. 1272 Malignant melanoma of conjunctiva in lower cul-de-sac arising from a lesion of acquired melanosis. (WU neg. 69-2211; from Zimmerman, L. E.: Discussion of Pigmented tumors of the conjunctiva; courtesy Registry of Ophthalmic Pathology, Armed Forces Institute of Pathology; AFIP 56-9886. In Boniuk, M., editor: Ocular and adnexal tumors, St. Louis, 1964, The C. V. Mosby Co.)

Malignant melanoma

Malignant melanoma of the conjunctiva and cornea may arise without an apparent precursor lesion, or it may be a sequela of a nevus or of acquired melanosis[63] (Figs. 1271 and 1272).

Nevus origin

Nevi of the conjunctiva, according to Reese,[66] seldom give rise to malignant melanoma. In his experience, precancerous melanosis has been a much more common precursor. In the Registry of Ophthalmic Pathology, however, there are many good examples of the occurrence of sudden growth during adult life of nevi known to

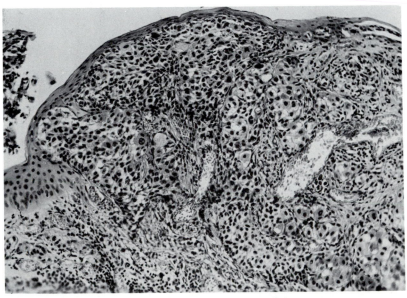

Fig. 1273 Malignant melanoma arising in nevus known to have been present since childhood. Patient, 59-year-old white woman, stated that lesion suddenly became quite large several months before it was excised. (×135; AFIP 643700.)

have been present since childhood (Fig. 1273).

Histologically, these tumors also have shown evidence of the occurrence of malignant change in previously benign compound nevi. Subsequent behavior of these histologically malignant melanomas has been difficult to predict. Many, particularly the pedunculated limbal lesions, have neither recurred nor metastasized even though removed by simple excision. Others have produced multiple recurrences, and at least one (Fig. 1274) has even metastasized without killing the patient.[64]

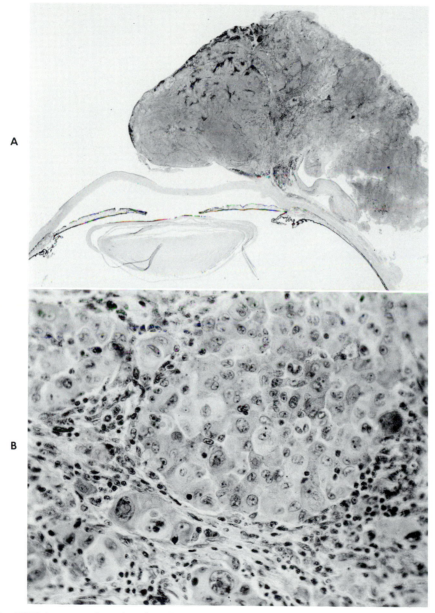

Fig. 1274 Large pedunculated malignant melanoma of limbus in 44-year-old black woman. Amputation of one leg because of metastasis was performed nine years after enucleation, but patient was living without other evidence of metastatic disease sixteen years later. (**A**, ×6; **B**, ×305; **A** and **B**, AFIP 35659.)

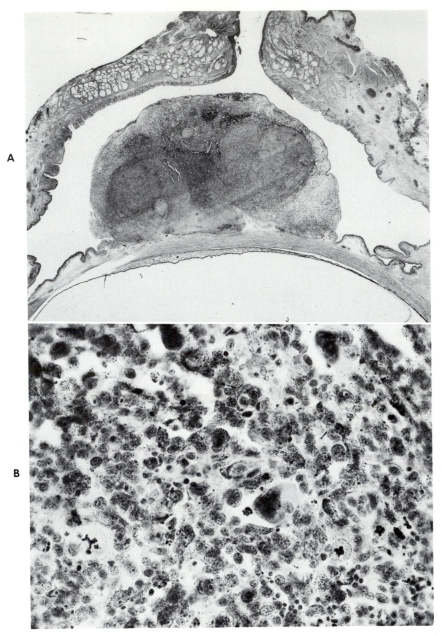

Fig. 1275 Malignant melanoma arising from acquired melanosis. Low-power view, **A,** and high-power view, **B,** of malignant melanoma that arose from limbus of eye with widespread acquired melanosis of conjunctiva (see Fig. 1276). (**A** and **B,** AFIP 897677.)

Acquired melanosis—benign and malignant

Acquired melanosis is also referred to as precancerous and cancerous melanosis.[67] The condition is characterized clinically by the insidious development (typically in the fifth decade) of a diffuse nonelevated granular pigmentation of the conjunctiva. It has a poor prognosis due to the frequency with which it gives rise to metastasizing malignant melanoma (Figs. 1275 and 1276).

Usually, a long period of five to ten years elapses between the onset of benign

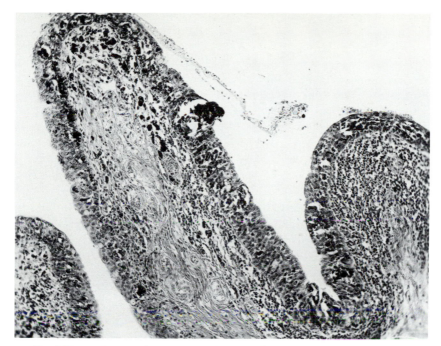

Fig. 1276 Widespread acquired melanosis of conjunctiva. (AFIP 897677.)

acquired melanosis and the development of malignant melanoma. During this interval, the extent of the lesion and the degree of pigmentation may fluctuate spontaneously or as a result of radiation therapy. The disease affects the bulbar conjunctiva most commonly, but associated lesions of the cornea, palpebral conjunctiva, and skin of the eyelids are not uncommon.

Because the term precancerous melanosis has led to the unwarranted assumption that the lesion will inevitably give rise to a malignant melanoma despite the fact that fewer than one in five cases actually progress to cancerous melanosis,[67] we believe this term should be dropped. We recommend Zimmerman's classification[68] which is based on the histopathologic appearance of the lesions.

Stage I—Benign acquired melanosis

A *With minimal junctional activity*—In some cases, the tissue shows only hyperpigmentation of the epithelium, while in others a few clusters of nevus cells (atypical melanocytes) also may be seen in the affected epithelium.

B *With marked junctional activity*—In addition

to hyperpigmentation, there are many nests of nevus cells, some of which appear rather disturbing, and there are engorged vessels and inflammatory cells in the substantia propria.

Stage II—Cancerous acquired melanosis

A *With minimal invasion*—This would correspond to the early malignant melanomas that other pathologists have variously designated as "superficial malignant melanoma" or "incipient malignant melanoma." In addition to changes indicated previously, there are focal areas in which the full thickness of the affected epithelium is replaced by extremely disturbing, very atypical melanocytes, often with mitotic activity in evidence. Often foci of invasion of the superficial substantia propria can be demonstrated.

B *With marked invasion*—A fully developed, frankly invasive malignant melanoma is present in addition to the other changes listed in Stage I and Stage IIA.

The transition from the benign to the cancerous state may not be apparent clinically, although usually there are areas that become elevated, nodular, ulcerated, and/or more deeply pigmented.

No therapy is recommended for most patients with benign acquired melanosis (Stage IA), and orbital exenteration is recommended for frank malignant melanoma arising in an extensive area of acquired melanosis (Stage IIB). Between these extremes lie the real therapeutic problems. We recommend careful follow-up plus antiinflammatory measures for Stage IB and wide excisional surgery for Stage IIA with preservation of the eye and eyelids when feasible.

Lymphoid tumors

Lymphomatous tumors analogous to those of the eyelid and the orbit (p. 1322) may present as an isolated focus in the conjunctiva. As with the lid and orbital lesions, they may range from obvious cancer to benign lymphoid hyperplasias.[65]

INTRAOCULAR TISSUES

Surgical pathology of the eye itself differs from most of the rest of surgical pathology for several important reasons.

In the first place, biopsies of intraocular tissues are rarely feasible. The only important exception is the iris, lesions of which often can be completely excised, or at least biopsied, by iridectomy.

In the second place, most of the eyes reaching the surgical pathology laboratory are obtained as a result of enucleation. Usually the globe is intact but free of such accessory tissues as the extraocular muscles and orbital fat. Much less often, the eye is eviscerated, and only fragments of the intraocular tissues are submitted for microscopic study. In such cases, it is rarely possible to arrive at a satisfactory diagnosis and clinicopathologic correlation. Eyes that are enucleated or eviscerated usually have been diseased for a long period of time and have become blind. Severe pain and unsightliness are the common immediate reasons for removing the eye. In these cases it is the responsibility of the pathologist not merely to arrive at a definitive diagnosis but also to reconstruct the sequence of events that took place from the onset of ocular disease to the final stages which led to enucleation.

This brings us to another distinctive characteristic of ophthalmic pathology. Frequently, the initial pathologic process becomes completely obscured by the subsequent series of events. For example, the patient may first complain of visual disturbance produced by a cataract. The lens opacification progresses, and cataract extraction is performed. Defective wound healing follows, and surface epithelium grows down into the anterior chamber. This leads to secondary glaucoma for which one or more additional surgical procedures are performed. These, in turn, may be complicated by hemorrhage, infection, or retinal detachment. Finally, the eye may become shrunken (phthisical) and disfiguring. A period of several years to a decade or more usually is required for such a series of events to take place.

Intraocular neoplasms represent an exception to the generalizations just given. Since only in the case of iris tumors is it ordinarily possible to excise the neoplasm, the procedure usually followed is to recommend early enucleation for other uveal and retinal neoplasms. The aim here is to arrive at a correct clinical diagnosis early, long before such secondary pathologic processes as cataract formation, massive retinal detachment, glaucoma, uveitis, or phthisis complicate the picture. Therefore, the pathologist often observes a much less confusing array of pathologic changes and has less difficulty making a diagnosis in eyes removed because of intraocular neoplasms than in other enucleated eyes. This, however, is not invariably the case for if the tumor has been present and growing for a long period of time, it, too, may lead to a wide assortment of secondary processes that sometimes confuse the pathologist as well as the clinician.

Congenital and developmental malformations

Many congenital and developmental malformations of the eye are rarely seen by the surgical pathologist but are seen only at postmortem examination.[75, 83] Congenital

abnormalities typify the point made earlier
—i.e., the initial pathologic process becomes completely obscured by the subsequent series of events occurring in that eye.

Congenital glaucoma

Congenital glaucoma is characterized by
an elevation in the intraocular pressure due
to a malformation of the tissues in the
region of the anterior chamber angle. The
precise nature of this malformation is still
not clear, but there seems to be either an
incomplete separation of the iris root from
the trabeculae or the retention of an embryonic membrane, or both.[76, 77, 81]

The increased intraocular pressure leads
to retinal and optic nerve degeneration,
corneal edema and scarring, and global
enlargement (buphthalmos). Unilateral
congenital glaucoma may occur in Recklinghausen's disease or in the Sturge-Weber
syndrome.

When there is a more obvious architectural distortion of the iris and angle of the
anterior chamber, it is referred to as the
anterior chamber cleavage syndrome[80] or
iridogoniodysgenesis. Depending upon the
degree of angle malformation, other various designations are used (e.g., Reiger's
syndrome and Axenfeld's syndrome). This
group of malformations is also often associated with a developmental glaucoma.

Retrolental fibroplasia

Retrolental fibroplasia, also called the
retinopathy of prematurity, is an acquired
form of developmental disorder resulting
from the unique sensitivity of retinal blood
vessels of the premature retina to oxygen.[79]

Much of the retinal periphery of a baby
born after only six or seven months of
gestation is completely avascular. If such
a premature infant is given high concentrations of oxygen (over 40%), normal
vascularization of the retinal periphery
may be inhibited. Vasoconstriction and
actual obliteration of the terminal vessels
may follow prolonged oxygen therapy.
Later, upon withdrawal of oxygen, pathologic neovascularization occurs. These

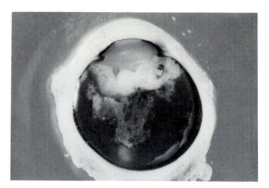

Fig. 1277 Retrolental fibroplasia (retinopathy of
premaurity) showing opaque mass consisting of
organized vitreous and completely detached
retina located immediately behind lens. (AFIP
597231.)

newly formed vessels frequently invade
the vitreous, leak serum or blood, and
eventually lead to organization of the vitreous, retinal detachment, and blindness
(Fig. 1277).

Phakoma

Phakomas are hamartomatous malformations often associated with extraocular
lesions as a part of well-defined clinicopathologic syndromes.[71] These include
Bourneville's syndrome (tuberous sclerosis), Recklinghausen's disease (neurofibromatosis), the Sturge-Weber syndrome
(encephalotrigeminal angiomatosis), and
Lindau–von Hippel disease (angioglioma-
tosis).

In tuberous sclerosis, the most characteristic intraocular lesions are glial plaques
and nodules in the nerve fiber layer of
the retina (Fig. 1278) and calcified giant
drusen of the optic disc (Fig. 1279).
Neurofibromas and melanotic tumors of
the uvea and gliomas of the optic nerve
(p. 1322) are observed in Recklinghausen's
disease.

Hemangioma of the choroid (Fig. 1242)
is the most common intraocular lesion of
the Sturge-Weber syndrome. Ipsilateral
glaucoma is often associated with the
Sturge-Weber syndrome or Recklinghausen's disease. Abnormally large tortuous
arteries and veins leading to a retinal

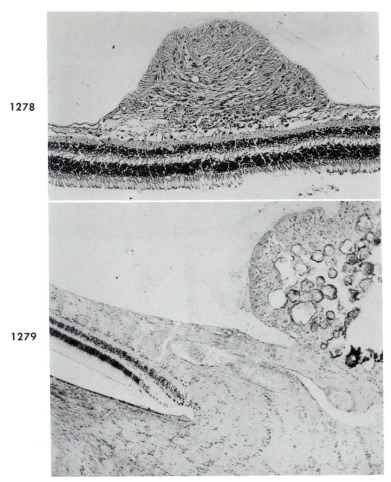

Fig. 1278 Tuberous sclerosis showing glial nodule or hamartoma projecting against vitreous body from nerve fiber layer of retina. (×90; AFIP 511046.)

Fig. 1279 Tuberous sclerosis. Large, partially calcified glial hamartoma (called giant *drusen*) projecting from optic disc that had been suspected clinically to be malignant tumor, and for this reason eye was enucleated. (×70; AFIP 511046; from Zimmerman, L. E., and Walsh, F. B.: Amer. J. Ophthalmol. **42**:737-747, 1956.)

nodule composed of vascular, endothelial, and glial tissues are characteristic of Lindau–von Hippel disease. Vitreous disturbance and retinal detachment are common complications.

Persistent hyperplastic primary vitreous

A congenital condition, persistent hyperplastic primary vitreous refers to the persistence and hyperplasia of the fibrovascular tunic of the lens and part of the hyaloid vascular system.[74] It is usually unilateral and occurs in a microphthalmic eye. Clinically, this anomaly is manifested by a white reflex behind the pupil (leukokoria). Therefore, the eyes usually are removed because of suspected retinoblastoma.

Histologically, there is a dense fibrovascular retrolental mass, and the elongated ciliary processes are enmeshed in this tissue. Remnants of the hyaloid artery system are present, and the retina may appear normal or show evidence of retinal dysplasia (Figs. 1280 and 1281).

Retinal dysplasia

A congenital anomaly, retinal dysplasia may occur as part of the 13-15 trisomy

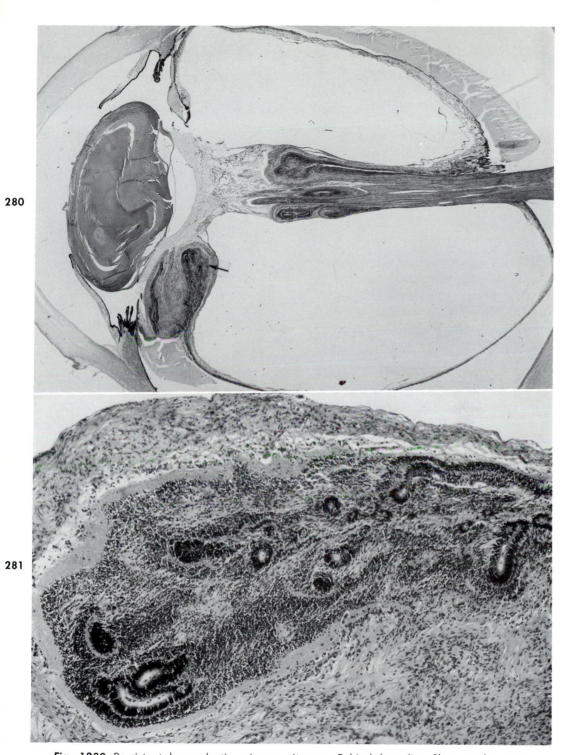

Fig. 1280 Persistent hyperplastic primary vitreous. Behind lens lies fibrovascular mass to which remnant of hyaloid system attaches. In some cases of persistent hyperplastic primary vitreous, there may be areas of retinal dysplasia (arrow). (×12; WU neg. 67-4230.)
Fig. 1281 Retinal dysplasia. Within retina are branching tubes composed of abortive elements of rod and cone layer. (×90; WU neg. 67-4229.)

syndrome or merely in a unilateral mal-
formed eye not associated with other
systemic anomalies.[70, 73] An example of the
latter situation would be in the case of
persistent hyperplastic primary vitreous, as
previously mentioned.

Dysplastic retina is characterized histologically by a series of straight branching tubes composed of abortive elements
of the rod and cone layers (Fig. 1281),
and it is believed that this represents disturbed differentiation of neural ectoderm.

Other congenital entities

Other congenital entities that are only
rarely seen by the surgical pathologist include the rubella syndrome,[69, 82] Lowe's
syndrome, Fabry's syndrome,[72] and aniridia, in which the nonfamilial case may
be associated with Wilms' tumor.[78]

Trauma

Severe trauma necessitating removal of
the globe is the most common reason for
eyes reaching the ophthalmic pathology
laboratory of a general hospital. Usually
the injury is penetration or perforation, but
at times severe contusion results in enough
intraocular change, especially hemorrhage
and fibrosis, to require enucleation.

Although some eyes are so extensively
damaged that immediate removal is necessary, most of the injured eyes are removed
at varying intervals because of secondary
changes such as organization of hemorrhage, glaucoma, retinal detachment, infections, inflammation, or complete atrophy
(phthisis bulbi) (Fig. 1282).

Histopathologic diagnosis is usually not
a problem, but a search should be made
for retained intraocular foreign bodies such
as metal, vegetation, and cilia. Retained
intraocular iron and copper may produce
siderosis and chalcosis, respectively.

Complications resulting from trauma include sympathetic ophthalmia, phacoanaphylactic endophthalmitis, postcon-
tusion angle deformity, and epithelializa-
tion of the anterior chamber. These entities will be considered subsequently.

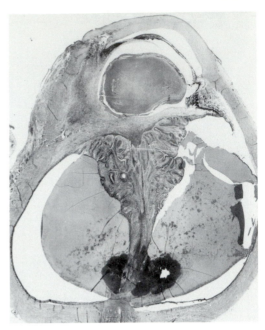

Fig. 1282 Penetrating wound of eye and multiple minute intraocular foreign bodies (palm
splinters) led to formation of dense mass of inflammatory tissue in anterior segment on one
side. Organization of vitreous has been complicated by retinal detachment. Blood clots are attached to stalk of detached retina near optic
disc. (×4; AFIP 737587.)

Inflammation

Inflammation of the eye, as elsewhere,
may be either acute or chronic, granulomatous or nongranulomatous.

Acute inflammation

Acute intraocular inflammation is often
infectious in origin. The causative organism is usually a bacterium or fungus and
is generally introduced through a perforating wound (Fig. 1283). Occasionally, however, the infection is hematogenous. There
have been reports of endogenous fungal
endophthalmitis,[86, 88] and metastatic endophthalmitis also has been reported after
injection of addictive drugs.[90]

Initially, there is a massive purulent reaction in the anterior and vitreous chambers, and the process is called endophthalmitis. As the infection spreads, other
intraocular tissues, such as the retina, uvea,
and eventually the cornea and sclera, may

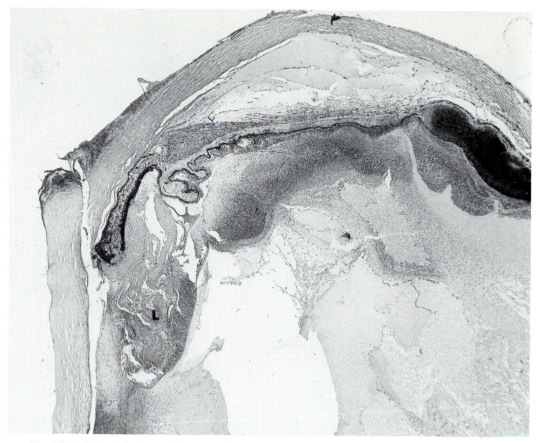

Fig. 1283 Endophthalmitis showing infiltration of all intraocular structures by acute inflammatory cells. Lens, **L**, is necrotic. Organism presumably gained entrance through corneal wound. (×15; WU neg. 67-4233.)

become involved. At this stage, the term panophthalmitis is applicable. Before the advent of antibiotic therapy, eyes affected by severe panophthalmitis were frequently eviscerated or enucleated early. Today the infection can often be controlled, but subsequent organization of the exudate leads to phthisis bulbi (p. 1347). A cause of noninfectious endophthalmitis or panophthalmitis that is not unusual is massive necrosis of a uveal malignant melanoma or a metastatic carcinoma.[87]

Chronic nongranulomatous inflammation

In chronic nongranulomatous inflammation of the eye, the uveal tract is primarily involved. In anterior uveitis (iridocyclitis), the tissues are typically infiltrated by plasma cells in a rather diffuse fashion (Fig. 1284), but occasionally we see nodular lymphocytic infiltrates. In posterior uveitis (choroiditis) the round cell infiltration also may be diffuse, but frequently it is focal or scattered as multiple discrete lesions. In choroiditis the overlying retina is usually involved by spread of the inflammatory reaction—hence the term chorioretinitis. In choroiditis, even if prolonged, enucleation is not often necessary, for the eyes do not become painful. However, with recurrent iridocyclitis, the inflammatory reaction often produces adhesions between the iris and the cornea (anterior synechiae) (Fig. 1285) or between the iris and the lens (posterior synechiae) (Fig. 1286), and secondary glaucoma results. If this condition is intractable, enucleation is almost inevitable. Often, the process is of such a long-term nature that when the eye is enucleated, all that is

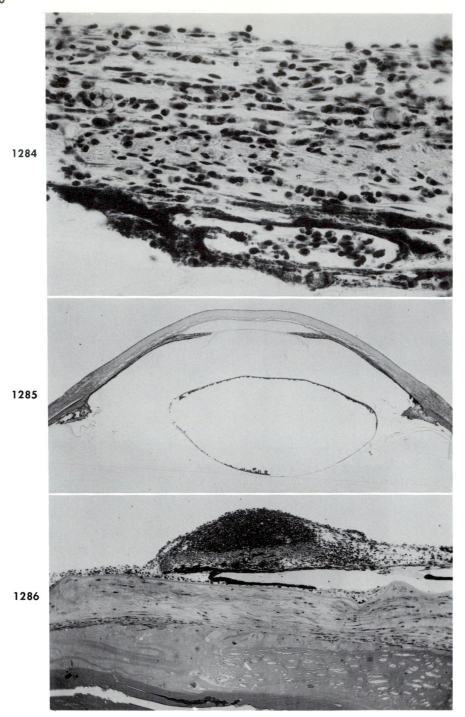

Fig. 1284 Nongranulomatous iritis in which atrophic iris is diffusely infiltrated by plasma cells and several Russell bodies are present. Irregular degenerative and proliferative changes may be observed in pigment epithelium. (×360; AFIP 698722.)

Fig. 1285 Same lesion illustrated in Fig. 1284 showing chronically inflamed iris almost completely adherent to cornea and anterior chamber virtually obliterated. (×8.)

Fig. 1286 Nongranulomatous iritis with posterior synechiae. Iris is firmly attached to lens, which reveals widespread degeneration of its cortex and fibrous metaplasia of its subcapsular epithelium. (×25; AFIP 184111.)

recognized is the massive scarring that is found in phthisis bulbi due to any cause.

The etiology and pathogenesis of nongranulomatous uveitis can rarely be ascertained clinically or pathologically. Occasionally, an entity presents a characteristic picture such as is seen in herpes zoster ophthalmicus in which there is a chronic inflammatory cell infiltration around the posterior ciliary nerves and vessels.[89] Behcet's disease produces an obliterative vasculitis of the retinal vessels.

Granulomatous inflammation

Granulomatous inflammation may be the result of a specific infection such as toxoplasmosis, tuberculosis, syphilis, nematodiasis, and cytomegalic inclusion disease. Also associated with granulomatous reactions are such entities as sarcoidosis and the collagen diseases. It should be kept in mind, however, that as with the nongranulomatous cases, the etiology often cannot be ascertained.

The inflammatory process in granulomatous uveitis may be diffuse, but often there is a more localized area of destruction in which the causative agent or otherwise diagnostic lesion will be found. It is of paramount importance, therefore, that the gross specimen be examined carefully with the dissecting microscope (×7 magnification) so that a small but important lesion will not be overlooked.

The term granulomatous uveitis is misleading, for often the most diagnostic lesions are not found in the iris, ciliary body, or choroid but rather in the retina, vitreous, or sclera. The diagnostic lesions of toxoplasmosis are found in the retina and choroid, those of nematodiasis in the vitreous or retina, and those of the rheumatoid group in the sclera between the limbus and the equator.

The studies of Wilder[91, 92] and other pathologists at the Armed Forces Institute of Pathology have established the fact that in enucleated eyes containing granulomatous lesions, toxoplasmosis and nematodiasis together account for more cases than all other infections combined.[94] This statement is based principally upon those cases in which the causative agents have been demonstrated within the ocular lesions by histopathologic study. Because of their relative importance, only the lesions of toxoplasmosis and nematodiasis will be described here.

Toxoplasmosis

Toxoplasmosis, whether congenital or acquired, tends to produce rather discrete chorioretinal lesions. The uveal tract, including the iris and ciliary body, often reveals diffuse infiltration by plasma cells and lymphocytes, but the destructive granulomatous lesions are typically restricted to the posterior half of the globe (Fig. 1287).

The morphologic pattern observed in these chorioretinal lesions is highly characteristic. Most important diagnostically is a focal, abruptly delineated area of coagulative necrosis of the retina (Fig. 1288). In this area of infarctlike retinal necrosis most of the nuclei of retinal cells have vanished or only their ghostly outlines remain. Very few inflammatory cells are present, but many pigment granules may be strewn about from the necrotic pigment epithelium. It is in this necrotic retinal tissue that the proliferative forms and cysts of *Toxoplasma gondii* will be found upon careful oil immersion microscopy (Fig. 1289). Occasionally, the cysts may be found in a completely uninvolved portion of the retina.

The choroid and sclera immediately adjacent to the area of retinal necrosis are typically thickened and massively infiltrated by epithelioid cells, lymphocytes, and plasma cells. In some cases there is also much episcleral reaction so that an epibulbar nodule is formed (Fig. 1287).

Nematodiasis

Nematodiasis is a broad term encompassing a variety of parasitic diseases. The one form of ocular nematodiasis that has been found with considerable frequency

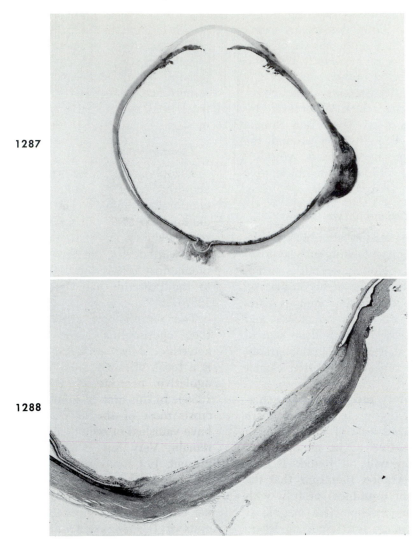

1287

1288

Fig. 1287 Granulomatous chorioretinitis, scleritis, and episcleritis due to toxoplasmosis. This type of segmental involvement of all ocular coats posterior to equator, with formation of epibulbar nodule of inflammatory tissue, is extremely characteristic of toxoplasmosis. (×2; AFIP 70313; from Wilder, H. C.: Toxoplasma chorioretinitis in adults, Arch. Ophthalmol. **48**:127-136, 1952; copyright 1952, American Medical Association.

Fig. 1288 Sharply outlined area of coagulative retinal necrosis with necrosis and granulomatous inflammation of immediately adjacent choroid, sclera, and episclera, which are typical of toxoplasmosis. It is in necrotic retina that parasites are found (Fig. 1289). (×7; AFIP 754058.)

in the United States and Great Britain[84] is a type of visceral larva migrans, probably produced in most cases by wandering larvae of *Toxocara canis*.[85] This is principally an infection of children between the ages of 3 and 14 years.[93]

Almost without exception, those children who have had ocular infection have not had clinical evidence of systemic visceral larva migrans, and those who have had the systemic form have not had ocular lesions. Typically, a single migrating larva finds its way, hematogenously, into the eye and comes to rest in the vitreous or on the inner surface of the retina (Fig. 1290).

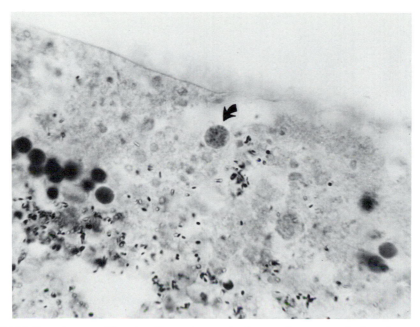

Fig. 1289 Encysting proliferative forms (arrows) of *Toxoplasma gondii* found in necrotic retina of lesion shown in Fig. 1288. Small particles are pigment granules from necrotic retinal pigment epithelium, whereas larger round structures represent pyknotic retinal nuclei. (×1000; AFIP 754058.)

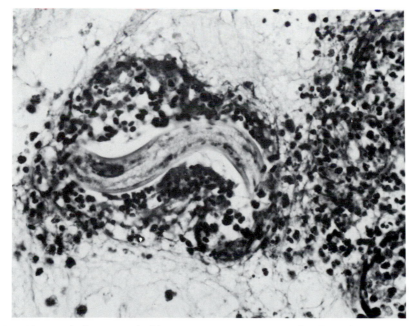

Fig. 1290 Nematode larva, probably *Toxocara canis*, surrounded by inflammatory cells in vitreous body. (×220; AFIP 298563.)

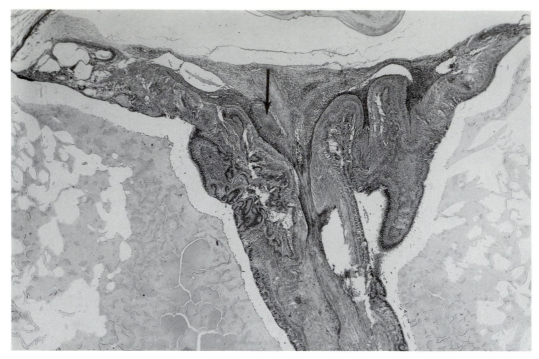

Fig. 1291 Nematode endophthalmitis in which inflammatory reaction in vitreous has led to retinal detachment. Parasite was found in area of necrosis (arrow). (×15; WU neg. 67-4234.)

A pronounced infiltration by acute and chronic inflammatory cells, often with intense eosinophilia, is observed in these tissues, but the uveal tract is often remarkably uninvolved. Presumably because of the freedom of uveal inflammation, the eye is usually asymptomatic.

Eventually, the inflammatory reaction in the vitreous leads to organization and contracture of this structure with consequent detachment of the retina (Fig. 1291). This leads to leukokoria, and the eye is enucleated because retinoblastoma cannot be ruled out.

As the nematode larvae die, they often stimulate the formation of a typical granulomatous inflammatory reaction about them. It is usually necessary to make serial sections to find these minute granulomas. The typical inflammatory reaction with intense eosinophilia observed in the vitreous is presumptive evidence of nematodiasis, but the larvae must be found to establish a definitive diagnosis.

Posttraumatic uveitis

Following penetrating injury of the eye, the development of a granulomatous uveitis always causes great concern because of the possibility of sympathetic uveitis, a dreaded disease in which injury to one eye gives rise to severe inflammation that sometimes progresses to blindness in the uninjured eye as well as in the injured eye. Fortunately, sympathetic uveitis is extremely rare today. Other causes of posttraumatic granulomatous inflammation are lens-induced endophthalmitis (phacoanaphylaxis), foreign bodies, and blood in the vitreous.

Sympathetic uveitis

Sympathetic uveitis is probably the best example of a pure granulomatous uveitis, for the significant lesion in this disease is confined to the uveal tissues. Typically, the process involves the entire uveal tract. There may, of course, be associated inflammatory lesions in other tissues due to the

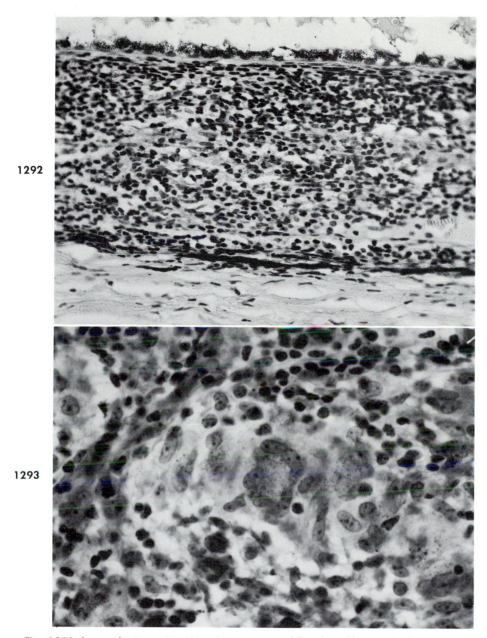

Fig. 1292 Sympathetic uveitis. Uveal tissues are diffusely infiltrated by lymphocytes, and there are small, irregular collections of pale-staining epithelioid cells. (×300; AFIP 731769.)
Fig. 1293 Epithelioid cells and giant cells containing finely dispersed uveal pigment granules that are characteristically present in sympathetic uveitis. (×655; AFIP 37381; from Friedenwald, J. S., et al.: Ophthalmic pathology: an atlas and textbook, Philadelphia, 1952, W. B. Saunders Co.

original trauma, the presence of foreign bodies, etc., but the reaction of sympathetic uveitis itself is purely uveal.

There is a dense, diffuse infiltration of the choroid by lymphocytes (Fig. 1292), and often the ciliary body and iris are similarly involved. Superimposed upon this lymphocytic infiltrate are small, irregular, patchy accumulations of large, pale-staining epithelioid cells which, upon high mag-

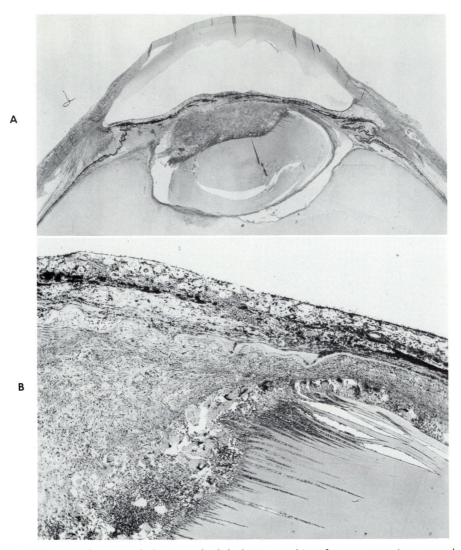

Fig. 1294   A, Phacoanaphylactic endophthalmitis resulting from penetrating wound that ruptured capsule of anterior lens. Dense infiltrate of acute and chronic inflammatory cells is present in area of lens damage. **B,** Higher magnification of lesion illustrated in **A.** Polymorphonuclear leukocytes are present in and about disintegrating lens fibers. Peripheral to them is wall of macrophages, epithelioid cells, and giant cells, and about entire lesion there is broad zone of granulation tissue. (**A,** ×10; AFIP 339621; **B,** ×53.)

nification, will often be found to contain finely dispersed melanin granules (Fig. 1293). Polymorphonuclear leukocytes are characteristically lacking, plasma cells are rare, but eosinophils are often included in moderate numbers.

The reaction involves the outer and middle coats of the choroid, extending into the scleral canals along ciliary vessels and nerves, sometimes to the episcleral sur-

face. The choriocapillaris, on the other hand, is typically uninvolved.

Phacoanaphylaxis

Phacoanaphylactic endophthalmitis usually follows penetrating injury to the lens, but a few cases have been observed following spontaneous rupture of a swollen cataractous lens. It is characterized by a granulomatous inflammatory reaction cen-

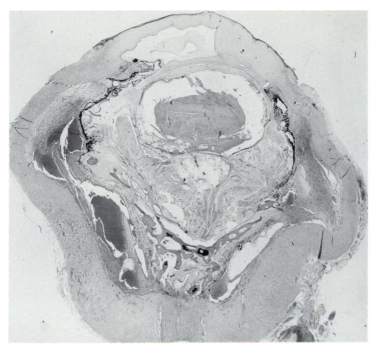

Fig. 1295 Phthisis bulbi in which globe is markedly shrunken, sclera is wrinkled, and all intraocular tissues reveal severe degenerative changes, including foci of ossification. (×7½; AFIP 276925.)

tered about an area of lens perforation. The process is believed to be the result of acquired hypersensitivity to lens protein.[96]

A typical zonal pattern of inflammatory reaction is observed in most cases (Fig. 1294, *A*). In the area in which the lens capsule is broken, there is a massive invasion of the lens by inflammatory cells. Centrally and immediately surrounding individual lens fibers are polymorphonuclear leukocytes. Peripheral to this is a wall of epithelioid and giant cells about which is a broader, more diffuse zone of granulation tissue and round cell infiltration (Fig. 1294, *B*). The iris reveals a variable degree of plasma cell infiltration, and posterior synechiae are commonly formed.

Ordinarily, the posterior uveal tract is not inflamed, but characteristically there is a perivasculitis of the retinal vessels. In a considerable number of cases, however, phacoanaphylactic endophthalmitis and sympathetic uveitis are coexistent.[95]

Degeneration

Degenerative changes are usually the result of other primary processes such as trauma or inflammation. The most advanced stage of ocular degeneration in which all tissues are involved is called phthisis bulbi.

Phthisis bulbi

Phthisis bulbi represents the final stage of ocular degeneration in which the production of aqueous humor is so markedly reduced that the intraocular pressure falls (hypotony) and the globe shrinks (Fig. 1295).

The causes of phthisis bulbi are myriad, but most phthisical eyes reaching the surgical pathology laboratory have been injured, either accidentally or as a result of surgical procedures.

Phthisical eyes are enucleated for several reasons. Many are enucleated because they are disfiguring and others because they become irritable because of periodic

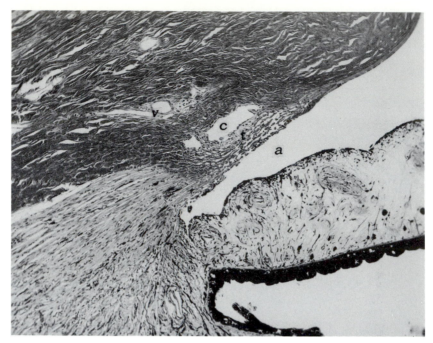

Fig. 1296 Normal outflow channels for passage of aqueous humor from anterior chamber angle, **a,** include corneoscleral trabecula, **t,** Schlemm's canal, **c,** and intrascleral plexus of veins, **v.** (Verhoeff–van Gieson; ×70; AFIP 630832.)

hemorrhages or bouts of uveitis. Some are enucleated for prophylactic reasons—the fear of sympathetic uveitis or of malignant melanoma, either of which may develop long after the eye has become blind and phthisical.

All tissues are affected to varying degrees in phthisis bulbi, and the degree of shrinkage is also variable. The eye may be soft and spongy or stony hard due to calcification and ossification. Typically, the media are opaque. Corneal scars, exudates in the anterior and posterior chambers, and advanced cataract formation prevent visualization of the inner eye. The vitreous is usually destroyed, and the retina is completely detached. Extensive areas of osseous metaplasia are frequently observed along the inner surface of the choroid posteriorly. The uvea is often edematous, and pools of serous exudate may separate it from the wrinkled sclera.

In phthisis bulbi which has followed extensive endophthalmitis or panophthalmitis, the various intraocular tissues often

are so necrotic and replaced by scar tissue that most of the internal architecture of the eye is effaced.

Glaucoma

Glaucoma is conveniently placed here, since it represents another condition of diverse etiology characterized by widespread degeneration of ocular tissues. The essential feature of the glaucomas is an unphysiologic state of increased intraocular pressure, due in almost all cases to impaired outflow of aqueous humor.[97] Aqueous humor is produced by the ciliary processes and discharged into the posterior chamber. It flows forward between the lens and the iris, through the pupil, into the anterior chamber. Aqueous humor leaves the anterior chamber via the trabecular meshwork, which is present in the deep layers of the peripheral cornea, just in front of the anterior chamber angle (Fig. 1296). After passing through the trabecula, aqueous humor enters the canal of Schlemm and leaves the eye via the

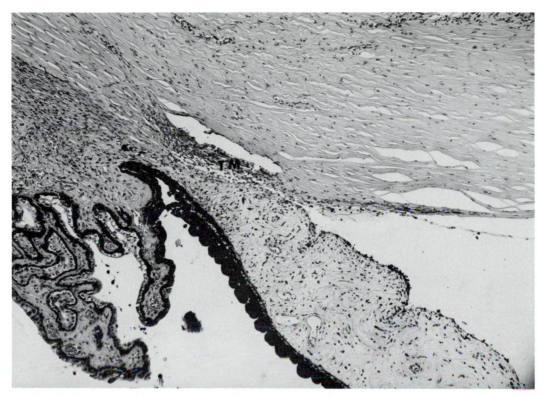

Fig. 1297 Peripheral aspect of iris lying against trabecular meshwork, **TM,** producing peripheral anterior synechia and blocking outflow of aqueous. (×90; WU neg. 67-4224.)

plexus of intrascleral and episcleral veins along the corneoscleral limbus. When the impaired aqueous drainage follows some known or suspected antecedent disease, we speak of secondary glaucoma. Here the surgical pathologist may play an important role in determining the antecedent disease.

Primary glaucoma

The primary glaucomas are not associated with antecedent disease but are either the "chronic simple" type or the "angle-closure" type. In the former, there are certain degenerative changes in the trabecular meshwork and the connective tissues about Schlemm's canal. The exact nature of these changes remains obscure. These eyes seldom reach the pathology laboratory since the process is usually insidious and often does not cause enough pain to necessitate enucleation.

Acute and chronic angle-closure glau-coma is due to anatomic and physiologic peculiarities of the tissues and the spaces of the anterior chamber that predispose to blockage of the outflow channels by the iris root. Chronic attacks of angle-closure glaucoma may lead to extensive adhesions of the iris root to the trabecular meshwork (peripheral anterior synechia, Fig. 1297), and if this glaucoma becomes intractable, it may necessitate enucleation because of pain.[100]

Secondary glaucoma

Secondary glaucoma may be a complication of numerous primary processes, including trauma, inflammation, neoplasia, and malformation. The sites of obstruction to the outflow of aqueous humor are numerous, but the most vulnerable areas are the pupil and the angle of the anterior chamber. Formation of pupillary membranes as a result of organization of hemorrhages and exudates or the development

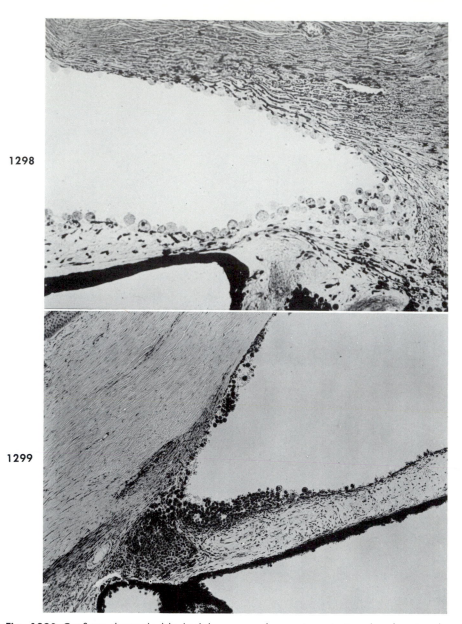

1298

1299

Fig. 1298 Outflow channels blocked by macrophages in anterior chamber in phacolytic glaucoma (glaucoma secondary to lysis and escape of lens protein into aqueous humor). (×75; AFIP 609920; from Flocks, M., Littwin, C. S., and Zimmerman, L. E.: Phacolytic glaucoma; clinicopathologic study of 138 cases of glaucoma associated with hypermature cataract, Arch. Ophthalmol. **54:**37-45, 1955; copyright 1955, American Medical Association.)

Fig. 1299 Anterior chamber angle and outflow channels filled with deeply pigmented cells dispersed into aqueous humor from malignant melanoma of iris. (×50; AFIP 176188.)

of extensive adhesions between the iris and the lens (posterior synechiae) as a consequence of iritis (Fig. 1286) are the usual mechanisms leading to pupillary obstruction.

The outflow channels in the anterior chamber angle may become obstructed by particulate matter or by the formation of extensive adhesions between the root of the iris and the peripheral cornea (anterior

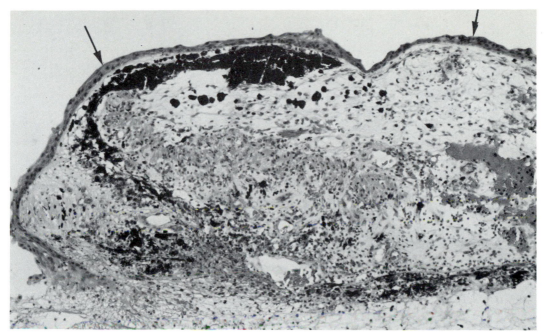

Fig. 1300 In this case of postcataract extraction, layer of epithelium has grown down the wound into anterior chamber to lie on surface of iris (arrows). (×100; WU neg. 72-3172.)

synechiae). Particulate matter clogging the passages between the anterior chamber and the canal of Schlemm is usually cellular—red blood cells after massive hemorrhage into the anterior chamber,[98] leukocytes in certain types of uveitis[99] (Fig. 1298), tumor cells, particularly with diffuse melanomas of the iris (Fig. 1299). Following accidental trauma or surgery, conjunctival and/or corneal epithelium may grow between the wound edges and eventually line the anterior chamber and iris, thus blocking the outflow of aqueous (Fig. 1300).

One of the common causes of secondary glaucoma encountered by the ophthalmic pathologist is the development of a neovascular membrane on the surface of the iris. This membrane, known as rubeosis iridis, is eventually associated with some degree of peripheral anterior synechia, thus causing blockage of the outflow channels (Fig. 1301).

Rubeosis iridis can occur following several different conditions. It occurs most commonly in diabetes or following occlusion of the central retinal artery or vein. Other conditions associated with rubeosis include carotid artery occlusion, long-standing retinal detachment, chronic uveitis, and intraocular neoplasms.

Damage to the outflow channels may occur as a result of blunt trauma to the eye and give rise to a chronic glaucoma. This situation is often associated with a recession of the anterior chamber angle. Histologically, the iris root insertion appears retrodisplaced, and there is atrophy of the ciliary body (Fig. 1302).

Regardless of the type and cause of glaucoma, certain degenerative changes are typically produced after periods of variable duration. When glaucoma begins in childhood, the tissues tend to stretch, and the globe may become greatly enlarged (buphthalmos). When its onset is in adult life, however, the tissues tend to resist stretching, and normal ocular dimensions are maintained.

The elevated intraocular pressure typically affects the inner retinal layers to a much more pronounced degree than it does the outer layers. A common observation is the presence of rather well-pre-

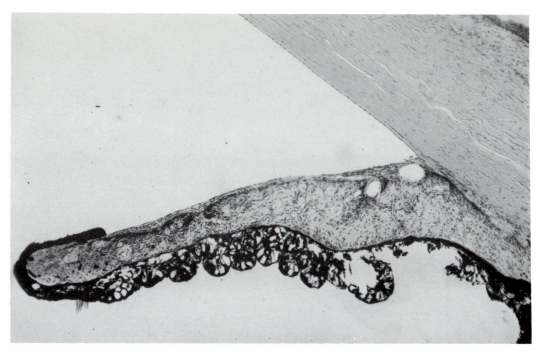

Fig. 1301 Rubeosis iridis in diabetes. Angle of anterior chamber is occluded by peripheral anterior synechia, and fibrovascular membrane (rubeosis iridis) covers anterior surface of iris. Contraction of this membrane has pulled pigment epithelium anteriorly to produce "ectropion uvea." There is marked diabetic vacuolization of pigment epithelial cells. (×90; WU neg. 67-4225.)

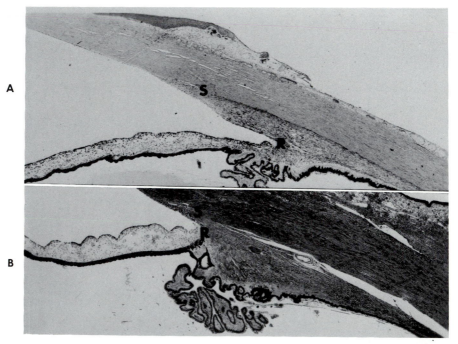

Fig. 1302 **A,** Recession of angle of anterior chamber. **B,** Normal angle. Iris root, **R,** is retro-displaced with reference to scleral spur, **S,** and contour of atrophic ciliary body is fusiform instead of normal wedge shape. (**A** and **B,** ×21; AFIP 58-7578.)

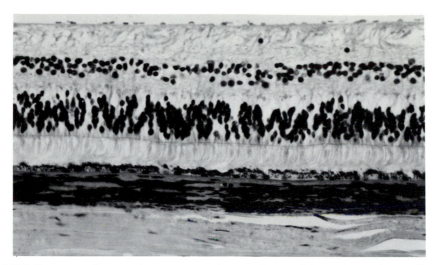

Fig. 1303 Retina in chronic glaucoma revealing widespread loss of ganglion cells and nerve fibers and reduction of cells in inner nuclear layer but relatively well-preserved visual cells. (×230; AFIP 49729; from Friedenwald, J. S., et al.: Ophthalmic pathology: an atlas and textbook, Philadelphia, 1952, W. B. Saunders Co.)

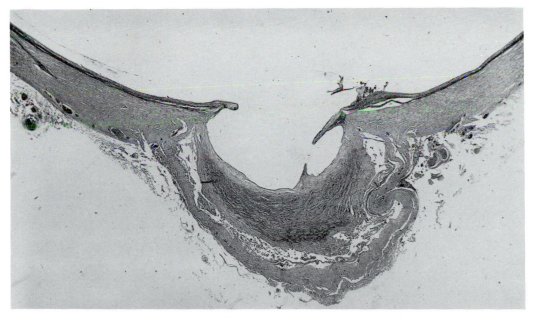

Fig. 1304 Deep excavation (cupping) of optic disc and severe atrophy of optic nerve, which are important complications of chronic glaucoma. (×12; WU neg. 67-4235.)

served rods and cones and an intact outer nuclear layer when virtually all ganglion cells have disappeared and the nerve fiber and inner nuclear layers have become reduced to one-half or one-third their normal thickness (Fig. 1303).

Degeneration of nerve fibers is especial-ly noteworthy in the region of the optic disc. This leads to excavation or cupping of the nerve head, posterior bowing of the lamina cribrosa, and severe atrophy of the optic nerve (Fig. 1304). Often, discrete areas of scleral ectasia are observed, particularly in the equatorial regions. These

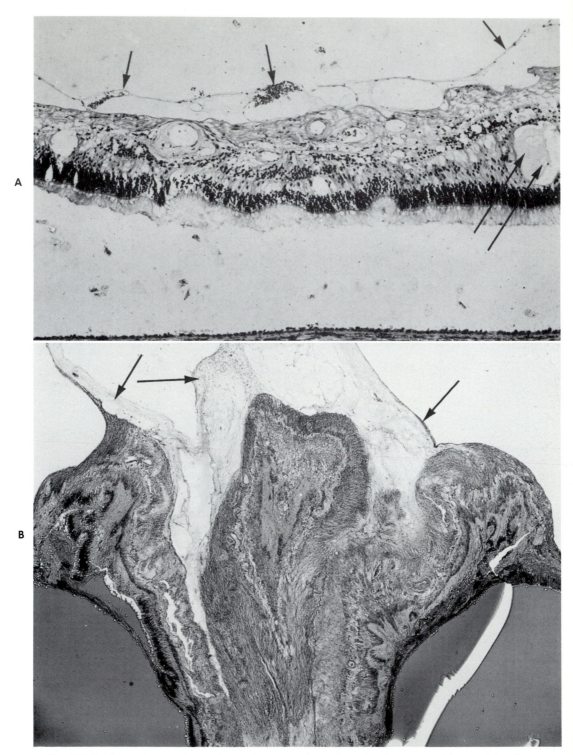

Fig. 1305 **A,** Diabetic retinopathy with scattered exudates in deep retinal layers (double arrows) and early neovascularization extending from inner surface of retina into vitreous (single arrows). **B,** Diabetic proliferative retinopathy (arrows) has caused complete retinal detachment. (**A,** ×90; WU neg. 72-3170; **B,** ×34; WU neg. 72-3171.)

are lined by uveal tissue and therefore have a bluish color—hence the name staphyloma (grapelike swelling).

Diabetes

Ocular diabetes is rapidly becoming one of the most common causes of blindness in western society. Diabetes can cause a variety of pathologic conditions within the eye. These conditions may lead to complete blindness and, if associated with pain, the eyes often do reach the pathology laboratory.[101]

The retina often shows scattered hemor-rhages and exudates, and there may be the development of neovascular tissue that grows from the inner surface of the retina into the vitreous (Fig. 1305, A). This condition, known as proliferative retinopathy, can cause a retinal detachment that usually does not respond well to surgical treatment (Fig. 1305, B).

As previously mentioned, secondary glaucoma may result from the development of diabetic rubeosis iridis with peripheral anterior synechia (Fig. 1301). Many eyes from diabetic patients will also manifest vacuolization of the iris pigment epithe-

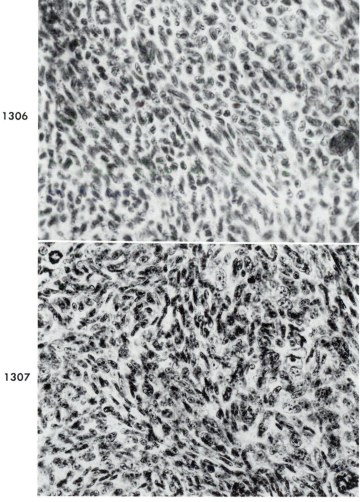

Fig. 1306 Spindle A type of melanoma cells. (×510; AFIP 49801.)
Fig. 1307 Spindle B type of melanoma cells that are larger and more pleomorphic than spindle A cells. Most of nuclei contain prominent nucleoli. (×305; AFIP 232296.)

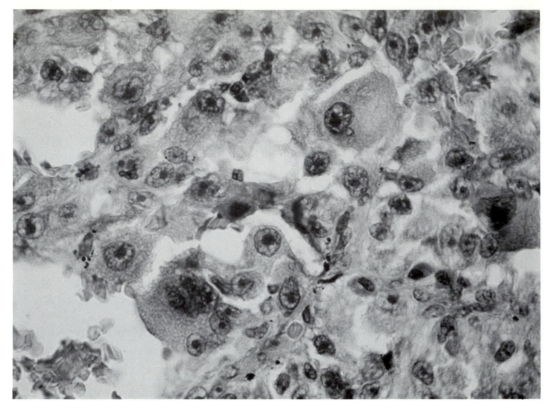

Fig. 1308 Epithelioid cells with abundant cytoplasm, large nuclei, and extremely prominent nucleoli. (×600; WU neg. 69-7517; from Ackerman, L. V., and del Regato, J. A.: Cancer, ed. 4, St. Louis, 1970, The C. V. Mosby Co.)

lium. These vacuoles have been demonstrated to contain glycogen (Fig. 1301).

Tumors and pseudotumors

Tumors of the intraocular tissues are neither numerous in type nor frequent in occurrence. From a practical standpoint, discussion may be limited to malignant melanomas, conditions confused with malignant melanomas of the uvea, retinoblastomas, pseudogliomas, and metastatic carcinomas.

Malignant melanoma

Melanomas arising from the pigmented or potentially pigment-producing cells of the uvea are by far the most frequent of all intraocular neoplasms except during the first decade. An extensive study of ocular melanomas and nevi has shown that virtually all malignant melanomas of the uveal tract appear to develop from preexisting nevi.[115-117] We have, therefore, continued to employ the Callender classification[104] which has stood the test of time in the Registry of Ophthalmic Pathology and elsewhere.

This classification is based primarily on the cytologic characteristics of the tumors. Its validity is derived from the differences in prognostic significance of each type of tumor. Three main cell types are recognized: spindle A, spindle B, and epithelioid. From their combinations and patterns six tumor types are defined.

Spindle A cells are rather slender, very benign-appearing spindle-shaped cells that have relatively small fusiform nuclei and no nucleoli (Fig. 1306). Frequently, the chromatin is arranged in a linear fashion along the central axis of the nucleus.

Spindle B cells are larger and more

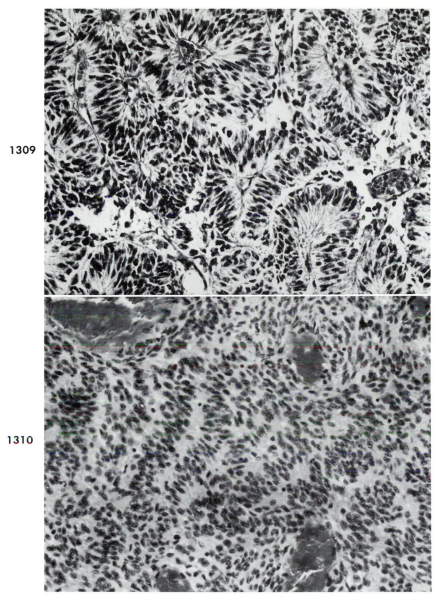

Fig. 1309 Fascicular type of melanoma composed of spindle cells arranged about dilated capillaries. (×250; AFIP 231963.)
Fig. 1310 Fascicular type of melanoma in which spindle-shaped cells are arranged with their nuclei in parallel rows. (×230; AFIP 48427.)

pleomorphic, merging on the one hand with spindle A cells and on the other with epithelioid cells. Typically, they possess large ovoid nuclei containing prominent nucleoli (Fig. 1307). Mitotic activity may be more marked.

Epithelioid cells are still larger and more irregular (Fig. 1308). They have an abun-

dance of cytoplasm and may be truly gigantic. Multinucleated forms are not unusual. The nuclei are large, and their nucleoli often are strikingly prominent. In some tumors, many bizarre nuclei may be seen.

As might be anticipated from the cytologic characteristics of these different

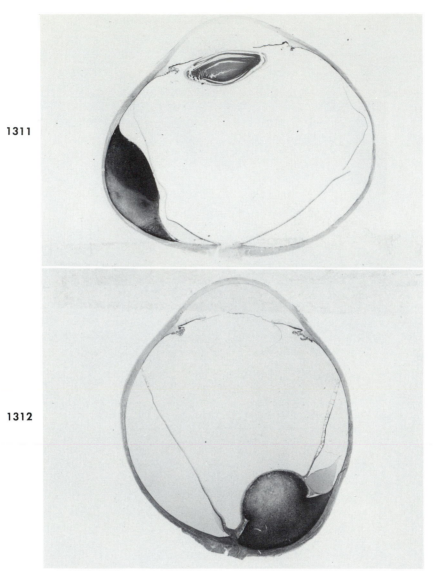

Fig. 1311 Malignant melanoma of choroid that has not broken through Bruch's membrane but has elevated retina. Most of retinal separation observed in this section is artifactitious. (×3; AFIP 79372; from Friedenwald, J. S., et al.: Ophthalmic pathology: an atlas and textbook, Philadelphia, 1952, W. B. Saunders Co.)

Fig. 1312 Malignant melanoma of choroid which, by erupting through Bruch's membrane, has formed mushroom-shaped subretinal mass. (×3; AFIP 289600.)

types of melanomatous tumors, the spindle A type is essentially a benign neoplasm, whereas the epithelioid tumors are much more prone to metastasize.[112]

It is rather unusual for these tumors to be composed of a single cell type. A mixture of spindle A and B cells or a mixture of spindle and epithelioid cells is very common. Certain of the spindle cell tumors present a fascicular pattern due to the palisading of nuclei (Figs. 1309 and 1310).

Table 55 presents the prognostic significance of the Callender classification.[104]

Melanomas of the uvea exhibit great differences in pigment formation. There is a definite tendency for the most benign spindle cell tumors to be virtually amel-anotic—another reason for believing them to be closely related to schwannian neo-plasms. Conversely, the most heavily pig-mented uveal tumors are often more pleo-morphic and more highly malignant. Un-fortunately, there are many exceptions to these generalizations.

Wilder and Callender[114] showed that the amount of reticulum about individual tumor cells is also of prognostic signifi-cance, for those with a heavy fiber content tend to be less malignant than do those with but little reticulum. Flocks et al.[107] showed that the size of choroidal and ciliary body melanomas at the time of enucleation is of considerable prognostic importance. Large tumors tend to contain epithelioid cells, and they have a decidedly worse prognosis than do small tumors that are typically pure spindle cell neoplasms.

Another extremely important fact con-cerning the prognosis of uveal tumors is the very benign behavior of almost all neoplasms of the iris. This is especially true of those iris tumors that are sufficiently small and localized to be excisable by iri-dectomy.[102, 118]

Choroidal melanomas, regardless of their cytologic characteristics, tend to grow in-ward as discoid, globular, or mushroom-shaped masses, first elevating and then de-taching the retina (Figs. 1311 and 1312). Less commonly, they spread diffusely and

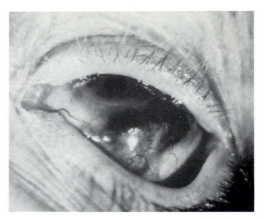

Fig. 1313 Malignant melanoma of choroid breaking through sclera and presenting under conjunctiva. (WU neg. 69-2213; from Ackerman, L. V., and del Regato, J. A.: Cancer, ed. 4, St. Louis, 1970, The C. V. Mosby Co.; courtesy Registry of Ophthalmic Pathology, Armed Forces Institute of Pathology.)

extend out along scleral canals into the orbit[108] (Figs. 1313 to 1315). Visual dis-turbance due to retinal detachment is therefore a much more frequent presenting complaint than is the formation of an orbital tumor. Not infrequently the patient remains asymptomatic until the tumor has grown sufficiently to become necrotic and produce such complications as en-dophthalmitis, massive intraocular hemor-rhage, and/or secondary glaucoma.

About 10% of all malignant melanomas of the posterior uvea are not discovered until the enucleated eye is examined in the laboratory. Iris tumors are much more often recognized early, for they can be seen by the patient and his family long before other symptoms appear (Figs. 1316 and 1317).

Conditions confused with malignant melanoma of uvea

Clinically, there are many lesions that simulate malignant melanoma, but his-topathologic problems in differential diag-nosis are infrequent.[105, 113] The latter consist primarily of differentiating nevi from spindle cell melanomas (especially in the case of iris tumors removed by iridec-tomy). Rarely, the problem concerns the

Table 55 Survival of 2,631 patients with malignant melanoma of choroid and ciliary body*

Cell type	Total cases	Actuarial survival rate	
		5 yr (%)	10 yr (%)
Spindle A	124	95	85
Spindle B and fascicular	1,027	89	80
Mixed and necrotic	1,389	60	46
Epithelioid	91	43	34
All tumors	2,631	71	60

*Based on data from Paul, E. V., Parnell, B. L., and Fraker, M.: Prognosis of malignant melanomas of the choroid and ciliary body, Int. Ophthalmol. Clin. 2:387-402, 1962.

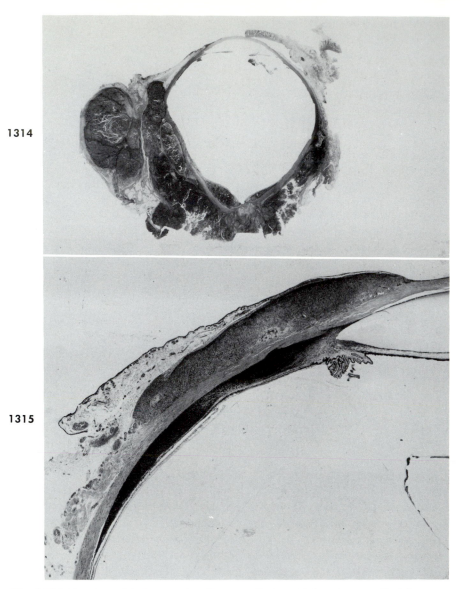

Fig. 1314 Massive orbital extension from small choroidal melanoma that has occurred as result of diffuse spread along natural passages through sclera and optic nerve. (×2; AFIP 159090; from Friedenwald, J. S., et al.: Ophthalmic pathology: an atlas and textbook, Philadelphia, 1952, W. B. Saunders Co.)

Fig. 1315 Diffuse malignant melanoma of ciliary body and choroid that extended forward through scleral canals to form large subconjunctival mass that encroached upon cornea. (×9; AFIP 824055.)

differentiation of amelanotic epithelioid melanomas from metastatic carcinoma or distinguishing certain amelanotic spindle cell melanomas with a fascicular pattern from neurofibromas, neurilemomas, or leiomyomas (especially in the ciliary body, where smooth muscle is so abundant).

Conditions that often present confusing clinical problems in differential diagnosis include metastatic carcinoma, retinal detachment secondary to holes or tears in the retina,[103] localized hemorrhage beneath the retina or between the pigment epithelium and choroid (Fig. 1318), cysts of the retina,

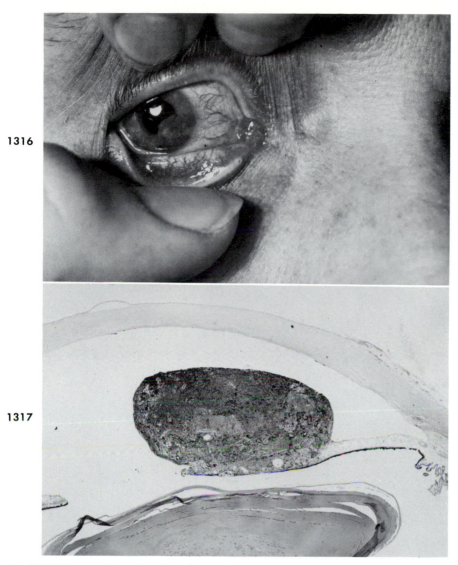

1316

1317

Fig. 1316 Tumor of iris that had been observed over period of ten years, during which time it became progressively larger and encroached upon pupil. Iridectomy revealed it to be of spindle A cell type. Tumor recurred and necessitated enucleation for secondary glaucoma fifteen years after iridectomy. (AFIP 749919; courtesy Dr. M. E. Nugent, Bismarck, N. D.)

Fig. 1317 Melanomas of iris frequently are clearly visible through cornea. Hence their duration and rate of growth often are known by patient or his family long before other subjective or objective manifestations appear. (×13; AFIP 272658.)

ciliary body, or iris, serous detachment of the ciliary body, staphylomas, focal areas of proliferation of the retinal pigment epithelium (Fig. 1319), and benign tumors such as nevi and hemangiomas. Melanocytomas are congenital benign pigmented tumors occurring in the disc or in the uveal tract that may be mistaken for melanomas.[111, 119]

To give some idea as to the difficulty that may attend the differential diagnosis of serous and neoplastic detachment of the retina, in a study of 204 eyes enucleated after one or more operations for reattach-

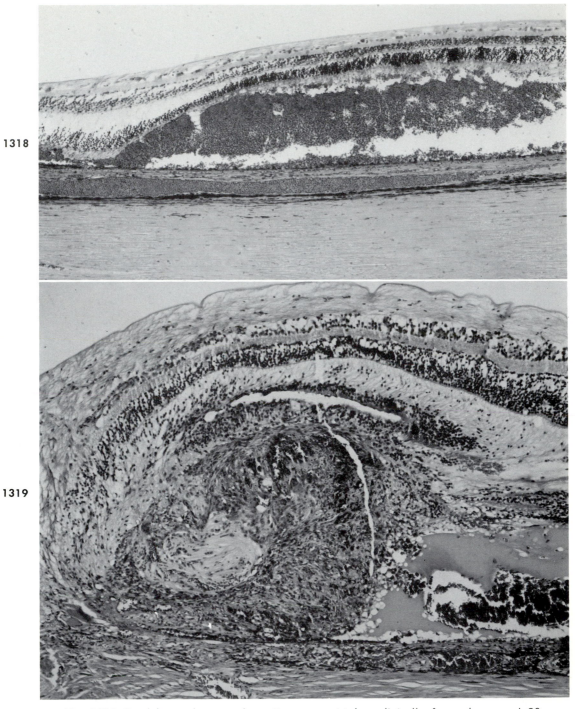

1318

1319

Fig. 1318 Focal hemorrhage under retina was mistaken clinically for melanoma. (×90; WU neg. 72-3167.)
Fig. 1319 Focal area of proliferation of retinal pigment epithelium that has elevated retina to simulate melanoma. (×90; WU neg. 72-3169.)

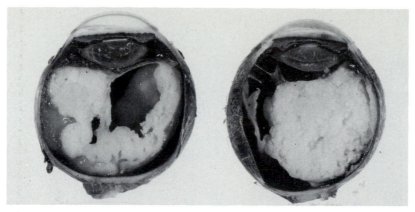

Fig. 1320 Bilateral retinoblastoma showing presence of white mass consisting of detached retina and neoplastic tissue immediately behind lens in each eye. (AFIP 635460.)

ment of the retina, sixty were found to contain intraocular tumors, fifty-six of which were malignant melanomas.[103] On the other hand, there were nine eyes that for one or another reason were suspected, postoperatively, of containing a tumor and, therefore, were enucleated. Histopathologic study failed to confirm the presence of a neoplasm. Scar tissue, proliferated pigment epithelium, hemorrhage, or other factors were responsible for the phantom tumor.

A later and more extensive study of eyes that were removed because of a clinical diagnosis of melanoma of the iris or choroid revealed some disturbing findings. In sixty-nine eyes removed with a diagnosis of melanoma of the iris, there was no tumor in 35%. In 529 eyes removed with a diagnosis of melanoma of the choroid, pathologic examination showed that malignant melanoma was not present in 19%.[106]

In recent years, the clinician has been aided by such techniques as fluorescein angiography,[109] and radioactive phosphorus uptake.[110]

Retinoblastoma

Retinoblastomas are the most common intraocular neoplasm of children. Generally believed to be congenital and derived from the incompletely differentiated retinal cells, they nevertheless are seldom recognized until considerable growth has taken place. They are usually diagnosed between the ages of 16 months and 2 years. Although most cases arise sporadically, the influence of heredity has been well shown in many. Bilaterality is present in 30% of all cases and in over 90% of the familial cases (Fig. 1320).

These tumors characteristically present as a leukocoria (white pupillary reflex) (Fig. 1321) or less often as a strabismus when the tumor is in the macula. Rarely, extraocular extension with the formation of an orbital mass is the presenting manifestation.

Retinoblastomas may be flat and diffuse or elevated and may show multicentric foci of origin. They may protrude into the vitreous (endophytic type) (Fig. 1322), often with vitreous seeding, or they may grow between the retina and the pigment epithelium (exophytic type). Since the tumors tend to outgrow their blood supply, necrosis is often extensive, and many minute foci of calcification are often

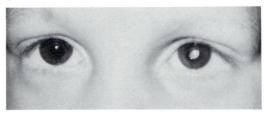

Fig. 1321 Prominent white reflex present in dilated pupil of left eye due to retinoblastoma.

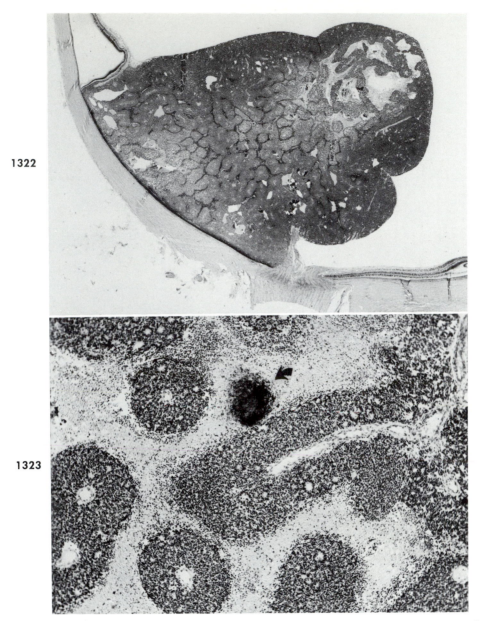

1322

1323

Fig. 1322 Retinoblastoma, highly cellular neoplasm with scanty stroma. Tumor tends to outgrow its blood supply, and irregular areas of necrosis are commonly observed. (×12; AFIP 747443.)

Fig. 1323 Retinoblastoma showing typical pattern of collar of viable cells about nutrient vessels. Foci of calcification (arrow) occur within areas of coagulation necrosis. (×80; AFIP 147292.)

present in these areas of necrosis (Fig. 1323). In fact, these areas of calcification may be appreciated by x-ray examination prior to enucleation.

Cytologically, the tumors are composed of dense masses of small round cells with hyperchromatic nuclei and scanty cytoplasm (Fig. 1324). In the more differentiated tumors, the cells are often arranged in rosettes (Fig. 1325) and fleu-

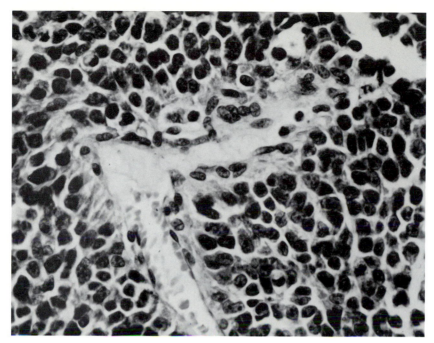

Fig. 1324 Undifferentiated retinoblastomas composed of relatively large anaplastic cells have less favorable prognosis than those that contain highly differentiated rosettes. (×400; AFIP 190088; from Friedenwald, J. S., et al.: Ophthalmic pathology: an atlas and text-book, Philadelphia, 1952, W. B. Saunders Co.)

rettes. Recent light and electron microscopic studies have confirmed that these tumors are neuronal neoplasms rather than gliomas as was suspected by many in years past.[124, 125]

A most important practical consideration for the surgical pathologist concerns examination of the optic nerve in order to determine the extent of invasion by the tumor (Fig. 1326). Ordinarily, the ophthalmic surgeon who suspects a retinoblastoma will try to obtain a long segment of optic nerve attached to the globe, usually 10 mm to 15 mm. Transverse sections of the nerve should be examined microscopically at the level of surgical transection and at various levels along the nerve. The prognosis is poor in tumors that have invaded the nerve and extended to the plane of transection or into the meninges. These tumors are very likely to extend along the nerve to the brain or be carried there by the subarachnoid fluid.

In most unilateral cases, the tumor is so large that the eye is no longer salvageable, and enucleation should be performed immediately. If tumor has extended to the surgically cut end of the nerve, radiation to the orbit should then be carried out. In patients with bilateral retinoblastoma, the less affected eye is treated with radiotherapy and at times in combination with chemotherapy. The success rate for life of the patient and for preservation of vision is quite good.[120] Tumor recurrences are then treated with photocoagulation, cryotherapy, and cobalt disks.[123]

Conditions confused with retinoblastoma

Any disease process (congenital malformations, developmental disorders, inflammatory processes, trauma, etc.) that leads to retinal detachment or a retrolental mass in a child under 6 years of age must be suspected as a possible retinoblastoma.[121] In a study of a series of 1,000 enucleations performed on children under 15 years of age, Kogan and Boniuk[122] found that eighty-four eyes were removed be-

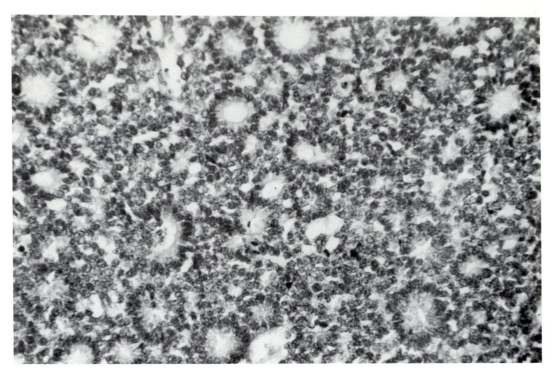

Fig. 1325 Retinoblastoma with typical rosettes. (×600; WU neg. 69-7513; from Ackerman, L. V., and del Regato, J. A.: Cancer, ed. 4, St. Louis, 1970, The C. V. Mosby Co.)

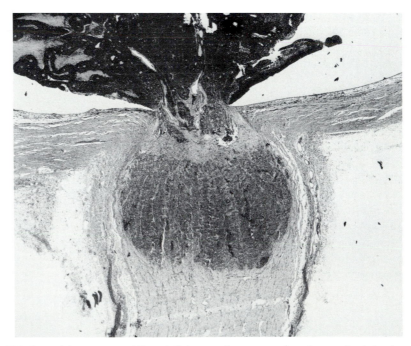

Fig. 1326 Retinoblastomas exhibit definite tendency to spread out of globe by way of optic nerve. It is therefore of utmost importance for surgical pathologist to determine whether such optic nerve extension has occurred and, if it has, to what extent. (×14; AFIP 57-344.)

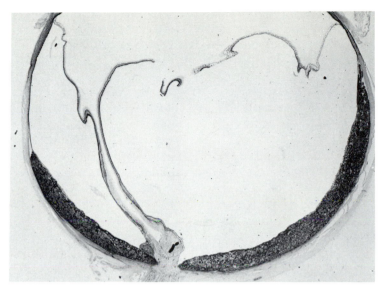

Fig. 1327 Metastatic carcinoma from breast producing diffuse thickening of choroid posteriorly. (×6; AFIP 638509.)

cause of nonneoplastic lesions that simulated retinoblastoma.

Lesions in this category include traumatic or idiopathic retinal detachments, retrolental fibroplasia, persistent hyperplastic primary vitreous, massive retinal gliosis, Coats' disease, nematodiasis, astrocytomas of tuberous sclerosis, and medulloepitheliomas.

Persistent hyperplastic primary vitreous and nematodiasis have already been discussed (pp. 1336 and 1341). Massive retinal gliosis is a relatively uncommon condition in which a large elevated scar develops near the disc and posterior pole following hemorrhage (e.g., in newborn infants) or inflammation.[126] Coats' disease is an exudative retinopathy associated with retinal detachment and foci of telangiectatic retinal vessels. It is usually unilateral and occurs in young children, more often in males. Medulloepitheliomas are rare tumors that resemble histologically the embryonic retina.[127]

Metastatic carcinoma

Although metastatic sarcomas to the eye are rare, metastatic carcinomas are actually the second most common intraocular tumors in adults. The most common primary lesions involved are the breast in the female and the lung in the male with the gastrointestinal next in frequency.[128, 129] Occasionally, the ocular metastasis may be the initial manifestation of the disease, and the primary lesion is discovered only after the eye has been enucleated.

The posterior choroid is most often affected by metastatic carcinoma (Fig. 1327). Anterior uveal involvement is much less common, and retinal metastases are rare. Although diffuse thickening of the choroid along both sides of the optic nerve is most characteristic, large, bulky tumor masses resembling malignant melanomas also may be observed.

Leukemia and malignant lymphoma

The eye is often involved in leukemic and lymphomatous processes, and the intraocular structures are no exception. In fact, ocular involvement is present in at least 50% of all patients who die of leukemia or allied disorders.[130] The histologic findings consist largely of leukemic infiltrations and hemorrhages, particularly in the vascular structures of the eye—i.e., the choroid and retina.[130, 132]

There is often confusion concerning these lesions as to whether they are true neoplasms of the reticuloendothelial system or merely benign lymphoid hyperplasias. It has been shown by Ryan et al.[131] that this unusual form of intraocular pseudotumor probably occurs more often than had been appreciated in the past.

Other tumors

Rare tumors include *leiomyomas* of the ciliary body and iris, pigmented and nonpigmented *neuroepitheliomas* of the iris, ciliary body, and retinal pigment epithelium, and hamartomatous lesions—e.g., hemangiomas, neurofibromas, and astrocytomas.

Juvenile xanthogranuloma can occur in the iris and can cause a spontaneous hyphema and/or secondary glaucoma. It occurs almost exclusively in young children and is associated with the same lesions of the skin from which a biopsy diagnosis can be made.[133]

TECHNIQUE FOR EXAMINATION AND OPENING OF ENUCLEATED EYES

It is very important that the eye be fixed well, oriented properly, examined with the aid of a dissecting microscope, and transilluminated before it is opened.

Good fixation is obtained by placing the intact surgical specimen in a pint of 10% aqueous formalin. It is not necessary to open the eye, to cut windows into the sclera, or to inject formalin into the vitreous in order to obtain good fixation for routine histopathologic techniques. After twenty-four hours in formalin, the globe should be washed in running tap water for several hours and then placed in 60% ethyl alcohol. Formalin is the fixative of choice because it penetrates readily, does not discolor and opacify the ocular tissues, and is generally very satisfactory for most staining procedures.

There is some evidence that glutaraldehyde may have some advantages over formalin for routine fixation.[135]

At the time of gross examination, it is imperative that the pathologist have a good summary of the clinical history and the results of ophthalmologic examination. If there have been accidental or surgical injuries to the globe, their sites should be determined before the eye is opened. Likewise, any particular lesion of interest observed in the fundus must be known so that the globe may be advantageously positioned when it is being opened.

Every effort should be made to open the eye in such a way that the plane of section will include the cornea, pupil, lens, and optic nerve, along with the lesion of principal clinical interest. If there is no focal lesion that requires a particular plane of section, the horizontal plane is used in order to obtain the macula in the block.

Many minute lesions of interest that would ordinarily be overlooked with the naked eye can be detected if the ×7 objective of a binocular dissecting microscope is used. Likewise, transillumination of the globe before it is opened will frequently reveal discrete shadows or areas of increased translucency. A substage microscope lamp in a darkened room is very satisfactory for this purpose. Rotation of the globe over the light source will often reveal in sharp outline the presence of intraocular tumors. Such shadows should then be delineated on the sclera with an indelible pencil.

When the presence of intraocular foreign bodies is suspected, it is good practice to examine the globe roentgenologically before it is opened.

The eye is opened with the aid of a double-edged razor blade. During sectioning, a right-handed individual holds the eye with the left hand, cornea down against the cutting block (Fig. 1328). The razor blade is held between the thumb and middle finger of the right hand. With a sawing motion, the eye is opened from back to front. The plane of section begins adjacent to the optic nerve and ends through the periphery of the cornea. After the interior of the globe is examined, a

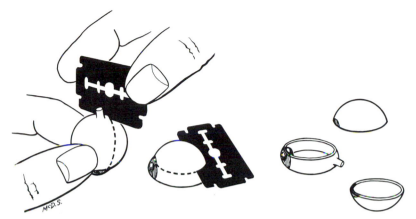

Fig. 1328 Steps used in opening whole eyes. See text for description.

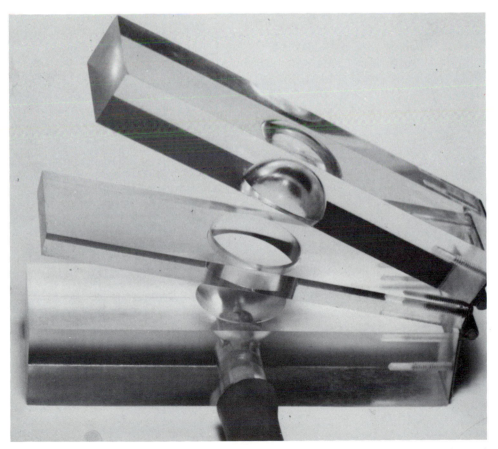

Fig. 1329 "Ophthalmotome" that can be used for cutting eyes. Model shown is fashioned after original instrument constructed by Herreman, de Buen, and Cortez. (WU neg. 67-4484.)

second plane of section, parallel to the first, is made, again passing from back to front. During this step, the eye is placed flat on its cut surface (Fig. 1328).

An alternate method of opening the globe is with the use of a plastic apparatus known as an "ophthalmotome" which was developed by Herreman, de Buen, and Cortez.[134] This device holds the eye within a compartment while the razor is passed through the different sections of the plastic block (Fig. 1329).

As a result of the two-step procedure, either with the "ophthalmotome" or by hand, a disc-shaped slab about 8 mm in thickness containing the cornea, pupil, lens, and optic nerve is obtained. This slab may be carried through the automatic tissue processor along with other surgical specimens that are to be embedded in paraffin. With experience, excellent paraffin sections may be cut on the rotary microtome, although it is technically easier to obtain good histologic preparations with celloidin embedding and use of a sliding microtome.

REFERENCES
GENERAL REFERENCES

 1 Boniuk, M., editor: Ocular and adnexal tumors, new and controversial aspects, St. Louis, 1964, The C. V. Mosby Co.
 2 Duke-Elder, W. S.: System of ophthalmology, vols. I-V, VII-XII, and XIV, St. Louis, The C. V. Mosby Co.
2a Ferry, A. P., editor: Ocular and adnexal tumors, Int. Ophthalmol. Clin. 12:1-269, 1972.
 3 Friedenwald, J. S., Wilder, H. C., Maumenee, A. E., Sanders, T. E., Keyes, J. E. L., Hogan, M. J., Owens, W. C., and Owens, E. U: Ophthalmic pathology: an atlas and textbook, Philadelphia, 1952, W. B. Saunders Co.
3a Henderson, J. W.: Orbital tumors, Philadelphia, 1973, W. B. Saunders Co.
 4 Hogan, M. J., and Zimmerman, L. E.: Ophthalmic pathology: an atlas and textbook, ed. 2, Philadelphia, 1962, W. B. Saunders Co.
 5 Hogan, M. J., Alvarado, J. A., and Weddell, J. E.: Histology of the human eye, Philadelphia, 1971, W. B. Saunders Co.
 6 Reese, A. B.: Tumors of the eye and adnexa. In Atlas of tumor pathology, Sect. X, Fasc. 38, Washington, D. C., 1956, Armed Forces Institute of Pathology.
 7 Reese, A. B.: Tumors of the eye, ed. 2, New York, 1963, Hoeber Medical Division, Harper & Row, Publishers.
 8 Salzmann, M.: The anatomy and histology of the human eyeball in the normal state (translated by E. V. L. Brown), Chicago, 1912, University of Chicago Press.
 9 Walsh, F., and Hoyt, W.: Clinical neuro-ophthalmology, ed. 3, Baltimore, 1969, The Williams & Wilkins Co.
10 Wolff, E.: The anatomy of the eye and orbit, ed. 5, London, 1961, H. K. Lewis & Co., Ltd.
11 Zimmerman, L. E.: Changing concepts concerning the malignancy of ocular tumors, Arch. Ophthalmol. 78:166-173, 1967.
12 Zimmerman, L. E.: Eye and ocular adnexa. In Saphir, O.: A text on systemic pathology, vol. 2, New York, 1958, Grune & Stratton, Inc., chap. 16, p. 1172.
13 Zimmerman, L. E., editor: Tumors of the eye and adnexa, Int. Ophthalmol. Clin. 2: 239-558, 1962.
14 Zimmerman, L. E., Font, R., and Ts'o, M.: Application of electron microscopy to histopathologic diagnosis, Trans. Am. Acad. Ophthalmol. Otolaryngol. 76:101-107, 1972.

EYELIDS
Developmental anomalies

15 Fitzpatrick, T. B., and others: Ocular and dermal melanocytosis, Arch. Ophthalmol. 56: 830-832, 1956.
16 Helmick, E. D., and Pringle, R. W.: Oculocutaneous melanosis or nevus of Ota, Arch. Ophthalmol. 56:833-838, 1956.
17 Henkind, P., and Friedman, A.: External ocular pigmentation, Int. Ophthalmol. Clin. 11:87-111, 1971.
18 Peterman, A. F., Hayles, A. B., and Dockerty, M. B.: Encephalotrigeminal angiomatosis (Sturge-Weber disease), J.A.M.A. 167:2169-2176, 1958.

Metabolic disorders

19 Smith, M. E., and Zimmerman, L. E.: Amyloidosis of the eyelid and conjunctiva, Arch. Ophthalmol. 75:42-56, 1966.

Tumors and tumorlike lesions

20 Aurora, A. L., and Blodi, F. C.: Lesions of the eyelids: a clinicopathologic study, Survey Ophthalmol. 15:94-104, 1970.
21 Boniuk, M.: Tumors of the eyelids, Int. Ophthalmol. Clin. 2:239-317, 1962.
22 Boniuk, M., and Zimmerman, L. E.: Pilomatrixoma (benign calcifying epithelioma) of the eyelids and eyebrow, Arch. Ophthalmol. 70:399-406, 1963.
23 Boniuk, M., and Zimmerman, L. E.: Eyelid tumors with reference to lesions confused

with squamous cell carcinoma. II. Inverted follicular keratosis, Arch. Ophthalmol. **69:** 698-707, 1963.

24 Boniuk, M., and Zimmerman, L. E.: Eyelid tumors with reference to lesions confused with squamous cell carcinoma. III. Keratoacanthoma, Arch. Ophthalmol. **77:**29-40, 1967.

25 Boniuk, M., and Zimmerman, L. E.: Sebaceous carcinomas of the eyelid, eyebrow, caruncle, and orbit, Trans. Am. Acad. Ophthalmol. Otolaryngol. **72:**619-642, 1968.

26 Font, R. L., and Zimmerman, L. E.: Nodular fasciitis of the eye and adnexa: a report of ten cases, Arch. Ophthalmol. **75:**475-481, 1966.

27 Forbis, R., Jr., and Helwig, E. G.: Pilomatrixoma (calcifying epithelioma), Arch. Dermatol. **83:**606-618, 1961.

28 Hood, C. I., Font, R., and Zimmerman, L. E.: Metastatic mammary carcinoma in the eyelid with histiocytoid appearance, Cancer **31:**793-800, 1973.

29 Kwitko, M. L., Boniuk, M., and Zimmerman, L. E.: Eyelid tumors with reference to lesions confused with squamous cell carcinoma. I. Incidence and errors in diagnosis, Arch. Ophthalmol. **69:**693-697, 1963.

30 Whorton, C. M., and Patterson, J. B.: Carcinoma of Moll's glands with extramammary Paget's disease of the eyelid, Cancer **8:**1009-1015, 1955.

31 Zimmerman, L. E.: Ocular lesions of juvenile xanthogranuloma: nevoxanthoendothelioma, Trans. Am. Acad. Ophthalmol. Otolaryngol. **69:**412-442, 1965.

LACRIMAL PASSAGES

32 Ryan, S. J., and Font, R. L.: Primary epithelial neoplasms of the lacrimal sac, Am. J. Ophthalmol. **76:**73-88, 1973.

LACRIMAL GLAND

33 Font, R. L., Yanoff, M., and Zimmerman, L. E.: Benign lymphoepithelial lesion of the lacrimal gland and its relationship to Sjögren's syndrome, Am. J. Clin. Pathol. **48:**365-376, 1967.

34 Godwin, J. T.: Benign lymphoepithelial lesion of the parotid gland (adenolymphoma, chonic inflammation, lymphoepithelioma, lymphocytic tumor, Mikulicz's disease), Cancer **5:** 1089-1103, 1952.

35 Meyer, D., Yanoff, M., and Hanno, H.: Differential diagnosis in Mikulicz syndrome, Mikulicz's disease, and similar disease entities, Am. J. Ophthalmol. **71:**516-524 1971.

36 Morgan, W. S., and Castleman, B.: A clinico-pathological study of "Mikulicz's disease," Am. J. Pathol. **29:**471-503, 1953.

37 Reese, A. B.: The treatment of expanding lesions of the orbit with particular regard to those arising in the lacrimal gland, Am. J. Ophthalmol. **41:**3-11, 1956.

38 Yanoff, M., Nix, R., and Swan, D.: Bilateral lacrimal gland enlargement associated with a diffuse gamma globulin elevation, Ophthalmol. Res. **1:**245-253, 1970.

Tumors

39 Sanders, T. E., Ackerman, L. V., and Zimmerman, L. E.: Epithelial tumors of the lacrimal gland; a comparison of the pathologic and clinical behavior with those of the salivary glands, Am. J. Surg. **104:**657-665, 1962.

40 Zimmerman, L. E., Sanders, T. E., and Ackerman, L. V.: Epithelial tumors of the lacrimal gland: prognostic and therapeutic significance of histologic types, Int. Ophthalmol. Clin. **2:**337-367, 1962.

ORBIT

41 Porterfield, J. F.: Orbital tumors in children: a report on 214 cases, Int. Ophthalmol. Clin. **2:**319-335, 1962.

42 Smith, M. E.: The differential diagnosis of unilateral exophthalmos, Int. Ophthalmol. Clin. **7:**911-933, 1967.

Congenital and developmental conditions

43 Ingalls, R. G.: Tumors of the orbit and allied pseudotumors; an analysis of 216 case histories, Springfield, Ill., 1953, Charles C Thomas, Publisher.

Inflammatory processes

44 Blodi, F., and Gass, D.: Inflammatory pseudotumor of the orbit, Trans. Am. Acad. Ophthalmol. Otolaryngol. **71:**303-323, 1967.

45 Reese, A. B.: Tumors of the eye, ed. 2, New York, 1963, Hoeber Medical Division, Harper & Row, Publishers.

46 Straatsma, B. R.: Ocular manifestations of Wegener's granulomatosis, Am. J. Ophthalmol. **44:**789-799, 1957.

Primary tumors
Connective tissue tumors

47 Ashton, N., and Morgan, G.: Embryonal sarcoma and embryonal rhabdomyosarcoma of the orbit, J. Clin. Pathol. **18:**699-714, 1965.

48 Font, R., and Zimmerman, L. E.: Nodular fasciitis of the eye and adnexa: a report of ten cases, Arch. Ophthalmol. **75:**475-481, 1966.

49 Forrest, A. W.: Tumors following radiation about the eye, Int. Ophthalmol. Clin. **2:**543-553, 1962.

50 Porterfield, J. F., and Zimmerman, L. E.: Rhabdomyosarcoma of the orbit; a clinico-

pathologic study of 55 cases, Virchows Arch. Pathol. Anat. **335**:329-344, 1962.

Lymphoid tumors

51 Burkitt, D., and O'Connor, G. T.: Malignant lymphoma in African children. I. A clinical syndrome, Cancer **14**:258-269, 1961.
52 Karp, L, Zimmerman, L., and Payne, T.: Intraocular involvement in Burkitt's lymphoma, Arch. Ophthalmol. **85**:295-298, 1971.
53 O'Connor, G. T.: Malignant lymphoma in African children. II. A pathologic entity, Cancer **14**:270-283, 1961.

Glioma of optic nerve

54 Davis, F. A.: Primary tumors of the optic nerve (a phenomenon of Recklinghausen's disease), Arch. Ophthalmol. **23**:735-821, 957-1022, 1940.
55 Verhoeff, F. A.: Tumors of optic nerve. In Penfield, W. C.: Cytology and cellular pathology of the nervous system, vol. 3, New York, 1932, Hoeber Medical Division, Harper & Row, Publishers, pp. 1029-1039.

Meningioma

56 Reese, A. B.: Tumors of the eye, ed. 2, New York, 1963, Hoeber Medical Division, Harper & Row, Publishers, pp. 169-175.

CONJUNCTIVA AND CORNEA
Congenital and
developmental lesions

57 Schulze, R.: Limbal dermoid with intraocular extension, Arch. Ophthalmol. **75**:803-805, 1966.
58 Schultz, G., Wendler, P., and Weseley, A.: Ocular dermoids and auricular appendages, Am. J. Ophthalmol. **63**:938-942, 1967.

Inflammation

59 Bornstein, J., Frank, M., and Radnec, D.: Conjunctival biopsy in the diagnosis of sarcoidosis, N. Engl. J. Med. **267**:60-64, 1962.
60 Chambers, J., Blodi, F., Golden, B., and McKee, A.: Ligneous conjunctivitis, Trans. Am. Acad. Ophthalmol. Otolaryngol. **73**:996-1004, 1969.

Tumors and related lesions

61 Carroll, I. M., and Kuwabara, T.: A classification of limbal epitheliomas, Arch. Ophthalmol. **73**:545-551, 1965.
62 Irvine, A. R., Jr.: Epibulbar squamous cell carcinoma and related lesions. In Ferry, A. P., editor: Ocular and adnexal tumors, Int. Ophthalmol. Clin. **12**:71-83, 1972.
63 Jay, B.: Naevi and melanomata of the conjunctiva, Br. J. Ophthalmol. **49**:169-204, 1965.

64 Lewis, P. M., and Zimmerman, L. E.: Delayed recurrence of malignant melanomas of the bulbar conjunctiva, Am. J. Ophthalmol. **45**:536-543, 1958.
65 Morgan, G.: Lymphocytic tumours of the conjunctiva, J. Clin. Pathol. **24**:585-595, 1971.
66 Reese, A. B.: Tumors of the eye, ed. 2, New York, 1963, Hoeber Medical Division, Harper & Row, Publishers.
67 Reese, A. B.: Precancerous and cancerous melanosis, Am. J. Ophthalmol. **61**:1272-1277, 1966.
68 Zimmerman, L. E.: Criteria for management of melanosis (correspondence), Arch. Ophthalmol. **76**:307-308, 1966.

INTRAOCULAR TISSUES
Congenital and
developmental malformations

69 Boniuk, M., and Zimmerman, L. E.: Ocular pathology in the rubella syndrome, Arch. Ophthalmol. **77**:455-473, 1967.
70 Cogan, D. G., and Kuwabara, T.: Ocular pathology of the 13-15 trisomy syndrome, Arch. Ophthalmol. **72**:246-247, 1964.
71 Font, R., and Ferry, A. P.: The phakomatoses. In Ferry, A. P., editor: Ocular and adnexal tumors, Int. Ophthalmol. Clin. **12**:1-50, 1972.
72 Font, R. L., and Fine, B. S.: Ocular pathology in Fabry's disease; histochemical and electron microscopic observations, Am. J. Ophthalmol. **73**:419-430, 1972.
73 Hunter, W. S., and Zimmerman, L. E.: Unilateral retinal dysplasia, Arch. Ophthalmol. **74**:23-30, 1965.
74 Jensen, O. A.: Persistent hyperplastic primary vitreous, Acta Ophthalmol. **46**:418-429, 1968.
75 Mann, I.: Developmental abnormalities of the eye, ed. 2, London, 1957, British Medical Association.
76 Maumenee, A. E.: The pathogenesis of congenital glaucoma, Trans. Am. Ophthalmol. Soc. **56**:507-570, 1958.
77 Maumenee, A. E.: Further observations on the pathogenesis of congenital glaucoma, Trans. Am. Ophthalmol. Soc. **60**:140-162, 1962.
78 Miller, R. W., Fraumeni, J. F., Jr., and Manning, M. D.: Association of Wilms' tumor with aniridia, hemihypertrophy, and other congenital malformations, N. Engl. J. Med. **270**:922-927, 1964.
79 Reese, A. B. (moderator): Symposium on retrolental fibroplasia, Trans. Am. Acad. Ophthalmol. Otolaryngol. **59**:7-41, 1955.
80 Reese, A. B., and Ellsworth, R. M.: The anterior chamber cleavage syndrome, Arch. Ophthalmol. **75**:307-318, 1968.

81 Worst, J. G. F.: Congenital glaucoma, Invest. Ophthalmol. **7**:127-137, 1968.

82 Zimmerman, L. E.: The histopathologic basis for ocular manifestations of the congenital rubella syndrome, Am. J. Ophthalmol. **65:** 837-862, 1968.

83 Zimmerman, L. E., and Font, R. L.: Some recent advances in the pathogenesis and histopathology of congenital malformations of the eye, J.A.M.A. **196**:684-696, 1966.

Inflammation
Acute inflammation/Chronic nongranulomatous inflammation/Granulomatous inflammation

84 Ashton, N.: Larval granulomatosis of the retina due to Toxocara, Br. J. Ophthalmol. **44**:129-148, 1960.

85 Beaver, P. C.: Larva migrans, Exp. Parasit. **5:** 587-621, 1956.

86 Fishman, L. S., Griffin, J. R., Sapico, F. L., and Hecht, R.: Hematogenous *Candida* endophthalmitis, N. Engl. J. Med. **286**:675-681, 1972.

87 Levine, R., and Williamson, D. E.: Metastatic carcinoma simulating a postoperative endophthalmitis, Arch. Ophthalmol. **83**:59-60, 1970.

88 Michelson, P. E., Stark, W., Reeser, F., and Green, W. R.: Endogenous *Candida* endophthalmitis. Report of 13 cases and 16 from the literature, Int. Ophthalmol. Clin. **11**:125-147, 1971.

89 Naumann, G., Gass, D., and Font, R.: Histopathology of herpes zoster opthalmicus, Am. J. Ophthalmol. **65**:533-541, 1968.

90 Sugar, S., Mandell, G., and Shaler, J.: Metastatic endophthalmitis associated with injection of addictive drugs, Am. J. Ophthalmol. **71**:1055-1058, 1971.

91 Wilder, H. C.: Nematode endophthalmitis, Trans. Am. Acad. Ophthalmol. Otolaryngol. **54**:99-109, 1950.

92 Wilder, H. C.: Toxoplasma chorioretinitis in adults, Arch. Ophthalmol. **48**:127-136, 1952.

93 Wilkinson, C., and Welch, R.: Intraocular Toxocara, Am. J. Ophthalmol. **71**:921-930, 1971.

94 Zimmerman, L. E., DeBuen, S., and Foerster, H. C.: Granulomatous inflammation within the eye, Transactions Fifth Pan-American Congress of Ophthalmology, Santiago, Chile, 1956, vol. 2, pp. 225-247.

Posttraumatic uveitis

95 Easom, H., and Zimmerman, L. E.: Sympathetic ophthalmia and bilateral phacoanaphylaxis, Arch. Ophthalmol. **72**:9-15, 1964.

96 Verhoeff, F. H., and Lemoine, A. N.: Endophthalmitis phacoanaphylactica, Transactions International Congress Ophthalmology, Washington, D. C., April 25, 1922.

Degeneration
Glaucoma

97 Bietti, G.: Recent experimental, clinical and therapeutic research on the problems of intraocular pressure and glaucoma, Am. J. Ophthalmol. **73**:475-500, 1972.

98 Fenton, R., and Zimmerman, L.: Hemolytic glaucoma, Arch. Ophthalmol. **70**:236-239, 1963.

99 Flocks, M., Littwin, C. S., and Zimmerman, L. E.: Phacolytic glaucoma, Arch. Ophthalmol. **54**:37-45, 1955.

100 Kolker, A. E., and Hetherington, J., Jr.: Becker-Shaffer's Diagnosis and therapy of the glaucomas, ed. 3, St. Louis, 1970, The C. V. Mosby Co.

Diabetes

101 Yanoff, M.: Ocular pathology in diabetes mellitus, Am. J. Ophthalmol. **67**:21-38, 1969.

Tumors and pseudotumors
Malignant melanoma

102 Ashton, N., and Wybar, K.: Primary tumours of the iris, Ophthalmologica **151**:97-113, 1966.

103 Boniuk, M., and Zimmerman, L. E.: Pathologic anatomy of complications of retinal surgery. In Schepens, C. L.: Controversial aspects of the management of retinal detachment, Boston, 1965, Little, Brown and Co.

104 Callender, G. R.: Malignant melanotic tumors of the eye: a study of histologic types in 111 cases, Trans. Am. Acad. Ophthalmol. Otolaryngol. **36**:131-142, 1931.

105 Ferry, A. P.: Lesions mistaken for malignant melanoma of posterior uvea, Arch. Ophthalmol. **72**:463-469, 1964.

106 Ferry, A. P.: Lesions mistaken for malignant melanoma of iris, Arch. Ophthalmol. **74**:9-18, 1965.

107 Flocks, M., Gerende, J. H., and Zimmerman, L. E.: The size and shape of malignant melanomas of the choroid and ciliary body in relation to prognosis and histologic characteristics—a statistical study of 210 tumors, Trans. Am. Acad. Ophthalmol. Otolaryngol. **59**:740-758, 1955.

108 Font, R., Spaulding, A., and Zimmerman, L. E.: Diffuse malignant melanoma of the uveal tract: a clinicopathologic report of 54 cases, Trans. Am. Acad. Ophthalmol. Otolaryngol. **72**:877-895, 1968.

109 Gass, J. D. M.: Fluorescein angiography; an aid in the differential diagnosis of intraocular tumors. In Ferry, A. P., editor: Ocular and adnexal tumors, Int. Ophthalmol. Clin. **12**:85-120, 1972.

110 Hagler, W., Jarrett, W., II, and Humphrey, W.: The radioactive phosphorus uptake test

in the diagnosis of uveal melanoma, Arch. Ophthalmol. **83**:548-557, 1970.

111 Howard, G. M., and Forrest, A. W.: Incidence and location of melanocytomas, Arch. Ophthalmol. **77**:61-66, 1967.

112 Paul, E. V., Parnell, B. L., and Fraker, M.: Prognosis of malignant melanomas of the choroid and ciliary body, Int. Ophthalmol. Clin. **2**:387-402, 1962.

113 Reese, A. B.: Tumors of the eye, ed. 2, New York, 1963, Hoeber Medical Division, Harper & Row, Publishers.

114 Wilder, H. C., and Callender, G. R.: Malignant melanoma of the choroid; further studies on prognosis by histologic type and fiber content, Am. J. Ophthalmol. **22**:851-855, 1939.

115 Yanoff, M., and Zimmerman, L. E.: Histogenesis of malignant melanomas of the uvea. I. Nevi of choroid and ciliary body, Arch. Ophthalmol. **76**:784-796, 1966.

116 Yanoff, M., and Zimmerman, L. E.: Histogenesis of malignant melanomas of the uvea. II. The relationship of uveal nevi to malignant melanoma, Cancer **20**:493-507, 1967.

117 Yanoff, M., and Zimmerman, L. E.: Histogenesis of malignant melanomas of the uvea. III. The relationship of congenital ocular melanocytosis and neurofibromatosis to uveal melanomas, Arch. Ophthalmol. **77**:331-336, 1967.

118 Zimmerman, L. E.: Clinical pathology of iris tumors, Am. J. Clin. Pathol. **39**:214-228, 1963.

119 Zimmerman, L. E.: Melanocytes, melanocytic nevi, and melanocytomas, Invest. Ophthalmol. **4**:11-41, 1965.

Retinoblastoma

120 Ellsworth, R.: Treatment of retinoblastoma, Am. J. Ophthalmol. **66**:49-51, 1968.

121 Howard, G. M., and Ellsworth, R. M.: Differential diagnosis of retinoblastoma; a statistical survey of 500 children, Am. J. Ophthalmol. **60**:610-612, 1965.

122 Kogan, L., and Boniuk, M.: Causes for enucleation in childhood with special reference to pseudogliomas and retinoblastomas, Int. Ophthalmol. Clin. **2**:507-524, 1962.

123 Stallard, H. B.: Retinoblastoma treated by radon seeds and radioactive disks, Ann. R. Coll. Surg. Engl. **16**:349-366, 1955.

124 Ts'o, M. O., Fine, B. S., and Zimmerman, L. E.: The nature of retinoblastoma. II. Photoreceptor differentiation: an electron microscopic study, Am. J. Ophthalmol. **69**:350-359, 1970.

125 Ts'o, M. O., Zimmerman, L. E., and Fine, B. S.: The nature of retinoblastoma. I. Photoreceptor differentiation: a clinical and histopathologic study, Am. J. Ophthalmol. **69**:339-349, 1970.

126 Yanoff, M., Zimmerman, L. E., and Davis, R.: Massive gliosis of the retina, Int. Ophthalmol. Clin. **11**:211-229, 1971.

127 Zimmerman, L. E.: Verhoeff's "teratoneuroma"; a critical appraisal in light of new observations and current concepts of embryonic tumors, Am. J. Ophthalmol. **72**:1039-1057, 1971.

Metastatic carcinoma

128 Albert, D. M., Rubenstein, R., and Scheie, H.: Tumor metastasis to the eye. Part I. Incidence in 213 adult patients with generalized malignancy, Am. J. Ophthalmol. **63**:724-726, 1967.

129 Ferry, A. P.: Metastatic carcinoma of the eye and ocular adnexa, Int. Ophthalmol. Clin. **7**:615-658, 1967.

Leukemia and malignant lymphoma

130 Allen, R., and Straatsma, B.: Ocular involvement in leukemia and allied disorders, Arch. Ophthalmol. **66**:490-508, 1961.

131 Ryan, S., Zimmerman, L. E., King, F. M.: Reactive lymphoid hyperplasia; an unusual form of intraocular pseudotumor, Trans. Am. Acad. Ophthalmol. Otolaryngol. **76**:652-671, 1972.

132 Vogel, M., Font, R., Zimmerman, L. E., and Levine, R.: Reticulum cell sarcoma of the retina and uvea, Am. J. Ophthalmol. **66**:205-215, 1968.

Other tumors

133 Zimmerman, L. E.: Ocular lesions of juvenile xanthogranuloma: nevoxanthoendothelioma, Trans. Am. Acad. Ophthalmol. Otolaryngol. **69**:412-442, 1965.

TECHNIQUE FOR EXAMINATION AND OPENING OF ENUCLEATED EYES

134 Herreman, R., De Buen, S., and Cortés, T.: Oftalmótomo: Un nuevo aparato para seccionar los ojos en el laboratorio de anatomía patológica, Rev. Fac. Med. (Mexico) **7**:157-167, 1965.

135 Yanoff, M., and Fine, B. S.: Glutaraldehyde fixation of routine surgical eye tissue, Am. J. Ophthalmol. **63**:137-140, 1967.

Index